Anesthesia and Co-Existing Disease

THIRD EDITION

Anesthesia and Co-Existing Disease

THIRD EDITION

Robert K. Stoelting, M.D.

Professor and Chairman
Department of Anesthesia
Indiana University School of Medicine
Indianapolis, Indiana

Stephen F. Dierdorf, M.D.

Professor
Department of Anesthesia
Indiana University School of Medicine
Indianapolis, Indiana

Churchill Livingstone
New York, Edinburgh, London, Madrid, Melbourne, Tokyo

Library of Congress Cataloging-in-Publication Data

Anesthesia and co-existing disease / [edited by] Robert K. Stoelting,
    Stephen F. Dierdorf. — 3rd ed.
        p.   cm.
    Includes bibliographical references and index.
    ISBN 0-443-08813-6
    1. Anesthesia—Complications. 2. Therapeutic, Surgical.
  I. Stoelting, Robert K. II. Dierdorf, Stephen F.
    [DNLM: 1. Anesthesia—adverse effects. 2. Anesthetics. WO 245
  A578 1993]
  RD87.A53 1993
  617.9'6041—dc20
  DNLM/DLC
  for Library of Congress   93-480
                                         CIP

Distributed in the United Kingdom by Churchill Livingstone, Robert Stevenson House, 1–3 Baxter's Place, Leith Walk, Edinburgh EH1 3AF, and by associated companies, branches, and representatives throughout the world.

Accurate indications, adverse reactions, and dosage schedules for drugs are provided in this book, but it is possible that they may change. The reader is urged to review the package information data of the manufacturers of the medications mentioned.

The Publishers have made every effort to trace the copyright holders for borrowed material. If they have inadvertently overlooked any, they will be pleased to make the necessary arrangements at the first opportunity.

Acquisitions Editor: *Toni M. Tracy*
Copy Editor: *Bridgett Dickinson*
Production Designer: *Patricia McFadden*
Production Supervisor: *Jeanine Furino*
Cover Design: *Paul Moran*

Printed in the United States of America

First published in 1993 7 6 5 4 3 2 1

Preface
to the Third Edition

This third edition of *Anesthesia and Co-Existing Disease* is published 10 years after the introduction of the first edition in 1983. As with the previous two editions, our goal is to provide the reader with a current and concise description of the pathophysiology of disease and the impact, if any, on the management of anesthesia. Common diseases are given detailed discussion, while rare diseases receive attention based on unique features that could be of importance in the perioperative period. Some chapter titles have been changed in an attempt to emphasize disease states more likely to occur in certain patient populations, including the parturient and the pediatric patient. Asthma is now a separate chapter, whereas topics such as artificial cardiac pacemakers, acid-base disturbances, and transfusion therapy are no longer free-standing chapters, but have been incorporated into appropriate areas of existing chapters. Numerous new figures and tables have been added to the third edition. Expanded sections dealing with peripheral nerve injury, anticoagulation and regional anesthesia, diabetes mellitus, and malignant hyperthermia are also included.

As with the second edition, this edition of *Anesthesia and Co-Existing Disease* is the product of the Editors. We believe this will provide a consistency in style and an absence of duplication or conflicting statements that the reader will find refreshing. As with the previous editions, we are confident that this newest edition can serve both as an introductory source of information and as a reference book for review. Therefore, this textbook should be equally valuable to the physician trainee and to the anesthesiologist.

We again wish to recognize the invaluable secretarial help of Deanna M. Walker in the preparation of the manuscript. Toni M. Tracy, President of Churchill Livingstone Inc., provided necessary resources and appropriate amounts of direction and encouragement to ensure a quality textbook. Bridgett Dickinson served as an efficient and understanding copy editor, for which we are greatly appreciative.

Robert K. Stoelting, M.D.
Stephen F. Dierdorf, M.D.

Preface
to the First Edition

Optimal management of anesthesia extends beyond an understanding of the pharmacology of drugs used during the intraoperative period and a dexterity in performance of technical procedures. Specifically, a knowledge of the pathophysiology of co-existing disease regardless of the reason for surgery and an understanding of the implications of concomitant drug therapy are mandatory for the optimal management of anesthesia in an individual patient. The goal of *Anesthesia and Co-Existing Disease* is to provide a concise description of the pathophysiology of disease states and their medical treatment that is relevant to the care of the patient in the perioperative period. Diseases or characteristics unique to the pediatric, geriatric, and pregnant patient are considered in separate chapters. There is a liberal use of illustrations and tables to reinforce written material. Discussions of disease states often include a section designated Management of Anesthesia. This section is designed to relate the impact of co-existing disease to the selection of drugs, techniques, and monitors to be employed in the perioperative period.

We feel that *Anesthesia and Co-Existing Disease* can serve both as an introductory source of information and as a reference for review. Therefore, this book should be equally valuable to the beginner or the individual with training and experience in the administration of anesthesia. Although several authors have contributed to this undertaking, a consistency in style is assured by virtue of the Editors' roles as the final "authors" so as to make the entire book read as if written by a single individual.

The Editors wish to recognize the invaluable secretarial help of Deanna Walker in preparation of manuscripts. We salute the contagious enthusiasm of Lewis Reines, President of Churchill Livingstone, in the initial formulation of the idea for this book. In addition, the superb cooperation of our copy editor, Donna Balopole, permitted us to continue to make important additions to the book as new information and references became available. As a result, we have been able to achieve our desire to provide a work which is current to within 6 months of publication. Finally, we are grateful to our colleagues and families for their understanding and support during the time the book was in preparation.

Robert K. Stoelting, M.D.
Stephen F. Dierdorf, M.D.

Contents

Ischemic Heart Disease

Ischemic heart disease (IHD), which reflects the presence of atherosclerosis in coronary arteries (coronary artery disease), is estimated to be present in 10 million adult Americans.[1] In any 12-month period, a new myocardial infarction develops in approximately 1.3 million patients. IHD is the number one cause of morbidity and mortality in the United States, with 500,000 deaths annually.[2] Acute myocardial infarction and sudden death are often the first manifestations of IHD. Indeed, greater than 50% of victims of sudden death have unexpected IHD. It appears that the prognosis for patients with IHD is related to the development and severity of cardiac dysrhythmias, myocardial infarction, and left ventricular dysfunction. Among the estimated 25 million patients in the United States who undergo surgery each year, approximately 7 million are considered to be at high risk of IHD.[3]

RISK FACTORS

The two most important risk factors for the development of atherosclerosis involving the coronary arteries are male gender and increasing age[4] (Table 1-1). Three additional risk factors are hypercholesterolemia, hypertension, and cigarette smoking.[1] Other proposed risk factors include diabetes mellitus, obesity, a sedentary life-style, and a family history of premature development of IHD.

Hypercholesterolemia

There is a linear correlation between the plasma concentration of cholesterol and the risk of development of IHD[4,5] (Fig. 1-1). An estimated one-third of adults in the United States have a plasma cholesterol level above 240 mg·dl^{-1} and therefore have a risk of IHD twice that of persons with a cholesterol level less than 180 mg·dl^{-1}. Acceleration of atherosclerosis is principally correlated with an increase in the plasma concentration of low-density lipoproteins, whereas high-density lipo-

proteins exert a protective effect, presumably by transporting cholesterol out of smooth muscle to its site of metabolism in the liver. The ratio of total cholesterol to high-density lipoprotein is a better predictor of IHD than is the level of either fraction alone.

Receptors for cholesterol-carrying low-density lipoproteins are genetically determined and represent the principal mechanism for removal of cholesterol from the plasma. These receptors are present mainly in the liver and to a lesser extent in other tissues. A patient who is heterozygous for the low-density lipoprotein receptor gene develops hypercholesterolemia and is susceptible to premature development of IHD. Familial heterozygous hypercholesterolemia occurs in about 1 in 500 persons. Less common is homozygous familial hypercholesterolemia, in which plasma cholesterol levels are about four times normal and premature atherosclerosis is frequent.

It has been proposed that the ideal plasma cholesterol concentration for an adult over 30 years of age is less than 200 mg·dl^{-1} and that attempts to lower the plasma concentration are indicated when the value exceeds about 240 mg·dl^{-1} (75th percentile).[6] Applying these criteria, 15% to 20% of the population has hypercholesterolemia. Diet (decreased overall fat intake and substitution of polyunsaturated fatty acids for saturated fatty acids) is the principal method for lowering the plasma concentration of cholesterol, although a diet sufficiently palatable to achieve patient acceptance typically lowers the plasma cholesterol concentration by only 10% or less. Drugs that lower the plasma cholesterol concentration by inhibiting the rate-limiting step in the synthesis of cholesterol (gemfibrozil, lovastatin, clofibrate) may be useful in treatment of nonfamilial hypercholesterolemia.[7] It is estimated that maintaining the plasma cholesterol concentration below 200 mg·dl^{-1} would decrease the incidence of IHD 30% to 50% in persons younger than 65 years of age.[8] Alternatively, a 1% decrease in a patient's total plasma cholesterol concentration yields a 2% to 3% reduction in the risk of IHD.[1]

Table 1-1.   Risk Factors for the Development of
Ischemic Heart Disease

Male gender
Increasing age
Hypercholesterolemia
Hypertension
Cigarette smoking
Diabetes mellitus
Obesity
Psychosocial characteristics
Sedentary life-style
Family history of premature development of ischemic heart disease

Hypertension

Hypertension may augment the risk of IHD by enhancing the process of arterial wall injury that leads to atherosclerosis. Furthermore, the ischemic effects of obstructive coronary artery lesions are increased by left ventricular pressure work and hypertrophy that may accompany sustained hypertension. Control of hypertension, however, is probably more important in prevention of stroke than of myocardial infarction. Nevertheless, the estimated decrease in the risk of myocardial infarction is 2% to 3% for every reduction of 1 mmHg in the diastolic blood pressure.[1]

Cigarette Smoking

Cigarette smoking is the only risk factor that has been consistently shown to increase the risk of IHD.[1,9] It is estimated that cigarette smoking is responsible for 30% of the 500,000 annual fatalities attributed to IHD. The addition of the risk factor of cigarette smoking is equivalent to increasing the plasma cholesterol concentration by 50 to 100 mg·dl^{-1}. Smoking acts synergistically with other risk factors, including diabetes mellitus and hypertension.[1] Coronary thrombosis and sudden cardiac death, rather than the atherosclerotic process, seem closely related to smoking. Enhancement of platelet aggregation, nicotine-induced coronary vasoconstriction, and arterial hypoxemia owing to inhalation of carbon monoxide are the principal physiologic disturbances related to smoking. Unlike lung cancer, in which the risk of smoking appears to be cumulative (pack years), the risk of IHD seems to be related to the concurrent level of smoking and to be reversible within 2 to 3 years when smoking is discontinued.

Sedentary Life-style

A sedentary life-style increases the risk of heart disease by nearly twofold.[2] It is estimated that less than 10% of adult Americans exercise at recommended levels.[10] There is no evidence, however, that exercise leads to the development of coronary collateral vessels or regression of atheromatous changes. Apart from changes in lipid levels related to weight reduction, there is little evidence that exercise alone can alter the plasma cholesterol concentration. A high level of physical activity improves the feeling of well-being and delays the onset of premature IHD but does not prolong the total life span.[11]

Medical Manifestations of Exercise

Bradycardia is the principal cardiac manifestation of exercise in the well-trained athlete, presumably reflecting increased vagal tone. Left ventricular hypertrophy is often suggested by the electrocardiogram (ECG), and either functional tricuspid or mitral regurgitation, or both, may be present. Cardiac dysrhythmias may be precipitated by exercise in the patient with IHD leading to sudden death. The most common cause of exercise-associated deaths in young athletes is unrecognized hypertrophic cardiomyopathy or a congenital anomaly of the coronary circulation. Exercise-induced asthma is the most common pulmonary complication of endurance training. Menstrual dysfunction is common in highly trained female athletes. In the female, 22% body fat is considered necessary to maintain normal menstrual function and endurance training decreases this percentage. Physical activity retards osteoporosis by increasing bone mineral content. Chronic endurance training may increase insulin sensitivity and thus improve control of diabetes mellitus.

An elevated plasma concentration of skeletal muscle enzymes, especially creatine kinase (CPK), usually accompany exercise. In addition, the plasma aspartate aminotransferase level may be increased. These elevated enzyme concentrations do not have any pathologic significance but may be misin-

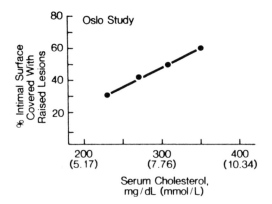

Fig. 1-1. Relationship of premortem serum cholesterol concentrations to severity of atherosclerosis discovered at autopsy. (From Grundy SM. Cholesterol and coronary artery disease. A new era. JAMA 1986;256:2849–58, with permission.)

terpreted in the absence of a history of exercise. Even the plasma concentration of CK-MB can be elevated after strenuous exercise; the source is presumed to be skeletal muscle, as cardiac damage does not occur. Mild albuminuria and even hematuria may be present in the first voided urine after strenuous exercise. Strenuous exertion is an infrequent cause of reversible neuropathy from nerve compression caused by hypertrophied skeletal muscles.

Other Risk Factors

Type A behavior (aggressive, compulsive, deadline conscious) has not been consistently correlated with IHD.[12] Diabetes mellitus is a prominent risk factor for the development of IHD. Apparently, the risk is not eliminated by control of hyperglycemia. A positive family history of IHD plus the presence of diabetes is associated with increased risk, especially in males younger than 60 years of age. Nevertheless, the role of diabetes as an independent risk factor is difficult to define, in view of the familial aggregation of diabetes, hypertension, and hypercholesterolemia. For the same reason, obesity is difficult to prove as an independent risk factor.

CARDIAC EVALUATION

History, physical examination, chest radiograph, and ECG are the basic components of the cardiac evaluation and diagnosis of the patient with known or suspected IHD (Table 1-2). More specialized and expensive noninvasive and invasive tests are employed selectively as adjuncts to the basic components of the cardiac evaluation. Left ventricular function can be classified as good or impaired based on the history, physical examination, and measurements obtained during cardiac catheterization (Table 1-3).

Table 1-2. Diagnosis of Ischemic Heart Disease

Initial Evaluation
  History
  Physical examination
  Laboratory data

Stress Testing If Initial Evaluation Suggestive
  Exercise electrocardiogram
  Radionuclide tests
    Exercise thallium
    Dipyridamole thallium

Stress Test Suggestive
  Coronary angiography

Table 1-3. Evaluation of Left Ventricular Function

Good Function	Impaired Function
History and Physical Examination	
Angina pectoris	Prior myocardial infarction
Essential hypertension	Evidence of congestive heart failure
No evidence of congestive heart failure	
Cardiac Catheterization	
Ejection fraction >0.55	Ejection fraction <0.4
Left ventricular end-diastolic pressure <12 mmHg	Left ventricular end-diastolic pressure >18 mmHg
Cardiac index >2.5 $L \cdot min^{-1} \cdot m^{-2}$	Cardiac index <2 $L \cdot min^{-1} \cdot m^{-2}$
No areas of ventricular dyskinesia	Multiple areas of ventricular dyskinesia

History

An important goal of the history is to elicit the severity, progression, and functional limitations introduced by IHD. Cardiac dysrhythmias, myocardial ischemia, and left ventricular dysfunction are usually responsible for the symptoms of IHD. Therefore, analysis of the symptoms of exercise tolerance, dyspnea, angina pectoris, and peripheral edema is the basic clinical method for detecting functional impairment owing to heart disease. Symptoms of cardiac disease may be absent at rest, emphasizing the need to evaluate the patient's response to various physical activities (walking up steps, walking at a known speed). Furthermore, a patient may remain asymptomatic despite 50% to 70% stenosis of a major coronary artery.

Exercise Tolerance

Limited exercise tolerance, in the absence of significant lung disease, is the most striking evidence of decreased cardiac reserve. If a patient can climb two to three flights of stairs without symptoms, it is likely that cardiac reserve is adequate. Dyspnea following the onset of angina pectoris suggests the presence of acute left ventricular dysfunction due to myocardial ischemia. It is important to identify the patient bordering on congestive heart failure (CHF), as the added stress of anesthesia, surgery, and fluid replacement may result in overt failure.

Angina Pectoris

Angina pectoris is the symptomatic manifestation of myocardial ischemia caused by an imbalance between myocardial oxygen supply and demand. Pain characterized as angina is typically substernal with occasional radiation to the neck, mandible, left shoulder, or left arm. Physical exertion typically evokes angina, whereas rest or sublingual nitroglycerin, or both, provides prompt relief.

A patient with aortic stenosis may experience angina despite a normal coronary angiogram, presumably reflecting excessive myocardial oxygen demands. A thickened and poorly compliant myocardium and the increased intraventricular pressure generated by the aortic obstruction may also interfere with subendocardial perfusion. Prognosis in these patients does not seem to be altered by their angina.

Esophageal spasm can result in substernal pain. Unlike angina, pain due to esophageal spasm is usually not related to exertion, does not radiate to the left arm, and is most likely to occur when the patient is supine. The pain of esophageal spasm, like that of angina, is relieved by nitroglycerin. Sharp pain exacerbated by deep breathing and coughing suggests pleural irritation or pericarditis.

Vasospastic angina (variant or Prinzmetal's angina) differs from classic angina in that it may occur at rest, owing to spasm of a coronary artery. This form of angina is often accompanied by cardiac dysrhythmias and about 85% of affected patients have a proximal fixed obstructive lesion in a major artery. The remaining 15% of patients have no evidence of IHD on angiography and presumably are experiencing vasospasm at the time of angina. An increased incidence of migraine headache and Raynaud's phenomenon has been observed in patients with vasospastic angina, suggesting that these conditions may be an expression of a basic vasospastic disease.

Treatment of angina is directed toward decreasing myocardial oxygen requirements with drugs such as beta antagonists, nitroglycerin, or calcium entry blockers. Preoperatively, it is important to determine that angina is stable. In this regard, angina is considered stable when there has been no change in the precipitating factors, frequency, and duration of pain for at least 60 days. Chest pain produced with less than normal activity or lasting for more prolonged periods than before is considered characteristic of unstable angina and may signal impending myocardial infarction. Most patients with unstable angina undergo coronary angiography.

Silent Myocardial Ischemia

Silent myocardial ischemia does not evoke angina and usually occurs at a heart rate and blood pressure substantially lower than that present during exercise-induced myocardial ischemia. Ambulatory and continuous monitoring of the ECG often demonstrates the occurrence of otherwise transient and asymptomatic evidence of myocardial ischemia on the ECG of the patient with IHD, especially with different forms of mental stress.[13] A history of IHD or an abnormal ECG suggestive of a prior myocardial infarction is associated with the highest incidence of silent myocardial ischemia, although similar changes may also occur in the absence of known IHD.[14] There seems to be an association between the presence of silent myocardial ischemia and an ejection fraction of less than 0.4.

Overall, it is estimated that about 70% of ischemic episodes in patients with symptomatic IHD are not associated with angina and that about 10% to 15% of acute myocardial infarctions are silent.[14] Mortality from myocardial infarction in the patient with silent myocardial ischemia is at least as great as that in patients with classic angina. Treatment of silent myocardial ischemia is the same as for classic angina.

Prior Myocardial Infarction

A history of a prior myocardial infarction is important information in the preoperative evaluation. Retrospective studies of large groups of adult patients have demonstrated that the incidence of myocardial reinfarction during the perioperative period is related to the time elapsed since the previous myocardial infarction[15-18] (Table 1-4). The incidence of perioperative myocardial reinfarction seems to stabilize at about 6% when the time elapsed after the prior myocardial infarction reaches about 6 months[15-18] (Table 1-4). This is the basis for the recommendation that an elective operation, especially a thoracic or upper abdominal procedure, be delayed for about 6 months after a myocardial infarction. Even after 6 months, the 6% incidence of myocardial reinfarction is about 50 times greater than the 0.13% incidence of perioperative myocardial infarction in the patient undergoing a similar operation but in the absence of a prior myocardial infarction.

Mortality from a myocardial reinfarction during the postoperative period exceeds 20%; more than 90% of these adverse cardiac events occur during the first 48 hours after operation.[17] By contrast, the incidence of myocardial infarction associated with coronary artery revascularization operations is substantial, but the mortality after these operations is usually less than 3%. Presumably, this low mortality reflects increased myocardial oxygen delivery to the heart after revascularization. This finding is in contrast with the lack of beneficial effects on the heart achieved with noncardiac surgery.

Hemodynamic monitoring using an intra-arterial and pulmonary artery catheter and prompt pharmacologic treatment or fluid infusion to treat hemodynamic alterations from a normal range may decrease the risk of perioperative myocardial rein-

Table 1-4.   Incidence of Perioperative Myocardial Reinfarction

Time Elapsed Since Prior Myocardial Infarction (mo)	Tarhan et al.[15] (%)	Steen et al.[16] (%)	Rao et al.[18] (%)	Shah et al.[17] (%)
0–3	37	27	5.7	4.3
4–6	16	11	2.3	0
>6	5	6		5.7

farction in high-risk patients.[17,18] For example, the reinfarction rate in intensely monitored and promptly treated patients was 5.7% and 2.3%, when the time elapsed since the prior infarction was up to 3 months and 4 to 6 months, respectively[15-18] (Table 1-4). Corresponding mortality rates were 5.3% and zero, substantially lower than that reported by others.[15-18]

The incidence of myocardial reinfarction is increased in the patient undergoing an intrathoracic or intra-abdominal operation lasting longer than 3 hours[16] (Table 1-5). A systolic blood pressure decrease greater than 30% lasting longer than 10 minutes is also associated with an increased incidence of myocardial reinfarction. Likewise, intraoperative hypertension and tachycardia are associated with an increased risk of myocardial reinfarction. There is evidence that intraoperative myocardial ischemia, most often associated with tachycardia, increases the likelihood of myocardial infarction.[19] The risk of postoperative myocardial infarction after noncardiac surgery is increased in the patient with known three-vessel coronary artery disease and in those with left main coronary artery disease.[20] Conversely, the risk of postoperative myocardial infarction after a noncardiac operation in a patient with one-vessel or two-vessel coronary artery disease appears to be relatively low. Likewise, the patient who has undergone a prior coronary artery bypass graft operation is not at increased risk when a subsequent noncardiac operation is performed.[20] Factors that have not been shown to predispose to myocardial reinfarction include the site of the previous myocardial infarction, the site of the operative procedure if the duration of the operation is less than 3 hours, and the drugs and/or techniques (regional versus general) used to produce anesthesia.[17] An attempt to develop a preoperative list of patient characteristics (age, prior myocardial infarction, aortic stenosis, evidence of CHF, cardiac dysrhythmias) that allows prediction of a life-threatening postoperative complication has not been shown to be superior to the physical status classification of the American Society of Anesthesiologists.[21,22]

Table 1-5. Incidence of Reinfarction

Duration of Operation (h)	Upper Abdominal or Intrathoracic Operation (%)	Other Operative Site (%)
<3	5.9	3.6
>3	15.9[a]	3.8

[a] $P < 0.05$ compared with other sites.

(Data from Steen PA, Tinker JH, Tarhan S. Myocardial reinfarction after anesthesia and surgery. An update: Incidence, mortality, and predisposing factors. JAMA 1978;239:2566–70.)

Co-Existing Noncardiac Diseases

The history obtained from the patient should elicit symptoms and information relevant to co-existing noncardiac diseases. For example, the patient with IHD is likely to exhibit peripheral vascular disease. Indeed, a history of stroke or syncope should suggest the presence of significant cerebrovascular disease. Chronic obstructive airway disease should be suspected in the patient with a history of cigarette smoking. Renal dysfunction may be associated with chronic hypertension. Diabetes mellitus is the most likely endocrine disease encountered in the patient with IHD.

Current Medications

An awareness of current medications used in the medical management of IHD is important, as these drugs may exert potential adverse effects during anesthesia. Medical therapy for IHD is designed to decrease myocardial oxygen requirements and to improve coronary blood flow. These goals are most often achieved by the combined use of beta antagonists, nitrates, and calcium entry blockers.

Beta Antagonists

A beta antagonist decreases myocardial oxygen requirements by decreasing the heart rate, blood pressure, and myocardial contractility. Effective beta blockade is probably present when the resting heart rate is 50 to 60 beats·min^{-1}. Routine physical activity should be expected to increase heart rate 10% to 20%. A patient on an optimal dose of beta antagonist should have no evidence of CHF or atrioventricular heart block on the ECG. Bronchospasm is less likely when a cardioselective beta antagonist is used. There is no evidence that beta antagonists adversely enhance negative inotropic effects of volatile anesthetics and the accepted practice is to continue the administration of these drugs throughout the perioperative period. Atropine (0.4 to 0.6 mg IV) is the initial treatment when excessive negative inotropic and/or chronotropic effects of a beta antagonist are manifested during the perioperative period. Atropine is effective because its vagolytic effects permit sympathetic nervous system innervation of the heart to emerge. Isoproterenol (2 to 5 μg·min^{-1} IV), as an initial infusion rate with adjustment to the desired heart rate, is the specific pharmacologic antagonist for excessive beta antagonist activity. Depending on the magnitude of beta blockade, a larger dose of isoproterenol may be necessary. Dobutamine is also an effective catecholamine for reversal of adverse cardiac effects due to beta antagonist therapy. High doses of dopamine, as may be required to antagonize beta blockade, could result in an undesirable increase in systemic vascular resistance due to relatively unopposed alpha stimulation. Calcium works at areas other than beta receptors to increase myocardial contractility in the presence of drug-induced beta blockade. For this reason, conventional doses of calcium (500 to 1000 mg

IV) will be effective. The postoperative period is a time when inadvertent acute withdrawal of beta antagonist therapy may occur, resulting in rebound increases in blood pressure and heart rate.

Nitrates

The ability of nitroglycerin to decrease myocardial oxygen requirements is the most likely mechanism by which this drug relieves angina in the patient with IHD. For example, nitroglycerin-induced venodilation and increased venous capacitance decreases venous return to the heart, resulting in a decreased ventricular end-diastolic pressure and volume, and therefore a decreased myocardial oxygen requirement. Nitroglycerin dilates coronary arteries, which may be an important mechanism in the relief of angina owing to vasospasm. The duration of sublingual nitroglycerin is about 30 minutes, limiting its usefulness to relief of individual anginal episodes rather than sustained prophylaxis. Transdermal preparations of nitroglycerin provide a sustained therapeutic effect, but tolerance often develops unless a nitrate-free interval such as during sleep is provided. Administered as a continuous intravenous infusion, nitroglycerin is titrated to produce a satisfactory physiologic response, reflected by relief of pain or a decrease in blood pressure and left ventricular filling pressure.

Calcium Entry Blockers

Calcium entry blockers decrease the influx of calcium into myocardial cells and vascular smooth muscle cells through slow calcium channels. Verapamil is the most depressant of the calcium entry blockers to conduction of the cardiac impulse through the atrioventricular node, accounting for its value in the treatment of atrial tachydysrhythmias. Nifedipine has the greatest vasodilating effect of the calcium entry blockers. It is often administered for the treatment of coronary artery vasospasm and angina. Diltiazem is useful for the treatment of vasospastic and classic angina. It seems to have a lower incidence of side effects (headache, flushing, paresthesia, weakness) than occurs with nifedipine.

Treatment of a patient with a calcium entry blocker may introduce the potential for adverse drug interactions during the perioperative period.[23] This prediction is based on the knowledge that calcium is necessary for the function of myocardial, skeletal, and vascular smooth muscle. For example, myocardial depression and peripheral vasodilation produced by a volatile anesthetic could be exaggerated by a similar action of the calcium entry blocker. Despite these theoretical concerns, only additive, and not synergistic, cardiac depression seems to occur when a patient with normal left ventricular function who is being treated chronically with a calcium entry blocker and beta antagonist receives a volatile anesthetic.[24–26] Because of the tendency to produce atrioventricular heart block, verapamil should be used cautiously in the patient re-

ceiving digitalis or a beta antagonist. Nevertheless, in the patient without preoperative evidence of a cardiac conduction abnormality, the chronic combined administration of a calcium entry blocker and beta antagonist is not associated with cardiac conduction abnormalities during the perioperative period.[27] Correction of hypotension or bradycardia due to a calcium entry blocker includes the intravenous administration of atropine, isoproterenol, and calcium. Calcium entry blockers may potentiate the effects of depolarizing and nondepolarizing muscle relaxants and exaggerate disease states associated with skeletal muscle weakness.[28] Antagonism of neuromuscular blockade may be impaired because of diminished presynaptic release of acetylcholine in the presence of a calcium entry blocker.[29]

Aspirin

Administration of aspirin (325 mg·d^{-1}) acts to inhibit platelet aggregation, which may be useful in preventing acute myocardial infarction, especially in the patient with unstable angina.[30] Indeed, there is evidence that this dose of aspirin decreases the risk of acute myocardial infarction in males over 50 years of age.[31] Mortality from cardiovascular disease is not altered by aspirin therapy, whereas the incidence of hemorrhagic stroke may be increased.[32] Heparin administered intravenously is an alternative to aspirin when surgery is imminent.

Combined Therapy

A beta antagonist and nitrate may be used in combination to achieve proper control of heart rate (less than 60 beats·min^{-1}) and blood pressure in the patient with IHD. The addition of a calcium entry blocker to this combination can produce further relief of angina in a patient who is refractory to the combination of a beta antagonist and nitrate. Nifedipine is likely to be selected for combination therapy because it does not add to inhibition of the sinus node produced by the beta antagonist. Because nifedipine dilates the coronary arteries by a different mechanism than that of nitrates, the two drugs complement each other in the treatment of coronary artery spasm.[33]

Physical Examination

The physical examination is often normal despite significant IHD. Nevertheless, signs of left ventricular failure (third heart sound, jugular venous distension) must be recognized (see Chapter 6). A carotid bruit may indicate previously unrecognized cerebrovascular disease. Orthostatic hypotension may reflect attenuated autonomic nervous system activity due to treatment with an antihypertensive drug. Evaluation of the upper airway and the anticipated ease of tracheal intubation, accessibility of peripheral venous sites, and determination of collateral blood flow if cannulation of a peripheral artery for intraoperative monitoring is planned are important aspects of the preoperative physical examination.

Chest Radiograph

Specific findings related to IHD are unlikely to be present on the chest radiograph, although evidence of cardiomegaly and CHF should be routinely sought. The earliest radiographic sign of pulmonary congestion is relative constriction of the pulmonary veins in the lower lung fields and dilation of pulmonary veins in the upper lung fields. This pattern reflects the redistribution of blood flow among the regions of the lung caused by elevated pulmonary venous pressure. Chronic pulmonary disease is suggested by the presence of lung hyperinflation and depression of the domes of the diaphragm.

Electrocardiogram

Review of the resting 12-lead ECG remains a cost-effective screening test in the cardiac evaluation of a patient with IHD. The preoperative ECG is reviewed for evidence of (1) myocardial ischemia, (2) prior myocardial infarction, (3) cardiac rhythm and/or conduction disturbances, (4) cardiomegaly, and (5) electrolyte abnormalities. It is important to remember that the resting ECG in the absence of angina may be normal despite extensive IHD. Furthermore, a prior myocardial infarction, especially if subendocardial, may not be accompanied by persistent changes on the ECG. The presence of premature ventricular beats may signal either their likely occurrence intraoperatively or the presence of myocardial ischemia. A P-R interval greater than 0.2 second on the ECG is most often related to digitalis therapy. A block in conduction of the cardiac impulse that occurs below the atrioventricular node is most likely to reflect a pathologic change, rather than a drug effect.

Myocardial Ischemia

The presence of ST segment depression greater than 1 mm on the resting ECG confirms the presence of subendocardial myocardial ischemia. Likewise, the accepted criterion for an ischemic response on the exercise ECG is ST segment depression of 1 mm or more in a patient in whom ST segments at rest were isoelectric. Furthermore, the ECG lead demonstrating evidence of myocardial ischemia can help determine the specific coronary artery that is diseased (Table 1-6). In this regard, the exercise ECG of a patient with narrowing of the left main coronary artery can show more than 2 mm of ST segment depression, often in association with angina, hypotension, and cardiac dysrhythmias. A decrease in blood pressure during exercise-induced ST segment depression suggests that a large portion of the myocardium is ischemic and increases the likelihood that three-vessel or left main coronary artery disease is present. It is estimated that narrowing of a major coronary artery by more than 50% (flow is proportional to the fourth power of the radius) will be associated with inadequate oxygen delivery during periods of increased myocardial oxygen demand, as associated with exercise-induced hyper-

Table 1-6. Relationship of the Electrocardiogram Lead to the Area of Myocardial Ischemia

Electrocardiogram Lead	Coronary Artery Responsible for Ischemia	Area of Myocardium That May Be Involved
II, III, aVF	Right coronary artery	Right atrium Right ventricle Sinoatrial node Atrioventricular node
I, aVL	Circumflex coronary artery	Lateral aspects of left ventricle
V3–V5	Left anterior descending coronary artery	Anterolateral aspects of left ventricle

tension and tachycardia. In 95% of females and 85% of males, the right coronary artery gives off the atrioventricular nodal artery; these persons are said to have a dominant right coronary artery. The remainder have a left dominant system in which the circumflex artery gives rise to the atrioventricular nodal artery.

The exercise ECG simulates sympathetic nervous system stimulation that may accompany perioperative events such as laryngoscopy and surgical stimulation. Interpretation of the exercise ECG is based on (1) the duration of exercise that the patient is able to perform, (2) the maximum heart rate that is achieved, (3) the time of onset of ST segment depression on the ECG, (4) the degree of ST segment depression, and (5) the time until resolution of the ST segment depression during the recovery period. Certainly, a normal exercise ECG indicates that the coronary circulation is reasonably adequate. Nevertheless, approximately 10% of the adult population with normal coronary arteries may develop ST segment changes on the exercise ECG that resemble changes observed in the patient with IHD. For this reason, use of the exercise ECG in an asymptomatic patient is of doubtful value.

Vasospastic angina is characterized by ST segment elevation on the ECG during periods of myocardial ischemia. The presence of ST segment elevation implies extensive transmural myocardial ischemia, in contrast to ST segment depression associated with subendocardial myocardial ischemia.

Advanced Diagnostic Methods

Advanced diagnostic methods used in the cardiac evaluation of the patient with suspected IHD may be categorized as noninvasive (ambulatory ECG monitoring, echocardiography, radioisotope imaging) and invasive (angiography and cardiac catheterization).

Ambulatory Electrocardiographic Monitoring

Electrocardiographic monitoring of ambulatory patients by tape recorder (Holter monitoring) is used principally to detect cardiac dysrhythmias, especially sustained episodes of paroxysmal tachycardia. Correlation of symptoms (palpitations, dizziness, syncope) is often the most valuable result of ambulatory recordings.

Echocardiography

Echocardiography provides dynamic images of the heart, including ventricular wall motion, wall thickness, cavity dimensions, intracardiac shunts, and cardiac value functions. Ejection fraction may also be estimated by echocardiography.

Radioisotope Imaging

Radioisotope imaging requires the intravenous injection of a gamma-emitting radiopharmaceutical that permits the imaging of blood within the heart and lungs. Thallium is the isotope most frequently used for myocardial imaging.[34] This isotope is almost completely extracted from the coronary circulation, providing a method of visualizing blood flow to the left ventricle. An area of decreased perfusion (cold spot) that appears only during exercise indicates myocardial ischemia, whereas a constant perfusion defect suggests an old myocardial infarction. An exercise thallium test complements the exercise ECG in diagnosing IHD.

Radionuclide angiocardiography using radioactive technetium bound to albumin permits imaging of blood within the heart and lungs. This technique is used to indicate the size and contractile function of the cardiac chambers, to detect abnormalities of left ventricular wall motion, and to calculate the ejection fraction.

Angiography

Coronary angiography and left ventricular angiography are highly specialized tests that are not routinely performed or even indicated in most patients before noncardiac surgery. When available, however, these data provide objective evidence of left ventricular function and facilitate prediction of the patient's response to the stress of anesthesia and surgery (Table 1-3). Digital subtraction angiography permits the injection of a small volume of radiopaque contrast material during cardiac catheterization so as to allow performance of a large number of angiographic studies during a single catheterization procedure. Although coronary angiography is the procedure that provides the most information about the condition of the coronary arteries, it is expensive and there is an associated risk (mortality 0.1%). The most compelling indication for coronary angiography is the presence of incapacitating angina in a patient receiving maximal medical therapy. A vessel is considered operable if it is of reasonable size, has a high-grade proximal stenosis, and is free of significant distal disease.

The most important determinant of the risk of death from IHD is the anatomic extent of disease as revealed by coronary angiography and the state of left ventricular function. For example, mortality over a 4- to 5-year period is greater in patients with left main coronary artery disease followed by three-vessel disease, two-vessel disease, and least with one-vessel disease.[35] Likewise, in patients with three-vessel disease, mortality over a 5-year period is greatest in those with left ventricular dysfunction, compared with those patients with normal left ventricular function.

Left ventricular angiography permits evaluation of the ejection fraction (stroke volume divided by the end-diastolic volume) and contractile patterns (hypokinetic, akinetic, dyskinetic). Ejection fraction can also be measured by echocardiography. A normally contracting left ventricle will eject 55% to 75% (ejection fraction 0.55 to 0.75) of its end-diastolic volume as stroke volume with each cardiac contraction. An ejection fraction of 0.4 to 0.55 is common in the patient with decreased myocardial contractility, owing to a prior myocardial infarction or increased left ventricular afterload in association with essential hypertension. A patient with an ejection fraction within this range is usually asymptomatic. Symptoms of decreased cardiac reserve are likely to manifest during exercise when the ejection fraction is 0.25 to 0.4. When the ejection fraction is less than 0.25, it is likely that the patient will be symptomatic at rest (New York Heart Association class IV). It is possible that the stress of anesthesia and operation will be poorly tolerated with this degree of left ventricular dysfunction.

Cardiac Catheterization

Normal left ventricular end-diastolic pressure (LVEDP) is less than 12 mmHg, whereas the corresponding value for the right ventricle is 5 mmHg or less. A resting LVEDP greater than 18 mmHg implies significantly decreased left ventricular contractility. Indeed, a failing left ventricle is unable to empty adequately in systole, leading to increased left ventricular end-diastolic volume and LVEDP. In addition to end-diastolic volume, LVEDP can be influenced by the compliance of the left ventricular muscle. Thus, an increased LVEDP may reflect increased end-diastolic volume or decreased compliance of the ventricle, or both. In the absence of mitral valve disease, mean left atrial pressure and pulmonary artery occlusion pressure reflect the LVEDP. Bed rest, fluid restriction, and diuretics may result in normalization of the LVEDP despite the continued presence of severe left ventricular dysfunction. Under these circumstances, a large increase in LVEDP pressure, following injection of the contrast medium during coronary angiography, may indicate poor left ventricular response to stress. Interpretation of the LVEDP must take into consideration the patient's exercise tolerance.

A normal resting cardiac index is 2.5 to 3.5 $L \cdot min^{-1} \cdot m^{-2}$. The patient with left ventricular dysfunction may have a normal resting cardiac output but be unable to increase flow in response to stress or exercise. A cardiac index of less than 2 $L \cdot min^{-1} \cdot m^{-2}$ in a patient with IHD suggests severe left ventricular dysfunction (Table 1-3). A decrease in cardiac output may be associated with an increase in the arterial-to-venous oxygen difference, as the tissues continue to require the same amount of oxygen but must extract this oxygen from a decreased blood flow.

ACUTE MYOCARDIAL INFARCTION

Acute myocardial infarction occurs in about 500,000 Americans annually, being more frequent in males until age 70. The incidence increases steeply with age in both sexes. The classic clinical syndrome consists of the sudden onset of characteristic symptoms, followed by serial ECG changes and a transient increase in the plasma concentration of myocardial enzymes. The first symptom of acute myocardial infarction is usually chest pain, typically similar to angina pectoris but more severe, persistent, and unrelieved by nitroglycerin. Pain simulating indigestion as well as diaphoresis and nausea are also common. Premonitory signs (change in characteristics of angina, fatigue) occur within 1 month before the onset of classic acute myocardial infarction in about two-thirds of patients. In many patients, especially the elderly, acute myocardial infarction is asymptomatic, being recognized only by the appearance of diagnostic Q waves on a routine ECG.

Pathogenesis

A sudden total occlusion of a major coronary artery by a thrombus causes infarction involving virtually the full thickness of the left ventricular wall in the specific region supplied by the artery. Coronary artery thrombosis nearly always occurs at the site of an atheromatous plaque, which undergoes ulceration, resulting in aggregation of platelets. These platelets release thromboxane, which promotes further platelet aggregation, coronary vasoconstriction, and ultimately the formation of a true thrombus. In some instances, the mere presence of severe narrowing of the coronary artery lumen, perhaps augmented by local vasospasm, may promote the initial platelet aggregation. Myocardial infarction may also arise from a sudden disparity between myocardial oxygen supply (hypotension) and demand (hypertension, tachycardia), as may occur during the perioperative period, and in the absence of an acute change in the caliber of the coronary arteries. Cocaine abuse

can produce a sudden increase in myocardial oxygen demand similar to that caused by catecholamines; it may also cause coronary artery vasospasm. Myocardial necrosis is largely completed in 3 to 6 hours and may be irreversible after an even shorter period, if the occlusion has been sudden and complete and there is no collateral circulation.

Diagnosis

The diagnosis of acute myocardial infarction is based on the patient's history plus supporting evidence of myocardial necrosis. Sympathetic nervous system overactivity (hypertension, tachycardia) is typically seen in a patient with an anterior wall myocardial infarction. This sympathetic nervous system overactivity can precipitate ventricular fibrillation during the first few hours after the onset of a myocardial infarction. Inferior wall myocardial infarction is often accompanied by bradycardia and hypotension owing to parasympathetic nervous system overactivity. Hypotension at the time of myocardial infarction may reflect parasympathetic nervous system overactivity or acute left ventricular failure from extensive cardiac muscle infarction. Ventricular premature beats occur in 90% of patients in whom acute myocardial infarction develops. Elevation of body temperature is common. Myocardial infarction that occurs in the perioperative period may be difficult to recognize because of concurrent medical circumstances, such as operation-related pain and administration of analgesics. Indeed, myocardial infarction may be silent, although the unexplained development of cardiac dysrhythmias, hypotension, or CHF during the perioperative period, especially in a patient considered at risk, should arouse suspicion of an acute myocardial infarction.

The development of pathologic Q waves and serial ST segment and T wave changes on the ECG are virtually diagnostic of acute myocardial infarction. Convex elevation of the ST segment in leads V1–V4 indicates occlusion of the left anterior descending coronary artery, whereas ST segment elevation in leads II, III, and aVF signals occlusion of the right coronary artery in about 80% of patients and of the left circumflex coronary artery in about 20% of patients. Evidence of a subendocardial myocardial infarction may be minimal, since the ECG only poorly reflects subendocardial electrical activity. Subendocardial myocardial infarction reflects damage to the inner third of the myocardium nearest the ventricular cavity. The subendocardium of the left ventricle is uniquely susceptible to myocardial ischemia because its nutrient vessels are occluded during systole by the high intramuscular pressure generated by the contracting heart. T waves become symmetrically and often deeply inverted as the ST segment begins to return to an isoelectric position. Persistent elevation of the ST segments beyond 2 to 4 days should arouse suspicion of the presence of a left ventricular aneurysm. Q waves do not develop unless the acute myocardial infarction involves the entire thickness (transmural) of the ventricular wall. Furthermore, Q waves do not develop immediately but are displayed only after sufficient time has passed for muscle necrosis to occur.

Necrosis of myocardial tissue results in the appearance of CPK and its MB molecular subtype (CK-MB) within 3 hours after an acute myocardial infarction. The peak concentration is in about 12 hours, followed by a decrease to a normal level after another 12 to 24 hours. The peak level of CK-MB correlates with the size of the infarct and therefore indicates the prognosis. Sampling of blood for CK-MB determination at 0, 12, and 24 hours is recommended. It is suggested that the upper normal limit of CK-MB is $13\,IU\cdot L^{-1}$ and that an increase of at least 50% in this level during the first 4 to 12 hours after the suspected event is necessary for the diagnosis of myocardial infarction.

Two-dimensional echocardiography is a useful bedside test that demonstrates abnormal wall motion of the left ventricle in the presence of an acute myocardial infarction. Magnetic resonance imaging may also demonstrate abnormal wall motion after an acute myocardial infarction. Radionuclide imaging with thallium (visualize myocardial perfusion) or technetium (selective uptake into an area of recent myocardial necrosis) may be helpful in the diagnosis of acute myocardial infarction.

Treatment

Treatment of an acute myocardial infarction is medical and surgical. Thrombolytic therapy instituted during the early postinfarction period (less than 6 hours after the onset of infarction) can reopen the occluded artery so as to restore perfusion and limit the extent of myocardial necrosis. As a result, ventricular function is preserved and mortality decreased. The principal risk of thrombolytic therapy is bleeding, with intracranial hemorrhage occurring in 0.5% to 1% of treated patients. Because the incidence of reocclusion after the administration of thrombolytic agents is relatively high (about 20%), antithrombotic therapy (aspirin and heparin) is usually initiated promptly after this procedure. A beta antagonist administered intravenously as soon as possible after the onset of acute myocardial infarction may decrease infarct size, whereas long-term oral administration of such a drug may decrease the incidence of myocardial reinfarction. Lidocaine administered in the early stages of acute myocardial infarction decreases the frequency of cardiac dysrhythmias but has no effect on mortality. If hemodynamically significant heart block accompanies a myocardial infarction, the insertion of an artificial cardiac pacemaker is indicated.

Emergency coronary arteriography and percutaneous transluminal coronary angioplasty (PTCA) may be utilized to treat an acute myocardial infarction. This treatment involves passage of a balloon-tipped catheter across an area of coronary artery stenosis followed by inflation of the balloon, causing dilation of the stenotic area. About 4% of patients undergoing PTCA require emergency surgical revascularization, for intractable myocardial ischemia. Restenosis occurs in 25% to 35% of treated patients, usually within 6 months of PTCA, and is often treated by repeat angioplasty.[36]

Emergency surgical revascularization may also be selected for treatment of an acute myocardial infarction, especially if the patency of the occluded vessel cannot be maintained. Intractable angina that is unresponsive to medical therapy is an indication for coronary artery bypass graft surgery. Surgical revascularization enhances survival in patients with high-grade stenosis of the left main coronary artery. Survival is also increased by revascularization surgery in patients with three-vessel disease and an ejection fraction of less than 0.5.[37] An enhanced quality of life, as reflected by an improved functional status, relief of angina, and decreased need for medical therapy, is provided by surgery. Operative mortality in a patient with good left ventricular function is 1% to 2%. Poor left ventricular function worsens prognosis, regardless of whether surgical or medical therapy is employed.

Rehabilitation after an acute myocardial infarction has focused on early ambulation after an uncomplicated myocardial infarction and exercise training. As little as 7 days of bed rest can produce deleterious physiologic changes, including decreased skeletal muscle mass and a decreased intravascular fluid volume, which in turn leads to orthostatic hypotension. Hemoconcentration also increases blood viscosity and the likelihood of thromboembolism. Exercise is typically in the form of walking, jogging, or stationary bicycling at an intensity sufficient to increase the heart rate to 70% to 85% of the maximum determined by exercise testing. Exercise enhances graft patency in the patient who has undergone surgical revascularization. The effects of exercise training on the natural history of IHD, however, remain uncertain. Nevertheless, postmyocardial infarction rehabilitation including exercise training decreases overall mortality by about 25%.[38]

Complications

Mortality after myocardial infarction may be as great as 60% for those patients in whom pulmonary edema develops and who show evidence of impaired organ perfusion (mental changes and oliguria). When only evidence of pulmonary congestion follows an acute myocardial infarction, the mortality is 11%, while mortality decreases to 1% for those without any clinical hemodynamic abnormalities. Patients with an ejection fraction of less than 0.30 have an increased late mortality. Ventricular premature beats after initial recovery correlate with an increased risk of mortality.

Cardiac Dysrhythmias and Conduction Disturbances

Acute myocardial infarction is frequently complicated by cardiac dysrhythmias and conduction disturbances. Ventricular premature beats occur in more than 90% of patients with an acute myocardial infarction, ventricular tachycardia in about 10% of patients, and ventricular fibrillation in about 15% of patients, emphasizing the value of monitoring in a coronary care unit. The most likely mechanism for production of ventricular dysrhythmias is a reentrant current resulting from delayed conduction in the ischemic area. The other explanation is enhanced automaticity (irritability) of injured cardiac cells. Hypokalemia from diuretic therapy or elevated circulating plasma concentrations of catecholamines may also contribute to the development of ventricular dysrhythmias. Lidocaine (50 to 100 mg IV, followed by 1 to 4 mg·min^{-1} IV) is the most useful drug for control of ventricular dysrhythmias that complicate an acute myocardial infarction. In about 20% of patients, ventricular premature beats persist despite lidocaine therapy necessitating treatment with procainamide (1000 mg IV over 1 hour, followed by 200 mg·h^{-1}). The dose of lidocaine and procainamide may need to be decreased in the patient in whom CHF with associated renal dysfunction develops after an acute myocardial infarction. Ventricular tachycardia may require electrical cardioversion.

Atrial premature beats, atrial flutter, and atrial fibrillation most often occur in the patient in whom CHF develops in association with an acute myocardial infarction. These atrial dysrhythmias may reflect an acute increase in atrial pressure owing to left ventricular failure or the presence of atrial ischemia or infarction. Treatment of a hemodynamically significant atrial dysrhythmia is directed at slowing the rapid heart rate with drugs (digoxin, verapamil), electrical cardioversion, or rapid atrial pacing.

Sinus bradycardia that occurs in the patient with an acute myocardial infarction may reflect increased parasympathetic nervous system activity or acute ischemia of the sinus node or atrioventricular node, especially if there is occlusion of the right coronary artery. Bradycardia that results in hypotension is treated initially with the intravenous administration of atropine; in resistant cases, a temporary transcutaneous or transvenous pacemaker may be used.

Pericarditis

Pericarditis is a frequent complication of an acute myocardial infarction and may cause anterior chest pain, which may be confused with continuing or recurring myocardial ischemia. In contrast to the pain of myocardial ischemia, discomfort associated with pericarditis is accentuated by inspiration. Diffuse ST segment elevation on the ECG may be present. Pericardial effusion occurs in about one-third of patients after an acute myocardial infarction. Specific treatment of pericarditis is rarely required, but corticosteroids will often dramatically relieve symptoms. Dressler syndrome (postmyocardial infarction syndrome) is a delayed form of acute pericarditis that develops in about 3% of patients anywhere between the first week and many months after an acute myocardial infarction.

Left Ventricular Thrombus

A mural thrombus may form on the endocardial surface of the left ventricle at the site of akinetic myocardium after an acute myocardial infarction. Echocardiography is used for detecting such emboli, although systemic arterial embolism develops in only a small proportion of patients.

Congestive Heart Failure and Cardiogenic Shock

Acute myocardial infarction is often complicated by some degree of left ventricular dysfunction (failure), as reflected by increased LVEDP, pulmonary congestion, decreased PaO$_2$, and the presence of a third heart sound. The term *cardiogenic shock* should be restricted to those instances of hypotension and oliguria that persist after the relief of pain, abatement of excess parasympathetic nervous system activity, correction of hypovolemia, and treatment of cardiac dysrhythmias. In this regard, cardiogenic shock is an advanced form of acute CHF in which the cardiac output is insufficient to maintain adequate perfusion to the kidneys and other vital organs. This clinical picture occurs in about 7.5% of patients who have experienced an acute myocardial infarction.[39] Systolic blood pressure is often less than 60 mmHg, and there may be associated pulmonary edema and arterial hypoxemia. Pulseless electrical activity (electromechanical dissociation) may also accompany cardiogenic shock. The patient in whom cardiogenic shock develops is likely to have experienced infarction of greater than 40% of the left ventricular myocardium. Mortality among patients in whom cardiogenic shock develops exceeds 70%.[39]

Treatment

Initial treatment of cardiogenic shock is to decrease left ventricular afterload with a vasodilator drug such as nitroglycerin during invasive monitoring of blood pressure and cardiac filling pressures. Dopamine and dobutamine may be administered in an attempt to improve cardiac output, whereas digitalis is probably of no value in the treatment of cardiogenic shock. An attempt to restore coronary blood flow in the infarct-related artery by means of thrombolytic therapy, PTCA, or surgical revascularization may be indicated. Circulatory assist devices may be considered as a means of sustaining viable cardiac output until surgical revascularization can be performed or the feasibility of cardiac transplantation established. In this regard, left ventricular assist devices provide a significantly greater cardiac output than the intra-aortic balloon. The intra-aortic balloon is programmed to the ECG so as to deflate just before systole and to inflate during diastole. Presystolic deflation of the balloon decreases systemic blood pressure and afterload, which decreases cardiac work and myocardial oxygen requirements. Inflation of the balloon during diastole increases diastolic blood pressure and thus improves coronary blood flow and myocardial oxygen delivery. The intravenous infusion of a combination of a catecholamine and vasodilator may serve as a pharmacologic alternative to mechanical counterpulsation with the intra-aortic balloon.

Surgically Treatable Complications

Ventricular septal rupture occurs in 0.5% to 1% of patients experiencing an acute myocardial infarction. Acute mitral regurgitation may reflect infarction of a papillary muscle and is likely to be accompanied by a V wave greater than 50 mmHg on the tracing of the pulmonary artery occlusion pressure. Ventricular dysrhythmias or intractable CHF, or both, may reflect the presence of a postinfarction left ventricular aneurysm. Cardiac rupture occurs in 2% to 3% of patients after an acute myocardial infarction, typically occurring 3 to 10 days after the initial infarction. There is usually little warning of impending cardiac rupture before the onset of sudden cardiovascular collapse accompanied by acute cardiac tamponade or pulseless electrical activity, or both.

ANESTHESIA FOR NONCARDIAC SURGERY

The goal of preoperative cardiac assessment is to identify the patient at increased risk of perioperative myocardial infarction and to identify a patient who already has such extensive IHD that the ability to compensate for any added stress is limited.[40] Anesthesia for elective noncardiac surgery in the patient with IHD may be associated with adverse cardiac events, especially myocardial infarction.[3] It is estimated that more than one-half of all adverse postoperative events have a cardiac etiology. In this regard, a recent preoperative myocardial infarction and current CHF have been observed to predict adverse postoperative cardiac events consistently. Specialized preoperative cardiac testing (exercise ECG, ambulatory ECG monitoring, dipyridamole-thallium imaging) may be useful in identifying those at increased risk of experiencing an adverse cardiac event during the postoperative period. Perhaps the most reliable indicator of adverse postoperative cardiac events in a patient undergoing noncardiac surgery is myocardial ischemia during the first 48 hours after surgery.[3] Preoperative predictors of postoperative myocardial ischemia include (1) left ventricular hypertrophy, (2) history of hypertension, (3) diabetes mellitus, (4) known ischemic heart disease, and (5) use of digoxin.[3] It is conceivable that postoperative outcome may be improved by monitoring and treating patients at known increased risk of myocardial ischemia after surgery.

Preoperative Medication

The principal goal of preoperative medication for the patient with IHD is to decrease anxiety. Anxiety can lead to the secretion of catecholamines manifesting as increased blood pressure and heart rate. As a result of these changes, myocardial oxygen requirements are increased predictably. Indeed, the patient with IHD often arrives in the operating room with evidence of myocardial ischemia on the ECG as compared with the preoperative ECG.[19] In most cases, changes on the ECG can be described as silent ischemia, as these changes are not associated with angina or hemodynamic abnormalities. In this regard, it is not clear whether these episodes of silent myocardial ischemia differ from those that occur in the same patients during their normal daily activity.[41] Indeed, it is suggested that about 90% of "new" myocardial ischemia observed during anesthesia is the manifestation of silent ischemia that is also present before operation.[42]

Anxiety reduction requires both psychological and pharmacologic approaches. A patient is more likely to arrive in the operating room in a relaxed state, if a preoperative visit has been performed and the anesthetic sequence explained in detail. Pharmacologic sedation can be achieved with wide variety of drugs or combinations of drugs. The drug used often depends on the personal preference of the person responsible for the management of anesthesia. The goal of drug administration is to produce maximum sedation and amnesia without an undesirable degree of circulatory and ventilatory depression. One useful approach to preoperative medication for the patient with IHD is administration of morphine (10 to 15 mg IM) plus scopolamine (0.4 to 0.6 mg IM), with or without a benzodiazepine. Scopolamine is valuable because of its profound sedative and amnesic effects without producing an undesirable change in heart rate. Drugs used in the medical management of a patient with IHD should be continued throughout the perioperative period, including, in some instances, administration of these drugs with the preoperative medication.[27,43] It is convincingly documented that abrupt withdrawal of a beta antagonist drug or antihypertensive drug may result in an excessive increase in sympathetic nervous system activity. This increased sympathetic nervous system activity is particularly undesirable in the patient with IHD. It may also be appropriate to apply nitroglycerin ointment at the same time that the preoperative medication is administered. Certainly, the patient with IHD should have access to sublingual nitroglycerin during the period preceding the induction of anesthesia. Administration of an H-2 receptor antagonist to increase the gastric fluid pH does not appear to produce an adverse effect in the patient with IHD, although these drugs have the theoretical ability to contribute to coronary artery vasoconstriction by virtue of leaving H-1 mediated coronary artery constricting effects relatively unopposed.

Intraoperative Management

The basic challenge during induction and maintenance of anesthesia for the patient with IHD is to prevent myocardial ischemia. This goal is logically achieved by maintaining the balance between myocardial oxygen delivery and myocardial oxygen requirements. Intraoperative events associated with persistent tachycardia, systolic hypertension, sympathetic nervous system stimulation, arterial hypoxemia, or diastolic hypotension can adversely influence this delicate balance (Table 1-7). An increase in heart rate is more likely than hypertension to produce signs of myocardial ischemia on the ECG. Indeed, in anesthetized patients, the incidence of myocardial ischemia on the ECG sharply increases in the patient who experiences a heart rate greater than 110 beats·min^{-1} (ischemic threshold)[44] (Fig. 1-2). When heart rate is less than 110 beats·min^{-1}, the incidence of myocardial ischemia is random and silent, being unrelated to heart rate. Conceptually, a rapid heart rate increases the myocardial oxygen requirement and decreases the time during diastole for coronary blood flow, and thus delivery of oxygen, to occur. Conversely, increased myocardial oxygen requirements produced by hypertension tend to be offset by improved perfusion through pressure-dependent atherosclerotic coronary arteries. Iatrogenic hyperventilation of the lungs that greatly decreases the PaCO$_2$ is avoided, as hypocapnia may evoke coronary artery vasoconstriction. In the final analysis, maintenance of the balance between myocardial oxygen requirements and myocardial oxygen delivery is probably more important than the specific technique or drugs chosen to produce anesthesia and skeletal muscle relaxation. Indeed, multiple studies of patients undergoing coronary artery bypass graft operations demonstrate that the incidence of intraoperative myocardial ischemia and postoperative outcome are not influenced by the choice of anesthetic drug (halothane, enflurane, isoflurane, opioid).[42,45,46] Furthermore, although isoflurane may cause a decrease in coronary vascular resistance and predispose to coro-

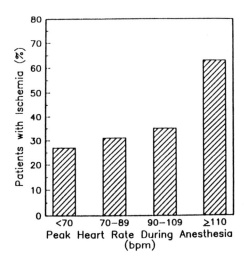

Fig. 1-2. The incidence of intraoperative myocardial ischemia is unrelated to heart rate (silent ischemia) until the heart rate exceeds about 110 beats·min^{-1}. (From Slogoff S, Keats AS. Does chronic treatment with calcium entry blocking drugs reduce perioperative myocardial ischemia? Anesthesiology 1988;68:676–80, with permission.)

nary artery steal, there is evidence that this drug does not increase the incidence of intraoperative myocardial ischemia when administered to patients with steal-prone coronary anatomy.[47]

It is important to avoid persistent and excessive changes in heart rate and blood pressure. A frequent recommendation is to maintain heart rate and blood pressure within 20% of the normal awake value for that patient. Nevertheless, most episodes of intraoperative myocardial ischemia on the ECG occur in the absence of hemodynamic changes, suggesting that it is unlikely that this form of myocardial ischemia will be preventable by the anesthesiologist.[42] In this regard, as many as 45% of patients show evidence of myocardial ischemia by thallium scan in the absence of hemodynamic changes during intubation of the trachea.[48] These episodes of silent myocardial ischemia are probably due to regional decreases in myocardial perfusion and oxygenation that are of doubtful significance and identical to episodes that occur in these patients during their daily activity in the absence of angina.

Induction of Anesthesia

Induction of anesthesia in the patient with IHD can be accomplished with the intravenous administration of nearly any of the available induction drugs. Ketamine is not popular, since an associated increase in heart rate and blood pressure may increase myocardial oxygen requirements. Intubation of the

Table 1-7. Intraoperative Events That Influence the Balance Between Myocardial Oxygen Delivery and Myocardial Oxygen Requirements

Decreased Oxygen Delivery	Increased Oxygen Requirements
Decreased coronary blood flow	Sympathetic nervous system stimulation
Tachycardia	Tachycardia
Diastolic hypotension	Systolic hypertension
Hypocapnia (coronary artery vasoconstriction)	Increased myocardial contractility
Coronary artery spasm	Increased afterload
Decreased oxygen content	
Anemia	
Arterial hypoxemia	
Shift of the oxyhemoglobin dissociation curve to the left	
Increased preload (wall tension)	

trachea is facilitated by the administration of succinylcholine or a nondepolarizing muscle relaxant.

Myocardial ischemia may accompany sympathetic nervous system stimulation that results from direct laryngoscopy and intubation of the trachea.[49] A short duration of laryngoscopy (15 seconds or less) may be useful in minimizing the magnitude and duration of circulatory stimulation associated with intubation of the trachea. When duration of direct laryngoscopy is not likely to be short, or when hypertension already exists, it is reasonable to consider additional drugs to minimize the pressor response produced by the intubation sequence. For example, laryngotracheal lidocaine (about 2 mg·kg^{-1}), administered just before placing the tube in the trachea, decreases the magnitude and duration of the blood pressure increase evoked by surgical stimulation. Likewise, lidocaine (1.5 mg·kg^{-1} IV), administered about 90 seconds before beginning direct laryngoscopy, may be efficacious in some patients. An alternative to lidocaine is nitroprusside (1 to 2 μg·kg^{-1} IV), administered about 15 seconds before beginning direct laryngoscopy.[50] This dose of nitroprusside is effective in attenuating the pressor, but not heart rate response to laryngoscopy, as well as in treating the hypertensive response that can follow intubation of the trachea. Continuous infusion of esmolol (100 to 300 μg·kg^{-1}·min^{-1} IV), before and during direct laryngoscopy, is useful for blunting the increase in heart rate evoked by intubation of the trachea.[51] A small dose of fentanyl (1 to 3 μg·kg^{-1} IV) (or an equivalent dose of sufentanil or alfentanil), administered before direct laryngoscopy, may also be useful for blunting the circulatory response evoked by intubation of the trachea. Although the rationale for these drug interventions is well founded, it must be recognized that the efficacy of any of these treatments remains undocumented.

The continuous infusion of nitroglycerin (0.25 to 1 μg·kg^{-1}·min^{-1} IV) has been used as prophylaxis against the development of coronary vasospasm in vulnerable patients. Despite the logic of this treatment, controlled studies have not consistently confirmed that this approach decreases the incidence of intraoperative myocardial ischemia.[52,53] The incidence of hypertension as produced by intubation of the trachea, however, is less in the patient receiving a continuous intravenous infusion of nitroglycerin.[53]

Maintenance of Anesthesia

Drugs selected for maintenance of anesthesia are often chosen on the basis of the patient's left ventricular function, as determined by the history and physical examination with or without data from cardiac catheterization (Table 1-3). For example, in the patient with IHD but normal left ventricular function, tachycardia and hypertension are likely to develop in response to intense stimulation, as during direct laryngoscopy or painful surgical stimulation. Controlled myocardial depression, using a volatile anesthetic, may be appropriate in such a patient, to minimize increased sympathetic nervous system activity and

a subsequent increase of myocardial oxygen requirements. Any of the currently popular volatile anesthetics are equally acceptable to produce controlled myocardial depression. Indeed, halothane and isoflurane produce similar changes in blood pressure and heart rate, when administered to the patient with IHD.[54] A volatile anesthetic can be used alone or in combination with nitrous oxide. Equally acceptable for maintenance of anesthesia is the use of a nitrous oxide–opioid technique, with the addition of a volatile anesthetic to treat an undesirable increase in blood pressure that may accompany painful stimulation. When used to control intraoperative hypertension, both isoflurane and halothane are equally effective, but the mechanism for lowering blood pressure is different, reflecting peripheral vasodilation produced by isoflurane and a decrease in cardiac output produced by halothane[55] (Fig. 1-3). In the final analysis, a volatile anesthetic may be beneficial in the patient with IHD because of a decrease in myocardial oxygen requirements, or it may be detrimental because it lowers blood pressure and thus coronary perfusion pressure. Despite the ability of isoflurane to cause coronary artery vasodilation there is no evidence that this drug increases the likelihood of myocardial ischemia, especially when coronary artery perfusion pressure is maintained.[47]

The patient with severely impaired left ventricular function, as associated with a prior myocardial infarction, may not tolerate anesthetic-induced myocardial depression. In these patients, the use of a short-acting opioid may be selected, rather than a volatile anesthetic. Indeed, high-dose fentanyl (50 to 100 μg·kg^{-1} IV) has been recommended for patients who cannot tolerate even minimal myocardial depression.[56] The addition of nitrous oxide to the opioid may be considered if the presence of total amnesia is uncertain. Although the combination of nitrous oxide with an opioid has an impressive record of safety in patients with impaired left ventricular function, nitrous oxide administered in the presence of an opioid may be associated with significant circulatory changes, including a decrease in blood pressure and cardiac output.[57] The combination of diazepam and fentanyl also produces a decrease in blood pressure that is not seen when either drug is administered alone.[58] Conversely, nitrous oxide added to background diazepam or a volatile anesthetic does not produce signs of myocardial depression.[59] Even nitrous oxide alone administered to the patient with IHD may produce evidence of myocardial depression.[60]

Regional anesthesia is an acceptable technique for the patient with IHD. Despite a decrease in myocardial oxygen requirements produced by peripheral sympathetic nervous system blockade, it is important to realize that flow through a coronary artery narrowed by atherosclerosis is pressure dependent. Therefore, a decrease in blood pressure associated with epidural or spinal anesthesia should not be allowed to persist on the mistaken notion that the patient is protected by a decrease in myocardial oxygen requirements. Prompt

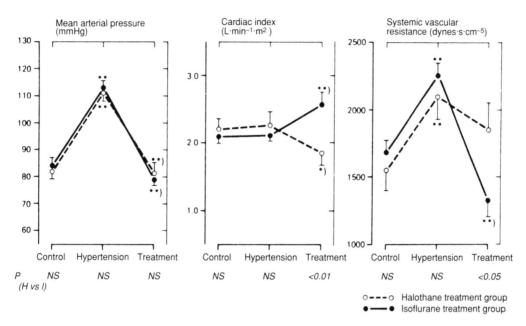

Fig. 1-3. Halothane (1% to 1.5% inspired) and isoflurane (1.5% to 2% inspired) were equally effective in returning mean arterial pressure to near control levels in patients who became hypertensive during surgical revascularization of the coronary circulation. Halothane lowers blood pressure principally by decreases in myocardial contractility (cardiac index), whereas decreases in blood pressure produced by isoflurane are due principally to decreases in systemic vascular resistance. (From Hess W, Arnold B, Schulte-Sasse U, Tarnow J. Comparison of isoflurane and halothane when used to control intraoperative hypertension in patients undergoing coronary artery bypass surgery. Anesth Analg 1983;62:15–20, with permission.)

treatment of a decrease in blood pressure that exceeds 20% of the preblock value, with the intravenous infusion of fluid and/or a sympathomimetic drug such as ephedrine or phenylephrine, is often recommended. A disadvantage of fluid infusion to correct hypotension is the time necessary for this treatment to be effective.

Choice of Muscle Relaxant

The choice of nondepolarizing muscle relaxant for administration to the patient with IHD is often influenced by the impact these drugs could have on the balance between myocardial oxygen delivery and requirements. In this regard, a muscle relaxant with minimal to absent effects on heart rate and blood pressure is an attractive selection for the patient with IHD.

Vecuronium, doxacurium, and pipecuronium are examples of muscle relaxants that have benign circulatory effects. Likewise, the blood pressure effects of atracurium are usually modest, especially if the drug is injected over a 30- to 45-second period, so as to minimize the likelihood of histamine release. Pancuronium has been used without apparent adverse effects for many years in patients with IHD despite its potential to increase myocardial oxygen requirements, owing

to modest increases in blood pressure and heart rate. Circulatory changes produced by pancuronium may be useful in offsetting negative inotropic and chronotropic effects of drugs used for anesthesia. This may be especially useful when opioid-induced bradycardia is considered excessive. The notion that co-existing beta antagonist therapy prevents pancuronium-induced increases in heart rate may not be valid, since this drug most likely increases heart rate by a vagolytic, and not a sympathomimetic, mechanism. Caution in the routine use of pancuronium in the patient with IHD is suggested by a report that evidence of myocardial ischemia on the ECG may occasionally accompany even the modest increases in heart rate produced by pancuronium when administered to patients with IHD.[61]

Reversal of nondepolarizing neuromuscular blockade with an anticholinesterase-anticholinergic drug combination can be safely accomplished in a patient with IHD. Glycopyrrolate, which is alleged to have a minimal chronotropic effect compared with atropine, may be selected as the anticholinergic drug when an excessive increase in heart rate is a possibility. Nevertheless, a marked increase in heart rate rarely occurs with the reversal of a nondepolarizing muscle relaxant, and atropine seems as acceptable as glycopyrrolate for inclusion with the anticholinesterase drug.

Monitoring

Perioperative monitoring is influenced by the complexity of the operative procedure and the severity of the IHD. An important goal in selecting monitors uniquely for the patient with IHD is early detection of myocardial ischemia (ECG) or decreased myocardial contractility (pulmonary artery catheter), or both. Most myocardial ischemia occurs in the absence of hemodynamic alterations; therefore, one should use caution in endorsing the routine use of expensive and complex monitors to detect myocardial ischemia.

Electrocardiogram

The ECG is a useful way to monitor the balance between myocardial oxygen delivery and myocardial oxygen requirements during general anesthesia. There is a predictable correlation between the lead of the ECG that reflects myocardial ischemia and the anatomic distribution of the diseased coronary artery (Table 1-6). For example, a V5 (precordial) lead (fifth interspace at the anterior axillary line) will reflect myocardial ischemia present in that portion of the left ventricle supplied by the left anterior descending coronary artery.[62] Therefore, it may be useful to monitor this lead or its equivalent during the perioperative period in patients with known disease of the left coronary artery. Using a three-lead electrode system, one can obtain the equivalent of a V5 lead by placing the left arm lead in the V5 position and selecting aVL on the ECG.[62]

Lead II is a better choice for detection of myocardial ischemia that occurs in the distribution of the right coronary artery. Furthermore, lead II is ideal for the identification of P waves and for the subsequent analysis of cardiac rhythm disturbances. Lead II, however, may not detect the more common occurrence of anterior or lateral wall myocardial ischemia specifically reflected by precordial leads. An esophageal ECG, by virtue of its position just posterior to the atrium and ventricle, results in augmented P waves and may facilitate intraoperative diagnosis of cardiac dysrhythmias or posterior wall myocardial ischemia.[63]

Significant myocardial ischemia is considered to be present when there is at least 1 mm downsloping of the ST segment from the baseline on the ECG. Cardiac dysrhythmias, cardiac conduction disturbances, digitalis therapy, electrolyte abnormalities, and hyperthermia can produce similar changes in the ST segment, in the absence of myocardial ischemia. An acute increase in the pulmonary artery occlusion pressure associated with the appearance of an abnormal wave form (an A wave greater than 15 mmHg or a V wave greater than 30 mmHg) may reflect the presence of myocardial ischemia.[64] Indeed, an abnormality in the tracing of the pulmonary artery occlusion pressure may precede a change on the ECG that suggests myocardial ischemia.

The appearance of signs of myocardial ischemia on the ECG supports prompt and aggressive pharmacologic treatment of associated adverse changes in heart rate or blood pressure, or both. A persistent elevation in heart rate is often treated with intravenous administration of a beta antagonist such as esmolol. An excessive increase in blood pressure without evidence of myocardial ischemia is often treated with nitroprusside. Nitroglycerin is a more appropriate choice when myocardial ischemia is associated with a normal to modestly elevated blood pressure. In this situation, nitroglycerin-induced decreases in preload will facilitate improvement in subendocardial blood flow, while not reducing blood pressure to the point that coronary perfusion pressure is jeopardized.

Hypotension should be treated with a sympathomimetic drug to restore perfusion through pressure-dependent atherosclerotic coronary arteries rapidly. A drug that increases blood pressure by increasing myocardial contractility, as well as systemic vascular resistance, is often chosen. In this regard, ephedrine may be superior to a relatively pure alpha drug such as phenylephrine. Nevertheless, co-existing beta blockade may convert ephedrine to a predominantly alpha agonist similar to phenylephrine. Furthermore, the dose of phenylephrine necessary to produce venoconstriction is less than the dose needed to constrict arteries, thus reducing the likelihood of drug-induced coronary artery vasoconstriction by stimulation of alpha receptors in coronary arteries.

In addition to drugs, intravenous infusion of fluid to restore blood pressure is useful, since myocardial oxygen requirements for volume work of the heart are less than those for pressure work. The risk of rapid infusion of fluid may be increased preload, leading to decreased subendocardial perfusion and ischemia. Regardless of the treatment, it is important to realize that prompt restoration of blood pressure is the goal, so as to maintain pressure-dependent blood flow through coronary arteries narrowed by atherosclerosis.

Pulmonary Artery Catheter

Monitoring the pulmonary artery occlusion pressure as a reflection of the left ventricular filling pressure may be helpful when a large intravascular fluid volume shift is expected intraoperatively. It is possible that a patient with IHD may manifest large volume requirements, reflecting a co-existing decreased intravascular fluid volume due to enhanced sympathetic nervous system activity. This volume deficit could be further exaggerated by preoperative fasting. Maintenance of the pulmonary artery occlusion pressure by the intravenous infusion of crystalloid or colloid solutions may contribute to cardiovascular stability during the operative period. In addition to guiding volume replacement, a pulmonary artery catheter allows measurement of cardiac output and calculation of systemic and pulmonary vascular resistance, information essential for evaluating the response to an inotropic or vasodilating drug. There should probably be a 10% to 15% change in thermodilution cardiac output before a significant change is accepted to have occurred. Even measurements of cardiac output considered to be significant changes should be considered within the context of the clinical status of the patient, as reflected by peripheral perfusion and urinary output. A sudden increase in pulmonary artery occlusion pressure may reflect acute myocardial ischemia. The appearance of a V wave component to the pulmonary artery occlusion pressure tracing may reflect mitral regurgitation due to papillary muscle ischemia, whereas an A wave is more likely to develop when ventricular compliance is decreased by myocardial ischemia.

The indications for placement of a pulmonary artery catheter are influenced by the information likely to be derived relative to the cost of the catheter. For example, outcome after coronary revascularization surgery cannot be shown to be influenced by the use of a pulmonary artery catheter compared with monitoring only the central venus pressure.[65,66] The central venous pressure and pulmonary artery occlusion pressure have been shown to correlate in patients with IHD when the ejection fraction is greater than 0.5 and there is no evidence of left ventricular dysfunction.[67] Conversely, when the ejection fraction is below 0.5, there is no longer a predictable correlation; changes in the filling pressures may even be in the opposite direction.

Transesophageal Echocardiography

Transesophageal echocardiography is a monitoring technique that may provide a useful method for continuous intraoperative assessment of left ventricular function.[68] Global left ventricular function is evaluated by measurements of end-diastolic and end-systolic dimensions. From these dimensions, estimates of ventricular volume, cardiac output, and ejection fraction are derived. As such, transesophageal echocardiography may be a useful monitor in the management of patients with IHD or those undergoing aortic cross-clamping who are at risk of acute ventricular dysfunction.[69,70] For example, regional deterioration in wall thickness or movement may permit early detection of myocardial ischemia, whereas reductions in myocardial contractility are reflected by decreases in the ejection fraction.[71]

Postoperative Period

Decreases in body temperature that occur intraoperatively may predispose to shivering on awakening, leading to abrupt and excessive increases in myocardial oxygen requirements. Attempts to minimize reductions in body temperature and provision of supplemental oxygen are of obvious importance. Postoperative pain may result in activation of the sympathetic nervous system, leading to increased myocardial oxygen requirements and myocardial ischemia. This emphasizes the unique importance of providing adequate postoperative pain relief to the patient with IHD. In this regard, it is of interest that postoperative myocardial reinfarction often occurs 48 to 72 hours postoperatively, a period that could correspond to discontinuation of supplemental oxygen and less aggressive treatment of pain.[15,16]

HEART TRANSPLANTATION

Heart transplantation is the only available treatment for returning a patient with end-stage heart disease (most often due to IHD or cardiomyopathy) to a functional life-style.[72] Organ damage related to heart disease must be reversible, and the likelihood of long-term survival (patients usually younger than 55 years of age) must be good. Preoperatively, the ejection fraction is typically less than 0.2; the prognosis for survival without a transplant is less than 12 months. Irreversible pulmonary hypertension is a contraindication to heart transplantation. In this regard, the principal indication for heart-lung transplantation is fixed pulmonary hypertension in a patient with end-stage cardiac disease. Heart-lung donors are scarce, as pulmonary injury is likely in victims of fatal accidents, and tracheal intubation may predispose to pneumonia.

Management of Anesthesia

Management of anesthesia for cardiac transplantation may include ketamine or a benzodiazepine, or both, for induction of anesthesia plus an opioid to provide analgesia during surgery.[73] Alternatively, an opioid may be used for induction and maintenance of anesthesia. A volatile anesthetic, especially in high doses, may produce unacceptable myocardial depression and vasodilation. Nitrous oxide is seldom used because of additive depressant effects in the presence of opioids and concern about enlargement of an accidental air embolus that may occur when large blood vessels are opened during the operation. Pancuronium or a muscle relaxant with minimal to absent effects on the blood pressure is useful. Airway equipment, including the anesthetic delivery tubing, is sterile and is handled with sterile gloves. Bacterial filters are often used on the inhaled and exhaled limbs of the anesthetic delivery tubing. Many patients undergoing cardiac transplantation have abnormal coagulation, reflecting passive congestion of the liver due to chronic CHF.

The operative technique consists of cardiopulmonary bypass and anastomosis of the aorta, pulmonary artery, and left and right atria. Immunosuppressive drugs are usually initiated during the preoperative period. Intravascular catheters are placed using an aseptic technique. It is necessary to withdraw a central venous catheter or pulmonary artery catheter back into the internal jugular vein when the recipient's heart is removed. The catheter is then repositioned when the donor heart is in place. Placement of these catheters into the central circulation through the left internal jugular vein leaves the right internal jugular vein available as an access site to perform cardiac biopsies during the postoperative period. An inotropic drug, especially isoproterenol, may be needed briefly to maintain myocardial contractility and heart rate of the donor heart after cardiopulmonary bypass. Therapeutic attempts to lower pulmonary vascular resistance may be necessary and include administration of isoproterenol and vasodilating prostaglandin preparations.[74] The denervated transplanted heart initially assumes an intrinsic heart rate of about 110 beats·min^{-1}, reflecting the absence of normal vagal tone. Stroke volume responds to augmented preload by the Frank-Starling mechanism, emphasizing that these patients tolerate hypovolemia poorly. Likewise, sudden vasodilation, as that due to spinal or epidural anesthesia, is undesirable in a patient with a cardiac transplant. The transplanted heart responds to direct-acting catecholamines (may be even more sensitive than the normal heart) but drugs that act by an indirect mechanism (ephedrine) have a less intense effect. The heart does not change in response to administration of anticholinergic or anticholinesterase drugs.

Complications

Early postoperative morbidity is linked to surgical complications (hemorrhage), sepsis, and rejection. The most frequent cause of death early after heart transplantation is opportunistic infection reflecting immunosuppressive therapy. Transvenous right ventricular endomyocardial biopsies are performed during the early post-transplant period to provide early warning of allograft rejection. Host rejection of the donor heart is signaled by a decrease in the amplitude of the QRS complexes on the ECG, echocardiographic demonstration of shortening of the isovolumic relaxation period, or onset of a restrictive pattern of left ventricular filling. The onset of CHF or cardiac dysrhythmias is a late sign of severe cardiac rejection.

It is presumed that the heart transplant recipient cannot experience angina because of persistent afferent denervation of the heart. In fact, limited sympathetic nervous system reinnervation of the transplanted heart occurs usually within 6 to 12 months, and angina is possible.[75] It is estimated that IHD develops within 3 years of heart transplantation in up to 40% of patients. This accelerated appearance of IHD may reflect a chronic rejection process taking place on the endothelium of the graft arteries. Cyclosporine-induced hypertension is present in more than 90% of heart transplant patients and is often resistant to control with antihypertensive drugs.[76] Cyclosporine is also associated with nephrotoxicity.

Long-term immunosuppressive therapy results in an increased incidence of lymphoproliferative malignancies.

Chronic use of corticosteroids is associated with skeletal demineralization (osteoporosis, aseptic necrosis of weight-bearing joints) and glucose intolerance.

REFERENCES

1. Manson JE, Tosteson H, Ridker PM, et al. The primary prevention of myocardial infarction. N Engl J Med 1992;326:1406–16
2. Cases of specified notifiable diseases, United States. MMWR 1987;35:813–4
3. Hollenberg M, Mangano DT, Browner WS, London MJ, Tubau JF, Tateo IM. Predictors of postoperative myocardial ischemia in patients undergoing noncardiac surgery. JAMA 1992;268:205–9
4. Grundy SM. Cholesterol and coronary heart disease. A new era. JAMA 1986;256:2849–58
5. Grundy SM. Cholesterol and coronary heart disease. Future directions. JAMA 1990;264:3053–9
6. Lowering blood cholesterol to prevent heart disease. Consensus Conference. JAMA 1985;253:2080–90
7. Therapeutic response to lovastatin (Mevinolin) in nonfamilial hypercholesterolemia. A multicenter study. JAMA 1986;256:2829–34
8. Stamler J, Wentworth D, Neaton J. Is the relationship between serum cholesterol and risk of death from coronary heart disease continuous and graded? JAMA 1986;256:2823–8
9. Barry J, Mead K, Nabel EG, et al. Effect of smoking on the activity of ischemic heart disease JAMA 1989;261:398–402
10. Harris SS, Caspersen CJ, DeFriese GH, et al. Physical activity counseling for healthy adults as a primary preventive intervention in the clinical setting: Report for the US Preventive Services Task Force. JAMA 1989;261:3590–5
11. Pekkaneu J, Marti B, Nissinen A, et al. Reduction of premature mortality by high physical activity: A 20-year follow-up of middle-aged Finnish men. Lancet 1987;1:1473–5
12. Dimsdale JE. A perspective on type A behavior and coronary disease. N Engl J Med 1988;318:110
13. Rozanski A, Bairey CN, Krantz DS, et al. Mental stress and the induction of silent myocardial ischemia in patients with coronary artery disease. N Engl J Med 1988;318:1005–12
14. Muir AD, Reeder MK, Foex P, Ormerod OJM, Sear JM, Johnston C. Perioperative silent myocardial ischemia: Incidence and predictors in a general surgical population. Br J Anaesth 1991;67:373–7
15. Tarhan S, Moffitt EA, Taylor WF, Giuliani ER. Myocardial infarction after general anesthesia. JAMA 1972;220:1451–4
16. Steen PA, Tinker JH, Tarhan S. Myocardial reinfarction after anesthesia and surgery. An update: Incidence, mortality, and predisposing factors. JAMA 1978;239:2566–70
17. Shah KB, Kleinman BS, Sami H, Patel J, Rao TLK. Reevaluation of perioperative myocardial infarction in patients with prior myocardial infarction undergoing noncardiac operations. Anesth Analg 1991;71:231–5
18. Rao TLK, Jacobs EH, El-Etr AA. Reinfarction following anesthesia in patients with myocardial infarction. Anesthesiology 1983;59:499–505
19. Slogoff S, Keats AS. Does perioperative myocardial ischemia lead

to postoperative myocardial infarction? Anesthesiology 1985;62: 107–14

20. Mahar LJ, Steen PA, Tinker JH, et al. Perioperative myocardial infarction in patients with coronary artery disease with and without aorto-coronary artery bypass grafts. J Thorac Cardiovasc Surg 1978;76:533–7

21. Goldman L, Caldera DL, Nussbaum SR, et al. Multifactorial index of cardiac risk in noncardiac surgical procedures. N Engl J Med 1977;297:845–50

22. Jeffrey CC, Kunsman J, Cullen DJ, Brewster DC. A prospective evaluation of cardiac risk index. Anesthesiology 1983;58:462–4

23. Reves JG, Kissin I, Lell WA, Tosone S. Calcium entry blockers: Uses and implications for anesthesiologists. Anesthesiology 1982;57:504–18

24. Schulte-Sasse U, Hess W, Markschies-Harnung A, Tarnow J. Combined effects of halothane anesthesia and verapamil on systemic hemodynamics and left ventricular myocardial contractility in patients with ischemic heart disease. Anesth Analg 1984;63: 791–8

25. Kapur PA, Bloor BC, Flacke WE, Olewine SK. Comparison of cardiovascular responses to verapamil during enflurane, isoflurane, or halothane anesthesia in the dog. Anesthesiology 1984;61: 156–60

26. Merin RG. Calcium channel blocking drugs and anesthetics: Is the drug interaction beneficial or detrimental? Anesthesiology 1987;66:111–13

27. Henling CE, Slogoff S, Kodali SV, Arlund C. Heart block after coronary artery bypass—effect of chronic administration of calcium-entry blockers and beta-blockers. Anesth Analg 1984;63: 515–20

28. Durant NN, Nguyen N, Katz R. Potentiation of neuromuscular blockade by verapamil. Anesthesiology 1984;60:298–303

29. Lawson NW, Kraynack BJ, Gintautas J. Neuromuscular and electrocardiographic responses to verapamil in dogs. Anesth Analg 1983;62:50–4

30. Cairns JA, Gent M, Singer J, et al. Aspirin, sulfinpyrazone, or both in unstable angina: Results of a Canadian multicenter trial. N Engl J Med 1985;313:1369–73

31. The Steering Committee of the Physicians Health Study Research Group. Final report on the aspirin component of the ongoing physicians' health study. N Engl J Med 1989;321:129–35

32. Peto R, Gray R, Collins R, et al. Randomized trial of prophylactic daily aspirin in British male doctors. Br Med J 1988;296:313–4

33. White HD, Polak JF, Wynne J, et al. Addition of nifedipine to maximal nitrate and beta-adrenoreceptor blocker therapy in coronary artery disease. Am J Cardiol 1985;55:1303–8

34. Beller GA. Pharmacologic stress imaging. JAMA 1991;265: 633–8

35. Mock MB, Ringqvist I, Fisher LD, et al. Survival of medically treated patients in the Coronary Artery Surgery Study (CASS) registry. Circulation 1982;66:562–6

36. McBride W, Lange RA, Hillis LD. Restenosis after successful coronary angioplasty. Pathophysiology and prevention. N Engl J Med 1988;318:1734–7

37. Passamani E, Davis KB, Gillespie MJ, et al. A randomized trial of coronary artery bypass surgery: Survival of patients with a low ejection fraction. N Engl J Med 1985;312:1665–8

38. Oldridge NB, Guyatt GH, Fischer ME, et al. Cardiac rehabilitation after myocardial infarction: Combined experience of randomized clinical trials. JAMA 1988;260:945–9

39. Goldberg RJ, Gore JM, Alpert JS, et al. Cardiogenic shock after acute myocardial infarction. Incidence and mortality from a community-wide perspective, 1975–1988. N Engl J Med 1991;325: 1117–22

40. deBono DP, Rose EL. Silent myocardial ischaemia in preoperative patients: What does it mean, and what should be done about it? Br J Anaesth 1991;67:367–8

41. Slogoff S, Keats AS. Further observations on perioperative myocardial ischemia. Anesthesiology 1986;65:539–42

42. Slogoff S, Keats AS. Randomized trial of primary anesthetic agents on outcome of coronary artery bypass operations. Anesthesiology 1989;70:179–88

43. Slogoff S, Keats AS, Ott E. Preoperative propranolol therapy and aorto-coronary bypass operation. JAMA 1978;240:1487–90

44. Slogoff S, Keats AS. Does chronic treatment with calcium entry blocking drugs reduce perioperative myocardial ischemia? Anesthesiology 1988;68:676–80

45. Tuman K, McCarthy R, Spies B, DaValle M, Dabir R, Ivankovich A. Does choice of anesthetic agent significantly affect outcome after coronary artery surgery? Anesthesiology 1989;70:189–98

46. Leung JM, Goehner P, O'Kelly BF, et al. Isoflurane anesthesia and myocardial ischemia: Comparative risk versus sufentanil anesthesia in patients undergoing coronary artery bypass graft surgery. Anesthesiology 1991;74:838–47

47. Slogoff S, Keats AS, Dear WE, et al. Steal-prone coronary anatomy and myocardial ischemia associated with four primary anesthetic agents in humans. Anesth Analg 1991;72:22–7

48. Kleinman B, Henkin RE, Glisson SN, et al. Qualitative evaluation of coronary flow during anesthetic induction using thallium-201 perfusion scans. Anesthesiology 1986;64:157–64

49. Roy WL, Edelist G, Gilbert B. Myocardial ischemia during noncardiac surgical procedures in patients with coronary artery disease. Anesthesiology 1979;51:393–7

50. Stoelting RK. Attenuation of blood pressure response to laryngoscopy and tracheal intubation with sodium nitroprusside. Anesth Analg 1979;58:116–9

51. Menkhaus PG, Reves JG, Kisson I, et al. Cardiovascular effects of esmolol in anesthetized humans. Anesth Analg 1985;64: 327–34

52. Thomson IR, Mutch WAC, Culligan JD. Failure of intravenous nitroglycerin to prevent intraoperative myocardial ischemia during fentanyl-pancuronium anesthesia. Anesthesiology 1984;61: 385–93

53. Gallagher JD, Moore RA, Jose AB, Botros SB, Clark DL. Prophylactic nitroglycerin infusions during coronary artery bypass surgery. Anesthesiology 1986;64:785–9

54. Bastard OG, Carter JG, Moyers JR, Bross BA. Circulatory effects of isoflurane in patients with ischemic heart disease: A comparison with halothane. Anesth Analg 1984;63:635–9

55. Hess W, Arnold B, Schulte-Sasse U, Tarnow J. Comparison of isoflurane and halothane when used to control intraoperative hypertension of patients undergoing coronary artery bypass surgery. Anesth Analg 1983;62:15–20

56. Lunn JK, Stanley TH, Eisele J, et al. High dose fentanyl anesthesia for coronary artery surgery: Plasma fentanyl concentrations

and influence of nitrous oxide on cardiovascular responses. Anesth Analg 1979;58:390–5

57. Stoelting RK, Gibbs PS. Hemodynamic effects of morphine and morphine–nitrous oxide in valvular heart disease and coronary artery disease. Anesthesiology 1973;38:45–52

58. Tomicheck RC, Rosow CE, Philbin DM, et al. Diazepam-fentanyl interaction—hemodynamic and hormonal effects in coronary artery surgery. Anesth Analg 1983;62:881–4.8

59. McCammon RL, Hilgenberg JC, Stoelting RK. Hemodynamic effects of diazepam and diazepam–nitrous oxide in patients with coronary artery disease. Anesth Analg 1980;59:438–41

60. Eisele JH, Smith NT. Cardiovascular effects of 40% nitrous oxide in man. Anesth Analg 1972;51:956–61

61. Thomson IR, Putnins CL. Adverse effects of pancuronium during high-dose fentanyl anesthesia for coronary artery bypass grafting. Anesthesiology 1985;62:708–13

62. Kaplan JA, King SB. The precordial electrocardiographic lead (V5) in patients who have coronary-artery disease. Anesthesiology 1976;45:570–4

63. Kates RA, Zaidan JR, Kaplan JA. Esophageal lead for intraoperative electrocardiographic monitoring. Anesth Analg 1982;61:781–5

64. Kaplan JA, Wells PH. Early diagnosis of myocardial ischemia using the pulmonary arterial catheter. Anesth Analg 1981;60:789–93

65. Tuman KJ, McCarthy RJ, Spiess BD, et al. Effect of pulmonary artery catheterization on outcome in patients undergoing coronary artery surgery. Anesthesiology 1989;70:199–206

66. Pearson KS, Gomez MN, Moyers JR, Carter JG, Tinker JH. A cost/benefit analysis of randomized invasive monitoring for patients undergoing cardiac surgery. Anesth Analg 1989;69:336–41

67. Mangano DT. Monitoring pulmonary artery pressure in coronary-artery disease. Anesthesiology 1980;53:364–70

68. Clements FM, deBruijn NP. Perioperative evaluation of regional wall motion by transesophageal two-dimensional echocardiography. Anesth Analg 1987;66:249–61

69. Konstadt SN, Thys D, Mindich BP, Kaplan JA, Goldman M. Validation of quantitative intraoperative transesophageal echocardiography. Anesthesiology 1986;65:418–21

70. LaMantia K, Lehmann K, Barash P. Echocardiography in the perioperative period. Acute Care 1985;11:106–16

71. Smith JS, Cahalan MK, Benefiel DJ. Intraoperative detection of myocardial ischemia in high risk patients. Circulation 1985;72:1015–21

72. Schroeder JS, Hunt S. Cardiac transplantation. Update 1987. JAMA 1987;258:3142–6

73. Demas K, Wyner J, Mihm FG, Samuels S. Anaesthesia for heart transplantation. A restrospective study and review. Br J Anaesth 1986;58:1357–64

74. Casella ES, Humphrey LS. Bronchospasm after cardiopulmonary bypass in a heart-lung transplant recipient. Anesthesiology 1988;69:135–8

75. Stark RP, McGinn AL, Wilson RF. Chest pain in cardiac-transplant recipients. Evidence of sensory reinnervation after cardiac transplantation. N Engl J Med 1991;324:1791–4

76. Scherrer U, Vissing SF, Morgan BJ, et al. Cyclosporine-induced sympathetic activation and hypertension after heart transplantation. N Engl J Med 1990;323:693–9

2

Valvular Heart Disease

Management of the patient with valvular heart disease during the perioperative period requires an understanding of the hemodynamic alterations that accompany dysfunction of the cardiac valves. The most frequently encountered cardiac valve lesions produce pressure overload (mitral stenosis, aortic stenosis) or volume overload (mitral regurgitation, aortic regurgitation) on the left atrium or left ventricle. Drug selections during the perioperative period for the patient with valvular heart disease are based on the likely effects a drug-induced change in cardiac rhythm, heart rate, blood pressure, systemic vascular resistance, and pulmonary vascular resistance will have relative to the pathophysiology of the heart disease.

PREOPERATIVE EVALUATION

Preoperative evaluation of the patient with valvular heart disease includes (1) assessment of the severity of the cardiac disease (2), the degree of impaired myocardial contractility, and (3) the presence of associated major organ disease (pulmonary, renal, hepatic). Recognition of compensatory mechanisms for maintaining cardiac output (increased sympathetic nervous system activity, cardiac hypertrophy) and consideration of drug therapy is needed. This information can be obtained from the history and physical examination and from a review of laboratory data.

Preoperative evaluation of the patient with a prosthetic heart valve includes (1) evaluation for paravalvular leak or other mechanical dysfunction, (2) determination of the presence of congestive heart failure (CHF), and (3) management of anticoagulation (see the section, Mitral Stenosis). Changes in cardiac valve sounds or the appearance of a new heart murmur are sought. Echocardiography and occasionally cardiac catheterization may be recommended in an attempt at further assessment of the performance of the prosthetic heart valve. Antibiotic prophylaxis is recommended when the patient with a prosthetic heart valve undergoes a dental or surgical procedure. Preoperative measurement of the plasma concentration of bilirubin and the reticulocyte count may be helpful in detecting occult hemolysis due to prosthetic valve dysfunction. Furthermore, the incidence of cholecystitis is increased in patients with prosthetic heart valves, presumably reflecting a chronic low-grade intravascular hemolysis.

History and Physical Examination

Questions designed to define the patient's exercise tolerance are useful for evaluating cardiac reserve in the presence of valvular heart disease. In this regard, it may be helpful to classify the patient according to the criteria established by the New York Heart Association (Table 2-1). CHF is a frequent companion of chronic valvular heart disease. When myocardial contractility is impaired, the patient may complain of dyspnea, orthopnea, and fatigability. A compensatory increase in sympathetic nervous system activity may be manifested as anxiety, diaphoresis, and resting tachycardia. In support of the diagnosis of CHF is the presence of basilar chest rales, jugular venous distension, and a third heart sound, as determined on physical examination (see Chapter 6). Ideally, elective surgery is deferred until CHF can be treated and myocardial contractility optimized.

Disease of a cardiac valve rarely occurs without an accompanying murmur reflecting turbulent blood flow across the valve. The character, location, intensity, and direction of radiation of a heart murmur provides a clue to the location and severity of the cardiac valve lesion[1] (Fig. 2-1). During systole, the aortic and pulmonic valves are open, and the mitral and tricuspid valves are closed. Therefore, a heart murmur occurring in systole is either due to stenosis of the aortic or pulmonic valves or to incompetence of the mitral or tricuspid valves. During diastole, the aortic and pulmonic valves are closed, and the mitral and tricuspid valves are open. Therefore, a heart murmur occurring in diastole is either due to stenosis of the mitral or tricuspid valves or to incompetence of the aortic or pulmonic valves.

Cardiac dysrhythmias are seen in all types of valvular heart

Table 2-1.   New York Heart Association Classification of Patients With Heart Disease

Class	Description
I	Asymptomatic
II	Symptoms with ordinary activity but comfortable at rest
III	Symptoms with minimal activity but comfortable at rest
IV	Symptoms at rest

disease. Atrial fibrillation is most common with rheumatic mitral valve disease associated with enlargement of the left atrium. Initially, atrial fibrillation is paroxysmal but, after several years, this cardiac dysrhythmia often becomes persistent.

Angina pectoris may occur in the patient with valvular heart disease, even in the absence of ischemic heart disease. This reflects an increased myocardial oxygen demand due to increased cardiac muscle mass that exceeds the ability of even normal coronary arteries to deliver adequate amounts of oxygen. Furthermore, valvular heart disease and ischemic heart disease frequently co-exist. Indeed, 50% of patients with aortic stenosis who are over 50 years of age have associated ischemic heart disease.

Drug Therapy

Drug therapy in the patient with valvular heart disease is likely to include a digitalis preparation and a diuretic. Digitalis is most often administered to increase myocardial contractility and to slow the ventricular heart rate response in the patient with atrial fibrillation. Slowing the ventricular heart rate response prolongs the duration of diastole and thus improves left ventricular filling. An adequate digitalis effect for heart

rate control is indicated by a ventricular rate of less than 80 beats·min^{-1} at rest that increases no more than 15 beats·min^{-1} with mild physical activity. In the absence of adequate preoperative heart rate control, activation of the sympathetic nervous system, as during intubation of the trachea or in response to surgical stimulation, may adversely increase the heart rate with a subsequent decrease in the diastolic filling time and stroke volume. Digitalis toxicity is suggested by prolongation of the P-R interval and the appearance of ventricular premature beats on the electrocardiogram (ECG), as well as by patient complaints related to gastrointestinal dysfunction. Vulnerability to the development of digitalis toxicity is increased when concomitant diuretic therapy has led to total body depletion of potassium.

Laboratory Data

The ECG often demonstrates characteristic changes due to valvular heart disease. For example, broad and notched P waves suggest the presence of left atrial enlargement typical of mitral stenosis. Ventricular hypertrophy is mirrored by the presence of left or right axis deviation. The size and shape of the heart and great vessels and vascular markings in the lung are evaluated on the chest radiograph. On a posterior-anterior chest radiograph, heart size should not exceed 50% of the internal width of the thoracic cage. The shadow of the left heart border from above downward represents the aorta, pulmonary artery, left atrium, and left ventricle; on the right side, the shadow is due to the superior vena cava and right atrium. Enlargement of the left atrium can result in elevation of the left bronchus and an increase in the angle of the carina to greater than 90 degrees. Vascular markings in the peripheral lung fields may be sparse in the presence of severe pulmonary hypertension.

Valvular heart disease can interfere with oxygenation and ventilation, as reflected by measurement of arterial blood gases. For example, a chronic increase in left atrial pressure will be reflected back into the pulmonary veins, and eventually into the lung interstitium. These changes can produce an alteration in the relationship of ventilation-to-perfusion matching, as well as the development of pulmonary edema, leading to a decrease in the PaO$_2$.

A transvalvular pressure gradient determined at the time of cardiac catheterization provides useful information as to the severity of valvular heart disease. Mitral and aortic stenosis are considered to be present when the transvalvular pressure gradient is greater than 10 mmHg and 50 mmHg, respectively.[2] These limits are valid only in the absence of CHF. For example, when CHF accompanies aortic stenosis, a transvalvular gradient of only 20 mmHg signifies severe valvular disease. Severity of valvular regurgitation can be estimated by visualizing the amount of angiographic dye that regurgitates

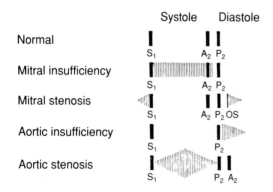

Fig. 2-1. Timing and characteristics of cardiac murmurs in relation to systole and diastole. (From Fishman MC, Hoffman AR, Klausner RD, Rockson SG, Thaler MS. Medicine. Philadelphia. JB Lippincott 1981;42, with permission.)

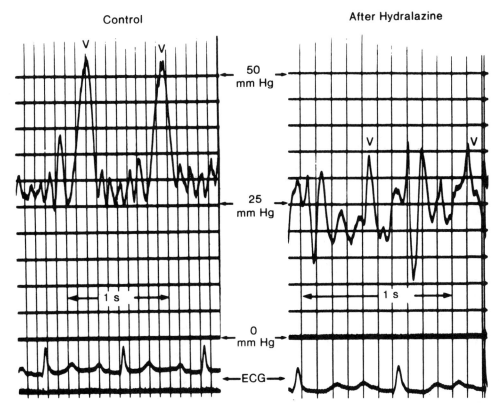

Fig. 2-2. Regurgitant blood flow into the left atrium produces a large V wave on the trace of the pulmonary artery occlusion pressure of a patient with mitral regurgitation. Administration of a vasodilator (hydralazine) decreases resistance to forward ejection of the left ventricular stroke volume. As a result, the volume of regurgitant flow into the left atrium is less, and the magnitude of the V wave is decreased. (From Greenberg BH, Rahimtoola SH. Vasodilator therapy for valvular heart disease. JAMA 1981;246: 269–72, with permission.)

back into the cardiac chamber distal to the diseased valve. Monitoring the magnitude of the V wave on a tracing of the pulmonary artery occlusion pressure can be a clinically useful measure of the severity of mitral regurgitation[3] (Fig. 2-2). In the patient with mitral stenosis or mitral regurgitation, measurement of pulmonary artery pressure and right ventricular filling pressure may indicate evidence of pulmonary hypertension and right ventricular failure. Coronary artery angiography may provide evidence of ischemic heart disease in the patient with valvular heart disease. Indeed, mitral regurgitation secondary to papillary muscle dysfunction may reflect myocardial ischemia or a prior myocardial infarction.

Doppler Echocardiography

Doppler echocardiography has revolutionized the noninvasive evaluation of valvular heart disease[4,5] (Table 2-2). Doppler techniques allow measurement of blood flow velocity in the heart and great vessels, thus permitting noninvasive hemody-namic measurements. Echocardiography is particularly useful in evaluating the significance of a systolic ejection murmur in suspected aortic stenosis and in detecting the presence of mitral stenosis. This technique permits both determination of the valve orifice area and assessment of the transvalvular

Table 2-2. Doppler Echocardiography and Valvular Heart Disease

Determine significance of cardiac murmurs (most often aortic stenosis)
Identify hemodynamic abnormalities associated with physical findings (most often mitral regurgitation)
Determine transvalvular pressure gradient
Determine orifice area of cardiac valve
Diagnose cardiac valve regurgitation
Evaluate prosthetic valve function

pressure gradient. Doppler echocardiography, especially with color flow mapping, is also useful for assessment of valvular regurgitation.

Treatment

Although commissurotomy or annuloplasty may be considered, the treatment for most forms of valvular heart disease is replacement of the damaged valve. The most frequently used prosthetic valves are the Starr-Edwards (caged ball), Bjork-Shiley (tilting disk), and St. Jude (two disks). A prosthetic heart valve is slightly stenotic (gradient 4 to 7 mmHg for a mitral valve prosthesis and 7 to 19 mmHg for an aortic valve prosthesis), but the greatest disadvantage is the tendency to promote thrombus formation and the subsequent risk of systemic embolization. Infection and rupture at the attachment points of the valve may also occur. The only tissue valve in current use is the porcine aortic valve. Its advantage over the prosthetic valve is that it is less likely to promote thrombosis and systemic embolism. The principal disadvantage associated with the porcine valve is structural deterioration with time.

The timing of cardiac valve replacement surgery depends on the projected natural history of the disease, with particular emphasis on left ventricular function. Advanced age is probably not a contraindication to valve replacement surgery. For most patients with valvular heart disease, the decision regarding surgical treatment can be provided by clinical evaluation and noninvasive tests. Cardiac catheterization is confirmatory in documenting the severity of the valvular heart lesion and the possible presence of ischemic heart disease.

Left ventricular dysfunction is often reversible after cardiac valve replacement, whereas in other cases CHF may persist or recur, presumably reflecting irreversible factors that were present before surgery. In most patients, increased pulmonary vascular resistance declines to normal after valve replacement. The preoperative degree of left ventricular dilation, ejection fraction, and the presence of ischemic heart disease are important determinants of overall success after prosthetic valve replacement.

MITRAL STENOSIS

Mitral stenosis is almost always due to fusion of the mitral valve leaflets at the commissures during the healing process of acute rheumatic fever. Initial symptoms (dyspnea on exertion, orthopnea, fatigue) due to a progressive decrease in the size of the mitral valve orifice do not usually develop until about 20 years after the first episode of rheumatic fever. The patient is likely to become symptomatic when the size of the mitral valve orifice (4 to 6 cm^2) has decreased at least 50%. When

the mitral valve area is less than 1 cm^2, a mean left atrial pressure of about 25 mmHg is necessary to maintain an adequate resting cardiac output. Measurement of the diastolic pressure gradient across the valve at cardiac catheterization provides the most definitive assessment of the degree of mitral stenosis with a gradient greater than 10 mmHg (normal less than 5 mmHg), suggesting severe stenosis. An average of 7 years separates the onset of initial symptoms from complete incapacity. When mitral stenosis is severe, the addition of stresses such as sepsis, atrial fibrillation, pulmonary embolism, or pregnancy may precipitate acute decompensation, most often manifested as pulmonary edema.

Clinically, mitral stenosis is recognized by the characteristic opening snap that occurs early in diastole and by a rumbling diastolic heart murmur best heard at the cardiac apex. The opening snap is caused by vibrations set in motion when the mobile but stenosed valve initially opens. Calcification of the valve may result in disappearance of the opening snap. Left atrial enlargement is often visible on the chest radiograph as straightening of the left heart border, widening of the carinal angle, and displacement of a barium-filled esophagus on a lateral view. There may be evidence of pulmonary edema on the chest radiograph. In the absence of atrial fibrillation, a large biphasic P wave on the ECG suggests left atrial enlargement. Atrial fibrillation is present in about one-third of patients with severe mitral stenosis, occurring most often when the left atrium is greatly enlarged.

Surgical replacement of the diseased mitral valve may ultimately be necessary. Indeed, when mitral stenosis produces total incapacity, 20% of patients die within 6 months without surgical correction. Dyspnea from pulmonary congestion is likely to be relieved by surgery, whereas chronic fatigue and cardiac dysrhythmias are unlikely to be altered. Catheter balloon valvuloplasty using a percutaneous venous introduction and a transeptal approach to the mitral valve may be used to decrease the degree of mitral stenosis in selected patients.[6]

Pathophysiology

Mitral stenosis is characterized by mechanical obstruction to left ventricular diastolic filling secondary to a progressive decrease in the orifice of the mitral valve. This valvular obstruction produces an increase in left atrial volume and pressure. Left ventricular filling and stroke volume in the presence of mild mitral stenosis are usually maintained at rest by the increased left atrial pressure. Stroke volume, however, may decrease during stress-induced tachycardia or when an effective atrial contraction is lost, as during atrial fibrillation.

Pulmonary venous pressure is increased in association with the increased left atrial pressure. The result is transudation of fluid into the pulmonary interstitial space, decreased pulmonary compliance, and increased work of breathing, leading to progressive dyspnea on exertion. Overt pulmonary edema is likely when the pulmonary venous pressure exceeds the oncotic pressure of plasma proteins. If the increase in this pressure is gradual, however, there is a concomitant increase in lymphatic drainage from the lungs, and a thickening of capillary basement membranes enables the patient to tolerate an increased pulmonary venous pressure without the development of pulmonary edema. For unknown reasons, in about 30% of patients, there is an accelerated increase in pulmonary artery pressure and pulmonary vascular resistance, leading to persistent pulmonary hypertension. Furthermore, pulmonary hypertension is likely when the left atrial pressure is chronically increased above 25 mmHg. Left ventricular dysfunction is uncommon in the presence of pure mitral stenosis. When aortic or mitral regurgitation, or both, accompany mitral stenosis, there is likely to be evidence of left ventricular dysfunction, as reflected by an increased left ventricular end-diastolic pressure.

Stasis of blood in the distended left atrium predisposes to the formation of thrombi, which can be displaced as systemic emboli, especially with the onset of atrial fibrillation. Furthermore, venous thrombosis is encouraged by the low cardiac output and decreased physical activity characteristic of these patients. For these reasons, the patient with mitral stenosis may be receiving chronic anticoagulant therapy.

Management of Anesthesia

Management of anesthesia for noncardiac surgery in the patient with mitral stenosis includes avoidance of events that may further decrease the cardiac output (Table 2-3). The development of atrial fibrillation with a rapid ventricular response rate may greatly decrease cardiac output and produce pulmonary edema. Treatment consists of cardioversion starting with 25 watt-sec or, alternatively, intravenous administration of a beta antagonist such as esmolol to decrease the heart rate below 110 beats·min^{-1}. Digoxin (0.25 to 0.5 mg IV over 10 minutes) is useful when a prolonged, but not immediate, heart rate control is desirable. An increase in central blood volume, as produced by excess volume administration, head-down position, or autotransfusion via a uterine contraction, can precipi-

Table 2-3. Anesthetic Considerations in the Patient With Mitral Stenosis

Avoid sinus tachycardia or rapid ventricular response rate during atrial fibrillation

Avoid marked increases in central blood volume as associated with overtransfusion or head-down position

Avoid drug-induced decreases in systemic vascular resistance

Avoid events, such as arterial hypoxemia and/or hypoventilation, that may exacerbate pulmonary hypertension and evoke right ventricular failure

tate CHF, pulmonary edema, or atrial fibrillation. In the patient with severe mitral stenosis, a sudden decrease in systemic vascular resistance may not be tolerated, since blood pressure can be maintained only by an increase in heart rate. If necessary, blood pressure and systemic vascular resistance may be maintained with a sympathomimetic drug, such as ephedrine or phenylephrine. The advantage of ephedrine is its beta agonist effect, which serves to increase myocardial contractility, whereas any drug-induced tachycardia would be undesirable. Phenylephrine eliminates the concern regarding heart rate, but increases in ventricular afterload that follow administration of this predominantly alpha agonist drug can decrease left ventricular stroke volume.[7] Pulmonary hypertension and right ventricular failure may be precipitated by multiple factors, including hypercarbia, hypoxemia, hyperinflation of the lungs, and increased lung water. If pulmonary hypertension and right ventricular failure develop, inotropic support with dopamine (3 to 10 μg·kg^{-1}·min^{-1} IV) and pulmonary vasodilation with nitroprusside (0.1 to 0.5 μg·kg^{-1}·min^{-1} IV) may be useful.

Preoperative preparation of the patient with mitral stenosis is designed to decrease anxiety as well as any associated likelihood of adverse circulatory responses produced by tachycardia. The best drug or drug combination for decreasing anxiety is not known, but it must be appreciated that such a patient can be more susceptible than a normal person to the ventilatory depressant effects of sedative drugs. Furthermore, the use of an anticholinergic drug is controversial because of concern that an adverse increase in heart rate could occur. Therefore, when an anticholinergic drug is included in the preoperative medication, it may be prudent to select scopolamine or glycopyrrolate, as these drugs have fewer chronotropic effects than those seen with atropine.

Prophylactic antibiotics instituted during the preoperative period for protection against the development of infective endocarditis are usually recommended for the patient with mitral stenosis scheduled for a dental or surgical procedure. For the patient taking digitalis for control of the ventricular heart rate response during atrial fibrillation, this drug should be continued until surgery. Since diuretic therapy is frequent, the plasma potassium concentration is often measured preoperatively. In addition, the presence of orthostatic hypotension may be evidence of diuretic-induced hypovolemia. The advisability of discontinuing anticoagulant medication before elective surgery is unclear. In one report, the incidence of thromboembolism was not increased when anticoagulant medication was gradually discontinued 1 to 3 days preoperatively, allowing the prothrombin time to return to within 20% of normal.[8]

Induction of anesthesia in the presence of mitral stenosis can be achieved with available intravenous induction drugs, with the possible exception of ketamine, which may be avoided because of its propensity to increase the heart rate. Intubation of the trachea is usually facilitated by administration of a muscle relaxant. In this regard, the incidence of ventricular dysrhythmias after administration of succinylcholine to patients taking digitalis has not been a consistent observation. Pancuronium is avoided because of its ability to increase the speed of transmission of the cardiac impulse through the atrioventricular node, which could lead to an excessive increase in heart rate.[9] Such an increase would seem particularly likely in the presence of atrial fibrillation, since the ventricular response to atrial impulses is determined by the degree of atrioventricular conduction. A muscle relaxant with minimal effects on heart rate, blood pressure, and systemic vascular resistance is useful in the patient with mitral stenosis. There is no reason to avoid pharmacologic reversal of a nondepolarizing muscle relaxant, although the adverse effects of any drug-induced tachycardia deserve consideration. Theoretically, combining the anticholinesterase drug with glycopyrrolate, rather than atropine, would be more appropriate as glycopyrrolate most

likely has fewer chronotropic effects than those produced by atropine.

Drugs used for maintenance of anesthesia should be associated with minimal changes in heart rate and in systemic and pulmonary vascular resistance. Furthermore, these drugs should not greatly decrease myocardial contractility. These goals are most closely achieved with the combination of nitrous oxide and an opioid or a low concentration of a volatile drug. Although nitrous oxide can evoke pulmonary vascular constriction and increase pulmonary vascular resistance, it seems unlikely the magnitude of this change would justify avoiding this drug in every patient with mitral stenosis[10,11] (Fig. 2-3). When co-existing pulmonary hypertension is severe, however, nitrous oxide may be more likely to increase pulmonary vascular resistance significantly.[12]

The use of invasive monitoring depends on the complexity of the operative procedure and the magnitude of physiologic

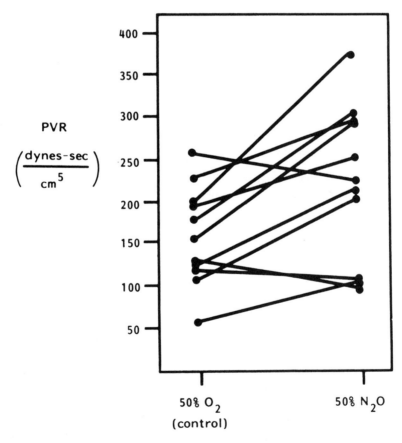

Fig. 2-3. The inhalation of 50% nitrous oxide modestly increased pulmonary vascular resistance in 8 of 11 patients with co-existing pulmonary hypertension due to mitral valve disease. (From Hilgenberg JC, McCammon RL, Stoelting RK. Pulmonary and systemic vascular responses to nitrous oxide in patients with mitral stenosis and pulmonary hypertension. Anesth Analg 1980;59: 323–6, with permission.)

impairment produced by mitral stenosis. Monitoring of an asymptomatic patient without evidence of pulmonary congestion is probably not different from that of the patient without valvular heart disease. Conversely, continuous monitoring of intra-arterial blood pressure and atrial filling pressures is useful when a major operative procedure is planned, particularly in the patient with mitral stenosis who is symptomatic at rest. These monitors are helpful in confirming the adequacy of ventilation, oxygenation, and intravascular fluid volume replacement and in assessing the efficacy of drug therapy on cardiac contractility. An increase in right atrial pressure could reflect nitrous oxide-induced pulmonary vasoconstriction, suggesting the need to discontinue inhalation of this drug. Intraoperative fluid replacement must be carefully titrated, as these patients are susceptible to volume overload and to the development of pulmonary edema. Likewise, the head-down position is not

well tolerated, since pulmonary blood volume is already increased.

Light anesthesia and surgical stimulation can lead to systemic hypertension and to decreased cardiac output, owing to the increased systemic and pulmonary vascular resistance. When this occurs, an intravenous infusion of nitroprusside may be effective in decreasing systemic vascular resistance, pulmonary artery pressure, and left atrial pressure.[13] Furthermore, a nitroprusside-induced decrease in systemic vascular resistance is also associated with increased left ventricular stroke volume, particularly when co-existing pulmonary hypertension is severe or when mitral regurgitation co-exists with mitral stenosis[13] (Fig. 2-4).

Postoperatively, the patient with mitral stenosis is at risk of the development of pulmonary edema and right heart failure. Pain, hypoventilation with respiratory acidosis, and arte-

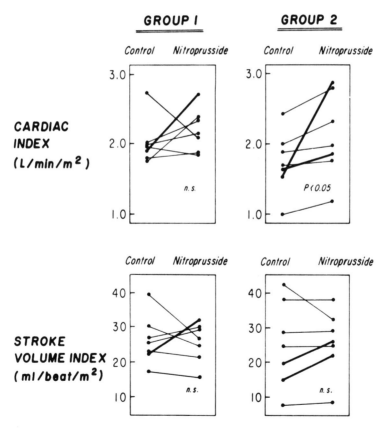

Fig. 2-4. The cardiovascular effects of nitroprusside (0.2–4.0 μg·kg^{-1}·min^{-1} IV) were evaluated in patients with pure mitral stenosis (group 1) and in patients with mixed mitral stenosis and mitral regurgitation (group 2) with (heavy lines) or without (fine lines) severe co-existing pulmonary hypertension. Nitroprusside-induced decreases in systemic vascular resistance were not detrimental in either group, with patients having severe co-existing pulmonary hypertension showing the most favorable responses. (From Stone JG, Hoar PF, Faltas AN, Khambata HF. Nitroprusside and mitral stenosis. Anesth Analg 1980;59:662–5, with permission.)

rial hypoxemia may be the events responsible for increasing heart rate or pulmonary vascular resistance. This emphasizes the usefulness of continuing cardiac monitoring during the postoperative period. Decreased pulmonary compliance and increased oxygen cost of breathing often accompany mitral stenosis. These changes may necessitate mechanical support of ventilation during the postoperative period, particularly after major thoracic or abdominal surgery.

MITRAL REGURGITATION

Mitral regurgitation is usually due to rheumatic fever and is almost always associated with mitral stenosis. Isolated mitral regurgitation in the absence of prior rheumatic fever is often acute. For example, acute mitral regurgitation may be due to papillary muscle dysfunction after a myocardial infarction or rupture of a chordae tendineae secondary to infective endocarditis. Another cause of mitral regurgitation is dilation of the mitral valve annulus owing to left ventricular hypertrophy. The cardinal feature of mitral regurgitation is a blowing pansystolic murmur, best heard at the cardiac apex, and often radiating to the left axilla. A ruptured chordae tendineae as a cause of acute mitral regurgitation is documented by echocardiography. Chronic mitral regurgitation is usually well tolerated, and patients may remain asymptomatic for 30 to 40 years. When CHF develops, however, a rapidly deteriorating course occurs, with a 5-year mortality rate approaching 50%. Surgical replacement of the diseased valve may ultimately become necessary. Vasodilator therapy with hydralazine or nitroprusside is particularly effective in increasing cardiac output (forward left ventricular stroke volume), when acute mitral regurgitation results in a sudden increase in left atrial pressure that can lead to pulmonary edema. When this regurgitation is due to papillary muscle dysfunction after a myocardial infarction, the use of vasodilator therapy may improve cardiac output to the extent that surgery for replacement of the mitral valve can be deferred until the patient is stabilized.

Pathophysiology

Left atrial volume overload is the principal pathophysiologic change produced by mitral regurgitation. Indeed, the basic hemodynamic derangement in mitral regurgitation is a decrease in the forward left ventricular stroke volume, as part of the stroke volume is regurgitated through the incompetent mitral valve back into the left atrium. A patient with a regurgitant fraction of greater than 0.6 is considered to have severe mitral regurgitation. This regurgitant flow is responsible for the V wave present on the recording of the pulmonary artery occlusion pressure[3] (Fig. 2-2). The size of the V wave correlates with the magnitude of the regurgitant flow.

The fraction of the left ventricular stroke volume that enters the left atrium depends on (1) the size of the mitral valve orifice; (2) the heart rate, which determines the duration of ventricular ejection; and (3) the pressure gradient across the mitral valve. For example, a mild increase in heart rate can improve forward left ventricular stroke volume, whereas bradycardia could result in acute volume overload of the left atrium. The pressure gradient across the mitral valve will depend on the compliance of the left ventricle and on the impedance of left ventricular ejection into the aorta. Pharmacologic interventions that increase or decrease systemic vascular resistance also have an important impact on the regurgitant fraction of the stroke volume.

The patient with isolated mitral regurgitation is less dependent on a properly timed left atrial contraction for left ventricular filling than is the patient with mitral or aortic stenosis. Indeed, conversion from atrial fibrillation (present in about one-third of patients with mitral regurgitation) to normal sinus rhythm produces a minimal change in cardiac output. The patient with rheumatic fever-induced mitral regurgitation is most likely to exhibit marked left atrial enlargement and associated atrial fibrillation. Myocardial ischemia is unlikely in the presence of mitral regurgitation because the increased ventricular wall tension is quickly dissipated as the stroke volume is rapidly ejected into both the aorta and left atrium. Furthermore, when mitral regurgitation develops gradually, the compliant left atrium is able to accommodate an increased regurgitant volume without an increase in left atrial pressure. Severe mitral regurgitation may be exhibited as left atrial and ventricular hypertrophy on the ECG and chest radiograph.

The frequent combination of mitral regurgitation and mitral stenosis results in increased volume and pressure work by the heart. In this situation, an increased flow rate across the stenotic valve secondary to regurgitation markedly increases the left atrial pressure. In these patients, atrial fibrillation, pulmonary edema, and pulmonary hypertension develop earlier than in the patient with isolated mitral regurgitation.

Management of Anesthesia

Management of anesthesia for noncardiac surgery in the patient with mitral regurgitation includes avoidance of events that may further decrease the cardiac output (Table 2-4). Maintenance of a normal to slightly increased heart rate is

Table 2-4.   Anesthetic Considerations in the Patient With Mitral Regurgitation

Avoid sudden decreases in heart rate
Avoid sudden increases in systemic vascular resistance
Minimize drug-induced myocardial depression
Monitor the size of the V wave as a reflection of regurgitant flow

recommended, as forward left ventricular stroke volume is likely rate dependent. In this regard, sudden bradycardia may result in abrupt left ventricular volume overload. Likewise, a sudden increase in systemic vascular resistance can cause acute decompensation of the left ventricle. Left ventricular failure due to this mechanism may benefit from drug-induced afterload reduction with nitroprusside combined with a cardiac inotrope such as dopamine to increase myocardial contractility. Because left ventricular dysfunction usually accompanies mitral regurgitation, even minimal drug-induced myocardial depression may be undesirable. Overall, the management of anesthesia is designed to avoid decreases in heart rate or increases in systemic vascular resistance that would potentially decrease forward left ventricular stroke volume. Conversely, cardiac output can be improved by a modest increase in heart rate and decrease in systemic vascular resistance.

Prophylactic antibiotics instituted during the preoperative period for protection against the development of infective endocarditis are usually recommended for the patient with mitral regurgitation who is scheduled for a dental or surgical procedure. General anesthesia is the usual choice for the patient with mitral regurgitation. Although a decrease in systemic vascular resistance is theoretically beneficial, the uncontrolled nature of this response with regional anesthesia detracts from the use of epidural or spinal anesthesia. Induction of anesthesia in the presence of mitral regurgitation can be achieved with available intravenous induction drugs, keeping in mind the importance of avoiding excessive and abrupt changes in systemic vascular resistance or decreases in heart rate. Bradycardia associated with the administration of succinylcholine would be undesirable, interventions to prevent this rare occurrence (increased heart rate the more common response) may be considered, including the prior administration of an anticholinergic drug.

In the absence of severe left ventricular dysfunction, maintenance of anesthesia is often provided with nitrous oxide plus a volatile anesthetic. A volatile anesthetic can be administered to attenuate an undesirable increase in blood pressure and systemic vascular resistance that can accompany surgical stimulation. Although a specific volatile anesthetic has not been demonstrated to be superior, the usual increase in heart rate and decrease in systemic vascular resistance with little evidence of direct myocardial depression characteristic of isoflurane makes selection of this drug attractive in these patients. When myocardial function is severely compromised, as in the presence of acute mitral regurgitation due to papillary muscle dysfunction or rupture of a chordae tendineae, the use of an opioid technique, which minimizes the likelihood of drug-induced myocardial depression, may be a consideration. The muscle relaxant selection is influenced by the likely circulatory effects associated with these drugs. In this regard, pancuronium, which generally produces a modest increase in heart

rate, would potentially contribute to maintenance of forward left ventricular stroke volume.

Ventilation of the lungs is often controlled and adjusted to maintain a near-normal $PaCO_2$. The pattern of ventilation should provide sufficient time between breaths for venous return to occur. Maintenance of intravascular fluid volume with prompt replacement of blood loss is important in maintaining cardiac filling volumes and ejection of an optimal forward left ventricular stroke volume.

A minor operation performed on a patient with asymptomatic mitral regurgitation probably does not require invasive monitoring. In the presence of severe mitral regurgitation, the use of invasive monitoring is helpful in detecting the onset of undesirable degrees of depression of myocardial contractility and in facilitating intravenous fluid replacement. Certainly, a pulmonary artery catheter is useful when a peripheral vasodilating drug is administered in an attempt to facilitate forward left ventricular stroke volume. Measurement of cardiac output by thermodilution confirms the response to a decrease in systemic vascular resistance produced by a drug such as nitroprusside. It should be appreciated that regurgitation of blood into the left atrium produces a V wave on the tracing of the pulmonary artery occlusion pressure. A change in the amplitude of the V wave can assist in estimating the magnitude of mitral regurgitation[3] (Fig. 2-2). The pulmonary artery occlusion pressure is a poor measure of the left atrial volume of left ventricular end-diastolic volume. With acute mitral regurgitation, however, the left atrium will be less compliant, and a change in the pulmonary artery occlusion pressure will more likely correlate with changes in left atrial and left ventricular end-diastolic pressure. An alternative to invasive monitoring is the use of Doppler echocardiography to monitor changes in mitral valve function.

MITRAL VALVE PROLAPSE

Mitral valve prolapse is the most common form of valvular heart disease, occurring in 5% to 10% of the general population. This abnormality is characterized by prolapse of the mitral valve leaflets into the left atrium during systole.[14] The presence of mitral valve prolapse is suggested by the auscultatory finding of a nonejection click cardiac murmur (click-murmur syndrome), best heard at the cardiac apex, which may or may not be associated with a late systolic murmur of mitral regurgitation. In view of the variability of the murmur and the high level of skill required to recognize the murmur, echocardiography has assumed increasing importance in diagnosis of mitral valve prolapse.[15]

The etiology of mitral valve prolapse is unclear, although there is definite familial incidence.[16] On physical examination, the person with mitral valve prolapse is often tall and thin, and there may be associated findings, such as a high arched palate, pectus excavatum, kyphoscoliosis, or hyperextensible joints. Indeed, the classic occurrence of this abnormality is in the patient with Marfan syndrome. There is also an increased incidence of mitral valve prolapse in the patient with von Willebrand syndrome.[17] Poor left ventricular contractility due to muscular dystrophy, cardiomyopathy, or ischemic heart disease is associated with mitral valve prolapse. This valvular abnormality may occur in the patient with an atrial septal defect or tricuspid regurgitation. Damage to the mitral valve from rheumatic fever can also result in mitral valve prolapse.

Complications

Despite the prevalence of mitral valve prolapse, most patients (85% or more) are asymtomatic, emphasizing the usual benign course of this abnormality. Nevertheless, potentially serious complications can result from mitral valve prolapse[14] (Table 2-5). For example, mitral valve prolapse is probably the most common cause of pure mitral regurgitation, which may progress to the need for surgical intervention. Infective endocarditis is a serious potential complication of mitral valve prolapse, accounting for 10% to 15% of these cases. Mitral valve prolapse without superimposed endocarditis is the underlying pathologic abnormality in most patients with ruptured chordae tendineae. This valvular abnormality is responsible for about 40% of the transient ischemic attacks that occur in persons younger than 45 years of age. It is postulated that a clot originates from the rough surface of the prolapsed mitral valve or the traumatized adjacent left atrial surface. For this reason, these patients may be treated with an anticoagulant. Atrial and ventricular dysrhythmias are common, with ventricular premature beats the most frequent. Beta antagonists are useful antidysrhythmic agents in these patients, perhaps reflecting the drug-induced increases in left ventricular end-diastolic volume that serve to decrease the degree of mitral valve prolapse. Supraventricular tachydysrhythmias may occur and are consistent with the occasional association of mitral valve prolapse with a pre-excitation syndrome. Bradycardia associated with atrioventricular heart block may be re-

Table 2-5. Complications Associated With Mitral Valve Prolapse

Mitral regurgitation
Infective endocarditis
Ruptured chordae tendineae
Transient ischemic attack
Cardiac dysrhythmias—ventricular premature beats
Atrioventricular heart block
ST segment and T wave changes on the electrocardiogram
Sudden death (rare)

sistant to atropine, requiring an intravenous infusion of isoproterenol and placement of an artificial cardiac pacemaker. The ECG, although usually normal, may reflect T wave flattening or inversion with or without ST segment depression.[16] It is estimated that as many as 4000 sudden deaths annually may be attributable to mitral valve prolapse.[15] Although this is a large number of patients, it represents a very small fraction of the estimated 7 million adults in the Untied States with mitral valve prolapse.

Management of Anesthesia

Management of anesthesia for noncardiac surgery in the patient with mitral prolapse includes those principles outlined for the patient with mitral regurgitation (Table 2-4). An important concept is the recognition that increased left ventricular emptying in these patients can accentuate mitral valve prolapse, leading to cardiac dysrhythmias or acute mitral regurgitation, or both.[17] Perioperative events that can increase left ventricular emptying include (1) increased sympathetic nervous system activity, (2) decreased systemic vascular resistance, and (3) assumption of the upright posture. A decrease in the level of anxiety is an important goal of the preanesthetic interview and premedication of these patients. The use of atropine in the preoperative medication is influenced by the realization that an increase in heart rate may be undesirable. Prophylactic antibiotics instituted during the preoperative period for protection against the development of infective endocarditis are usually recommended for the patient with mitral valve prolapse who is scheduled for a dental or surgical procedure.

Induction of anesthesia in the presence of mitral valve prolapse can be achieved with available intravenous induction drugs, keeping in mind the need to avoid sudden and prolonged decreases in systemic vascular resistance. For this reason, it is important to optimize the intravascular fluid volume during the preoperative period. Ketamine is an unlikely selection for the induction of anesthesia in the patient with mitral valve prolapse, considering its ability to stimulate the sympathetic nervous system. Maintenance of anesthesia is designed to minimize sympathetic nervous system activation secondary to painful intraoperative stimulation. A volatile anesthetic, combined with nitrous oxide or an opioid, or both, is useful in attenuating sympathetic nervous system activity, keeping in mind the importance of titrating the drug doses to minimize the likelihood of undesirable decreases in systemic vascular resistance. Maintenance of skeletal muscle paralysis is often provided with a nondepolarizing muscle relaxant that lacks significant circulatory effects. Pancuronium may be avoided if there is concern that this drug could enhance left ventricular emptying by increasing the heart rate and myocardial contractility. Decreased systemic vascular resistance is a consideration when epidural anesthesia or spinal anesthesia is proposed for the patient with mitral valve prolapse.

Unexpected cardiac dysrhythmias may occur during anesthesia, emphasizing the importance of monitoring the ECG in the patient with mitral valve prolapse.[18] Ventricular cardiac dysrhythmias are particularly likely to occur during an operation performed in the head-up or sitting position, presumably reflecting increased left ventricular emptying and accentuation of mitral valve prolapse. Lidocaine and a beta antagonist such as esmolol or propranolol are useful for treatment of cardiac dysrhythmias. Prompt replacement of blood loss and generous intravenous fluid maintenance (5 ml·kg^{-1}·h^{-1}) will tend to optimize intravascular fluid volume and decrease the likelihood of adverse effects produced by positive-pressure ventilation of the lungs. Furthermore, a high normal intravascular fluid volume helps maintain forward left ventricular stroke volume, should acute mitral regurgitation occur intraoperatively. If a vasopressor is needed, an alpha agonist such as phenylephrine is acceptable. Production of controlled hypotension with a vasodilator drug is an unlikely technique, since the associated decrease in systemic vascular resistance could enhance mitral valve prolapse.

AORTIC STENOSIS

Isolated nonrheumatic aortic stenosis usually results from progressive calcification and stenosis of a congenitally abnormal bicuspid valve. By contrast, aortic stenosis due to rheumatic fever almost always occurs in association with mitral valve disease. In either situation, the natural history of aortic valve disease includes a long latent period, often 30 years or more before symptoms occur. Clinically, aortic stenosis is recognized by its characteristic systolic murmur, best heard in the second right intercostal space with transmission into the neck. Since many patients with aortic stenosis are asymptomatic, it is important to listen for this heart murmur in patients scheduled for surgery. Echocardiography shows thickening and calcification of the aortic valve and decreased mobility of the valve leaflets in nearly every patient with calcific aortic stenosis. A chest radiograph may show a prominent ascending aorta due to poststenotic dilation, whereas the ECG demonstrates evidence of left ventricular hypertrophy.

The characteristic triad of symptoms associated with aortic stenosis includes angina pectoris, dyspnea on exertion, and a history of syncope. Syncope characteristically occurs with effort, presumably reflecting inability of the heart to maintain an adequate cardiac output and systemic blood pressure in the presence of peripheral vasodilation associated with exercise. The incidence of sudden death is increased in the patient with aortic stenosis. Indeed, when any of the triad of symptoms is present, the patient's life expectancy without surgery is less

than 5 years, and 15% to 20% of these patients experience sudden death. Surgical replacement of the diseased valve is usually indicated when symptoms of angina pectoris, syncope, and left ventricular failure have appeared and when the stenosis is severe, as demonstrated by a transvalvular pressure gradient greater than 50 mmHg or an aortic valve orifice area less than 1 cm^2. Even if symptoms are mild, surgery may be recommended, in view of the risk of sudden death. Nevertheless, even in the presence of severe aortic stenosis, there is no evidence that elective noncardiac surgery is associated with an increased risk.[19] Percutaneous transluminal valvuloplasty may be an alternative to surgery in selected patients.

Pathophysiology

Obstruction to ejection of blood into the aorta due to a decrease in the area of the aortic valve orifice necessitates an increase in left ventricular pressure, in order to maintain forward stroke volume. Hemodynamically significant aortic stenosis is normally associated with a transvalvular pressure gradient greater than 50 mmHg and an aortic valve orifice area less than 1 cm^2 (normal 2.5 to 3.5 cm^2). Furthermore, aortic stenosis is almost always associated with some degree of aortic regurgitation. Determination of the pressure gradient across the valve is noninvasively depicted by echocardiography, whereas cardiac catheterization is the definitive method of measuring the systolic pressure gradient across the aortic valve.

Angina pectoris often occurs in the patient with aortic stenosis despite the absence of coronary artery atherosclerosis. This reflects an increased myocardial oxygen requirement, owing to the increased amount of ventricular muscle associated with concentric myocardial hypertrophy. Furthermore, myocardial oxygen delivery is decreased, due to compression of subendocardial coronary blood vessels by the increased left ventricular systolic pressure.

Management of Anesthesia

Management of anesthesia for noncardiac surgery in the patient with aortic stenosis includes avoidance of events that may further decrease the cardiac output (Table 2-6). Preservation of normal sinus rhythm is important, since the left ven-

Table 2-6. Anesthetic Considerations in the Patient With Aortic Stenosis

Maintain normal sinus rhythm
Avoid bradycardia
Avoid sudden increases or decreases in systemic vascular resistance
Optimize intravascular fluid volume to maintain venous return and left ventricular filling

tricle is dependent on a properly timed atrial contraction to ensure an optimal left ventricular end-diastolic volume. Indeed, loss of the normal arterial contraction, as during junctional rhythm or atrial fibrillation, may produce a significant decrease in stroke volume and blood pressure. Monitoring the heart rate is important, as it determines the time available for filling of the ventricles and ejection of forward left ventricular stroke volume. For example, a marked and sustained increase in heart rate can decrease the time for left ventricular filling and ejection, leading to an undesirable decrease in stroke volume. Likewise, a sudden decrease in heart rate can lead to acute overdistension of the left ventricle. In view of the obstruction to left ventricular ejection, it is important to recognize that decreased systemic vascular resistance may be associated with a large decrease in blood pressure and subsequent decrease in coronary blood flow. Conversely, increased systemic vascular resistance and blood pressure can lead to a decrease in stroke volume. It is important to have available a direct current defibrillator whenever anesthesia is administered to the patient with aortic stenosis. External cardiac massage is unlikely to be effective, should cardiac arrest occur, as it is difficult to create an adequate stroke volume across a stenotic valve using mechanical compression of the sternum.

Prophylactic antibiotics instituted during the preoperative period for protection against the development of infective endocarditis are usually recommended for the patient with aortic stenosis who is scheduled for a dental or surgical procedure. Preoperative medication is tailored to minimize the likelihood of a decrease in systemic vascular resistance. General anesthesia is often selected in preference over epidural anesthesia or spinal anesthesia, since peripheral sympathetic nervous system blockade produced by regional anesthesia can lead to an undesirable decrease in systemic vascular resistance. If a regional anesthetic is selected, it may be useful to consider the more likely gradual onset of peripheral sympathetic nervous system blockade after epidural anesthesia, as compared with spinal anesthesia.

Induction of anesthesia in the presence of aortic stenosis can be achieved with available intravenous induction drugs. Intubation of the trachea is facilitated by the administration of a muscle relaxant. Bradycardia associated with the administration of succinylcholine would be undesirable. Interventions to prevent this rare occurrence (increased heart rate the more common response) may be considered, including the prior administration of an anticholinergic drug. Maintenance of anesthesia is most often accomplished with a combination of nitrous oxide plus a volatile anesthetic or an opioid. A disadvantage of volatile drugs (especially halothane) is depression of sinoatrial node automaticity, which may lead to a junctional rhythm and loss of properly timed atrial contractions. Furthermore, when left ventricular function is severely impaired by aortic stenosis, it is useful to avoid any additional depression of myocardial contractility with a volatile anesthetic. Decreased systemic

vascular resistance produced by isoflurane would be undesirable, although clinical experience using low concentrations of this anesthetic has not been recognized as a hazard. Maintenance of anesthesia with nitrous oxide plus an opioid or with an opioid alone in a high dose (fentanyl, 50 to 100 $\mu g \cdot kg^{-1}$ IV or an equivalent dose of sufentanil or alfentanil) has been recommended for the patient with marked left ventricular dysfunction attributable to aortic stenosis. A nondepolarizing muscle relaxant with a minimal effect on the circulation is useful, although the modest increase in blood pressure and heart rate typically produced by pancuronium are acceptable. Intravascular fluid volume is maintained by prompt replacement of blood loss and liberal administration (5 ml·kg^{-1}·h^{-1}) of intravenous fluids.

Intraoperative monitoring of the patient with aortic stenosis often includes an ECG lead that will reflect left ventricular ischemia. The use of an arterial and pulmonary artery catheter depends on the magnitude of the surgery and the severity of the aortic stenosis. These monitors help determine whether intraoperative hypotension is due to hypovolemia or CHF. It should be remembered that the pulmonary artery occlusion pressure may overestimate left ventricular end-diastolic pressure because of the decreased compliance of the left ventricle that accompanies chronic aortic stenosis.

The onset of junctional rhythm or bradycardia during anesthesia and surgery will usually require prompt treatment with the intravenous administration of atropine. A persistent tachycardia can be treated with a beta antagonist such as esmolol or propranolol. A large dose of beta antagonist should probably be avoided, since these patients may be dependent on endogenous beta activity to maintain stroke volume, particularly in the presence of increased systemic vascular resistance that occurs in response to surgical stimulation. Supraventricular tachycardia should be promptly terminated with electrical cardioversion. Lidocaine is kept available, as these patients have a propensity toward the development of ventricular cardiac dysrhythmias.

AORTIC REGURGITATION

Aortic regurgitation may be acute or chronic. Acute aortic regurgitation is most often due to infective endocarditis, trauma, or dissection of a thoracic aneurysm. Treatment of acute aortic regurgitation usually consists of prompt surgical replacement of the aortic valve. Chronic aortic regurgitation is usually due to prior rheumatic fever or persistent systemic hypertension. Aortic regurgitation is recognized by its characteristic diastolic murmur, best heard in the second right intercostal space, widened pulse pressure, decreased diastolic pressure, and bounding peripheral pulses. There is evidence of left ventricular enlargement on the chest radiograph and

ECG and by echocardiography. Cardiac catheterization with angiography is the most definitive means of assessing the severity of aortic regurgitation. In contrast to aortic stenosis, sudden death related to aortic regurgitation is rare. Surgical replacement of the diseased valve may ultimately become necessary. Delay of surgery until after the onset of CHF introduces the risk of irreversible cardiac damage.

Pathophysiology

The basic hemodynamic problem in aortic regurgitation is a decrease in forward left ventricular stroke volume because of regurgitation of part of the ejected stroke volume from the aorta back into the left ventricle. The magnitude of the regurgitant volume depends on (1) the duration for the regurgitant flow to occur, which is determined by the heart rate; and (2) the pressure gradient across the aortic valve, which is dependent on systemic vascular resistance. The magnitude of aortic regurgitation will be decreased by an increased heart rate and a decreased systemic vascular resistance.

The left ventricle usually tolerates a chronic increase in left ventricular volume overload. When left ventricular failure does occur, however, left ventricular end-diastolic volume increases precipitously, and evidence of pulmonary edema is likely. Indeed, a helpful indicator of left ventricular function in the presence of aortic regurgitation is the echocardiographic determination of end-systolic volume and ejection fraction, both of which remain normal until left ventricular function becomes impaired. A gradual onset of aortic regurgitation is associated with a marked increase in left ventricular muscle mass. Increased myocardial oxygen requirements secondary to left ventricular hypertrophy, plus a characteristic decrease in aortic diastolic pressure, which decreases coronary blood flow, can be manifested as angina pectoris due to subendocardial ischemia, in the absence of ischemic heart disease. Compared with the patient with chronic aortic regurgitation, the patient with acute aortic regurgitation experiences a sudden increase in ventricular volume before left ventricular hypertrophy can occur. This limits the effectiveness of compensatory mechanisms, such as increased heart rate and myocardial contractility, with the end result often being decreased cardiac output and blood pressure. An intravenous infusion of nitroprusside may be useful in improving forward left ventricular stroke volume when acute aortic regurgitation results in left ventricular volume overload and decreased cardiac output.

Management of Anesthesia

Management of anesthesia for noncardiac surgery in the patient with aortic regurgitation is designed to maintain forward left ventricular stroke volume (Table 2-7). In this regard, it is useful to maintain the heart rate above 80 beats·min^{-1}, as bradycardia, by increasing the duration of ventricular dias-

Table 2-7. Anesthetic Considerations in the Patient With Aortic Regurgitation

Avoid sudden decreases in heart rate
Avoid sudden increases in systemic vascular resistance
Minimize drug-induced myocardial depression

tole, will lead to acute left ventricular volume overload. An abrupt increase in systemic vascular resistance can precipitate left ventricular failure, requiring treatment with a peripheral vasodilator such as nitroprusside. Aortic regurgitation usually produces left ventricular impairment, and anesthetic-induced depression of myocardial contractility may be undesirable. Left ventricular failure may be treated with afterload reduction provided by nitroprusside and a cardiac inotrope such as dopamine, to increase myocardial contractility. Overall, a slight increase in heart rate and a modest decrease in systemic vascular resistance are reasonable goals for management of anesthesia. Still, it should be recognized that these patients may be exquisitely sensitive to peripheral vasodilation.

Prophylactic antibiotics instituted during the preoperative period for protection against the development of endocarditis are usually recommended for the patient with aortic regurgitation who is scheduled for a dental or surgical procedure. General anesthesia is the usual choice for the patient with aortic regurgitation. Although decreased systemic vascular resistance is theoretically beneficial, the uncontrolled nature of this response with regional anesthesia detracts from the use of epidural or spinal anesthesia. Induction of anesthesia in the presence of aortic regurgitation can be achieved with available intravenous induction drugs. Ketamine may be advantageous by virtue of its ability to accelerate heart rate, but the accompanying increase in resistance to ejection of forward left ventricular stroke volume due to increased systemic vascular resistance could be undesirable. Nevertheless, when intravascular fluid volume is judged to be decreased, the use of ketamine for induction of anesthesia is an acceptable choice. Bradycardia associated with the administration of succinylcholine would be undesirable; interventions to prevent this rare occurrence (increased heart rate the more common response) may be considered, including the prior administration of an anticholinergic drug.

In the absence of severe left ventricular dysfunction, maintenance of anesthesia is often provided with nitrous oxide plus a volatile anesthetic or an opioid. Although a specific volatile anesthetic has not been demonstrated to be superior, the usual increased heart rate and decreased systemic vascular resistance with little evidence of direct myocardial depression characteristic of isoflurane make selection of this drug attractive in these patients. When myocardial function is severely compromised, the use of an opioid technique (fentanyl, 50 to

$100 \ \mu g \cdot kg^{-1}$ IV, or an equivalent dose of sufentanil or alfentanil) as the sole drug for maintenance of anesthesia may be the best choice for providing adequate amnesia without producing additional cardiac depression. It is important to consider the possibility of exaggerated myocardial depression that may occur when nitrous oxide is added to opioids or when benzodiazepines are added to opioids.[20,21] The muscle relaxant selection is influenced by the likely circulatory effects produced by these drugs. A drug with minimal to absent effects on blood pressure and heart rate may be the most attractive selection, although the modest increase in heart rate associated with pancuronium could contribute to the maintenance of forward left ventricular stroke volume.

Ventilation of the lungs is often controlled and adjusted to maintain the $PaCO_2$ near normal. The pattern of ventilation should provide sufficient time between breaths for venous return to occur. Maintenance of intravascular fluid volume with prompt replacement of blood loss is important in maintaining cardiac filling and ejection of an optimal forward left ventricular stroke volume. Preoperative fluid loading and an intravenous infusion of nitroprusside may be useful for maintaining cardiac output during surgery[22] (Fig. 2-5). Bradycardia and junctional rhythm are undesirable and may require prompt treatment with the intravenous administration of atropine.

A minor operation performed in a patient with asymptomatic aortic regurgitation probably does not require invasive monitoring. In view of the possibility of myocardial ischemia, it is useful to monitor an appropriate ECG lead. In the presence of severe aortic regurgitation, the use of invasive monitoring is helpful in detecting the onset of undesirable degrees of depression of myocardial contractility and in facilitating intravenous fluid replacement. Certainly, a pulmonary artery catheter is useful when a peripheral vasodilating drug is administered in an attempt to facilitate forward left ventricular stroke volume. Measurement of cardiac output by thermodilution confirms the response to decreased systemic vascular resistance produced by a drug such as nitroprusside.

TRICUSPID REGURGITATION

Tricuspid regurgitation is usually functional, reflecting dilation of the right ventricle due to pulmonary hypertension. Indeed, tricuspid regurgitation often accompanies pulmonary hypertension and right ventricular volume overloading due to left ventricular failure produced by aortic or mitral valve disease. A significant incidence of tricuspid regurgitation secondary to infective endocarditis is also associated with intravenous drug abuse. Tricuspid regurgitation is invariably associated with tricuspid stenosis when valve dysfunction is the result of prior rheumatic fever.

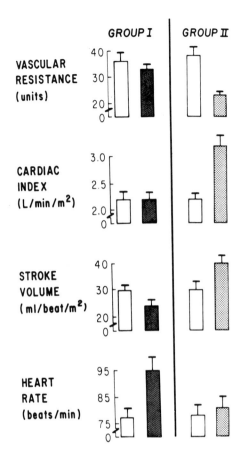

Fig. 2-5. The cardiovascular effects of nitroprusside (1.3–3.7 $\mu g \cdot kg^{-1} \cdot min^{-1}$ IV) (dark bars) compared with control (clear bars) were determined in patients with mitral and/or aortic regurgitation with (group II) or without (group I) preoperative fluid loading. The combination of afterload reduction and preload augmentation (group II) produced more desirable circulatory responses than afterload reduction alone (group I). Preoperative fluid loading was with approximately 2 L of lactated Ringer's solution. (From Stone JG, Hoar PF, Calabro JR, et al. Afterload reductions and preload augmentation of patients with cardiac failure and valvular regurgitation. Anesth Analg 1980;59:737–42, with permission.)

Pathophysiology

The basic hemodynamic consequence of tricuspid regurgitation is right atrial volume overload that is well tolerated. The high compliance of the right atrium and vena cavae result in a minimal increase in right atrial pressure, even in the presence of a large regurgitant volume. Even surgical removal of the tricuspid valve, as in the patient with infective endocarditis, is usually well tolerated. Although pure tricuspid regurgitation is relatively benign, the addition of right ventricular pressure overload as produced by left ventricular failure or pulmonary hypertension will often lead to right ventricular failure. Right ventricular failure causes an increased magnitude of regurgitation through an incompetent tricuspid valve, further decreasing left ventricular stroke volume due to decreased pulmonary blood flow. The combination of right ventricular failure and left ventricular underloading can cause the right atrial pressure to exceed the left atrial pressure, potentially leading to a right-to-left intracardiac shunt through an incompletely closed foramen ovale. Annuloplasty, rather than tricuspid valve replacement, is often the preferred surgical treatment of tricuspid regurgitation.

Management of Anesthesia

Management of anesthesia in the patient with tricuspid regurgitation is similar, whether the regurgitation is isolated or associated with aortic or mitral valve disease. Intravascular fluid volume and central venous pressure are maintained in a high normal range, to facilitate an adequate right ventricular stroke volume and left ventricular filling. High intrathoracic pressure due to positive-pressure ventilation of the lungs or drug-induced venodilation will decrease venous return and eventually compromise left ventricular stroke volume. Likewise, any event known to increase pulmonary vascular resistance, such as arterial hypoxemia and hypercarbia, should be avoided.

A specific anesthetic drug combination or technique cannot be uniquely recommended for management of anesthesia in the patient with tricuspid regurgitation. Nevertheless, a volatile anesthetic that could produce pulmonary vasodilation is a consideration, whereas ketamine is useful by virtue of its ability to maintain venous return. Nitrous oxide is a weak pulmonary vasoconstrictor, when combined with an opioid, and could increase the magnitude of tricuspid regurgitation by this mechanism. If nitrous oxide is administered, it may be helpful to monitor central venous pressure and consider the possible role of nitrous oxide, should an unexpected increase in right atrial pressure occur. Intraoperative monitors should include measurement of right atrial filling pressure to guide intravenous fluid replacement and to detect adverse effects of the anesthetic drugs or technique on the magnitude of tricuspid regurgitation. Intravenous infusion of air through the tubing used to deliver intravenous fluids must be guarded against, in view of the possibility of a right-to-left intracardiac shunt through an incompletely closed foramen ovale.

REFERENCES

1. Fishman MC, Hoffman AR, Klausner RD, Rockson SG, Thalar MS. Medicine. Philadelphia. JB Lippincott 1981;42
2. Rapaport E. Natural history of aortic and mitral valve disease. Am J Cardiol 1975;35:221–7
3. Greenberg BH, Rahimtoola SH. Vasodilator therapy for valvular heart disease. JAMA 1981;246:269–72
4. Clements FM, deBruijn NP. Perioperative evaluation of regional wall motion by transesophageal two-dimensional echocardiography. Anesth Analg 1987;66:249–61
5. Lee RT, Bhatia SJS, Sutton MG. Assessment of valvular heart disease with Doppler echocardiography. JAMA 1989;262:2131–5
6. McKay CR, Kawanishi DT, Rahimtoola SH. Catheter balloon valvuloplasty of the mitral valve in adults using a double-balloon technique. JAMA 1987;257:1753–61
7. Bolen JL, Lopes MG, Harrison DC, Alderman EL. Analysis of left ventricular function in response to afterload changes in patients with mitral stenosis. Circulation 1975;52:894–900
8. Tinker JH, Tarhan S. Discontinuing anticoagulant therapy in surgical patients with cardiac prosthesis. JAMA 1978;239:738–9
9. Geha DG, Rozelle BC, Raessler KL, et al. Pancuronium bromide enhances atrioventricular conduction in halothane-anesthetized dogs. Anesthesiology 1977;46:342–5
10. Hilgenberg JC, McCammon RL, Stoelting RK. Pulmonary and systemic vascular responses to nitrous oxide in patients with mitral stenosis and pulmonary hypertension. Anesth Analg 1980;59:323–6
11. Konstadt SN, Reich DL, Thys DM. Nitrous oxide does not exacerbate pulmonary hypertension or ventricular dysfunction in patients with mitral valvular disease. Can J Anaesth 1990;37:613–7
12. Schulte-Sasse U, Hess W, Tarnow J. Pulmonary vascular responses to nitrous oxide in patients with normal and high pulmonary vascular resistance. Anesthesiology 1982;57:9–13
13. Stone JG, Hoar PF, Baltas AN, Khambatta HJ. Nitroprusside and mitral stenosis. Anesth Analg 1980;59:662–5
14. Jeresaty RM. Mitral valve prolapse: An update. JAMA 1985;254:793–5
15. Devereux RB. Diagnosis and prognosis of mitral valve prolapse. N Engl J Med 1989;320:1077–9
16. Kowalski SE. Mitral valve prolapse. Can Anaesth Soc J 1985;32:138–41
17. Krantz EM, Viljoen JF, Schermer R, Canas MS. Mitral valve prolapse. Anesth Analg 1980;59:379–83
18. Berry FA, Lake CL, Johns RA, Rogers BM. Mitral valve prolapse—another cause of intraoperative dysrhythmias in the pediatric patient. Anesthesiology 1985;62:662–4
19. O'Keefe JH, Shub C, Rettke SR. Risk of noncardiac surgical procedures in patients with aortic stenosis. Mayo Clin Proc 1989;64:400–5
20. Stoelting RK, Gibbs PS. Hemodynamic effects of morphine and morphine-nitrous oxide in valvular heart disease and coronary-artery disease. Anesthesiology 1973;38:45–52
21. Tomicheck RC, Rosow CE, Philbin DM, Moss J, Teplick RS, Schneider RC. Diazepam-fentanyl interaction—hemodynamic and hormonal effects in coronary artery surgery. Anesth Analg 1983;62:881–4
22. Stone JG, Hoar PF, Calabro JR, Khambata HJ. Afterload reduction and preload augmentation improve the anesthetic management of patients with cardiac failure and valvular regurgitation. Anesth Analg 1980;59:737–42

3

Congenital Heart Disease

Congenital heart disease is present in about 1% of newborn infants.[1] Causes of congenital heart disease are idiopathic, genetic, or environmental (rubella in the first trimester, lithium ingestion, fetal alcohol syndrome). A child born to a parent with congenital heart disease has an increased likelihood of having a similar congenital lesion. Prematurity, multiple gestations, and the presence of noncardiac congenital anomalies are also associated with an increased incidence of cardiac defects. Signs and symptoms of congenital heart disease most often include dyspnea and slow physical development; there is also a significant recognizable cardiac murmur in association with abnormalities on the electrocardiogram (ECG) and chest radiograph (Table 3-1). The diagnosis of congenital heart disease is apparent during the first week of life in about 50% of afflicted neonates and before 5 years of age in virtually all remaining patients. Echocardiography is the initial diagnostic test recommended if congenital heart disease is suspected. Doppler ultrasound provides further information in demonstrating valvular dysfunction and septal defects. Computed tomography offers advantages over echocardiography in demonstrating anomalies involving the great vessels. Magnetic resonance imaging provides information similar to that provided by computed tomography but offers better resolution without the need for radiopaque contrast media. Cardiac catheterization and selective angiocardiography are the most definitive diagnostic techniques available for use in patients with congenital heart disease. The major unsolved problem in management of congenital heart disease is treatment of pulmonary vascular disease and associated pulmonary hypertension. In some patients, heart-lung transplantation may be the only hope for survival.

Certain general problems may afflict the patient with congenital heart disease (Table 3-2). For example, infective endocarditis is a complication of most congenital cardiac anomalies, especially in the patient with a ventricular septal defect (VSD) or patent ductus arteriosus (PDA). The patient with a congenital heart lesion that predisposes to infective endocarditis should receive prophylactic antibiotics before undergoing any dental or surgical procedure. Cardiac dysrhythmias are usually not a prominent feature of congenital heart disease, except for atrial fibrillation, which often develops in the patient older than 40 years of age with an atrial septal defect (ASD). A surgical procedure in the area of the atrioventricular node as for closure of a VSD may result in heart block and in the need for insertion of an artificial cardiac pacemaker. Sudden cardiac death that is probably related to a cardiac dysrhythmia occasionally occurs in a patient who has previously undergone surgical correction of congenital heart disease, presumably reflecting myocardial scarring or damage to the cardiac conduction system. Indeed, surgical repair of most congenital heart defects is associated with lingering cardiac mortality.[2] Hypertension is likely in the patient with coarctation of the aorta. This may persist even after surgical repair, which in some patients reflects a recurrence of the aortic narrowing. In the patient with cyanotic congenital heart disease, secondary polycythemia reflecting a physiologic response to chronic arterial hypoxemia results in a risk of thromboembolism, especially when the hematocrit exceeds 70%. Phlebotomy may be a useful treatment but can result in exaggeration of dyspnea. The patient with secondary polycythemia may exhibit coagulation defects, most likely owing to deficiencies in the synthesis of vitamin K-dependent clotting factors in the liver and defective platelet aggregation. The development of a brain abscess is a major risk in the patient with cyanotic congenital heart disease. The onset of a brain abscess often mimics the onset of stroke both clinically and by its appearance on computed tomography. The blood uric acid concentration is often increased in the patient with cyanotic congenital heart disease, accounting for the occasional prophylactic administration of allopurinol to these patients.

Although more than 100 different congenital heart lesions are known, nearly 90% of all cardiac defects can be placed in 1 of 10 categories (Table 3-3). Management of anesthesia for patients with congenital heart disease requires thorough knowledge of the pathophysiology of each cardiac defect. In this respect, it is convenient to categorize congenital heart

Table 3-1. Signs and Symptoms of Congenital Heart Disease

Infants	Children
Tachypnea	Dyspnea
Failure to gain weight	Slow physical development
Heart rate >200 beats·min^{-1}	Decreased exercise tolerance
Heart murmur	Heart murmur
Congestive heart failure	Congestive heart failure
Cyanosis	Cyanosis
	Clubbing of digits
	Squatting
	Hypertension

Table 3-3. Common Congenital Heart Defects

	Total (%)
Ventricular septal defect	28
Secundum atrial septal defect	10
Patent ductus arteriosus	10
Tetralogy of Fallot	10
Pulmonic stenosis	10
Aortic stenosis	7
Coarctation of the aorta	5
Transposition of the great arteries	5
Primum atrial septal defect	3
Total anomalous pulmonary venous return	1

defects as those lesions that result in (1) a left-to-right intracardiac shunt, (2) a right-to-left intracardiac shunt, (3) separation of the pulmonary and systemic circulation, (4) mixing of blood between the pulmonary and systemic circulation, (5) increased myocardial work, and (6) mechanical obstruction of the airway.

LEFT-TO-RIGHT INTRACARDIAC SHUNT

A left-to-right intracardiac shunt or its equivalent can occur at the atrial, ventricular, or arterial level (Table 3-4). The ultimate result of this shunt, regardless of its location, is increased pulmonary blood flow with pulmonary hypertension, right ventricular hypertrophy, and eventually congestive heart failure. The younger the patient at the time of operation, the greater the likelihood that pulmonary vascular resistance will normalize. In the older patient, if pulmonary vascular resistance is one-third or less of systemic vascular resistance, progressive pulmonary vascular disease after operation is unlikely.[3] The onset and severity of clinical symptoms vary with the site and magnitude of the vascular shunt.

Secundum Atrial Septal Defect

A secundum ASD is most often located in the center of the interatrial septum and can vary from a single opening to a fenestrated septum (Fig. 3-1). Isolated defects are usually

Table 3-2. Common Problems Associated With Congenital Heart Disease

Infective endocarditis	Thromboembolism
Cardiac dysrhythmias	Coagulopathy
Complete heart block	Brain abscess
Hypertension	Increased plasma uric acid concentration
Polycythemia	

Table 3-4. Congenital Heart Defects Resulting in a Left-to-Right Intracardiac Shunt or Its Equivalent

Secundum atrial septal defect
Primum atrial septal defect (endocardial cushion defect)
Ventricular septal defect
Aorticopulmonary fenestration

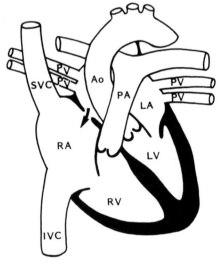

Fig. 3-1. Schematic diagram of a secundum atrial septal defect located in the center of the interatrial septum. Blood flows along a pressure gradient from the left atrium (LA) to the right atrium (RA). The resulting left-to-right intracardiac shunt is associated with an increased flow through the pulmonary artery (PA). A decrease in systemic vascular resistance or an increase in pulmonary vascular resistance will decrease the pressure gradient across the defect, leading to a decrease in the magnitude of the shunt. Ao, aorta; RV, right ventricle; LV, left ventricle; SVC, superior vena cava; IVC, inferior vena cava; PV, pulmonary vein.

well tolerated in childhood and often produce symptoms only after the second or third decade of life. Indeed, ASD is the most common congenital heart lesion recognized in the adult.

Signs and Symptoms

The presence of a secundum ASD is occasionally first suspected when there is a history of frequent pulmonary infections or when a systolic murmur is noted over the area of the pulmonic valve during a routine physical examination. For example, less than 20% of newborns with an ASD have a characteristic cardiac murmur. The incidence of a systolic ejection murmur over the pulmonic valve area, however, increases to 80% by 5 years of age. The second heart sound in the presence of an ASD is widely split. The cardiac murmur and fixed splitting of the second heart sound reflect the increased pulmonary blood flow characteristic of an ASD. The two principal complications of an ASD are pulmonary hypertension and right ventricular failure, reflecting the chronic increase in pulmonary blood flow. A chest radiograph may indicate signs of increased pulmonary blood flow, characterized by an enlarged pulmonary artery trunk and hypertrophy of the right atrium and ventricle. The ECG typically shows a pattern of right bundle branch block and right axis deviation. First-degree atrioventricular heart block may be present. Echocardiography often demonstrates an increased right ventricular dimension and paradoxical motion of the atrial septum. Mitral valve prolapse, which occurs in about 30% of patients with this cardiac defect, can also be detected with echocardiography. Cardiac catheterization usually demonstrates increases in venous oxygen saturation at the right atrial level. This increase in oxygen saturation may not be apparent until the ventricular level if streaming of the shunted blood occurs.

Treatment

Surgical closure of a secundum ASD is indicated when pulmonary blood flow is at least twice the systemic blood flow. Surgery is not indicated when pulmonary hypertension has progressed to the point that pulmonary vascular pressure is near systemic vascular pressure, as closure of the defect under these circumstances is associated with high mortality.

Primum Atrial Septal Defect

A primum ASD (endocardial cushion defect) is characterized by a large opening in the interatrial septum. This defect frequently involves the mitral and tricuspid valves; mitral regurgitation in association with a cleft anterior leaflet of the mitral valve is present in about 50% of patients. Physiologically, a primum and secundum ASD are similar.

Signs and Symptoms

A primum ASD defect usually becomes evident in infancy or early childhood, characterized by frequent pulmonary infections, failure to thrive, tachycardia, and congestive heart fail-

ure. Physical findings differ from those observed in the presence of a secundum ASD only if mitral or tricuspid regurgitation, or both, are present. Findings on the chest radiograph and the ECG are similar to those observed in the presence of a secundum ASD. Echocardiography and angiocardiography are important for defining the placement of the mitral and tricuspid valves. Cardiac catheterization usually demonstrates an increase in venous oxygen saturation at both the atrial and ventricular levels, as well as the presence of pulmonary hypertension.

Treatment

Surgical repair of a primum ASD is usually necessary in the first decade of life, to prevent pulmonary hypertension from becoming irreversible. Initially, palliative banding of the pulmonary artery may be selected in an attempt to reduce the magnitude of the left-to-right intracardiac shunt. Mortality with banding, however, remains high; for this reason, some favor a complete repair, even at a very young age. Nevertheless, complete surgical repair is often unsuccessful because of the inability to produce adequately functioning mitral and tricuspid valves from the rudimentary leaflets that are present. A residual cleft mitral valve might be vulnerable to infective endocarditis. Residual pulmonary hypertension that occurs after surgical correction of this defect assumes importance during the postoperative period, as it can lead to tricuspid regurgitation and right ventricular failure. Surgical repair of a low-lying defect also carries the risk of third-degree atrioventricular heart block since this defect is near the conduction system necessary for propagation of the cardiac impulse. Sinoatrial node or atrioventricular node dysfunction or atrial fibrillation may be manifested years after successful surgical repair.

Management of Anesthesia

An ASD associated with a left-to-right intracardiac shunt has only minor implications for the management of anesthesia. For example, as long as systemic blood flow remains normal, the pharmacokinetics of inhaled drugs will not be significantly altered despite increased pulmonary blood flow.[4] Conversely, increased pulmonary blood flow could dilute drugs that are injected intravenously. It is unlikely, however, that this potential dilution will alter the clinical response to these drugs, since pulmonary circulation time is very short. Another effect of increased pulmonary blood flow is that positive-pressure ventilation of the lungs is well tolerated.

Any change in systemic vascular resistance during the perioperative period could have important implications for the patient with an ASD. For example, drugs or events that produce prolonged increases in systemic vascular resistance should be avoided, as this change will favor an increase in the magnitude of the left-to-right shunt at the atrial level. This is particularly true with a primum ASD defect associated with mitral regurgitation. Conversely, a decrease in systemic vascular resistance, as produced by a volatile anesthetic, or increases in pulmonary vascular resistance due to positive-pressure ventilation of the lungs will tend to decrease the magnitude of the left-to-right shunt.

Other considerations for the management of anesthesia in the presence of an ASD include the need to provide antibiotics during the preoperative period to protect against the development of infective endocarditis. In addition, meticulous avoidance of the entrance of air into the circulation, as can occur through the tubing used to deliver intravenous solutions, is imperative. Transient supraventricular dysrhythmias and atrioventricular conduction defects are common during the early postoperative period after surgical repair of an ASD.

Ventricular Septal Defect

A VSD is the most common congenital cardiac abnormality in infants. It is rarely seen in adults because defects that are not corrected surgically are associated with a high mortality (Table 3-2). In addition, the incidence of spontaneous VSD closure is relatively high. The incidence of VSD in premature births is about four times that in term infants. About 90% of these defects are located below the crista supraventricularis, a muscular ridge that separates the body of the right ventricle from the pulmonary artery outflow tract (Fig. 3-2). These defects may be single openings in the muscular portion of the ventricular septum or multiple lesions giving rise to a fenestrated septum.

Signs and Symptoms

Manifestations of a VSD depend on the size of the defect and on the pulmonary vascular resistance. The patient with a small defect is usually asymptomatic but has a loud pansystolic murmur of maximum intensity along the left sternal border. A chest radiograph and the ECG typically show no abnormal findings. The magnitude of the left-to-right intracardiac shunt is usually minimal, such that the ratio of pulmonary to systemic blood flow is less than 1.5:1. As a result, pulmonary hypertension and congestive heart failure are unlikely.

The patient with a moderate-size VSD may be asymptomatic, but a chest radiograph typically indicates biventricular enlargement and evidence of increased pulmonary blood flow. Cardiac catheterization usually demonstrates a pulmonary blood flow exceeding systemic blood flow by 1.5 to 3 times. Pulmonary vascular resistance may be moderately elevated. A 15 to 20 mmHg gradient across the pulmonary artery outflow tract may develop, as right ventricular hypertrophy results in obstruction to blood flow at this site.

A large VSD is characterized by a left-to-right intracardiac shunt that results in pulmonary blood flow exceeding systemic

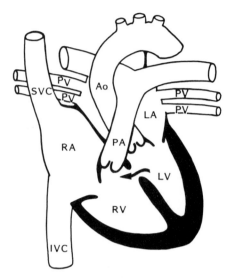

Fig. 3-2. Schematic diagram of a ventricular septal defect located just below the muscular ridge that separates the body of the right ventricle (RV) from the pulmonary artery (PA) outflow tract. Blood flow is along a pressure gradient from the left ventricle (LV) to the RV. The resulting left-to-right intracardiac shunt is associated with a pulmonary blood flow that exceeds the stroke volume of the LV. A decrease in systemic vascular resistance will decrease the pressure gradient across the defect and reduce the magnitude of the shunt.

blood flow by three to five times. Symptoms appear early in life (often at about 4 weeks of age) and are characterized by tachypnea, failure to gain weight, recurrent pneumonia, and congestive heart failure. A chest radiograph and the ECG will likely show evidence of pulmonary hypertension. When pulmonary vascular resistance exceeds systemic vascular resistance, right-to-left shunting will occur, producing cyanosis.

A VSD that opens into the pulmonary outflow portion of the right ventricle may be complicated by aortic regurgitation owing to prolapse of an aortic cusp into the defect. A left ventricular-to-right atrial septal defect (Gerbode defect) is associated with cardiac conduction disturbances and tricuspid regurgitation.

Treatment

About 25% of all VSDs will close spontaneously without surgical intervention, whereas about one-half of infants in whom congestive heart failure develops due to a VSD will improve with medical management. When medical management is not successful, a palliative surgical procedure such as pulmonary artery banding should be considered. Placement of a constricting band around the pulmonary artery serves to increase resistance to right ventricular ejection, thereby decreasing the magnitude of the left-to-right shunt at the ventricular level.

This procedure may also prevent development of irreversible pulmonary hypertension. Elevation of pulmonary vascular resistance seems to be reversible when banding is performed in patients younger than 2 years of age.

Management of Anesthesia

Administration of antibiotics to provide prophylaxis against bacterial endocarditis is indicated when noncardiac surgery is planned in the patient with a VSD. The pharmacokinetics of inhaled and injected drugs are not significantly altered by a VSD. As with an ASD, acute and persistent increases in systemic vascular resistance or decreases in pulmonary vascular resistance are undesirable, as these changes could accentuate the magnitude of the left-to-right shunt at the ventricular level. In this regard, a volatile anesthetic that decreases systemic vascular resistance and positive-pressure ventilation of the lungs, which increases pulmonary vascular resistance, are well tolerated. However, there maybe increased delivery of depressant drugs to the heart if coronary blood flow is increased to supply the hypertrophied ventricles. Conceivably, increasing the inspired concentration of a volatile anesthetic to achieve rapid induction of anesthesia, as is often done in normal children, could result in excessive depression of the heart before the central nervous system is anesthetized.

Right ventricular infundibular hypertrophy may be present in the patient with a VSD. Normally, this is a beneficial change, as it increases the resistance to right ventricular ejection, leading to a decrease in the magnitude of the left-to-right intracardiac shunt. Nevertheless, perioperative events that exaggerate this obstruction to right ventricular outflow, such as increased myocardial contractility or hypovolemia, must be minimized. Therefore, these patients are often anesthetized with a volatile anesthetic. In addition, intravascular fluid volume should be maintained by prompt replacement of blood loss.

Anesthesia for placement of a pulmonary artery band is often achieved with a drug that provides minimum cardiac depression. Muscle relaxants are used to prevent patient movement. If bradycardia or hypotension develops during surgery, it may be necessary to remove the pulmonary artery band promptly. Continuous monitoring of blood pressure with an intra-arterial catheter is helpful. Positive end-expiratory pressure may be useful in the presence of congestive heart failure but should be discontinued when the pulmonary artery band is in place. The high mortality associated with pulmonary artery banding has led to attempts at complete surgical correction at an early age using cardiopulmonary bypass. Third-degree atrioventricular heart block may follow surgical closure if the cardiac conduction system is near the VSD. Premature ventricular beats may reflect the electrical instability of the ventricle due to surgical ventriculotomy. The risk of ventricular tachycardia, however, is low if postoperative ventricular filling pressures are normal.

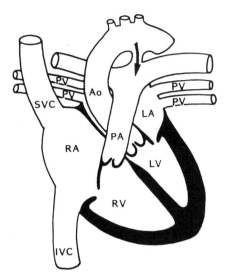

Fig. 3-3. Schematic diagram of a patent ductus arteriosus connecting the arch of the aorta (Ao) with the pulmonary artery (PA). Blood flow is from the high pressure Ao into the PA. The resulting aorto-to-pulmonary artery shunt (left-to-right shunt) leads to increased pulmonary blood flow. A decrease in systemic vascular resistance or increase in pulmonary vascular resistance will decrease the magnitude of the shunt through the ductus arteriosus.

Patent Ductus Arteriosus

Failure of the ductus arteriosus to close after birth results in passage of oxygenated blood from the aorta into the pulmonary artery (Fig. 3-3). The ratio of pulmonary to systemic blood flow depends on (1) the pressure gradient from the aorta to the pulmonary artery, (2) the ratio of pulmonary to systemic vascular resistance, and (3) the diameter and length of the ductus arteriosus.

Signs and Symptoms

Most patients with a PDA are asymptomatic and have only a moderate left-to-right shunt. This cardiac defect is often detected during a routine physical examination, when a characteristic continuous systolic and diastolic murmur is heard. If the magnitude of the left-to-right shunt is large, there may be evidence of left ventricular hypertrophy and increased pulmonary blood flow on the chest radiograph and the ECG.

Treatment

Treatment is by surgical ligation of the PDA through a left thoracotomy incision. Ideally, surgery is performed in patients older than 2 years of age. Without surgical correction, most patients remain asymptomatic until adolescence, when pulmonary hypertension and congestive heart failure can intervene.

Administration of indomethacin may result in closure of a PDA present in premature infants with respiratory distress syndrome.

Management of Anesthesia

Antibiotics for protection against the development of infective endocarditis should be administered to a patient with a PDA who is scheduled for noncardiac surgery. When surgical closure of the PDA is planned, appropriate preparations must be taken, in anticipation of the possibility of a large blood loss, should control of the PDA be lost during attempted ligation. Anesthesia with a volatile drug is useful, as these drugs tend to lower blood pressure, lessening the danger that the PDA will escape from the vascular clamp or tear as it is being divided. Furthermore, the decreased systemic vascular resistance produced by a volatile anesthetic may improve systemic blood flow by decreasing the magnitude of the left-to-right shunt. Likewise, positive-pressure ventilation of the lungs is well tolerated, as increased airway pressure increases pulmonary vascular resistance, reducing the pressure gradient across the PDA. Conversely, an increase in systemic vascular resistance or a decrease in pulmonary vascular resistance should be avoided, as these changes would increase the magnitude of the left-to-right shunt. Continuous monitoring of blood pressure by a catheter placed in a peripheral artery is helpful during the intraoperative period.

Ligation of the PDA is often associated with significant systemic hypertension during the early postoperative period. This hypertension can be managed with continuous infusion of a vasodilator drug such as nitroprusside. Long-acting antihypertensive drugs, such as hydralazine, can be gradually substituted for nitroprusside if hypertension persists.

Aorticopulmonary Fenestration

Aorticopulmonary fenestration is characterized by a communication between the left side of the ascending aorta and the right wall of the main pulmonary artery, just anterior to the origin of the right pulmonary artery. This communication is due to a failure of the aorticopulmonary septum to fuse and separate completely the aorta from the pulmonary artery. Clinical and hemodynamic manifestations of an aorticopulmonary communication are similar to those associated with a large PDA. The correct diagnosis is made by angiocardiography. Treatment is surgical and requires the use of cardiopulmonary bypass. Management of anesthesia entails the same principles as outlined for the patient with a PDA.

RIGHT-TO-LEFT INTRACARDIAC SHUNT

A variety of congenital heart defects result in a right-to-left intracardiac shunt, with associated decreases in pulmonary blood flow and the development of arterial hypoxemia (Table

Table 3-5. Congenital Heart Defects Resulting in a Right-to-Left Intracardiac Shunt

Tetralogy of Fallot
Eisenmenger syndrome
Ebstein's malformation of the tricuspid valve
Pulmonary atresia with a ventricular septal defect (pseudotruncus)
Tricuspid atresia
Foramen ovale

3-5). Survival in the presence of a right-to-left shunt requires a communication between the systemic and pulmonary circulation and obstruction to blood flow from the right ventricle. The time of onset and severity of symptoms usually depend on the degree of obstruction. Tetralogy of Fallot is the prototype of these defects. Principles for management of anesthesia are the same for all defects in this group.

Tetralogy of Fallot

Tetralogy of Fallot is the most common congenital heart defect producing a right-to-left intracardiac shunt with decreased pulmonary blood flow and arterial hypoxemia. Anatomic defects, which characterize this tetralogy, are a VSD, an aorta that overrides the pulmonary artery outflow tract, obstruction of the pulmonary artery outflow tract, and right ventricular hypertrophy (Fig. 3-4). The VSD is typically large and single. Infundibular pulmonary artery stenosis is prominent, and about 70% of patients have bicuspid aortic valves. The distal pulmonary artery may be hypoplastic or even absent. In general, the greater the stenosis of the pulmonary artery, the greater the overriding of the aorta. Right ventricular hypertrophy occurs because the large VSD permits continuous exposure of the right ventricle to the high pressures present in the left ventricle.

Signs and Symptoms

Manifestations of tetralogy of Fallot depend on the size of the right ventricular outflow tract. In general, cyanosis due to arterial hypoxemia will be apparent by 6 months of age. Clubbing of the distal ends of the digits is rarely seen before 6 months of age. The most common auscultatory finding is an ejection murmur heard along the left sternal border, resulting from blood flow across the infundibular pulmonic stenosis. Congestive heart failure rarely develops because the large VSD permits equilibration of intraventricular pressures and cardiac workload. A chest radiograph typically shows decreased vascularity of the lungs. The ECG is characterized by changes of right axis deviation and right ventricular hypertrophy. Arterial blood gases and pH are likely to demonstrate a normal $PaCO_2$ and pH and a markedly decreased PaO_2 (usually below 50 mmHg), even when breathing 100% oxygen.

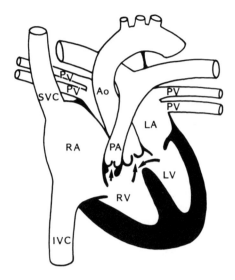

Fig. 3-4. Schematic diagram of the anatomic cardiac defects associated with tetralogy of Fallot. Defects include (1) ventricular septal defect, (2) aorta (Ao) overriding the pulmonary artery (PA) outflow tract, (3) obstruction to blood flow through a narrowed PA or stenotic pulmonic valve, and (4) right ventricular hypertrophy. Obstruction to PA outflow results in a pressure gradient that favors blood flow across the ventricular septal defect from the right ventricle (RV) to the left ventricle (LV). The resulting right-to-left intracardiac shunt combined with obstruction to ejection of the stroke volume from the RV leads to a marked decrease in pulmonary blood flow and the development of arterial hypoxemia. Any event that increases pulmonary vascular resistance or that decreases systemic vascular resistance will increase the magnitude of the shunt and accentuate arterial hypoxemia.

Squatting is a common feature of children with tetralogy of Fallot. It is speculated that squatting increases the systemic vascular resistance by kinking the large arteries in the inguinal area. The resulting increase in systemic vascular resistance tends to decrease the magnitude of the right-to-left intracardiac shunt. This leads to increased pulmonary blood flow and a subsequent improvement in arterial oxygenation and carbon dioxide elimination.

Hypercyanotic Attacks

About 35% of children with tetralogy of Fallot develop hypercyanotic attacks or "tet spells." These attacks can occur without obvious provocation but are often associated with crying or exercise. Hyperventilation and syncope may accompany these periods of increased arterial hypoxemia. The mechanism for the attack is unknown. The most likely explanation, however, is a sudden decrease in pulmonary blood flow due either to a spasm of the infundibular cardiac muscle or to decreased systemic vascular resistance. The treatment of a

hypercyanotic attack is influenced by the cause of pulmonary outflow obstruction.[5] When symptoms reflect a dynamic infundibular obstruction (spasm), an appropriate treatment is administration of a beta antagonist such as esmolol or propranolol. Indeed, chronic oral propranolol therapy is indicated in the patient who has recurrent attacks caused by spasm of the outflow tract muscle. If the cause is a decrease in systemic vascular resistance, treatment is with intravenous administration of fluids or phenylephrine, or both. Sympathomimetic drugs that display beta agonist properties are not chosen, as they may accentuate spasm of the infundibular cardiac muscle. Recurrent hypercyanotic attacks are an indication for surgical correction of abnormalities associated with tetralogy of Fallot.

Cerebrovascular Accident

Cerebrovascular accident is common in children with severe tetralogy of Fallot. Cerebrovascular thrombosis or severe arterial hypoxemia may be the explanations for these adverse responses. Dehydration and polycythemia may contribute to thrombosis. A hemoglobin concentration exceeding 20 $g \cdot dl^{-1}$ is common in these patients.

Cerebral Abscess

A cerebral abscess is suggested by the abrupt onset of headache, fever, and lethargy, followed by persistent emesis and the appearance of seizure activity. The most likely cause is bacterial seeding into areas of prior cerebral infarction.

Infective Endocarditis

Infective endocarditis is a constant danger in the patient with tetralogy of Fallot. This complication is associated with a high mortality. Antibiotics should be administered to protect against this serious possibility whenever a dental or surgical procedure is planned in these patients.

Treatment

Surgical treatment of tetralogy of Fallot is initially with a palliative procedure designed to increase pulmonary blood flow by virtue of the anastomosis of a systemic artery to a pulmonary artery. After successful systemic-to-pulmonary artery shunt procedure, the pulmonary vasculature usually enlarges, PaO_2 increases, and polycythemia regresses. Complete correction of the cardiac defects is subsequently accomplished using cardiopulmonary bypass, when the patient is 3 to 6 years old.

Palliative surgical procedures designed to increase pulmonary blood flow include (1) the Potts operation, (2) the Waterston shunt, and (3) the Blalock-Taussig shunt. The Potts operation consists of a direct anastomosis between the descending thoracic aorta and the left pulmonary artery. This operation is no longer popular because an excessive increase in pulmonary blood flow can result in pulmonary hypertension and congestive heart failure. Furthermore, takedown of this anastomosis during subsequent complete surgical correction is difficult.

The Waterston shunt is a direct anastomosis between the ascending thoracic aorta and the right pulmonary artery. Takedown of this anastomosis at the time of complete surgical correction is easier than with the Potts operation. The proper sizing of the anastomosis produced by a Waterston shunt is difficult, however, and an excessive increase in pulmonary blood flow and pulmonary hypertension can result. Furthermore, the right pulmonary artery may thrombose after this procedure in occasional patients.

The Blalock-Taussig shunt consists of an anastomosis between a branch of the thoracic aorta and one of the pulmonary arteries. A popular approach is an end-to-side anastomosis between the subclavian artery and the pulmonary artery on the side opposite the aortic arch. The long length of the subclavian artery limits pulmonary blood flow through the shunt and minimizes the likelihood of an excessive increase in pulmonary blood flow and the development of pulmonary hypertension. The major complications associated with this vascular anastomosis include thrombosis of the shunt and the development of subclavian steal syndrome. The use of prosthetic shunts has become increasingly popular, as it avoids some of the problems inherent with use of the patient's arteries.

Complete surgical repair of tetralogy of Fallot typically consists of closure of the VSD with a Dacron patch and enlargement of the pulmonary artery outflow tract by placement of a synthetic graft. Pulmonic regurgitation due to an incompetent pulmonic valve usually results from surgical correction of the cardiac defects but poses no major hazard unless the distal pulmonary arteries are hypoplastic, in which case volume overload of the right ventricle secondary to regurgitant blood flow may result. Major complications of complete surgical repair include third-degree atrioventricular heart block and difficulty in achieving hemostasis. Platelet dysfunction and hypofibrinogenemia are common in these patients and may contribute to postoperative bleeding problems. Right-to-left intracardiac shunting often develops through the foramen ovale during the postoperative period. Shunting through the foramen ovale acts as a safety valve if the right ventricle is unable to function at the same efficiency as the left ventricle.

Management of Anesthesia

Management of anesthesia for the patient with tetralogy of Fallot requires a thorough understanding of those events and drugs that can alter the magnitude of the right-to-left intracardiac shunt. For example, when shunt magnitude is acutely increased, there are associated decreases in pulmonary blood flow and PaO_2. Furthermore, the magnitude of the right-to-left shunt may alter the pharmacokinetics of both inhaled and injected drugs.

The magnitude of a right-to-left intracardiac shunt can be increased by (1) decreased systemic vascular resistance, (2) increased pulmonary vascular resistance, and (3) increased myocardial contractility that accentuates infundibular obstruction to ejection of blood by the right ventricle. In many respects, resistance to ejection of blood into the pulmonary artery outflow tract is relatively fixed, and hence the magnitude of the shunt is inversely proportional to the systemic vascular resistance. Pharmacologically induced responses that decrease systemic vascular resistance (volatile anesthetics, histamine release, ganglionic blockade, and alpha blockade) will increase the magnitude of the right-to-left shunt and accentuate arterial hypoxemia. Pulmonary blood flow can be decreased by increases in pulmonary vascular resistance that accompany such intraoperative ventilatory maneuvers as intermittent positive airway pressure or positive end-expiratory pressure. Furthermore, the loss of negative intrapleural pressure on opening the chest will increase pulmonary vascular resistance and the magnitude of the shunt. Nevertheless, the advantages of controlled ventilation of the lungs during operations usually offset this potential hazard. Indeed, arterial oxygenation does not predictably deteriorate in patients with tetralogy of Fallot, either with the institution of positive-pressure ventilation of the lungs or after the opening of the chest.

Preoperatively, it is important to avoid dehydration by maintaining oral feedings in the very young patient or by providing intravenous fluids before the patient's arrival in the operating room. Crying associated with intramuscular administration of drugs used for preoperative medication can lead to a hypercyanotic attack. For this reason, it may be prudent to avoid administration of drugs by this route until the patient is in a highly supervised environment and the ability to treat a hypercyanotic attack is optimal (see the section, Hypercyanotic Attacks). Beta antagonists should be continued until the induction of anesthesia in the patient receiving these drugs for prophylaxis against hypercyanotic attacks.

Induction of anesthesia in the patient with tetralogy of Fallot is often accomplished with ketamine (3 to 4 mg·kg^{-1} IM or 1 to 2 mg·kg^{-1} IV). The onset of anesthesia after injection of ketamine may be associated with improved arterial oxygenation, presumably reflecting increased pulmonary blood flow due to ketamine-induced increases in systemic vascular resistance, which can lead to decreases in the magnitude of the right-to-left intracardiac shunt. Ketamine has also been alleged to increase pulmonary vascular resistance, which would be undesirable in the patient with a right-to-left shunt. The efficacious response to ketamine of patients with tetralogy of Fallot, however, suggests that this concern is not clinically significant. Intubation of the trachea is facilitated by administration of a muscle relaxant. It should be remembered that the onset of action of drugs administered intravenously may be more rapid in the presence of a right-to-left shunt, since the dilutional effect in the lungs is decreased. For this reason, it may be prudent to decrease the rate of intravenous injection of depressant drugs in these patients.

Induction of anesthesia with a volatile anesthetic, such as halothane, is acceptable but must be done with caution and careful monitoring of systemic oxygenation.[6] Although decreased pulmonary blood flow will speed the achievement of an anesthetic concentration, the hazard of decreased blood pressure and systemic vascular resistance is great. Indeed, hypercyanotic attacks can occur during administration of low concentrations of a volatile anesthetic.

Maintenance of anesthesia is often achieved with nitrous oxide combined with ketamine. The advantage of this combination is the preservation of the systemic vascular resistance. Nitrous oxide may also increase pulmonary vascular resistance, but this potential adverse effect is more than offset by the beneficial effects of the inhaled anesthetic on the systemic circulation. The principal disadvantage of using nitrous oxide is the associated decrease in the inspired oxygen concentration. Theoretically, an increased inspired oxygen concentration could decrease pulmonary vascular resistance, leading to increased pulmonary blood flow and an improved PaO_2. Therefore, it would seem prudent to limit the inspired concentration of nitrous oxide to 50%. The use of opioids or benzodiazepines may also be considered during the maintenance of anesthesia, but the doses and rate of administration must be adjusted to minimize decreased blood pressure or systemic vascular resistance.

Intraoperative skeletal muscle paralysis is often provided by pancuronium, as this drug maintains blood pressure and systemic vascular resistance. An increase in heart rate associated with administration of pancuronium is helpful in maintaining left ventricular cardiac output. Vecuronium, atracurium, pipecuronium, and doxacurium would also be acceptable but could not be expected to produce beneficial hemodynamic stimulation.

Ventilation of the lungs should be controlled, but it must be appreciated that excessive positive airway pressure may adversely increase resistance to blood flow through the lungs. Intravascular fluid volume must be maintained with intravenous fluid administration, since acute hypovolemia will tend to increase the magnitude of the right-to-left intracardiac shunt. In view of co-existing polycythemia, it is probably not necessary to consider blood replacement until about 20% of the blood volume has been lost. It is crucial that meticulous care be taken to avoid infusion of air through the tubing used to deliver intravenous solutions, as this could lead to systemic embolization of air. An alpha-agonist drug such as phenylephrine must be promptly available to treat undesirable decreases in systemic blood pressure caused by decreased systemic vascular resistance.

Eisenmenger Syndrome

Eisenmenger syndrome describes a situation in which the left-to-right intracardiac shunt is reversed as a result of increased pulmonary vascular resistance to a level that equals or exceeds the systemic vascular resistance. Shunt reversal occurs in about 50% of untreated patients with a large VSD but in only about 10% of patients with a large ASD. Manifestations of intracardiac shunt reversal reflect decreases in pulmonary blood flow, with resulting arterial hypoxemia. The presence of this syndrome contraindicates surgical correction of the congenital cardiac defect, as pulmonary vascular resistance is irreversibly increased.

Management of Anesthesia

Management of anesthesia for noncardiac surgery in the patient with Eisenmenger syndrome is as outlined for tetralogy of Fallot. Despite the potential for undesirable decreases in blood pressure and systemic vascular resistance, the successful management of anesthesia using epidural anesthesia has been described in patients undergoing tubal ligation and cesarean section.[7] If epidural anesthesia is selected, however, it would seem prudent not to add epinephrine to the local anesthetic solution injected into the epidural space. This recommendation is based on the observation that a peripheral beta effect produced by the epinephrine absorbed from the epidural space into the systemic circulation could exaggerate the decreases in blood pressure and systemic vascular resistance associated with epidural anesthesia.

Ebstein's Malformation of the Tricuspid Valve

Ebstein's malformation of the tricuspid valve occurs in less than 1% of patients with congenital heart disease. The major anatomic abnormality of this malformation is the downward displacement of the tricuspid valve into the right ventricle. The mitral valve may also have abnormal placement of leaflets. The right atrium is almost always enlarged. Frequently, there is a right-to-left shunt through a patent foramen ovale or an associated ASD. Malformation of the tricuspid valve causes obstruction to right ventricular filling, a decrease in the size of the right ventricle, and tricuspid regurgitation, leading to right heart failure. Enlargement of the right atrium can be so massive that the apical portions of the lungs are compressed, resulting in restrictive pulmonary disease. Fatigue, dyspnea, and cardiac tachydysrhythmias are frequently observed in these patients. Hazards during anesthesia include the development of cardiac tachydysrhythmias and arterial hypoxemia due to increases in the magnitude of a right-to-left intracardiac shunt.[8] Indeed, 5% to 10% of these patients have Wolff-Parkinson-White syndrome (see Chapter 4). Elevated right atrial pressure may indicate the presence of right ventricular failure. The delayed onset of effects after intravenous administration of drugs most likely reflects pooling and dilution in an enlarged right atrium.

Tricuspid Atresia

Tricuspid atresia is characterized by arterial hypoxemia, a small right ventricle, a large left ventricle, and markedly decreased pulmonary blood flow. Poorly oxygenated blood from the right atrium passes through an ASD into the left atrium, mixes with oxygenated blood, and then enters the left ventricle, from which it is ejected into the systemic circulation. Pulmonary blood flow is via a VSD, PDA, or bronchial vessels.

Treatment

A Fontan procedure (anastomosis of the right atrial appendage to the right pulmonary artery so as to bypass the right ventricle and provide a direct atriopulmonary communication) is used for the treatment of tricuspid atresia. This operation is also used for the treatment of pulmonary artery atresia.

Management of Anesthesia

Management of anesthesia for the patient undergoing a Fontan procedure has been successfully achieved with opioids or volatile anesthetics.[9] Immediately after cardiopulmonary bypass and continuing into the early postoperative period, it is important to maintain an elevated right atrial pressure (16 to 20 mmHg) to facilitate pulmonary blood flow. An increase in pulmonary vascular resistance due to acidosis, hypothermia, peak airway pressures above 15 cm H_2O, or a reaction to the tracheal tube may cause right-sided heart failure. Early extubation of the trachea and spontaneous ventilation are desirable. A positive inotropic drug (dopamine) with or without a vasodilator (nitroprusside) is often required to optimize cardiac output and maintain low pulmonary vascular resistance. Pleural effusion, ascites, and edema of the lower extremities are not uncommon postoperatively but usually resolve within a few weeks. Right atrial pressure equal to pulmonary artery pressure remains elevated after this operation, averaging 15 mmHg.[10]

Although the absence of a contractile right ventricle is compatible with long-term survival, the adaptability of the circulatory system is restricted. This decreased capacity of a single ventricle to respond to an increased workload may have a significant impact on the management of these patients for another operation. In this regard, the subsequent management of anesthesia in a patient who has undergone a Fontan procedure is facilitated by monitoring central venous pressure (equal to pulmonary artery pressure in these patients) for assessment of intravascular fluid volume and detection of sudden impairment of left ventricular function, as well as increases in pulmonary vascular resistance.[11] The value of monitoring central venous pressure reflects the absence of a contractile right ventricle and the impaired ability of a single ventricle to adapt to an acute increase in afterload that may necessitate prompt administration of a positive inotropic drug. Insertion of a thermodilution pulmonary artery catheter in a patient after a Fontan repair may be technically difficult secondary to the unusual anatomy. Furthermore, no information is available regarding the accuracy of thermodilution cardiac output measurements in such a patient.

Foramen Ovale

The foramen ovale is mechanically closed by a left atrial pressure that exceeds the pressure in the right atrium. Eventually, the foramen ovale becomes permanently closed. In about 30% of normal patients, however, the foramen ovale remains probe patent.[12] In these patients, an increase in the right atrial pressure above the pressure in the left atrium can lead to a right-to-left intracardiac shunt through the foramen ovale. Unexplained arterial hypoxemia or paradoxical air embolism during the perioperative period may be due to the shunting of blood or air through a previously closed foramen ovale.[13]

SEPARATION OF THE PULMONARY AND SYSTEMIC CIRCULATIONS

Transposition of the great arteries is an example of a cardiac defect that results in separation of the pulmonary and systemic circulations.

Transposition of the Great Arteries

Transposition of the great arteries results from failure of the truncus arteriosus to spiral (Fig. 3-5). As a result, the aorta arises from the right ventricle, and the pulmonary artery arises from the left ventricle. Anatomically, transposition means that the left and right ventricles are not connected in series. As a result, the pulmonary and systemic circulations function independently, causing profound arterial hypoxemia. Survival is not possible unless there is mixing of blood between the two circulations through an ASD, VSD, or PDA. About 10% of infants with preductal coarctation of the aorta also have transportation of the great arteries.

Signs and Symptoms

Persistent cyanosis at birth is often the first clue to the presence of transposition of the great arteries. Congestive heart failure occurs early in life. The ECG is normal at birth but, in the presence of transposition of the great arteries, neonatal patterns of right ventricular hypertrophy persist beyond the

Previously, complete surgical correction of transposition of the great arteries was most often accomplished by removing the atrial septum and replacing it with a baffle made of pericardium. This baffle is placed so as to redirect superior and inferior vena caval blood toward the mitral valve, whereas pulmonary venous return is directed toward the tricuspid valve. This surgically produced reversal of flow at the atrial level is known as the Mustard procedure.[15] Complications of this operation include third-degree atrioventricular heart block and obstruction of the vena cava. In addition, the long-term ability of the right ventricle to perform as a left ventricle in terms of coronary perfusion, as well as the function of the tricuspid valve, is unknown. Currently, the most definitive surgical treatment of transposition of the great vessels is an arterial switch procedure. This operation requires surgical translocation and reanastomosis of the aorta and main pulmonary artery with reimplantation of the coronary arteries.

Transposition of the great arteries plus left ventricular outlet obstruction has been treated by closing the VSD and creating a pulmonary outflow tract with a Dacron conduit that contains an artificial valve. This operation is known as the Rastelli procedure.[16] Unlike the Mustard procedure, the Rastelli operation restores the normal anatomic relationship, with the left ventricle pumping systemic blood and the right ventricle pumping pulmonary blood. The Fontan procedure may also be used in the treatment of these patients (see the section, Tricuspid Atresia).

Management of Anesthesia

Management of anesthesia in the presence of transposition of the great arteries must take into account separation of the pulmonary and systemic circulations. Drugs administered intravenously will be distributed with minimal dilution to organs such as the heart and brain. Therefore, doses and rate of injection of intravenously administered drugs may need to be reduced. Conversely, onset of anesthesia produced by inhaled drugs will be delayed, as only small amounts of the inhaled drug reach the systemic circulation. In the final analysis, induction and maintenance of anesthesia are often accomplished with ketamine, combined with a muscle relaxant to facilitate intubation of the trachea. Ketamine can be supplemented with an opioid or benzodiazepine, for maintenance of anesthesia. Nitrous oxide has limited application, as it is important to administer a high inspired oxygen concentration to these patients. The potential cardiac depressant effects of volatile anesthetics detract from the use of these drugs. Pancuronium is useful if intraoperative skeletal muscle paralysis is indicated.

Dehydration must be avoided during the perioperative period. These patients may have a hematocrit in excess of 70%, which may contribute to the high incidence of cerebral venous thrombosis. This finding suggests that oral fluids should not be withheld from these patients for prolonged periods. If fluids cannot be ingested orally, intravenous infusion of fluids should

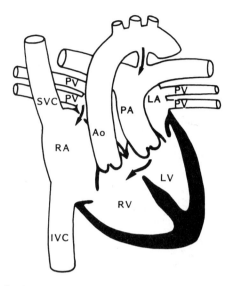

Fig. 3-5. Schematic diagram of transposition of the great arteries. The right ventricle (RV) and left ventricle (LV) are not connected in series. Instead, the two ventricles function as parallel and independent circulations, with the aorta (Ao) arising from the RV and the pulmonary artery (PA) arising from the LV. Survival is not possible unless mixing of blood between the two circulations occurs through an atrial septal defect, ventricular septal defect, or patent ductus arteriosus.

newborn period. Cardiac catheterization demonstrates normal systemic and pulmonary artery pressures and severe arterial hypoxemia. Echocardiography may demonstrate the pulmonary valve opening earlier and closing later than the aortic valve, which is the reverse of the normal sequence.

Treatment

Initial treatment of transposition of the great arteries includes a palliative procedure designed to increase mixing of blood between the two circulations so as to improve systemic oxygenation. The procedure is performed at cardiac catheterization as soon as the diagnosis of transposition of the great arteries is confirmed. Complete surgical correction is then performed, using cardiopulmonary bypass, when the patient is 6 to 9 months of age. The most common palliative procedure is the creation of an ASD by passing a ballooned catheter across the foramen ovale, inflating the balloon, and then pulling the entire catheter through the foramen ovale to enlarge the opening. This balloon atrial septostomy is known as the Rashkind procedure.[14] Third-degree atrioventricular heart block may follow a balloon septotomy. Therefore, chronotropic drugs such as atropine and isoproterenol should be available for prompt intravenous infusion. It may be necessary to perform pulmonary artery banding to prevent the development of intractable congestive heart failure when a large VSD accompanies transposition of the great arteries.

be started during the operative period. Atrial dysrhythmias and conduction disturbances may occur postoperatively.

MIXING OF BLOOD BETWEEN THE PULMONARY AND SYSTEMIC CIRCULATIONS

Several uncommon congenital heart defects result in mixing of oxygenated and unoxygenated blood. As a result of this mixing, pulmonary arterial blood has a higher oxygen saturation than that of systemic venous blood, and systemic arterial blood has a lower oxygen saturation than that of pulmonary venous blood. Arterial hypoxemia varies in severity, depending on the magnitude of pulmonary blood flow.

Truncus Arteriosus

Truncus arteriosus refers to the situation in which a single arterial trunk gives rise to the aorta and pulmonary artery (Fig. 3-6). This single arterial trunk overrides both ventricles, which are connected through a VSD. Mortality is high, with a median age of survival of about 5 to 6 weeks.

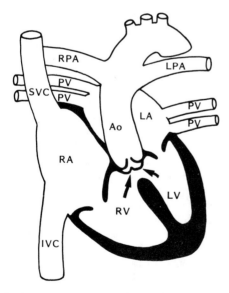

Fig. 3-6. Schematic diagram of truncus arteriosus in which the pulmonary artery (RPA, right pulmonary artery; LPA, left pulmonary artery) and aorta (Ao) arise from a single trunk that overrides the left ventricle (LV) and right ventricle (RV). This trunk receives blood from both ventricles by virtue of a ventricular septal defect.

Signs and Symptoms

Presenting signs and symptoms of truncus arteriosus include failure to thrive, arterial hypoxemia, and congestive heart failure soon after birth. Peripheral pulses may be accentuated due to the rapid diastolic runoff of blood into the pulmonary bed. Auscultation of the chest and evaluation of the ECG do not give predictable information and are not diagnostic. A chest radiograph indicates cardiomegaly and increased vascularity of the lung fields. The diagnosis is confirmed by angiocardiography performed during cardiac catheterization.

Treatment

Surgical treatment of truncus arteriosus includes banding of the right and left pulmonary arteries if pulmonary blood flow is excessive. In addition, an associated VSD can be closed, so only left ventricular output enters the truncus arteriosus. When this is done, a Dacron conduit with a valve is also placed between the right ventricle and pulmonary artery.

Management of Anesthesia

Management of anesthesia in the presence of truncus arteriosus is influenced by the magnitude of pulmonary blood flow. When pulmonary blood flow is increased, the use of positive end-expiratory pressure is beneficial and may serve to decrease the symptoms of congestive heart failure. Increased pulmonary blood flow may be associated with evidence of myocardial ischemia on the ECG. When myocardial ischemia that occurs intraoperatively does not respond to either intravenous administration of phenylephrine or fluids or the use of positive end-expiratory pressure, consideration may be given to temporary banding of the pulmonary artery, so as to increase systemic and coronary blood flow.[17] Patients with decreased pulmonary blood flow and arterial hypoxemia should be managed as described for tetralogy of Fallot.

Partial Anomalous Pulmonary Venous Return

Partial anomalous pulmonary venous return is characterized by the presence of left or right pulmonary veins that empty into the right side of the circulation, rather than the left atrium. In about one-half of cases, the aberrant pulmonary veins drain into the superior vena cava. In the remaining cases, pulmonary veins enter the right atrium, inferior vena cava, azygous vein, or coronary sinus. Partial anomalous pulmonary venous return may be more common than appreciated, as suggested by the presence of this anomaly in about 0.5% of routine autopsies.

The onset and severity of symptoms produced by this abnormality depend on the amount of pulmonary blood flow routed through the right side of the heart. Fatigue and exertional dyspnea are the most frequent initial manifestations, usually appearing in early adulthood. Cyanosis and congestive heart failure are likely if more than 50% of the pulmonary venous flow enters the right side of the circulation.

Angiography is the most useful technique for confirming the diagnosis of partial anomalous pulmonary venous return. Cardiac catheterization usually demonstrates normal intracardiac pressures and increased oxygen saturation of blood in the right side of the heart. Treatment is by surgical repair.

Total Anomalous Pulmonary Venous Return

Total anomalous pulmonary venous return is characterized by drainage of all four of the pulmonary veins into the systemic venous system. The most common presentation of this defect, accounting for about one-half of cases, is drainage of the four pulmonary veins into the left innominate vein, in association with a left-sided superior vena cava. Oxygenated blood reaches the left atrium by way of an ASD. A PDA is present in about one-third of cases.

Signs and Symptoms

Total anomalous pulmonary venous return presents clinically as congestive heart failure in 50% of patients by 1 month of age and in 90% by 1 year. The definitive diagnosis is by angiocardiography. Mortality is about 80% by 1 year of age, unless surgical correction using cardiopulmonary bypass is performed.

Management of Anesthesia

Management of anesthesia in the presence of total anomalous pulmonary venous return may include positive end-expiratory pressure applied to the airways in an attempt to decrease excessive pulmonary blood flow. The patient who presents with pulmonary edema should be given positive-pressure ventilation to the lungs through a tube placed in the trachea before cardiac catheterization. Operative manipulation of the right atrium, which would be tolerated by a normal patient, may result in obstruction to flow into the right atrium, manifested as a sudden decrease in blood pressure and the onset of bradycardia. Intravenous transfusions may be hazardous, as any increase in right atrial pressure is transmitted directly to the pulmonary veins, leading to the possibility of pulmonary edema.

Hypoplastic Left Heart Syndrome

Hypoplastic left heart syndrome occurs in about 7.5% of infants with congenital heart disease. It is characterized by left ventricular hypoplasia, mitral valve hypoplasia, aortic valve atresia, and hypoplasia of the ascending aorta.[18] Extracardiac congenital anomalies do not usually accompany this syndrome. There is complete mixing of pulmonary venous and systemic

venous blood in a single ventricle, which is connected in parallel to both the pulmonary and systemic circulations. Systemic blood flow is dependent on a PDA. In addition to ductal patency, infant survival is also dependent on a balance between systemic vascular resistance and pulmonary vascular resistance, since both circulations are supplied from a single ventricle in a parallel fashion. An abrupt decrease in pulmonary vascular resistance after delivery results in increased pulmonary blood flow at the expense of systemic blood flow (pulmonary steal phenomena). When this occurs, coronary and systemic blood flow are inadequate, leading to metabolic acidosis, high-output cardiac failure, and ventricular fibrillation, despite increasingly high PaO_2 levels[18] (Fig. 3-7). Alternatively, any postnatal event that leads to an increase of pulmonary vascular resistance can decrease pulmonary blood flow so severely that arterial hypoxemia worsens, leading to progressive metabolic acidosis and circulatory collapse[18] (Fig. 3-7). Because rapid changes in pulmonary vascular resistance occur during the postnatal period, the necessary fine balance between pulmonary vascular resistance and systemic vascular resistance is unstable and difficult to maintain.

Treatment

Treatment of hypoplastic left heart syndrome is surgical, beginning with a palliative procedure that eliminates the need for continued patency of the ductus arteriosus. Preoperatively, a continuous intravenous infusion of prostaglandin E-1 may be necessary to prevent physiologic closure of the ductus arteriosus. In addition, administration of cardiac inotropes and sodium bicarbonate may be necessary.

The palliative procedure consists of reconstruction of the ascending aorta, using the proximal pulmonary artery[18] (Fig. 3-8). A systemic-to-pulmonary shunt to provide pulmonary blood flow is placed between the reconstructed aorta and distal pulmonary artery. Typically, the infant is placed on cardiopulmonary bypass to permit the production of whole-body hypothermia; reconstruction of the aorta is then accomplished during 40 to 60 minutes of circulatory arrest. The central shunt is placed after reinstitution of cardiopulmonary bypass and during rewarming. The completed palliative procedure leaves the single right ventricle connected in parallel to the systemic circulation and pulmonary circulations. The stage is set, however, for later correction with a Fontan procedure when pulmonary vascular resistance has decreased to an adult level (see the section, Tricuspid Atresia). The Fontan procedure, plus elimination of the systemic-to-pulmonary shunt, separates the two circulations and facilitates development of normal arterial oxygen saturations.

Management of Anesthesia

An umbilical artery and intravenous catheter is usually placed before the arrival of the infant in the operating room. After institution of monitoring, induction of anesthesia is often ac-

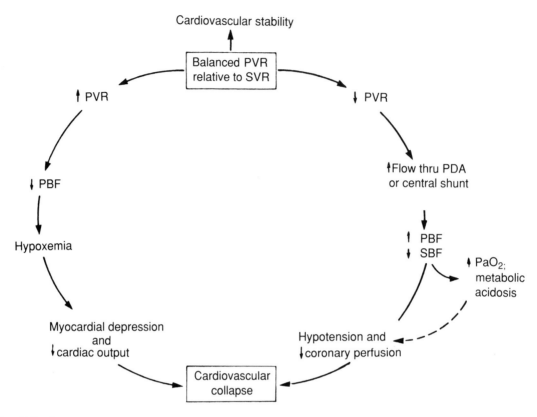

Fig. 3-7. Cardiovascular stability in the presence of hypoplastic left heart syndrome requires a balance between pulmonary vascular resistance (PVR) relative to systemic vascular resistance (SVR). An abrupt decrease in PVR after delivery can result in excessive pulmonary blood flow (PBF) relative to systemic blood flow (SBF) with cardiovascular collapse despite the absence of arterial hypoxemia. Conversely, postnatal changes that elevate PVR can lead to cardiovascular collapse in the presence of arterial hypoxemia. (From Hansen DD, Hickey PR. Anesthesia for hypoplastic left heart syndrome: Use of high-dose fentanyl in 30 neonates. Anesth Analg 1986;65:127–32, with permission.)

complished with fentanyl (50 to 75 μg·kg^{-1} IV) administered simultaneously with pancuronium (0.1 to 0.15 mg·kg^{-1} IV).[18] There is also a suggestion that deep anesthesia with an opioid continued for 24 hours postoperatively is effective in attenuating the hormonal and metabolic responses to stress in these critically ill neonates leading to decreased morbidity and mortality, compared with neonates receiving lighter anesthesia (halothane plus morphine).[19] Nevertheless, it would be inappropriate to conclude from these limited data that deep anesthesia is always safer than light anesthesia in such critically ill patients.[20]

These infants are vulnerable to the development of ventricular fibrillation due to inadequate coronary blood flow before the palliative procedure. The danger of ventricular fibrillation and borderline cardiac status argues against the use of a volatile anesthetic in these infants. The lungs are ventilated with 100% oxygen, and the trachea is intubated. Crystalloid solu-

tions (10 to 15 ml·kg^{-1} IV) are often infused before cardiopulmonary bypass is performed. After induction of anesthesia and intubation of the trachea, ventilation of the lungs is adjusted on the basis of arterial blood gases. A high PaO$_2$ implies excessive pulmonary blood flow at the expense of the systemic circulation. Indeed, if the initial PaO$_2$ is greater than 100 mmHg, maneuvers to increase pulmonary vascular resistance and decrease pulmonary blood flow are instituted. For example, a decrease in the volume of ventilation leads to an increase in the PaCO$_2$ and to a decrease in pH, resulting in increased pulmonary vascular resistance and decreased pulmonary blood flow. If the PaO$_2$ still remains unacceptably elevated, the institution of positive end-expiratory pressure leads to increased lung volumes and a further increase in pulmonary vascular resistance. In extreme cases, temporary occlusion of one pulmonary artery serves to decrease the PaO$_2$.

Dopamine or isoproterenol is administered when necessary

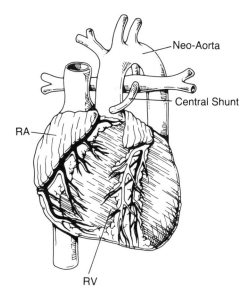

Fig. 3-8. Anatomy after the first-stage palliative procedure for hypoplastic left heart syndrome during the neonatal period. The ascending aorta has been reconstructed from the proximal pulmonary artery to form a neo-aorta. (From Hansen DD, Hickey PR. Anesthesia for hypoplastic left heart syndrome: Use of high-dose fentanyl in 30 neonates. Anesth Analg 1986;65:127–32, with permission.)

for inotropic support at the conclusion of cardiopulmonary bypass. The selection of specific inotropic drugs is influenced by pulmonary vascular resistance. The most frequent problem after cardiopulmonary bypass is too little pulmonary blood flow with associated arterial hypoxemia (PaO_2 less than 20 mmHg).[18] Attempts directed at improving the PaO_2 include hyperventilation of the lungs to produce a low $PaCO_2$ (20 to 25 mmHg) and elevated pH and infusion of isoproterenol to decrease pulmonary vascular resistance. A PaO_2 above 50 mmHg after cardiopulmonary bypass may indicate inadequate systemic blood flow and the likely occurrence of progressive metabolic acidosis, unless steps are taken to decrease pulmonary blood flow.

Double-Outlet Right Ventricle

Double-outlet right ventricle is characterized by the origin of the aorta from the posterior wall of the right ventricle. Left ventricular outflow is through a VSD that permits blood flow into the right ventricle. Arterial hypoxemia does not occur unless there is an obstruction to pulmonary outflow. This cardiac defect is rare, accounting for only about 0.5% of patients with congenital heart disease.

Clinically, most of these patients present with congestive heart failure. Presentation is indistinguishable from that of a patient with a large VSD. Angiocardiography performed at cardiac catheterization is usually required to establish the diagnosis, since the chest radiograph and ECG are nonspecific.

Surgical treatment may include banding of the pulmonary artery or a Blalock-Taussig shunt, depending on the magnitude of the pulmonary blood flow. Complete repair may be attempted by placing a tunnel of synthetic material from the VSD to the aorta. Management of anesthesia is dependent on the magnitude of pulmonary blood flow.

INCREASED MYOCARDIAL WORK

Aortic stenosis, coarctation of the aorta, and pulmonic stenosis are examples of congenital cardiac defects characterized by increased cardiac work due to obstruction to ejection of blood from the left or right ventricle. These lesions require the myocardium to produce considerably more hydraulic work than normal.

Aortic Stenosis

Aortic stenosis is the most common cause of obstruction to ejection of the left ventricular stroke volume. The site of this obstruction can be valvular, subvalvular (hypertrophic cardiomyopathy), or supravalvular (see Chapters 2 and 7). Cardiac catheterization is necessary to determine the site of obstruction, as well as the pressure gradient across the aortic valve. Regardless of the type of aortic stenosis, the myocardium must generate an intraventricular pressure that is two to three times normal, while the pressure in the aorta remains within a physiologic range. The resulting concentric myocardial hypertrophy leads to increased myocardial oxygen requirements. Furthermore, the high velocity of blood flow through the stenotic area predisposes to the development of infective endocarditis and is associated with poststenotic dilation of the aorta.

Signs and Symptoms

Auscultation of the chest in the presence of aortic stenosis indicates a systolic ejection murmur best heard at the second right intercostal space and radiating to the neck. Most patients with congenital aortic stenosis are asymptomatic until adulthood. Infants with severe aortic stenosis, however, may present with signs of congestive heart failure. Most infants with aortic stenosis severe enough to produce symptoms will also have endocardial fibroelastosis involving the left side of the heart. Subvalvular aortic stenosis rarely presents in infancy. The ECG in the presence of congenital aortic stenosis typically shows left ventricular hypertrophy. Depression of the ST segment is likely during exercise, particularly if the pressure gradient across the aortic valve is greater than 50 mmHg. A chest radiograph will likely show left ventricular hypertrophy, with or without poststenotic dilation of the aorta. Calcification of the aortic valve will not usually be apparent before 15 years of age.

Sudden death, rare in children with aortic stenosis, can occur in adult patients and is presumably due to a cardiac dysrhythmia. Likewise, angina pectoris is uncommon in the very young but reaches an incidence of about 20% between the ages of 15 and 30 years. Angina pectoris in the absence of coronary artery disease reflects the inability of coronary blood flow to meet increased myocardial oxygen requirements of the hypertrophied left ventricle. Syncope can occur when the pressure gradient across the aortic valve exceeds 50 mmHg.

Findings in the patient with supravalvular stenosis may include a characteristic appearance in which the facial bones are prominent, the forehead is rounded, and the upper lip is pursed. Strabismus, inguinal hernia, dental abnormalities, and moderate mental retardation are commonly present. Blood pressure readings taken in the upper extremities may be unequal, depending on how the high-velocity jet stream of blood ejected through the stenotic aortic valve strikes the innominate artery.

Treatment

Medical treatment is not predictably successful in the management of patients with congenital aortic stenosis. The exception is the patient with subvalvular stenosis in whom decreased myocardial contractility produced by a beta antagonist may be useful until surgical correction can be undertaken.

Surgical treatment is indicated in the patient with a pressure gradient greater than 50 mmHg across the aortic valve at rest or in the patient who has experienced syncope or angina pectoris. A pressure gradient of 40 mmHg due to supravalvular aortic stenosis is considered an indication for surgery, since high pressures in the coronary arteries may lead to premature development of atherosclerosis. Children with congenital aortic stenosis at the level of the valve are usually treated with valvulotomy performed during cardiopulmonary bypass. Aortic valve replacement is often necessary at a later age. Subvalvular aortic stenosis is treated by resection of the abnormal musculature. Supravalvular aortic stenosis is corrected by widening the lumen of the aorta with an artificial patch. Management of anesthesia for the patient with aortic stenosis is as described in Chapters 2 and 7.

Coarctation of the Aorta

Coarctation of the aorta accounts for about 5% of patients with congenital heart disease. Depending on the position of the narrowing in the aorta in relationship to the ductus arteriosus, this abnormality is designated as preductal (infantile) or postductal (adult).

Preductal

Anatomically, the preductal form of coarctation of the aorta is most often characterized by a localized constriction, just proximal to the ductus arteriosus, or diffuse narrowing of the arch of the aorta. Associated cardiac defects include PDA in about two-thirds, VSD in one-third, and bicuspid aortic valve in about one-fourth of patients. Transposition of the great arteries is present in about 10% of cases. Cardiac catheterization is necessary to detect associated defects. A chest radiograph often shows biventricular enlargement. A prominent fluctuation in the quality of the femoral pulse is characteristic.

Congestive heart failure as a result of this cardiac defect is usually manifest within the first weeks of life. Treatment is initially with digitalis and diuretics. If rapid improvement does not occur, surgical repair should be undertaken. Surgical treatment includes resection of the stenotic portion of the aorta and closure of the ductus arteriosus if it has remained patent. The pulmonary artery may need to be banded at the same operation if a VSD is also present.

Management of Anesthesia

Management of anesthesia in the patient with the preductal form of coarctation of the aorta may be mainly resuscitative, as these infants are often critically ill. Positive end-expiratory pressure can be helpful in the presence of left ventricular failure and at the same time can serve to decrease excessive pulmonary blood flow if there is an associated VSD. Surgically, a PDA must be ligated before the coarctation is repaired. This initial ligation can eliminate most of the blood flow to the lower half of the body until repair of the narrowed portion of the aorta is completed. As a result, metabolic acidosis, requiring therapy with sodium bicarbonate, may develop during this phase of the operation. Monitoring of arterial blood pressure is best achieved with a catheter in the right radial artery, as the left subclavian artery may be clamped during the operation.

Postductal

Coarctation of the aorta manifested in a young adult characteristically involves that portion of the aorta immediately distal to the left subclavian artery. The diagnosis often depends on a chance finding on routine physical examination, when either hypertension or a systolic murmur is detected. Characteristically, hypertension is present in the upper extremities, decreased blood pressure in the legs, and a palpable delay in the femoral pulse. Hypertension presumably reflects ejection of the left ventricular stroke volume into the fixed resistance created by the narrowed aorta. Arterial pulses are prominent in the upper extremities and weak or absent in the legs. A systolic murmur is best heard over the stenotic area of the aorta in the left paravertebral area. If obstruction to blood flow is severe, blood reaches the lower part of the body through the development of an extensive collateral system involving the internal mammary and intercostal arteries. A continuous murmur over these enlarged collateral vessels may be audible.

A chest radiograph may demonstrate left ventricular hypertrophy and notching along the lower borders of the ribs, reflecting the development of collateral circulation through the intercostal arteries. The ECG usually shows changes associated with left ventricular hypertrophy. Cardiac catheterization and angiocardiography are necessary to determine pressure gradients across the coarctation and to define the anatomic characteristics of the narrowing. Echocardiography is also helpful in defining the site and severity of the coarctation. About one-half of these patients have a bicuspid aortic valve as well.

Complications associated with a postductal coarctation of the aorta include cerebral hemorrhage, cerebral thrombosis, rupture of the aorta, and necrotizing arteritis. A bicuspid aortic valve is vulnerable to the development of infective endocarditis. Therefore, these patients should be treated with antibiotics before undergoing a dental or surgical procedure.

Treatment

Surgical intervention is indicated when systolic hypertension exceeds 180 mmHg or when the resting pressure gradient across the coarctation is greater than 40 mmHg. Surgical repair is accomplished by resection of the stenotic portion of the aorta and end-to-end anastomosis. A synthetic graft may be necessary to approximate the aorta, if the resected stenotic portion is unusually long.

Management of Anesthesia

Management of anesthesia for correction of coarctation of the aorta must consider (1) the adequacy of perfusion of the lower portion of the body during cross-clamping of the aorta, (2) the propensity for systemic hypertension during cross-clamping of the aorta, and (3) the risk of neurologic sequelae due to ischemia of the spinal cord. Blood flow to the anterior spinal artery is augmented by radicular branches of the intercostal arteries and may be compromised during cross-clamping of the aorta. Indeed, the incidence of paraplegia after coarctation repair is estimated to be 0.41%.[21] Continuous monitoring of arterial blood pressure both above and below the level of the coarctation is achieved by placement of a catheter in the right radial artery and right femoral artery. By monitoring these pressures simultaneously, it is possible to evaluate the adequacy of collateral circulation during periods of aortic cross-clamping. Mean arterial pressures in the lower extremities should probably be at least 40 mmHg to ensure adequate blood flow to the kidneys and spinal cord. If blood pressure in the lower portion of the body cannot be maintained above this

level, it may be necessary to use partial circulatory bypass. Somatosensory evoked potentials are useful for monitoring spinal cord function and the adequacy of its blood flow during cross-clamping of the aorta. Nevertheless, case reports of paraplegia despite normal somatosensory evoked potentials suggest that monitoring of posterior (sensory) cord function does not ensure adequacy of blood flow to the anterior (motor) portion of the spinal cord.[22,23] An excessive increase in systolic blood pressure during cross-clamping of the aorta may adversely increase the work of the heart and make surgical repair more difficult. In this situation, the use of a volatile anesthetic is helpful in maintaining a normal blood pressure. If hypertension persists, a continuous intravenous infusion of nitroprusside should be considered. A disadvantage of lowering blood pressure to a normal level may be an excessive decrease in blood pressure in the lower part of the body and subsequent ischemia of the spinal cord or kidneys.

Postoperatively, there may be a paradoxical increase in blood pressure. Baroreceptor reflexes, activation of the renin-angiotensin-aldosterone system, and excessive release of catecholamines have all been implicated as possible causes. Regardless of the etiology, intravenous administration of nitroprusside with or without propranolol or esmolol works well to control systemic hypertension during the early postoperative period. A longer-acting antihypertensive drug, such as hydralazine or labetalol, can be administered if hypertension persists. Abdominal pain may occur during the postoperative period and is presumably due to a sudden increase in blood flow to the gastrointestinal tract, leading to increased vasoactivity. Intraoperative ischemic damage to the spinal cord due to prolonged hypotension or ligation of collateral vessels will be manifested during the postoperative period as paraplegia. Hypertension may persist chronically, even after successful correction of the coarctation. In this regard, the younger the patient at the time of surgical correction, the more likely it is that blood pressure will normalize.[3] Premature coronary artery disease may reflect the effects of hypertension before surgery. The risks of a bicuspid aortic valve persist after the surgery and include infective endocarditis and the development of aortic regurgitation.

Pulmonic Stenosis

Pulmonic stenosis accounts for about 10% of all patients with congenital heart disease. Congenital pulmonic stenosis is valvular in 90% of cases and infundibular in the remainder. About three-fourths of these patients will have a probe-patent foramen ovale, and 10% will have an associated ASD. Infundibular pulmonic stenosis is often associated with a VSD.

Signs and Symptoms

Manifestations of congenital pulmonic stenosis vary with the degree of obstruction to ejection of right ventricular stroke volume. Mild to moderate degrees of pulmonic stenosis are usually not associated with symptoms. The detection of a systolic ejection murmur, best heard at the second left intercostal space, is often the first clue that this stenosis is present. The intensity and duration of the cardiac murmur parallel the severity of the stenosis. Right atrial and ventricular hypertrophy and right ventricular failure can occur when pulmonic stenosis is severe. Arterial hypoxemia and congestive heart failure may be manifestations of severe pulmonic stenosis in neonates. Onset of symptoms in the neonate may correspond to closure of the ductus arteriosus. Patients presenting at older ages may have episodes of syncope and angina pectoris. Sudden death can also occur and is thought to be due to infarction of the right ventricle. A chest radiograph and the ECG show evidence of right atrial and ventricular enlargement. Pulmonic stenosis is considered to be severe when the gradient measured across the valve during cardiac catheterization is greater than 50 mmHg.

Treatment

Surgical treatment of congenital pulmonic stenosis is often a valvulotomy performed during cardiopulmonary bypass. Alternatively, catheter balloon valvuloplasty may be effective therapy. Infundibular pulmonic stenosis is treated by resection of excess ventricular muscle.

Management of Anesthesia

Management of anesthesia is designed to avoid an increase in right ventricular oxygen requirements. Therefore, an excessive increase in heart rate and myocardial contractility are undesirable. The impact of a change in pulmonary vascular resistance is minimized by the presence of the fixed obstruction at the pulmonic valve. As a result, an elevation in pulmonary vascular resistance due to positive-pressure ventilation of the lungs is unlikely to produce a significant increase in right ventricular afterload and oxygen requirements. These patients are extremely difficult to resuscitate if cardiac arrest occurs, because external cardiac compression is not highly effective in forcing blood across a stenotic pulmonic valve. Therefore, a decrease in blood pressure should be promptly treated with a sympathomimetic drug. Likewise, cardiac dysrhythmias or an increase in heart rate that becomes hemodynamically significant should be rapidly corrected, using such drugs as lidocaine, propranolol, or esmolol. An electrical defibrillator should be available when anesthesia is administered to the patient with pulmonic stenosis.

MECHANICAL OBSTRUCTION OF THE TRACHEA

The trachea can be obstructed by circulatory anomalies that produce a vascular ring or by dilation of the pulmonary artery secondary to the absence of the pulmonic valve. These lesions

must be considered when evaluating a child with unexplained stridor or other evidence of upper airway obstruction. The possibility of an undiagnosed vascular ring should always be considered in the differential diagnosis of airway obstruction after placement of a nasogastric tube or an esophageal stethoscope.

Double Aortic Arch

Double aortic arch results in a vascular ring that can produce pressure on the trachea and esophagus. Compression resulting from this pressure can be manifested as inspiratory stridor, difficulty in mobilizing secretions, and dysphagia. A patient with this cardiac defect usually prefers to lie with the neck extended, as flexion of the neck often accentuates compression of the trachea.

Surgical transection of the smaller aortic arch is the treatment of choice in a symptomatic patient. During surgery, the tube in the trachea should be placed beyond the area of tracheal compression, if this can be safely accomplished without producing an endobronchial intubation. It must be appreciated that an esophageal stethoscope or nasogastric tube can cause occlusion of the trachea, if the tracheal tube remains above the level of vascular compression. Clinical improvement after surgical transection is often prompt. Tracheomalacia from prolonged compression of the trachea, however, can jeopardize the patency of the trachea.

Aberrant Left Pulmonary Artery

Tracheal or bronchial obstruction can occur when the left pulmonary artery is absent and the arterial supply to the left lung is derived from a branch of the right pulmonary artery passing between the trachea and esophagus. This anatomic arrangement has been referred to as a vascular sling, since a complete ring is not present. The sling can cause obstruction of the right mainstem bronchus, the distal trachea, or rarely the left mainstem bronchus.

Clinical manifestations of an aberrant left pulmonary artery include stridor, wheezing, and occasionally arterial hypoxemia. In contrast to a true vascular ring, esophageal obstruction is rare, and the stridor produced by this defect is usually present during exhalation rather than inspiration. A chest radiograph may demonstrate an abnormal separation between the esophagus and trachea. Hyperinflation or atelectasis of either lung may be present. Angiography is the most accurate approach for confirming the diagnosis.

Surgical division of the aberrant left pulmonary artery at its origin and redirection of its course anterior to the trachea, with anastomosis to the main pulmonary artery, is the treatment of choice. During the first months of life, surgical correction using deep hypothermia without cardiopulmonary bypass has been described.[24] Theoretically, continuous positive airway pressure or positive end-expiratory pressure should relieve airway obstruction and associated stridor in these cases.

Absent Pulmonic Valve

Absence of the pulmonic valve results in dilation of the pulmonary artery, which can result in compression of the trachea and left mainstem bronchus. This lesion can occur as an isolated defect or in conjunction with tetralogy of Fallot. Symptoms include signs of tracheal obstruction and occasionally the development of arterial hypoxemia and congestive heart failure. Any increase in pulmonary vascular resistance, as may occur with arterial hypoxemia or hypercarbia, will accentuate airway obstruction. Intubation of the trachea and maintenance of 4 to 6 mmHg of continuous positive airway pressure can be used to keep the trachea distended, reducing the magnitude of airway obstuction. Definitive treatment consists of insertion of a tubular graft with an artificial pulmonic valve.

REFERENCES

1. Nora JJ, Nora AH. Genetic epidemiology of congenital heart diseases. Prog Med Genet 1983;5:91–6
2. Morris CD, Menashe VD. 25 year mortality after surgical repair of congenital heart defect in childhood. A population-based cohort study. JAMA 1991;266:3447–52
3. Perloff JK. Adults with surgically treated congenital heart disease. JAMA 1983;250:2033–6
4. Eger EI II. Effect of ventilation/perfusion abnormalities. In: Eger EI II, ed. Anesthetic Uptake and Action. Baltimore. Williams & Wilkins 1974;146–59
5. Greeley WJ, Stanley TE, Ungerleider RM, Kisslo JA. Intraoperative hypoxemic spells in tetralogy of Fallot, an echocardiographic analysis of diagnosis and treatment. Anesth Analg 1989;68:815–9
6. Greeley WJ, Bushman GA, Davis DP, Reves JG. Comparative effects of halothane and ketamine on systemic arterial oxygen saturation in children with cyanotic heart disease. Anesthesiology 1986;65:666–8
7. Spinnato JA, Kraynack BJ, Cooper MW. Eisenmenger's syndrome in pregnancy: Epidural anesthesia for elective cesarean section. N Engl J Med 1981;304:1215–6
8. Elsten JL, Kim YD, Hanowell ST, Macnamara TE. Prolonged

9. Fyman PN, Goodman K, Casthely PA, et al. Anesthetic management of patients undergoing Fontan procedure. Anesth Analg 1986;65:516–9
10. Laks H, Milliken JC, Perloff JK, et al. Experience with the Fontan procedure. J Thorac Cardiovasc Surg 1984;88:934–51
11. Hosking MP, Beynen F. Repair of coarctation of the aorta in a child after a modified Fontan's operation: Anesthetic implications and management. Anesthesiology 1989;71:312–15
12. Hagen PT, Scholtz DG, Edwards WD. Incidence and size of patent foramen ovale during the first 10 decades of life: An autopsy study of 965 normal hearts. Mayo Clin Proc 1984;59:17–20
13. Moorthy SS, LoSasso AM. Patency of the foramen ovale in the critically ill patient. Anesthesiology 1974;41:405–7
14. Rashkind WJ, Miller WW. Creation of an atrial septal defect without thoracotomy. JAMA 1966;196:991–2
15. Mustard WT, Keith JD, Trusler GA, et al. The surgical management of transposition of the great vessels. J Thorac Cardiovasc Surg 1964;48:953–8
16. Rastelli GC, McGoon DC, Wallace RB. Anatomic correction of the great arteries with ventricular septal defect and subpulmonary stenosis. J Thorac Cardiovasc Surg 1969;58:545–52
17. Wong RS, Baum VC, Sangivan S. Truncus arteriosus: Recognition and therapy of intraoperative cardiac ischemia. Anesthesiology 1991;74:378–80
18. Hansen DD, Hickey PR. Anesthesia for hypoplastic left heart syndrome: Use of high-dose fentanyl in 30 neonates. Anesth Analg 1986;65:127–32
19. Anand KJS, Hickey PR. Halothane-morphine compared with high-dose sufentanil for anesthesia and postoperative analgesia in neonatal cardiac surgery. N Engl J Med 1992;326:1–9
20. Larson CP. Anesthesia in neonatal cardiac surgery. N Engl J Med 1992;327:124
21. Brewer LA, Fosburg RG, Mulder GA, Berska JJ. Spinal cord complication following surgery for coarctation of the aorta. A study of 66 cases. J Thorac Cardiovasc Surg 1972;64:368–78
22. Takaki O, Okumura F. Application and limitation of somatosensory evoked potential monitoring during thoracic aortic aneurysm surgery. A case report. Anesthesiology 1985;63:700–3
23. Ginsburg HH, Shelter AG, Raudzens PA. Postoperative paraplegia with preserved intraoperative somatosensory evoked potentials. J Neurosurg 1985;63:296–300
24. McLeskey CH, Martin WE. Anesthesia for repair of a pulmonary-artery sling in an infant with severe tracheal stenosis. Anesthesiology 1977;46:368–70

4

Abnormalities of Cardiac Conduction and Cardiac Rhythm

Cardiac dysrhythmias that occur during the perioperative period can usually be explained on the basis of abnormalities of cardiac impulse conduction (reentry) or impulse formation (automatic or ectopic). Reentry excitation accounts for most premature beats and tachydysrhythmias. Conditions necessary for reentry include two pathways over which the cardiac impulse is conducted at different velocities[1] (Fig. 4-1). One pathway conducts the cardiac impulse forward (antegrade), whereas the other pathway conducts the reentering cardiac impulse backward (retrograde). In the retrograde pathway, antegrade conduction is usually blocked or delayed, but retrograde conduction remains intact. Pharmacologic or physiologic events may alter the crucial balance between conduction velocities and refractory periods of dual pathways, resulting in initiation or termination of reentry cardiac dysrhythmias (Table 4-1). Automatic cardiac dysrhythmias are due to enhanced automaticity of a focus in the heart capable of undergoing spontaneous depolarization (repetitive firing) analogous to that of the sinus node. Automaticity refers to the slope of phase 4 depolarization of the cardiac action potential (Fig. 4-2). Increasing the slope of phase 4 depolarization or decreasing the resting membrane potential leads to enhanced automaticity manifested as an accelerated heart rate and ventricular irritability (Table 4-2). Conversely, a decrease in the slope of phase 4 depolarization slows the heart rate (Table 4-2). Examples of automatic cardiac dysrhythmias are bradydysrhythmias and disturbances of atrioventricular or intraventricular conduction. Factors that determine how a patient tolerates a cardiac dysrhythmia include the heart rate, duration of the dysrhythmia, and the presence and severity of any underlying cardiac disease. The importance of cardiac dys-

rhythmias in the management of anesthesia relates to the effects of the specific rhythm disturbance on cardiac output and possible interactions of antidysrhythmic drugs with drugs administered to produce anesthesia and skeletal muscle relaxation.

DIAGNOSIS

The electrocardiogram (ECG) is the cornerstone for the diagnosis of cardiac conduction and rhythm disturbances. The normal ECG consists of three waveforms designated the P wave (atrial depolarization), QRS complex (ventricular depolarization), and T wave (ventricular repolarization) (Fig. 4-2). The P-R interval is the time necessary for the cardiac impulse to pass through the atrioventricular (AV) node. Transmission of the cardiac impulse is through a specialized conduction system present in the atria and ventricles (Fig. 4-3). The following questions should be asked when interpreting the ECG:

1. What is the heart rate?
2. Are P waves present? What is their relationship to the QRS complex?
3. What is the duration of the P-R interval?
4. What is the duration of the QRS complex?
5. Is the ventricular rhythm regular?
6. Are there early cardiac beats or abnormal pauses after the QRS complex?

It is important to confirm the presence of a P wave for each QRS complex. Lead II of the ECG reflects P waves most

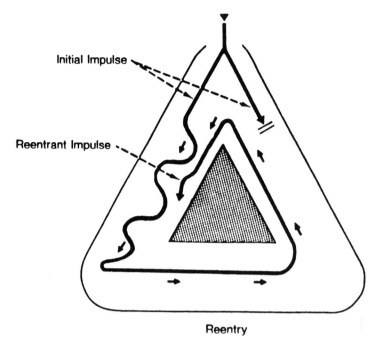

Reentry

Fig. 4-1. The essential requirement for initiation of reentry excitation is a unilateral block that prevents uniform anterograde propagation of the initial cardiac impulse. Under appropriate conditions, this same cardiac impulse can traverse the area of blockade in a retrograde direction and become a reentrant cardiac impulse. (From Akhtar M. Management of ventricular tachyarrhythmias. JAMA 1982;247:671–4, with permission.)

Table 4-1. Events Associated With Initiation of Cardiac Dysrhythmias During the Perioperative Period

Arterial hypoxemia

Electrolyte disturbances
  Potassium
  Magnesium

Acid-base disturbances

Altered activity of the autonomic nervous system

Increased myocardial fiber stretch
  Hypertension
  Intubation of the trachea

Myocardial ischemia

Drugs
  Catecholamines
  Volatile anesthetics

Co-existing cardiac disease
  Pre-excitation syndrome
  Prolonged Q-T interval syndrome

predictably and is the lead most often selected for analysis of cardiac dysrhythmias during the perioperative period. Inverted P waves are present when an abnormal pathway exists for the conduction of the cardiac impulse or when atrial (ectopic) sites other than the sinoatrial (SA) node exist. The P-R interval is 0.12 to 0.2 second when the heart rate is normal. This interval is prolonged when there is increased delay of conduction of the cardiac impulse through the AV node and is shortened in the presence of a junctional rhythm. The QRS complex is normally 0.05 to 0.1 second in duration. Abnormal intraventricular conduction of the cardiac impulse is suggested

Table 4-2. Events That Alter the Slope of Phase 4 Depolarization

Increase Slope	Decrease Slope
Arterial hypoxemia	Vagal stimulation
Hypercarbia	Positive airway pressure
Catecholamines	Acute hyperkalemia
Sympathomimetic drugs	Hypothermia
Acute hypokalemia	
Hyperthermia	
Hypertension	

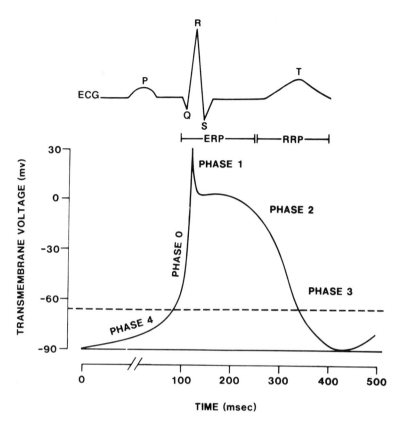

Fig. 4-2. Schematic diagram of a transmembrane action potential generated by an automatic cardiac cell, and of the relationship of this action potential to events depicted on the electrocardiogram (ECG). Phase 4 undergoes spontaneous depolarization from the resting membrane potential (-90 mV) until the threshold potential (broken line) is reached. Depolarization (phase 0) occurs when the threshold potential is reached and corresponds to the QRS complex on the ECG. Phases 1 through 3 represent repolarization with phase 3 corresponding to the T wave on the ECG. The effective refractory period (ERP) is that time during which cardiac impulses cannot be conducted, regardless of the intensity of the stimulus. During the relative refractory period (RRP), a stronger than normal stimulus can initiate an action potential. The action potential from a contractile cardiac cell differs from an automatic cardiac cell, in that phase 4 does not undergo spontaneous depolarization.

by a QRS complex that exceeds 0.12 second. A pathologic Q wave is present when its duration exceeds 0.04 second. The ST segment is normally isoelectric but can be elevated up to 1 mm in standard and precordial leads in the absence of any cardiac abnormality. The ST segment, however, is never normally depressed. The T wave is in the same direction as the QRS complex and should not exceed 5 mm in amplitude in standard leads or 10 mm in precordial leads. The Q-T interval must be corrected for heart rate but normally should be less than one-half the preceding R-R interval.

Ambulatory Electrocardiographic Monitoring

Ambulatory ECG monitoring (Holter monitoring) is most useful in (1) documenting the occurrence of a life-threatening cardiac dysrhythmia, (2) assessing the efficacy of antidys-

rhythmic drug therapy, and (3) detecting the occurrence of silent (asymptomatic) myocardial ischemia.[2] Transtelephone transmission of the ECG may be used to delineate the nature of a cardiac dysrhythmia that occurs infrequently. Semiautomated analysis of several hours of recordings facilitates rapid interpretation.

TREATMENT

It is important to consider and correct events responsible for evoking a cardiac dysrhythmia before initiating antidysrhythmic drug therapy or placing an artificial cardiac pacemaker (Table 4-1). In this regard, establishment of physiologic values for PaO_2, $PaCO_2$, pH, plasma concentrations of potassium and magnesium, and normalization of autonomic nervous system

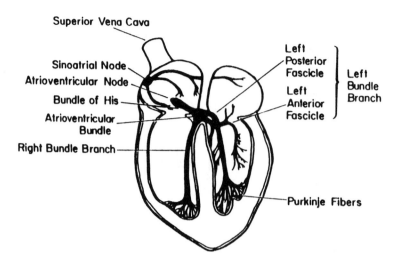

Fig. 4-3. Anatomy of the conduction system for conduction of cardiac impulses.

activity is essential. It is not commonly appreciated that alkalosis is even more likely than acidosis to produce ventricular dysrhythmias. Bradycardia can result in ventricular dysrhythmias by causing a temporal dispersion of refractory periods among Purkinje fibers.

Antidysrhythmic Drugs

Antidysrhythmic drugs are administered when correction of identifiable precipitating events is not sufficient to suppress the cardiac dysrhythmia (Table 4-3). These drugs act by altering electrophysiologic characteristics of the myocardial cells. For example, most antidysrhythmic drugs suppress automaticity in pacemaker cells by decreasing the slope of phase 4 depolarization. Quinidine, procainamide, and propranolol slow conduction of the cardiac impulse and prolong the effective refractory period of the cardiac action potential. Prolongation of the effective refractory periods serves to eliminate reentry circuits by converting unidirectional blockade to total bidirectional blockade. Conversely, lidocaine and phenytoin facilitate conduction of the cardiac impulse, eliminating unidirectional blockade and thereby preventing cardiac dysrhythmias due to a reentry circuit. Antidysrhythmic drugs may also produce characteristic changes (increased P-R interval, prolonged QRS duration) on the ECG.

The effectiveness of a specific antidysrhythmic drug is determined by the underlying cardiac conduction or rhythm disturbance (Table 4-3). Quinidine (50 to 75 mg·h^{-1} IV) is an effective drug for the control of atrial and ventricular tachydysrhythmias and for the chemical conversion of atrial flutter or fibrillation to normal sinus rhythm. Quinidine can produce direct myocardial depression, peripheral vasodilation, and hypotension. Normal neuromuscular transmission is altered, resulting in the potential for accentuation of the effects of nondepolarizing muscle relaxants.[3,4] Paradoxical ventricular tachycardia can occur occasionally and is usually preceded by prolongation of the Q-T interval on the ECG. Procainamide (100 mg IV every 5 minutes, to a maximum of about 500 mg) is as effective as quinidine for the treatment of ventricular tachydysrhythmias and ventricular premature beats but is not very effective in the treatment of atrial tachydysrhythmias. Hypotension most likely reflects direct myocardial depression. Monitoring the ECG during intravenous infusion of procainamide is important, as this drug can prolong the Q-T interval. In animals, large doses of procainamide can potentiate nondepolarizing muscle relaxants.[3,4] Disopyramide effectively suppresses atrial and ventricular tachydysrhythmias but is associated with significant direct myocardial depression, prolongation of the Q-T interval on the ECG, and anticholinergic effects (dry mouth, urinary hesitancy). Propranolol (0.1 to 0.2 mg·min^{-1} IV, usually not to exceed 50 μg·kg^{-1}) by slowing conduction of the cardiac impulse through the AV node is effective in slowing the ventricular response rate in the presence of atrial fibrillation or flutter. This drug is also useful in the treatment of digitalis-induced ventricular dysrhythmias. The principal toxic effects of propranolol are related to its beta blocking activity, manifested as sinus bradycardia, congestive heart failure, or bronchoconstriction in the patient with obstructive airway disease. Esmolol (100 to 300 μg·kg^{-1}·min^{-1} IV) is an alternative to propranolol for the perioperative control of atrial tachydysrhythmias. Verapamil (75 to 150 μg·kg^{-1} IV, over about 5 minutes) exerts a depressant effect on the AV node, accounting for its value in terminating paroxysmal supraventricular tachycardia and slowing the ventricular re-

Table 4-3.   Cardiac Antidysrhythmic Drugs

	Indication	Side Effects
Quinidine	Atrial tachydysrhythmias Ventricular tachydysrhythmias Ventricular premature beats Atrial fibrillation Atrial flutter	Direct myocardial depression Peripheral vasodilation Hypotension Paradoxical ventricular tachycardia Thrombocytopenia Diarrhea Hepatitis Potentiates nondepolarizing muscle relaxants
Procainamide	Ventricular tachydysrhythmias Ventricular premature beats	Direct myocardial depression Peripheral vasodilation Hypotension Paradoxical ventricular tachycardia Lupus erythematosus-like syndrome Accumulation with renal dysfunction Potentiates nondepolarizing muscle relaxants
Disopyramide	Ventricular tachydysrhythmias Atrial tachydysrhythmias	Direct myocardial depression Anticholinergic effects Paradoxical ventricular tachycardia Accumulation with renal dysfunction Potentiates nondepolarizing muscle relaxants
Propranolol	Atrial fibrillation Atrial flutter Paroxysmal atrial tachycardia Ventricular tachydysrhythmias Digitalis-induced ventricular dysrhythmias	Sinus bradycardia Direct myocardial depression Bronchoconstriction Lethargy
Verapamil	Paroxysmal supraventricular tachycardia Atrial fibrillation Atrial flutter	Direct myocardial depression Bradycardia Hypotension Potentiates depolarizing and nondepolarizing muscle relaxants Impairs antagonism of nondepolarizing neuromuscular blockade
Digoxin	Atrial tachydysrhythmias Atrial fibrillation Atrial flutter	Toxicity, especially with renal dysfunction and/or hypokalemia
Adenosine	Paroxysmal supraventricular tachycardia, including that associated with accessory tracts	Peripheral vasodilation Heart block
Phenytoin	Digitalis-induced supraventricular and ventricular dysrhythmias Paradoxical ventricular tachycardia	Hypotension Heart block Sedation Ataxia Hyperglycemia Gingival hyperplasia
Bretylium	Recurrent ventricular fibrillation Recurrent ventricular dysrhythmias	Initial hypertension Peripheral vasodilation Hypotension Accumulation with renal dysfunction Aggravates digitalis toxicity

Continued

Table 4-3.   (*Continued*)

	Indication	Side Effects
Amiodarone	Supraventricular tachydysrhythmias Ventricular tachydysrhythmias	Prolonged elimination half-time Bradycardia Hypotension Pulmonary fibrosis Postoperative ventilatory failure Skeletal muscle weakness Peripheral neuropathies Hepatitis Thyroid dysfunction Cyanotic discoloration of the face Corneal deposits
Lidocaine	Ventricular premature beats Recurrent ventricular fibrillation	Accumulation with decreased hepatic blood flow Central nervous system toxicity, direct cardiac depression, and peripheral vasodilation with excessive plasma concentrations

sponse rate in the presence of atrial flutter or fibrillation. Like digitalis, this drug does not exert a depressant effect on accessory conduction pathways. Caution is recommended when verapamil and propranolol are administered simultaneously, as both drugs depress AV conduction, SA node automaticity, and myocardial contractility. In the presence of co-existing left ventricular dysfunction, verapamil may potentiate the negative inotropic effects of volatile anesthetics.[5] The response to muscle relaxants is potentiated, similar to that seen with mycin antibiotics.[6] Digoxin (0.25 mg IV every 20 to 30 minutes, to a total dose of 0.5 to 0.75 mg), slows conduction of the cardiac impulse through the AV node and is thus effective in slowing the ventricular response rate in the presence of atrial fibrillation or flutter as well as in the prevention of atrial tachydysrhythmias. Adenosine (3 to 12 mg IV) is useful for the conversion of paroxysmal supraventricular tachycardia, including that associated with accessory pathways to normal sinus rhythm. Hypotension and flushing rarely accompany this dose of adenosine. Phenytoin (10 mg IV every 5 minutes, to a maximum dose of about 500 mg) is uniquely effective in treating ventricular cardiac dysrhythmias, owing to digitalis toxicity and may be effective in the management of paradoxical ventricular tachycardia (torsade de pointes) associated with a prolonged Q-T interval on the ECG. Among the antidysrhythmic drugs, phenytoin is the most effective in shortening the Q-T interval on the ECG, while effects on the ST segment and T wave are absent. Bretylium (5 mg·kg^{-1} IV, over 5 minutes) may be a useful drug in the treatment of recurrent ventricular fibrillation and of ventricular dysrhythmias that do not respond to lidocaine or procainamide. Amiodarone (5 mg·kg^{-1} IV, over about 5 minutes) is effective in the treatment of supraventricular and ventricular tachydysrhythmias. The antiadrenergic effects of amiodarone may be enhanced in the presence of general anesthesia, manifested as

atropine-resistant bradycardia and hypotension.[7] Pulmonary fibrosis and the need for postoperative mechanical support of ventilation have been observed in patients treated with this drug.[7]

Lidocaine

Most ventricular cardiac dysrhythmias that require pharmacologic treatment during the perioperative period are responsive to lidocaine. Lidocaine decreases the automaticity of ectopic cardiac pacemakers and increases the threshold for ventricular fibrillation. Supraventricular tachydysrhythmias are not suppressed by lidocaine. Treatment of ventricular premature beats is with a loading dose of lidocaine (1 to 2 mg·kg^{-1} IV), followed by a continuous intravenous infusion of 1 to 4 mg·min^{-1}, to maintain a therapeutic plasma concentration of 2 to 5 µg·ml^{-1}. In the presence of decreases in hepatic blood flow as associated with general anesthesia, it may be necessary to decrease the lidocaine dose. In usual therapeutic doses, lidocaine does not alter the P-R, QRS, or Q-T intervals on the ECG and has minimal negative inotropic effects. An excessive plasma concentration of lidocaine may decrease the conduction of the cardiac impulse through the AV node and His-Purkinje system and evoke seizures followed by coma. Large doses of lidocaine (5 mg·kg^{-1}) administered to animals may increase the intensity and duration of neuromuscular blockade produced by nondepolarizing muscle relaxants.[4]

Electrical Cardioversion

Cardiac dysrhythmias most responsive to electrical cardioversion are atrial flutter, atrial fibrillation, and ventricular tachycardia, although any ectopic tachydysrhythmia that is unresponsive to antidysrhythmic drug therapy can often be successfully terminated with cardioversion. The only exception is treatment of digitalis-induced cardiac dysrhythmias, as these dysrhythmias are refractory to cardioversion, and cardioversion can trigger more serious ventricular dysrhythmias. Cardioversion carries the risk of systemic embolization in the patient with atrial fibrillation. This accounts for the recommendation that elective cardioversion be preceded by anticoagulation if the dysrhythmia has been present for more than 48 hours.[8]

Elective cardioversion is performed with intravenous sedation (methohexital, etomidate, propofol), and resuscitation equipment should be immediately available. Drugs such as atopine and lidocaine (ventricular ectopy is common after treatment, as well as equipment for emergency artificial cardiac pacing, should be available in case underlying SA node dysfunction manifests after successful cardioversion. The electrical discharge is delivered by means of two chest electrodes (one placed anteriorly and one placed posteriorly), beginning at 50 to 100 joules and increasing in increments of 50 to 100 joules as necessary. High energy levels may be needed in the patient with a thickened thorax, a problem often seen in association with pulmonary emphysema. Even with repeated shocks, there does not appear to be a major risk of inflicting damage to the myocardium. Because of the short duration of the electrical current required (2 to 3 msec), it is possible to program the device delivering the current (cardioverter), to be discharged by the R wave of the ECG. Thus, the current is delivered during the QRS complex, and the discharge will not occur during the relative refractory period of the cardiac action potential (R on T phenomena), when an electrical stimulus might evoke ventricular tachycardia or ventricular fibrillation.

Artificial Cardiac Pacemakers

Placement of an artificial cardiac pacemaker is the treatment of choice for disturbances of cardiac impulse conduction characterized as AV heart block. Temporary artificial cardiac pacing is often required when transient heart block follows cardiopulmonary bypass. A pulmonary artery catheter with a pacing electrode may be selected if simultaneous pressure monitoring and pacing capabilities are required. The physiologic basis for the effectiveness of an artificial cardiac pacemaker is that the myocardium will contract when stimulated.

An artificial cardiac pacemaker can be inserted intravenously (endocardial lead) or by the subcostal approach (epicardial or myocardial lead). Tranvenous insertion sites include the internal jugular, external jugular, femoral, and antecubital veins. All pacemakers consist of two components, designated the pulse generator and pacing electrode leads[9] (Table 4-4). Electrical impulses are formed in the pulse generator and are transmitted to the endocardial or myocardial surface of the heart, resulting in a mechanical contraction. A five-letter generic code is used to describe the various pacing modalities of

Table 4-4.   Definition of Terms Used in Describing Artificial Cardiac Pacemakers

Term	Definition
Pulse generator	Consists of the energy source (battery) and electrical circuits necessary for pacing and sensory functions
Implanted or external	Anatomic placement of the pulse generator relative to the skin
Lead	Insulated wire connecting the pulse generator to the electrode
Electrode	Exposed metal end of electrode in contact with endocardium or epicardium (myocardium)
Endocardial pacing	Right atrium or right ventricle stimulated by contact of electrode with the endocardium after transvenous insertion of the lead
Epicardial pacing	Right atrium or right ventricle stimulated by insertion of electrode through the epicardium into the myocardium under direct vision
Unipolar pacing	Describes placement of the negative (stimulating) electrode in the atrium or ventricle and the positive (ground) electrode distant from the heart (metallic portion of the pulse generator or subcutaneous tissue)
Bipolar pacing	Describes placement of the negative and positive electrodes in the cardiac chamber being paced
Stimulation threshold	Minimal amount of current (amperes) or voltage (volts) necessary to cause contraction of the chamber that is being paced
Resistance	Measure of the combined resistance of the electrode-lead-myocardial interface as calculated using Ohm's law with values for current and voltage thresholds; normal value 350–1000 ohms
R wave sensitivity	Minimal voltage of intrinsic R wave necessary to activate the sensing circuit of the pulse generator and thus inhibit or trigger the pacing circuit (an R wave sensitivity of about 3 mV on an external pulse generator will maintain ventricle-inhibited pacing)
Hysteresis	Difference between intrinsic heart rate at which pacing begins (about 60 beats·min^{-1}) and pacing rate (72 beats·min^{-1})

Table 4-5. Generic Code for Identification and Description of Pacemaker Function

First Letter	Second Letter	Third Letter	Fourth Letter	Fifth Letter
Cardiac chamber paced	Cardiac chamber in which electrical activity is sensed	Response of generator to sensed R wave and P wave	Programmable functions of the generator	Antitachycardia functions of the generator
V—Ventricle	V—Ventricle	T—Triggering	P—Programmable (rate and/or output only)	B—Bursts
A—Atrium	A—Atrium	I—Inhibited	M—Multiprogrammable	N—Normal rate competition[a]
D—Dual (atrium and ventricle)	D—Dual	D—Dual	C—Communicating[b]	S—Scanning
	O—None (asynchronous)	O—None (asynchronous)	O—None (fixed function)	E—External

[a] Stimuli delivered at normal rates upon sensing of tachycardia (underdrive pacing).
[b] Capability of being noninvasively interrogated.

artificial cardiac pacemakers (Table 4-5). The first three letters of this code describe the various types of artificial cardiac pulse generators (Table 4-6). A standard ventricular demand pacemaker is classified as VVI, whereas an AV pacemaker with two pacing electrodes is classified as DVI. A dual-chamber pacemaker that paces and senses in both the atrium and ventricle and that is triggered by an atrial event and inhibited by a ventricular event is classified as DDD. Artificial cardiac pacing that preserves the atrial and ventricular contraction sequence is described as physiologic pacing. The atrial contribution to ventricular filling may result in a 20% to 30% increase in cardiac output compared with ventricular pacing. Measurement of cardiac output may be necessary to establish the optimal atrial heart rate.

Early pacemaker failures are usually due to electrode displacement or breakage, whereas failures that occur more than 6 months after implantation are most often due to premature battery depletion or a faulty pulse generator. The development of lithium batteries with a projected longevity of 8 to 20 years has greatly decreased the need to replace pacemakers for battery failure. Cardiac dysrhythmias may be evoked by artificial cardiac pacemakers, especially dual-chamber devices. Improved shielding of artificial cardiac pacemakers has largely eliminated earlier problems related to external electrical fields (microwaves, electrocautery, magnetic resonance imaging), manifested as inhibition of ventricular-inhibited pacemakers. Many artificial cardiac pacemakers are now designed such that external electrical fields will change the pacemaker rhythm to an asynchronous mode rather than shut off the unit. Many functions of an artificial cardiac pacemaker can be adjusted by using a magnetically activated potentiometer held externally in proximity to the pulse generator. A demand pacemaker may be overridden by the intrinsic heart rate if this rate is more rapid or if the pacemaker can be momentarily converted to an

Table 4-6. Types of Artificial Cardiac Pulse Generators

Letter Number[a]			Description
I	II	III	
A	O	O	Asynchronous (fixed rate) atrial pacing
V	O	O	Asynchronous (fixed rate) ventricular pacing
A	A	I	Noncompetitive (demand) atrial pacing, electrical output inhibited by intrinsic atrial depolarization (P wave)
V	V	I	Noncompetitive (demand) ventricular pacing, electrical output inhibited by intrinsic ventricular depolarization (R wave)
A	A	T	Triggered atrial pacing, electrical output triggered by intrinsic atrial depolarization (P wave)
V	V	T	Triggered ventricular pacing, electrical output triggered by intrinsic ventricular depolarization (R wave)
D	V	I	Paces (sequential) in atrium and ventricle, does not sense P waves, does sense R waves
D	D	D	Paces and senses in atrium and ventricle
V	D	D	Paces in ventricle, senses in atrium and ventricle, synchronized with atrial activity and paces ventricle after a preset atrioventricular interval

[a] See Table 4-5 for definitions of letter numbers.

asynchronous mode by placing a magnet externally over the pulse generator. An acute myocardial infarction near the site of electrode placement may interfere with the electrode-tissue interface and result in pacemaker failure.

Noninvasive Transcutaneous Cardiac Pacing

An alternative to emergency transvenous artificial cardiac pacemaker placement is noninvasive transcutaneous cardiac pacing (NTP).[10] Judicious placement of cutaneous chest and back electrodes over areas of minimal skeletal muscle mass and delivery of low-density constant-current impulses permits effective cardiac stimulation with little or no skeletal muscle or cutaneous activation. Hemodynamic responses to NTP are similar to those produced by right ventricular cardiac pacing. NTP is rapidly becoming the treatment of choice in clinical situations (bradydysrhythmias, cardiac arrest owing to asystole) requiring emergency cardiac pacing. NTP may be of value when applied early in witnessed bradyasystolic arrest, whereas transvenous pacing does not improve outcome after cardiac arrest.[10] This form of cardiac pacing may be useful for elective overdrive suppression of hemodynamically stable tachydysrhythmias. It may also become useful for prophylaxis in the patient with a co-existing artificial cardiac pacemaker or for the patient with left bundle branch block who is undergoing central hemodynamic monitoring.

Preoperative Evaluation

Preoperative evaluation of the patient with an artificial cardiac pacemaker in place includes determination of the reason for placing the pacemaker and an assessment of its present function (Table 4-5). A preoperative history of vertigo or syncope may reflect dysfunction of the artificial cardiac pacemaker. The rate of discharge of an atrial or ventricular asynchronous cardiac pacemaker (usually 70 to 72 beats·min^{-1}) is a useful indicator of pulse generator function. A 10% decrease in heart rate from the initial fixed discharge rate may reflect battery failure. An irregular heart rate may reflect competition of the pulse generator with the patient's intrinsic heart rate or failure of the pulse generator to sense R waves. The ECG is evaluated to confirm one-to-one capture, as evidenced by a pacemaker spike for every palpated peripheral pulse. The ECG is not a diagnostic aid in the patient in whom the intrinsic heart rate is greater than the preset pacemaker rate. In such cases, the proper function of a ventricular synchronous or sequential artificial cardiac pacemaker can be confirmed by demonstrating the appearance of captured beats on the ECG when the pacemaker is converted to the asynchronous mode by placement of an external converter magnet over the pulse generator. An attempt to slow the heart rate by massaging the carotid sinus is not recommended, as dislodgment of an arteriosclerotic plaque is a risk, whereas the Valsalva maneuver may not lower the intrinsic heart rate sufficiently to confirm the function of the artificial cardiac pacemaker. A chest radiograph is useful to confirm the absence of a break in the pacemaker's electrodes.

Management of Anesthesia

Management of anesthesia in the patient with an artificial cardiac pacemaker includes monitoring to confirm continued function of the pulse generator and ready availability of equipment and drugs to maintain an acceptable intrinsic heart rate, should the artificial cardiac pacemaker unexpectedly fail (Table 4-7). If electrocautery interferes with the ECG, the placement of a finger on a peripheral pulse or auscultation through an esophageal stethoscope, or both, confirms continued cardiac activity. Insertion of a pulmonary artery catheter will not disturb epicardial electrodes but might become entangled in, or dislodge, a recently placed transvenous (endocardial) electrode. Dislodgment of endocardial electrodes, however, has not been observed when these electrodes have been in place for more than 4 weeks.[9] The choice of drugs to produce anesthesia is not altered by the presence of a properly functioning artificial cardiac pacemaker. An artificial cardiac pacemaker that is functioning normally preoperatively should continue to function intraoperatively without incident.

Improved shielding of the artificial cardiac pacemaker has largely eliminated the problem of electromagnetic interference from electrocautery in which the electrical artifact was sensed as an intrinsic myocardial potential (R wave) by the pacemaker, resulting in inhibition of the pulse generator. Nevertheless, the possibility of this problem still exists, necessitating a high index of suspicion and the availability of drugs (atropine, isoproterenol) for prompt administration, in the event that the artificial cardiac pacemaker fails.[11] An external converter magnet may be used to convert the pacemaker to an asynchronous mode. Despite improved shielding of the artificial cardiac pacemaker, it is still a reasonable recommendation to place the ground plate for the electrocautery as far as possible from the pulse generator, to minimize detection of the current by the pulse generator. Furthermore, it is useful to keep the electrocautery current as low as possible and to apply electrocautery in short bursts no more frequently than about every 10 seconds, especially when the current is being applied close to the pulse generator.[12] Paradoxically, the use

Table 4-7. Management of Anesthesia in the Patient With an Artificial Cardiac Pacemaker

Continuous monitoring of the electrocardiogram
Continuous monitoring of a peripheral pulse
Electrical defibrillator present
External converter magnet available
Drugs prepared—atropine, isoproterenol

of a repetitive electrical stimulus delivered by a peripheral nerve stimulator (twitch mode at a frequency of 2 Hz) placed ipsilateral to the artificial cardiac pacemaker generator, has been used intraoperatively for deliberate suppression of a malfunctioning ventricular-inhibited pacemaker.[13]

Ventricular fibrillation in a patient with a permanent artificial cardiac pacemaker is managed in the conventional manner, with the exception that the defibrillator paddles should not be placed directly over the pulse generator. An acute increase in stimulation threshold may follow external defibrillation, causing a loss of capture and the need for prompt insertion of a transvenous artificial cardiac pacemaker or use of NTP.[14] Presumably, electrical defibrillation results in endocardial burns and fibrosis at the electrode-endocardial interface, resulting in an increased stimulation threshold and emphasizing the need to administer the lowest effective dose of electrical energy.

There is no evidence that anesthetic drugs or events likely to be associated with the perioperative period alter the stimulation threshold of an artificial cardiac pacemaker (Table 4-8). Nevertheless, it would seem prudent to avoid events that acutely increase or decrease (hyperventilation of the lungs, diuretic-induced diuresis) the plasma potassium concentration. Conceivably, succinylcholine could increase the stimulation threshold by virtue of an acute increase in the plasma potassium concentration or inhibit a normal-functioning artificial cardiac pacemaker by causing contraction of skeletal muscle groups (myopotential inhibition) interpreted as intrinsic R waves by the pulse generator. For example, a unipolar pulse generator of an artificial cardiac pacemaker system may be inhibited by skeletal muscle myopotentials (fasciculations) produced by succinylcholine.[14] For this reason, it has been recommended that when succinylcholine is to be administered to a patient with unipolar demand pacemaker that the pacemaker be switched to an asynchronous mode using a precordial magnet.[14] Nevertheless, such use of a precordial magnet may increase the risk of cardiac dysrhythmias secondary to the "R on T" phenomenon and may allow unintentional reprogramming of certain pacemakers. It is unclear whether attenuation of succinylcholine-induced skeletal muscle fasciculations by prior administration of a nonparalyzing dose of a nondepolarizing muscle relaxant decreases the risk of myopotential inhibition of the pulse generator. Clinical experience suggests that succinylcholine is usually a safe drug in the pacemaker patient; if myopotential inhibition does occur, it is generally transient and asymptomatic. A rare occurrence is a transvenous pacemaker failure associated with positive-pressure ventilation of the lungs, which may reflect an abrupt volume change in the heart and cardiac septal deviation causing loss of electrode contact with the endocardial surface of the myocardium.[15]

Anesthesia for Pacemaker Insertion

A functioning transvenous artificial cardiac pacemaker should be in place or NTP available before induction of anesthesia for permanent artificial cardiac pacemaker placement, as there is a risk that third-degree AV heart block will deteriorate to cardiac arrest. The patient's arm should not be placed in hyperextension when the brachial vein has been used for insertion of the transvenous pacemaker. The presence of a transvenous pacemaker creates a situation in which there is a direct connection between any external electrical source and the endocardium, predisposing the patient to the risk of ventricular fibrillation from microshock levels of electrical current.

DISTURBANCES OF CARDIAC IMPULSE CONDUCTION

Disturbances of cardiac impulse conduction are classified according to the site of the conduction block relative to the AV node (Table 4-9). Heart block that occurs above the AV node is usually benign and transient, whereas heart block that

Table 4-8.   Factors That Could Alter Stimulation Threshold of an Artificial Cardiac Pacemaker

Hyperkalemia (succinylcholine?)
Hypokalemia (hyperventilation)
Arterial hypoxemia
Myocardial ischemia/infarction
Catecholamines

Table 4-9.   Classification of Heart Block

First-Degree AV Heart Block
Second-Degree AV Heart Block
Mobitz type 1 (Wenckebach)
Mobitz type 2
Unifascicular Heart Block
Left anterior hemiblock
Left posterior hemiblock
Right Bundle Branch Block
Left Bundle Branch Block
Bifascicular Heart Block
Right bundle branch block plus left anterior hemiblock
Right bundle branch block plus left posterior hemiblock
Third-Degree (Trifascicular, Complete) AV Heart Block
Nodal
Infranodal

AV, atrioventricular.

develops below the AV node tends to be progressive and permanent.

First-Degree Atrioventricular Heart Block

First-degree AV heart block is arbitrarily defined as a P-R interval on the ECG that is greater than 0.2 second at a heart rate of 70 beats·min^{-1}. This prolonged P-R interval reflects a delay in passage of the cardiac impulse through the AV node. Commonly, a prolonged P-R interval is the result of degeneration of the cardiac conduction system that accompanies aging. Other causes are digitalis, ischemia of the AV node as may occur with a diaphragmatic myocardial infarction, and enhanced parasympathetic nervous system activity. Aortic regurgitation is commonly accompanied by first-degree heart block. This form of heart block is usually asymptomatic. Intravenous administration of atropine is effective in speeding conduction of the cardiac impulse through the AV node.

Second-Degree Atrioventricular Heart Block

Second-degree AV heart block is categorized as Mobitz type 1 block (Wenckebach) or Mobitz type 2 block. Mobitz type 1 block is caused by delayed conduction of the cardiac impulse through the AV node. There is progressive prolongation of the P-R interval until a beat is entirely blocked (dropped beat), followed by a repeat of this sequence. By contrast, Mobitz type 2 block reflects disease of the His-Purkinje conduction system (infranodal block), characterized by a sudden interruption of the conduction of a cardiac impulse without prior prolongation of the P-R interval on the ECG. Type 2 block has a more serious prognosis than type 1 block, as it frequently progresses to third-degree AV heart block. Treatment of type 2 block may include placement of an artificial cardiac pacemaker, even in the absence of symptoms such as syncope.[16]

Unifascicular Heart Block

Block of conduction of the cardiac impulse over the left anterior or posterior fascicle of the left bundle branch is characterized as unifascicular heart block or hemiblock. Block of the left anterior fascicle of the left bundle branch is designated left anterior hemiblock. Left posterior hemiblock is uncommon, as the posterior fascicle of the left bundle branch is larger and better perfused than the anterior fascicle. Although hemiblock is a form of intraventricular block, the duration of the QRS complex is normal or only minimally prolonged.

Right Bundle Branch Block

Right bundle branch block (RBBB) is due to block of conduction of the cardiac impulse over the right bundle branch, which is present in about 1% of hospitalized adult patients.[17] On the ECG, RBBB is recognized by QRS complexes that exceed 0.1 second in duration and by broad RSR complexes in leads V1 and V3. RBBB does not always imply cardiac disease and is often of no clinical significance. Incomplete RBBB (QRS complex duration 0.09 to 0.1 second) is frequently present in the patient with an increased right ventricular pressure, as produced by chronic pulmonary disease or an atrial septal defect.

Left Bundle Branch Block

Left bundle branch block (LBBB) is recognized on the ECG as a QRS complex greater than 0.12 second in duration and by wide notched R waves in all leads. Incomplete LBBB is present when the duration of the QRS complex on the ECG is 0.1 to 0.12 second in duration. LBBB, in contrast to RBBB, is often associated with ischemic heart disease or may reflect left ventricular hypertrophy that accompanies chronic hypertension or cardiac valve disease. The appearance of LBBB has been observed to occur during anesthesia (especially when the heart rate exceeds 115 beats·min^{-1} or in the presence of hypertension) and may signal an acute myocardial infarction.[18–20] It is difficult to diagnose a myocardial infarction on the ECG in the presence of LBBB. The wide QRS complexes characteristic of LBBB can be mistaken for ventricular tachycardia.

The presence of LBBB may have special implications for the insertion of a pulmonary artery catheter.[21] For example, RBBB occurs during insertion of a pulmonary artery catheter in about 5% of patients with ischemic heart disease. Theoretically, third-degree AV heart block could occur if catheter-induced RBBB occurred in a patient with co-existing LBBB. Nevertheless, clinical experience has not confirmed an increased incidence of third-degree AV heart block in such patients during insertion of a pulmonary artery catheter.

Bifascicular Heart Block

Bifascicular heart block is present when RBBB is associated with block of one of the fascicles of the left bundle branch. RBBB plus left anterior hemiblock (anterior fascicle of the left bundle) is the most frequent combination, present on about 1% of all the ECGs recorded from adults.[22] Each year, about 1% to 2% of these patients progress to third-degree AV heart block.[16] The combination of RBBB and left posterior hemiblock (posterior fascicle of the left bundle branch) is infrequent but, in contrast to left anterior hemiblock, it often progresses to third-degree AV heart block. Insertion of an artificial cardiac pacemaker, however, is recommended only when symptomatic bradydysrhythmias occur.

A theoretical concern in the patient with bifascicular heart block is that perioperative events (changes in blood pressure, arterial oxygenation, or electrolyte concentrations) might compromise conduction of the cardiac impulse in the one remaining intact fascicle, leading to the sudden onset of third-degree AV heart block. There is no evidence, however, that surgery performed with general or regional anesthesia predisposes the patient with a co-existing bifascicular heart block to the development of third-degree AV heart block.[22–24] For this reason, prophylactic placement of an artificial cardiac pacemaker is not recommended before anesthesia for elective surgery. This recommendation is based on the clinical course of patients with co-existing bifascicular heart block who had normal preoperative P-R intervals on the ECG and who denied a history of unexplained syncope that might suggest the prior occurrence of transient third-degree AV heart block. Conceivably, a temporary transvenous artificial cardiac pacemaker should be placed before a major surgical procedure, when the preoperative ECG shows a prolonged P-R interval or when there is a history of unexplained syncope. Nevertheless, even symptomatic patients with bifascicular heart block have undergone uneventful surgery without prior placement of an artificial cardiac pacemaker.[22–24]

Third-Degree Atrioventricular Heart Block

Third-degree AV heart block is characterized by complete absence of the conduction of the cardiac impulse from the atria to the ventricles. Continued activity of the ventricles is due to stimulation from an ectopic cardiac pacemaker distal to the site of the conduction block. When the conduction block is near the AV node, the heart rate is 45 to 55 beats·min^{-1}, and the QRS complex on the ECG appears normal. When conduction block is below the AV node (infranodal), the heart rate is 30 to 40 beats·min^{-1}, and the QRS complex on the ECG is wide. The onset of third-degree AV heart block may be signaled by an episode of vertigo and syncope. Syncope associated with a seizure is designated an Adams-Stokes attack. Congestive heart failure may occur when stroke volume is unable to offset the decreased cardiac output produced by the bradycardia accompanying third-degree AV heart block. The most common cause of third-degree AV heart block in adults is primary fibrous degeneration of the cardiac conduction system associated with aging (Lenegre's disease) (Table 4-10). Degenerative changes in tissues adjacent to the mitral annulus can also interrupt the cardiac conduction system (Lev's disease). Congenital third-degree AV heart block is almost always at the level of the AV node.

Treatment

Treatment of third-degree AV heart block consists of placement of a permanent artificial cardiac pacemaker. Prior placement of a transvenous pacemaker or availability of NTP is common before induction of anesthesia for insertion of a per-

Table 4-10. Causes of Third-Degree Atrioventricular Heart Block

Primary fibrous degeneration of the cardiac conduction system (Lenegre's disease, Lev's disease)
Ischemic heart disease (acute myocardial infarction)
Cardiomyopathy
Myocarditis
Ankylosing spondylitis
Iatrogenic after cardiac surgery
Congenital
Increased parasympathetic nervous system activity
Drugs (digitalis, beta adrenergic antagonists, quinidine)
Electrolyte derangements (hyperkalemia)

manent artificial cardiac pacemaker. Isoproterenol (1 to 4 μg·min^{-1} IV) may be useful along with atropine, to maintain a viable ventricular heart rate (chemical pacemaker) until the permanent pacemaker is functional. An antidysrhythmic drug may suppress ectopic ventricular pacemakers. For this reason, an antidysrhythmic drug should probably not be administered to the patient with third-degree AV heart block, in the absence of an artificial cardiac pacemaker.

DISTURBANCES OF CARDIAC RHYTHM

Cardiac dysrhythmias that arise in the atria or AV node are defined as supraventricular dysrhythmias. Cardiac dysrhythmias that arise below the AV node are defined as ventricular dysrhythmias.

Sinus Tachycardia

Sinus tachycardia is defined as a heart rate of greater than 120 beats·min^{-1}. It is due to an acceleration of the normal discharge rate of the SA node. An increased heart rate during the preoperative period may reflect anxiety, pain, sepsis, hypovolemia, fever, or congestive heart failure. Light anesthesia relative to the surgical stimulus may produce tachycardia. Intraoperative causes of tachycardia other than light anesthesia include arterial hypoxemia, hypoglycemia, hyperthyroidism, and malignant hyperthermia. Treatment of sinus tachycardia depends on the cause of the increased heart rate. When sinus tachycardia results in myocardial ischemia, the intravenous administration of a beta antagonist such as propranolol or esmolol is useful.

Sinus Bradycardia

Sinus bradycardia is defined as a heart rate of less than 60 beats·min^{-1}. It is due to a deceleration of the normal discharge rate of the SA node. This can be a normal finding in the physically active patient with a high degree of parasympathetic nervous system activity (athletic heart syndrome). Unexpected cardiac arrest has been described in a well-trained athlete during spinal anesthesia, perhaps reflecting parasympathetic nervous system predominance enhanced by anesthesia-induced blockade of the cardioaccelerator nerves.[25] An acute diaphragmatic myocardial infarction or the presence of severe pain represent conditions in which discharge of the SA node can be normally slow. Halothane may decrease heart rate by decreasing the automaticity of the SA node.[26] Other factors that slow heart rate by depression of SA node automaticity, rather than by vagal stimulation, include beta antagonist drugs, hypothermia, hypothyroidism, and icterus. In the presence of carotid sinus hypersensitivity, prolonged asystole can follow even minimal pressure on the carotid sinus. Reflex bradycardia may occur with traction on ocular muscles (oculocardiac reflex) and with traction on abdominal mesentery (celiac plexus stimulation); it can also occur during laryngoscopy, laparoscopy, and electroconvulsive therapy.[26] Drugs associated with reflex bradycardia include opioids and succinylcholine. Intravenous administration of atropine is the treatment of choice when heart rate slowing becomes hemodynamically significant.

Sick Sinus Syndrome

Sick sinus syndrome (bradycardia-tachycardia syndrome) is characterized by bradycardia punctuated by episodes of supraventricular tachycardia, most often observed in the elderly patient. In an afflicted patient, the SA node seems to be depressed and more vulnerable to other exogenous influences, such as vagal stimulation and certain drugs. Many patients are asymptomatic, although syncope and palpitations are often described. Bradycardia may contribute to the development of congestive heart failure, whereas tachycardia can precipitate angina pectoris in the patient with ischemic heart disease. Systemic embolism occurs in up to 20% of afflicted patients.[27]

Placement of an artificial cardiac pacemaker is the treatment of choice for bradycardia that accompanies this syndrome, although suppression of tachydysrhythmias is less predictable. If AV node conduction is normal, artificial cardiac pacing may be initiated from the atrium versus ventricular or AV sequential pacing if the AV node is diseased. Digitalis, quinidine, and beta antagonists are effective in suppressing tachydysrhythmias, but the presence of an artificial cardiac pacemaker is recommended considering the known depressant effects of those drugs on SA node activity. When tachycardia is incapacitating, surgical ablation of the common bundle and insertion of an artificial ventricular pacemaker may be indicated. Acute treatment of bradycardia is with atropine (0.5 to 1 mg IV) or isoproterenol (1 to 4 μg·min^{-1} IV). Long-term anticoagulation is favored by some, in view of the high incidence of systemic embolism.

Atrial Premature and Junctional Premature Beats

Atrial premature and junctional premature beats arise from an ectopic cardiac pacemaker in the atria or near the AV node. These premature beats are recognized on the ECG by the presence of early and abnormal-shaped P waves. The duration of the corresponding QRS complex is normal because activation of the ventricles occurs by a normal conduction pathway. When aberrant conduction of a cardiac impulse occurs, however, the configuration of the QRS complex is widened and can mimic a ventricular premature beat. A distinguishing feature is that an atrial premature beat, unlike a ventricular premature beat, is generally not followed by a compensatory pause. An atrial premature beat can occur in the patient with or without heart disease. It is usually insignificant, except when it precedes the onset of a tachydysrhythmia. Acceleration of the heart rate as produced by the intravenous administration of atropine usually abolishes atrial premature beats. Quinidine is effective in the rare patient who requires chronic suppression of atrial premature beats.

Paroxysmal Supraventricular Tachycardia

Paroxysmal supraventricular tachycardia (atrial or junctional) is characterized by sudden onset and termination. The initiating event is often a supraventricular premature beat.[28,29] The cardiac rhythm is absolutely regular, at a rate of 130 to 220 beats·min^{-1}. Paroxysmal supraventricular tachycardia is commonly seen in patients with a pre-excitation syndrome and in association with congenital abnormalities such as atrial septal defect and Ebstein's anomaly of the tricuspid valve. Paroxysmal supraventricular tachycardia is usually well tolerated, but occasionally it may precipitate congestive heart failure or hypotension. Polyuria is common during this dysrhythmia.

Treatment

Initial treatment of paroxysmal supraventricular tachycardia consists of maneuvers to increase vagal tone, particularly carotid sinus massage. The carotid sinus is located below the site of maximum pulsation of the carotid artery in the neck, usually immediately lateral to the thyroid cartilage. In the absence of detectable carotid bruits by auscultation, firm external pressure is applied over the carotid sinus for 10 to 20 seconds during constant monitoring of the ECG. Application of pressure over the right carotid sinus is more likely to be successful than is compression applied over the left carotid sinus. Under no circumstances should both carotid sinuses be compressed simultaneously. Additional vagal maneuvers include stimulation of the posterior pharynx or performance of a Valsalva maneuver.

If vagal maneuvers fail to terminate supraventricular tachycardia promptly, pharmacologic treatment or electrical cardioversion is necessary. In this regard, adenosine (3 to 12 mg IV) is useful for conversion of paroxysmal supraventricular tachycardia, including that associated with accessory pathways to normal sinus rhythm. Verapamil (75 to 150 μg·kg^{-1} IV, over 1 to 3 minutes) produces conversion to normal sinus rhythm, usually within 10 minutes. Esmolol as a rapid injection (1 to 2 mg·kg^{-1} IV) and/or continuous infusion (100 to 300 μg·kg^{-1}·min^{-1} IV) may be effective in slowing the heart rate.[30,31] Electrical cardioversion is the initial treatment in the patient in whom paroxysmal supraventricular tachycardia produces hypotension or angina pectoris. Long-term suppression of this dysrhythmia is achieved with drugs (verapamil, digitalis, beta antagonists, quinidine, procainamide) or by electrical ablation of the AV node plus placement of a permanent artificial cardiac pacemaker.

Paroxysmal supraventricular tachycardia with varying degrees of AV heart block is most often due to digitalis toxicity, especially in the patient with chronic obstructive pulmonary disease. In this situation, carotid sinus massage has no beneficial effect and may even increase the degree of AV block. Treatment includes normalization of the plasma potassium concentration and administration of phenytoin (100 mg IV, over 5 minutes to a maximum of about 600 mg). Treatment of digitalis-induced supraventricular tachycardia with electrical cardioversion can lead to the development of ventricular dysrhythmias.

Atrial Flutter

Atrial flutter is characterized on the ECG by an absolutely regular atrial rate at 250 to 320 beats·min^{-1} with varying degrees of AV block, often 2:1. The baseline of the ECG reveals flutter waves (F waves), resulting in a sawtooth pattern. This dysrhythmia differs from paroxysmal supraventricular tachycardia in that the atrial rate is faster and carotid sinus massage is ineffective or increases the degree of AV block. Initial treatment of this dysrhythmia is often with digoxin (0.25 to 0.75 mg IV) with or without a beta antagonist or verapamil. If drug therapy is not promptly effective, electrical cardioversion is usually effective. Chronic suppression of this dysrhythmia is often with digoxin combined, if necessary, with quinidine or procainamide.

Atrial Fibrillation

Atrial fibrillation is the most common sustained cardiac dysrhythmia, present in about 0.4% of all Americans and in approximately 10% of the population older than 60 years of age. This dysrhythmia is characterized on the ECG as totally chaotic atrial activity at a rate of 350 to 500 beats·min^{-1}, with a corresponding irregular but slower ventricular response. In the absence of treatment designed to slow conduction of the cardiac impulse through the AV node, the ventricular response can be greater than 140 beats·min^{-1}. P waves are not discernible on the ECG. Aberrant conduction of a beat with the configuration of RBBB (Ashman's phenomenon) may be confused with a ventricular premature beat. This is an important distinction, since digitalis toxicity may be manifested initially as a ventricular dysrhythmia. The absence of a synchronized atrial contraction combined with a rapid ventricular response rate can decrease cardiac output to the point of congestive heart failure, in some patients. An increased incidence of systemic embolization reflects the formation of thrombi in the atria due to stasis of blood in these cardiac chambers, associated with loss of a coordinated atrial contraction. Atrial fibrillation is frequently part of the sick sinus syndrome, is common in the patient with mitral valve or ischemic heart disease, and is not infrequent after thoracic or cardiac surgery.

Treatment

Initial treatment of atrial fibrillation is often with drugs (digitalis compounds, beta antagonists, calcium entry blockers) intended to slow the ventricular response rate by blocking conduction of cardiac impulses in an anterograde direction through the AV node.[32] In the past, digoxin (0.25 to 0.75 mg IV) was administered for this purpose, but it has been partially replaced by the faster-acting beta antagonists and calcium entry blockers. Verapamil (75 to 150 μg·kg^{-1} IV) administered over about 5 minutes promptly slows the heart rate, but the response is transient and control of the ventricular response rate is usually lost within 90 minutes. Verapamil also has negative inotropic effects and may aggravate congestive heart failure. Diltiazem administered intravenously is an alternative to verapamil when negative inotropic effects are considered hazardous. A beta antagonist, such as esmolol, administered most often as a continuous intravenous infusion, may also be selected to slow the ventricular response rate. A beta antagonist will likely have additive effects with digoxin. An alternative to initial drug therapy designed to slow the ventricular response rate in the presence of atrial fibrillation is electrical cardioversion. The principal disadvantage of electrical cardioversion is the need for general anesthesia. Anticoagulation is recommended to decrease the risk of emboli at the time of cardioversion.

Procainamide has been used to restore sinus rhythm in patients with atrial fibrillation of recent onset. When restoration of normal sinus rhythm is not urgent, oral therapy, most often with quinidine, is a consideration. Quinidine is also useful for maintaining normal sinus rhythm after successful cardioversion.

For patients with disabling symptoms of atrial fibrillation that cannot be controlled with drug therapy, surgical or radiofrequency catheter-induced ablation of the AV node is effective therapy. The irreversible nature of this procedure and the need for permanent artificial cardiac pacing limit the application of this approach. Alternatively, surgical procedures are being developed that maintain normal sinus rhythm by connecting the SA node to the AV node by a corridor of tissue (atrial corridor procedure) that electrically isolates the conduction system from the remainder of the atrium. The "maze procedure" involves making multiple small incisions in the atrium to disrupt pathways that lead to the development of reentrant cardiac impulses that may lead to atrial fibrillation.[33]

Junctional Rhythm

Junctional (nodal) rhythm is due to the activity of an ectopic cardiac pacemaker in the tissues surrounding the AV node. The cardiac impulse initiated by this pacemaker travels to the ventricles in a normal manner but is also conducted retrograde into the atria. Depending on the site of the junctional pacemaker, the P wave (1) precedes the QRS complex, but the P-R interval is less than 0.1 second; (2) follows the QRS complex; or (3) is obscured by the QRS complex. A junctional rhythm leading to decreased cardiac output and blood pressure is not infrequent during general anesthesia, especially when halothane is being administered. Intravenous administration of atropine is the initial treatment for a hemodynamically significant junctional rhythm.

Wandering Atrial Pacemaker

The wandering atrial pacemaker reflects the presence of multiple atrial ectopic pacemakers. The ECG shows P waves with different configurations, and the P-R intervals vary with each QRS complex. Treatment is necessary only when the loss of a coordinated atrial contraction leads to decreased blood pressure; when this occurs, intravenous administration of atropine is usually effective.

Ventricular Premature Beats

Ventricular premature beats arise from single (unifocal) or multiple (multifocal) ectopic cardiac pacemaker sites located below the AV node. Characteristic findings on the ECG serve to identify a ventricular premature beat (Table 4-11). A vul-

Table 4-11. Characteristic Appearance of a Ventricular Premature Beat on the Electrocardiogram

Premature occurrence
Absence of a P wave preceding the QRS complex
Wide and often bizarre appearing QRS complex
ST segment in a direction opposite to the QRS complex
Inverted T wave
Compensatory pause after the premature beat

Table 4-12. Conditions Associated With the Appearance of Ventricular Premature Beats

Normal heart
Arterial hypoxemia
Myocardial ischemia
Myocardial infarction
Myocarditis
Sympathetic nervous system activation
Hypokalemia
Hypomagnesemia
Digitalis toxicity
Caffeine
Cocaine
Alcohol
Mechanical irritation (central venous or pulmonary artery catheter)

nerable period exists in diastole, corresponding to the relative refractory period of the cardiac action potential (roughly the middle third of the T wave) (R-on-T phenomena), during which time a ventricular premature beat may initiate repetitive ventricular responses, including ventricular tachycardia or ventricular fibrillation (Fig. 4-2). Ventricular premature beats may occur in the patient without heart disease, especially with advancing age; nevertheless, they most often reflect a cardiac abnormality (Table 4-12). For example, ventricular premature beats occur in as many as 95% of patients with an acute myocardial infarction. In the patient with chronic myocardial ischemia, the presence of ventricular premature beats is directly correlated with the severity of ischemic heart disease and left ventricular dysfunction. The most common conditions in which ventricular premature beats predispose to life-threatening ventricular dysrhythmias include myocardial ischemia, valvular heart disease causing pressure or volume overload on the ventricles, cardiomyopathies, a prolonged Q-T interval on the ECG, and the presence of electrolyte abnormalities, especially hypokalemia. Typically, benign ventricular premature beats tend to disappear with exercise, whereas an increase in frequency with exercise is often considered to reflect underlying cardiac disease.

Treatment

Ventricular premature beats should be treated when they are frequent (more than 6 beats·min^{-1}), are multifocal, occur in salvos of three or more, or take place during the vulnerable period of the T wave (R-on-T phenomena), as these characteristics are associated with an increased incidence of ventricular tachycardia and fibrillation. The first step in the treatment of ventricular premature beats is elimination of the underlying cause such as arterial hypoxemia or other events associated with excessive sympathetic nervous system activity. If ventricular premature beats persist despite correction of the underlying cause, or are hemodynamically significant, the initial drug therapy of choice is administration of lidocaine (1 to 2 mg·kg^{-1} IV). This initial dose of lidocaine may be followed with a continuous infusion (1 to 4 mg·min^{-1} IV), to maintain a therapeutic blood level and continued suppression of the ectopic ventricular pacemaker. Lidocaine is not effective in suppressing ventricular premature beats due to mechanical irritation of the heart, as by an intracardiac catheter. Chronic suppression of ventricular premature beats may be achieved with several drugs, including quinidine, procainamide, disopyramide, and amiodarone (Table 4-3).

Ventricular Tachycardia

Ventricular tachycardia is defined as three or more consecutive ventricular premature beats at a calculated heart rate of greater than 120 beats·min^{-1}. The QRS complexes on the ECG are widened, reflecting aberrant intraventricular conduction of the cardiac impulse, and there are no discernible P waves. Without the aid of His bundle electrocardiography, it may be difficult to distinguish paroxysmal supraventricular tachycardia with aberrant conduction from reentrant ventricular tachycardia. Ventricular tachycardia is common after an acute myocardial infarction and in the presence of inflammatory or infectious diseases of the heart. Digitalis toxicity may be manifested as ventricular tachycardia. Torsade de pointes is an unusual form of ventricular tachycardia that is initiated by a ventricular premature beat in the setting of abnormal ventricular repolarization characterized by prolongation of the Q-T interval on the ECG (see the section, Prolonged Q-T Interval Syndrome).

Treatment

Treatment of hemodynamically significant ventricular tachycardia consists of prompt electrical cardioversion. If ventricular tachycardia is well tolerated, it is acceptable to use lidocaine (1 to 2 mg·kg^{-1} IV) as a rapid injection followed by a continuous infusion (1 to 4 mg·min^{-1} IV), to maintain an effective plasma concentration. Procainamide (100 mg IV every 2 minutes, to a maximum dose of 2 g) is also effective in converting this dysrhythmia to a supraventricular rhythm. When lidocaine and procainamide are ineffective, bretylium (5 mg·kg^{-1} IV) may be effective. Surgical resection of endocardium using electrode catheter-mapping studies may be successful in removing the ectopic focus (often in scar tissue or a ventricular aneurysm) that is the site of initiation of ventricular tachycardia.

Ventricular Fibrillation

Ventricular fibrillation is characterized by chaotic asynchronous contraction of the ventricles with no visible QRS complexes on the ECG. There is no effective associated stroke volume, emphasizing the need for prompt institution of cardiopulmonary resuscitation. Electrical defibrillation is the only effective treatment for converting ventricular fibrillation to a rhythm capable of generating a spontaneous cardiac output. This electrical treatment should be instituted as soon as possible, as cardiac output, coronary blood flow, and cerebral blood flow are very low despite properly performed external cardiac compression. For example, cerebral blood flow and coronary blood flow may be less than 10% of normal during external cardiac compression.[34] When ventricular fibrillation is refractory to treatment, intravenous injection of lidocaine or bretylium may improve the response to electrical defibrillation.

Automatic Implantable Cardioverter Defibrillator

Recurrent ventricular tachycardia or ventricular fibrillation that can result in sudden death in the survivor of cardiac arrest may be treated with an automatic implantable cardioverter defibrillator (AICD) that senses the onset of these ventricular dysrhythmias and delivers a synchronized 25-joule electrical discharge.[35] Electrophysiologic testing is required before implantation of an AICD, to demonstrate the presence of inducible ventricular tachycardia or ventricular fibrillation that is unresponsive to antidysrhythmic drug therapy. Implantation of an AICD requires general anesthesia for surgical placement of epicardial electrodes, demonstration that the ventricular dysrhythmia can be induced and electrically converted, and placement of the pulse generator in a subcutaneous periumbilical pocket. Periodic follow-up with the aid of a magnet determines the number of shocks that have been delivered to the patient, the battery strength, the status of the pulse generator, and the integrity of the sensing function.

PRE-EXCITATION SYNDROMES

Pre-excitation syndromes are characterized by premature activation of a portion of the ventricles by a cardiac impulse traveling in an accessory (anomalous) pathway that bypasses the AV node. This accessory pathway functions as an electrically active muscular bridge. In the absence of the usual delay in conduction of the cardiac impulse across the AV node, activation of the ventricles occurs earlier than when the cardiac impulse reaches the ventricles by the usual internodal pathway. The accessory pathways providing this abnormal electrical continuity between the atria and ventricles are congenital, most likely reflecting remnants of fetal atrioventricular muscular connections left in place by incomplete development of the annulus fibrosis. It is estimated that these accessory tracts are present in 0.1% to 0.3% of the population.[36] By far, the most common accessory pathway is an atrioventricular pathway (Kent's bundle). The other abnormal connections are

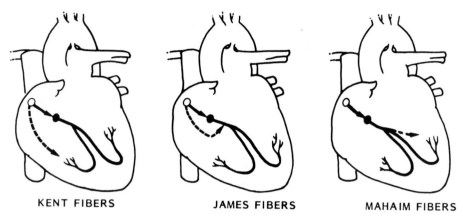

KENT FIBERS   JAMES FIBERS   MAHAIM FIBERS

Fig. 4-4. Schematic diagram of the three most common accessory atrioventricular conduction pathways associated with pre-excitation syndromes. Kent fibers bridge the atrium and ventricle without passing through the atrioventricular node. James fibers bypass the atrioventricular node and attach to the bundle of His. Mahaim fibers shunt cardiac impulses from the bundle of His or either bundle branch into the intraventricular septal myocardium. Clear circle, sinoatrial node; solid circle, atrioventricular node.

rare; their demonstration requires sophisticated intracardiac stimulation techniques and recordings (Fig. 4-4, Table 4-13). The most common cardiac dysrhythmias in these patients are paroxysmal supraventricular tachycardia, atrial fibrillation, and atrial flutter. These dysrhythmias are generally sporadic and well tolerated because they occur in the young patient where heart is otherwise normal. At times, however, these dysrhythmias are disabling, and sudden death is possible.[37]

Wolff-Parkinson-White Syndrome

Wolff-Parkinson-White (WPW) syndrome is the most common of the pre-excitation syndromes, reflecting conduction of the cardiac impulse simultaneously from the SA node down a normal conduction pathway through the AV node and through an accessory pathway (Kent's bundle) that bypasses the AV node (Fig. 4-4). The absence of a physiologic delay in the AV node

for the cardiac impulse that travels along Kent's bundle is manifested on the ECG as a short P-R interval (less than 0.12 second), followed by a wide QRS complex (greater than 0.12 second) and a delta wave. The wide QRS complex and delta wave reflect the fact that ventricular excitation is a composite of cardiac impulses conducted by a normal and accessory pathway. The delta wave is caused by early activation of the ventricle by a cardiac impulse traveling through an accessory pathway. Paroxysmal supraventricular tachycardia is the most frequent cardiac dysrhythmia associated with WPW syndrome. Ebstein's malformation of the tricuspid valve is present in 5% to 10% of patients with WPW syndrome (see Chapter 3). Atrial septal defect may also be associated with the WPW syndrome. In extreme cases, syncope or congestive heart failure, or both, result from the rapid heart rate. The incidence of sudden death in WPW syndrome is reported to be 1 in 700 to 1 in 1000.[38,39] The first manifestation of WPW

Table 4-13. Pathophysiology of Pre-excitation Syndromes

Nomenclature	Accessory Pathway Connections	Electrocardiographic Manifestations
Kent's bundle (accessory atrioventricular pathway; Wolff-Parkinson-White syndrome)	Atrium to ventricle	Short P-R interval (<0.12 sec) Wide QRS complex (>0.12 sec) Delta wave
James fibers (intranodal bypass tract, Lown-Ganong-Levine syndrome)	Intranodal bypass	Short P-R interval Normal QRS complex No delta wave
Mahaim fiber (nodoventricular or fasciculoventricular pathway)	Atrioventricular node to ventricle His bundle or bundle branch to ventricle	Normal to short P-R interval Wide QRS complex Delta wave

syndrome in 12% of patients is cardiac arrest.[40] The first manifestation of WPW syndrome may also appear during the perioperative period.[41]

Treatment

The initial treatment in the patient with WPW syndrome who is experiencing the abrupt onset of supraventricular tachycardia is performance of maneuvers designed to increase parasympathetic nervous system activity at the heart[36,42] (Table 4-14). These maneuvers should be performed promptly, as any delay is likely to be associated with increasing sympathetic nervous system activity and a decreased likelihood that vagal stimulation will be successful. If vagal stimulation fails to terminate the supraventricular tachycardia, the intravenous injection of a drug that abruptly prolongs the refractory period of the AV node (adenosine) or that lengthens the refractory period of the accessory pathways (procainamide) should be considered.[36,42] Electrical pacing or cardioversion is rarely required. An increased incidence of asystole may occur in the patient treated with verapamil and a beta antagonist, followed by cardioversion, emphasizing the importance of having an artificial cardiac pacemaker available. To prevent recurrent supraventricular tachycardia, a drug, such as amiodarone, that depresses conduction of the cardiac impulse and that increases the relative refractory period in both the AV node and accessory pathways is often effective. The most effective drug for prophylaxis is often determined by trial and error.

Initial treatment of atrial fibrillation in the patient with WPW syndrome is influenced by the ventricular response rate and hemodynamic consequences of the cardiac dysrhythmia[32,36,42] (Table 4-14). Electrical cardioversion is necessary if a rapid ventricular response during atrial fibrillation results in life-threatening hypotension. If atrial fibrillation is tolerated, a drug that prolongs the refractory period of the accessory pathways

(procainamide, quinidine, encainide) is administered. Verapamil or a digitalis preparation may decrease the relative refractory period of accessory pathways responsible for atrial fibrillation, resulting in an increased ventricular response rate. Likewise, increased sympathetic nervous system activity after the onset of atrial fibrillation tends to decrease the refractory periods of accessory pathways. Prophylaxis against recurrence of atrial fibrillation in the patient with WPW syndrome is with a drug that lengthens the refractory period of accessory pathways, often combined with a beta antagonist.

Treatment options for the patient with WPW syndrome who is resistant to medical management of life-threatening cardiac dysrhythmias includes antidysrhythmic surgery (division or cryoablation of accessory pathways as located by endocardial or epicardial electrophysiologic mapping) or catheter ablation techniques.[43] Antidysrhythmic surgery, while likely to be curative, requires a median sternotomy and often the use of cardiopulmonary bypass. Radiofrequency current is highly effective in ablating accessory pathways with low morbidity and mortality.[44,45] As an energy source, radiofrequency current produces a discrete lesion without causing hemodynamic effects, cardiac dysrhythmias, or neuromuscular stimulation, thereby eliminating the need for general anesthesia. Mapping studies have shown that the most common accessory pathways are those connecting the left atrium with the left ventricle.

Management of Anesthesia

The goal during management of anesthesia in the patient with WPW syndrome is to avoid any event (increased sympathetic nervous system activity, hypovolemia) or drug (digoxin) that would enhance conduction of the cardiac impulse through the accessory pathways.[46] All cardiac antidysrhythmic drugs should be continued throughout the perioperative period. Logic would suggest the avoidance of preoperative medications that are known to increase heart rate. Although atropine has been used in preoperative medication without adverse heart rate responses, scopolamine or glycopyrrolate may be equally acceptable choices, if administration of an anticholinergic drug is deemed necessary. Reduction of anxiety with preoperative medication is desirable, but no specific drug has proved superior.

Induction of anesthesia can be achieved with a variety of drugs (barbiturates, benzodiazepines, opioids) administered intravenously.[47–49] Droperidol increases the refractory period of accessory pathways, but the large dose (200 to 600 $\mu g \cdot kg^{-1}$ IV) required renders this a clinically impractical use of the drug[49] (Fig. 4-5). Thiopental has been alleged to increase aberrant conduction of the cardiac impulse, but this has not been susbstantiated by clinical use of the drug. The electrophysiologic effects of propofol, etomidate, and ketamine have not been determined, and clinical experience with these drugs in the patient with WPW syndrome is too limited

Table 4-14. Management of Cardiac Dysrhythmias in the Patient With Wolff-Parkinson-White Syndrome

Paroxysmal Supraventricular Tachycardia
  Vagal maneuvers
    Valsalva
    Gag reflex (finger in the throat)
    Immersion of face in cold water (diving reflex)
  Adenosine 3–12 mg IV
  Verapamil 2.5–10 mg IV
  Esmolol 50–100 mg IV
  Procainamide 500 mg IV
  Artificial cardiac (overdrive) pacing (transvenous)
  Electrical cardioversion

Atrial Fibrillation
  Electrical cardioversion (hemodynamically unstable)
  Procainamide (hemodynamically stable)

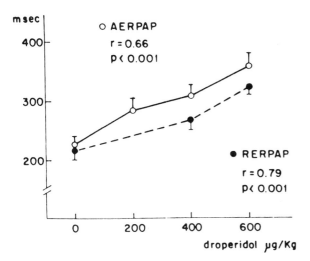

Fig. 4-5. Droperidol produces dose-dependent prolongation of the antegrade effective refractory period of accessory pathways (From Gomez-Arnau J, Marques-Montes J, Avello F. Fentanyl and droperidol effects on the refractoriness of the accessory pathway in the Wolff-Parkinson-White syndrome. Anesthesiology 1983;58:307–13, with permission.)

for a recommendation. Sympathomimetic stimulating effects of ketamine would detract from its use in the patient with WPW syndrome.

Intubation of the trachea and maintenance of anesthesia should be achieved with drugs selected to minimize the likelihood of increased sympathetic nervous system activity, as may occur in response to direct laryngoscopy or surgical stimulation. Volatile anesthetics in appropriate concentrations decrease sympathetic nervous system activity and also depress conduction of the cardiac impulse through accessory pathways.[50,51] Indeed, nitrous oxide combined with a volatile anesthetic has been administered without incident to patients with WPW syndrome.[47–49,52] Concentrations of a volatile anesthetic sufficient to prevent sympathetic nervous system responses produced by intense stimulation are recommended. In this regard, it seems logical to establish an adequate depth of anesthesia with either a volatile drug or injected drug, or both, before intubation of the trachea is attempted.

Succinylcholine has been used without incident, although the selection of a muscle relaxant lacking significant cardiovascular side effects would seem logical. Pancuronium has a vagolytic effect and increases the rate of cardiac impulse conduction through the AV node, and possibly through the accessory pathways.[53] Pharmacologic antagonism of a nondepolarizing muscle relaxant using an anticholinesterase drug should not introduce a risk since, historically, edrophonium, has been used to treat supraventricular tachycardia. Conceivably, a large intravenous dose of an anticholinergic drug, as combined with the anticholinesterase drug, could increase conduction of the cardiac impulse through the SA and AV node, placing the patient with WPW syndrome at increased risk of atrial tachydysrhythmia. The decision to antagonize a nondepolarizing muscle relaxant pharmacologically with an anticholinesterase-anticholinergic drug combination must be individualized, as clinical experience is too limited to offer a recommendation.

The degree of invasive monitoring is determined by the complexity of the surgery and the presence of concomitant cardiac disease. An intra-arterial catheter is often useful, whereas monitoring of cardiac filling pressures is usually not required for noncardiac surgery. Indeed, placement of a central venous or pulmonary artery catheter could theoretically predispose to an atrial tachydysrhythmia. Nevertheless, in selected patients, a pulmonary artery catheter with the ability to deliver artificial cardiac pacing may be indicated. Prompt electrical cardioversion and artificial cardiac pacing should be immediately available. Drugs known to be effective in the management of acute atrial tachydysrhythmias should be prepared and be rapidly available (Table 4-14). Maintenance of normothermia is especially important when electrophysiologic mapping is planned.

Lown-Ganong-Levine Syndrome

Lown-Ganong-Levine syndrome is due to accessory pathways designated as the James fibers. These fibers bypass the AV node and insert directly into the bundle of His (Fig. 4-4). As a result, the normal physiologic delay in conduction of the cardiac impulse at the AV node is absent. This syndrome is characterized on the ECG by a short P-R interval and a normal-appearing QRS complex, without a delta wave. Atrial flutter or atrial fibrillation is the cardiac dysrhythmia most often associated with this syndrome, although these patients are frequently asymptomatic. Treatment and management of anesthesia is the same as described for the patient with the WPW syndrome.

Mahaim Pathway

The Mahaim pathway is a variant of the pre-excitation syndrome, characterized by a normal to slightly short P-R interval, wide QRS complex, and delta wave on the ECG. This pattern may be misdiagnosed as a bundle branch block pattern on the ECG. This syndrome results from conduction of the cardiac impulse over accessory pathways known as Mahaim fibers, which arise below the AV node and insert directly into ventricular muscle (Fig. 4-4). Treatment and management of anesthesia is the same as described for the patient with the WPW syndrome.

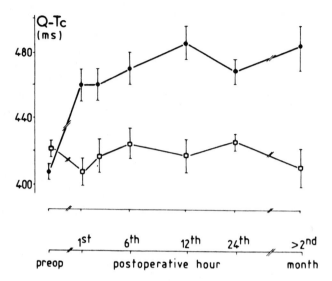

Fig. 4-6. Corrected Q-T intervals (Q-Tc) in milliseconds were prolonged after right radical neck dissections (solid symbols) but not after left radical neck dissections (clear symbols). Mean ± SE. (From Otenni JC, Pottecher T, Bronner G, Flesch H, Diebolt JR. Prolongation of the Q-T interval and sudden cardiac arrest following right radical neck dissection. Anesthesiology 1983;59: 358–61, with persmission.)

PROLONGED Q-T INTERVAL SYNDROME

Prolonged Q-T interval syndrome can be congenital (Jervell and Lange-Nielsen syndrome when nerve deafness is present and Romano-Ward without deafness) or acquired (quinidine, disopyramide, tricyclic antidepressants, subarachnoid hemorrhage, hypokalemia, hypomagnesemia). Right radical neck dissection, but not left neck dissection, may result in an increase in the Q-T interval and cardiac dysrhythmias in the postoperative period[54] (Fig. 4-6). The diagnostic feature is a prolonged Q-T interval (greater than 0.44 second) on the ECG, even when corrected for heart rate. Syncope associated with the prolonged Q-T interval syndrome may be confused with a seizure disorder if an ECG is not obtained. A syncopal attack may be triggered by sympathetic nervous system stimulation, as produced by exercise or fright. Occasional sudden death in a patient with this syndrome is most likely due to ventricular tachycardia.[55] The most accepted congenital mechanism for the prolonged Q-T interval syndrome is asymmetric sympathetic nervous system innervation of the heart caused by increased left cardiac sympathetic nerve activity or decreased right cardiac sympathetic nerve activity. Delayed repolarization of the ventricle as reflected by a prolonged Q-T interval on the ECG increases the susceptibility of the heart to the development of ventricular dysrhythmias.

Treatment

Treatment of the prolonged Q-T interval syndrome is empirical, often directed at pharmacologic and surgical attempts to decrease cardiac sympathetic nervous system activity. For example, treatment with a beta antagonist shortens the Q-T interval on the ECG of the affected patient, decreases sympathetic nervous system activity, and increases the threshold for ventricular fibrillation. In the absence of a response to drug therapy, a left stellate ganglion block may be considered for temporary abolishment of the sympathetic nervous system imbalance that exists between the left and right cardiac nerves.[56] A successful stellate ganglion block is indicated by a shortening of the Q-T interval on the ECG. The effect of a left stellate ganglion block is only transient; therefore, it is used only to control acute cardiac dysrhythmias, to assess whether surgical ganglionectomy will be successful, and as preoperative preparation of the patient not on medical treatment requiring emergency surgery.

Management of Anesthesia

A preoperative ECG to rule out prolonged Q-T interval syndrome is useful in a child with congenital deafness or in a family with a history of sudden death, as the physical examination is likely to be otherwise unremarkable. Likewise, members of the family of afflicted patients should be evaluated by ECG.

General anesthesia may trigger a life-threatening ventricular dysrhythmia and cardiac arrest in the patient with prolonged Q-T interval syndrome.[55,57] For this reason, consideration may be given to establishment of beta blockade or performance of a prophylactic left stellate ganglion block prior to induction of anesthesia in the patient believed to be at risk. Events known to prolong the Q-T interval, such as an abrupt increase in sympathetic nervous system activity associated with preoperative anxiety or with noxious stimulation that can occur intraoperatively and acute hypokalemia due to iatrogenic hyperventilation of the lungs, are avoided. In this regard, it seems logical to provide pharmacologic preoperative medication to decrease anxiety. Inclusion of an anticholinergic drug in the preoperative medication, however, is questionable, in view of the possible alteration in the balance of sympathetic and parasympathetic nervous system activity that can accompany the administration of such a drug.

Induction of anesthesia has been safely accomplished with thiopental despite the ability of this drug to prolong the Q-T interval on the ECG of an otherwise normal patient. Ketamine is an unlikely selection because of its sympathetic nervous system-stimulating effects. Intubation of the trachea is attempted only after establishment of a depth of anesthesia deemed sufficient to blunt the effect of noxious stimulation has been established. Prior administration of an opioid or a volatile anesthetic, or both, may facilitate this goal. The choice of volatile anesthetic is influenced not only by the ability of the anesthetic to suppress sympathetic nervous system responses to painful stimulation but also by the necessity to avoid sensitizing the heart to the arrhythmogenic effects of catecholamines. In this regard, isoflurane, enflurane, or desflurane with or without nitrous oxide are acceptable.[55,57,58] Halothane is an unlikely selection, in view of its ability to increase the likelihood of cardiac dysrhythmias in the presence of elevated plasma concentrations of epinephrine. Extubation of the trachea may be considered when the patient is still anesthetized, to minimize sympathetic nervous system stimulation associated with this event.

The choice of muscle relaxant is guided by the desire to avoid any drug that could stimulate the sympathetic nervous system or evoke the release of histamine. Succinylcholine has been administered without incident to at-risk patients. Pancuronium has been administered without incident despite its sympathomimetic activity. Pharmacologic reversal of nondepolarizing neuromuscular blockade does not seem to have an adverse effect on the Q-T interval in these patients.

An electrical defibrillator should be promptly available, as the likelihood of perioperative ventricular fibrillation is increased. A beta antagonist (esmolol, propranolol) is useful for the treatment of an acute ventricular dysrhythmia that develops intraoperatively. Lidocaine, procainamide, and quinidine are not recommended for management of an acute ventricular dysrhythmia in these patients, as these drugs prolong the Q-T interval on the ECG of normal patients.[54] Nevertheless, lidocaine was reported to be effective in reversing intraoperative ventricular tachycardia in a patient with prolonged Q-T interval syndrome. The ability of phenytoin to shorten the Q-T interval on the ECG is the rationale for administering this drug orally during the postoperative period.

REFERENCES

1. Akhtar M. Management of ventricular tachyarrhythmias. JAMA 1982;247:671–4
2. Campbell S, Barry J, Rebacca GS, et al. Active transient myocardial ischemia during daily life in asymptomatic patients with positive exercise tests and coronary artery disease. Am J Cardiol 1986;57:1010–6
3. Miller RD, Way WL, Katzung BG. The potentiation of neuromuscular blocking agents by quindine. Anesthesiology 1967;28:1036–41
4. Harrah MD, Way WL, Katzung BG. The interaction of d-tubocurarine with antiarrhythmic drugs. Anesthesiology 1970;33:406–10
5. Schulte-Sasse U, Hess W, Markschies-Harnung A, Tarnow J. Combined effects of halothane anesthesia and verapamil on systemic hemodynamics and left ventricular myocardial contractility in patients with ischemic heart disease. Anesth Analg 1984;63:791–8
6. Durant NN, Nguyen N, Katz R. Potentiation of neuromuscular blockade by verapamil. Anesthesiology 1984;60:298–303
7. Chassard D, George M, Guiraud M, et al. Relationship between preoperative amiodarone treatment and complications observed during anesthesia for valvular cardiac surgery. Can J Anaesth 1990;37:151–4
8. Dunn M, Alexander J, deSilva R, et al. Antithrombotic therapy in atrial fibrillation. Chest 1986;89:68S–72S
9. Zaidan JR. Pacemakers. Anesthesiology 1984;60:319–34
10. Kelly JS, Royster RL. Noninvasive transcutaneous cardiac pacing. Anesth Analg 1989;69:229–38
11. Mangar D, Atlas GM, Kane PG. Electrocautery-induced pacemaker malfunction during surgery. Can J Anaesth 1991;38:616–8
12. Domino KB, Smith TC. Electrocautery-induced reprogramming of a pacemaker using a precordial magnet. Anesth Analg 1983;62:609–12
13. Ducey JP, Fincher CW, Baysinger CL. Therapeutic suppression of a permanent ventricular pacemaker using a peripheral nerve stimulator. Anesthesiology 1991;75:533–6
14. Finer SR. Pacemaker failure on induction of anaesthesia. Br J Anaesth 1991;66:509–12
15. Thiagarajah S, Azar I, Agres M, Lear E. Pacemaker malfunction associated with positive-pressure ventilation. Anesthesiology 1983;58:565–6
16. Phibbs B, Friedman HS, Graboys TB, et al. Indications for pacing in the treatment of bradyarrhythmias. Report of an independent study group. JAMA 1984;252:1307–11
17. Mulcahy R, Hickey N, Mauser B. An etiology of bundle branch block. Br Heart J 1968;30:34–7

18. Rorie DK, Muldoon SM, Krabill DR. Transient bundle branch block occurring during anesthesia. Anesth Analg 1972;51:633–7

19. Pratila M, Pratilas V, Dimich I. Transient left-bundle branch block during anesthesia. Anesthesiology 1979;51:461–3

20. Edelman JD, Hurlbert BJ. Intermittent left bundle branch block during anesthesia. Anesth Analg 1981;59:628–30

21. Thomson IR, Dalton BC, Lappas DG, Lowenstein E. Right bundle-branch block and complete heart block caused by the Swan-Ganz catheter. Anesthesiology 1979;51:359–62

22. Rooney S-M, Goldiner PL, Muss E. Relationship of right bundle-branch block and marked left axis deviation to complete heart block during general anesthesia. Anesthesiology 1976;44:64–6

23. Venkataraman K, Madias JE, Hood WB. Indications for prophylactic preoperative insertion of pacemakers in patients with right bundle branch block and left anterior hemiblock. Chest 1975;68:501–6

24. Coriat P, Harari A, Ducardonet A, et al. Risk of advanced heart block during extradural anaesthesia in patients with right bundle branch block and left anterior hemiblock. Br J Anaesth 1981;53:545–8

25. Kreutz JM, Mazuzan JE. Sudden asystole in a marathon runner: The athletic heart syndrome and its anesthetic implications. Anesthesiology 1990;73:1266–8

26. Doyle DJ, Mark PWS. Reflex bradycardia during surgery. Can J Anaesth 1990;37:219–22

27. Fairfax AJ, Lambert CD, Latham A. Systemic embolism in chronic sinoatrial disorder. N Engl J Med 1976;295:190–6

28. Jones RM, Broadbent MP, Adams AP. Anaesthetic considerations in patients with paroxysmal supraventricular tachycardia. A review and report of cases. Anaesthesia 1984;39:307–13

29. Sprague DH, Mandel SD. Paroxysmal supraventricular tachycardia during anesthesia. Anesthesiology 1977;46:75–7

30. Oxorn D, Knox JWD, Hill J. Bolus doses of esmolol for the prevention of perioperative hypertension and tachycardia. Can J Anaesth 1990;37:206–9

31. Menkhaus PG, Reves JG, Kisson I, et al. Cardiovascular effects of esmolol in anesthetized humans. Anesth Analg 1985;64:327–34

32. Pritchett ELC. Management of atrial fibrillation. N Engl J Med 1992;326:1264–71

33. Cox JL, Boineau JP, Schuessler RB, et al. Successful surgical treatment of atrial fibrillation. Review and clinical update. JAMA 1991;266:1976–80

34. White BC, Wiegenstein JG, Winegar CD. Brain ischemic anoxia. Mechanisms of injury. JAMA 1984;251:1586–90

35. Goldsmith MF. Implanted defibrillators slash sudden death rate in study, thousands more may get them in future. JAMA 1991;266:3400–2

36. Wellens HJJ, Brugada P, Penn OC. The management of preexcitation syndromes. JAMA 1987;257:2325–33

37. Klein GJ, Bashore TM, Sellers TD, Pritchett ELC, Smith WW, Gallagher JJ. Ventricular fibrillation in the Wolff-Parkinson-White syndrome. N Engl J Med 1979;301:1080–5

38. Gallagher JJ, Pritchett ELC, Sealy WC, Kasell J, Wallace AG. The preexcitation syndrome. Prog Cardiovasc Dis 1978;20:285–327

39. Gillette PC. Concealed anomalous cardiac conduction pathways: A frequent cause of supraventricular tachycardia. Am J Cardiol 1977;40:848–54

40. Berkman NL, Lamb LE. The Wolff-Parkinson-White syndrome electrocardiogram: A follow-up study of 5 to 28 years. N Engl J Med 1968;278:492–4

41. Lubarsky D, Kaufman B, Turndorf H. Anesthesia unmasking benign Wolff-Parkinson-White syndrome. Anesth Analg 1989;68:172–4

42. Camm AJ, Garratt CJ. Adenosine and supraventricular tachycardia. N Engl J Med 1991;325:1621–9

43. Ruskin JN. Catheter ablation for supraventricular tachycardia. N Engl J Med 1991;324:1660–2

44. Jackman WM, Wang X, Friday KJ, et al. Catheter ablation of accessory atrioventricular pathways (Wolff-Parkinson-White syndrome) by radiofrequency current. N Engl J Med 1991;324:1605–11

45. Calkins H, Sousa J, El-Atassi R, et al. Diagnosis and cure of the Wolff-Parkinson-White syndrome or paroxysmal supraventricular tachycardias during a single electrophysiologic test. N Engl J Med 1991;324:1612–8

46. Irish CL, Murkin JM, Guiraudon GM. Anaesthetic management for surgical cryoablation of accessory conducting pathways; a review and report of 181 cases. Can J Anaesth 1988;35:634–40

47. vanderStarre PJA. Wolff-Parkinson-White syndrome during anesthesia. Anesthesiology 1978;48:369–72

48. Sadowski AR, Moyers JR. Anesthetic management of the Wolff-Parkinson-White syndrome. Anesthesiology 1979;51:553–6

49. Gomez-Arnau J, Marques-Montes J, Avello F. Fentanyl and droperidol effects on the refractoriness of the accessory pathway in the Wolff-Parkinson-White syndrome. Anesthesiology 1983;58:307–13

50. Sharpe JM, Murkin WB, Dobkowski C, et al. Halothane depresses conduction of normal and accessory pathways during surgery for Wolff-Parkinson-White syndrome. Anesth Analg 1990;70:S365

51. Dobkowski WB, Murkin JM, Sharpe MD, Sharma Yee R, Guiraudon GM. The effect of isoflurane on the normal AV conduction system and accessory pathways. Anesth Analg 1990;70:S86

52. Hunnington-Kiff JG. The Wolff-Parkinson-White syndrome and general anaesthesia. Br J Anaesth 1968;40:791–5

53. Ghea DG, Rozella BC, Raessler KL, et al. Pancuronium bromide enhances atrioventricular conduction in halothane anesthetized dogs. Anesthesiology 1977;46:342–5

54. Otteni JC, Pottecher T, Bronner G, Flesch H, Diebold JR. Prolongation of the Q-T interval and sudden cardiac arrest following right radical neck dissection. Anesthesiology 1983;59:358–61

55. Adu-Gyamfi Y, Said A, Chowdhary UM, Abomelha A, Sanyal SK. Anaesthetic-induced ventricular tachyarrhythmia in Jervell and Lange-Nielsen syndrome. Can J Anaesth 1991;38:345–6

56. Moss AJ. Prolonged QT interval syndromes. JAMA 1986;256:2985–8

57. Galloway PA, Glass PSA. Anesthetic implications of prolonged QT interval syndromes. Anesth Analg 1985;64:612–20

58. Wilton NCT, Hantler CB. Congenital long QT syndrome: Changes in QT interval during anesthesia with thiopental, vecuronium, fentanyl and isoflurane. Anesth Analg 1989;66:357–60

5

Hypertension

Hypertension is the most common circulatory derangement, affecting an estimated 60 million Americans.[1] Increased systemic blood pressure is a significant risk factor for the development of ischemic heart disease and is a major cause of congestive heart failure, renal failure, and cerebrovascular accident (stroke) (Fig. 5-1). Blood pressure is normally regulated by a series of feedback loops (baroreceptors) and by the secretion of vasoactive hormones (renin, angiotensin, aldosterone, catecholamines) (Fig. 5-2). Any derangement in this system can lead to hypertension. Essential (primary) hypertension accounts for more than 90% of afflicted patients and has no identifiable cause, whereas secondary hypertension has a demonstrable etiology (Table 5-1). In this regard, renal disease is the most common cause of secondary hypertension, whereas pheochromocytoma is a rare cause.

There is no critical level of blood pressure that appears to delineate excess risk; therefore, the definition of hypertension remains arbitrary. It is generally agreed that a systolic blood pressure greater than 160 mmHg or diastolic blood pressure greater than 90 mmHg, or both, constitutes hypertension, regardless of age.[2] Morbidity and mortality increase linearly with increasing levels of either systolic or diastolic blood pressure. The risk of myocardial infarction is increased in males with isolated systolic hypertension (greater than 160 mmHg)[3,4] (Fig. 5-3). The prevalence of hypertension increases progressively with age, with nearly two-thirds of persons older than 65 years of age exhibiting systolic or diastolic hypertension (greater than 160/90 mmHg)[3] (Fig. 5-4).

TREATMENT

Drug therapy is often recommended when diastolic blood pressure exceeds 90 mmHg, whereas isolated systolic hypertension (greater than 160 mmHg) may respond initially to nonpharmacologic therapy such as low sodium diet and weight loss.[2] Vigorous exercise and weight loss can significantly decrease systolic and diastolic blood pressure in some patients with borderline hypertension. When diastolic blood pressure exceeds 105 mmHg, aggressive therapy is indicated, as lowering the blood pressure decreases morbidity and mortality from myocardial infarction, congestive heart failure, stroke, and renal failure. Large clinical trials demonstrate that patients with diastolic blood pressures ranging from 90 to 104 mmHg benefit from treatment, with a decreased incidence of congestive heart failure and stroke. The indications for pharmacologic treatment of systolic hypertension in the absence of diastolic hypertension are less clear. The presence of risk factors for the development of cardiovascular complications (hypercholesterolemia, glucose intolerance, left ventricular hypertrophy, cigarette smoking) lowers the threshold at which the hypertensive patient should be treated.

Drugs

Drugs used for the treatment of hypertension include diuretics, angiotensin-converting enzyme (ACE) inhibitors, calcium entry blockers, vasodilators, and sympatholytics (Table 5-2). Initial drug therapy for hypertension may be with a diuretic, ACE inhibitor, or beta antagonist. Ventricular irritability may accompany diuretic-induced hypokalemia and is particularly undesirable in the patient who is receiving digitalis or who has ischemic heart disease. ACE inhibitors are useful as initial treatment of hypertension, being associated with minimal side effects and high patient compliance.[5] Hyperkalemia is a risk of treatment with these drugs, especially in the patient with renal insufficiency or in those being treated with potassium-sparing diuretics. Urticaria or angioedema occurs in less than 0.1% of patients treated with ACE inhibitors. However, it can cause dyspnea and upper airway obstruction, requiring prompt treatment with epinephrine. Single-drug therapy with a beta antagonist seems to be most effective in the patient younger than 40 years of age. A selective beta-1 antagonist such as atenolol is less likely to exacerbate obstructive airway disease or interfere with the beta-mediated response to hypoglycemia. Calcium entry blockers have been particularly useful in the treatment of hypertension in the elderly.

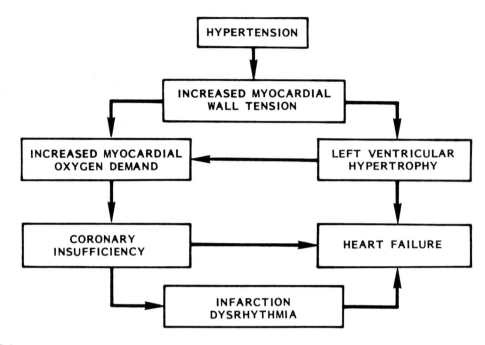

Fig. 5-1. Chronic increases in systemic blood pressure initiate a series of pathophysiologic changes that may culminate in congestive heart failure.

Combination drug therapy is often used based on the observation that the efficacy of a single drug is often offset by homeostatic compensation. For example, diuretics frequently evoke a compensatory increase in renin activity, presumably reflecting a depletion in intravascular fluid volume. Conversely, drugs that decrease sympathetic nervous system activity can lead to increased intravascular fluid volume. Vasodilators, which do not attenuate baroreceptor reflex activity, typically produce an increase in heart rate that tends to offset the blood pressure-lowering effects of these drugs. With this in mind, one can prescribe a combination of antihypertensive drugs that both lower blood pressure and offset undesirable compensatory responses associated with individual drugs.

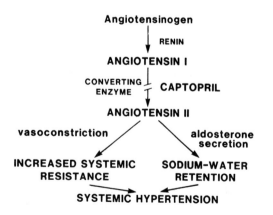

Fig. 5-2. Captopril competitively inhibits the activity of the converting enzyme that normally converts angiotensin I to angiotensin II. As a result, the formation of angiotensin II and subsequent events that can contribute to hypertension are attenuated.

Table 5-1. Causes of Secondary Hypertension

Etiology	Screening Test
Renal disease (pyelonephritis, glomerulonephritis, diabetic nephropathy, vascular disease)	Pyelogram Renin activity Angiography
Coarctation	Chest radiograph
Hyperadrenocorticism (Cushing's disease)	Plasma cortisol after dexamethasone suppression
Pheochromocytoma	Urine metanephrine or vanillylmandelic acid Clonidine suppression test Plasma catecholamines
Primary aldosteronism	Plasma and urine potassium
Drugs	Drug screen
Intracranial hypertension	

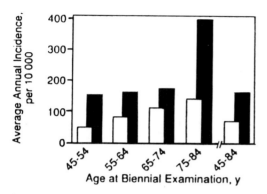

Fig. 5-3. Risk of myocardial infarction among males with (solid bars) and without (clear bars) systolic blood pressure greater than 160 mmHg. (From Tjoa HI, Kaplan NM. Treatment of hypertension in the elderly. JAMA 1990;264:1015–8, with permission.)

Furthermore, combination drug therapy permits maximum therapeutic effects with a decreased dose of a single drug. This approach decreases the likelihood of dose-related side effects. Nevertheless, it is estimated that one-half or more of all patients with mild hypertension can achieve a blood pressure of less than 140/90 mmHg with a single drug and more than 90% can be controlled with two drugs.[6]

MANAGEMENT OF ANESTHESIA

Considerations for the perioperative management of the patient with essential hypertension who is scheduled for elective or emergency surgery are outlined in Table 5-3. Despite

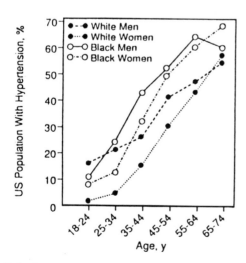

Fig. 5-4. Prevalence of hypertension (greater than 160/90 mmHg) among adult Americans. (From Tjoa HI, Kaplan NM. Treatment of hypertension in the elderly. JAMA 1990;264:1015–8, with permission.)

Table 5-2. Drugs Used in the Treatment of Hypertension

Diuretics
   Thiazides
   Potassium-sparing diuretics
   Combination of thiazide and potassium-sparing diuretic
   Loop diuretic

Angiotensin-Converting Enzyme Inhibitors
   Captopril
   Enalapril
   Lisinopril

Calcium Entry Blockers
   Diltiazem
   Nifedipine
   Verapamil

Vasodilators
   Hydralazine
   Minoxidil

Sympatholytics
   Beta antagonists
   Combined alpha and beta antagonist
     Labetalol
   Clonidine
   Guanabenz
   Methyldopa
   Guanadrel
   Prazosin

Table 5-3. Management of Anesthesia for the Hypertensive Patient

Preoperative Evaluation
   Determine adequacy of blood pressure control
   Review pharmacology of antihypertensive drugs
   Detect associated organ dysfunction
     Orthostatic hypotension
     Ischemic heart disease
     Cerebrovascular disease
     Peripheral vascular disease
     Renal dysfunction

Induction of Anesthesia
   Expect exaggerated blood pressure changes
   Perform short-duration laryngoscopy

Maintenance of Anesthesia
   Administer volatile anesthetic to control blood pressure
   Monitor for myocardial ischemia

Postoperative Management
   Anticipate hypertension
   Maintain intraoperative monitoring

earlier suggestions that antihypertensive drugs should be discontinued preoperatively, it is now accepted that drugs showing efficacy in controlling blood pressure in an individual patient should be continued throughout the perioperative period to ensure optimum medical control of blood pressure. Emergency surgery in the patient with uncontrolled hypertension introduces the added question of the safe level for maintenance of blood pressure during the perioperative period. In this situation, systemic blood pressure may be safely lowered to about 140/90 mmHg, assuming that this blood pressure is not associated with evidence of cerebral ischemia or renal dysfunction.

Preoperative Evaluation

Preoperative evaluation of the patient with essential hypertension should determine the adequacy of blood pressure control. Antihypertensive drug therapy that has rendered the patient normotensive preoperatively should be continued throughout the perioperative period. Ideally, hypertensive patients should be rendered normotensive before undergoing elective surgery. This recommendation is based on the observation that the incidence of hypotension and evidence of myocardial ischemia on the electrocardiogram during the maintenance of anesthesia is increased in the patient who remains hypertensive before the induction of anesthesia.[7-9] Furthermore, the decrease in blood pressure during anesthesia is likely to be greater in the hypertensive than in the normotensive patient.[10] An increase in blood pressure during the intraoperative period is more likely to occur in a patient with a history of hypertension regardless of the degree of blood pressure control before the induction of anesthesia[10] (Table 5-4).

Table 5-4. Risk of General Anesthesia and Elective Surgery in the Hypertensive Patient

Blood Pressure Status Before Operation	Incidence of Perioperative Hypertensive Episodes (%)	Incidence of Postoperative Cardiac Complications (%)
Normotensive	8[a]	11
Treated and rendered normotensive	27	24
Treated but remain hypertensive	25	7
Untreated and hypertensive	20	12

[a] $P < 0.5$ compared with other groups in same column.
(Data from Goldman L, Caldera DL. Risk of general anesthesia and elective operation in the hypertensive patient. Anesthesiology 1979; 50:285–92.)

There is no evidence, however, that the incidence of postoperative cardiac complications is increased when a hypertensive patient undergoes an elective operation, as long as the preoperative diastolic blood pressure does not exceed 110 mmHg[10] (Table 5-4). Nevertheless, in specific situations, such as the patient undergoing carotid endarterectomy, the co-existence of inadequately controlled hypertension may be associated with an increased incidence of neurologic deficits.[11] Furthermore, co-existing hypertension may increase the incidence of postoperative myocardial reinfarction in a patient with a prior history of myocardial infarction.[12] There is no evidence that antihypertensive drug therapy adversely alters the course or conduct of anesthesia.

It is not uncommon for the blood pressure taken on admission to the hospital to be elevated. Subsequent blood pressure recordings are often normal, and the initial elevated reading is regarded as a normal response to hospital admission. This subset of patients, however, are likely to display an exaggerated pressor response to direct laryngoscopy for intubation of the trachea and are more likely than other patients to experience perioperative myocardial ischemia or to require vasodilator therapy intraoperatively.[13] This subset of patients can be identified by preoperative review of the medical record.

It is important to review the pharmacology and potential side effects of the drugs being used to treat hypertension[14] (Table 5-5). Indeed, many drugs used in the treatment of essential hypertension interfere with autonomic nervous system function. Preoperatively, this may be manifested as orthostatic hypotension. During anesthesia, an exaggerated decrease in blood pressure as associated with blood loss, positive airway pressure, or a sudden change in body position could reflect impaired compensatory peripheral vascular vasoconstriction due to inhibitory effects of antihypertensive drugs on the sympathetic nervous system. Indeed, in animals, large doses of antihypertensive drugs attenuate the blood pressure response evoked by ephedrine.[15] Despite the possible presence of drug-induced impairment of sympathetic nervous system activity, there is reassuring evidence in patients, supported by clinical experience, that the administration of a vasopressor, such as ephedrine, results in predictable and acceptable responses in the treated patient.[16] Bradycardia may be a manifestation of selective impairment of sympathetic nervous system activity that results in a predominance of parasympathetic nervous system activity. There is no evidence, however, that heart rate responses to surgical stimulation or blood loss are absent in the treated patient. Likewise, clinical experience does not support the theoretical possibility that an exaggerated decrease in heart rate could occur when a drug that normally increases parasympathetic nervous system activity, such as an anticholinesterase agent, is administered during anesthesia. Sedation accompanying treatment with antihypertensive drugs may result in decreased anesthetic requirements during the intraoperative period. In this regard,

Table 5-5. Potential Side Effects of Antihypertensive Drugs

Thiazide Diuretics	
Hypokalemia	Hyperglycemia
Hypomagnesemia	Hypercholesterolemia
Hyperuricemia	Decreased lithium clearance
Hypercalcemia	Dermatitis
Alkalosis	Photosensitivity
Potassium-Sparing Diuretics	
Hyperkalemia	
Hyponatremia	
Megaloblastic anemia	
Dermatitis	
Angiotensin-Converting Enzyme Inhibitors	
Hyperkalemia	Fetal death
Proteinuria	Dermatitis
Cough	Angioedema
Beta Antagonists	
Congestive heart failure	Raynaud's phenomenon
Bradycardia	Sedation
Bronchospasm	Angina pectoris with abrupt
Masking of hypoglycemia	discontinuation
	Paresthesias
Calcium Entry Blockers	
Bradycardia	Weakness
Tachycardia	Hepatic dysfunction
Heart block	Syncope
Congestive heart failure	
Clonidine	
Sedation	Heart block
Orthostatic hypotension	Dry mouth
Rebound hypertension	Impaired glucose tolerance
Bradycardia	
Methyldopa	
Sedation	Positive Coombs test
Orthostatic hypotension	Exacerbation of parkinsonism
Rebound hypertension	
Hepatotoxicity	
Prazosin	
Sedation	
Weakness	
Orthostatic hypotension	
Tachycardia	
Hydralazine	
Tachycardia	
Lupus-like syndrome	
Fever	
Minoxidil	
Orthostatic hypotension	Sodium and water retention
Tachycardia	Hemodiluition
Congestive heart failure	Pericardial effusion
Hypertrichosis	Nonspecific T wave changes

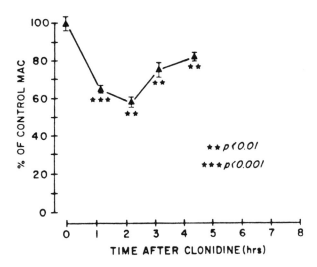

Fig. 5-5. Change in halothane MAC (mean ± SE) after administration of clonidine (5 μg·kg⁻¹ IV) to dogs. (From Bloor BC, Flacke WE. Reduction in halothane anesthetic requirement by clonidine, an alpha-adrenergic agonist. Anesth Analg 1982;61:741–5, with permission.)

clonidine is associated with a significantly decreased requirement for inhaled and injected anesthetics[17,18] (Fig. 5-5). Sudden withdrawal of central-acting antihypertensive drugs and beta antagonists can result in rebound hypertension. Rebound hypertension is most likely to occur in the patient receiving more than 1.2 mg of clonidine daily; it may occur before the induction of anesthesia, as well as after surgery, while still in the postanesthesia recovery room.[19,20] Antihypertensive drugs acting independent of the autonomic nervous system, such as ACE inhibitors, do not seem to be associated with rebound hypertension. A plasma potassium concentration of less than 3.5 mEq·L⁻¹ occurs in 20% to 40% of hypertensive patients treated with diuretics despite potassium supplementation. Nevertheless, this drug-induced hypokalemia has not been documented to increase the incidence of cardiac dysrhythmias in either the awake or anesthetized patient.[21,22] Hyperkalemia is a consideration in the patient treated with an ACE inhibitor who is also receiving potassium supplementation or experiencing renal dysfunction. Bradycardia, heart block, and congestive heart failure are risks of excessive beta blockade.

The presence of associated organ dysfunction (end-organ damage) is evaluated preoperatively by routine tests, including measurement of electrolytes, blood urea nitrogen, and creatinine, and the electrocardiogram. Incipient congestive heart failure is a consideration that must be evaluated preoperatively. The patient with essential hypertension should be presumed to have ischemic heart disease until proved otherwise.

Evidence of peripheral vascular disease may influence the placement site of an intra-arterial catheter for intraoperative monitoring of blood pressure. Symptoms of cerebrovascular disease may be reflected as dizziness or syncope with changes in head position, as may be necessary for direct laryngoscopy during intubation of the trachea and subsequent positioning for surgery. Essential hypertension is associated with a shift to the right of the curve for autoregulation of cerebral blood flow. This shift suggests that, in such cases, cerebral blood flow is more dependent on perfusion pressure than in the normotensive adult. Renal dysfunction, secondary to longstanding hypertension, places the patient at increased risk and signals a widespread hypertensive disease process.

Induction of Anesthesia

Induction of anesthesia with rapidly acting intravenous drugs is acceptable, recognizing that an exaggerated decrease in blood pressure may occur, particularly if hypertension is present preoperatively. This most likely reflects drug-induced peripheral vasodilation in the presence of a decreased intravascular fluid volume, as is likely in the presence of diastolic hypertension. Ketamine is rarely selected for induction of anesthesia in a hypertensive patient, as its circulatory stimulant effects could theoretically exaggerate blood pressure increases in response to painful stimulation.

Direct laryngoscopy and intubation of the trachea may result in exaggerated increases in blood pressure in the patient with a history of hypertension, even if the patient has been rendered normotensive before surgery.[8] Evidence of myocardial ischemia on the electrocardiogram of a patient with ischemic heart disease is most likely to occur in association with increases in blood pressure and heart rate that accompany the intubation sequence.[9,23] The increased incidence of myocardial ischemia is consistent with increased diastolic intracavitary pressure in the left ventricle that compresses subendocardial arteries, as well as increased myocardial oxygen requirements attributable to tachycardia. It is possible that drugs administered for the intravenous induction of anesthesia will not adequately or predictably suppress circulatory responses evoked by intubation of the trachea. For this reason, it may be prudent to increase the level of anesthesia with the inhalation of a volatile anesthetic or injection of an opioid (fentanyl 50 to 150 μg IV, sufentanil 10 to 30 μg IV) prior to initiating direct laryngoscopy. There are data suggesting that sympathetic nervous system responses to painful stimulation are not blocked until a concentration equivalent to about 1.5 MAC for the volatile anesthetic is established.[24] During the short period available during the typical anesthetic induction, it is unlikely that a 1.5 MAC of a volatile anesthetic can be reliably achieved. In addition to anesthetic depth, the duration of direct laryngoscopy is important in limiting the pressor response that occurs to this noxious stimulus. Direct laryngoscopy that does not exceed 15 seconds in duration is helpful in minimizing the blood pressure elevation evoked by this painful stimulus.[25] In addition, administration of laryngotracheal lidocaine (2 mg·kg^{-1}) immediately before placement of the tracheal tube may attenuate any additional pressor response produced by tracheal intubation.[26] Alternatively, lidocaine (1.5 mg·kg^{-1} IV) administered about 1 minute before induction of anesthesia may be useful for attenuating the pressor response. When the duration of direct laryngoscopy is likely to exceed 15 seconds, it may be useful to inject nitroprusside (1 to 2 μg·kg^{-1} IV) just before beginning direct laryngoscopy in an attempt to attenuate the blood pressure response produced by intubation of the trachea.[27] Injection of esmolol (100 to 200 mg IV, 15 seconds before the induction of anesthesia) is an alternative to nitroprusside and has the advantage of attenuating both the heart rate and blood pressure response produced by intubation of the trachea.[28] Regardless of the drugs administered before attempting intubation of the trachea, it should be appreciated that an excessive drug effect can produce hypotension that could be more undesirable than the stimulation responses evoked by direct laryngoscopy and intubation of the trachea.

Maintenance of Anesthesia

The goal during maintenance of anesthesia is to adjust the depth of anesthesia in an appropriate direction to minimize wide fluctuations in blood pressure. In this regard, a technique that includes a volatile anesthetic is useful for permitting a rapid adjustment in depth of anesthesia in response to a change in blood pressure. Indeed, management of intraoperative blood pressure lability with the anesthetic technique may be more important than preoperative control of hypertension.[10]

The most likely intraoperative change in blood pressure is hypertension produced by painful stimulation. Indeed, the incidence of perioperative hypertensive episodes is increased in patients diagnosed as having essential hypertension, even in those previously rendered normotensive with drug therapy[10] (Table 5-4). A volatile anesthetic is useful for attenuating the activity of the sympathetic nervous system, which is responsible for the pressor response. Halothane, enflurane, and isoflurane produce dose-dependent decreases in blood pressure. Although each drug lowers blood pressure by a different primary mechanism (halothane by decreased cardiac output and isoflurane by peripheral vasodilation), there is no evidence that one drug is preferable over another[29] (see Fig. 1-3). Desflurane may exert a more rapid blood pressure lowering effect due to the ability to promptly increase the alveolar concentration of this poorly soluble volatile anesthetic.

A nitrous oxide–opioid technique is also acceptable for maintaining anesthesia. If this approach is selected, however, it is likely that a volatile anesthetic will be needed at various times to control undesirable increases in blood pressure, as are likely during periods of maximal surgical stimulation. A continuous intravenous infusion of nitroprusside is an alternative to the use of a volatile anesthetic for maintaining normotension during the perioperative period. There is no evidence that a specific muscle relaxant is the best selection in the hypertensive patient. Although pancuronium can modestly increase blood pressure, there is no evidence that this pressor response is exaggerated by co-existing hypertension.

Hypotension that occurs during the maintenance of anesthesia may be treated by decreasing the delivered concentration of volatile anesthetic and by increasing the infusion rate of crystalloid or colloid solutions. A sympathomimetic drug such as ephedrine or phenylephrine may be necessary to restore vital organ perfusion pressure, until the underlying cause of hypotension can be corrected. Despite the predictable suppressant effect of many antihypertensive drugs on the autonomic nervous system, extensive clinical experience has confirmed that the response to sympathomimetic drugs is both appropriate and predictable. Another cause of an abrupt decrease in blood pressure may be the sudden onset of a junctional cardiac rhythm. In this regard, avoidance of a marked decrease in $PaCO_2$ and of high delivered concentrations of the volatile anesthetic (particularly halothane) will minimize the likelihood that this cardiac rhythm will occur. A persistent junction rhythm associated with a decrease in blood pressure may be treated with the intravenous administration of atropine.

The selection of monitors for the patient with co-existing hypertension is influenced by the complexity of the surgery. The electrocardiogram is particularly useful in recognizing the occurrence of myocardial ischemia during painful stimulation, such as direct laryngoscopy. Invasive monitoring using an intra-arterial and pulmonary artery catheter may be useful if extensive surgery is planned and there is preoperative evidence of left ventricular dysfunction. Invasive monitoring is useful when emergency surgery is required in the presence of uncontrolled hypertension.

Regional anesthesia is an acceptable selection for the hypertensive patient recognizing that a need for high sensory levels of anesthesia and associated sympathetic nervous system denervation could unmask unsuspected hypovolemia. It is important to recognize that chronic hypertension is often associated with hypovolemia and ischemic heart disease, which means that decreases in blood pressure are more likely to result in myocardial ischemia.

Postoperative Management

Hypertension during the early postoperative period is not an unexpected response in the patient with preoperative hypertension. The mechanism is not known but likely reflects exaggerated sympathetic nervous system activity with or without a relative hypervolemia related to intraoperative fluid replacement. The development of postoperative hypertension warrants prompt assessment and treatment to decrease the risks of myocardial ischemia, cardiac dysrhythmias, conges-

Table 5-6. Causes of a Hypertensive Crisis

Chronic essential hypertension
Renovascular hypertension
Sudden withdrawal from antihypertensive therapy (central acting and beta antagonists)
Drug ingestion (cocaine, LSD, amphetamine, tricyclic antidepressants)
Pregnancy-induced hypertension (eclampsia)
Head injury
Pheochromocytoma
Guillain-Barré syndrome
Spinal cord injury
Collagen vascular diseases
Thoracic aorta dissection

tive heart failure, stroke, and bleeding. If hypertension persists despite adequate analgesia, it may be necessary to administer a peripherally acting vasodilator drug such as hydralazine (2.5 to 10 mg IV, every 10 to 20 minutes) or nitroprusside. If nitroprusside is selected, the dose is titrated (0.5 to 10 $\mu g \cdot kg^{-1} \cdot min^{-1}$ IV) to produce the desired systolic blood pressure with the aid of continuous intra-arterial blood pressure monitoring. Alternatively, labetalol (0.1 to 0.25 $mg \cdot kg^{-1}$ IV, every 10 minutes) may be a useful drug for controlling acute postoperative hypertension.[30]

HYPERTENSIVE CRISIS

Hypertensive crisis is arbitrarily defined as a sudden increase of the diastolic blood pressure above 130 mmHg.[1] Causes of a hypertensive crisis are multiple but occur most often in the patient with chronic hypertension, presumably reflecting activation of the renin-angiotensin-aldosterone system (Table 5-6). A hypertensive emergency is considered present when hypertension is accompanied by evidence of encephalopathy, congestive heart failure, or renal dysfunction (oliguria, proteinuria). These patients require prompt but controlled reduction in blood pressure with administration of nitroprusside (0.5 to 10 $\mu g \cdot kg^{-1} \cdot min^{-1}$ IV) during continuous monitoring of intra-arterial pressure and urine output.[1,31] The goal is to decrease the diastolic blood pressure to 100 to 110 mmHg over a period of several minutes to several hours. A precipitous decrease in blood pressure may provoke end-organ ischemia.

REFERENCES

1. Calhoun DA, Oparil S. Treatment of hypertensive crisis. N Engl J Med 1990;323:1177–83
2. 1989 Guidelines for the management of mild hypertension: Memorandum from a WHO/ISH meeting. J Hypertens 1989;7:689–93

3. Tjoa HI, Kaplan NM. Treatment of hypertension in the elderly. JAMA 1990;264:1015–8
4. Kannel WB. Risk factors in hypertension. J Cardiovasc Pharmacol 1989;13:S4–10
5. Croog SH, Levine S, Testa MA, et al. The effects of antihypertensive therapy on the quality of life. N Engl J Med 1986;314:1657–64
6. Chobanian AV. Antihypertensive therapy in evolution. N Engl J Med 1986;314:1701–2
7. Prys-Roberts C. Anaesthesia and hypertension. Br J Anaesth 1984;56:711–24
8. Prys-Roberts C, Meloche R, Foex P. Studies of anaesthesia in relation to hypertension. I. Cardiovascular responses to treated and untreated patients. Br J Anaesth 1971;43:122–37
9. Stone JG, Foex P, Sear JW, Johnson LL, Khambatta HJ, Triner L. Risk of myocardical ischaemia during anaesthesia in treated and untreated hypertensive patients. Br J Anaesth 1988;61:675–9
10. Goldman L, Caldera DL. Risks of general anesthesia and elective operation in the hypertensive patient. Anesthesiology 1979;50:285–92
11. Asiddas CB, Donegan JH, Whitesell RC, Kalbfleisch JH. Factors associated with perioperative complications during carotid endarterectomy. Anesth Analg 1982;61:631–7
12. Steen PA, Tinker JH, Tarhan S. Myocardial reinfarction after anesthesia and surgery. An update: Incidence, mortality and predisposing factors. JAMA 1978;239:2566–70
13. Bedford RF, Feinstein B. Hospital admission blood pressure: A predictor for hypertension following endotracheal intubation. Anesth Analg 1980;59:367–70
14. Husserl FE, Messerli FH. Adverse effects of antihypertensive drugs. Drug 1981;22:188–210
15. Miller RD, Way WL, Eger EI. The effects of alpha-methyldopa, reserpine, guanethidine, and iproniazid on minimum alveolar anesthetic requirement (MAC). Anesthesiology 1969;29:1153–8
16. Katz RL, Weintraub HD, Papper EM. Anesthesia, surgery, and rauwolfia. Anesthesiology 1964;25:142–7
17. Bloor BC, Flacke WE. Reduction in halothane anesthetic requirements by clonidine, an alpha-adrenergic agonist. Anesth Analg 1982;61:741–5
18. Ghignone M, Quintin L, Duke PC, et al. Effects of clonidine on narcotic requirements and hemodynamic response during induction of fentanyl anesthesia and endotracheal intubation. Anesthesiology 1986;64:36–42
19. Bruce DL, Croley TF, Lee JS. Preoperative clonidine withdrawal syndrome. Anesthesiology 1979;51:90–2
20. Brodsky JB, Bravo JJ. Acute postoperative clonidine withdrawal syndrome. Anesthesiology 1976;44:519–20
21. Papademetrious V, Burris J, Kukich S, Freis ED. Effectiveness of potassium chloride or triameterene in thiazide hypokalemia. Arch Intern Med 1985;145:1986–90
22. Vitez TS, Soper LE, Wong KC, Soper P. Chronic hypokalemia and intraoperative dysrhythmias. Anesthesiology 1985;63:130–3
23. Roy WL, Edelist G, Gilbert B. Myocardial ischemia during noncardiac surgical procedures in patients with coronary artery disease. Anesthesiology 1979;51:393–7
24. Roizen MF, Horrigan RW, Frazer BM. Anesthetic doses blocking adrenergic (stress) and cardiovascular responses to incision-MAC BAR. Anesthesiology 1981;54:390–8
25. Stoelting RK. Blood pressure and heart rate changes during short duration laryngoscopy for tracheal intubation: Influence of viscous or intravenous lidocaine. Anesth Analg 1978;57:197–9
26. Stoelting RK. Circulatory changes during direct laryngoscopy and tracheal intubation: Influence of duration of laryngoscopy with or without prior lidocaine. Anesthesiology 1977;47:381–3
27. Stoelting RK. Attenuation of blood pressure response to laryngoscopy and tracheal intubation with sodium nitroprusside. Anesth Analg 1979;58:116–9
28. Sheppard S, Eagle CJ, Strunin L. A bolus dose of esmolol attenuates tachycardia and hypertension after tracheal intubation. Can J Anaesth 1990;37:202–5
29. Hess W, Arnold B, Schulte-Sasse UWE, Tarnow J. Comparison of isoflurane and halothane when used to control intraoperative hypertension in patients undergoing coronary artery bypass surgery. Anesth Analg 1983;62:15–20
30. Leslie JB, Kalayjian RW, Sirgo MA, Plachetka JR, Watkins WD. Intravenous labetalol for treatment of postoperative hypertension. Anesthesiology 1987;67:413–6
31. Gifford RW. Management of hypertensive crises. JAMA 1991;266:829–35

6

Congestive Heart Failure

Congestive heart failure (CHF) is most often due to (1) cardiac valve abnormalities, (2) impaired myocardial contractility secondary to ischemic heart disease or cardiomyopathy, (3) systemic hypertension, or (4) pulmonary hypertension (cor pulmonale). The most common cause of right ventricular failure is left ventricular failure. The pathophysiologic hallmarks of CHF are (1) decreased cardiac output, (2) increased ventricular end-diastolic pressure, (3) peripheral vasoconstriction, and (4) metabolic acidosis. Conceptually, left ventricular failure results in symptoms and signs of pulmonary edema, whereas right ventricular failure results in systemic venous hypertension and associated peripheral edema.

The incidence of CHF increases with increasing age and is the most common DRG diagnosis. The presence of CHF during the preoperative period is the most important single abnormality shown to contribute to postoperative cardiac morbidity and mortality.[1]

ADAPTIVE PHYSIOLOGIC MECHANISMS

A heart with properly functioning valves can adequately accept venous return (preload) and eject it against systemic vascular resistance (afterload). The heart can be overloaded either by an increase in the volume of blood it has to eject forward (aortic or mitral regurgitation) or by an increase in the resistance against which it must eject blood (systemic hypertension, aortic stenosis). Adaptive mechanisms that allow the heart to maintain its cardiac output with changes in physiology include the (1) Frank-Starling relation, (2) inotropic state, (3) afterload, (4) heart rate, and (5) myocardial hypertrophy and dilation. In addition, alterations in sympathetic nervous system activity and humoral-mediated responses occur in the presence of CHF.

Frank-Starling Relation

The Frank-Starling relation describes an increase in stroke volume that accompanies progressive increases in the left or right ventricular end-diastolic volume, which is closely related to the end-diastolic pressure[2] (Fig. 6-1). Increased stroke volume occurs because the tension developed by contracting muscle is greater when the resting length of that muscle is increased. The magnitude of stroke volume increase produced by the increased resting tension of ventricular muscle fibers depends on the state of myocardial contractility. For example, when myocardial contractility is decreased, as in the presence of CHF, a lower stroke volume is achieved relative to any given left ventricular end-diastolic filling pressure (Fig. 6-1). Constriction of venous capacitance vessels shifts blood centrally, which helps maintain cardiac output by the Frank-Starling relation.

Inotropic State

The inotropic state describes myocardial contractility, as reflected by the velocity of contraction developed by cardiac muscle. Maximum velocity of contraction is referred to as V_{max}. When the inotropic state of the heart is increased, as in the presence of catecholamines, V_{max} is increased. Conversely, V_{max} is decreased when myocardial contractility is impaired. Volatile anesthetics have been shown to decrease V_{max}, and this effect is additive to the decrease produced by CHF alone[3] (Fig. 6-2). In clinical practice, the rate of increase in interventricular pressure (dp/dt) simulates V_{max} and is used as an approximation of the inotropic state of the heart.

CHF is associated with a depletion of catecholamines in the heart with a subsequent decrease in myocardial contractility. In contrast to depletion of myocardial catecholamines, plasma concentrations, as well as urinary excretion of catecholamines, are invariably increased in patients in CHF.[4] Furthermore, there is a decrease in the density of beta receptors in the muscle of failing hearts and decreased inotropic responses to beta agonist stimulation. Drugs such as digitalis and cate-

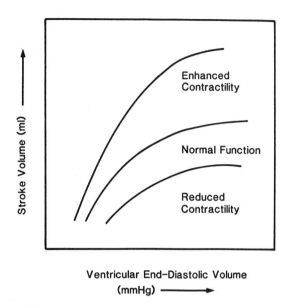

Fig. 6-1. The Frank-Starling relation states that stroke volume is directly related to the ventricular end-diastolic pressure.

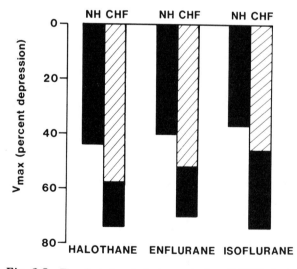

Fig. 6-2. The effect of equipotent concentrations (1 MAC) of volatile anesthetics on maximal velocity of shortening (V_{max}) of isolated papillary muscles taken from adult cats with normal hearts (NH) or experimentally induced congestive heart failure (CHF) was studied. The presence of CHF had an additive depressant effect on V_{max} in the presence of a volatile anesthetic. (Data from Kemmotsu O, Hashimoto Y, Shimosato S. The effects of performance of isolated papillary muscles from failing hearts. Anesthesiology 1974;40:252–60.)

cholamines that increase myocardial contractility are useful in the treatment of CHF (see the section, Treatment of Congestive Heart Failure).

Afterload

Afterload is the tension the ventricular muscle must develop to open the aortic or pulmonic valve. As defined by the law of Laplace, the afterload presented to the left ventricle is increased in the presence of systemic hypertension. Forward left ventricular stroke volume in a patient with CHF can be increased by administration of a vasodilator (see the section, Treatment of Congestive Heart Failure).

Heart Rate

In the normal heart, ventricular filling time parallels heart rate such that changes in heart rate are associated with the opposite change in stroke volume, and cardiac output is unlikely to change. Conversely, in the presence of CHF and low basal cardiac output, the stroke volume is relatively fixed, and an increase in heart rate often increases stroke volume. Increases in myocardial contractility that accompany increases in heart rate are known as the rate-treppe phenomenon. Tachycardia is an expected finding in the presence of CHF, reflecting activation of the sympathetic nervous system.

Myocardial Hypertrophy and Dilation

Myocardial hypertrophy represents compensatory mechanisms that develop in response to chronic pressure overload (mitral stenosis, aortic stenosis, systemic hypertension, pulmonary hypertension), whereas cardiac dilation occurs in response to volume overload (mitral regurgitation, aortic regurgitation). Myocardial hypertrophy helps overcome pressure loads on the heart but has limitations, since hypertrophied cardiac muscles function at lower inotropic states than does normal cardiac muscle. Cardiac dilation leads to compensatory increases in cardiac output by the Frank-Starling relation. Increased cardiac wall tension, however, produced by the enlarged ventricular radius is also associated with an increased myocardial oxygen requirement and decreased cardiac efficiency.

Sympathetic Nervous System Activity

Arteriolar and venous constriction occur in the presence of CHF. Arteriolar constriction serves to maintain blood pressure despite a decreased cardiac output, whereas increased venous tone shifts blood from peripheral sites to the central circulation, thus enhancing venous return and maintaining cardiac output by the Frank-Starling relation. Furthermore, arteriolar constriction causes redistribution of blood from the kidneys, splanchnic organs, skeletal muscles, and skin so as to maintain coronary and cerebral blood flow despite an overall decrease in cardiac output. Decreased renal blood flow (as low as 25% of normal) evokes increased renal tubular absorption of sodium and water, resulting in increased blood volume and enhancement of cardiac output by the Frank-Starling relation. These compensatory peripheral responses, although effective in compensating for hypovolemic states such as acute blood loss, can contribute to a vicious circle in the presence of CHF. For example, fluid retention, increased venous return, and increased afterload all impose more work on the failing myocardium and can further decrease cardiac output. Interruption of this vicious circle is the rationale for treatment of CHF with vasodilators and angiotensin-converting enzyme (ACE) inhibitors (see the section, Treatment of Congestive Heart Failure).

Humoral-Mediated Responses

Atrial natriuretic factor is stored in atrial muscle and released in response to an increase in atrial pressure, as produced by tachycardia or hypervolemia. This hormone increases the glomerular filtration rate, leading to natriuresis and diuresis. In addition, it suppresses aldosterone secretion and the release of antidiuretic hormone.

HEMODYNAMIC PARAMETERS OF VENTRICULAR FUNCTION

Hemodynamic parameters of ventricular function likely to be altered by CHF include (1) cardiac output, (2) ejection fraction, and (3) ventricular end-diastolic pressure.

Cardiac Output

Cardiac output is the product of stroke volume and heart rate. Stroke volume is determined by myocardial contractility, synchronous contraction of all portions of the ventricle, afterload, and, most importantly, venous return. In the presence of left ventricular dysfunction, the resting cardiac output may be normal but unable to increase in response to exercise, whereas more severe CHF is associated with a decreased cardiac output (less than 2.5 $L \cdot min^{-1} \cdot m^{-2}$). When cardiac output cannot increase, any enhanced extraction of oxygen by peripheral tissues lowers the oxygen content of venous blood, leading to an increased arterial to venous oxygen content difference.

Ejection Fraction

Normally, the heart ejects 56% to 75% of its volume during systole resulting in an ejection fraction (ratio of stroke volume to end-diastolic volume) of 0.56 to 0.78. The ejection fraction,

as measured by angiographic techniques, radioisotope imaging, or echocardiography, is decreased by decreased myocardial contractility, increased afterload, or asynchrony of left ventricular contraction.

End-Diastolic Pressure

End-diastolic pressure that parallels end-diastolic volume is increased in the presence of CHF. In addition, end-diastolic pressure can also be increased in the presence of a poorly compliant (stiff) ventricle, even in the absence of an increase in ventricular volume. Left ventricular end-diastolic pressure is normally less than 12 mmHg, whereas right ventricular end-diastolic pressure is normally less than 5 mmHg. In the absence of mitral valve disease, mean left atrial pressure parallels left ventricular end-diastolic pressure. Likewise, in the absence of increased pulmonary vascular resistance or mitral valve disease, pulmonary artery end-diastolic pressure reflects left ventricular end-diastolic pressure. Manifestations of left atrial enlargement on the electrocardiogram (P wave lasts longer than 0.1 second and has an M-shaped configuration on lead II) correlates with an acute increase in left atrial pressure.

MANIFESTATIONS OF LEFT VENTRICULAR FAILURE

Manifestations of left ventricular failure are elicited by the preanesthetic history and physical examination and interpretation of laboratory tests. Insomnia, skeletal muscle wasting, and fatigue may be due to left ventricular failure. Indeed, the hallmark of decreased cardiac reserve and low cardiac output is fatigue at rest or with minimal exertion. Associated decreases in cerebral blood flow may produce confusion, while decreases in renal blood flow may lead to prerenal azotemia characterized by a disproportionate increase in blood urea nitrogen concentration relative to the serum creatinine concentration.

Dyspnea

Dyspnea, which reflects increased work of breathing owing to stiffness of the lungs produced by interstitial pulmonary edema, is one of the earliest subjective symptoms of left ventricular failure. Initially, this symptom occurs only with exertion. It can be quantitated by asking the patient how many flights of stairs can be climbed or the distance that can be walked at a normal pace before dyspnea occurs. Patients experiencing angina pectoris may interpret substernal discomfort as breathlessness.

Orthopnea

Orthopnea reflects the inability of a failing left ventricle to handle increased venous return associated with the recumbent position. A dry nonproductive cough that develops with the assumption of the supine position and that is relieved by sitting up is the equivalent of orthopnea owing to pulmonary congestion. The orthopneic cough differs from the productive morning cough characteristic of patients with chronic bronchitis.

Paroxysmal Nocturnal Dyspnea

Paroxysmal nocturnal dyspnea is shortness of breath that awakens the patient from sleep. This symptom must be differentiated from anxiety-provoked hyperventilation or wheezing owing to accumulation of secretions in patients with chronic bronchitis. Wheezing caused by pulmonary congestion (cardiac asthma) is typically accompanied by radiographic evidence of pulmonary congestion, which serves to distinguish this response from that due to sputum accumulation in the airways.

Acute Pulmonary Edema

Acute pulmonary edema reflecting movement of fluid into the alveoli is the ultimate manifestation of left ventricular failure. Blood pressure is often increased. Other signs of sympathetic nervous system stimulation such as tachycardia and vasoconstriction are often present. Bubbling rales are diffusely present with or without wheezes. Pulmonary artery occlusion pressure is likely to be greater than 30 mmHg in the presence of acute pulmonary edema. When the left atrial pressure remains normal, pulmonary edema is characterized as noncardiogenic, reflecting direct damage to the alveolar epithelium or pulmonary capillary walls, or both. The ratio of the colloid osmotic pressure of the edema fluid relative to that of the plasma serves to differentiate pulmonary edema due to left ventricular failure (ratio less than 0.6) from that due to noncardiogenic causes (ratio approaching 1.0, reflecting a high protein content).

Treatment

Initial treatment of acute pulmonary edema includes placement of the patient in a head-up position, delivery of humidified oxygen by a face mask, and administration of morphine (5 to 10 mg IV), to decrease venous return to the heart. A rapid-acting diuretic such as furosemide (10 to 40 mg IV) is administered, whereas digoxin is reserved early in therapy only for the control of atrial tachydysrhythmias. Dopamine is probably the preferred initial inotrope because it maintains systemic vascular resistance and enhances renal blood flow. In patients who have high systemic vascular resistance, however, dobutamine, which has relatively little effect on systemic vascular resistance, may be selected. The determination of arterial blood gases and pH is useful, and monitoring systemic and pulmonary arterial pressures may be indicated.

Physical Signs

The most prominent physical sign in patients experiencing left ventricular failure is moist rales in the lungs, often associated with tachypnea. These extraneous sounds may be confined to lung bases in mild degrees of left ventricular failure or generalized in acute pulmonary edema. Compensatory increases in sympathetic nervous system activity are manifested as resting tachycardia and peripheral vasoconstriction, which help maintain blood pressure and blood flow to the heart and brain despite a decrease in cardiac output. An associated decrease in renal blood flow can be manifested as an increased blood urea nitrogen concentration and oliguria. Unexplained resting tachycardia during the preoperative period should suggest CHF, particularly if the patient is elderly or is known to have co-existing heart disease. A third heart sound (S3 gallop or ventricular diastolic gallop) indicates significant left ventricular dysfunction and may be the first sign of CHF. This heart sound is due to blood entering and distending a relatively noncompliant left ventricle.

Chest Radiograph

The earliest radiographic sign of left ventricular failure and associated pulmonary venous hypertension is evidence of distension of the pulmonary veins in the upper lobes of the lungs. Perivascular edema appears as a hilar and perihilar haze. The hilus appears large, with ill-defined margins. Septal edema on the chest radiograph is described as Kerley's lines, reflecting edematous interlobular septa in the upper lung fields (Kerley A lines), lower lung fields (Kerley B lines) or basilar regions of the lungs producing a honeycomb pattern (Kerley C lines). Subpleural edema indicates extension of interstitial pulmonary edema to the periphery of the lungs. Alveolar edema typically produces homogeneous densities in the lung fields, resembling a butterfly pattern when the distribution is central, bilateral, and symmetric. Pleural effusion and pericardial effusion may accompany CHF, particularly if it is biventricular. Radiographic changes of pulmonary edema may lag behind acute elevations of left atrial pressure by up to 12 hours. Likewise, radiographic patterns of pulmonary congestion may persist for 1 to 4 days after normalization of cardiac filling pressures.

MANIFESTATIONS OF RIGHT VENTRICULAR FAILURE

Manifestations of right ventricular failure include systemic venous congestion with associated organomegaly and peripheral edema.

Systemic Venous Congestion

The hallmark of right ventricular failure is systemic venous congestion, classically evidenced by jugular venous distension. For example, distension of the external jugular veins above the clavicles of a patient in the sitting position suggests right ventricular failure. In the presence of normal right ventricular function, the increased venous return produced by inspiration and associated negative intrathoracic pressure is easily propelled into the pulmonary circulation. By contrast, in the presence of right ventricular failure, any increase in venous return causes a further increase, rather than a normal decrease, in jugular venous pressure. This distension of neck veins with inspiration is known as Kussmaul's sign. A similar response may be seen in the patient with constrictive pericarditis or cardiac tamponade.

Organomegaly

The liver is typically the first organ to become engorged with blood in the presence of right ventricular failure. If the engorgement is rapid, right upper quadrant pain and tenderness may occur, reflecting distension of the liver against its capsule. When moderate liver congestion is present, the results of liver function tests may be mildly elevated, whereas prothrombin times may be prolonged when liver engorgement is severe. Ascites is a late manifestation of right ventricular failure and is most likely to occur in the patient with CHF owing to constrictive pericarditis or tricuspid stenosis.

Peripheral Edema

Peripheral edema, which is usually dependent and often characterized as pitting, is an early sign of right ventricular failure. It reflects a combination of venous congestion, sodium, and water retention. Ankle edema caused by local venous or lymphatic obstruction, cirrhosis of the liver, or hypoalbuminemia is differentiated from similar edema attributable to right ventricular failure by the absence of jugular venous distension with inspiration.

TREATMENT OF CONGESTIVE HEART FAILURE

The treatment of CHF begins with correction of reversible causes (systemic hypertension, valvular heart disease, anemia, beta blockade). When symptoms persist despite correction of reversible causes, the three cornerstones of the pharmacologic treatment of CHF are digitalis, diuretics, and vasodilators.[5] The present trend in treatment of CHF is to optimize cardiac function by manipulating the peripheral circulation with a vasodilator.[2] In this regard, ACE inhibitors are emerging as the treatment of choice for chronic CHF. Nevertheless, digitalis and diuretics remain the initial therapy for most patients with left ventricular failure, and vasodilators serve as adjunctive drugs.[6] With the advent of potent di-

uretics, marked sodium restriction is necessary only in the most severe cases.

Digitalis

Digitalis is the only orally effective positive inotropic drug in common use, having a long history of efficacy (more than 200 years) in the treatment of CHF.[6] This drug increases myocardial contractility, decreases heart size, and increases cardiac output in patients with CHF in whom systemic vascular resistance is increased owing to increased sympathetic nervous system activity. Drug-induced increases in cardiac output result in a lessening of peripheral vasoconstriction. Enhanced parasympathetic nervous system activity produced by a therapeutic concentration of digitalis is useful in slowing a rapid heart rate, especially in a patient with atrial fibrillation.

Several preparations of digitalis are available, but a detailed knowledge of digoxin is sufficient for most situations (Table 6-1). Digoxin is excreted principally by the kidneys. Its clearance (normally about one-third the daily dose) is closely related to creatinine clearance. In this regard, daily doses of digoxin should be adjusted to replace that drug that is eliminated by the kidneys. Clearly, sensitivity to digoxin can be increased during the perioperative period if there are associated decreases in renal function.

Table 6-1. Characteristics of Frequently Used Digitalis Preparations

	Digoxin	Ouabain	Digitoxin
Absorption from the gastrointestinal tract	Good	Erratic	Excellent
Onset of action after intravenous administration (min)	15–30	5–10	30–120
Peak effects (h)	1.5–5	0.5–2	4–12
Elimination half-time (h)	31–33	21	120–168
Principal route of elimination	Kidneys	Kidneys	Hepatic
Average digitalizing dose (mg)			
Intravenous	0.75–1.0	0.3–0.5	0.7–1.0
Oral (during 12–24 h)	0.75–1.5		0.7–1.2
Average daily maintenance dose (adults with normal liver and renal function)			
Oral (mg)	0.125–0.5		0.05–0.2
Therapeutic plasma concentration (ng·ml^{-1})	1–1.5	0.5	15–25

Prophylactic Use of Digitalis

Prophylactic administration of digitalis to a patient scheduled for an elective operation without evidence of CHF is controversial. The disadvantage of such prophylaxis is administration of a drug with a small therapeutic-to-toxic dose difference to a patient with no clinical indication for the drug. Furthermore, differentiation of anesthetic-induced cardiac dysrhythmias from those due to digitalis toxicity may be difficult.[7] Indeed, such events as increased sympathetic nervous system activity, decreased plasma potassium concentration, and decreased renal function are likely to occur intraoperatively, thereby enhancing the chances of increased pharmacologic effects from circulating digitalis. Despite these theoretical disadvantages, there is evidence that patients with limited cardiac reserve may benefit from the prophylactic administration of digitalis. For example, preoperative administration of digoxin (0.75 mg orally in divided doses the day before surgery and 0.25 mg before the induction of anesthesia) decreases the incidence of atrial fibrillation in elderly patients undergoing thoracic or abdominal surgery.[8] Prophylactic digoxin also decreases evidence of impaired cardiac function in patients with ischemic heart disease who are recovering from anesthesia[9] (Fig. 6-3). Therefore, it may be reasonable to conclude that the beneficial effects of prophylactic digitalis administered to selected patients during the preoperative period outweigh any potential risks of digitalis toxicity. Certainly, there are no data to support discontinuing digitalis preoperatively, especially if the drug is being administered for the control of heart rate.

Digitalis Toxicity

Digitalis toxicity is always a hazard in the patient being treated with this drug. Factors that predispose to digitalis toxicity are hypokalemia, hypercalcemia, hypomagnesemia, and arterial hypoxemia. During the preoperative period, digitalis toxicity should be suspected in the patient who complains of anorexia or nausea, especially if hypokalemia is also present.

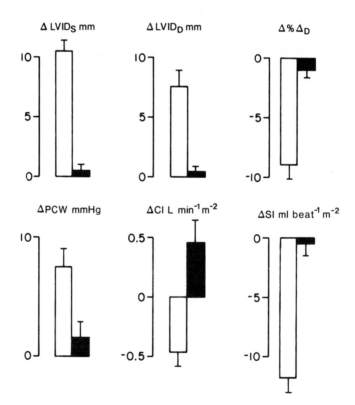

Fig. 6-3. M-Mode echocardiograms and systemic hemodynamics were measured in patients with ischemic heart disease and receiving digoxin (10 μg·kg^{-1} IV) 48, 24, and 3 hours before surgery (solid bars) or not receiving digoxin (clear bars). Values represent differences in preoperative and postoperative measurements. LVID, left ventricular dimension in systole (S) or diastole (D); PCW, pulmonary capillary wedge; CI, cardiac index; SI, stroke index. (Redrawn from Pinaud MLF, Blanboeil YAG, Souron RJ. Preoperative prophylactic digitalization of patients with coronary artery disease—a randomized echocardiographic and hemodynamic study. Anesth Analg 1983;62:865–9, with permission.)

Cardiac Manifestations of Digitalis Toxicity

Cardiac dysrhythmias are the first evidence of digitalis toxicity in about one-third of patients. Although no specific cardiac dysrhythmia is pathognomonic for digitalis toxicity, ventricular premature beats (particularly bigeminy) and various forms of atrioventricular heart block are common. Depression of ST segments and T waves on the electrocardiogram are nonspecific changes that do not necessarily indicate digitalis toxicity. Ventricular fibrillation is the most frequent cause of death from digitalis toxicity.

Plasma Digitalis Concentration

The wide range of overlap between the therapeutic and toxic plasma concentration of digitalis preparations has cast doubt on the usefulness of the plasma concentration as the sole indicator of digitalis toxicity (Table 6-1). Nevertheless, a plasma digoxin concentration above 3 ng·ml^{-1} usually reflects a toxic level of the drug.[10]

Treatment of Digitalis-Induced Cardiac Dysrhythmias

Treatment of digitalis toxicity includes the correction of predisposing events (especially hypokalemia), administration of drugs (lidocaine, phenytoin, atropine) to treat cardiac dysrhythmias, and insertion of a temporary transvenous cardiac pacemaker if complete heart block is present.[11]

Surgery in the Presence of Digitalis Toxicity

Proceeding with anesthesia and surgery in the presence of suspected or confirmed digitalis toxicity depends entirely on the urgency of the surgery. Certainly, elective operations should be delayed until digitalis toxicity subsides. When the surgical disease is life-threatening, it will be necessary to proceed with the operative procedure despite digitalis toxicity. In this situation, events or drugs, such as ketamine, that stimulate the autonomic nervous system should be avoided. Halothane (and, by inference, other volatile anesthetics) has been shown to antagonize cardiac effects of digitalis in animals.[12] This finding suggests that volatile anesthetics would be reasonable choices in the presence of digitalis toxicity. Hyperventilation of the lungs, which can acutely lower the plasma potassium concentration, must be avoided. Drugs to treat digitalis-induced cardiac dysrhythmias must be readily available (see the section, Treatment of Digitalis-Induced Cardiac Dysrhythmias). Potassium decreases binding of digitalis to cardiac tissue and thus directly antagonizes cardiotoxic effects of these drugs. Conversely, potassium will intensify digitalis-induced heart block and depress the automaticity of an ectopic pacemaker in the ventricle, leading to complete heart block, em-

phasizing the importance of measuring the plasma potassium concentration before administering supplemental potassium. If renal function is normal and heart block is not present, it is acceptable to administer potassium (0.025 to 0.05 mEq·kg^{-1} IV) to suppress the life-threatening cardiac dysrhythmias associated with digitalis toxicity.

Lidocaine (0.5 to 1 mg·kg^{-1} IV), is useful as the initial treatment of digitalis-induced ventricular irritability not accompanied by hypokalemia.[9] Therapeutic plasma concentrations of lidocaine suppress ectopic ventricular cardiac pacemakers without affecting myocardial contractility or prolonging conduction of cardiac impulses through the atrioventricular node. Lidocaine is not highly effective in the management of digitalis-induced supraventricular dysrhythmias. For the treatment of these cardiac dysrhythmias, the drug of choice is phenytoin (20 mg·min^{-1} IV), until the cardiac dysrhythmias disappears or a total dose of 1000 mg is reached.[7] Atropine can be used to increase heart rate by offsetting excessive parasympathetic nervous system activity produced by a toxic plasma concentration of digitalis. Propranolol is effective in suppressing increased cardiac automaticity produced by digitalis toxicity, but its tendency to slow conduction of cardiac impulses through the atrioventricular node limits its usefulness when conduction block is present. When heart rate remains slow despite appropriate drug therapy, it may be necessary to insert a temporary transvenous cardiac pacemaker.

Life-threatening digitalis toxicity can be treated by administering antibodies (Fab fragments) to the drug, thereby decreasing the plasma concentration of digitalis available to attach to cardiac cell membranes.[13] External electrical cardioversion must be used with caution in the treatment of digitalis-induced supraventricular dysrhythmias, as even more severe cardiac dysrhythmias, including ventricular fibrillation, have occurred after this treatment in the presence of digitalis toxicity.

Diuretics

Chlorothiazide and hydrochlorothiazide are the most commonly used thiazide diuretics. Hypokalemia, which may produce cardiac dysrhythmias, is the most frequent side effect. These drugs may also cause hypomagnesemia, which can cause cardiac dysrhythmias. Thiazide diuretics may exacerbate hyperglycemia. The plasma potassium concentration should be determined periodically when thiazide diuretics are administered chronically, especially if the patient is also to be treated with a digitalis preparation.

Chronic oral administration of loop diuretics (ethacrynic acid, furosemide, bumetanide) can result in hypovolemia, orthostatic hypotension, hypokalemia, and azotemia. An increase in the blood urea nitrogen concentration is one of the earliest indications that hypovolemia is responsible for poor renal perfusion.

Potassium-sparing diuretics (spironolactone, triamterene, amiloride), when combined with other diuretics, enhance the diuretic action of these other drugs and counteract the kaliuretic effects of both thiazide and loop diuretics. These drugs also conserve magnesium. Hyperkalemia is a risk of treatment with these drugs, especially in patients with marked renal dysfunction.

Vasodilators

The present trend in the pharmacologic treatment of CHF is to optimize cardiac output by manipulating the peripheral circulation with vasodilators[2] (Table 6-2). Vasodilators increase cardiac output by decreasing impedance to the forward ejection of left ventricular stroke volume. Previously, treatment was based on increasing myocardial contractility with inotropes or decreasing preload by drug-induced diuresis, or both. It now appears acceptable to reserve inotropes for those patients in whom afterload reduction yields less than optimal results.

Vasodilators administered to treat CHF may act as venodilators (nitroglycerin), arteriolar dilators (hydralazine), combined venous and arteriolar dilators (prazosin, nitroprusside), or ACE inhibitors (captopril, enalapril, lisinopril)[2] (Table 6-2). the effectiveness of ACE inhibitors in treating CHF emphasizes the potential detrimental role of the renin-angiotensin system (peripheral vasoconstriction, sodium, and water retention) in these patients. Vasodilator therapy is particularly effective in treating CHF, owing to the sudden onset of mechanical abnormalities, such as (1) acute mitral regurgitation from myocardial infarction, ruptured chordae tendineae, and infective endocarditis; (2) acute aortic regurgitation from dissection of the aorta or infective endocarditis; and (3) acute perforation of the ventricular septum secondary to myocardial infarction.

The limiting factor in the treatment of CHF with vasodilators is hypotension. It is unlikely that treatment of CHF with a vasodilator can be continued if mean arterial pressure decreases more than 20% below the predrug value. Under most circumstances, administration of a vasodilator requires a device to regulate its continuous intravenous infusion. Furthermore, invasive monitoring, including an arterial and pulmonary artery catheter, is useful for determining changes in cardiac filling pressures and cardiac output and for calculating systemic and pulmonary vascular resistance.

Beta Agonists

Dopamine has dose-dependent effects on dopaminergic, beta, and alpha receptors, with stimulation of renal dopaminergic receptors occurring at principally low doses (less than $3 \mu g \cdot kg^{-1} \cdot min^{-1}$) and stimulation of alpha receptors at high doses (greater than $10 \mu g \cdot kg^{-1} \cdot min^{-1}$). Dobutamine produces dose-dependent effects on myocardial contractility by virtue of relatively selective stimulation of beta-1 receptors, whereas the effects on systemic vascular resistance are minimal. Combinations of dopamine and dobutamine provide the desirable renal effects of dopamine and the beta effects of dobutamine at doses that are unlikely to increase afterload by virtue of alpha receptor stimulation. Intravenous infusions of dopamine or dobutamine, or both, are commonly used during the perioperative period, when it is important to improve myocardial contractility. In these instances, it is useful to monitor the effects of the drug on cardiac output and cardiac filling pressures using a pulmonary artery catheter.

Phosphodiesterase Inhibitors

Phosphodiesterase inhibitors produce positive inotropic effects by enhancing the intracellular concentrations of cAMP, as well as producing arterial and venous dilation. Amrinone can be administered intravenously for the treatment of acute CHF, but oral administration for a prolonged period of time

Table 6-2. Vasodilator Drugs Used in Therapy for Congestive Heart Failure

	Effect on Venous System	Effect on Arterial System	Peak Action (h)	Duration of Effect (h)	Usual Dose and Route
Nitroglycerin	+ + +	+			$0.5–5 \mu g \cdot kg^{-1} \cdot min^{-1}$ IV
Hydralazine	0	+ + +	1–2	4–6	25–100 mg PO
Nitroprusside	+ + +	+ + +			$0.5–5 \mu g \cdot kg^{-1} \cdot min^{-1}$ IV
Prazosin	+ +	+ +	1–2	4–6	1–5 mg PO
Captopril	+ +	+ + +	1–2	4–8	25–75 mg PO
Enalapril	+ +	+ + +	4–8	18–30	5–40 mg PO
Lisinopril	+ +	+ + +	2–6	18–30	5–40 mg PO

is not recommended. Milrinone resembles amrinone but, for unknown reasons, when administered chronically, is associated with increased morbidity and mortality in patients with severe chronic CHF.[14]

SURGERY IN THE PRESENCE OF CONGESTIVE HEART FAILURE

Elective operations are not recommended in patients with evidence of CHF. In fact, the presence of CHF has been described as the single most important factor for predicting postoperative cardiac morbidity.[1] If surgery cannot be deferred, drugs and techniques chosen to provide anesthesia are often selected with the goal of optimizing cardiac output.

General Anesthesia

Ketamine is a useful drug for the induction of anesthesia in the presence of CHF. Administration of a volatile anesthetic must be done cautiously, in view of the dose-dependent cardiac depressant effects produced by these drugs. The cardiac depression produced by the combined effects of a volatile anesthetic and CHF is greater than that present in the absence of CHF[3] (Fig. 6-2). Opioids, benzodiazepines, and possibly etomidate are acceptable considerations, since they produce little or no direct myocardial depression. It must be remembered, however, that the addition of nitrous oxide to opioids or the combination of benzodiazepines and opioids is associated with significant depression of cardiac output and blood pressure.[15,16] Conversely, nitrous oxide added to diazepam does not seem to produce predictable cardiac depression.[17] In the presence of severe CHF, the use of opioids as the only drug for maintenance of anesthesia may be justified. Positive-pressure ventilation of the lungs may be beneficial by decreasing pulmonary congestion and improving arterial oxygenation. Monitoring is adjusted to the complexity of the operation. Invasive monitoring of arterial pressure, as well as cardiac filling pressures, is justified when major operations are necessary in the presence of CHF. Support of cardiac output with drugs such as dopamine or dobutamine may be necessary during the perioperative period.

Drug interactions in patients treated with digitalis should be anticipated. For example, succinylcholine, or any other drug that can abruptly increase parasympathetic nervous system activity, could theoretically have additive effects with digitalis. Nevertheless, clinical experience does not support the occurrence of an increased incidence of cardiac dysrhythmias in patients treated with digitalis and receiving succinylcholine.[18] Sympathomimetics with beta agonist effects, as well as pancuronium, may increase the likelihood of cardiac dysrhythmias in patients treated with digitalis. Calcium may accentuate the effects of a previously therapeutic plasma concentration of digitalis. Hyperventilation of the lungs, which acutely lowers the plasma concentration of potassium, must be avoided in patients treated with digitalis.

Regional Anesthesia

Regional anesthesia is an acceptable selection to provide anesthesia for a peripheral operation in the presence of CHF. In fact, modest decreases in systemic vascular resistance secondary to peripheral sympathetic nervous system blockade may permit an increased cardiac output. Nevertheless, decreased systemic vascular resistance produced by epidural or spinal anesthesia is not reliably predictable or easy to control. Therefore, regional anesthesia should probably not be selected over general anesthesia if the only reason is the belief that regional anesthesia will improve cardiac output.

REFERENCES

1. Goldman L, Caldera DL, Nussbaum SR, et al. Multifactorial index of cardiac risk in noncardiac surgical procedures. N Engl J Med 1977;297:845–50
2. Fyman PN, Cottrell JE, Kushins L, Casthely PA. Vasodilator therapy in the perioperative period. Can Anaesth Soc J 1986;33:629–43
3. Kemmotsu O, Hashimoto Y, Shimosato S. The effects of fluroxene and enflurane on contractile performance of isolated papillary muscles from failing hearts. Anesthesiology 1974;40:252–60
4. Francis GS, Goldsmith SR, Ziesche SM, Cohn JN. Response of plasma norepinephrine and epinephrine to dynamic exercise in patients with congestive heart failure. Am J Cardiol 1982;49:1152–6
5. Braunwald E. ACE inhibitors—cornerstone of the treatment of heart failure. N Engl J Med 1991;325:351–3
6. Kulick DL, Rahimtoola SH. Current role of digitalis therapy in patients with congestive heart failure. JAMA 1991;265:2995–7
7. Chung DC. Anaesthetic problems associated with the treatment of cardiovascular disease. I. Digitalis toxicity. Can Anaesth Soc J 1981;28:6–16
8. Chee TP, Prakash NS, Desser KB, Benchimol A. postoperative supraventricular arrhythmias and the role of prophylactic digoxin in cardiac surgery. Am Heart J 1982;104:974–7
9. Pinaud MLJ, Blanloeil YAG, Souron RJ. Preoperative prophylactic digitalization of patients with coronary artery disease—a randomized echocardiographic and hemodynamic study. Anesth Analg 1983;62:865–9
10. Doherty JA. How and when to use digitalis serum levels. JAMA 1978;239:2594–6
11. Mason DT, Zelis R, Lee G, et al. Current concepts and treatment of digitalis toxicity. Am J Cardiol 1971;27:546–59
12. Morrow DH, Townley NT. Anesthesia and digitalis toxicity: An experimental study. Anesth Analg 1964;43:510–19

13. Ochs HR, Smith TW. Reversal of advanced digitoxin toxicity and modification of pharmacokinetics by specific antibodies and Fab fragments. J Clin Invest 1977;60:1303–13

14. Packer M, Carver JR, Rodeheffer RJ, et al. Effect of oral milrinone on mortality in severe chronic heart failure. N Engl J Med 1991;325:1468–75

15. Stoelting RK, Gibbs PS. Hemodynamic effects of morphine and morphine-nitrous oxide in valvular heart disease and coronary artery disease. Anesthesiology 1973;38:45–52

16. Tomicheck RC, Rosow CE, Philbin DM, et al. Diazepam-fentanyl interaction-hemodynamic and hormonal effects in coronary artery surgery. Anesth Analg 1983;62:881–4

17. McCammon RL, Hilgenberg JC, Stoelting RK. Hemodynamic effects of diazepam and diazepam–nitrous oxide in patients with coronary artery disease. Anesth Analg 1980;59:438–41

18. Bartolone RS, Rao TLK. Dysrhythmias following muscle relaxant administration in patients receiving digitalis. Anesthesiology 1983;58:567–9

7
Cardiomyopathies

Cardiomyopathies are a diverse group of disorders characterized by myocardial dysfunction unrelated to the usual causes of heart disease, such as coronary atherosclerosis, valvular abnormalities, or hypertension. Common to all cardiomyopathies is progressive and life-threatening congestive heart failure. The etiologic classification of cardiomyopathies includes many diverse causes (Table 7-1). Alternatively, cardiomyopathies may be classified on a morphologic and hemodynamic basis as (1) dilated, (2) hypertrophic, (3) restrictive, and (4) obliterative (Table 7-2). In an individual patient, features of more than one type of cardiomyopathy may be present.

DILATED CARDIOMYOPATHY

Dilated cardiomyopathy is characterized by decreased myocardial contractility, usually involving both ventricles, manifested as decreased cardiac output and increased ventricular filling pressures (Table 7-2). Ventricular dilation may be so marked that functional mitral or tricuspid regurgitation, or both, occurs. The electrocardiogram is likely to show evidence of left ventricular hypertrophy, ST and T wave abnormalities, first-degree atrioventricular heart block, and bundle branch block. Cardiac dysrhythmias are frequent and include ventricular premature beats and atrial fibrillation. The chest radiograph may show evidence of cardiac enlargement involving all four chambers and signs of interstitial pulmonary edema. Echocardiographic criteria for the diagnosis of dilated cardiomyopathy include an ejection fraction of less than 0.4, a dilated and hypokinetic left ventricle, and mild to moderate mitral regurgitation. Systemic embolization is common, reflecting the formation of mural thrombi in dilated and hypokinetic cardiac chambers.

Multiple myocardial infarctions caused by diffuse coronary artery disease are the most common cause of dilated cardiomyopathy.[1] A striking association exists between alcohol abuse and dilated cardiomyopathy. Dilated cardiomyopathy may occur in peripartum patients, most often manifesting 1 to 6 weeks after delivery. A viral etiology in some patients is suggested by the frequent occurrence of a febrile illness preceding the onset of cardiac dysfunction.

Prognosis is poor, with only 25% to 40% of patients surviving 5 years after the definitive diagnosis. The most common complication of dilated cardiomyopathy is progressive congestive heart failure, the cause of death in 75% of these patients. Angina pectoris may be prominent. Sudden death as a result of cardiac dysrhythmia is frequent, and evidence of systemic or pulmonary embolism, or both, is present in more than 50% of these patients at autopsy.

Treatment

The avoidance of unnecessary physical activity and total abstinence from alcohol is recommended for all patients with dilated cardiomyopathy. Treatment of congestive heart failure is initially with digoxin and diuretics. Vasodilator therapy or, alternatively, administration of an inotrope that possesses vasodilator properties, such as amrinone, may be useful. Ventricular cardiac dysrhythmias may be suppressed with procainamide or quinidine. Because of the frequency of systemic and pulmonary embolism, patients with dilated cardiomyopathy are often treated with anticoagulants such as warfarin.

Immunosuppressive therapy (corticosteroids, azathioprine) may be useful in the occasional patient with dilated cardiomyopathy associated with collagen vascular disease, sarcoidosis, or evidence of active inflammation on endomyocardial biopsy. Surprisingly, beta antagonist therapy may be beneficial in some patients in whom tachydysrhythmias develop. Occasionally, in patients with dilated cardiomyopathy and ischemic heart disease, coronary revascularization may result in improved left ventricular function. When congestive heart failure is advanced, the possibility of cardiac transplantation is a consideration in the patient who does not have pulmonary hypertension or other systemic diseases.

Table 7-1. Etiology of Cardiomyopathies

Infectious
  Viral
  Bacterial

Toxic
  Alcohol
  Daunorubicin
  Doxorubicin
  Cocaine

Systemic
  Muscular dystrophy
  Myotonic dystrophy
  Collagen vascular diseases
  Sarcoidosis
  Pheochromocytoma
  Acromegaly
  Thyrotoxicosis
  Myxedema

Infiltrative
  Amyloidosis
  Hemochromatosis
  Primary or metastatic tumors

Nutritional

Ischemic

Idiopathic

Management of Anesthesia

Goals during the management of anesthesia in the patient with dilated cardiomyopathy include (1) avoidance of drug-induced myocardial depression, (2) maintenance of normovolemia, and (3) prevention of increases in ventricular afterload. Excessive cardiovascular depression in response to induction of anesthesia in the patient with a history of alcohol abuse may reflect unsuspected dilated cardiomyopathy.[2] Conversely, failure of the expected sedative response to the intravenous injection of an induction drug may reflect a slow circulation time, making the patient vulnerable to a drug overdose if additional drug is administered on the mistaken assumption that an inadequate dose was injected. During maintenance of anesthesia, the dose-dependent direct myocardial depression produced by volatile anesthetics must be considered, although the vasodilating properties of isoflurane would theoretically be desirable. Opioids are associated with benign effects on cardiac contractility but, when used alone, may not produce unconsciousness. Administration of an opioid with nitrous oxide or benzodiazepine may result in unexpected depression of myocardial contractility. Surgical stimulation that produces undesirable increases in heart rate or systemic vascular resistance may be treated with a beta antagonist such as esmolol, keeping in mind the potential for these drugs to cause cardiac depression. Skeletal muscle paralysis is provided with nondepolarizing muscle relaxants that lack significant cardiovascular effects. Intravenous infusion of crystalloid solutions or blood should be guided by cardiac filling pressures, to decrease the likelihood of volume overload. By permitting determination of cardiac output and cardiac filling pressures, a pulmonary artery catheter facilitates early recognition of the need for inotropic support or administration of peripheral vasodilating drugs. Prominent A waves on the venous pressure tracing reflect decreased ventricular compliance, whereas prominent V waves reflect the functional incompetence of the tricuspid or mitral valves, owing to cardiac dilation. Intraoperative hypotension is logically treated with drugs such as ephedrine, which provide some degree of beta stimulation. Conversely, predominant alpha stimulation, as produced by phenylephrine, could theoretically evoke adverse increases in ventricular afterload, owing to increased systemic vascular resistance.

Table 7-2. Classification of Cardiomyopathies on Morphologic and Hemodynamic Basis

Factors	Type of Cardiomyopathy			
	Dilated	Restrictive	Hypertrophic	Obliterative
Morphology	Biventricular dilation	Decreased ventricular compliance	Hypertrophy of left ventricle and usually interventricular septum	Thickened endocardium or mural thrombi
Ventricular volume	↑ ↑	Normal or ↑	Normal or ↓	↓
Ejection fraction	↓ ↓	Normal or ↓	↑ ↑	Normal or ↓
Ventricular compliance	Normal or ↓	↓ ↓	↓ ↓	↓ ↓
Ventricular filling pressure	↑ ↑	↑ ↑	Normal or ↑	↑
Stroke volume	↓ ↓	Normal or ↓	Normal or ↑	Normal or ↓

Regional anesthesia may be an alternative to general anesthesia in selected patients with dilated cardiomyopathy.[3] For example, epidural anesthesia produces changes in preload and afterload that mimic pharmacologic goals in the treatment of this disease. Nevertheless, clinical experience is limited, and caution is indicated for avoiding an abrupt onset of blockade of sympathetic nervous system innervation.

RESTRICTIVE CARDIOMYOPATHY

Restrictive cardiomyopathy is characterized by impaired diastolic filling, which produces a clinical and hemodynamic picture (increased filling pressures and decreased cardiac output) that mimics constrictive pericarditis (see Chapter 9). In contrast to the eventual equalization of filling pressures that characterize constrictive pericarditis, restrictive cardiomyopathy tends to cause greater impairment of left than right ventricular filling. As a result, left heart filling pressures are almost always higher than those recorded on the right side of the heart. Infiltration of the myocardium by abnormal material (amyloidosis, hemochromatosis, glycogen storage diseases) is consistent with the noncompliant characteristics of the ventricles. There is no effective treatment for restrictive cardiomyopathy, and death is usually due to cardiac dysrhythmias or intractable congestive heart failure. Management of anesthesia invokes the same principles outlined for patients with cardiac tamponade (see Chapter 9).

HYPERTROPHIC CARDIOMYOPATHY

Hypertrophic cardiomyopathy is often hereditary; it is transmitted as an autosomal dominant characteristic.[4] The age distribution at diagnosis of the disease is bimodal, with a peak incidence early in the fifth decade and a second peak early in the seventh decade. Most elderly patients are females. Sporadic cases of hypertrophic cardiomyopathy may be related to chronic hypertension or to abnormal responses by cardiac muscle to prolonged catecholamine stimulation.

The basic genetic defect seems to be in the contractile elements of the heart (increased density of calcium channels). It is manifested as unexplained myocardial hypertrophy, usually with greater thickening of the interventricular septum compared with that of the free wall of the left ventricle. For this reason, the disease has been termed asymmetric septal hypertrophy, although it is now recognized that the ventricular hypertrophy may be concentric. Furthermore, echocardiography indicates a large variation in the location and extent of the

Table 7-3. Factors That Influence Left Ventricular Outflow Obstruction in Patients With Hypertrophic Cardiomyopathy

Events That Increase Outflow Obstruction	Events That Decrease Outflow Obstruction
Increased myocardial contractility	Decreased myocardial contractility
Beta stimulation (catecholamines)	Beta blockade (propranolol, esmolol)
Digitalis	Volatile anesthetics (halothane)
Tachycardia	Calcium entry blockers
Decreased preload	Increased preload
Hypovolemia	Hypervolemia
Vasodilators (nitroglycerin, nitroprusside)	Bradycardia
Tachycardia	
Positive-pressure ventilation	
Decreased afterload	Increased afterload
Hypotension	Alpha stimulation (phenylephrine)
Hypovolemia	Hypervolemia
Vasodilators	

hypertrophy. The preferred terminology is therefore hypertrophic cardiomyopathy with or without left ventricular outflow obstruction. There is general agreement that known afflicted patients should not participate in competitive sports because of the risk of sudden death.

In its severest form, there is hypertrophy of the left ventricular chamber, which becomes elongated and slitlike (Table 7-2). Even in the presence of severe left ventricular outflow obstruction, the ejection fraction is usually greater than 0.8, reflecting the hypercontractile condition of the heart. Mitral regurgitation reflects interference with movement of the septal leaflet of the mitral valve by the hypertrophied interventricular septum. Alternatively, septal hypertrophy may result in left ventricular outflow obstruction that is constant or intermittent (dynamic). The degree of left ventricular outflow obstruction is influenced by (1) myocardial contractility, (2) preload, and (3) afterload (Table 7-3).

Clinical Features

The principal symptoms of hypertrophic cardiomyopathy are angina pectoris, syncope, tachydysrhythmias, and congestive heart failure. Angina relieved by the assumption of the recumbent position is virtually pathognomonic for hypertrophic cardiomyopathy, presumably because the increase in left ventricular size in recumbency acts to decrease the outflow obstruction. Marked left ventricular hypertrophy makes these patients particularly vulnerable to myocardial ischemia, especially when subendocardial blood flow is decreased because of excessive pressure in the left ventricle. Furthermore, the incidence of ischemic heart disease is increased in these patients; this may subsequently increase the risk of anesthesia and surgery.[5]

Because the left ventricle is so massively hypertrophied, the presystolic atrial contraction is extremely important for the preservation of cardiac output. Consequently, the onset of atrial fibrillation is often poorly tolerated, while an associated rapid heart rate also impairs diastolic filling time and further enhances the deleterious effect of this cardiac dysrhythmia. Systemic embolism is a common complication of atrial fibrillation in this disease. Sudden unexpected death, presumably caused by acute left ventricular outflow obstruction or a cardiac dysrhythmia such as ventricular tachycardia, is possible even in asymptomatic patients.[6] Such fatal cardiac dysrhythmias are especially likely to occur in young patients between the ages of 10 and 30 years.[4]

Cardiac murmurs may reflect the presence of left ventricular outflow obstruction or mitral regurgitation in patients with hypertrophic cardiomyopathy. Indeed, hypertrophic cardiomyopathy may be confused with aortic or mitral valve disease. Characteristic of these murmurs is their marked variation with different maneuvers. For example, the Valsalva maneuver decreases left ventricular chamber size, which increases left ventricular outflow obstruction. In addition, since left ventricular systolic pressure increases, the murmur of mitral regurgitation intensifies as well. Nitroglycerin and standing versus recumbency likewise increases the loudness of the murmur. Hypertrophic cardiomyopathy should be considered in an otherwise asymptomatic patient in whom a systolic murmur develops during long-standing hypertension.[7] Furthermore, previously unrecognized hypertrophic cardiomyopathy may be manifested intraoperatively as hypotension and as a sudden increase in the intensity of a systolic murmur, typically in association with acute hemorrhage or drug-induced vasodilation.[8,9]

The chest radiograph and the electrocardiogram typically depict left ventricular hypertrophy. In an asymptomatic patient, marked unexplained left ventricular hypertrophy may be the only sign of the disease. Because of massive hypertrophy of the interventricular septum, abnormal Q waves resembling those of myocardial infarction may be present. The diagnosis of hypertrophic cardiomyopathy should be considered in any young patient whose electrocardiogram suggests a prior myocardial infarction. Nevertheless, as many as 15% of patients with hypertrophic cardiomyopathy show no evidence of left ventricular hypertrophy on the electrocardiogram.

Echocardiography is useful in demonstrating asymmetric hypertrophy of the interventricular septum, as well as estimating the pressure gradient across the left ventricular outflow tract. When the ratio of septal thickness to left ventricular free wall thickness exceeds 1.3:1, the diagnosis of hypertrophic cardiomyopathy should be considered.

Cardiac catheterization may demonstrate evidence of mitral regurgitation or the presence of increased left ventricular end-diastolic pressure as a consequence of decreased left ventricular compliance. Decreased left ventricular compliance produces an increase in the height of the A wave on the venous pressure tracing that may exceed 30 mmHg. If left ventricular outflow obstruction is present, there is a demonstrable pressure gradient between the left ventricle and aorta. Provocative measures such as the Valsalva maneuver may be required to evoke evidence of left ventricular outflow obstruction during echocardiography or cardiac catheterization, emphasizing the dynamic nature of this obstruction. Left ventricular angiography characteristically shows a small hyperdynamic chamber.

Treatment

Treatment of hypertrophic cardiomyopathy is directed at relieving the obstruction to left ventricular outflow, which may be fixed or dynamic (Table 7-3). Beta antagonists designed to decrease heart rate and myocardial contractility are the preferred initial therapy for the patient with hypertrophic cardiomyopathy. Evidence that suggests an increased density of myocardial calcium channels in afflicted patients suggests a possible beneficial role for calcium entry blockers.[10] Indeed, verapamil has been effective, although drug-induced hypotension and negative inotropic effects would be particularly undesirable in patients with severe left ventricular outflow obstruction. Nitroglycerin should not be administered to the patient with hypertrophic cardiomyopathy and angina. Treatment of congestive heart failure is difficult. This is because diuretics can cause hypovolemia and digoxin can enhance myocardial contractility, with both changes possibly increasing left ventricular outflow obstruction. Cardioversion may be considered in an attempt to maintain normal sinus rhythm. Patients with sustained atrial fibrillation are at increased risk of systemic embolization and, for this reason, may be treated prophylactically with anticoagulants. Infective endocarditis is a risk necessitating appropriate antibiotic prophylaxis for dental or other surgical procedures. Amiodarone may be administered to patients considered at risk of sudden death attributable to cardiac dysrhythmias, usually ventricular tachycardia.

Approximately 10% to 15% of patients with hypertrophic cardiomyopathy undergo myotomy or myomectomy of the left ventricular outflow tract, using cardiopulmonary bypass. In some patients, mitral valve replacement may be necessary. The objective of surgical therapy is relief of left ventricular outflow obstruction with a concomitant decrease in left ventricular systolic pressure. Mortality may approach 8%; for this reason, surgical therapy is usually reserved for symptomatic patients with outflow gradients exceeding 50 mmHg.[4] Symptomatic relief is likely after surgical therapy, but the incidence of sudden cardiac death remains unaltered.[11]

Management of Anesthesia

Management of anesthesia in a patient with hypertrophic cardiomyopathy is directed toward minimizing left ventricular outflow obstruction.[5] In this regard, any drug or event that decreases myocardial contractility or that increases preload or afterload will decrease left ventricular outflow obstruction (Table 7-3). For example, dose-dependent cardiac depression produced by volatile anesthetics and expansion of the intravascular fluid volume will distend the left ventricle and increase stroke volume. Conversely, intraoperative events associated with increased myocardial contractility are not desirable, as these events may increase left ventricular outflow obstruction (Table 7-3). Overall, the risk associated with general anesthesia seems acceptable in patients with hypertrophic cardiomyopathy.[5]

Preoperative Medication

Ideally, preoperative medication should decrease anxiety and associated activation of the sympathetic nervous system. Administration of an anticholinergic such as atropine is questionable, since tachycardia may increase left ventricular outflow obstruction. Conversely, scopolamine produces desirable sedation when used in conjunction with other central nervous system depressant drugs. Changes in heart rate are unlikely after administration of scopolamine. Expansion of intravascular fluid volume during the preoperative period is important in maintaining intraoperative stroke volume and in minimizing adverse effects of positive-pressure ventilation of the lungs.

Induction of Anesthesia

Induction of anesthesia with intravenous drugs is acceptable, remembering the importance of avoiding sudden drug-induced decreases in systemic vascular resistance. Modest degrees of direct myocardial depression are acceptable. In this regard, ketamine is not a likely selection, since increased myocardial contractility will enhance left ventricular outflow obstruction and decrease stroke volume. The duration of direct laryngoscopy should be brief, to minimize activation of the sympathetic nervous system. Administration of a volatile anesthetic or beta antagonist before directly initiating laryngoscopy is a consideration in attempts to blunt the response to intubation of the trachea.

Maintenance of Anesthesia

Maintenance of anesthesia is designed to produce mild depression of myocardial contractility and, at the same time, preserve intravascular fluid volume and systemic vascular resistance. Nitrous oxide combined with a volatile anesthetic such as halothane is acceptable. Theoretically, other volatile anesthetics would be less ideal choices than halothane, as these drugs decrease systemic vascular resistance more than halothane. Nevertheless, enflurane has been administered to these patients without apparent detrimental effects.[5] Opioids are not likely choices for maintenance of anesthesia, as these drugs do not produce myocardial depression and at the same time can decrease systemic vascular resistance. The combination of an opioid with nitrous oxide, however, may be associated with direct myocardial depression and a modest increase in systemic vascular resistance.[12] Hemodynamic changes (hypotension, decreased venous return) that may accompany high levels of sensory anesthesia produced by spinal or epidural anesthesia could contribute to increases in left ventricular outflow obstruction.[13]

Nondepolarizing muscle relaxants that have minimal to no effects on the circulation are useful choices for the production of skeletal muscle paralysis. Increased heart rate as may accompany the administration of pancuronium is not desirable.[5] Likewise, drug-induced histamine release and hypotension that may occur in response to rapid intravenous injection of large doses of atracurium are to be avoided.

Invasive monitoring of arterial and cardiac filling pressures is helpful. Transesophageal echocardiography and Doppler color flow imaging may provide useful information regarding intraoperative left ventricular function and mitral valve function.[14] When intraoperative hypotension occurs in response to decreased preload or afterload, a drug with predominant alpha activity such as phenylephrine (50 to 100 μg IV) is useful for normalizing blood pressure. Drugs with beta agonist activity such as ephedrine, dopamine, or dobutamine are not recommended for treatment of hypotension, since drug-induced increases in myocardial contractility and heart rate can increase left ventricular outflow obstruction.[9] Prompt replacement of blood loss and titration of intravenous fluid administration by measurement of cardiac filling pressures is important in maintaining blood pressure. Pulmonary edema has been observed in parturients with hypertrophic cardiomyopathy after delivery, emphasizing the delicate fluid requirements of these patients.[15] Increased delivered concentrations of a volatile anesthetic are useful for the treatment of persistent hypertension. Vasodilators, such as nitroprusside or nitroglycerin, are not used to lower blood pressure in these patients, since decreased systemic vascular resistance could accentuate left ventricular outflow obstruction (Table 7-3).

Maintenance of normal sinus rhythm in the patient with hypertrophic cardiomyopathy is important, since ventricular filling is dependent on left atrial contraction. A change from sinus rhythm to junctional rhythm is treated with a decrease in the delivered concentration of the volatile anesthetic. If this cardiac dysrhythmia persists, the intravenous administration of atropine may be helpful. A beta antagonist, such as propranolol or esmolol, is indicated to slow a persistently elevated heart rate.

Parturients at term with hypertrophic cardiomyopathy present a major anesthetic challenge, since events such as catecholamine release and "bearing down" (Valsalva maneuver) may increase left ventricular outflow obstruction. Many clinicians believe that regional anesthesia should be avoided in these patients; instead, they recommend general anesthesia with halothane, in the event that cesarean section is needed. Nevertheless, epidural anesthesia has been successfully administered to these patients.[15]

As with the parturient, a patient with hypertrophic cardiomyopathy and an intracranial lesion requiring surgery facilitated by controlled hypotension produces several conflicting therapeutic goals for anesthetic management.[16] Although experience is limited, administration of a beta antagonist, such as esmolol, and the utilization of invasive monitoring, are useful to permit the application of techniques (osmotic diuresis, controlled hypotension) that facilitate intracranial surgery but that are usually avoided in the presence of hypertrophic cardiomyopathy.

OBLITERATIVE CARDIOMYOPATHY

Obliterative cardiomyopathy is considered by some to be a variant of restrictive cardiomyopathy, characterized by marked decreases in ventricular compliance (Table 7-2). This cardiomyopathy may occur in association with hypereosinophilic syndromes that are accompanied by the eosinophilic infiltration of multiple organs. Cardiac dysrhythmias, cardiac conduction disturbances, systemic embolization, and tricuspid and mitral regurgitation are common. Medical therapy may include corticosteroids.

REFERENCES

1. Johnson RA, Palacios I. Dilated cardiomyopathies of the adult. N Engl J Med 1982;307:1051–8
2. Hanson CW. Asymptomatic cardiomyopathy presenting as cardiac arrest in the day surgical unit. Anesthesiology 1989;71:982–4
3. Amaranath L, Eskandiari S, Lockrem J, Rollins M. Epidural analgesia for total hip replacement in a patient with dilated cardiomyopathy. Can Anaesth Soc J 1986;33:84–8
4. Maron BJ, Bonow RO, Canon RO, et al. Hypertrophic cardiomyopathy. Interrelations of clinical manifestations, pathophysiology and therapy. N Engl J Med 1987;316:780–90; 844–51
5. Thompson RC, Liberthson RR, Lowenstein E. Perioperative anesthetic risk of noncardiac surgery in hypertrophic obstructive cardiomyopathy. N Engl J Med 1989;320:755–61
6. Nicod P, Polikar R, Peterson KL. Hypertrophic cardiomyopathy and sudden death. N Engl J Med 1988;318:1255–7
7. Petrin TJ, Tavel ME. Idiopathic hypertrophic subaortic stenosis as observed in a large community hospital. Relation to age and history of hypertension. J Am Geriatr Soc 1979;27:43–6
8. Lanier W, Prough DS. Intraoperative diagnosis of hypertrophic obstructive cardiomyopathy. Anesthesiology 1984;60:61–3
9. Pearson J, Reves JG. Unusual cause of hypotension after coronary artery bypass grafting: Idiopathic hypertrophic subaortic stenosis. Anesthesiology 1984;60:592–4
10. Wagner JA, Sax FL, Weisman HF, et al. Calcium-antagonist receptors in atrial tissue of patients with hypertrophic cardiomyopathy. N Engl J Med 1989;320:755–61
11. McIntosh CL, Maron BJ. Current operative treatment of obstructive hypertrophic cardiomyopathy. Circulation 1988;78:487–93
12. Stoelting RK, Gibbs PS. Hemodynamic effects of morphine and morphine-nitrous oxide in valvular heart disease and coronary artery disease. Anesthesiology 1973;38:45–52
13. Loubser P, Suh K, Cohen S. Adverse effects of spinal anesthesia in a patient with idiopathic hypertrophic subaortic stenosis. Anesthesiology 1984;60:228–30
14. Stanley TE, Rankin JS. Idiopathic hypertrophic subaortic stenosis and ischemic mitral regurgitation: The value of intraoperative transesophageal echocardiography and Doppler color flow imaging in guiding operative therapy. Anesthesiology 1990;72:1083–5
15. Tessler MJ, Hudson R, Naugler-Colville MA, Biehl DR. Pulmonary oedema in two parturients with hypertrophic obstructive cardiomyopathy (HOCM). Can J Anaesth 1990;37:469–73
16. Freilich JD, Jacobs BR. Anesthetic management of cerebral aneurysm resection in a patient with idiopathic hypertrophic subaortic stenosis. Anesth Analg 1990;71:558–60

8

Cor Pulmonale

Cor pulmonale is right ventricular enlargement that develops secondary to pulmonary hypertension.[1] In persons older than 50 years of age, cor pulmonale is the third most common cardiac disorder, after ischemic heart disease and hypertensive heart disease. Males are afflicted five times more often than females. It is estimated that 10% to 30% of patients admitted to the hospital with congestive heart failure exhibit cor pulmonale.

Chronic obstructive pulmonary disease (COPD) with associated loss of pulmonary capillaries and arterial hypoxemia leading to pulmonary vascular vasoconstriction is the most likely cause of cor pulmonale. If this pulmonary vascular vasoconstriction is sustained, it produces hypertrophy of vascular smooth muscle and irreversible increases in the pulmonary vascular resistance. Alveolar hypoxia, when generalized, is the most potent known stimulus for pulmonary vasoconstriction. When alveolar hypoxia is localized, the associated pulmonary vasoconstriction (hypoxic pulmonary vasoconstriction) acts to divert blood flow to better oxygenated alveoli, thereby optimizing ventilation-to-perfusion relationships and arterial oxygenation. Systemic acidosis also promotes pulmonary vasoconstriction and acts synergistically with arterial hypoxemia.

Prognosis for patients with cor pulmonale is determined by the pulmonary disease responsible for initiating the increase in pulmonary vascular resistance. In patients with COPD in whom arterial oxygenation can be maintained at near-normal levels, the prognosis for longevity is favorable. Prognosis is poor in those patients in whom cor pulmonale is the result of gradual destruction of pulmonary vessels by intrinsic pulmonary vascular disease or pulmonary fibrosis. These anatomic changes produce irreversible alterations in the pulmonary vasculature, resulting in fixed elevations of pulmonary vascular resistance.

SIGNS AND SYMPTOMS

Clinical manifestations of cor pulmonale are often nonspecific and tend to be obscured by co-existing COPD. As right ventricular function becomes more impaired, dyspnea increases and effort-related syncope can occur. Right heart catheterization demonstrates elevated mean pulmonary artery pressure (greater than 20 mmHg) and normal pulmonary artery occlusion pressure. Pulmonary hypertension is considered moderate when mean pulmonary artery pressure exceeds 35 mmHg. Accentuation of the pulmonic component of the second heart sound and a diastolic murmur due to incompetence of the pulmonic valve connote severe pulmonary artery hypertension. The A wave of the right atrial pressure tracing becomes prominent, reflecting enhanced right atrial contraction in response to decreased right ventricular compliance. Doppler ultrasonography usually demonstrates some evidence of tricuspid regurgitation, even in the absence of an audible murmur. Overt right ventricular failure is evidenced by an elevated jugular venous pressure, hepatosplenomegaly, and peripheral dependent edema. Patients with COPD are often cigarette smokers and are therefore likely to have ischemic heart disease that may result in left ventricular dysfunction along with right ventricular failure.

The rate at which right ventricular dysfunction develops depends on the magnitude of pressure increase in the pulmonary circulation and on the rapidity with which this increase occurs. For example, pulmonary embolism may produce right ventricular failure with a mean pulmonary artery pressure as low as 30 mmHg. By contrast, when pulmonary hypertension develops gradually, as with COPD, and the right ventricle has time to compensate, congestive heart failure (CHF) rarely occurs until mean pulmonary artery pressure exceeds 50 mmHg.[2] In patients with COPD, acute right ventricular failure may develop during pulmonary infections. This CHF may reverse spontaneously with successful treatment of the pulmonary infection, presumably reflecting a concomitant decrease in pulmonary vascular resistance.

Chest Radiograph

Right ventricular hypertrophy is reflected by a decrease in the retrosternal space seen on the lateral projection of the chest radiograph. Prominence of the main pulmonary artery and decreased pulmonary vascular markings are suggestive of pulmonary hypertension. In patients with COPD, dramatic changes in heart size may characteristically occur between episodes of acute pulmonary dysfunction and recovery.

Electrocardiogram

The electrocardiogram in the presence of cor pulmonale may show signs of right atrial and ventricular hypertrophy. Right atrial hypertrophy is suggested by peaked P waves in leads II, III, and aVF. Right axis deviation and a partial or complete right bundle branch block are often seen on the electrocardiogram when right ventricular hypertrophy is present.

TREATMENT

Treatment of cor pulmonale is intended to decrease the workload of the right ventricle by decreasing pulmonary vascular resistance (Table 8-1). This goal is best achieved by returning the PaO_2, $PaCO_2$, and pH to a normal range, assuming that pulmonary artery and arteriolar vasoconstriction are reversible. This assumption is likely to be valid in the presence of COPD, particularly during an exacerbation caused by an acute pulmonary infection. By contrast, pulmonary vascular resistance is unlikely to be responsive to treatment when anatomic occlusive lesions are responsible for pulmonary artery hypertension.

Supplemental administration of oxygen to maintain the PaO_2 greater than 60 mmHg or a SaO_2 above 90%, decreases the mortality from cor pulmonale and improves cognitive function and quality of life.[1] Uncontrolled oxygen administration entails some risk, especially if hypoxic stimulation is necessary to maintain alveolar ventilation. An alternative to supplemental oxygen may be the administration of almitrine, a carotid body stimulant that improves ventilation-to-perfusion matching without affecting minute ventilation.[1]

Long-term anticoagulation with warfarin-type drugs or the administration of antiplatelet drugs is often recommended as prophylaxis against thrombus formation that may result in pulmonary emboli. Indeed, low cardiac output and a sedentary life-style are consistent with the increased incidence of thrombus formation in patients with cor pulmonale. A small pulmonary embolism that would likely have little effect on a normal patient could have catastrophic consequences in a patient with pulmonary hypertension.

Diuretics and digitalis may be administered for treatment of CHF that does not respond to correction of arterial blood gases. Diuretics have to be given with care, as drug-induced metabolic alkalosis may aggravate ventilatory insufficiency by depressing the effectiveness of carbon dioxide as a stimulus to breathing. Moreover, diuresis may increase blood viscosity by further increasing the hematocrit. Digitalis must be used cautiously, since the risk of drug toxicity is increased in the presence of arterial hypoxemia, acidosis, and electrolyte imbalance, which are common in patients with cor pulmonale.

Despite the initial enthusiasm for vasodilator therapy, only about one-third of treated patients experience improvement, and even this may be transient. Calcium entry blockers, notably nifedipine or diltiazem, have met with some success. Unfortunately, vasodilators often affect the systemic circulation more than the pulmonary circulation. If vasodilation affects primarily the systemic circulation without an adequate increase in cardiac output, systemic hypotension will result. In addition to hypotension, acute administration of vasodilators may aggravate arterial hypoxemia by attenuating hypoxic vasoconstriction, worsening the homogeneity of ventilation-to-perfusion matching. In an animal model of pulmonary hypertension, nitroglycerin, but not nitroprusside, lowered both pulmonary artery pressure and pulmonary vascular resistance.[3]

Prompt treatment with antibiotics will minimize an additional increase in pulmonary vascular resistance associated with a pulmonary infection. Invading organisms are most often strains of *Haemophilus* or *Pneumococcus,* which are usually sensitive to ampicillin or, alternatively, to a cephalosporin. When cor pulmonale is progressive despite maximum medical therapy, transplantation of either a single lung or of two lungs, or a heart-lung block, can provide dramatic relief of cardiorespiratory failure.[1]

MANAGEMENT OF ANESTHESIA

It is recommended that elective operations in patients with cor pulmonale be postponed until the reversible components of co-existing COPD are treated. Preoperative preparation is directed toward (1) elimination and control of acute or chronic pulmonary infections, or both; (2) reversal of bronchospasm; (3) improvement of secretion clearance; (4) expansion of collapsed or poorly ventilated alveoli; (5) hydration; and (6) correction of any electrolyte imbalance. Arterial blood gases and pH should be determined to provide guidelines for management of the patient, both intraoperatively and postoperatively.

Table 8-1. Treatment of Cor Pulmonale

Supplemental oxygen	Anticoagulants
Diuretics	Antibiotics
Digitalis	Heart-lung transplantation
Vasodilators	

Preoperative Medication

Preoperative medication should not include drugs that are likely to produce excessive depression of ventilation. Although opioids are the most potent in this regard, any medication that produces sedation can result in depression of ventilation. Often, a preoperative interview will serve to allay the patient's apprehension, eliminating the need for pharmacologic premedication.

The depressant effects of anticholinergic drugs on mucociliary activity and the possible impairment of clearance of secretions may outweigh the advantages of including these drugs in the preoperative medication. If a specific case requires anticholinergic drugs, an alternative is to administer these drugs intravenously, just before the induction of anesthesia.

Induction of Anesthesia

Induction of anesthesia is usually accomplished with the intravenous injection of rapidly acting induction drugs, taking care to avoid an abrupt decrease in systemic vascular resistance in the presence of a fixed increase in pulmonary vascular resistance. An adequate depth of anesthesia should be present before a tube is placed in the trachea, as this stimulus in a lightly anesthetized patient can elicit reflex bronchospasm. Furthermore, an increase in systemic and pulmonary vascular resistance may accompany intubation of the trachea, especially when the concentration of anesthetic drugs is minimal.[4]

Maintenance of Anesthesia

Maintenance of anesthesia is usually with a combination of inhalation anesthetics. Enflurane and isoflurane are probably as effective as halothane as bronchodilators, in the patient with co-existing reversible bronchospasm.[5] Large doses of opioids are not recommended, as they could contribute to prolonged depression of ventilation during the postoperative period. Nitrous oxide may produce pulmonary artery vasoconstriction and a further increase in pulmonary vascular resistance.[6,7] For this reason, it may be prudent to monitor right atrial pressure to provide an early warning that nitrous oxide is causing enhanced and undesirable degrees of pulmonary hypertension. Conversely, there are also data demonstrating that administration of nitrous oxide does not exacerbate pulmonary hypertension.[8] The choice of nondepolarizing muscle relaxants is not critical, although histamine release with administration of certain of these drugs might have adverse effects on airway and pulmonary vascular resistance.

Intermittent positive-pressure breathing is most often selected for the intraoperative management of ventilation in a patient with cor pulmonale. Although positive pressure applied to the airways and alveoli can increase pulmonary vascular resistance, this potential adverse effect is usually more than offset by improved arterial oxygenation. Improved oxygenation during positive-pressure ventilation of the lungs presumably reflects better distribution of ventilation-to-perfusion. An excessive decrease in the $PaCO_2$ during controlled ventilation of the lungs should be avoided, since metabolic alkalosis could produce hypokalemia. This is particularly important in the patient being treated with digitalis, since an acute decrease in the plasma potassium concentration can predispose to digitalis toxicity. Humidification of the inhaled gases helps maintain hydration and liquefaction of secretions.

Regional anesthetic techniques are appropriate considerations for superficial surgery or operations on the extremities of a patient with cor pulmonale. Operations that would require a high sensory level of anesthesia are not optimally performed with regional anesthesia in patients with pulmonary hypertension, since any decrease in systemic vascular resistance in the presence of a fixed increase in pulmonary vascular resistance could produce undesirable degrees of systemic hypotension.

Monitoring

Intraoperative monitoring of a patient with cor pulmonale is influenced by the invasiveness of the operation. An intra-arterial catheter permits frequent determination of arterial blood gases and subsequent adjustments in inspired concentrations of oxygen. Continuous monitoring of SaO_2 and $P_{ET}CO_2$ decreases the need for frequent analysis of arterial blood gases. A right atrial catheter provides useful information regarding right ventricular function and the safety of intravenous infusions of fluids. Abrupt increases in right atrial pressure during the intraoperative period signal right ventricular dysfunction that mandates a search for a sudden increase in pulmonary vascular resistance, as can be produced by unrecognized arterial hypoxemia, hypoventilation, or drugs such as nitrous oxide. Furthermore, maintenance of an adequate right heart filling pressure is necessary to ensure an optimal right ventricular stroke volume. When left ventricular dysfunction accompanies cor pulmonale and the magnitude of the surgery includes the likelihood of large fluid volume replacement, it may be helpful to place a pulmonary artery catheter, which facilitates regulation of intravascular fluid volume and cardiac output with volume infusions and inotropic drugs.

PRIMARY PULMONARY HYPERTENSION

Primary pulmonary hypertension is a rare disorder that is diagnosed when cor pulmonale develops in the absence of a recognizable cause (pulmonary embolism, COPD) for elevated pressures in the pulmonary circulation.[1,12] In this regard, primary pulmonary hypertension is a diagnosis of exclusion. The mean age at diagnosis is 33 years with females predominating. A high prevalence of antinuclear antibodies in patients with primary pulmonary hypertension raises the possibility that some of these patients have collagen vascular disease and associated vasculitis confined to the pulmonary vasculature. Further evidence of a generalized vasospastic disease is the frequency of Raynaud's phenomenon, Prinzmetal's angina, and migraine headache in patients with primary pulmonary hypertension. The occurrence of pulmonary hypertension in patients with advanced liver disease implicates vasoactive compounds that bypass liver degradation. Familial cases of pulmonary hypertension may occur. Primary pulmonary hypertension may present for the first time during pregnancy when cardiovascular demands increase.

The time from onset of symptoms (dyspnea, fatigue, exertional syncope) to diagnosis (elevated pulmonary artery pressures in association with normal left heart filling pressures) of pulmonary hypertension is about 2 years. Syncope presumably reflects the inability of the right ventricular stroke volume to increase in the presence of a fixed elevation of pulmonary vascular resistance. Events leading to sudden peripheral vasodilation (strenuous exercise, standing after a hot bath, drug-induced hypotension) may also lead to syncope.

Chest pain similar to angina pectoris may occur in primary pulmonary hypertension, probably because increased myocardial oxygen demand by the right ventricle cannot be adequately met by the limited capacity of the coronary arteries that supply the right ventricle. The natural history of primary pulmonary hypertension is unpredictable, with the average survival after the diagnosis being 2 years, although occasional patients survive 15 to 20 years. Treatment of primary pulmonary hypertension is as described for cor pulmonale. The goals in the management of anesthesia are to prevent sudden and sustained decreases in systemic vascular resistance or a further increase in pulmonary vascular resistance.

Some degree of pulmonary hypertension is present in all high-altitude residents, including persons born at sea level. Most patients with primary pulmonary hypertension will be adversely affected by even modest altitude elevation (1500 m). Exertional dyspnea is intensified, presumably reflecting a hypoxia-induced increase in pulmonary vascular resistance.

REFERENCES

1. Palevsky HI, Fishman AP. Chronic cor pulmonale. Etiology and management. JAMA 1991;263:2347–53
2. Robotham JL. Cardiovascular disturbance in chronic respiratory insufficiency. Am J Cardiol 1981;47:941–9
3. Pearl RG, Rosenthal MH, Ashton JPA. Pulmonary vasodilator effects of nitroglycerin and sodium nitroprusside in canine oleic acid-induced pulmonary hypertension. Anesthesiology 1983;58:514–8
4. Sorensen MB, Jacobsen E. Pulmonary hemodynamics during induction of anesthesia. Anesthesiology 1977;46:246–51
5. Hirshman CA, Edelstein G, Peetz S, et al. Mechanism of action of inhalational anesthesia on airways. Anesthesiology 1982;56:107–111
6. Hilgenberg JC, McCammon RL, Stoelting RK. Pulmonary and systemic vascular responses to nitrous oxide in patients with mitral stenosis and pulmonary hypertension. Anesth Analg 1980;59:323–6
7. Schulte-Sasse U, Hess W, Tarnow J. Pulmonary vascular responses to nitrous oxide in patients with normal and high pulmonary vascular resistance. Anesthesiology 1982;57:9–13
8. Konstadt SN, Reich DL, Thys DM. Nitrous oxide does not exacerbate pulmonary hypertension or ventricular dysfunction in patients with mitral valvular disease. Can J Anaesth 1990;37:613–7
9. Rich S, Dantzker DR, Ayres SM, et al. Primary pulmonary hypertension: A national prospective study. Ann Intern Med 1987;107:216–23

9

Pericardial Diseases

Pericardial disease results from diverse causes that evoke responses described as acute pericarditis, pericardial effusion, or chronic constrictive pericarditis. Cardiac tamponade is a possibility when pericardial fluid accumulates under pressure. Management of anesthesia in patients with pericardial disease requires an understanding of alterations in cardiovascular function produced by specific pericardial diseases.[1]

ACUTE PERICARDITIS

Acute pericarditis is an inflammatory process of the pericardium that may be due to a variety of causes but most often reflects a viral infection[2] (Table 9-1). Dressler syndrome is a delayed form of acute pericarditis that may follow an acute myocardial infarction. The clinical diagnosis of acute pericarditis is suggested by the sudden onset of severe chest pain exaggerated by inspiration and diffuse ST segment elevation on the electrocardiogram, which presumably reflects extension of the inflammatory reaction from the pericardium to the surface of the heart. Auscultation of the chest often indicates a friction rub described as "to-and-fro," leathery in quality, and of increased intensity during exhalation. Sinus tachycardia and a low-grade temperature elevation are usually present. In some instances, pain of acute pericarditis can radiate to the abdomen and mimic surgical disease. Treatment of acute pericarditis is symptomatic, including analgesics and corticosteroids. Acute pericarditis in the absence of an associated pericardial effusion does not alter cardiac function.

PERICARDIAL EFFUSION

The inflammatory reaction characteristic of acute pericarditis may be associated with the accumulation of fluid in the pericardial space. Normally, the pericardial space contains 20 to 25 ml of pericardial fluid (an ultrafiltrate of plasma); intraper-icardial pressure is subatmospheric, decreasing on inspiration and increasing on exhalation. The clinical effects of a pericardial effusion depend on whether the fluid is under increased pressure and producing cardiac tamponade (see the section, Cardiac Tamponade). If the effusion develops gradually, the pericardium can stretch to accommodate a large volume of fluid without a significant increase in pressure. By contrast, even a small volume of fluid (100 to 200 ml) that accumulates rapidly can cause acute cardiac tamponade. Echocardiography is the most useful method for clinical detection of pericardial effusion. Computed tomography is also highly reliable in detecting pericardial effusion and pericardial thickening.

CHRONIC CONSTRICTIVE PERICARDITIS

Chronic constrictive pericarditis resembles cardiac tamponade, in that both processes impede diastolic filling of the heart, increase venous pressure, and decrease stroke volume. Most cases of chronic constrictive pericarditis are idiopathic, although chronic renal failure, radiation therapy, rheumatoid arthritis, and cardiac surgery may be predisposing events. The characteristic fibrous scarring and adhesion of both pericardial layers have been likened to a rigid shell around the heart.

The diagnosis of constrictive pericarditis depends on the recognition of increased venous pressure in a patient who does not have other obvious signs or symptoms of heart disease. Although constrictive pericarditis involves both sides of the heart, the dominant manifestations are often those of right ventricular failure with venous congestion, hepatosplenomegaly, and ascites. Elevation and eventual equalization of right atrial pressure, pulmonary artery end-diastolic pressure, and pulmonary artery occlusion pressure may occur in the presence of both chronic constrictive pericarditis and cardiac tamponade. Atrial dysrhythmias (atrial fibrillation or flutter) are common in patients with chronic constrictive pericarditis, pre-

Table 9-1.   Causes of Acute Pericarditis With or Without Pericardial Effusion

Infectious
    Viral
    Bacterial
    Fungal
    Tuberculosis (often associated with acquired immunodeficiency
        syndrome)
Postmyocardial infarction (Dressler syndrome)
Post-traumatic (cardiac surgery, pacemaker, or pressure monitoring
    catheters)
Metastatic disease
Drug-induced (minoxidil, procainamide)
Mediastinal radiation
Systemic disease
    Rheumatoid arthritis
    Systemic lupus erythematosus
    Scleroderma

sumably reflecting involvement of the sinoatrial node by the disease process. Exaggerated distension of neck veins during inspiration (Kussmaul sign) is commonly present, whereas accentuated decreases in systolic blood pressure during inspiration (pulsus paradoxus) are seen more frequently in patients with cardiac tamponade. A chest radiograph reveals a normal to small heart, and calcium is often visible in the pericardium. The electrocardiogram may reveal low-voltage QRS complexes, inversion of T waves, and notched P waves. Computed tomography is superior to echocardiography in demonstrating pericardial thickening.

Treatment

Treatment of chronic constrictive pericarditis consists of surgical removal of the constricting adherent pericardium, which may result in massive bleeding from the epicardial surface of the heart. Cardiopulmonary bypass may be used to facilitate the procedure, especially if hemorrhage is difficult to control. Unlike cardiac tamponade, in which hemodynamic improvement occurs promptly, surgical removal of constricting pericardium is not immediately followed by decreases in right atrial pressure or by increases in cardiac output. Typically, right atrial pressure returns to normal levels within 3 months after surgery. The absence of immediate hemodynamic improvement may reflect disuse atrophy from prolonged constriction of myocardial muscle fibers or persistent constrictive effects from sclerotic epicardium, which is not removed with the parietal pericardium. In general, myocardial function is normal in patients with constrictive pericarditis.

Management of Anesthesia

In the absence of hypotension caused by increased intrapericardial pressure, anesthetic drugs that do not excessively (1) depress myocardial contractility, (2) decrease blood pressure,

(3) slow heart rate, or (4) interfere with venous return are most often selected. Combinations of benzodiazepines, opioids, and nitrous oxide with or without low doses of volatile anesthetics are acceptable for maintenance of anesthesia. Muscle relaxants with minimal circulatory effects are often selected, although modest increases in heart rate as associated with pancuronium are acceptable. Preoperative optimization of intravascular fluid volume is important in these patients. When hemodynamic compromise from elevated intrapericardial pressure is present, treatment and management of anesthesia are as described for cardiac tamponade (see the section, Cardiac Tamponade).

Invasive monitoring of arterial and venous pressures is useful, as removal of adherent pericardium may be tedious and may be associated with decreases in blood pressure and cardiac output. Cardiac dysrhythmias are common during surgical removal of adherent pericardium, presumably reflecting direct mechanical stimulation of the heart. In this regard, cardiac antidysrhythmic drugs and an electrical defibrillator should be promptly available. Venous access and appropriate fluids are necessary to treat the occasional massive blood loss associated with pericardectomy.

Postoperative ventilatory insufficiency may necessitate continued mechanical ventilation of the lungs. Cardiac dysrhythmias and low cardiac output may require treatment during the postoperative period. An infrequent complication of subtotal pericardectomy is pneumopericardium.

CARDIAC TAMPONADE

Cardiac tamponade results from an accumulation of fluid in the pericardial space that elevates intrapericardial pressure, leading to (1) impaired diastolic filling of the heart, (2) decreased stroke volume, and (3) hypotension. Accumulation of pericardial fluid leading to cardiac tamponade may follow a variety of events. Cardiac tamponade may be a cause of low cardiac output syndrome during the early postoperative period after cardiac surgery, necessitating an urgent return to the operating room.[1] Cardiac tamponade has been observed in up to 6% of patients in renal failure and in 15% to 55% of patients with uremic pericarditis.[3] Echocardiography is the most useful method for detecting the presence of pericardial fluid. The cardiac silhouette on a chest radiograph does not change until about 250 ml of fluid is present in the pericardial space.

Signs and Symptoms

A high index of suspicion is necessary for the prompt diagnosis of cardiac tamponade (Table 9-2). As the intrapericardial fluid pressure increases, there is a corresponding increase in central venous pressure, emphasizing that monitoring right atrial pressure may be used to determine whether cardiac

Table 9-2.   Signs and Symptoms of Cardiac Tamponade

Increased central venous pressure
Activation of the sympathetic nervous system
Equalization of atrial filling pressures and pulmonary artery end-diastolic pressure
Decreased voltage and electrical alternans on the electrocardiogram
Paradoxical pulse
Hypotension

tamponade is present. Activation of the sympathetic nervous system occurs in an attempt to maintain cardiac output and blood pressure, by virtue of tachycardia and peripheral vasoconstriction. Indeed, cardiac output and blood pressure are maintained as long as pressure in central veins exceeds right ventricular end-diastolic pressure. A persistent and progressive elevation of intrapericardial fluid pressure eventually result in equalization at about 20 mmHg of right and left atrial pressures and right ventricular end-diastolic filling pressures, as measured with a pulmonary artery catheter.[4] It should be remembered that accumulation of blood and blood clots over the right ventricle, as often occurs after cardiac surgery, may result in an elevated right atrial pressure, although the pulmonary artery occlusion pressure remains normal. Compensatory mechanisms may ultimately fail, and profound hypotension is likely. Many of the initial manifestations of cardiac tamponade mimic pulmonary embolism.

The electrocardiogram in the presence of cardiac tamponade may show decreased voltage, owing to a short-circuiting effect of pericardial fluid. Evidence of myocardial ischemia may be present if elevated transmural pressure on the ventricles interferes with coronary blood flow. Electrical alternans is present in 10% to 15% of patients with cardiac tamponade, reflecting a beat-to-beat oscillation of the heart within the pericardial sac.[1]

A paradoxical pulse (pulsus paradoxus) is an exaggerated decrease in systolic blood pressure (greater than 10 mmHg) during inspiration in the presence of increased intrapericardial pressure (Fig. 9-1). Nevertheless, 10 mmHg is an arbitrary value and should not be regarded as a definitive finding in establishing the presence of cardiac tamponade. The physiology of paradoxical pulse is not clear but most likely involves selective impairment of left ventricular filling during inspiration. Kussmaul sign is increased venous pressure with inspiration that occurs only in cases of cardiac tamponade associated with constrictive pericarditis.

Treatment

Percutaneous subxiphoid pericardiocentesis performed with local anesthesia is the most commonly used surgical method for the treatment of cardiac tamponade. Echocardiography or a monitoring electrocardiogram is useful in guiding the needle into the pericardial space.[5] Removal of only small amounts of pericardial fluid often results in a dramatic decrease in intrapericardial pressure. A pericardiotomy performed in the operating room under local or general anesthesia is the recommended treatment when cardiac tamponade results from trauma or develops after cardiac surgery.

Temporary measures designed to maintain stroke volume until definitive treatment of cardiac tamponade can be insti-

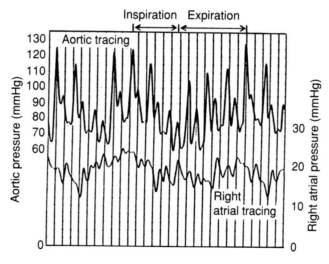

Fig. 9-1. In the presence of cardiac tamponade, the arterial blood pressure decreases greater than 10 mmHg during inspiration, as a reflection of a concomitant decrease in left ventricular stroke volume. This contrasts with the opposite response observed during inspiration in the absence of cardiac tamponade, accounting for its designation as a paradoxical pulse (pulsus paradoxus).

Table 9-3.   Effects of Volume Expansion and Pericardiocentesis in Patients With Acute Cardiac Tamponade (Mean $\pm$ SE)

	Cardiac Tamponade	Cardiac Tamponade Plus Volume Expansion With 500 ml Normal Saline	After Pericardiocentesis
Mean arterial pressure (mmHg)	83 ± 16	82 ± 19	80 ± 13
Right atrial pressure (mmHg)	15 ± 3	17 ± 4	8 ± 4[a]
Pulsus paradoxus (mmHg)	25 ± 12	25 ± 15	8 ± 4[a]
Cardiac output (L·min^{-1})	5.1 ± 2.6	5.5 ± 2.6	9.1 ± 3[a]
Heart rate (beats·min^{-1})	118 ± 11	112 ± 11	121 ± 16

[a] $P < 0.05$ versus other condition.

(Data from Kerber RE, Gascho JA, Litchfield R, et al. Hemodynamic effects of volume expansion and nitroprusside compared with pericardiocentesis in patients with acute cardiac tamponade. N Engl J Med 1982;307:929–31.)

tuted include (1) expansion of intravascular fluid volume, (2) administration of a catecholamine to increase myocardial contractility, and (3) correction of metabolic acidosis.[1]

Expansion of intravascular fluid volume can be achieved by intravenous infusion of a colloid or crystalloid solution (500 ml over 5 to 10 minutes). Volume infusion that increases right atrial pressure to 25 to 30 mmHg may be necessary to offset the effect of increased intrapericardial pressure on venous return.[6] Despite the time-honored acceptance of intravascular fluid volume expansion for the emergency treatment of cardiac tamponade, improvement in hemodynamic function may be limited, and pericardiocentesis should not be delayed[7] (Table 9-3).

Continuous intravenous infusion of isoproterenol or another catecholamine may be an effective temporizing measure for increasing myocardial contractility and heart rate, although the beneficial effects of these drugs in animals with experimentally induced cardiac tamponade has not been reproduced in patients.[8] High doses of dopamine that increase systemic vascular resistance could be undesirable. Vasodilator drugs, such as nitroprusside or hydralazine, could theoretically improve cardiac output, but their use should be considered only when intravascular fluid replacement is achieved. As with intravascular fluid volume replacement, pericardiocentesis should never be delayed in preference for drug therapy.

Metabolic acidosis owing to low cardiac output is appropriately treated with administration of sodium bicarbonate (0.5 to 1 mEq·kg^{-1} IV). Correction of metabolic acidosis is important, as an increased hydrogen ion concentration can depress myocardial contractility and attenuate the positive inotropic effects of catecholamines. Atropine may be necessary to treat bradycardia that results from vagal reflexes, as intrapericardial pressures increase.[9]

Management of Anesthesia

Institution of general anesthesia and positive-pressure ventilation of the lungs in the presence of cardiac tamponade that is hemodynamically significant can lead to life-threatening hy-

potension. Reasons for hypotension include anesthetic-induced peripheral vasodilation, direct myocardial depression, and decreased venous return. In this regard, pericardiocentesis performed with local anesthesia is often preferred for the initial management of a patient who is hypotensive, owing to low cardiac output produced by cardiac tamponade.[10] Ketamine, administered intravenously, can provide sedation in selected patients.[1]

After hemodynamic status has been improved by percutaneous pericardiocentesis, it may be considered more acceptable to induce general anesthesia and institute positive-pressure ventilation of the lungs to permit surgical exploration and more definitive treatment of cardiac tamponade. Induction and maintenance of anesthesia are often with ketamine or a benzodiazepine plus nitrous oxide. The circulatory effects of pancuronium make this a useful drug for the production of skeletal muscle paralysis in these patients. Monitors should include intra-arterial and central venous pressure catheters.

When it is not possible to relieve intrapericardial pressure causing cardiac tamponade before the induction of anesthesia, the goal must be to maintain cardiac output. Anesthetic-induced decreases in myocardial contractility, systemic vascular resistance, and heart rate must be avoided. Increased intrathoracic pressure caused by straining or coughing during induction of anesthesia or by controlled ventilation of the lungs may further reduce venous return in the presence of increased intrapericardial pressure[11] (Fig. 9-2). For this reason, it may be prudent to avoid vigorous positive-pressure ventilation of the lungs until the chest is opened and drainage of the pericardial space is imminent. Ketamine is useful for induction and maintenance of anesthesia, as this drug can increase myocardial contractility, systemic vascular resistance, and heart rate. Induction of anesthesia with diazepam, followed by maintenance of anesthesia with nitrous oxide plus fentanyl and pancuronium for skeletal muscle relaxation, has also been successfully used in these patients.[12] Continuous monitoring of central venous pressure and systemic blood pressure should be initi-

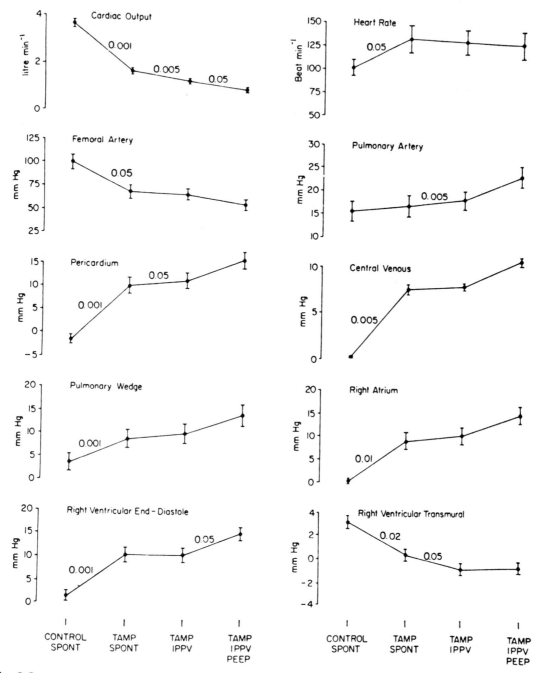

Fig. 9-2. Cardiac output and pleural, pericardial, arterial, and cardiac filling pressures (mean ±SE), as measured in animals during different modes of ventilation in the presence of acute cardiac tamponade. SPONT, spontaneous breathing; TAMP, cardiac tamponade; IPPV, intermittent positive-pressure ventilation; PEEP, positive end-expiratory pressure. (From Moller CT, Schoonbee CG, Rosendorff C. Haemodynamics of cardiac tamponade during various modes of ventilation. Br J Anaesth 1979;51: 409–15, with permission.)

ated before the induction of anesthesia. Maintenance of elevated central venous pressure with generous administration of intravenous fluids is indicated to maintain venous return. A continuous intravenous infusion of catecholamines, such as isoproterenol, dopamine, or dobutamine, may be necessary to maintain cardiac output until the pericardial space can be surgically drained. In addition, personnel and equipment should be available to perform an emergency pericardiocentesis, in case circulatory collapse occurs after induction of anesthesia.

REFERENCES

1. Lake CL. Anesthesia and pericardial disease. Anesth Analg 1983; 62:431–43
2. Permanyer-Miralda G, Sagrista-Sauleda J, Soler-Soler J: Primary acute pericardial disease: A prospective series of 231 consecutive patients. Am J Cardiol 1985;56:623–6
3. Singh S, Newmark K, Ishikawa I. Pericardectomy in uremia, treatment of choice for cardiac tamponade in chronic renal failure. JAMA 1974;228:1132–5
4. Weeks KR, Chatterjee K, Block S, et al. Bedside hemodynamic monitoring: Its value in the diagnosis of tamponade complicating cardiac surgery. J Thorac Cardiovasc Surg 1976;71:250–2
5. Callahan JA, Seward JB, Nishimura RA, et al. Two-dimensional echocardiographically guided pericardiocentesis: Experience in 117 consecutive patients. Am J Cardiol 1985;55:476–80
6. DeCrestofaro D, Liu CK. The hemodynamics of cardiac tamponade and blood volume overload in dogs. Cardiovasc Res 1969;3: 292–8
7. Kerber RE, Gascho JA, Litchfield R, et al. Hemodynamic effects of volume expansion and nitroprusside compared with pericardiocentesis in patients with acute cardiac tamponade. N Engl J Med 1982;307:929–31
8. Martins JB, Manuel JB, Marcus ML, Kerber RE. Comparative effects of catecholamines in cardiac tamponade: Experimental and clinical studies. Am J Cardiol 1980;46:59–66
9. Friedman HS, Lajam F, Gomes JA, et al. Demonstration of a depressor reflex in acute cardiac tamponade. J Thorac Cardiovasc Surg 1977;73:278–86
10. Stanley TH, Weidauer HE. Anesthesia for the patient with cardiac tamponade. Anesth Analg 1973;52:110–4
11. Moller CT, Schoonbee CG, Rosendorff C. Haemodynamics of cardiac tamponade during various modes of ventilation. Br J Anaesth 1979;51:409–15
12. Konchigere HN, Levitsky S. Anesthetic considerations for pericardectomy in uremic pericardial effusion. Anesth Analg 1976;55: 378–82

10

Aneurysms of the Thoracic and Abdominal Aorta

Diseases of the aorta are most often aneurysmal, whereas occlusive disease is more likely to occur in the peripheral arteries. Aneurysms of the aorta may involve the ascending or descending portions of the thoracic aorta or the portion of the aorta below the diaphragm. The initiating event in aortic dissection is a tear in the intima. Blood surges through the tear into a false lumen separating the intima from the adventitia for various distances.[1] The origin of side branches arising from this portion of the aorta may be compromised and the aortic valve rendered incompetent. Blood in the false lumen can reenter the true lumen anywhere along the course of the dissection. Alternatively, rupture of the aorta occurs most frequently into the pericardial space and the left pleural cavity.

ANEURYSMS OF THE THORACIC AORTA

Dissection of the aorta can originate anywhere along the length of the aorta, but the most common point of origin is the ascending aorta within a few centimeters of the aortic valve. The second most common location is the descending thoracic aorta just distal to the origin of the left subclavian artery in the region of the insertion of the ligamentum arteriosum.

Classification

The traditional classification of aortic dissection recognizes three anatomic types[2] (Fig. 10-1). Type I and II aortic dissections both originate in the ascending aorta. Type I dissections may extend either retrograde around the arch of the aorta or anterograde toward the abdominal aorta, or both, whereas type II dissections are confined to the ascending aorta. Type I dissections account for about 70% of all aneurysms of the

thoracic aorta. Type III dissections originate in the descending thoracic aorta, with type IIIA stopping above the diaphragm and type IIIB extending below the diaphragm. Alternatively, aortic dissections can be classified as those that involve the ascending aorta (type A) and those that are limited to the descending aorta (distal to the left subclavian artery) (type B)[3] (Fig. 10-2). Type A dissections may involve the descending aorta as well. Aortic dissection is categorized as "acute" if presentation occurs within 14 days of onset and as "chronic" if more than 14 days have elapsed. The importance of this temporal distinction is the 65% to 75% mortality in patients with untreated dissection of the aorta within the first 14 days after onset.

Etiology

Classically, aortic dissection has been associated with degeneration of the media of the aorta (cystic medial necrosis). Hypertension is the most important predisposing factor for aortic dissection, being present in 70% to 90% of afflicted patients. Although arteriosclerosis frequently co-exists with aortic dissection, especially distal dissection, its etiologic role is unclear. Other factors predisposing to aortic dissection, especially of the ascending aorta, are congenital disorders of connective tissue, such as Marfan syndrome, and, to a lesser extent, Ehlers-Danlos syndrome. Deceleration injuries, as result from automobile accidents, are another cause of aortic dissection, most often involving the distal descending thoracic aorta at its site of fixation to the thorax by the ligamentum arteriosum just distal to the origin of the left subclavian artery. Blunt trauma to the thoracic aorta or the heart, or both, must be considered in any patient with severe chest injury (see the section, Myocardial Contusion). Chest trauma may seem so trivial that associated injury to the thoracic aorta is not suspected. Aortic dissection predominates in males, but there is an association with pregnancy. For example, about one-half of all aortic dissections in females younger than 40 years of age occur during pregnancy, usually in the third trimester.[4] Iatrogenic aortic dissection may occur as a complication of cardiopulmonary bypass at the site of aortic cannulation. Aortic dissection may also arise where the aorta has been cross-clamped or incised, as for aortic valve replacement or proximal anastomosis of a vein bypass graft.

Signs and Symptoms

Acute dissection of the thoracic aorta is usually heralded by the onset of excruciating chest pain (tearing or ripping sensation), in contrast to the crescendo nature of angina pectoris, which is of maximal intensity at its inception. Pain often

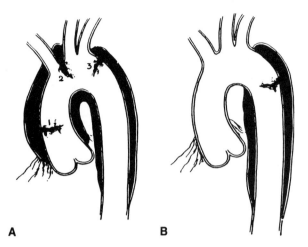

A   **B**

Fig. 10-2. Aortic dissections may be classified as (**A**) those that involve the ascending aorta (type A) and (**B**) those that are limited to the descending aorta (type B). The intimal tear in type A dissection is usually at position 1, whereas the intimal tear for a type B dissection is usually within 2 to 5 cm of the left subclavian artery. (From Daily PO, Trueblood W, Stinson EB, Wuerflein RD, Shumway NE. Management of acute aortic dissections. Ann Thorac Surg 1970;10: 237–47, with permission.)

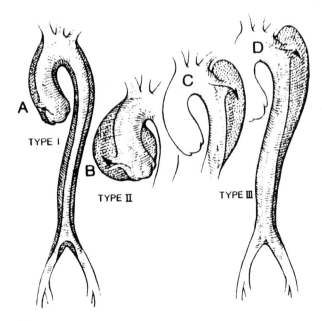

Fig. 10-1. Schematic depiction of three types of dissecting aneurysms of the aorta. Arrows indicate the most common site of the intimal tear. (**A**) Type I dissections arise from a tear in the intima of the ascending aorta. The resulting dissection (shaded area) can extend retrograde, to involve the aortic valve or produce cardiac tamponade. Likewise, type I dissections can extend anterograde and involve side branches of the aorta. (**B**) Type II dissections differ from type I only in the limitation of the extension to the arch of the aorta. (**C & D**) Type III dissections arise from a tear in the intima of the descending thoracic aorta, usually just distal to the left subclavian artery. (From DeBakey ME, McCollum CH, Crawford ES, et al. Dissection and dissecting aneurysms of the aorta: Twenty year follow-up of five hundred twenty patients treated surgically. Surgery 1982;92: 1118–34, with permission.)

migrates as the dissection advances along the aorta. Neurologic complications of aortic dissection include stroke caused by occlusion of a carotid artery, ischemic peripheral neuropathy associated with obvious ischemia of the limb, and paraparesis or paraplegia owing to impairment of the blood supply to the spinal cord. Patients with aortic dissection often appear as if they are in shock (vasoconstricted), yet the blood pressure is elevated in one-half to two-thirds of cases, especially in those with distal dissection. Diminution or absence of peripheral pulses is an important clue to aortic dissection. Recent onset of aortic regurgitation with or without associated congestive heart failure is an important sign of proximal aortic dissection, being present in approximately two-thirds of these patients. Myocardial infarction may reflect occlusion of the coronary arteries by proximal aortic dissection. Retrograde dissection into the sinus of Valsalva with rupture into the pericardial space leading to cardiac tamponade is a major cause of early mortality. Renal artery obstruction is manifested as an increase in the blood creatinine level.

Diagnosis

A noninvasive diagnostic strategy using magnetic resonance imaging in hemodynamically stable patients and transthoracic color flow Doppler echocardiography for patients who are too unstable to be moved may be the optimal approach for detecting dissection of the thoracic aorta. Magnetic resonance imaging in the acutely ill patient is limited because of the time required and because patients with life-support systems cannot be subjected to the magnetic field. Chest radiography usually shows moderate widening of the thoracic aorta (mediastinal shadow), the result of bleeding into the mediastinum.

Treatment

Treatment of aortic dissection has developed by means of empirical evolution in the absence of randomized controlled studies contrasting medical and surgical therapy for comparable patients.[1,5] In this regard, treatment of aortic dissection can be considered in two phases: early short-term therapy and subsequent definitive therapy. The early survival rate of patients treated medically and surgically for aortic dissection is greater than 90%.[5]

Early Short-term Treatment

Clinical suspicion of aortic dissection mandates institution of medical therapy, often before initiation of diagnostic procedures such as emergency aortography. The objective of early medical therapy is (1) to decrease the blood pressure to the lowest level compatible with maintenance of adequate cerebral, coronary, and renal perfusion pressure; (2) to diminish the velocity of ventricular contraction; and (3) to relieve pain. The first two objectives are accomplished by a continuous intravenous infusion of nitroprusside (lower systolic blood pressure to about 100 mmHg, urine output at least 25 ml·h^{-1}) and a beta adrenergic antagonist such as esmolol (decrease velocity of ventricular contraction and decrease heart rate to about 60 beats·min^{-1}). Administration of nitroprusside in the absence of a beta antagonist may increase the velocity of ventricular contraction. Trimethaphan is an alternative drug, if coexisting diseases (obstructive pulmonary disease, heart block) limit the usefulness of a beta antagonist. Prolonged use of trimethaphan may result in paralytic ileus and tachyphylaxis. Responses to drug therapy are most often monitored by continuous measurement of blood pressure, ventricular filling pressures, and urine output. In this regard, early treatment includes placement of a right radial artery catheter, a pulmonary artery catheter, and urinary bladder catheter. As soon as the diagnosis is confirmed, the appropriate subsequent definitive (medical or surgical) treatment is instituted.

Subsequent Definitive Treatment

It is generally agreed that acute proximal aortic dissections (type A dissection) should be treated surgically, whenever possible, even in the presence of serious complications such as myocardial infarction or stroke. Mortality after surgery for acute type A dissection is less than 10%.[5] The objective of surgical treatment is to excise the intimal tear, whenever possible; to obliterate entry into the false channel proximally and distally; and to reconstitute the aorta, usually with the placement of a synthetic sleeve graft. Concomitant aortic valve repair or replacement may be necessary in proximal aortic dissection. A composite valve-graft conduit is an alternative to the separate insertion of a prosthetic graft and aortic valve. The ostia of the coronary arteries are reimplanted into the composite graft. Another surgical approach is the use of an intraluminal prosthesis consisting of a Dacron sleeve inserted into the aortic lumen so that the ends are proximal and distal to the sites of dissection. The prosthesis is fixed in place by encircling tapes around the outside of the aorta, and the arterial branches are anastomosed to the prosthesis.

The definitive treatment of acute distal thoracic aortic dissection (type B dissection) is controversial. Medical treatment of acute stable distal aortic dissection has generally been associated with an in-hospital survival rate of 80%, whereas others recommend surgical treatment for uncomplicated type B dissection.[1] These dissections are most commonly anterograde, extending below the diaphragm, such that aortic regurgitation or cardiac tamponade is unlikely. The surgical approach is generally used for type B dissection in patients with (1) Marfan syndrome; (2) dissections complicated by leaking, rupture, or compromise of an arterial trunk sufficient to cause limb ischemia; (3) continued or recurrent pain; and (4) inability to control blood pressure medically.[6] Patients with distal thoracic aortic dissection tend to be elderly, to be hypertensive with generalized arteriosclerosis, and to have a history of smoking with associated chronic obstructive pulmonary disease. In addition, chronic renal disease is often present. This patient profile may increase the risk of surgery and favor at least initial attempts at medical management. An uncommon but devastating complication of surgery for distal aortic dissection is ischemic damage to the spinal cord. A brief period of aortic cross-clamping (less than 30 minutes) and the use of partial circulatory assistance or a shunt may decrease the likelihood of this complication.[7]

Patients who present with chronic thoracic aortic dissection have survived the most hazardous period and are most often treated medically, unless surgery for treatment of a complication is necessary. The most common complication is aortic regurgitation. Long-term medical treatment usually includes a beta antagonist and antihypertensive drug other than hydralazine or minoxidil, which can increase the velocity of ventricular contraction. A calcium entry blocker may also be useful in these patients.

The 10-year survival of treated patients who leave the hospital is approximately 60%, regardless of the site of aortic dissection, degree of acuteness, or type of treatment. Redissection is a significant risk in these patients.[8]

Management of Anesthesia

Cross-clamping of the thoracic aorta at the suprarenal or supraceliac level, as necessary for surgical therapy of a descending thoracic aortic aneurysm, is associated with a marked increase in systemic vascular resistance, mean arterial pressure, central venous pressure, and pulmonary artery occlusion pressure, while the cardiac output decreases.[9] Echocardiography often indicates abnormal wall motion of the left ventricle, suggesting myocardial ischemia. Intestinal ischemia and release of vasoactive substances may contribute to the hemodynamic effects of supraceliac cross-clamping of the thoracic aorta. Compared with the more benign hemodynamic effects of cross-clamping of the infrarenal aorta, as necessary for abdominal aortic aneurysm resection, the marked changes evoked by cross-clamping of the thoracic aorta are not surprising, considering the portion of the cardiac output that normally goes to the renal vessels (22%) and to the superior mesenteric vessels and celiac trunk (27%).

Operations on the descending thoracic aorta that require supraceliac cross-clamping may be complicated by spinal cord ischemia and paraplegia.[7] Hypotension and surgical interruption of the blood supply to the anterior spinal cord are the presumed mechanism for this complication. The principal radicular arterial supply of the caudad spinal cord (artery of Adamkiewicz) has its origin at T9–T12 in most patients. Experimental studies have reported no relationship between spinal cord damage and arterial blood pressure or intraspinal pressure.[10] Despite an initial favorable report, there is no evidence that intraoperative monitoring of somatosensory evoked potentials permits recognition of spinal cord ischemia and avoidance of postoperative neurologic damage.[11,12] This should not be surprising, as somatosensory evoked potential monitoring principally reflects dorsal column (sensory tracts) function, such that ischemic changes of anterior cord function (motor tracts) are not detected.[13] For this reason, monitoring of somatosensory evoked potentials has limited value in surgery for thoracic aortic aneurysm.[12] Monitoring of motor evoked potentials would reflect anterior spinal cord function but remains impractical, since, if monitored, neuromuscular blockade would not be possible.

Proper monitoring is more important than the actual drugs selected for anesthesia in a patient undergoing resection of a thoracic aortic aneurysm. Monitoring of blood pressure above (right radial artery or left radial artery if the aneurysm involves the innominate artery) and below (femoral artery) the aneurysm is essential. This approach permits assessment both of cerebral perfusion pressure and of the perfusion pressure to the kidneys during aortic cross-clamping. Somatosensory evoked potentials or electroencephalography are methods of evaluating central nervous system viability during the period of aortic cross-clamping. Agents such as sympathomimetics or vasodilators, or both, may be required to adjust perfusion pressure above and below the aortic dissection. Esmolol may be used to provide blood pressure control comparable to that achieved with nitroprusside, but without the potential for reflex tachycardia or decreased PaO_2 associated with a vasodilator.[14] Attempts should be made to maintain the mean arterial pressure near 100 mmHg in the upper part of the body and above 50 mmHg distal to the aneurysm. The use of a vasodilator to treat blood pressure elevations above the aortic cross-clamp must be balanced against the likely undesirable decreases in perfusion pressure below the clamp. The use of a temporary external heparinized shunt to bypass the occluded thoracic aorta (proximal aorta to femoral artery) may be considered in attempting to maintain distal circulation to the kidneys and spinal cord. Alternatively, left heart bypass may be performed, but the need for systemic heparinization is a possible disadvantage. A pulmonary artery catheter is placed to permit monitoring of cardiac function and adequacy of fluid and blood replacement. Diuresis should be established preoperatively and maintained intraoperatively with mannitol or furosemide, or both, if necessary. Nevertheless, data from animals show that profound decreases in glomerular filtration rate and renal blood flow are not attenuated by mannitol or dopamine, suggesting that efforts to protect renal function should be directed toward improving blood flow in the post pump period.[15]

Induction of anesthesia and intubation of the trachea must minimize undesirable increases in blood pressure that could exacerbate the aortic dissection. Selective endobronchial intubation permitting collapse of the left lung facilitates surgical exposure during resection of a thoracic aortic aneurysm. Nevertheless, the use of an endobronchial tube is not mandatory for these operations. Indeed, a disadvantage of one-lung ventilation is the production of an iatrogenic intrapulmonary shunt that can lead to arterial hypoxemia despite a maximum delivered concentration of oxygen. The magnitude of this iatrogenic intrapulmonary shunt can be decreased by minimizing pulmonary blood flow through the collapsed left lung. The application of 5 to 10 cm H_2O continuous positive airway pressure to the nondependent unventilated lung may improve arterial oxygenation as well. If this does not improve arterial oxygenation, it may be beneficial to apply continuous positive airway pressure to the dependent ventilated lung. General anesthesia, including a volatile anesthetic and opioid, is a frequent selection for maintenance of anesthesia that takes advantage of the cerebral metabolic suppression produced by this approach. A long-acting nondepolarizing muscle relaxant is useful, bearing in mind the likely dependence of these drugs on renal clearance mechanisms.

Postoperative Management

The patient recovering from a thoracic aneurysm resection is at risk of the development of cardiac, ventilatory, and renal failure during the immediate postoperative period. Cerebrovascular accidents may be produced by air or thrombotic emboli that occur during surgical resection of the diseased aorta. A patient with co-existing cerebrovascular disease is probably more vulnerable to the development of central nervous system complications. The possibility of postoperative central nervous system dysfunction emphasizes the importance of documenting any preoperative abnormalities. Spinal cord injury during the postoperative period may be manifested as paresis or flaccid paralysis.

Hypertension is not uncommon and may jeopardize the vascular integrity of the surgical repair, predisposing to myocardial ischemia. The role of pain in the etiology of hypertension must be considered; priority should be given to provide adequate analgesia, as with a neuraxial opioid with or without a local anesthetic, or patient-controlled analgesia, or both. Institution of antihypertensive therapy with such drugs as nitroglycerin, nitroprusside, hydralazine, or labetalol may be appropriate. Some patients may benefit from administration of a beta antagonist to attenuate the manifestations of a hyperdynamic circulation.

CARDIAC CONTUSION

In addition to causing acute dissection of the descending thoracic aorta, deceleration injuries involving the anterior chest wall are also the most frequent cause of myocardial contusion.[16] Sudden impact of the anterior chest against the steering wheel in an automobile accident is a common preceding event in the patient with myocardial contusion. Sudden deceleration from speeds as low as 33 km·h^{-1} may injure the heart without displaying any obvious external signs of trauma. Because of its immediate substernal location, the right ventricle is more likely than the left ventricle to be injured. Chest pain resembling angina pectoris but unrelieved by nitroglycerin may be present. Thrombosis of a coronary artery may result from blunt chest trauma. The presence of chest pain, as well as changes on the electrocardiogram resembling myocardial infarction, especially in a young patient, should prompt questions about recent chest trauma that might have seemed trivial at the time of its occurrence.

Cardiac dysrhythmias and congestive heart failure are the two most important consequences of myocardial contusion. Continuous monitoring of the electrocardiogram is necessary to detect life-threatening ventricular cardiac dysrhythmias, ST and T wave abnormalities, and bundle branch block.[16] Right ventricular contusion may be associated with right bundle branch block and selective right ventricular failure. Noninvasive diagnostic techniques for determining the presence of cardiac trauma include echocardiography, radionuclide angiocardiography, and determination of the MB fraction of creatine kinase (CK-MB).

Treatment

Treatment of cardiac contusion is directed toward the symptoms and anticipation of possible complications. Serial electrocardiograms should be considered in accident victims who have incurred chest trauma. Suppression of ventricular dysrhythmias is important. Temporary artificial cardiac pacing may be required if heart block is present. Right ventricular failure usually requires maintenance of high right-sided filling pressures. Inotropic support may be necessary, although these drugs may increase pulmonary artery pressure or may accentuate injury-related pulmonary hypertension. Most patients who survive the acute episode of myocardial contusion eventually regain normal myocardial function.

ANEURYSMS OF THE ABDOMINAL AORTA

Aneurysms of the abdominal aorta are most often due to atherosclerosis, although a genetic predisposition may be present.[17] Clinically, an abdominal aneurysm can usually be detected as a pulsating abdominal mass in the absence of any other symptoms. Ultrasound examination identifies virtually all abdominal aneurysms and accurately indicates their size. Magnetic resonance imaging is also useful in the diagnosis.

Treatment

Elective resection of an abdominal aortic aneurysm and replacement with a prosthetic graft has a mortality of less than 5%, death is usually related to myocardial infarction.[18] Considering the low mortality associated with elective resection of an abdominal aneurysm, surgery is a consideration for all aneurysms greater than 5 cm in diameter.[19] Smaller aneurysms are less likely to rupture, but the removal of any clinically detectable abdominal aortic aneurysm may be justified in patients considered at low operative risk.[20] Patients at significant operative risk may be identified preoperatively on the basis of history (angina pectoris, evidence of generalized atherosclerosis), supplemented by treadmill exercise testing, radionuclide scanning, and coronary arteriography, when indicated. Serial ultrasound examinations are useful for following changes in the size of an abdominal aneurysm. Long-term oral treatment with a beta antagonist may be useful in slowing the expansion of an abdominal aneurysm.[21] Emergency surgery to repair a leaking or ruptured abdominal aortic aneurysm is associated with a perioperative mortality of 25% to 50%. About 5% of abdominal aortic aneurysms exhibit a dense fibrotic periaortic inflammatory reaction that may cause obstruction of the renal veins, ureters, or duodenum.[22]

Infrarenal aortic cross-clamping and unclamping is an integral component of abdominal aortic surgery. The hemodynamic response to infrarenal aortic cross-clamping will be influenced by (1) preoperative cardiac status, (2) intravascular fluid volume, and (3) anesthetic drugs and techniques selected. The anticipated consequences of an abrupt aortic cross-clamp include increased resistance to ventricular ejection (afterload) and decreased venous return (preload). Nevertheless, myocardial performance and circulatory variables usually remain within an acceptable range after the aorta is occluded at an infrarenal level, even in patients with co-existing cardiac dysfunction.[23] Deepening anesthesia or administration of a vasodilator at the time of infrarenal aortic occlusion may be necessary in some patients, to maintain myocardial performance at an acceptable level. Despite these reassuring observations, some reports suggest that patients with ischemic heart disease are more vulnerable to the development of myocardial ischemia and left ventricular failure after abrupt increases in afterload.[18,24]

Small bowel evisceration and mesenteric traction associated with abdominal aortic aneurysm resection may evoke the release of prostaglandin I-2 (prostacyclin), manifested as peripheral vasodilation, decreased blood pressure, and facial flushing. Even aortic cross-clamping may evoke the release of vasodilating prostaglandins. Conversely, unclamping the aorta may evoke the release of prostaglandins that attenuate hypotension. Cyclo-oxygenase inhibition with aspirin or ibuprofen before surgery may prevent decreased myocardial contractility and maintain a stable cardiac output after cross-clamping of the aorta in patients with adequate intravascular fluid volume.[25]

Despite the negligible cardiovascular effects of infrarenal aortic cross-clamping, hypotension still may occur when the cross-clamp is removed. Severe hypotension is unlikely, but transient decreases in systolic blood pressure of about 40 mmHg are not uncommon. Prevention of declamping hypotension and maintenance of a stable cardiac output are often achieved by volume loading to a higher level than that of the preoperative pulmonary capillary wedge pressure before cross-clamp release. Likewise, gradual removal of the aortic cross-clamp may minimize decreases in blood pressure by allowing pooled venous blood to return to the central circulation. The role of the washout of acid metabolites from the ischemic extremities when the clamp is released has been discredited as a cause of declamping hypotension.[9,26] If hypotension persists for more than about 4 minutes after removal

of the cross-clamp, the presence of unrecognized bleeding or inadequate volume replacement must be considered. Echocardiography at this time may be helpful in determining the adequacy of volume replacement and cardiac output.

Acute renal failure may follow infrarenal aortic cross-clamping for resection of an abdominal aortic aneurysm. Nevertheless, even patients with mild renal dysfunction (serum creatinine less than 4 mg·dl^{-1}) can generally undergo elective abdominal aneurysm resection without additional mortality.[18] Preoperative hydration with a balanced salt solution and prompt intraoperative hydration and blood loss replacement guided by data obtained from a pulmonary artery catheter are considered useful in attempting to maintain intravascular fluid volume and thus renal function after abdominal aortic surgery. Spinal cord damage is more likely to occur after resection of a thoracic aortic aneurysm than with an abdominal aortic aneurysm (see the section, Aneurysms of the Thoracic Aorta, Management of Anesthesia).

Ischemic colitis is a well-recognized complication of abdominal aortic surgery, presumably reflecting the need to ligate the inferior mesenteric artery. Nitroglycerin, but not nitroprusside, as administered for afterload reduction, may exacerbate the decrease in intestinal blood flow by shunting blood flow from the colonic mucosa.

Management of Anesthesia

Management of anesthesia for resection of an abdominal aortic aneurysm must consider the high incidence of associated ischemic heart disease, hypertension, chronic obstructive pulmonary disease, diabetes mellitus, and renal dysfunction, in these usually elderly patients. Indeed, myocardial infarction is responsible for 40% to 70% of the mortality associated with abdominal aortic surgery.[18,25] Preoperative evaluation of cardiac function may include monitored exercise testing, echocardiography, radionuclide angiography, and dipridamole-thallium imaging.

In view of the many complications associated with surgical resection of an abdominal aortic aneurysm, it is important to monitor carefully the intravascular fluid volume and cardiac, pulmonary, and renal function, during the perioperative period. Blood pressure is monitored continuously by an intraarterial catheter. Pulmonary artery catheterization is indicated in most patients, as it is not always possible to predict whether central venous pressure will parallel left heart filling pressure. This is particularly true in the patient with a history of previous myocardial infarction or angina pectoris or who exhibits signs of congestive heart failure. The appearance of an abnormal V wave on the tracing of the pulmonary capillary occlusion pressure may reflect myocardial ischemia, even before ischemic changes are displayed on the electrocardiogram. Echocardiography has been popularized as a useful monitor of the cardiac response to aortic cross-clamping and unclamping, providing an assessment of left ventricular filling volume and regional and global myocardial contractility. Urine output is monitored continuously. Warming of fluids and blood helps maintain body temperature.

No single anesthetic drug or technique is ideal for all patients undergoing elective surgical resection of an abdominal aortic aneurysm. Overall, an anesthetic technique that produces low blood pressure and low myocardial oxygen demand is probably preferable.[25] Combinations of a volatile drug and opioid are frequently used with or without nitrous oxide. The clinical implications of isoflurane-induced coronary arteriolar dilation in a patient with ischemic heart disease (possible coronary artery steal) are controversial. Skeletal muscle relaxation may be provided with an intermediate- or long-acting nondepolarizing muscle relaxant, keeping in mind the dependence on renal clearance characteristic of some of these drugs. The prophylactic use of a vasodilator to prevent hemodynamic changes is also controversial, although intravenous infusion of nitroglycerin seems reasonable if hypertension (greater than 20% of baseline), decreased myocardial contractility, or signs of myocardial ischemia develop. Nitroprusside may be more likely than nitroglycerin to cause myocardial ischemia when perfusion pressure is reduced by this drug. Dopamine or dobutamine may be indicated if evidence of decreased myocardial contractility accompanies aortic cross-clamping.

Patients undergoing abdominal aortic surgery usually experience major functional extracellular fluid and blood loss. A combination of balanced salt and colloid solutions guided by appropriate monitoring of cardiac and renal function will facilitate maintenance of an adequate intravascular fluid volume, cardiac output, and urine formation. A balanced salt solution, with or without a colloid solution, should be infused during aortic cross-clamping. In this way, the pulmonary artery occlusion pressure will be maintained 3 to 5 mmHg above the preclamp value, thereby minimizing declamping hypotension and decreased cardiac output. If urine output is unsatisfactory (less than 50 ml·h^{-1}) despite adequate fluid and blood replacement, diuretic therapy with mannitol or furosemide may be considered. Low-dose dopamine (approximately 3 μg·kg^{-1}·min^{-1} IV) may also be administered, to improve renal function. Nevertheless, transient decreases in glomerular filtration rate have been demonstrated to follow removal of the infrarenal aortic cross-clamp. This response is not altered by volume expansion beginning before induction of anesthesia, with or without administration of mannitol and dopamine.[27] Furthermore, intraoperative urine output in the presence of normal blood pressure and filling pressures does not correlate with postoperative renal dysfunction in patients undergoing abdominal aortic reconstruction[28] (Fig. 10-3). Rather, co-existing renal disease seems to be the greatest risk factor.

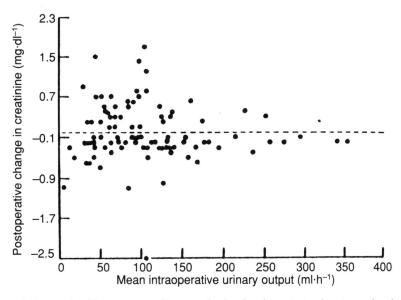

Fig. 10-3. No correlation was found between mean intraoperative hourly urine output and postoperative changes in the plasma creatinine concentrations in 137 patients undergoing elective abdominal aortic aneurysm resection. (From Alpert RA, Roizen MF, Hamilton WK, et al. Intraoperative urinary output does not predict postoperative renal function in patients undergoing abdominal aortic revascularization. Surgery 1984;95:701–11, with permission.)

Adequacy of coagulation should be confirmed preoperatively, as many patients presenting for abdominal aortic surgery have elevation of fibrin split products.[29] The greatest blood loss during elective abdominal aortic aneurysm resection usually occurs when the aneurysm is opened and the lumbar arteries are backbleeding. Intraoperative blood salvage and reinfusion and acceptance of modest degrees of hemodilution have decreased the need for homologous blood transfusion during elective abdominal aneurysm surgery.

Continuous epidural anesthesia, alone or combined with general anesthesia and tracheal intubation, provides the advantages of decreased depressant drug requirements, attenuation of increased systemic vascular resistance with aortic cross-clamping, and significant alleviation of postoperative pain. Nevertheless, there is no evidence that the combination technique decreases postoperative cardiac or pulmonary morbidity compared with similar high-risk patients undergoing the same abdominal aortic surgery with general anesthesia.[30] There remains, however, the possibility that postoperative epidural analgesia may favorably influence the postoperative course. Anticoagulation during abdominal aortic surgery introduces the controversy regarding the placement of an epidural catheter and the remote risk of epidural hematoma formation. Nevertheless, the relative safety of anticoagulation after epidural catheter insertion is well described in patients experiencing atraumatic placement of the catheter and subsequent heparin administration based on monitoring the activated clotting time.[31]

Postoperative Management

Patients recovering from resection of an abdominal aortic aneurysm are at risk of the development of cardiac, ventilatory, and renal failure during the immediate postoperative period. Assessment of graft patency and lower extremity blood flow is important. Provision of adequate analgesia as with neuraxial opioids with or without local anesthetics or patient-controlled analgesia, or both, should be given priority. Pain relief may permit early tracheal extubation and resumption of spontaneous breathing.

Hypertension is a potentially serious complication during the postoperative period that seems more likely in patients with preoperative hypertension. Overzealous intraoperative hydration or postoperative hypothermia with compensatory vasoconstriction, or both, may contribute to postoperative hypertension. Treatment of postoperative hypertension consists of the exclusion of contributing causes and of prompt institution of antihypertensive therapy with such drugs as nitroglycerin, nitroprusside, labetalol, or hydralazine. Preoperative administration of clonidine may attenuate hyperdynamic responses during the postoperative period.[32]

REFERENCES

1. DeSanctis RW, Doroghazi RM, Austen WG, Buckley MJ. Aortic dissection. N Engl J Med 1987;317:1060–8
2. Debakey ME, McCollum CH, Crawford ES, et al. Dissection and dissecting aneurysms of the aorta: Twenty year followup of five hundred twenty patients treated surgically. Surgery 1982;92: 1118–34
3. Daily PO, Trueblood W, Stinson EB, Wuerflein RD, Shumway NE. Management of acute aortic dissections. Ann Thorac Surg 1970;237–47
4. Williams GM, Gott VL, Brawley RK, et al. Aortic disease associated with pregnancy. J Vasc Surg 1988;8:470–5
5. Crawford ES. The diagnosis and management of aortic dissection. JAMA 1990;264:2537–41
6. Carlson DE, Karp RB, Kouchoukas NT. Surgical treatment of aneurysms of the desceding thoracic aorta: An analysis of 85 patients. Ann Thorac Surg 1983;35:58–63
7. Katz NM, Blackstone EH, Kirklin JW, Karp RB. Incremental risk factors for spinal cord injury following operation for acute traumatic aortic transection. J Thorac Cardiovasc Surg 1981;81: 669–74
8. Yamaguchi T, Guthaner DF, Wexler L. Natural history of the false channel of Type A aortic dissection after surgical repair: CT study. Radiology 1989;170:743–8
9. Kouchoukos NT, Lell WA, Karp RB, et al. Hemodynamic effects of aortic clamping and decompression with a temporary shunt for resection of the descending thoracic aorta. Surgery 1979;85: 25–32
10. Wadouh F, Lindemann EM, Arndt CF, et al. The arteria radicularis magna anterior as a decisive factor influencing spinal cord damage during aortic occlusion. J Thorac Cardiovasc Surg 1984; 88:1–10
11. Crawford ES, Mizrahi EM, Hess KR, Coselli JS, Safi RJ, Patel VM. The impact of distal aortic perfusion and somatosensory evoked potential monitoring on prevention of paraplegia after aortic aneurysm operation. J Thorac Cardiovasc Surg 1988;95: 357–67
12. Takaki O, Okumura F. Application and limitation of somatosensory evoked potential monitoring during thoracic aortic aneurysm surgery: A case report. Anesthesiology 1985;63:700–3
13. Loughman BA, Hall GM. Spinal cord monitoring 1989. Br J Anaesth 1989;63:587–94
14. Fenner SG, Mahoney A, Cashman JN. Repair of traumatic transection of the thoracic aorta: Esmolol for intraoperative control of arterial pressure. Br J Anaesth 1991;67:483–7
15. Pass LJ, Eberhart RC, Brown JC, Rohn GN, Estrera AS. The effect of mannitol and dopamine on the renal response to thoracic aortic cross-clamping. J Thorac Cardiovasc Surg 1988;95:608–12
16. Rothstein RJ. Myocardial contusion. JAMA 1983;250:2189–91
17. Johansen K, Loepsell T. Familial tendency for abdominal aortic aneurysms. JAMA 1986;256:1934–6
18. Cunningham AJ. Anaesthesia for abdominal aortic surgery—a review. Part 1. Can J Anaesth 1989;36:426–44
19. Nevitt MP, Ballard DJ, Hallett JW. Prognosis of abdominal aortic aneurysms: A population-based study. N Engl J Med 1989;321: 1009–11

20. Crawford ES, Hess KR. Abdominal aortic aneurysm. N Engl J Med 1989;321:1040–1

21. Leach SD, Toole AL, Stern H, et al. Effect of beta adrenergic blockade on the growth rate of abdominal aortic aneurysms. Arch Surg 1988;123:606–10

22. Moosa HH, Pietzman AB, Steed DL, et al. Inflammatory aneurysms of the abdominal aorta. Arch Surg 1989;124:673–8

23. Roizen MG, Beaupre PN, Alpert RN, et al. Monitoring with two dimensional transesophageal echocardiography: Comparison of myocardial function in patients undergoing supraceliac, suprarenal-infraceliac, or infrarenal aortic occlusion. J Vasc Surg 1984;1:300–11

24. Attia RR, Murphy JD, Snider MT, et al. Myocardial ischemia due to infrarenal aortic cross clamping during aortic surgery in patients with severe coronary artery disease. Circulation 1976;53:961–5

25. Cunningham AJ. Anaesthesia for abdominal aortic surgery—a review. Part II. Can J Anaesth 1989;36:568–77

26. Bush HL, LoGerfo RW, Weisel RD, et al. Assessment of myocardial performance and optimal volume loading during elective abdominal aortic aneurysm resection. Arch Surg 1977;112:1301–6

27. Paul MD, Mazer CD, Byrick RJ, Rose DK, Goldstein MB. Influence of mannitol and dopamine on renal function during elective infrarenal aortic clamping in man. Am J Nephrol 1986;6:427–34

28. Alpert RA, Roizen MF, Hamilton WK, et al. Intraoperative urinary output does not predict postoperative renal function in patients undergoing abdominal aortic revascularization. Surgery 1984;95:707–11

29. Fisher DF, Yawn DH, Crawford ES. Preoperative disseminated intravascular coagulation associated with aortic aneurysms. Arch Surg 1983;118:1252–5

30. Baron J-F, Bertrand M, Barre E, et al. Combined epidural and general anesthesia versus general anesthesia for abdominal aortic surgery. Anesthesiology 1991;75:611–8

31. Rao TKL, El-Etr AA. Anticoagulation following placement of epidural and subarachnoid catheters: An evaluation of neurologic sequelae. Anesthesiology 1981;55:618–20

32. Flacke JW, Bloor BC, Flacke WE, et al. Reduced narcotic requirement by clonidine with improved hemodynamic and adrenergic stability in patients undergoing coronary bypass surgery. Anesthesiology 1987;67:11–9

11

Peripheral Vascular Disease

Peripheral vascular disease may be manifested as systemic vasculitis or arterial occlusive disease (Table 11-1). Clinical syndromes involving inflammation of the blood vessels present in nonspecific ways that may suggest connective tissue disease, sepsis, or malignancy[1] (Table 11-2). The diagnosis of systemic vasculitis may be facilitated by biopsy of an involved organ and by detection of autoantibodies directed against cytoplasmic (extranuclear) components of neutrophils. An immune mechanism generated in response to one or more factors is the most likely cause of systemic vasculitis. Acute peripheral arterial occlusion is most often due to an embolus, whereas chronic occlusion likely reflects atherosclerosis.

TAKAYASU'S ARTERITIS

Takayasu's arteritis (pulseless disease) primarily affects young Asian females, often presenting as upper extremity claudication and minimal to no palpable arterial pulsation in the arms and neck. The lack of peripheral pulses reflects chronic inflammation of the aorta and its major branches. The definitive diagnosis is made on the basis of contrast angiography.

Signs and symptoms of Takayasu syndrome manifest on multiple organ systems (Table 11-3). Decreased perfusion to the brain owing to involvement of the carotid arteries by occlusive inflammatory and thrombotic processes can be manifested as vertigo, visual disturbances, seizures, and cerebrovascular accidents with hemiparesis or hemiplegia. Bruits are often audible over stenosed carotid or subclavian vessels. Hyperextension of the head may decrease carotid blood flow by shortening the arteries. Indeed, patients often hold their heads in a flexed (drooping) position to prevent syncope.

Involvement of the pulmonary arteries by vasculitis occurs in about 50% of patients and can be manifested as pulmonary hypertension. Ventilation-to-perfusion abnormalities owing to occlusion of small pulmonary arteries by the inflammatory process may contribute to unexpected decreases in the PaO_2. Myocardial ischemia can reflect inflammation of the coronary arteries. There may be involvement of the cardiac valves and cardiac conduction system. Renal artery stenosis can lead to decreased renal function as well as to initiation of events producing renal hypertension. Ankylosing spondylitis and rheumatoid arthritis may accompany this syndrome.

Treatment of Takayasu's arteritis is with corticosteroids. Inhibitors of platelet aggregation or oral anticoagulants may be instituted in selected patients. Hypertension may be treated with calcium entry blockers or angiotensin-converting enzyme inhibitors. Life-threatening or incapacitating arterial occlusions are sometimes amenable to surgical intervention.

Management of Anesthesia

Takayasu's arteritis may be encountered in patients presenting for obstetric anesthesia, incidental surgery, or such corrective vascular procedures as carotid endarterectomy. Formulation of a plan for the management of anesthesia must take into account the drugs used for treatment of this syndrome, as well as multiple organ system involvement by vasculitis.[2,3] For example, chronic corticosteroid therapy may result in suppression of adrenocortical function, indicating the need for supplemental exogenous corticosteroids during the perioperative period. Regional anesthesia may be a controversial selection in the presence of anticoagulation. Associated musculoskeletal changes can make performance of lumbar epidural or spinal anesthesia difficult. Nevertheless, lumbar epidural anesthesia has been described for vaginal delivery and tubal ligation in these patients.[3]

Blood pressure may be difficult to measure noninvasively in the upper extremities. Indeed, blood pressure is predictably

123

Table 11-1. Peripheral Vascular Disease

Systemic Vasculitis
    Takayasu's arteritis (pulseless disease)
    Thromboangiitis obliterans (Buerger's disease)
    Wegener's granulomatosis
    Temporal arteritis
    Polyarteritis nodosa
    Schönlein-Henoch purpura
    Raynaud's phenomenon
    Moyamoya disease
    Kawasaki disease

Acute Peripheral Arterial Occlusive Disease (Embolism)

Chronic Peripheral Arterial Occlusive Disease (Atherosclerosis)
    Distal abdominal aorta or iliac arteries
    Femoral arteries
    Subclavian steal syndrome
    Coronary-subclavian steal syndrome

Table 11-2. Signs and Symptoms of Systemic Vasculitis

Fever	Increased erythrocyte sedimentation rate
Fatigue	Anemia
Weight loss	Hypoalbuminemia
Neuropathy	

Table 11-3. Signs and Symptoms of Takayasu's Arteritis

Central Nervous System
    Vertigo
    Visual disturbances
    Syncope
    Seizures
    Cerebral ischemia or infarction

Cardiovascular System
    Multiple occlusions of peripheral arteries
    Ischemic heart disease
    Cardiac valve dysfunction
    Cardiac conduction defects

Lungs
    Pulmonary hypertension
    Ventilation-to-perfusion mismatch

Kidneys
    Renal artery stenosis

Musculoskeletal System
    Ankylosing spondylitis
    Rheumatoid arthritis

decreased in the upper extremities because of narrowing of the arterial lumen. There is a theoretical but undocumented concern regarding cannulation of arteries that may be involved by the inflammatory process characteristic of this syndrome. Nevertheless, a catheter placed in the radial artery is useful for confirming the presence of an adequate perfusion pressure during major operations. Monitoring blood pressure from a catheter placed in the femoral artery is an option, but it should be recognized that systolic blood pressure in the legs will be higher than that present in the central aorta. In addition, constant monitoring of the electrocardiogram and of urine output provides an index of the adequacy of perfusion of the heart and kidneys, respectively. Placement of a pulmonary artery catheter is acceptable if the magnitude of the surgery dictates.[2] In patients with known compromise of carotid blood flow, intraoperative monitoring of the electroencephalogram may be useful in detecting cerebral ischemia.

It is important to recognize that hyperextension of the head, as during direct laryngoscopy for intubation of the trachea, may compromise blood flow through the carotid arteries shortened as a result of the vascular inflammatory process associated with this disease. Indeed, during the preoperative evaluation of the patient, it is useful to establish the effect of changes in head position on cerebral function.

Regardless of the drugs selected to producce anesthesia, the priority must be to maintain an adequate arterial perfusion pressure during the intraoperative period. Therefore, anesthetic-induced decreased blood pressure caused by decreased cardiac output or systemic vascular resistance must be recognized promptly and treated by either reducing the concentration of anesthetic drugs or expanding the intravascular fluid volume, or both. The administration of a sympathomimetic to maintain perfusion pressure may be helpful until the underlying cause of the decrease in blood pressure can be corrected. Avoidance of excessive hyperventilation of the lungs, as well as the selection of a volatile anesthetic, perceived to favor maintenance of cerebral blood flow, is a reasonable goal, especially in patients in whom the disease process involves the carotid arteries.[2]

THROMBOANGIITIS OBLITERANS

Thromboangiitis obliterans (Buerger's disease) is an inflammatory and occlusive disease that involves arteries and veins. This disease has its greatest incidence in Jewish males between 20 and 40 years of age. There is an undeniable association with cigarette smoking, and exposure to cold temperatures or trauma is also recognized as exacerbating the disease process.

The most prominent early clinical finding of thromboangiitis obliterans is vasospasm alternating with periods of quiescence. Vascular changes are typically present in the extremities, although the cerebral, coronary, and mesenteric vessels are involved on rare occasions. Intermittent claudication reflects accumulation of pain-producing metabolites owing to poor skeletal muscle blood flow. Migratory thrombophlebitis, usually involving the lower extremities, occurs in a high percentage of patients. The diagnosis of thromboangiitis obliterans can be confirmed only by the biopsy of an active vascular lesion.

Treatment of thromboangiitis obliterans consists of cessation of smoking and avoidance of exposure to cold ambient temperatures and trauma to ischemic extremities. Corticosteroids and peripheral vasodilating drugs have been administered with unpredictable success. A surgical sympathectomy (removal of L1–L3 ganglia of the sympathetic chain) can be considered if medical treatment is unsatisfactory.

Management of Anesthesia

Management of anesthesia in the presence of thromboangiitis obliterans requires avoidance of the events that might damage the already ischemic extremities. Positioning during surgery must ensure attempts to avoid pressure points on the extremities. It would seem prudent to increase the ambient temperature of the operating room and to warm and humidify the inspired gases in order to maintain body temperature. Noninvasive monitoring of blood pressure is preferred, as placement of a catheter in a diseased artery is at least of theoretical concern. The presence of pulmonary disease and the presence of elevated carboxyhemoglobin levels must be considered, as many of these patients are cigarette smokers (see Chapter 13).

The possible interaction of anesthetic drugs with peripheral vasodilators used to treat thromboangiitis obliterans, as well as the potential need for supplemental corticosteroids, is considered preoperatively. In the final analysis, regional or general anesthesia can be administered to these patients. If a regional anesthetic technique is selected, it may be prudent to omit epinephrine from the local anesthetic solution so as to avoid any possibility of accentuating co-existing vasospasm.

WEGENER'S GRANULOMATOSIS

Wegener's granulomatosis is characterized by pathophysiologic changes owing to the formation of necrotizing granulomas in inflamed vessels as present in the central nervous system, airways and lungs, cardiovascular system, and kidneys (Table 11-4). In this regard, patients may present with sinusitis, pneumonia, or renal failure. Laryngeal mucosa may be replaced by granulation tissue, resulting in narrowing of the glottic opening. Vasculitis may result in occlusion of pulmonary vessels. There may be random interstitial distribution of pulmonary granulomas with surrounding infection and hemorrhage. Progressive renal failure is the most frequent cause of death in patients with Wegener's granulomatosis. Tests for

Table 11-4.   Signs and Symptoms of Wegener's Granulomatosis

Central Nervous System
  Cerebral arterial aneurysms
  Peripheral neuropathy

Respiratory Tract and Lungs
  Sinusitis
  Laryngeal stenosis
  Epiglottic destruction
  Ventilation-to-perfusion mismatch
  Pneumonia
  Hemoptysis
  Bronchial destruction

Cardiovascular System
  Cardiac valve destruction
  Disturbances of cardiac impulse conduction
  Myocardial ischemia
  Infarction of the tips of digits

Kidneys
  Hematuria
  Azotemia
  Renal failure

antineutrophil cytoplasmic antibodies have a high degree of specificity for Wegener's granulomatosis, suggesting a role of immunologic dysfunction and hypersensitivity to an unidentified antigen in the etiology of this vasculitis. Treatment of Wegener's granulomatosis with cyclophosphamide produces dramatic remission in nearly every case.

Management of Anesthesia

Management of anesthesia in patients with Wegener's granulomatosis requires an appreciation of the widespread organ involvement associated with this disease.[4] The potential depressant effect of cyclophosphamide on the immune system, as well as the association of hemolytic anemia and leukopenia with administration of this drug, should be considered. Cyclophosphamide may evoke a decrease in plasma cholinesterase activity, but prolonged skeletal muscle paralysis after the administration of succinylcholine has not been observed.[5]

Avoidance of trauma during direct laryngoscopy is important, as bleeding from granulomas and dislodgment of friable ulcerated tissues can occur. A smaller than expected endotracheal tube may be required if the glottic opening is narrowed by granulomatous changes. Suctioning of the airway may be required, to remove necrotic debris. The likely presence of lung disease emphasizes the need for supplemental oxygen during the perioperative period. Arteritis that is likely to involve peripheral vessels may limit the placement of an indwelling arterial catheter to monitor blood pressure or the frequency with which arterial punctures can be performed to analyze arterial blood gases and pH. A careful neurologic examination to detect the presence of peripheral neuropathies should be performed before the decision is made to recommend regional anesthesia to the patient. The choice and doses of neuromuscular blocking drugs may be influenced by the magnitude of renal dysfunction produced by the disease. Implications for the use of succinylcholine in the presence of skeletal muscle atrophy owing to neuritis should also be considered. Conceivably, volatile anesthetic drugs could be associated with exaggerated myocardial depression when the disease process involves the myocardium and cardiac values. Monitoring of the electrocardiogram is helpful in detecting disturbances of cardiac conduction. Ultimately, the rational administration of anesthesia to patients with Wegener's granulomatosis is based on the magnitude and type of organ system dysfunction produced by the disease.

TEMPORAL ARTERITIS

Temporal arteritis is an inflammation of arteries in the head and neck, manifesting most often as headache, tenderness of the scalp, or jaw claudication. Any patient older than 50 years of age complaining of a unilateral headache is suspect for this diagnosis. Superficial branches of the temporal arteries are often tender and enlarged. Arteritis of branches of the ophthalmic artery may lead to ischemic optic neuritis and sudden unilateral blindness. Indeed, prompt initiation of treatment with corticosteroids is indicated in patients with visual symptoms, to prevent blindness. Evidence of arteritis on a biopsy of the temporal artery is present in about 90% of patients.

POLYARTERITIS NODOSA

Polyarteritis nodosa (formerly termed periarteritis nodosa) is a vasculitis that most often occurs in females 20 to 60 years of age, commonly in association with hepatitis B antigenemia and allergic reactions to drugs. Small and medium-size arteries are involved with inflammatory changes, resulting in glomerulitis, myocardial ischemia, peripheral neuropathies, and seizures. Hypertension is frequent, presumably reflecting renal disease. Renal failure is the most common cause of death. A polyarteritis-like vasculitis may accompany acquired immunodeficiency syndrome (AIDS).

The diagnosis of polyarteritis nodosa depends on histologic evidence of vasculitis on biopsy, and arteriography demonstrating characteristic aneurysms. Treatment is empirical and usually includes corticosteroids and cyclophosphamide, removal of an offending drug, and treatment of an underlying disease such as cancer. Potential adverse effects of cyclophosphamide in patients treated with this drug should be considered (see the section, Wegener's Granulomatosis).

Management of anesthesia in patients with polyarteritis nodosa should take into consideration the likelihood of renal and cardiac disease and the implications of co-existing hypertension. Supplemental corticosteroids are appropriate in patients who have been receiving these drugs preoperatively for treatment of their underlying disease.

SCHÖNLEIN-HENOCH PURPURA

Schönlein-Henoch purpura principally affects arterioles and capillaries in the skin, kidneys, gastrointestinal tract, and large joints of children. The disease is usually benign. Corticosteroids may be administered to patients with renal dysfunction.

RAYNAUD'S PHENOMENON

Raynaud's phenomenon is regarded as a complication of organic arterial disease in the extremities with superimposed cold-induced vasospasm. Adult females are affected most often, and an underlying disease (scleroderma, systemic lupus erythematosus) is nearly always associated with this disease. Primary pulmonary hypertension may also accompany Raynaud's phenomenon. Ultimately, the prognosis depends on the progression of the associated underlying disease. Often Raynaud's phenomenon is characterized by a slow progression that may consist of stationary periods lasting years.

The initial clinical manifestations of Raynaud's phenomenon are pallor and cyanosis of the digits, followed by erythema and edema. Arterial vasoconstriction of the digital arteries is responsible for the initial pallor; stasis of blood leads to cyanosis. Erythema and edema occur when the arteries suddenly reopen. Burning and throbbing pain typically follow the ischemic episode.

Treatment

Treatment of Raynaud's phenomenon consists of avoiding the precipitating causes, that is, exposure to cold ambient temperatures and abstaining from cigarette smoking. Arterial spasm and pain may be relieved on occasion by the intravenous administration of reserpine or guanethidine into a tourniquet-isolated extremity.[6,7] In severe cases with trophic changes, surgical interruption of the sympathetic nervous system supply to the hand (transection of preganglionic fibers in the sympathetic chain at T2 and T3) may be considered but has not produced consistently predictable favorable responses.

Management of Anesthesia

There are no specific recommendations as to choices of drugs to produce general anesthesia in patients with Raynaud's phenomenon. Maintenance of body temperature and increasing the ambient temperature of the operating room would seem logical. Blood pressure is most often monitored by a noninvasive technique, in view of the theoretical risk of placing a catheter in a peripheral artery supplying a potentially ischemic extremity.

Regional anesthesia is acceptable for peripheral operations in patients with Raynaud's phenomenon. Indeed, regional anesthetic techniques that interrupt the sympathetic nervous system innervation to an extremity are often selected for diagnostic purposes. If a regional anesthetic technique is chosen, it may be prudent not to include epinephrine in the local anesthetic solution, as the catecholamine could provoke undesirable vasoconstriction.

MOYAMOYA DISEASE

Moyamoya disease is a rare neurovascular disease characterized by narrowing or occlusion of both internal carotid arteries. Children and adults are affected, and a familial tendency may be present. The most common presentation in children is transient ischemic attacks, whereas the most common presentation in adults is intracerebral hemorrhage. The incidence of intracranial aneurysms associated with Moyamoya disease has been estimated to be 14% in adults but is rare in children. Medical management of these patients includes the use of antiplatelet (aspirin) and cerebral vasodilating (verapamil) drugs. Surgical treatment has included bypass (superficial temporal to middle cerebral artery anastomosis) and revascularization procedures.

Management of Anesthesia

Management of anesthesia must recognize the importance of preserving a balance between cerebral blood flow and cerebral oxygen consumption. Isoflurane has been recommended because of its mild cerebral vasodilating effects and ability to produce a greatly decreased cerebral metabolic rate.[8] Normocapnia is maintained to avoid any possible detrimental effect of an altered $PaCO_2$ on cerebral blood flow. The presence of neurologic changes may limit the use of succinylcholine. Increased intraoperative bleeding may reflect the effects of therapy with antiplatelet drugs. Cardiac rhythm disturbances have been reported in these patients during anesthesia and surgery. Patients with a history of seizures should be maintained on anticonvulsant medications. Seizures and temporary hemiparesis have been described after administration of spinal anesthesia to a child with Moyamoya disease.[9] It is possible that circulatory changes induced by spinal anesthesia altered cerebral blood flow sufficiently to produce cerebral focal ischemia in the presence of co-existing cerebrovascular disease.

KLIPPEL-TRENAUNAY SYNDROME

Klippel-Trenaunay syndrome is characterized by a port-wine hemangioma (neck, trunk, extremities) associated with spinal cord arteriovenous malformations. Spinal cord lesions may bleed spontaneously after straining or coughing. Spinal or epidural anesthesia is not recommended for use in these patients.[10]

BEHÇET'S DISEASE

Behçet's disease is a chronic relapsing syndrome of oral ulceration, painful genital ulcers, and uveitis. In Japan, the incidence is about 1 per 1000, whereas the prevalence in the United States is less than 1 per 15,000 persons. The most effective treatment is with chlorambucil, whereas corticosteroids are only modestly effective.

KAWASAKI DISEASE

Kawasaki disease (mucocutaneous lymph node syndrome) occurs primarily in children, manifesting as fever, conjunctivitis, inflammation of the mucous membranes, swollen erythematous hands and feet, trunkal rashes, and cervical lymphadenopathy. Vasculitis appears early in the disease and subsequently the walls of coronary arteries and other medium-size muscular arteries may show evidence of focal segmental destruction, with coronary artery aneurysms or ectasia developing in about 15% to 25% of affected children. Complications have included pericarditis, myocarditis, angina pectoris, myocardial infarction, and cerebral hemorrhage. The syndrome may be caused by a retrovirus, although there is no evidence of person-to-person transmission. Treatment is with gamma globulin and aspirin.

ACUTE PERIPHERAL ARTERIAL OCCLUSIVE DISEASE

Acute peripheral arterial occlusive disease affecting the extremities most often reflects embolism that originate in the heart. These emboli can originate from (1) thrombi in the akinetic portion of the left ventricle in patients with a prior myocardial infarction, (2) an enlarged and often fibrillating left atrium, (3) prosthetic heart valves, (4) vegetations of infective endocarditis, and (5) left atrial myxomas. Alternatively, emboli may originate from an atheromatous lesion in the abdominal aorta or ileofemoral artery. Emboli commonly lodge at arterial bifurcations, such as the distal abdominal aorta or the femoral artery bifurcation, causing a syndrome of sudden pain, sharply demarcated skin color changes, numbness, and decreased skin temperature below the level of the arterial occlusion. Surgical embolectomy and adjunctive heparin therapy is recommended when an acute embolism lodges in a large peripheral artery and causes persistent ischemia. Surgically removed emboli should be examined microscopically for myxomatous material to detect the presence of a previously unsuspected atrial myxoma (see Chapter 2).

Atheromatous embolism to the lower extremities produces a characteristic syndrome of abrupt ischemic symptoms in the lower leg or foot. In most cases of atheromatous embolism, severe pain is present, the area of ischemia is sharply demarcated cutaneously, and the proximal extremity pulses are still palpable. Embolectomy is usually not feasible.

CHRONIC PERIPHERAL ARTERIAL OCCLUSIVE DISEASE

Chronic peripheral arterial occlusive disease of the extremities is nearly always due to atherosclerosis. Indeed, many patients with symptomatic chronic occlusive disease of the lower extremities (claudication, ulcers, gangrene) have clinically evident coronary or cerebral atherosclerotic disease as well. Peripheral atherosclerosis may be diffuse, especially in the elderly or in patients with diabetes mellitus, or it may be distributed in characteristic segments of large arteries. Occlusion of the distal abdominal aorta or iliac arteries tends to occur in males less than 60 years of age, manifested as claudication in the hips and buttocks. Occlusion of the common femoral or superficial femoral arteries is the most common form of segmental peripheral atherosclerosis, especially in elderly patients, producing a syndrome of claudication in or below the calf. Doppler recordings of the arterial pulse wave show a monophasic velocity profile distal to sites of arterial obstruction, whereas normal recordings show two phases of forward flow separated by a brief period of backflow.

Treatment

Vasodilator drugs and thrombolytic therapy are generally ineffective in treating peripheral atherosclerotic occlusive disease. Transluminal angioplasty with a balloon catheter, combined with an exercise program and cessation of smoking, is particularly useful in treatment of peripheral arterial stenosis.[11] The arterial system of patients with segmental large artery disease can usually be satisfactorily reconstructed by surgery, if the smaller vessels below the knees are still patent. Arteriography is used to determine the appropriateness of revascularization surgery. Unilateral iliac occlusive disease can be managed by constructing a bypass from the opposite

femoral artery (femorofemoral bypass). In the surgical management of femoropopliteal disease, a saphenous vein bypass graft may be preferred over the use of either a synthetic graft or endarterectomy. Lumbar sympathectomy does not improve the long-term viability of femoropopliteal vein bypass grafts, but it may aid in maintaining graft patency during the early postoperative period. Aspirin and dipyridamole may be useful in patients undergoing prosthetic or saphenous vein femoropopliteal operations. Antiplatelet therapy should be begun preoperatively with dipyridamole, whereas aspirin should be initiated postoperatively. Dextran 40 need not be administered routinely to prevent postoperative thrombosis after revascularization of the lower extremities. Revascularization surgery for vessels distal to the popliteal artery is seldom successful.

Management of Anesthesia

Management of anesthesia for surgical revascularization of the lower extremities incorporates many of the same principles described for management of patients with abdominal aneurysms.[12] For example, the principal risk in reconstructive peripheral vascular surgery is associated atherosclerosis, particularly ischemic heart disease. Coronary artery bypass graft operations are usually performed before peripheral vascular surgery in patients who have both angina pectoris and claudication. Because patients with claudication are often unable to perform a treadmill exercise test, a thallium perfusion scan during intravenous dypyridamole infusion is a useful method for detecting ischemic heart disease. Ambulatory electrocardiographic monitoring for detection of evidence of myocardial ischemia, which is often asymptomatic (silent), is an alternative method for evaluating ischemic heart disease.

There is often reluctance to select epidural or spinal anesthesia for patients undergoing surgical revascularization procedures of the legs, despite some perceived advantages (increased graft blood flow, less increase in systemic vascular resistance with aortic cross-clamping, postoperative pain relief) when this technique is used alone or in combination with general anesthesia. The popularity of general anesthesia is in part due to the controversy surrounding the performance of regional anesthesia, especially placement of a lumbar epidural catheter, in the presence of drug-induced anticoagulation (see Chapter 25). Nevertheless, placement of an epidural catheter before the institution of heparin anticoagulation in patients undergoing revascularization of the lower extremity is not associated with untoward neurologic events.[13] Furthermore, provision of epidural analgesia after this type of surgery attenuates postoperative stress-induced hypercoagulability and may beneficially influence outcome in high-risk patients who have undergone major peripheral vascular surgery.[14]

Infrarenal aortic cross-clamping in the presence of peripheral vascular occlusive disease, but good collateral circulation as verified on the preoperative arteriogram, is associated with

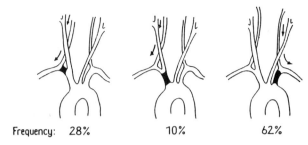

Fig. 11-1. Comparison of the frequency of occurrence of left, right, and bilateral subclavian steal syndrome. (From Heidrich H, Bayer O. Symptomatology of the subclavian steal syndrome. Angiology 1969;20:406–13, with permission.)

fewer hemodynamic derangements than occur in patients undergoing resection of an abdominal aortic aneurysm. Likewise, minimal hemodynamic changes associated with declamping of the aorta may reflect, in part, the beneficial role of collateral circulation in preventing marked increases in lactate during the aortic cross-clamp period. In view of the decreased likelihood of major hemodynamic alterations associated with aortic cross-clamping, it may be acceptable to use a central venous pressure catheter in lieu of a pulmonary artery catheter, especially in the absence of symptomatic left ventricular dysfunction or ischemic heart disease, or both.

Heparin is commonly administered before the application of the aortic cross-clamp, presumably to decrease the risk of thromboembolic complications. It is now recognized, however, that distal emboli, especially to the kidneys, most likely reflect dislodgment of atheroembolic debris from the diseased aorta. Thus, in the absence of major distal occlusive disease, care in manipulation and clamping of the aorta to minimize the likely dislodgment of potentially embolic debris may be more important than administration of heparin. Spinal cord damage associated with surgical revascularization of the legs is unlikely; special monitoring for this complication is not necessary. Postoperative management includes the provision of analgesia, such as with neuraxial opioids, and treatment of fluid and electrolyte derangements.

Subclavian Steal Syndrome

Occlusion of the subclavian or innominate artery proximal to the origin of the vertebral artery by an atherosclerotic lesion may result in reversal of flow through the ipsilateral vertebral artery into the distal subclavian artery[15,16] (Fig. 11-1). Reversal of flow diverts blood flow from the brain to supply the arm (subclavian steal syndrome). Symptoms of central nervous system ischemia (syncope, vertigo, ataxia, hemiplegia) or arm ischemia, or both, are usually present. Exercise of the ipsilateral arm accentuates these hemodynamic changes and may

evoke neurologic symptoms. There is often an absent or diminished pulse in the ipsilateral arm and the systolic blood pressure is likely to be at least 20 mmHg lower in the ipsilateral arm.[16] Physical examination may demonstrate a bruit over the subclavian artery. Stenosis of the left subclavian artery is responsible for this syndrome in about 70% of patients. Subclavian endarterectomy may be curative.

Coronary-Subclavian Steal Syndrome

A rare complication of using the internal mammary artery for coronary revascularization is the coronary-subclavian steal syndrome. This syndrome occurs when the development of a proximal incomplete stenosis in the left subclavian artery produces reversal of blood flow through the patent internal mammary artery graft[17] (Fig. 11-2). This steal syndrome is

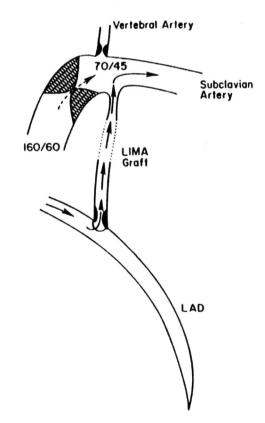

Fig. 11-2. Development of subtotal stenosis of the left subclavian artery may produce reversal of flow through a patent internal mammary graft (LIMA), thus diverting flow (coronary-subclavian steal syndrome) destined for the left anterior descending coronary artery (LAD). (From Martin JL, Rock P. Coronary-subclavian steal syndrome: Anesthetic implications and management in the perioperative period. Anesthesiology 1988;68:933–6, with permission.)

characterized by angina pectoris, signs of central nervous system ischemia, and decreased systolic blood pressure of at least 20 mmHg in the ipsilateral arm. Bilateral upper extremity brachial artery blood pressure measurements may be useful in the preoperative evaluation of patients with internal mammary artery to coronary artery bypass grafts. Angina pectoris associated with coronary-subclavian steal syndrome require surgical bypass grafting. Management of anesthesia in these patients includes the application of the same principles recommended for patients with ischemic heart disease owing to atherosclerosis.

REFERENCES

1. Conn DL. Update on systemic necrotizing vasculitis. Mayo Clin Proc 1989;64:535–46
2. Warner MA, Hughes DR, Messick JM. Anesthetic management of a patient with pulseless disease. Anesth Analg 1983;62:532–5
3. McKay RSF, Dillard SR. Management of epidural anesthesia in a patient with Takayasu's disease. Anesth Analg 1992;74:297–9
4. Lake CL. Anesthesia and Wegener's granulomatosis: Case report and review of the literature. Anesth Analg 1978;57:353–9
5. Dillman JF. Safe use of succinylcholine during repeated anesthetics in a patient treated with cyclophosphamide. Anesth Analg 1987;66:351–3
6. Gorsky BH. Intravenous perfusion with reserpine for Raynaud's phenomenon. Reg Anaesth 1977;2:5
7. Holland AJC, Davies KH, Wallace DH. Sympathetic blockade of isolated limbs by intravenous guanethidine. Can Anaesth Soc J 1977;24:597–602
8. Brown SC, Lam AM. Moyamoya disease—a review of clinical experience and anaesthetic management. Can J Anaesth 1987; 34:71–5
9. Yasukawa M, Yasukawa K, Akawaga S, Nakagawa Y, Miyasaka K. Convulsions and temporary hemiparesis following spinal anesthesia in a child with Moyamoya disease. Anesthesiology 1988; 69:1023–4
10. deLeon-Casasola OA, Lema MJ. Epidural anesthesia in patients with Klippel-Trenaunay syndrome. Anesth Analg 1992;74:470
11. Widlus DM, Osterman FA. Evaluation and percutaneous management of atherosclerotic peripheral vascular disease. JAMA 1989; 261:3148–55
12. Cunningham AJ. Anaesthesia for abdominal aortic surgery—a review. Can J Anaesth 1989;36:426–44;568–77
13. Baron HC, LaRaja RD, Rossi G, Atkinson D. Continuous epidural analgesia in the heparinized vascular surgical patient: A retrospective review of 912 patients. J Vasc Surg 1987;6:144–6
14. Tuman KJ, McCarthy RJ, March RJ, DeLaria GA, Patel RV, Ivankovich AD. Effects of epidural anesthesia and analgesia on coagulation and outcome after major vascular surgery. Anesth Analg 1991;73:696–704
15. Heidrich H, Bayer O. Symptomatology of the subclavian steal syndrome. Angiology 1969;20:406–13
16. Killen DA, Fostert JH, Gobbel WG, et al. The subclavian steal syndrome. J Thorac Cardiovasc Surg 1966;60:539–60
17. Martin JL, Rock P. Coronary-subclavian steal syndrome: Anesthetic implications and management in the perioperative period. Anesthesiology 1988;68:933–6

12

Deep Vein Thrombosis and Pulmonary Embolism

Deep vein thrombosis and associated pulmonary embolism are among the leading causes of postoperative morbidity and mortality.[1,2] The formation of clot inside a blood vessel is designated a thrombus, to distinguish it from normal extravascular clotting of blood. An embolus is a fragment of the thrombus that breaks off and travels in the blood until it lodges at a site of vascular narrowing. For this reason, an embolus originating in a vein commonly lodges in the pulmonary vasculature, whereas an embolus originating in an artery usually occludes a more distal and smaller artery (see Chapter 11).

Factors that predispose to thromboembolism are multiple but often include events likely to be associated with anesthesia and surgery (Table 12-1). For example, venous stasis as associated with postoperative immobility or pregnancy results in failure to dilute or promptly clear activated clotting factors, thus predisposing to thrombus formation. Any condition that causes a roughened endothelial vessel wall, such as infection, trauma, or drug-induced irritation, predisposes to thrombus formation. In addition to venous embolism, pulmonary embolism can also result from fat, air, amniotic fluid, and, on rare occasions, cells from a tumor.

DEEP VEIN THROMBOSIS

Studies employing radiolabeled fibrinogen show deep vein thrombosis in the legs of 20% to 30% of patients older than 50 years or age who have undergone herniorrhaphy and in more than 50% of patients who have undergone prostatectomy or hip surgery.[1] Most of these venous thromboses are subclinical and resolve completely when mobility is restored, although some produce damage to venous valves with resulting chronic venous insufficiency. A few, however, may travel to the lungs and produce pulmonary embolism. Venous stasis,

endothelial damage, and hypercoagulability as may accompany anesthesia and surgery predispose to venous thrombosis. Venous thrombi formed below the knees or in the arms rarely give rise to significant pulmonary emboli, whereas thrombi that extend into the iliofemoral venous system can produce life-threatening pulmonary embolism. Likewise, thrombi formed in the right atrium of a patient in atrial fibrillation are common sources of pulmonary embolism.

Diagnosis and Treatment

Superficial thrombophlebitis as may follow an intravenous infusion or drug injection is rarely associated with pulmonary embolism. Indeed, intense inflammation that accompanies superficial thrombophlebitis leads to rapid total occlusion of the vein making subsequent embolism unlikely. Typically the vein can be palpated as a cord-like structure surrounded by an area of erythema, warmth, and edema. The presence of fever suggests bacterial infection. Treatment of superficial vein thrombosis is usually conservative, consisting of elevation of the affected site, local application of heat, and administration of antibiotics for suspected bacterial infection.

The diagnosis of deep vein thrombosis by clinical signs is unreliable. For example, throbbing pain, edema, and associated skeletal muscle spasm characteristic of thrombophlebitis may be absent, even after pulmonary embolism has occurred. Ultimately, the diagnosis of deep vein thrombosis depends on specific tests. The most reliable of these tests is venography, demonstrating the presence of a filling defect on a venogram. Nevertheless, lower extremity venography is negative in about one-third of patients who subsequently experience pulmonary embolism. Furthermore, venography is an invasive and expensive test, negating its value for routine clinical use. The fibrinogen uptake test uses radiolabeled fibrinogen injected before operation, and a scan is used noninvasively to

131

Table 12-1.   Predisposing Factors to Thromboembolism

Venous Stasis
   Trauma (including surgery)
   Lack of ambulation
   Pregnancy
   Low cardiac output (congestive heart failure, myocardial infarction)

Abnormality of the Venous Wall
   Varicose veins
   Drug-induced irritation

Hypercoagulable State
   Estrogen therapy (oral contraceptives)
   Cancer (Trousseau syndrome)
   Deficiencies of endogenous anticoagulants (antithrombin III, protein C, protein S)
   Stress response associated with surgery

History of Previous Thromboembolism

Morbid Obesity

Advanced Age

detect incorporation of fibrinogen into newly formed thrombus. This test is accurate for clots below midthigh but in hip surgery is associated with a false-positive rate greater than 30%. As such, its role is that of a screening technique. The risk of transmission of disease is a further hazard of the fibrinogen uptake test. In addition, this test is of little use in the detection of existing thrombi. Impedance plethysmography and duplex ultrasound are highly sensitive noninvasive methods for detecting proximal deep vein thrombi (iliofemoral) and are used for determining the need for institution of anticoagulant therapy.[3,4] Conversely, the current view is that distal deep vein thrombi (below the knees) rarely result in clinically significant pulmonary emboli, therefore, anticoagulant therapy is probably not necessary.

Heparin

Treatment of proximal deep vein thrombosis is with heparin (5000 units IV) as a single injection, followed by a continuous intravenous infusion of heparin adjusted to maintain the activated partial thromboplastin time 1.5 to 2 times normal.[5] Alternatively, subcutaneous low-molecular-weight heparin administered once daily may be as effective and safe as intravenous heparin; another advantage is that it can be administered on an outpatient basis.[6] Heparin works promptly to prevent both further thrombus formation and the release of serotonin and thromboxane from platelets adherent to thrombi that embolize to the lungs. These vasoactive substances are suspected to be mediators of the intense pulmonary arteriolar vasoconstriction that results in severe pulmonary hypertension. Intravenous heparin therapy is usually continued for 10 days (based on animal data that it takes as long as 7 to 10 days for thrombus to become firmly adherent to the vein wall), although a 5-day course may be equally effective.[7]

Oral anticoagulation with warfarin sufficient to prolong the prothrombin time to 1.2 to 1.5 times normal is eventually instituted to replace heparin therapy. The proper duration of oral anticoagulant therapy is not established, although treatment is usually continued for 3 to 6 months. Cimetidine, third-generation cephalosporins, and aspirin are examples of drugs that may potentiate the anticoagulant effects of warfarin. Heparin, which, in contrast to warfarin, does not cross the placenta, is the preferred drug for anticoagulation during pregnancy.

Complications

Heparin-induced bleeding usually occurs after about 48 hours; it is especially hazardous when intracranial. Nevertheless, the only absolute contraindication to the use of heparin is the presence of a known coagulation disorder or active hemorrhage. Hemoptysis from pulmonary infarction is not a contraindication to therapy with heparin. Thrombocytopenia develops in up to 30% of patients receiving therapeutic doses of heparin, typically occurring 3 to 15 days (median 10 days) after institution of heparin therapy.[5] Hyperkalemia, presumably reflecting heparin-induced hypoaldosternism, is an unusual complication that seems more likely to occur in the patient with diabetes mellitus or renal insufficiency. Elevated serum aminotransferases occur in most patients who receive heparin, tending to peak after about 7 days of therapy. Intravenous infusion of nitroglycerin may induce heparin resistance, and discontinuation of nitroglycerin is followed by a period of increased sensitivity to heparin.[8]

Prophylaxis

Venous stasis is minimized by exercises that include flexion and extension at the knees, ankles, and feet. A useful practice is to teach these exercises to the patient before an elective surgical procedures is performed. The application of elastic stockings preoperatively provides graded compression from the ankle to thigh and decreases the incidence of deep vein thrombosis in patients undergoing major surgery. These stockings need not be custom made, and their protective effect appears to be additive to that of low-dose heparin. Proper fit and positioning of these stockings are important, as arterial thrombosis may occur when stockings are applied incorrectly. Stockings are inexpensive and, in many instances, are the most cost-effective prophylactic measure against the development of deep vein thrombosis during the postoperative period.[9] External pneumatic calf compression may be useful in patients undergoing neurosurgical procedures or total hip replacement.[10]

Subcutaneous Heparin

Perioperative administration of subcutaneous heparin (5000 units every 12 hours) has been demonstrated to prevent about two-thirds of all deep vein thromboses and about one-half of all pulmonary emboli among patients undergoing urologic, orthopaedic, or general surgical procedures.[1,5] As such, perioperative subcutaneous heparin prophylaxis may be viewed as a cost-effective means of decreasing postoperative mortality from pulmonary embolism in selected patients. This does not mean that some other method of prophylaxis (elastic stockings, oral anticoagulants) could be used in addition to, or instead of, subcutaneous heparin. Aspirin has not proved efficacious in the prevention of deep vein thrombosis.

Institution of subcutaneous heparin therapy introduces concern regarding the subsequent use of regional anesthesia and the possibility of hematoma formation, especially in the epidural space. In this regard, a suggestion that the start of subcutaneous heparin therapy can be delayed until after surgery would be attractive.[1] The use of low-dose heparin is associated with an increased incidence of wound hematomas but not in an increase in major hemorrhage.

Although low-dose heparin is effective in decreasing deep venous thrombosis after hip surgery, the risk of thrombosis remains substantial at 25% to 30%. It is possible that low-dose warfarin is more effective than a fixed low dose of heparin in patients undergoing major orthopaedic procedures.[5]

Regional Anesthesia

The incidence of postoperative deep vein thrombosis and pulmonary embolism in patients who have undergone total hip replacement or knee replacement is decreased by greater than 50% in patients receiving epidural or spinal anesthesia compared with those undergoing the same surgery but with general anesthesia.[11-14] Nevertheless, deep vein thrombosis still occurs, and long-term outcome is not affected by the choice of anesthesia.[15]

Presumably, the beneficial effect of regional anesthesia compared with general anesthesia is due to vasodilation that maximizes venous blood flow and to the ability to provide optimal postoperative analgesia with associated early ambulation. Furthermore, patients given regional anesthesia are often given fluid loads that could decrease viscosity of blood and offset venous stasis. Local anesthetics may even exert a beneficial effect by inhibition of platelet aggregation.[12] By contrast, general anesthesia may contribute to an increased incidence of deep vein thrombosis by virtue of decreased leg blood flow, estimated to be as much as 50%. Theoretically, controlled ventilation of the lungs would further impede venous return from the legs, but the incidence of deep vein thrombosis is not influenced by the method of ventilation.[16]

PULMONARY EMBOLISM

Clinical manifestations of pulmonary embolism are nonspecific, and the diagnosis is often difficult to establish on clinical grounds alone (Table 12-2). A high index of suspicion is important in recognizing the patient with pulmonary embolism. The most consistent manifestation is an acute onset of dyspnea that most likely reflects a sudden increase in alveolar dead space and a decrease in pulmonary compliance. Often dyspnea and associated apprehension seem out of proportion to the degree and extent of the objective abnormal findings. Typically, breathing is rapid and shallow. Wheezing may be heard on auscultation of the lungs. Substernal chest pain, which may be indistinguishable from angina pectoris, often accompanies a large pulmonary embolus. Hypotension, tachycardia, and increased central venous pressure are consistent with the diagnosis of a life-threatening pulmonary embolus resulting in cor pulmonale. Nevertheless, right-sided filling pressures may not be elevated until at least 50% of the pulmonary circulation has been occluded by clot. Conversely, in the patient with co-existing cardiopulmonary disease, a relatively small volume of clot may abruptly elevate pulmonary artery pressure and produce signs of cor pulmonale. When pulmonary infarction occurs (typically manifested hours to days after the initial event), the triad of cough, hemoptysis, and pleuritic pain is often present. In addition, body temperature elevation often accompanies the signs of consolidation and effusion. Fever makes it difficult to distinguish a pulmonary infarction from pneumonia. Indeed, an isolated pulmonary infiltrate may be interpreted radiographically as pneumonia.

Arterial blood gases that accompany pulmonary embolism are characterized by decreased PaO_2 and $PaCO_2$ and a normal to increased alveolar-to-arterial difference for oxygen (A-

Table 12-2.   Signs and Symptoms of Pulmonary Embolism

Sign/Symptom	Patients (%)
Acute dyspnea	80–85
Tachypnea (>20 breaths·min^{-1})	75–85
Pleuritic chest pain	65–70
Nonproductive cough	50–60
Accentuation of pulmonic valve second sound	50–60
Rales	50–60
Tachycardia (>100 beats·min^{-1})	45–65
Fever (38°–39°C)	40–50
Hemoptysis	30

aDO$_2$). Changes on the electrocardiogram (ECG) are unlikely in the absence of a pulmonary embolism sufficient to cause acute cor pulmonale (peaked P waves, atrial fibrillation, right bundle branch block). The ECG is mainly used to help distinguish between massive pulmonary embolism and myocardial infarction. A delayed nonspecific increase in the serum concentration of an isoenzyme fraction of lacate dehydrogenase occurs in about 80% of patients experiencing pulmonary embolism. Serum aspartate aminotransferase and the myocardial fraction of creatine kinase tend to remain normal in the presence of pulmonary embolism but are often increased in the patient experiencing myocardial ischemia or an acute myocardial infarction. Leukocytosis and an increased erythrocyte sedimentation rate are common changes associated with a pulmonary infarction.

Manifestations of pulmonary embolism during anesthesia are nonspecific and often transient.[17] Changes suggestive of pulmonary embolism during anesthesia include unexplained arterial hypoxemia, hypotension, tachycardia, and bronchospasm. The ECG and central venous pressure may reflect an abrupt onset of pulmonary hypertension and right ventricular dysfunction. Monitoring the $P_{ET}CO_2$ will demonstrate an increased alveolar-to-arterial difference for carbon dioxide (A-aDCO$_2$) owing to ventilation of unperfused alveoli. Transeosphageal echocardiography demonstrating acute dilation of the right atrium, right ventricle, and pulmonary artery may aid in the diagnosis of an intraoperative pulmonary embolus.[18]

Diagnosis

The definitive diagnosis of pulmonary embolism may require both invasive and noninvasive diagnostic tests. Ventilation-to-perfusion scans are noninvasive, using gamma-emitting isotopes to delineate pulmonary blood flow. Although considered highly sensitive, about 4% of normal or near-normal scans are subsequently demonstrated to be associated with pulmonary embolism.[19] If the diagnosis remains in doubt, the method of greatest sensitivity and specificity for pulmonary embolism is pulmonary arteriography. The cost and morbidity (cardiac dysrhythmias, allergic reaction to the contrast media) associated with pulmonary arteriography prohibit routine use of this diagnostic technique. Should suspected pulmonary embolism occur in the patient monitored with a pulmonary artery catheter, it is permissible to use this catheter for pulmonary arteriography.[20] Contrast media is injected through the distal port, with the catheter placed in a proximal pulmonary artery. Digital subtraction arteriography may replace the need for direct pulmonary artery injection of contrast medium. Nonspecific chest radiograph abnormalities develop in about 45% of patients with pulmonary embolism, proved by pulmonary arteriography. The abnormalities appear an average of about 2 days after the initial event. Computed tomography may detect evidence of pulmonary embolism not apparent on a conventional chest radiograph.

Treatment

Treatment of pulmonary embolism is intended to support cardiopulmonary function and to prevent extension or recurrence of the embolus. Intravenous administration of heparin works promptly to prevent extension of venous thrombus or recurrence of additional embolization to the lungs and improves outcome (see the section, Heparin). Thrombolytic drugs may be considered, but lysis of previously formed clots outside the lungs may be undesirable in the postoperative patient.[21] Hypotension caused by a low cardiac output may require treatment with a catecholamine such as isoproterenol, dopamine, or dobutamine. Isoproterenol is an attractive choice, as it is more likely than other catecholamines to decrease pulmonary vascular resistance. Nevertheless, the value of a pulmonary vasodilator in the management of pulmonary embolism has not been established. Intubation of the trachea and institution of controlled ventilation of the lungs with positive end-expiratory pressure may be necessary. An analgesic to treat pain associated with pulmonary embolism is important but must be prescribed bearing the underlying instability of the cardiovascular system in mind.

Pulmonary arteriography may indicate the need for pulmonary embolectomy and interruption of the inferior vena cava. Since more than 90% of pulmonary emboli originate from thrombi in the legs, surgical treatment may include the placement of an umbrella filter in the inferior vena cava, using fluoroscopy. Migration of this umbrella filter is a serious hazard in about 5% of patients treated in this manner. Pulmonary artery embolectomy using cardiopulmonary bypass is reserved for the patient with a massive pulmonary embolism documented by pulmonary arteriography and who is unresponsive to medical therapy.

Management of Anesthesia

Management of anesthesia for the surgical treatment of life-threatening pulmonary embolism is designed to support vital organ function and to minimize anesthetic-induced myocardial depression. Most patients will arrive in the operating room with a tracheal tube in place and with ventilation of the lungs being controlled with an increased inspired concentration of oxygen. Monitoring of arterial and cardiac filling pressures is important. It is important to monitor right atrial filling pressure and to adjust the rate of intravenous fluid administration, in an effort to optimize right ventricular stroke volume in the presence of a marked increase in afterload. It may be necessary to support cardiac output with the continuous infusion of a catecholamine during the operative procedure. In this regard, isoproterenol increases myocardial contractility and may decrease pulmonary vascular resistance. The disadvantage of isoproterenol is a decrease in diastolic blood pressure, which may jeopardize coronary blood flow. Dopamine or dobutamine are acceptable alternative drugs to isoproterenol, but neither of these catecholamines is likely to decrease pulmonary vascular resistance. In fact, large doses of dopamine may increase pulmonary vascular resistance.

Induction and maintenance of anesthesia should avoid accentuation of co-existing arterial hypoxemia, systemic hypotension, and pulmonary hypertension. Among the intravenous induction drugs, the potential adverse effects of ketamine on the pulmonary vascular resistance must be considered. Maintenance of anesthesia can be achieved with any drug or combination of drugs that does not produce excessive myocardial depression. Nitrous oxide is not a likely selection, considering the need to administer high concentrations of oxygen and the potential of this drug to increase pulmonary vascular resistance. Pancuronium is an acceptable drug for the production of skeletal muscle paralysis. Likewise, nondepolarizing muscle relaxants with little or no effect on heart rate or blood pressure are acceptable selections.

Removal of emboli fragments from the distal pulmonary arteries may be facilitated by the application of positive-pressure ventilation of the lungs when the surgeon applies suction through the arteriotomy placed in the pulmonary trunk. Although the cardiopulmonary status of these patients is perilous before surgery, significant hemodynamic improvement usually occurs postoperatively.

FAT EMBOLISM

The syndrome of fat embolism to the lungs typically appears 12 to 48 hours (rarely more than 72 hours) after a long bone fracture, especially of the femur or tibia.[22] Associated pulmonary dysfunction may be limited to arterial hypoxemia (always present) or may be fulminant, progressing from tachypnea to alveolar capillary leak and adult respiratory distress syndrome. Central nervous system dysfunction ranges from confusion to seizures and coma. Petechiae, especially over the neck, shoulders, and chest, occur in at least 50% of patients with clinical evidence of fat embolism. Coagulopathy and thrombocytopenia are probably related to other complications of severe trauma, including disseminated intravascular coagulation. An increased plasma lipase concentration or the presence of lipiduria is suggestive of fat embolism but may also occur after trauma in the absence of this problem. Temperature increases up to 42°C and tachycardia are often present.

The source of fat producing fat embolism is undocumented but may represent disruption of the adipose architecture of bone marrow. Treatment of the fat embolism syndrome includes management of adult respiratory distress syndrome and immobilization of long bone fractures. Prophylactic administration of corticosteroids for patients at risk may be useful, but the efficacy of corticosteroids for the established syndrome has not been documented.[23]

REFERENCES

1. Collins R, Scrimgeour A, Yusuf S, Peto R. Reduction in fatal pulmonary embolism and venous thrombosis by perioperative administration of subcutaneous heparin. Overview of results of randomized trials in general, orthopedic, and urologic surgery. N Engl J Med 1988;318:1162–73
2. McKenzie PJ. Deep vein thrombosis and anaesthesia. Br J Anaesth 1991;66:4–7
3. Huisman MV, Buller HR, tenCate JW. Utility of impedance plethymography in the diagnosis of recurrent deep-vein thrombosis. Arch Intern Med 1988;148:681–6
4. White RH, McGahan JP, Dashbach MM, et al. Diagnosis of deep-vein thrombosis using duplex ultra sound. Ann Intern Med 1989;111:297–303
5. Hirsh J. Heparin. N Engl J Med 1991;324:1565–73
6. Hull RD, Raskob GE, Pineo GF, et al. Subcutaneous low-molecular weight heparin compared with continuous intravenous heparin in the treatment of proximal-vein thrombosis. N Engl J Med 1992;326:975–82
7. Hull RD, Raskob GE, Rosenbloom D, et al. Heparin for 5 days as compared with 10 days in the initial treatment of proximal venous thrombosis. N Engl J Med 1990;322:1260–6
8. Habbab MA, Haft JI. Heparin resistance induced by intravenous nitroglycerin: A word of caution when both drugs are used concomitantly. Arch Intern Med 1987;147:857–61
9. Oster G, Tuden RL, Colditz GA. Prevention of venous thromboembolism after general surgery: Cost-effectiveness of alternative approaches to prophylaxis. Am J Med 1987;82:889–93
10. Hull RD, Raskob GE, Gent M, et al. Effectiveness of intermittent pneumatic leg compression for preventing deep vein thrombosis after total hip replacement. JAMA 1990;263:2313–7
11. Modig J, Maripuu E, Sahlstedt B. Thromboembolism following total hip replacement. A prospective investigation of 94 patients with emphasis on efficacy of lumbar epidural anaesthesia in prophylaxis. Reg Anaesth 1986;11:72–9
12. McKenzie PJ, Wishart HY, Gray I, Smith G. Effects of anaesthetic technique on deep vein thrombosis. A comparison of subarachnoid and general anesthesia. Br J Anaesth 1985;57:853–7
13. Jorgensen LN, Rasmussen LS, Neilsen PT, Leffers A, Albrecht-Beste E. Antithrombotic efficacy of continuous extradural analgesia after knee replacement. Br J Anaesth 1991;66:8–12
14. Modig J, Borg T, Karlstrom G, Maripuu E, Sahlstedt B. Thromboembolism after total hip replacement: Role of epidural and general anesthesia. Anesth Analg 1983;62:174–80
15. Davis FM, Woolner DF, Frampton C, et al. Prospective, multicentre trial of mortality following general or spinal anaesthesia for hip fracture surgery in the elderly. Br J Anaesth 1987;59:1080–8

16. Coleman SA, Boyce WJ, Cosh PH, McKenzie PJ. Outcome after general anaesthesia for repair of fractured neck of femur: A randomized trial of spontaneous v. controlled ventilation. Br J Anaesth 1988;60:43–7

17. Divekan VM, Kamdar BM, Pansare SN. Pulmonary embolism during anaesthesia: Case report. Can Anaesth Soc J 1981;28: 277–9

18. Langeron O, Goarin J-P, Pansard J-L, Riou B, Viars P. Massive intraoperative pulmonary embolism: Diagnosis with transesophageal two-dimensional echocardiography. Anesth Analg 1992;74: 148–50

19. The PIOPED Investigators: Value of the ventilation/perfusion scan in acute pulmonary embolism: Results of the prospective investigation of pulmonary embolism diagnosis (PIOPED). JAMA 1990;263:2753–59

20. Berry AJ. Pulmonary embolism during spinal anesthesia: Angiographic diagnosis via a flow-directed pulmonary artery catheter. Anesthesiology 1982;57:57–9

21. Sasahara AA, Sharma GVRK, Tow DE, et al. Clinical use of thrombolytic agents in venous thromboembolism. Arch Intern Med 1982;142:684–8

22. Gossling HR, Donahue TA. The fat embolism syndrome. JAMA 1979;241:2740–6

23. Schonfeld SA, Ploysongsang Y, DiLisio R, et al. Fat embolism prophylaxis with corticosteroids: A prospective study in high-risk patients. Ann Intern Med 1983;99:438–43

13
Chronic Obstructive Pulmonary Disease

Chronic obstructive pulmonary disease (COPD) affects an estimated 10 million Americans and is the fifth leading cause of death in the United States.[1] Chronic bronchitis and emphysema are the most common causes of COPD, and virtually all these cases are secondary to tobacco abuse. These diseases are characterized by permanent or minimally reversible obstruction to airflow during exhalation. At diagnosis, most patients have significant cough or dyspnea that affects daily living. Exercise limitation is typically characterized by dyspnea that occurs while climbing one flight of stairs or less. Cor pulmonale is usually present to some degree. These patients are extraordinarily vulnerable to development of acute respiratory failure from insults (acute respiratory infections, surgery) that would not affect normal persons significantly (see Chapter 16). Asthma is distinguished from COPD on the basis of a reversible component of airway obstruction (see Chapter 14).

CHRONIC BRONCHITIS AND PULMONARY EMPHYSEMA

Chronic bronchitis follows prolonged exposure of the airway to irritants, manifested as hypersecretion of mucus and a productive cough. Acute bronchitis differs from chronic bronchitis in that it is usually self-limited and is caused by an infectious agent. The clinical features of chronic bronchitis can resemble or contrast with findings present in patients with pulmonary emphysema (Table 13-1). The prognosis of chronic bronchitis is poor, with death often occurring within 5 years after the first episode of acute respiratory failure.

Pulmonary emphysema is characterized by a destructive process involving the lung parenchyma that results in loss of elastic recoil of the lungs (Table 13-1). As a result, airway collapse occurs during exhalation, leading to increased airway

resistance. Obstruction to expiratory airflow can also lead to the formation of bullae with compression of adjacent lung tissue. Dyspnea is severe, reflecting increased work of breathing due to loss of elastic recoil of the lungs.

Epidemiology

Cigarette smoking is the major predisposing factor to the development of COPD. The risk of death from chronic bronchitis or emphysema is 30 times greater for heavy smokers (at least 25 cigarettes daily). Environmental pollution appears to play some role, but its effects are minor compared with those of cigarette smoke. Most smokers have slightly decreased expiratory flow rates, and about 10% exhibit chronic airflow obstruction (forced exhaled volume in 1 second [FEV_1], less than 65% of predicted). The usefulness of the forced expiratory flow between 25% and 75% of vital capacity is limited. The specific pathogenic substances in cigarette smoke have not been identified with certainty, but it is likely that particle size and gas solubility determine which toxic substances are deposited in the trachea and large bronchi, causing bronchitis, and which are deposited in the bronchioles and alveoli, causing emphysema. Virtually all cigarette smokers older than 60 years of age exhibit some evidence of emphysema.

The dominant feature of the natural history of COPD is progressive airflow obstruction, as reflected by decreases in FEV_1. Respiratory tract infections do not influence the overall course of the disease. It seems likely that lung damage is irreversible by the time chronic airflow obstruction is present in patients with chronic bronchitis and emphysema and the FEV_1 has decreased below the normal range. Smoking cessation at this point serves only to slow the rate of further loss of lung function.

Emphysema may develop in some patients because of an

Table 13-1.   Comparative Features of Chronic Obstructive Pulmonary Disease

Feature	Chronic Bronchitis	Pulmonary Emphysema
Mechanism of airway obstruction	Decreased airway lumen due to mucus and inflammation	Loss of elastic recoil
Dyspnea	Moderate	Severe
Forced exhaled volume in 1 second	Decreased	Decreased
PaO_2	Marked decrease ("blue bloater")	Modest decrease ("pink puffer")
$PaCO_2$	Increased	Normal to decreased
Diffusing capacity	Normal	Decreased
Hematocrit	Increased	Normal
Cor pulmonale	Marked	Mild
Prognosis	Poor	Good

imbalance between protease and antiprotease activities in the lungs. Indeed, alpha-1-antitrypsin deficiency results in unopposed degradation of pulmonary interstitial elastin fibers by the enzyme elastase and the early development of emphysema. The genetic absence of alpha-1-antitrypsin activity is present in about 0.1% of the population; emphysema develops in about 80% of these people. Wide variability exists in the tendency toward the development of emphysema in patients with the deficiency but those who smoke cigarettes become disabled 15 to 20 years earlier in those who do not smoke.[2] Liver disease, most often cirrhosis, occurs in 5% to 10% of adults with alpha-1-antitrypsin deficiency. Heterozygotes for alpha-1-antitrypsin whose enzymatic activity is equal to or greater than 40% of normal probably are protected against the development of emphysema.[3] Most cigarette smokers have normal plasma concentrations of alpha-1-antitrypsin, but chronic inhalation of cigarette smoke can increase elastase activity in the lungs. Furthermore, oxidants in cigarette smoke can inactivate alpha-1-antitrypsin.

Clinical Features and Diagnosis

Chronic productive cough and progressive exercise limitation are the hallmarks of persistent expiratory airflow obstruction characteristic of COPD (Table 13-1). Pulmonary function tests are useful for confirming the presence, severity, and reversibility of airflow obstruction, as well as monitoring for the progression of the disease. COPD is most often diagnosed and assessed by spirometric measurements (Fig. 13-1). Characteristic of expiratory airflow obstruction on spirometry is a decrease in the ratio of the FEV_1 to the forced vital capacity (FVC). FEV_1 is typically less than 80% of the FVC in the presence of COPD. Measurement of the FEV_1 alone may be misleading, as this value may be low if the vital capacity is also low or if the patient is uncooperative. Measurement of lung

volumes demonstrates an increased residual volume and often an increased functional residual capacity (FRC) (Fig. 13-1). Slowing of expiratory flow and gas trapping behind prematurely closed airways is responsible for the increase in residual volume (RV). The advantage of increased RV and FRC in the patient with significant COPD is an enlarged airway diameter with greater radial support and elastic recoil for exhalation. The cost to the patient is greater work of breathing incurred at the higher lung volumes.

Radiographic abnormalities may be minimal even in the presence of advanced COPD. Hyperlucency of the lungs owing to arterial vascular deficiency in the lung periphery and hyperinflation (flattening of the diaphragm with loss of the normal domed appearance and a vertically oriented cardiac silhouette) suggest the diagnosis of emphysema. If bullae are also present, the diagnosis of emphysema is virtually certain, except only a small percentage of patients affected with emphysema have bullae. Chronic bronchitis is rarely recognized on the chest radiograph.

Arterial blood gases in the presence of advanced COPD are commonly used to categorize the patient as a "pink puffer" (PaO_2 usually greater than 60 mmHg and $PaCO_2$ normal) or a "blue bloater" (PaO_2 less than 60 mmHg, $PaCO_2$ greater than 45 mmHg, cor pulmonale) (Table 13-1). The pink puffer usually has severe emphysema, whereas chronic bronchitis is more likely to be the diagnosis in the blue bloater. The common denominator is chronic cigarette smoking, and many patients have features of both emphysema and chronic bronchitis. Pulmonary artery hypertension and ultimately cor pulmonale are likely developments in patients in whom arterial hypoxemia and hypercarbia develop. Conversely, the loss of pulmonary capillaries owing to destroyed alveoli characteristic of emphysema is manifested as decreased diffusing capacity for carbon monoxide. Since arterial hypoxemia is not prominent in these patients, pulmonary vasoconstriction is minimal,

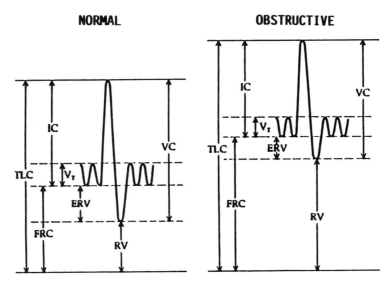

Fig. 13-1. Lung volumes in chronic obstructive pulmonary disease compared with normal values. In the presence of obstructive lung disease, the VC is normal to decreased, the RV and FRC are increased, the TLC is normal to increased, and the RV/TLC ratio is increased. TLC, total lung capacity; FRC, functional residual capacity; RV, residual volume; VC, vital capacity; V_T, tidal volume; IC, inspiratory capacity; ERV, expiratory reserve volume.

secondary erythropoiesis does not develop, and cor pulmonale is unlikely.

Treatment

The only useful treatment of COPD is cessation of smoking and chronic administration of supplemental oxygen to those patients with arterial hypoxemia. Supplemental inspired oxygen is usually recommended when the PaO_2 is less than 60 mmHg, the hematocrit is greater than 55%, or there is evidence of cor pulmonale. The goal is an arterial hemoglobin saturation with oxygen (SaO_2) greater than 90% (PaO_2 60 to 80 mmHg), which can usually be achieved with supplemental oxygen delivered at a rate of 2 $L \cdot min^{-1}$ through a nasal cannula. Ultimately, the rate of oxygen administration is titrated to the individual patient's needs according to arterial blood gas measurements. In some patients experiencing an acute exacerbation of COPD, the delivery of inspiratory positive airway pressure by means of a tight-fitting face mask may obviate the need for intubation of the trachea and mechanical ventilation of the lungs.[4]

Bronchodilators rarely improve expiratory airflow greater than 10%. In contrast to asthma, anticholinergic therapy seems more effective in the treatment of chronic bronchitis and emphysema. Intermittent broad-spectrum antibiotic therapy (ampicillin, cephalosporin, erythromycin, tetracycline) is indicated for acute episodes of clinical deterioration characterized by increased dyspnea, sputum production, and sputum purulence.[5] Annual vaccination against influenza may be beneficial in selected patients.

Drug-induced diuresis may be considered for patients with cor pulmonale and right ventricular failure. Attempts to produce pulmonary artery vasodilation with drugs such as hydralazine and nifedipine are not of any proven benefit and may produce systemic hypotension and decreased renal blood flow.[5] In fact, relief of arterial hypoxemia with supplemental inspired oxygen is more effective than any other drug therapy in decreasing pulmonary vascular resistance and in preventing excessive erythrocytosis with associated increases in blood viscosity. Physical training programs can increase the exercise capacity of patients with COPD despite the absence of a detectable effect on the FEV_1. Prompt deconditioning occurs when the exercise program is abandoned.

Preoperative Evaluation

Preoperative evaluation of patients with COPD should determine the severity of the disease and elucidate any reversible components such as bronchospasm or infection. Treatment of COPD preoperatively will decrease the incidence and severity of postoperative pulmonary complications.[6,7] The history, pulmonary function studies, and measurement of arterial blood gases and pH are useful in evaluating the severity and significance of COPD before elective surgery.[8]

Dyspnea, especially at rest, as well as cough and sputum production suggest the possible value of pulmonary function tests and arterial blood gas measurement. Measurement of the ratio of the FEV_1 to the FVC may be helpful in predicting the severity of COPD and the ability of cough to clear secretions from the airways. It is unusual for carbon dioxide retention to occur until the ratio of FEV_1/FVC is less than 0.35. The presence of a $PaCO_2$ greater than 50 mmHg preoperatively should caution against elective surgery, as the risk of postoperative respiratory failure may be increased.[9] Preoperative recognition that cor pulmonale is present and treatment with supplemental inspired oxygen in an attempt to decrease pulmonary vascular resistance may be useful. Drug-induced diuresis and positive inotropic drugs may improve cardiac function, although cor pulmonale is not due to intrinsic dysfunction of the heart.

Eradication of acute bacterial infection with appropriate antibiotics is important, particularly if infection is contributing to carbon dioxide retention. Production of purulent sputum suggests active infection and is an indication for treatment with antibiotics. The use of antibiotics, however, to sterilize the sputum is to be avoided, as this practice can lead to an overgrowth of resistant bacteria or fungi. Chest physiotherapy combined with adequate hydration of the patient is a useful approach for facilitating removal of secretions from the airways.

Steps to improve preoperative strength of skeletal muscles used for breathing include good nutrition and treatment of hypokalemia. Familiarization during the preoperative period with the respiratory therapy equipment and techniques to be used during the postoperative period is important for optimal patient cooperation after surgery. Preoperative use of intermittent positive-pressure breathing (IPPB) has not been shown to decrease the incidence of postoperative pulmonary complications.[10]

Pulmonary function studies and arterial blood gas measurements should be repeated after antibiotic and bronchodilator therapy. Ideally, prolonged expiratory flow rates and increased $PaCO_2$ values should return toward normal, and sputum production should be decreased. Wheezing should also be less or absent. Presumably, these changes reflect a beneficial response to therapy and place patients with COPD at decreased risk of the development of postoperative pulmonary complications.

Cessation of Cigarette Smoking

Postoperative pulmonary complications are increased in those who smoke cigarettes.[11] Therefore, cessation of cigarette smoking during the perioperative period would seem prudent, although sufficient time for reversible changes to occur may not always be possible. Nevertheless, the adverse effects of carbon monoxide on oxygen-carrying capacity and of nicotine on the cardiovascular system are short-lived. For example, the elimination half-time of carbon monoxide is about 4 to 6 hours, such that smoke-free intervals of 12 to 18 hours should

result in substantial decreases in carboxyhemoglobin levels, reversal of tissue hypoxia, and normalization of the oxyhemoglobin dissociation curve. Indeed, within 12 hours after cessation of smoking, the P_{50} increases from 22.9 mmHg to 26.4 mmHg, and plasma levels of carboxyhemoglobin decrease from 6.5% to 1.1%.[12] Increased plasma concentrations of carboxyhemoglobin can cause the pulse oximeter to overestimate the SaO_2. It seems unlikely, however, that the relatively low plasma carboxyhemoglobin concentrations associated with cigarette smoking will produce significant overestimations. Carbon monoxide may also have negative inotropic effects. Sympathomimetic effects of nicotine on the heart are transient, lasting only 20 to 30 minutes. Despite the favorable effects on plasma carboxyhemoglobin concentrations, short-term abstinence from cigarettes has not been proven to decrease the incidence of postoperative pulmonary complications.

Cigarette smoking causes mucous hypersecretion, impairment of mucociliary transport activity, and narrowing of the small airways. In contrast to favorable effects on short-term abstinence from smoking on levels of carboxyhemoglobin, improved ciliary and small airway function and decreased sputum production occur slowly over periods of weeks after cigarette smoking is stopped. Indeed, the incidence of postoperative pulmonary complications after coronary artery surgery decreases only when abstinence from cigarette smoking is greater than 8 weeks[13] (Fig. 13-2).

Cigarette smoke may interfere with normal immune responses and could exaggerate suppression of these responses associated with anesthesia and surgery. Return of normal immune function may require at least 6 weeks of abstinence from smoking.[9] Some components of cigarette smoke may stimulate hepatic enzymes, which could influence perioperative analgesic requirements. Again, a period of 6 to 8 weeks of abstinence is necessary before hepatic enzymatic activity returns to normal. Paradoxically, the incidence of deep vein thrombosis after myocardial infarction and lower abdominal surgery is dramatically reduced in smokers, as compared with nonsmokers.[14,15] This is even more surprising considering that chronic cigarette smoking is often associated with an elevated hematocrit and an associated increase in blood viscosity. Although evidence is not available, it is possible that deprived smokers are more restless and move about more than nonsmokers, thereby minimizing venous stasis.[15]

Logic supports a strong recommendation to patients to cease cigarette smoking before they undergo elective surgery. Even brief periods of abstinence will improve the oxygen-carrying capacity of the blood. Arguments that the time available is too brief to be useful are nonconvincing. It seems illogical to sacrifice the proven advantages of cessation of smoking for theoretical concerns that sputum may become more viscous and difficult to clear when patients abruptly stop smoking.

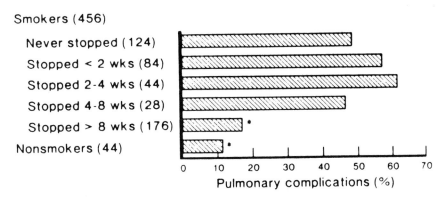

Fig. 13-2. Preoperative duration of smoking cessation and pulmonary complication rates after coronary artery bypass graft surgery. The incidence of postoperative complications in the patient population was decreased only when abstinence from cigarette smoking was greater than 8 weeks. (From Warner MA, Divertie MB, Tinker JH. Preoperative cessation of smoking and pulmonary complications in coronary artery bypass graft patients. Anesthesiology 1984;60:380–3, with permission.)

Management of Anesthesia

The preoperative presence of COPD does not dictate the use of specific drugs or techniques for the management of anesthesia. Regional anesthesia is most suited for operations that do not invade the peritoneum or surgical procedures performed on the extremities.[7,16] Lower abdominal surgery can be performed using regional techniques, but general anesthesia is equally acceptable.[16] General anesthesia is the usual choice for upper abdominal and intrathoracic operations.

More important than the drugs or techniques selected is the realization that these patients are susceptible to the development of acute respiratory failure during the postoperative period. Therefore, continued intubation of the trachea and mechanical ventilation of the lungs may be necessary, particularly after major surgery. Alternatively, postoperative analgesia with neuraxial opioids that permit pain-free breathing during the postoperative period may permit early tracheal extubation and also decrease systemic analgesic requirements with their associated depressant effects on ventilation and consciousness.

Regional Anesthesia

Regional anesthesia remains a useful selection in the patient with COPD only when sedative drugs are not needed. For example, it must be appreciated that such a patient may be extremely sensitive to the ventilatory depressant effects of sedative drugs used for systemic medication. If patient anxiety is substantial, however, small doses of a benzodiazepine, such as midazolam, in increments of 1 to 2 mg IV, can be administered with minimal likelihood of producing undesirable degrees of ventilatory depression. Elderly patients may be uniquely susceptible to depression of ventilation after being adminis-

tered drugs intended to allay anxiety. Regional anesthetic techniques that produce sensory anesthesia above T6 are not recommended, as this level can lead to a decrease in expiratory reserve volume. The most important adverse effect produced by this decrease is gas flow inadequate to produce an effective cough that leads to reduced clearance of secretions from airways.

General Anesthesia

General anesthesia in the patient with COPD is often provided with a volatile anesthetic, using humidification of the inspired gases and mechanical ventilation of the lungs. A volatile anesthetic is useful because of the patient's ability to eliminate it rapidly through the lungs and thereby minimize residual ventilatory depression during the early postoperative period. Furthermore, a volatile anesthetic may produce beneficial effects secondary to drug-induced bronchodilation. Halothane, enflurane, isoflurane, and desflurane would seem to be equally acceptable selections for administration to patients with COPD.

Nitrous oxide is frequently administered in combination with a volatile anesthetic. When using nitrous oxide, one should consider the potential passage of this gas into pulmonary bullae associated with pulmonary emphysema. Conceivably, nitrous oxide could lead to enlargement and rupture of bullae, resulting in development of a tension pneumothorax.[17] Another potential disadvantage of nitrous oxide is the limitation on the inspired concentration of oxygen introduced by the use of this anesthetic. In this regard, it is important to remember that inhaled anesthetics may attenuate regional hypoxic pulmonary vasoconstriction, leading to increased degrees of right-to-left intrapulmonary shunting. It is conceivable that increased inspired concentrations of oxygen might be necessary to offset the potential adverse consequences of this anesthetic-induced change. Nevertheless, not all studies confirm an anesthetic-induced inhibition of regional hypoxic pulmonary vasoconstriction.

Opioids, although acceptable, may be less useful than inhaled anesthetics for maintenance of anesthesia in the patient with COPD. For example, opioids can be associated with prolonged depression of ventilation, reflecting their slow rate of inactivation by the liver or elimination by the kidneys, or both. Even the duration of depression of ventilation produced by such drugs as thiopental and midazolam may be prolonged in patients with COPD, as compared with normal patients.[18] A high inspired concentration of nitrous oxide may be required to ensure amnesia when an opioid is used for the maintenance of anesthesia. In this regard, administration of an adequate inspired concentration of oxygen may be compromised by the need to administer high concentrations of nitrous oxide.

Humidification of inspired gases during anesthesia is important to prevent drying of secretions in the airways. It should be remembered that placement of a tube in the trachea results in bypass of nearly the entire airway humidification system. Furthermore, high flows of dry anesthetic gases will intensify the need for humidification of inhaled gases. Systemic dehydration due to inadequate fluid administration during the perioperative period can result in excessive drying of secretions in the airways, despite humidification of inhaled gases.

Controlled ventilation of the lungs is useful for optimizing arterial oxygenation in patients with COPD who are undergoing operations requiring general anesthesia.[9] A large tidal volume (10 to 15 ml·kg^{-1}) combined with a slow inspiratory flow rate minimizes the likelihood of turbulent airflow through airways and maintains optimal ventilation-to-perfusion matching. A slow breathing rate (6 to 10 breaths·min^{-1}) allows sufficient time for venous return to the heart and is less likely to be associated with undesirable degrees of hyperventilation, as reflected by the PaCO$_2$. Furthermore, a slow rate of breathing provides sufficient time for complete exhalation to occur, which is particularly important if air trapping is to be minimized in patients with COPD. The hazard of pulmonary barotrauma in the presence of pulmonary bullae should be appreciated, particularly if high positive airway pressures are required to provide adequate ventilation of the lungs. Overall, the intraoperative use of a large tidal volume and slow breathing rate is often as efficacious as positive end-expiratory pressure with respect to arterial oxygenation, without the detrimental cardiovascular effects produced by sustained positive airway pressure. If spontaneous ventilation is permitted during anesthesia, it should be appreciated that depression of ventilation produced by halothane, and presumably other volatile anesthetics, is greater in patients with COPD, as compared with patients with normal lungs.[9] Regardless of the method of ventilation of the lungs selected during surgery, objective adjustments in the mode of ventilation or in ventilator settings can be made only on the basis of (1) measurements of arterial blood gases and pH, (2) continuous monitoring of SaO$_2$ by pulse oximetry, and (3) continuous monitoring of the exhaled carbon dioxide concentration by capnography.

Postoperative Care

Postoperative care of the patient with COPD is intended to minimize the incidence and severity of pulmonary complications, recognizing that these patients are at increased risk of the development of acute respiratory failure. The likelihood of postoperative pulmonary complications is increased in the patient with COPD, associated with sputum production, decreased vital capacity, or decreased FEV$_1$, as documented preoperatively. The incidence of postoperative pulmonary complications is difficult to determine because there is no general agreement as to what represents pulmonary morbidity. Postoperatively, decreased lung volumes (vital capacity, FRC) interfere with the generation of an effective cough and clearance of secretions as well as contributing to the collapse of alveoli. Indeed, postoperative pulmonary complications are most often characterized by atelectasis, followed by pneumonia and decreases in the PaO$_2$ (Fig. 13-3).

As would be expected from changes in pulmonary mechanics, the frequency of postoperative pulmonary complications is greatest after upper abdominal surgery.[19] Vital capacity is decreased about 40% from the preoperative value on the day of upper abdominal surgery and does not return to near preoperative levels for 10 to 14 days. In contrast to vital capacity, the FRC does not decrease until about 16 hours after upper abdominal surgery, suggesting that altered breathing patterns during the postoperative period are responsible for this delayed change. Complete relief of postoperative pain, however, does not restore vital capacity or FRC, further suggesting that trauma from the surgical procedure itself, in addition to an altered breathing pattern, contributes to decreased lung volumes after upper abdominal surgery.[20]

Residual effects of anesthetic drugs may contribute to decreased PaO$_2$ and increased PaCO$_2$ during the immediate postoperative period. For example, anesthetics may impair regional hypoxic pulmonary vasoconstriction and blunt the ventilatory responses both to carbon dioxide and to hypoxemia[21] (Fig. 13-4). Decreases in the PaO$_2$ that persist beyond the early postoperative period most likely reflect mechanical abnormalities of the lungs, as reflected by a decrease in the FRC.[19] Upper abdominal surgery has the greatest effect on FRC and is followed by the largest decreases in the PaO$_2$. Arterial oxygenation associated with a decrease in the FRC may not return to preoperative levels until 10 to 14 days after surgery. With respect to abdominal operations, there is no evidence that the type of abdominal incision (transverse versus vertical) alters the incidence of postoperative pulmonary complications.[22]

The choice of drugs or techniques used to produce anesthesia does not seem to alter predictably the incidence of postoperative pulmonary infections.[19] Studies in patients with COPD

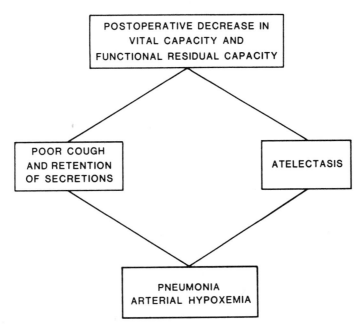

Fig. 13-3. Pathogenesis of postoperative pulmonary complications.

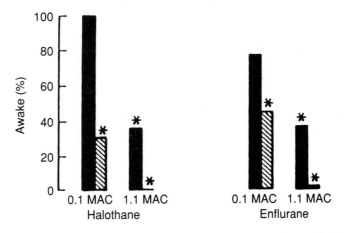

Fig. 13-4. Dose-related effects of halothane and enflurane on the ventilatory response to hypercarbia (solid bars) and hypoxemia (slash bars). *$P < 0.05$ compared with awake values. (Adapted from Knill RL, Clement JL. Variable effects of anesthetics on the ventilatory response to hypoxemia in man. Can Anaesth Soc J 1982;29:93–9, with permission.)

that suggest a higher incidence of postoperative acute respiratory failure in patients who receive general anesthesia might reflect the fact that the operative site dictated selection of general anesthesia rather than regional anesthesia. Whether there is a relationship between the duration of anesthesia and the incidence of postoperative pulmonary complications is not clear, although some reports describe a positive correlation between duration of surgery and the subsequent development of pulmonary complications.[19]

Prophylaxis Against Pulmonary Complications

Prophylaxis against development of postoperative pulmonary complications in the patient with COPD is based on restoring decreased lung volumes and facilitating the production of an effective cough so as to remove secretions from the airways. Identification of the FRC as the most important lung volume during the postoperative period provides a specific goal of therapy. Indeed, treatment regimens that maintain or improve the FRC can be expected to improve both pulmonary mechanics and gas exchange (Table 13-2). The large number of therapeutic approaches designed to provide prophylaxis against the development of postoperative pulmonary infections suggests that no single treatment is superior. Often, the best clinical response is obtained using a combination of treatments. Furthermore, factors such as site and duration of surgery contribute to postoperative morbidity in these patients.[23]

Mechanical Ventilation

Continued intubation of the trachea and mechanical ventilation of the lungs during the immediate postoperative period may be necessary in the patient with severe COPD undergoing major upper abdominal or intrathoracic surgery.[19] For example, it is likely that a patient with a preoperative ratio of FEV_1/FVC less than 0.5 will need continued mechanical support of ventilation of the lungs during the early postoperative period after upper abdominal or thoracic surgery.[6] The presence of a preoperative $PaCO_2$ above 50 mmHg is likely to be associated with the need for postoperative mechanical ventilation. It should be appreciated that the measured $PaCO_2$ during the preoperative period may be falsely low if the arterial puncture

Table 13-2.   Postoperative Treatments to Decrease the Incidence of Pulmonary Complications

Continued mechanical ventilation of the lungs
Analgesia with neuraxial opioids and/or nerve blocks
Transcutaneous electrical nerve stimulation
Chest physiotherapy
Voluntary deep breathing
Incentive spirometry

was painful and produced hyperventilation. An increased plasma concentration of bicarbonate in the presence of a low or normal $PaCO_2$ suggests that acute hyperventilation is masking chronic carbon dioxide retention. When the $PaCO_2$ has been chronically elevated, it is important not to correct the hypercarbia too quickly. This is because sudden decreases can result in alkalemia, since the kidneys cannot instantly excrete the excess bicarbonate. This alkalemia can be associated with cardiac dysrhythmias and central nervous system stimulation, culminating in seizures.

When continued mechanical ventilation of the lungs is necessary during the postoperative period, the inspired concentration of oxygen and ventilator settings should be adjusted to maintain the PaO_2 between 60 to 100 mmHg and the $PaCO_2$ in the range that maintains the arterial pH 7.35 to 7.45. Until these values can be confirmed during the postoperative period, it is customary to administer at least 50% oxygen, using a tidal volume of 10 to 15 $ml \cdot kg^{-1}$ and a breathing rate of 6 to 10 $breaths \cdot min^{-1}$. Institution of positive end-expiratory pressure may be necessary if the PaO_2 cannot be maintained above 60 mmHg breathing 50% oxygen. It must be remembered that positive end-expiratory pressure may be associated with increased air trapping in the patient with COPD. The decision to discontinue mechanical support of ventilation of the lungs and to extubate the trachea is based on the patient's clinical status and measurement to indices of pulmonary function (see Chapter 16).

Analgesia

Relief of postoperative pain with neuraxial opioids permits extubation of the trachea in patients who would otherwise require systemic opioids and sedatives to permit mechanical ventilation of the lungs and tolerance of the tracheal tube.[24] Sympathetic nervous system blockade and loss of proprioception as produced by a local anesthetic placed in the epidural space does not accompany neuraxial opioids. Therefore, early ambulation is possible in patients treated with neuraxial opioids. Ambulation serves to increase FRC and improve arterial oxygenation, presumably by improving ventilation-to-perfusion matching. Neuraxial opioids administered after intrathoracic and upper abdominal surgery help restore FEV_1 toward preoperative values.[24] Breakthrough pain may occur requiring treatment with an opioid administered intravenously. In this regard, patient-controlled analgesia may serve as a useful adjunct to neuraxial opioids. Sedation may accompany neuraxial opioid administration, and delayed depression of ventilation 6 to 12 hours after epidural opioid placement is a rare problem. Presumably, the opioid is absorbed into the subarachnoid space, ultimately diffusing into the area of the fourth cerebral ventricle, where it can depress the medullary ventilatory center. This delayed depression is more likely to occur in (1) elderly patients, (2) patients considered naive to opioids, (3) patients receiving systemic opioids as well, and (4) patients in whom a lipid soluble opioid is used.

Analgesia provided by injection of a local anesthetic into the epidural space provides intense analgesia, but associated sympathetic nervous system blockade and sensory nerve blockade can produce orthostatic hypotension and interfere with ambulation during the early postoperative period. Placement of local anesthetic through a catheter into the pleural space provides analgesia after thoracic or upper abdominal surgery.[25] Systemic absorption of the local anesthetic is substantial and a recognized disadvantage of this technique.

Direct intrathoracic block of intercostal nerves at the conclusion of thoracic surgery is an effective technique for providing analgesia. Occasional decreases in blood pressure and the production of total spinal anesthesia have been observed after direct intrathoracic block.[26,27] The mechanism for the decrease in blood pressure is not clear; total spinal anesthesia most likely reflects passage of the local anesthetic along nerve sheaths into the subarachnoid space. The picture resulting from a total spinal anesthetic is difficult to distinguish from unrecognized cerebral hypoxia, as patients are flaccid and apneic, and their pupils are widely dilated and unreactive to light, during the postoperative period. It is possible that bilateral intercostal nerve blocks could impair the ability to cough and effectively clear secretions from the airways.

Transcutaneous electrical nerve stimulation, as a method for providing postoperative analgesia and decreasing the incidence of pulmonary complications, is attractive because of its simplicity. This form of analgesia attenuates the decreased vital capacity and FRC that develops after upper abdominal surgery.[28]

Chest Physiotherapy

A combination of chest physiotherapy and postural drainage plus deep breathing exercises taught during the preoperative period have been reported to reduce the incidence of radiographic findings of atelectasis after performance of cholecystectomy.[19] Presumably, vibrations produced on the chest wall by physiotherapy result in displacement of mucus plugs from peripheral airways. Appropriate positioning facilitates elimination of loosened mucus from the airways. Close observation by the therapist is necessary to see how much sputum is produced and to ensure that the patient is taking deep breaths.

Ultrasonic nebulizers produce a dense aerosol of distilled water that is irritating to the larynx and upper trachea. This creates involuntary coughing and helps clear secretions from the airways. Patients must have an intact cough mechanism to benefit from this treatment. Furthermore, the aerosol produced can cause bronchoconstriction in patients with hyperreactive airways. Some patients are refractory and do not cough even during the first treatment, while others become resistant to the treatment.

Voluntary Deep Breathing

Voluntary deep breathing with slow inspiration and maintenance of inspiration at peak inflation for 3 to 5 seconds creates a large transpulmonary pressure gradient and facilitates reexpansion of collapsed alveoli and restoration of lung volumes.[29] This mode of treatment requires a motivated patient and relief of pain, to permit maximal inspiration.

Incentive Spirometry

Incentive spirometry is a type of voluntary deep breathing in which the patient is given inspired volumes as a goal to achieve. This treatment also emphasizes holding the inhaled volume to provide sustained inflation important for expanding collapsed alveoli. The major disadvantage is the need for patient cooperation to accomplish the treatment.

Expiratory maneuvers, such as inflating balloons, the use of blow bottles, or performing a FVC, are not recommended, since performance of these events causes patients to exhale to below the FRC. For example, to inflate a balloon, the patient must generate pleural pressures that exceed airway pressures, causing alveoli to become smaller or to collapse. Indeed, the only therapeutic benefit elicited by expiratory maneuvers is the deep breath that must be taken initially.

Intermittent Positive-Pressure Breathing

IPPB as a treatment to decrease the incidence of postoperative pulmonary complications is controversial. It is speculated that IPPB will expand collapsed alveoli, leading to a restoration of lung volumes with improvement in the elimination of secretions from the airways and an increase in the PaO_2. Nevertheless, studies of the efficacy of IPPB have been inconclusive.[10] Part of the failure of IPPB may be due to emphasis on peak pressures achieved at the apparatus used to deliver the treatment, rather than insisting on achievement of an optimal tidal volume. Particularly in an uncooperative patient, the peak pressure and tidal volume do not correlate. Ideally, the patient should inhale three to six times the predicted tidal volume, for the IPPB treatment to be effective. This inhaled tidal volume should be monitored with a spirometer placed on the exhalation valve.

BRONCHIECTASIS

Bronchiectasis is characterized by a localized and irreversible dilation of a bronchus caused by destructive inflammatory processes involving the bronchial walls. Untreated or inadequately treated bronchopneumonia may be the cause of bronchiectasis. Affected bronchi frequently contain purulent secretions, predictably leading to a productive cough with purulent sputum. In addition, affected bronchi often contain highly vascularized granulation tissue, which may be the source of recurrent hemoptysis. The most important consequence of bronchiectasis is increased susceptibility to recurrent or persistent bacterial infections, reflecting impaired ciliary activity and pooling of mucus in dilated airways. Clubbing of the digits is a common observation in affected patients. Pulmonary function changes are unpredictable, ranging from no change to alterations characteristic of COPD or restrictive lung disease. Computed tomography provides excellent images of bronchiectatic airways and can be used to confirm the presence and extent of the disease.

Treatment of bronchiectasis, regardless of its cause, is with oral administration of antibiotics and postural drainage. Hemoptysis is usually controlled by antibiotic therapy, although bronchial artery embolization may be useful in severe cases. Surgical resection may be considered if bronchiectasis is present distal to an obstructive bronchial lesion.

Management of anesthesia in patients with bronchiectasis should include consideration of the use of a double-lumen endobronchial tube, to prevent spillage of purulent sputum into normal areas of the lungs. Instrumentation of the nares may not be prudent, in view of the high incidence of chronic sinusitis in these patients.

CYSTIC FIBROSIS

Cystic fibrosis is the most common potentially lethal autosomal recessive disease among whites, affecting approximately 1 in every 2500 newborns.[30,31] The disease is due to mutation of a gene on chromosome 7 that functions as a chloride channel.[30] As a result of this mutation, there is a defect in exocrine gland secretion, leading to the production of chemically abnormal sweat and viscous mucus. Abnormal regulation of chloride transport across epithelial cell membranes is the fundamental biochemical defect in these patients.[31] Indeed, sweat chloride concentrations exceed 60 mEq·L^{-1} in nearly every patient with cystic fibrosis. It is likely that impaired tracheobronchial clearance of secretions leads to widespread mucous plugging of the airways with secondary bacterial infection and development of bronchiectasis. Obstruction to expiratory airflow is present in nearly all patients. Dyspnea and a chronic cough productive of purulent sputum are hallmarks of cystic fibrosis. Nasal polyposis and chronic sinusitis are frequent upper respiratory tract complications, whereas hemoptysis and pneumothorax are manifestations of lower respiratory tract complications of cystic fibrosis.

Extrapulmonary manifestations of cystic fibrosis include pancreatic insufficiency owing to mucous obstruction of pancreatic ducts. Hepatic cirrhosis and portal hypertension may develop with progressive obstruction of bile ducts by viscous mucus, gastrointestinal obstruction manifested as meconium ileus may be a manifestation of cystic fibrosis at birth. Infants with cystic fibrosis may be at increased risk of hemorrhage arising from vitamin K deficiency related to malabsorption of fat-soluble vitamins.

Management of Anesthesia

Management of anesthesia in the patient with cystic fibrosis invokes the same principles as outlined for the patient with COPD. Elective surgical procedures should be delayed until optimal pulmonary function can be ensured by control of bronchial infection and by facilitation of the removal of secretions from the airways. Vitamin K treatment may be necessary if hepatic function is poor or if absorption of fat-soluble vitamins from the gastrointestinal tract is impaired. Preoperative medication is probably unnecessary, as sedation may lead to undesirable ventilatory depression, and anticholinergic drugs may further increase the viscosity of secretions. Maintenance of anesthesia with a volatile anesthetic permits the use of a high inspired concentration of oxygen and can decrease airway resistance by decreasing the tone of bronchial smooth muscles. Furthermore, volatile anesthetics are helpful in reducing the responsiveness of hyperreactive airways characteristic of cystic fibrosis. Humidification of inspired gases is important for maintaining secretions in a less viscous state. Frequent suctioning of the trachea is often necessary during the operative period.

KARTAGENER SYNDROME

Kartagener syndrome consists of situs inversus, chronic sinusitis, and bronchiectasis.[32,33] This syndrome is inherited as an autosomal recessive trait and accounts for about 0.5% of cases of dextrocardia. These patients experience repeated pulmonary infections and chronic otitis media, beginning in childhood. A productive cough and hemoptysis are common, as bronchiectasis is the most prominent feature of the syndrome. Isolated dextrocardia is almost always associated with congenital heart disease.

The principal defect in patients with this syndrome is a generalized abnormality of ciliary function (primary ciliary dyskinesia) with failure to transport mucus toward the glottic opening at normal rates. This defect in ciliary motility extends to spermatozoa, and most males with this disease are sterile.

Management of Anesthesia

Preoperative preparation is directed at treating any active pulmonary infection and determining the presence of cor pulmonale. Drugs that depress ventilation or ciliary activity may be avoided in the preoperative medication. In the presence of dextrocardia, it is necessary to reverse the electrocardiogram leads, to permit accurate interpretation. Inversion of the great vessels is a reason to select the left internal jugular vein for cannulation so as to avoid the thoracic duct and to ensure more direct access to the right atrium. Uterine displacement in a parturient is logically to the right in these patients. Should use of a double-lumen endobronchial tube be considered, it is useful to appreciate the altered anatomy introduced by pulmonary inversion. For example, a left-sided tube is inserted, with the bronchial tube on the right. In view of the high incidence of sinusitis, the use of a nasopharyngeal airway is a questionable selection.

BRONCHIOLITIS OBLITERANS

Bronchiolitis obliterans as a cause of chronic airflow obstruction in adults may accompany viral pneumonia, collagen vascular disease (especially rheumatoid arthritis), and inhalation of nitrogen dioxide (silo-fillers' disease), or may be a sequela of graft-versus-host disease after bone marrow transplantation.[34] Nitrogen dioxide may accumulate above fresh silage and cause dyspnea, nonproductive cough, and noncardiogenic pulmonary edema. The treatment of bronchiolitis obliterans is usually ineffective, although corticosteroids may be administered in an attempt to suppress the inflammatory reaction involving the bronchioles. Symptomatic improvement may accompany the use of bronchodilators.

TRACHEAL STENOSIS

Tracheal stenosis is an extreme example of COPD that typically develops after mechanical ventilation of the lungs requiring prolonged translaryngeal intubation of the trachea or tracheostomy. Tracheal mucosal ischemia that may progress to the destruction of cartilaginous rings and subsequent circumferential constricting scar formation is minimized by the use of high residual volume cuffs on tracheal tubes, in an effort to avoid excessive pressure on the underlying mucosa. Infection and systemic hypotension may contribute to events that culminate in tracheal stenosis.

Tracheal stenosis becomes symptomatic when the lumen of the adult trachea is decreased to less than 5 mm. Symptoms may not develop until several weeks after extubation of the trachea. Dyspnea is prominent even at rest, as these patients must use accessory muscles of breathing during all phases of the breathing cycle. Ineffective cough is present, and stridor may be audible. A patient with tracheal stenosis breathes slowly because of an inability to increase the tidal volume despite additional muscular efforts. Peak flow rates are re-

duced during exhalation. A flow-volume loop is likely to display flattened exhaled and inhaled portions (see Fig. 14-2). Tomograms of the trachea demonstrate tracheal narrowing in these patients.

Tracheal dilation may be useful in some patients, but surgical resection of the stenotic tracheal segment with primary anastomosis is often required.[35] Anesthesia for tracheal resection may be complicated by total airway obstruction during surgical mobilization of the trachea. Initially, a translaryngeal tube is placed in the trachea. After surgical exposure, the distal normal trachea is opened and a sterile cuffed tube inserted and attached to the anesthetic breathing system. Maintenance of anesthesia with a volatile anesthetic is useful for ensuring a maximum inspired concentration of oxygen. In selected patients, high frequency ventilation may be useful. The addition of helium (50% to 75%) to the inspired gases decreases the density of these gases and may improve flow through the area of tracheal narrowing.

REFERENCES

1. Schmidt GA, Hall JB. Acute or chronic respiratory failure. Assessment and management of patients with COPD in the emergent setting. JAMA 1989;261:3444–53
2. Pierce JA. Antitrypsin and emphysema: Perspective and prospects. JAMA 1988;259:2890–6
3. Bruce RM, Cohen BH, Diamond EL, et al. Collaborative study to assess risk of lung disease in Pi MZ phenotype subjects. Am Rev Respir Dis 1984;130:386–92
4. Brochard L, Isabey D, Piquet J, et al. Reversal of acute exacerbations of chronic obstructive lung disease by inspiratory assistance with a face mask. N Engl J Med 1990;323:1523–30
5. Anthonisen NR, Manfreda J, Warren CPW, et al. Antibiotic therapy in exacerbations of chronic obstructive pulmonary disease. Ann Intern Med 1987;106:196–202
6. Stenin M, Cassara EL. Preoperative pulmonary evaluation and therapy for surgery patients. JAMA 1970;211:878–90
7. Tarhan S, Moffitt EA, Sessler AD, et al. Risk of anesthesia and surgery in patients with chronic bronchitis and chronic obstructive pulmonary disease. Surgery 1973;74:720–6
8. Nunn JF, Milledge JS, Chen D, Dore C. Respiratory criteria of fitness for surgery and anaesthesia. Anaesthesia 1988;43:543–51
9. Pietak S, Weenig CS, Hickey RF, Fairley HB. Anesthetic effects on ventilation in patients with chronic obstructive pulmonary disease. Anesthesiology 1975;42:160–6
10. Cottrell JE, Siker ES. Preoperative intermittent positive pressure breathing therapy in patients with chronic obstructive lung disease: Effect on postoperative pulmonary complications. Anesth Analg 1973;52:258–62
11. Pearce AC, Jones RM. Smoking and anesthesia: Preoperative abstinence and perioperative morbidity. Anesthesiology 1984;61:576–84
12. Kambam JR, Chen LH, Hyman SA. Effect of short-term smoking halt on carboxyhemoglobin levels and P_{50} values. Anesth Analg 1986;65:1186–8

13. Warner MA, Divertie MB, Tinker JH. Preoperative cessation of smoking and pulmonary complications in coronary artery bypass patients. Anesthesiology 1984;60:380–3

14. Clayton JK, Anderson JA, McNicol GP. Effect of cigarette smoking on subsequent postoperative thromboembolic disease in gynaecological patients. Br Med J 1978;2:402–3

15. Bucknall TE, Bowker T, Leaper DJ. Does increased movement protect smokers from postoperative deep vein thrombosis? Br Med J 1980;1:447–8

16. Ravin MB. Comparison of spinal and general anesthesia for lower abdominal surgery in patients with chronic obstructive pulmonary disease. Anesthesiology 1971;35:319–22

17. Gold MI, Joseph SI. Bilateral tension pneumothorax following induction of anesthesia in two patients with chronic obstructive airway disease. Anesthesiology 1973;38:93–6

18. Gross JB, Zebrowski ME, Carel WD, et al. Time course of ventilatory depression after thiopental and midazolam in normal subjects and in patients with chronic obstructive pulmonary disease. Anesthesiology 1983;58:540–4

19. Craig DB. Postoperative recovery of pulmonary function. Anesth Analg 1981;60:46–52

20. Spence AA, Smith G. Postoperative analgesia and lung function: A comparison of morphine with extradural block. Br J Anaesth 1971;43:144–8

21. Knill RL, Clement JL. Variable effects of anaesthetics on the ventilatory response to hypoxemia in man. Can Anaesth Soc J 1982;29:93–9

22. Williams CD, Brenowitz JB. Ventilatory patterns after vertical and transverse upper abdominal incisions. Am J Surg 1975;130:725–8

23. Kroenke K, Lawrence VA, Theroux JF, Tuley MR. Operative risk in patients with severe obstructive pulmonary disease. Arch Intern Med 1992;152:967–71

24. Shulman M, Sandler AN, Bradley JW, Young PS, Brebner J. Postthoracotomy pain and pulmonary function following epidural and systemic morphine. Anesthesiology 1984;61:569–75

25. Ferrante FM, Chan VWS, Arthur R, Rocco AG. Interpleural analgesia after thoracotomy. Anesth Analg 1991;72:105–9

26. Brodsky JB, James MBD. Hypotension from intraoperative intercostal nerve blocks. Reg Anaesth 1979;4:17–8

27. Benumof JL, Semenza J. Total spinal anesthesia following intrathoracic intercostal nerve blocks. Anesthesiology 1975;43:124–5

28. Ali J, Yaffe C, Serrette C. The effect of transcutaneous electric nerve stimulation on postoperative pain and pulmonary function. Surgery 1981;89:507–12

29. Bartlett RH, Gazzaniga AB, Geraghty TR. Respiratory maneuvers to prevent postoperative pulmonary complications. JAMA 1973;224:1017–21

30. Collins FS. Cystic fibrosis: Molecular biology and therapeutic implications. Science 1992;256:774–9

31. Fizzell RA, Rechkemmer G, Shoemaker RL. Altered regulation of airway epithelial cell chloride channels in cystic fibrosis. Science 1986;233:558–60

32. Woodring JH, Royer JM, McDonagh D. Kartagener's syndrome. JAMA 1982;247:2814–6

33. Ho AM-H, Friedland MJ. Kartagener's syndrome: Anesthetic considerations. Anesthesiology 1992;77:386–8

34. Ralph DD, Springmeyer SC, Sullivan KM, et al. Rapidly progressive airflow obstruction in marrow transplant recipients: Possible association between obliterative bronchiolitis and chronic graft-versus-host disease. Am Rev Respir Dis 1984;129:641–6

35. Boyan CP, Privitera PA. Resection of stenotic trachea: A case presentation. Anesth Analg 1976;55:191–4

14

Bronchial Asthma

Bronchial asthma is a disease defined by the presence of (1) increased responsiveness of the airways to various stimuli, (2) reversible expiratory airflow obstruction, and (3) chronic inflammatory changes in the submucosa of the airways. Airway hyperreactivity is present even in asymptomatic patients, and is characterized by the development of bronchoconstriction in response to stimuli (allergens, exercise) that have little or no impact on normal airways. The degree of airway hyperreactivity probably parallels the extent of inflammation of the airways and the numbers of eosinophils in the peripheral blood.[1] The reversibility of expiratory airflow obstruction is distinct from the more fixed airflow obstruction characteristic of patients with chronic obstructive pulmonary disease (chronic bronchitis, emphysema, bronchiectasis) (see Chapter 13). Nevertheless, this definition must remain flexible, as airway hyperreactivity and reversible airflow obstruction are not unique to asthma. For example, many patients with chronic obstructive pulmonary disease also demonstrate increased responsiveness of the airways, whereas some patients with asthma show the development of irreversible expiratory airflow obstruction. Current cigarette smokers, or ex-smokers, with chronic bronchitis who demonstrate episodic wheezing and dyspnea mimicking asthma may be diagnosed as having asthmatic bronchitis. These ambiguous situations reflect the deficiencies in the definition of a disease for which there is no pathognomonic feature or definitive diagnostic test. Nevertheless, a greater than 15% increase in expiratory airflow in response to bronchodilator therapy is supportive evidence when asthma is suspected on clinical grounds. Sputum examination in patients with asthma often contains eosinophils, whereas neutrophils are characteristic of bronchitis or pneumonia.

It is estimated that 3% to 6% of the United States population is affected by asthma.[2] In about two-thirds of these patients, symptoms develop before 5 years of age and males outnumber female patients by approximately 2:1. Complete remission of asthma is relatively common among children but not among adults. Severe attacks of asthma can end fatally and, in some instances, may reflect toxicity of drugs used to treat asthma.[3,4] In patients dying from asthma, there is often evidence of widespread occlusion of airways with mucous plugs.

PATHOGENESIS

The pathogenesis of asthma may reflect the explosive release of chemical mediators (histamine, leukotrienes, prostaglandins) from mast cells in atopic persons. An alternative hypothesis implicates abnormalities of the regulation of airway function by the autonomic nervous system. This hypothesis is supported by increased expiratory airflow obstruction in patients with asthma being treated with a nonselective beta antagonist (propranolol), suggesting the presence of an imbalance between excitatory (bronchoconstrictor) and inhibitory (bronchodilator) neural input. It is likely that chemical mediators released from mast cells interact with the autonomic nervous system. For example, some chemical mediators can stimulate airway irritant receptors to trigger reflex bronchoconstriction, while other mediators sensitize bronchial smooth muscle to the effects of acetylcholine. In addition, stimulation of muscarinic receptors facilitates mediator release from mast cells, providing another positive feedback loop for sustained inflammation and bronchoconstriction. Stimuli that trigger an acute asthma attack vary from person to person (Table 14-1). The chronic inflammatory response present in the airways also most likely plays an important role in the pathogenesis of asthma.

SIGNS AND SYMPTOMS

During periods of normal to near-normal pulmonary function, patients are likely to have no physical findings referable to their asthma. As expiratory airflow obstruction increases, a number of signs and symptoms may manifest and offer clues

Table 14-1. Precipitating Factors for Acute Asthma

Inhaled or ingested antigens
Strenuous exercise
Viral upper respiratory tract infections
Inhaled irritants
Reflux of gastric acid into the lower esophagus

as to the severity of the asthmatic attack. The classic clinical presentation of asthma is wheezing, cough, and dyspnea.

Wheezing, the most common finding during an acute asthma attack, is the term used to describe the expiratory sound produced by turbulent gas flow through narrowed airways. As obstruction becomes more severe, wheezing becomes more prominent and is audible during earlier phases of exhalation. Forced exhalation may demonstrate wheezing that was not audible during quiet breathing. The degree of airway obstruction may change abruptly; the absence of wheezing in severe cases may reflect a parallel absence of airflow to create an expiratory sound. In contrast to the random monophasic wheezes of asthma, the presence of a single monophasic wheeze that occurs repetitively with consistent timing suggests a focal airway obstruction, such as bronchus narrowed by an aspirated foreign body or by a neoplasm.

The characteristic cough of asthma ranges from nonproduc-

tive to the production of copious amounts of sputum that is typically mucoid and often very tenacious. Dyspnea associated with asthma tends to parallel the severity of expiratory airflow obstruction; in severe cases, patients may insist on breathing in a sitting position. Chest discomfort is a frequent accompaniment of dyspnea in patients with asthma and may mimic angina pectoris.

The forced exhaled volume in 1 second (FEV_1) and the maximum midexpiratory flow rate are direct reflections of the severity of expiratory airflow obstruction[5] (Fig. 14-1 and Table 14-2). These measurements provide objective data that can be used to assess the severity and monitor the course of an exacerbation of asthma. The typical patient with asthma who presents at the hospital for treatment of an asthmatic attack has an FEV_1 that is less than 35% of normal and a maximum midexpiratory flow rate that is 20% of normal or lower.[6] The flow-volume loop shows a characteristic downward scooping of the expiratory limb of the loop[5] (Fig. 14-2). A flow-volume loop in which the inhaled and exhaled portions of the loop are flat helps distinguish wheezing owing to upper airway obstruction (foreign body, tracheal stenosis, mediastinal mass) from asthma (see Fig. 15-2). In moderate to severe attacks of asthma, the functional residual capacity may increase as much as 1 to 2 L, whereas total lung capacity usually remains within the normal range. Diffusing capacity of the lungs for carbon monoxide is not decreased in patients with

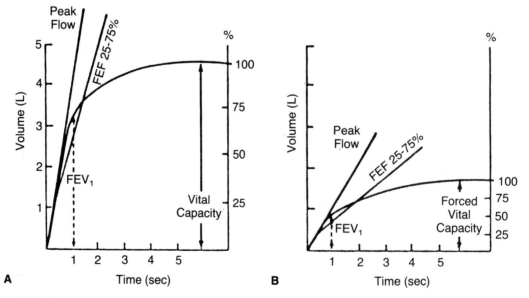

Fig. 14-1. Spirogram changes of (**A**) a normal subject and (**B**) a patient in bronchospasm. The forced exhaled volume in 1 second (FEV_1) is typically less than 80% of the vital capacity in the presence of obstructive airway disease. Peak flow and maximum midexpiratory flow rate (FEF 25–75%) are also decreased in these patients (Fig. B). (From Kingston HGG, Hirshman CA. Perioperative management of the patient with asthma. Anesth Analg 1984;63:844–55, with permission.)

Table 14-2.   Severity of Expiratory Airflow Obstruction

	FEV$_1$[a] (% Predicted)	FEF$_{25-75\%}$[a] (% Predicted)	PaO$_2$[b] (mmHg)	PaCO$_2$[b] (mmHg)
Mild (asymptomatic)	65–80	60–75	>60	<40
Moderate	50–64	45–59	>60	<45
Marked	35–49	30–44	<60	>50
Severe (status asthmaticus)	<35	<30	<60	>50

[a] See Fig. 14-1 for definitions.
[b] Values are estimates.
(Data from Kingston HGG, Hirshman CA. Perioperative management of the patient with asthma. Anesth Analg 1984;63:844–55.)

asthma. Residual abnormalities as detected by pulmonary function tests may persist for several days after an acute asthmatic attack despite the absence of symptoms.

Mild asthma is usually accompanied by a normal PaO$_2$ and PaCO$_2$. Tachypnea and hyperventilation observed during an acute asthmatic attack, therefore, do not reflect arterial hypoxemia but, rather, neural reflexes within the lungs. Indeed, hypocarbia and respiratory alkalosis are the most common arterial blood gas findings in the presence of asthma. As the severity of airflow obstruction increases, the associated ventilation-to-perfusion mismatching may result in a PaO$_2$ less than 60 mmHg while breathing room air. The PaCO$_2$ is likely to increase when the FEV$_1$ is less than 25% of the predicted value. Fatigue of the skeletal muscles necessary for breathing may contribute to the development of hypercarbia.

A chest radiograph may demonstrate hyperinflation of the lungs but is more useful in ruling out pneumonia or congestive heart failure that may be associated with asthma. The electrocardiogram may show evidence of acute right heart failure and ventricular irritability during an acute asthmatic attack.

CLASSIFICATION

Asthma is not a single disease; rather, it comprises a group of disorders with various etiologies.

Allergen-Induced Asthma

Allergen-induced (immunoglobulin E-mediated) asthma is the most common form of reversible expiratory airflow obstruction. Patients with allergen-induced asthma commonly have other atopic diseases, such as allergic rhinitis and allergic dermatitis. A genetic predisposition is suggested by the common presence of a family history of asthma. Peripheral blood eosinophilia and an increased plasma concentration of immunoglobulin E support the diagnosis of atopic disease. Presumably, inhalation of antigens evokes the release of vasoactive substances from mast cells, leading to bronchoconstriction, edema of the bronchial mucosa, and secretion of viscous mucus.

Exercise-Induced Asthma

Exercise-induced asthma is characterized by bronchoconstriction that accompanies increased physical activity. Patients typically describe exercise in cold weather as more likely to

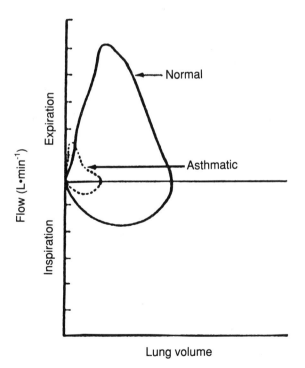

Fig. 14-2. A flow-volume curve of both a normal and an asthmatic individual. (From Kingston HGG, Hirshman CA. Perioperative management of the patient with asthma. Anesth Analg 1984;63:844–55, with permission.)

evoke symptoms. A decrease in airway wall temperature when exercise-induced increases in airflow expose the airways to cold and dry air may be responsible for symptoms in susceptible patients.[7]

Nocturnal Asthma

Nocturnal exacerbations of asthma may reflect sleep-related changes in airway tone, circadian variations in circulating catecholamine concentrations, gastroesophageal reflux related to the supine position, or retained airway secretions resulting from a depressed cough reflex. An increased incidence of asthmatic deaths after midnight and before morning may reflect this phenomenon.

Aspirin-Induced Asthma

An idiosyncratic reaction to ingestion of even small doses of aspirin characterized by bronchoconstriction, rhinorrhea, and conjunctional injection occurs in 10% to 20% of patients with asthma. Nasal polyps, although common among aspirin-sensitive asthmatics, are also often present in the absence of aspirin sensitivity. It is possible that aspirin triggers bronchoconstriction in susceptible patients by blocking the cyclo-oxygenase-mediated conversion of arachidonic acid to prostaglandins, thus diverting arachidonic acid toward the formation of leukotrienes, which are intense bronchoconstrictors. The high incidence of cross-reactivity with other nonsteroidal anti-inflammatory drugs favors a mechanism that involves cyclo-oxygenase inhibition.

An estimated 5% of patients with asthma are sensitive to bisulfite and metabisulfite, as used for preservatives and antioxidants by the food-processing industry. These substances are also present in a large number of medications, including some bronchodilator solutions. In view of this sensitivity to derivatives of benzoic acid, there is a theoretical but unsubstantiated concern for the use of ester local anesthetics in these patients.

Occupational Asthma

Persons with asthma may be susceptible to exacerbation of expiratory airflow obstruction when exposed to irritant dusts, animal dander, or fumes in the environment. These irritants produce bronchoconstriction by direct effects on the airway, and not by an immunologic mechanism.

Infectious Asthma

Infectious asthma is increased airway resistance caused by acute inflammatory disease of the bronchi. Causative agents can be viruses, bacteria, or *Mycoplasma* organisms. Eradica-

tion of the infectious organisms results in a rapid subsidence of bronchoconstriction.

TREATMENT

The traditional treatment of asthma has been directed at the prevention and control of bronchospasm with bronchodilator drugs. Recent recognition of the consistent presence of inflammation in the airways of patients with asthma emphasizes the importance of therapy designed to prevent and control bronchial inflammation as well.[8–10] In fact, bronchodilator therapy is unlikely to influence inflammatory changes in the airways but could mask underlying inflammation by relieving the symptoms and thus allowing greater exposure to allergens, irritants, and other environmental triggers. Regular use of anti-inflammatory drugs, preferably inhaled corticosteroids, is recommended as the first line of therapy for anything more than occasional mild asthma.[9] Bronchodilator therapy with beta-2 agonists is endorsed only for pretreatment of exercise-induced asthma and for the symptomatic relief of acute exacerbations of asthma when anti-inflammatory therapy is insufficient.[9]

Conceptually, treatment of asthma is with drugs classified as bronchodilators and anti-inflammatory drugs. Serial determinations of pulmonary function are useful for monitoring the response to treatment. When the FEV_1 returns to about 50% of normal, patients usually have minimal to no symptoms.

Bronchodilator Drugs

Bronchodilator drugs used in the treatment of asthma include beta-2 agonists, theophylline, and anticholinergics. Selective beta-2 agonists are the most effective bronchodilators available, emphasizing the exclusive presence of beta-2 receptors on human airway smooth muscle. Presumably, the activation of beta-2 receptors stimulates adenylate cyclase, with a subsequent increase in intracellular cyclic adenosine monophosphate.

Beta-2 Agonists

Albuterol is a selective beta-2 agonist that is becoming the standard for the bronchodilator treatment of asthma and other forms of bronchospasm. Using a metered dose inhaler, the drug is delivered by two to three deep inhalations spaced 1 to 5 minutes apart. This may be repeated every 4 to 6 hours. Inhaled beta-2 agonists are indicated for the short-term relief of bronchoconstriction and are the treatment of choice for acute exacerbations of asthma. These drugs are also useful for the prevention of bronchoconstriction precipitated by exercise. Administered orally, beta-2 agonists provide long-term effects. Side effects, although minimal with inhaled delivery, resemble sympathetic nervous system stimulation and include tachycardia, cardiac dysrhythmias, and intracellular shifts of potassium. The use of beta-2 agonists and an increased risk of death or near death from asthma has not been conclusively established as a drug-induced effect. A theoretical concern with chronic administration of a beta agonist is the development of tolerance as a result of a decreased number of beta receptors (down-regulation) in the cell membrane. Nevertheless, most evidence suggests that tolerance to the bronchodilator effects of a beta agonist does not occur.

Theophylline

Theophylline is a less effective bronchodilator than beta-2 agonists, although this drug historically was often considered the first choice of asthma therapy. There is now a trend toward introducing theophylline as a secondary bronchodilator drug, as it may have a synergistic effect with beta-2 agonists. Theophylline produces bronchodilation principally by virtue of its anti-adenosine effect, since only modest inhibition of phosphodiesterase activity is present at therapeutic plasma concentrations of 10 to 20 $mg \cdot L^{-1}$. Aminophylline (the ethylenediamine salt of theophylline) is the preparation used for intravenous administration, its bronchodilator activity is entirely due to theophylline. The starting intravenous dose of aminophylline is 5 $mg \cdot kg^{-1}$ administered over about 15 minutes, followed by 0.5 to 1 $mg \cdot kg^{-1} \cdot h^{-1}$ as a continuous infusion.

The principal disadvantages of theophylline are its ineffectiveness by the inhalation route and the risk of side effects, including cardiac dysrhythmias and seizures when the plasma concentration is greater than about 20 $mg \cdot L^{-1}$. The relatively narrow therapeutic range combined with highly variable clearance rates has necessitated measurement of plasma theophylline concentrations, especially when maximum bronchodilator effects are sought. Conditions contributing to increased plasma concentrations of theophylline are acute viral infections, congestive heart failure, and the administration of certain drugs such as cimetidine and hepatic disease. Acute but not chronic administration of aminophylline decreases the dose of epinephrine necessary to produce cardiac dysrhythmias in animals anesthetized with halothane.[11] Aminophylline readily crosses the placenta and may produce toxicity in infants of mothers receiving this drug during labor. This risk is accentuated in premature infants, as a greater proportion of aminophylline is converted to caffeine.[5] In animals, aminophylline partially antagonizes barbiturate anesthesia, presumably by its ability to antagonize adenosine receptors, which facilitates release of norepinephrine. A change in the depth of anesthesia may be an important consideration in asthmatic patients because of the risk of provoking bronchospasm in lightly anesthetized patients. This potential drug interaction may deserve consideration when determining the dose of drugs, especially barbiturates, to be administered for induction of anesthesia in patients being treated with aminophylline. Likewise, aminoph-

ylline-induced reductions in anesthetic requirements for a volatile anesthetic could result in unexpected light levels of anesthesia. Nevertheless, halothane MAC is not altered in animals acutely treated with aminophylline.[12]

Anticholinergics

By blocking muscarinic receptors in airway smooth muscle, anticholinergics inhibit vagal cholinergic tone, resulting in bronchodilation. Ipratroprium is a synthetic derivative of atropine administered by metered dose inhaler. This drug is most useful in the treatment of bronchoconstriction caused by chronic bronchitis and pulmonary emphysema or bronchospasm due to a beta antagonist. In patients with asthma, ipratropium is less effective than a beta-2 agonist but in selected patients may be ueful as combination therapy. Compared with the prompt bronchodilator effect produced by beta-2 agonists, the onset of peak bronchodilator effect produced by ipratropium is 15 to 30 minutes. The quaternary structure of ipratropium limits its systemic absorption and production of anticholinergic side effects.

Anti-inflammatory Drugs

Since chronic inflammation appears to be central to the pathogenesis of asthma, it is logical to use drugs such as corticosteroids and cromolyn to suppress inflammation.[8] These drugs are regarded as prophylactic therapy, since they neither provide rapid bronchodilator effects nor evoke prompt relief of symptoms.

Corticosteroids

Corticosteroids delivered by metered dose inhaler should be the first line of therapy for chronic asthma.[8] Inhaled corticosteroids such as beclomethasone and triamcinolone decrease airway reactivity but tend to be underutilized because patients are accustomed to rapid relief provided by an inhaled beta-2 agonist. The delivery of corticosteroids by inhalation does not produce systemic effects or adrenal suppression, although oropharyngeal candidiasis, glossitis, and dysphonia may occur. Oral administration of corticosteroids (prednisone, prednisolone, methylprednisolone) is necessary in a few patients, to control symptoms. In this patient group, the well-known side effects of corticosteroids (osteoporosis, hypertension, diabetes, myopathy, adrenal suppression) are possible, especially when the daily dose exceeds 10 mg. Methotrexate may decrease the dose of corticosteroids needed for control of asthma.[13]

Cromolyn

Cromolyn administered by metered dose inhaler is the anti-inflammatory drug of first choice in children, whereas corticosteroids are preferred in adults. Nevertheless, adults may also respond to cromolyn. The mechanism of action of cromolyn is unknown but probably includes inhibition of release of chemical mediators from mast cells, macrophages, and eosinophils by virtue of a membrane-stabilizing effect. Inhibition of sensory airway nerves may explain the occasional dramatic effectiveness of cromolyn in suppressing coughing associated with asthma. Side effects of cromolyn are rare. Cromolyn is used as prophylaxis against bronchoconstriction because it is ineffective once bronchospasm is present. Typically, the drug is delivered by inhalation 10 to 20 minutes before an anticipated provoking stimulus, such as exercise.

Emergency Treatment

Emergency treatment of asthma (status asthmaticus) includes repetitive administration of a beta-2 agonist by inhalation or subcutaneous injection. Corticosteroids are a fundamental component of the treatment of status asthmaticus, having been conclusively shown to shorten hospitalization and decrease morbidity.[14] Two commonly employed regimens are (1) cortisol (2 mg·kg^{-1} IV, followed by 0.5 mg·kg^{-1}·h^{-1}); and (2) methylprednisolone (60 to 125 mg IV every 6 hours). In selected patients, oral administration of methylprednisolone is as effective as the intravenous route.[15] Patients whose FEV_1 or peak expiratory flow rate is decreased to 25% of normal or less are at risk of the development of hypercarbia. The presence of hypercarbia ($PaCO_2$ greater than 50 mmHg) despite aggressive bronchodilator and anti-inflammatory therapy may require tracheal intubation and mechanical support of ventilation. When patients are resistant to therapy, it is likely that airflow obstruction is caused predominantly by edema and inflammation of the airways and by intraluminal secretions. Indeed, patients experiencing near-fatal exacerbations of asthma are at risk of asphyxia, owing to the presence of mucus plugged airways.[16] In this regard, undertreatment rather than overtreatment may contribute to an increase in mortality from asthma.

Under rare circumstances in which life-threatening status asthmaticus persists despite aggressive pharmacologic therapy, it may be acceptable to consider general anesthesia in an attempt to produce bronchodilation. In this regard, halothane, enflurane, and isoflurane have been described as effective therapy in selected patients.[17,18] Clearly, this hazardous approach is reserved for the desperately ill patient and can only be considered when the potential benefits are judged to merit the risks.

MANAGEMENT OF ANESTHESIA

Management of anesthesia for the patient with asthma requires an understanding of the pathophysiology of the disease and the pharmacology of the drugs being used for treatment.[5]

Preoperative Evaluation

The preoperative absence of wheezing during auscultation of the chest or complaints of dyspnea suggest that the patient is not experiencing an acute exacerbation of asthma. The observation that the blood eosinophil count may parallel the degree of airway inflammation and airway hyperreactivity provides an indirect preoperative assessment of the status of the disease. Performance of pulmonary function studies (especially FEV_1) before and after bronchodilator therapy may be indicated in the patient with known bronchial asthma who is scheduled for a major elective operation. Chest physiotherapy, systemic hydration, appropriate antibiotics, and bronchodilator therapy during the preoperative period will often improve reversible components of asthma, as evidenced by pulmonary function tests. Comparison of a chest radiograph with a previous radiograph is helpful in evaluating the status of the disease process. Measurement of arterial blood gases before undertaking elective surgery is indicated if there are any questions about the adequacy of ventilation or arterial oxygenation.

Preanesthetic Medication

No studies confirm a preferred drug or combination of drugs for use as preanesthetic medication in patients with asthma. In addition, there is no evidence that opioids, in doses used for preanesthetic medication, produce direct or reflex bronchoconstriction or stimulate release of vasoactive substances from mast cells. A more important consideration is the possible ventilatory depressant effects of opioids. The use of anticholinergic drugs should be individualized, remembering that these drugs can increase the viscosity of secretions, making it difficult to remove them from the airway. Furthermore, achievement of a decrease in airway resistance by inhibition of postganglionic cholinergic receptors is unlikely with intramuscular doses of anticholinergic drugs used for preanesthetic mediation. The use of an H-2 receptor antagonist, such as cimetidine, in patients with asthma is questionable. This concern is based on evidence that histamine mediates bronchoconstriction by H-1 receptors, during which bronchodilation is mediated by H-2 receptors.[19] Conceivably, antagonism of H-2 receptors by antagonist drugs would unmask histamine-mediated H-1 receptor bronchoconstriction, leading to acute increases in airway resistance in patients with asthma.

Bronchodilator drugs used in the treatment of asthma should be continued to the time of induction of anesthesia. For example, cromolyn does not interact adversely with drugs used during anesthesia and thus can be safely continued during the immediate preoperative period. Supplementation with exogenous corticosteroids may be indicated before major surgery, if adrenal cortex suppression by drugs used to treat asthma is a possibility.

Induction and Maintenance of Anesthesia

The goal during induction and maintenance of anesthesia in the patient with asthma is to depress airway reflexes with anesthetic drugs so as to avoid bronchoconstriction of the hyperreactive airways in response to mechanical stimulation. Indeed, stimuli that do not cause problems in the absence of asthma can precipitate life-threatening bronchoconstriction in the patient with this disease.

Regional anesthesia is an attractive choice when the site of operation is superficial or on the extremities or when avoidance of intubation of the trachea is considered desirable. In most patients, however, a general anesthetic will be necessary. Induction of anesthesia with a barbiturate, benzodiazepine, propofol, or etomidate is acceptable, but it must be remembered that these drugs are unlikely to depress airway reflexes adequately, increasing the likelihood of bronchospasm if the trachea is intubated at this time. Ketamine, presumably reflecting its sympathomimetic effects, has been shown to be superior to thiopental in preventing increased airway resistance[20] (Fig. 14-3). Therefore, ketamine (1 to 2 mg·kg^{-1} IV), may be a useful drug for induction of anesthesia. Increased secretions associated with administration of ketamine may detract from the use of this drug in the patient with asthma.

After unconsciousness is produced by intravenous injection of drugs, the lungs are often ventilated with a gas mixture containing a volatile anesthetic. The goal is to establish a depth of anesthesia that will depress hyperreactive airway reflexes sufficiently to permit intubation of the trachea without precipitating bronchospasm. Indeed, the one factor shown to precipitate bronchospasm in patients with asthma is the introduction of a tube into the trachea without previously establishing a sufficient depth of anesthesia to suppress airway reflexes.[21] Halothane is most often selected because of its ability to produce bronchodilation of the constricted airway. Nevertheless, halothane is not an ideal drug, since it sensitizes the myocardium to the cardiac dysrhythmic effects of beta stimulation as produced by beta agonist drugs and aminophylline. Cardiac dysrhythmias during administration of aminophylline would seem less likely with other volatile anesthetics, which do not sensitize the myocardium. Consistent with this speculation is the report that induction of enflurance anesthesia in animals treated with aminophylline does not cause cardiac dysrhythmias.[22] It is likely that enflurane and isoflurane are equally acceptable alternatives to halothane for administration to patients with increased airway resistance caused by asthma. Indeed, both enflurane and isoflurane have been observed to produce beneficial airway effects in patients with status asthmaticus. Furthermore, enflurane and isoflurane are as effective as halothane in reversing allergen-induced bronchospasm in a dog model[23] (Fig. 14-4).

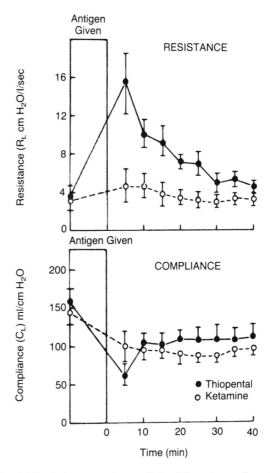

Fig. 14-3. Pulmonary resistance (R_L) and dynamic compliance before and after Ascaris antigen aerosal challenge during thiopental and ketamine anesthesia in dogs. (From Hirshman CA, Downes H, Farbood A, Bergman NA. Ketamine block of bronchospasm in experimental canine asthma. Br J Anaesth 1979;51:713–8, with permission.)

The rate of intravenous infusion of aminophylline may have to be decreased during the intraoperative period because of decreased inactivation of aminophylline by the liver owing to decreased hepatic blood flow. Indeed, a continuous intravenous infusion rate associated with a therapeutic plasma concentration of aminophylline in the awake patient may result in a toxic plasma concentration when hepatic blood flow is decreased during anesthesia. Therefore, it may be prudent to decrease the infusion rate by approximately 30%, to offset a similar decrease in hepatic blood flow as is likely during anesthesia and surgical stimulation, particularly during upper abdominal operations.

An alternative to the administration of a volatile anesthetic to suppress airway reflexes before intubation of the trachea

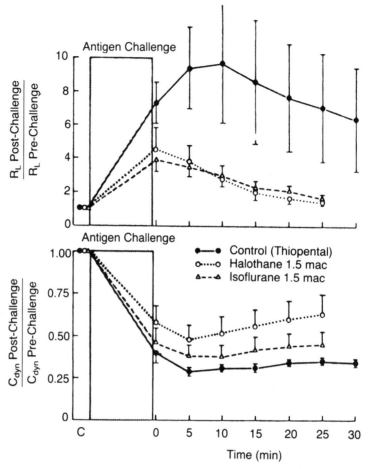

Fig. 14-4. Pulmonary resistance (R_L) and dynamic compliance (C_{dyn}) in dogs before and after Ascaris antigen challenge during thiopental, halothane, or isoflurane anesthesia in dogs. Halothane and isoflurane are equally effective in attenuating antigen-induced increases in R_L. (From Hirshman CA, Edelstein G, Peetz S, et al. Mechanisms of action of inhalation anesthesia on airways. Anesthesiology 1982;56:107–11, with permission.)

may be the intravenous injection of lidocaine.[24] Lidocaine (1.5 mg·kg^{-1} IV) given about 1 minute before intubation of the trachea, is useful in preventing reflex bronchoconstriction provoked by instrumentation of the airway. Furthermore, the continuous administration of lidocaine (1 to 3 mg·kg^{-1}·h^{-1} IV) can be used in place of a volatile anesthetic in patients with limited cardiac reserve, in whom deep anesthesia may be needed to suppress the reflex activity of hyperreactive airways. The decision to administer intratracheal lidocaine just before the placement of a tube in the trachea must consider both the beneficial effect of topical anesthesia and the possible initiation of bronchospasm by placement of the solution into hyperreactive airways. Although specific data are not available to support a recommendation for use of intratracheal lidocaine in the patient with asthma, clinical experience suggests that,

in the presence of adequate anesthesia, bronchospasm does not follow the intratracheal administration of lidocaine.

Skeletal muscle relaxation during maintenance of anesthesia is often provided with a nondepolarizing muscle relaxant. In this regard, drugs with limited ability to evoke the release of histamine are likely to be selected. For example, severe bronchospasm following the administration of atracurium has been reported in patients with asthma.[25] Nevertheless, in large comparative studies, the incidence of bronchospasm following administration of atracurium or other nondepolarizing muscle relaxants is not different.[26] Although histamine release has been attributed to succinylcholine, there is no evidence that this drug is associated with the appearance of increased airway resistance when administered to a patient with asthma.

Theoretically, antagonism of nondepolarizing neuromuscular blockade with an anticholinesterase drug could precipitate bronchospasm secondary to stimulation of postganglionic cholinergic receptors in airway smooth muscle. That bronchospasm does not predictably occur after the administration of an anticholinesterase drug may reflect the protective effects provided by the simultaneous administration of an anticholinergic drug.

Intraoperatively, the desirable level of arterial oxygenation and ventilation are best provided by mechanical ventilation of the lungs. A slow inspiratory flow rate provides optimal distribution of ventilation relative to perfusion. Sufficient time for passive exhalation to occur is necessary to prevent air trapping in the presence of expiratory airflow obstruction characteristic of asthma. In this respect, positive end-expiratory pressure may not be ideal because of the likelihood that it will impair adequate exhalation in the presence of narrowed airways. Humidification and warming of inspired gases would seem logical, particularly in the patient with a history of exercise-induced asthma, in whom bronchospasm is presumed to be due to transmucosal loss of heat. Nevertheless, it must be appreciated that particulate humidification, as produced by ultrasonic nebulizers and pneumatic aerosols, can produce bronchospasm. Liberal intravenous administration of crystalloid solutions during the perioperative period is important in maintaining adequate hydration and ensuring the presence of less viscous secretions, which can be expelled more easily from the airways.

At the conclusion of anesthesia for elective surgery, it is prudent to remove the tube from the trachea while anesthesia is still sufficient to suppress hyperreactive airway reflexes. When it is deemed unwise to remove the tube from the trachea until the patient is awake, it would seem reasonable to attempt to minimize the likelihood of airway stimulation due to the tracheal tube. Therefore, continuous intravenous infusion of lidocaine (1 to 3 $mg \cdot kg^{-1} \cdot h^{-1}$ IV) may be useful.

Intraoperative Bronchospasm

Bronchospasm that occurs intraoperatively is usually due to factors other than an acute asthmatic attack (Table 14-3). Indeed, treatment with drugs appropriate for the management of bronchospasm caused by asthma should not be instituted until more likely causes for wheezing, such as mechanical obstruction to the breathing circuit and the patient's airway, are considered. In this regard, fiberoptic bronchoscopy may be useful to rule out mechanical obstructive causes of bronchospasm. Bronchospasm that occurs intraoperatively in the presence of a patent anesthetic delivery system and upper airway, but in the absence of an acute exacerbation of asthma, is most logically treated by optimizing the depth of anesthesia with a volatile anesthetic or instituting skeletal muscle paralysis. Bronchospasm owing to asthma may respond to deepening of anesthesia with a volatile anesthetic, but not to skeletal

Table 14-3. Differential Diagnosis of Intraoperative Bronchospasm and Wheezing

Mechanical Obstruction of Tracheal Tube
  Kinking
  Secretions
  Overinflation of cuff

Inadequate Depth of Anesthesia
  Active expiratory efforts
  Decreased functional residual capacity

Endobronchial Intubation

Pulmonary Aspiration

Pulmonary Edema

Pulmonary Embolus

Pneumothorax

Acute Asthmatic Attack

muscle paralysis produced by administration of a muscle relaxant. Should bronchospasm due to asthma persist despite adjustment of the depth of anesthesia, the institution of beta agonist therapy should be considered. In this regard, albuterol may be delivered into the patient's airway by attaching the metered dose inhaler to the anesthesia delivery system by a T connector. The efficiency of delivery can be improved using a small-bore catheter placed near the distal end of the tracheal tube.[27] Each actuation of the metered dose inhaler delivers about 90 μg of albuterol. The effect of albuterol in attenuating bronchospasm is additive to the effects of a volatile anesthetic.[28] When bronchospasm persists despite beta-2 agonist therapy, the addition of aminophylline and corticosteroids to the treatment regimen may be indicated (see the sections, Theophylline and Corticosteroids).

REFERENCES

1. Taylor KJ, Luksza AR. Peripheral blood eosinophil counts and bronchial responsiveness. Thorax 1987;42:452–6
2. Weiss KB, Gergen PJ, Hodgson TA. An economic evaluation of asthma in the United States. N Engl J Med 1992;326:862–6
3. Benatar SR. Fatal asthma. N Engl J Med 1986;314:423–6
4. Drislane FW, Samuels MA, Kozakewich H, et al. Myocardial contraction band lesions in patients with fatal asthma: Possible neurocardiologic mechanisms. Am Rev Respir Dis 1987;135:498–506
5. Kingston HGG, Hirshman CA. Perioperative management of the patient with asthma. Anesth Analg 1984;63:844–55
6. McFadden ER. Clinical physiologic correlates in asthma. J Allergy Clin Immunol 1986;77:1–6
7. Deal EC, McFadden ER, Ingram RH, et al. Airway responsive-

ness to cold air and hyperpnea in normal subjects and in those with hay fever and asthma. Am Rev Respir Dis 1980;121:621–8

8. Barnes PJ. A new approach to the treatment of asthma. N Engl J Med 1989;321:1517–27

9. Randall T. International consensus report urges sweeping reform in asthma treatment. JAMA 1992;267:2153–4

10. Larsen GL. Asthma in children. N Engl J Med 1992;326:1540–5

11. Prokocimer PG, Nichols F, Gaga DM, Maze M. Epinephrine arrhythmogenicity is enhanced by acute, but not by chronic aminophylline administration during halothane anesthesia in dogs. Anesthesiology 1986;65:13–8

12. Nichols EA, Louie GL, Prokocimer PG, Maze M. Halothane anesthetic requirements are not affected by aminophylline treatment in rats and dogs. Anesthesiology 1986;65:637–41

13. Mullarkey MF, Blumenstine BA, Andrade WP, et al. Methotrexate in the treatment of corticosteroid-dependent asthma: A double blind crossover study. N Engl J Med 1988;318:603–8

14. Fanta CH, Rossing TH, McFadden ER. Glucocorticoids in acute asthma. A critical controlled trial. Am J Med 1983;74:845–51

15. Ratto D, Alfaro C, Sipsey J, Glovsky MM, Sharma OP. Are intravenous corticosteroids required in status asthmaticus? JAMA 1988;260:527–9

16. Molfino NA, Nannine LJ, Martelli AN, Slutsky AS. Respiratory arrest in near-fatal asthma. N Engl J Med 1991;324:285–8

17. Parnass SM, Feld JM, Chamberlin WH, Segil LJ. Status asthmaticus treated with isoflurane and enflurane. Anesth Analg 1987; 66:193–5

18. Schwartz SH. Treatment of status asthmaticus with halothane. JAMA 1984;151:2688–9

19. Nathan R, Segall N, Schocket A. A comparison of the actions of H-1 and H-2 antihistamine on histamine-induced bronchoconstriction and cutaneous wheal response in asthmatic patients. J Allergy Clin Immunol 1981;67:171–7

20. Hirshman CA, Downes H, Farbood A, Bergman NA. Ketamine block of bronchospasm in experimental canine asthma. Br J Anaesth 1979;51:713–8

21. Shnider SM, Papper EM. Anesthesia for the asthmatic patient. Anesthesiology 1961;22:886–92

22. Stirt JA, Berger JM, Roe SD, et al. Safety of enflurane following administration of aminophylline in experimental animals. Anesth Analg 1981;60:871–3

23. Hirshman CA, Edelstein G, Peetz S, et al. Mechanism of action of inhalational anesthesia on airways. Anesthesiology 1982;56: 107–11

24. Downes H, Gerber N, Hirshman CA. I.V. lidocaine in reflex and allergic bronchoconstriction. Br J Anaesth 1980;52:873–8

25. Oh TE, Horton JM. Adverse reactions to atracurium. Br J Anaesth 1989;62:467–70

26. Lawson DH, Paice GM, Glavin RJ, et al. Atracurium—a post-marketing surveillence study: UK. Study and discussion. Br J Anaesth 1989;62:596–600

27. Taylor RH, Lerman J. High-efficiency delivery of salbutamol with a metered-dose inhaler in narrow tracheal tubes and catheters. Anesthesiology 1991;74:360–3

28. Tobias JD, Hirshman CA. Attenuation of histamine-induced airway constriction by albuterol during halothane anesthesia. Anesthesiology 1990;72:105–110

15

Restrictive Lung Disease

Restrictive lung disease is characterized by a decrease in total lung capacity, most often reflecting an intrinsic disease process that alters the elastic properties of the lung, causing the lungs to stiffen (Fig. 15-1 and Table 15-1). Intrinsic restrictive lung disease may be categorized as pulmonary edema and chronic intrinsic restrictive lung disease. In pulmonary edema, water and solutes accumulate in the interstitial tissues, causing the lungs to become stiff. In chronic restrictive lung disease, changes in the elastic tissue elements of the lung cause the lungs to stiffen. Destruction of pulmonary vasculature by some disease processes may result in pulmonary hypertension, ultimately leading to cor pulmonale. In a small group of patients, chronic extrinsic restrictive lung disease develops, in which processes affecting the thoracic cage, pleura, or abdominal contents decrease total lung capacity. Disorders of the pleura and mediastinum may also contribute to restrictive lung disease.

The classic evidence of restrictive lung disease is decreased vital capacity (normal greater than 70 ml·kg^{-1}); in these cases, expiratory flow rates, in contrast to obstructive airway disease, are normal. Also, in contrast to the patient with obstructive lung disease, the ratio of the forced exhaled volume in 1 second to the forced vital capacity (FEV_1/FVC) is preserved in the presence of restrictive lung disease. Patients with restrictive lung disease complain of dyspnea, reflecting the increased work of breathing necessary to expand the poorly compliant lungs. A rapid shallow pattern of breathing is characteristic, acting as a compensatory response that minimizes the work of breathing in the presence of decreased lung compliance. A decrease in the $PaCO_2$ reflects hyperventilation produced by the rapid, shallow pattern of breathing. Indeed, the $PaCO_2$ is usually maintained at a decreased to normal value, until restrictive lung disease is far advanced.

Changes in the elastic properties of the lungs can be quantitated by determining lung compliance, defined as the change in lung volume per unit change in pressure. Compliance is 0.1 to 0.2 L·cm H_2O^{-1} in normal persons, but it may be as low as 0.02 L·cm H_2O^{-1} in patients with restrictive lung disease. Pressure-volume curves are shifted downward and to the right

in patients with increased lung stiffness[1] (Fig. 15-2). The diffusing capacity of the lungs for carbon monoxide is often decreased, attributable most often to an uneven ventilation-to-perfusion distribution, rather than to impaired movement of gases across the alveolar capillary membrane.

Table 15-1. Causes of Restrictive Lung Disease

Pulmonary Edema (Acute Intrinsic Restrictive Lung Disease)
  Adult respiratory distress syndrome
  Aspiration
  Neurogenic
  Opioid overdose
  High altitude
  Negative pressure
  Congestive heart failure

Chronic Intrinsic Restrictive Lung Disease
  Sarcoidosis
  Hypersensitive pneumonitis
  Eosinophilic granuloma
  Alveolar proteinosis
  Drug-induced pulmonary fibrosis

Chronic Extrinsic Restrictive Lung Disease
  Obesity
  Ascites
  Pregnancy
  Kyphoscoliosis
  Ankylosing spondylitis
  Deformities of the sternum
  Neuromuscular disorders
    Spinal cord transection
    Guillain-Barré syndrome
    Myasthenia gravis
    Eaton-Lambert syndrome
    Muscular dystrophies
    Pleural fibrosis
    Flail chest

Disorders of the Pleura and Mediastinum
  Pleural effusion
  Pneumothorax
  Mediastinal mass
  Pneumomediastinum

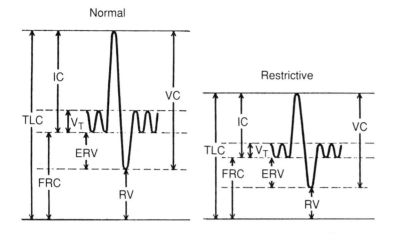

Normal

Restrictive

Fig. 15-1. Lung volumes in restrictive lung disease compared with normal values. In the presence of restrictive lung disease, VC, RV, FRC, and TLC are decreased. TLC, total lung capacity; FRC, functional residual capacity; RV, residual volume; VC, vital capacity; V_T, tidal volume; IC, inspiratory capacity; ERV, expiratory reserve volume.

PULMONARY EDEMA

Pulmonary edema as a result of leakage of intravascular fluid into the interstitium of the lungs and into the alveoli is the most common cause of acute intrinsic restrictive lung disease. Loss of intravascular fluid into the lungs can reflect increased pulmonary capillary endothelial permeability or increased pulmonary capillary pressure (congestive heart failure).

Adult Respiratory Distress Syndome

Adult respiratory distress syndrome (ARDS) is characterized by abnormal permeability of pulmonary capillary endothelium, leading to leakage of fluid containing high concentrations of protein into the pulmonary parenchyma and alveoli.[2] Along with the pulmonary edema, there are associated decreases in functional residual capacity and lung compliance, as well as increased perfusion of unventilated alveoli, resulting in venous admixture and severe arterial hypoxemia. Despite improvements in supportive therapy the mortality rate associated with ARDS over the last 25 years remains unchanged at 60% to 70%.[3]

Causes

ARDS is most often associated with shock or sepsis (Table 15-2). Complement activation that predisposes to leukocyte aggregation in the lungs may accompany sepsis. Proteinases and lipases released during acute pancreatitis may damage the pulmonary capillary endothelium. In vulnerable patients, oxygen may injure the alveolar and pulmonary epithelium,

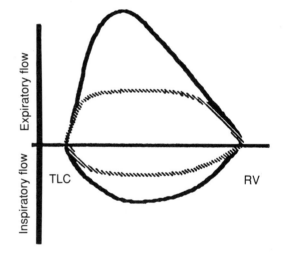

Fig. 15-2. Flow-volume loop in a normal patient (solid line) and in the presence of an intrathoracic (mediastinal) mass (hatched line). TLC, total lung capacity, RV, residual volume. (From Pullerits J, Holzman R. Anaesthesia for patients with mediastinal masses. Can J Anaesth 1989;36:681–8, with permission.)

Table 15-2.   Causes of Adult Respiratory Distress Syndrome

Shock	Drug-induced
Sepsis	Aspiration
Multisystem organ failure	Fat embolism
Acute pancreatitis	Pulmonary contusion
Oxygen toxicity	Cardiopulmonary bypass
Smoke inhalation	Near-drowning
Disseminated intravascular coagulation	

leading to the recommendation that inspired oxygen concentrations be limited to that compatible with acceptable arterial oxygenation. Chemotherapeutic drugs such as bleomycin and busulfan and the antidysrhythmic drug, amiodarone, have been associated with dose-related pulmonary fibrosis and development of ARDS (see Chapters 4 and 28). Phosgene and oxides of nitrogen in the inhaled smoke from fires may injure the lung structure. Disseminated intravascular coagulation damages pulmonary capillaries, as well as the endothelium of other vascular beds. Pulmonary contusion frequently manifests as ARDS. Even when trauma involves only one lung, both lungs may be affected, suggesting that mechanical forces are transmitted bilaterally. In patients who seem to make an uneventful recovery from near-drowning, diffuse pulmonary edema may subsequently develop, with all the features of ARDS. This edema appears to be the result of direct osmotic damage to the lungs by hyperosmotic or hypoosmotic fluid.

Manifestations

Classically, patients in whom ARDS develops manifest progressive tachypnea; chest radiographs will show bilateral and diffuse pulmonary infiltrates. This radiographic picture resembles that of pulmonary edema, progressing in some patients to complete opacification ("whiteout"). Pulmonary capillary occlusion pressure is normal or even decreased in patients with ARDS, except in cases complicated by congestive heart failure. Pulmonary hypertension may be due in part to obliteration of capillaries by fibrotic changes. Compliance of the lungs becomes progressively decreased, requiring increased positive airway pressures to generate the tidal volume. Initially, the PaO_2 can be maintained with supplemental oxygen, and the $PaCO_2$ is decreased. As ARDS worsens, even 100% oxygen may not prevent arterial hypoxemia, and the $PaCO_2$ increases. Nosocomial pneumonia is present in more than 50% of patients with ARDS. Thrombocytopenia may be prominent, and superinfections with bacterial and fungal pathogens often ensue. Multisystem organ failure may develop. In fact, more than 75% of patients dying with ARDS now die of multisystem organ failure and systemic hemodynamic instability, rather than lung dysfunction.[4]

Treatment

Treatment of ARDS begins with the delivery of supplemental inspired oxygen, intended to maintain acceptable oxygenation (see Chapter 16). One recommendation is to institute mechanical ventilation of the lungs through a tracheal tube, using a volume-cycled ventilator whenever greater than 50% inspired oxygen is required to maintain PaO_2 above about 60 mmHg. In the event of further deterioration of lung function, as indicated by decreasing pulmonary compliance and increasing arterial hypoxemia, the addition of positive end-expiratory pressure (PEEP) and a trial of diuretics and a decrease in intravenous fluid administration may be considered, in an attempt to improve the PaO_2. If hypotension and oliguria are present, the administration of an inotrope (dopamine, dobutamine) may be useful. Likewise, high levels of PEEP may decrease venous return to the point that a cardiac inotrope plus increased fluid administration are needed to maintain cardiac output. Pulmonary artery occlusion pressure may be falsely increased when PEEP is being applied, reflecting transmission of intra-alveolar pressure to the pulmonary capillaries. Keeping this in mind, patients with increased pulmonary artery occlusion pressures may be treated with a diuretic, whereas those with decreased pulmonary artery occlusion pressures may be treated with administration of intravenous fluids. The therapeutic goal is to maintain the lowest pulmonary artery occlusion pressure consistent with an acceptable cardiac output and blood pressure.

Despite the frequent administration of high doses of corticosteroids in the treatment of ARDS, there is no evidence this treatment improves survival.[3] Short-term infusion of prostacyclin has been used to treat pulmonary artery hypertension during ARDS.[5] Extracorporeal membrane oxygenation may be considered in desperate situations.

Post-traumatic Multisystem Organ Failure

The syndrome of multisystem organ failure may affect critically ill or injured patients. It is characterized initially by a hyperdynamic and hypermetabolic state similar to sepsis.[4] In most patients, the lungs are the first organs to fail, followed progressively by hepatic and then renal failure. Failure of the gastrointestinal mucosa to act as a barrier to systemic access of luminal bacteria is common. Cardiac dysfunction manifests as ventricular wall motion abnormalities despite a paradoxical increase in cardiac output. Central nervous system dysfunction may reflect effects of catabolic byproducts. Mortality approaches 100% if three or more organ systems become involved.

Aspiration Pneumonitis

Inhaled acidic gastric fluid is rapidly distributed throughout the lungs, leading to destruction of surfactant-producing cells and damage to the pulmonary capillary endothelium. As a result, atelectasis occurs, and intravascular fluid leaks into the lungs, producing a clinical picture similar to that of ARDS. Arterial hypoxemia is the most consistent manifestation of aspiration pneumonitis. In addition, there may be tachypnea, bronchospasm, and pulmonary vascular vasoconstriction, with associated pulmonary hypertension. The chest radiograph may not demonstrate evidence of aspiration pneumonitis for

6 to 12 hours after the event. Evidence of aspiration, when it does appear, is most likely to manifest in the right lower lobe.

Treatment

Assuming a tracheal tube is placed promptly after inhalation of gastric fluid, it is reasonable to inject small volumes of saline (5 ml) through the tracheal tube. It must be appreciated, however, that gastric fluid is rapidly distributed to peripheral areas of the lungs and that lavage with large volumes of fluid could exaggerate this spread. Measurement of the gastric fluid pH is useful, as it reflects the pH of the aspirated fluid. Measurement of tracheal aspirate is of doubtful value, since inhaled gastric fluid is likely to be rapidly diluted by airway secretions.

The most effective treatment of aspiration pneumonitis is delivery of supplemental inspired oxygen and institution of PEEP. Inhalation of a nebulized mist (metered dose inhaler) containing a beta-2 agonist such as albuterol may be effective in relieving bronchospasm. Although acid-injured lungs may be susceptible to bacterial infection, there is no evidence that antibiotics administered prophylactically decrease the incidence of infection or alter outcome after aspiration of gastric fluid. The use of corticosteroids for the treatment of aspiration pneumonitis is controversial. There is animal evidence that corticosteroids administered promptly after inhalation of acidic gastric fluid may be effective in decreasing pulmonary damage.[6] Conversely, other data show no beneficial effects or suggest that their use may enhance the development of gram-negative pneumonia.[7] Despite the absence of confirmatory evidence that corticosteroids are beneficial, it is not uncommon for the treatment of aspiration pneumonitis to include the empirical use of pharmacologic doses of methylprednisolone (30 mg·kg^{-1} IV) or dexamethasone (1 mg·kg^{-1} IV). Hypoalbuminemia, resulting from extravasation of protein-containing fluids into the lungs, is logically treated with albumin solutions. This approach, however, must be tempered by the possibility that these solutions will also leak across damaged pulmonary capillary endothelium and draw additional fluid into the lungs.

Neurogenic Pulmonary Edema

Neurogenic pulmonary edema develops in a small proportion of patients experiencing brain injury, especially in the area of the medulla. Typically, this form of pulmonary edema occurs a few hours after central nervous system injury and may occur during the perioperative period.[8] There is a massive outpouring of sympathetic nervous system impulses from the injured central nervous system, resulting in generalized vasoconstriction and a shift of blood volume into the pulmonary circulation. Presumably, increased pulmonary capillary pressures lead to transudation of fluid into the interstitial portions of the lungs and alveoli. In addition, pulmonary hypertension and hypervolemia can injure blood vessels of the lung. As a

result of this injury, altered pulmonary capillary permeability can persist after normalization of systemic and pulmonary vascular pressures. Treatment of neurogenic pulmonary edema is directed at decreasing intracranial pressure and support of oxygenation and ventilation. Digitalis is not indicated in the treatment of neurogenic pulmonary edema, as cardiac function is normal.

Opioid-Induced Pulmonary Edema

Opioid overdose, particularly with heroin, can lead to fulminant pulmonary edema. Altered pulmonary capillary permeability is suggested by the protein-rich nature of the pulmonary edema fluid. As in patients with neurogenic pulmonary edema, the function of the left ventricle is not impaired as reflected by a normal pulmonary artery occlusion pressure.

High-Altitude Pulmonary Edema

High-altitude pulmonary edema (above 2400 m or 8000 ft) is primarily a disorder of the pulmonary circulation induced by a relatively sustained alveolar hypoxia. The initiating event is presumed to be hypoxic pulmonary vasoconstriction, which elevates pulmonary vascular pressures. Treatment of high-altitude pulmonary edema is prompt descent from altitude to near sea level and administration of supplement inspired oxygen. The prophylactic administration of nifedipine is effective in lowering pulmonary artery pressure and preventing pulmonary edema in susceptible patients.[9] A portable hyperbaric chamber (Gamow bag) can be used for rapid simultation of descent.

Negative-Pressure Pulmonary Edema

Pulmonary edema associated with acute upper airway obstruction has been described as negative pressure pulmonary edema.[10] Presumably, the negative intrapleural pressure that occurs in the presence of airway obstruction is the principal mechanism responsible for this form of pulmonary edema. Indeed, most of the affected patients have experienced laryngospasm or epiglottitis. Pulmonary edema typically presents within minutes of either the development of acute upper airway obstruction or relief of the obstruction. Resolution is typically rapid, and rarely is anything more required for management than maintenance of a patent upper airway and administration of supplement inspired oxygen. Occasionally, mechanical ventilation of the lungs with PEEP may be required.

CHRONIC INTRINSIC RESTRICTIVE LUNG DISEASE

Chronic intrinsic restrictive lung disease is characterized by changes in the intrinsic properties of the lung, most often owing to pulmonary fibrosis. Pulmonary hypertension and cor pulmonale are likely, as progression of pulmonary fibrosis results in loss of pulmonary vasculature. Pneumothorax is common when pulmonary fibrosis is far advanced. Dyspnea is prominent, and breathing is rapid and shallow. Examples of chronic intrinsic restrictive lung disease are sarcoidosis, hypersensitivity pneumonitis, eosinophilic granuloma, and alveolar proteinosis.

Sarcoidosis

Sarcoidosis is a systemic granulomatous disorder that involves many tissues but that has a marked predilection for the thoracic lymph nodes and lungs. Laryngeal sarcoid occurs in 1% to 5% of patients and may interfere with the passage of an adult-size tracheal tube.[11] Cor pulmonale owing to sarcoidosis may develop. Parotid gland, facial nerve, and optic nerve involvement may occur. Myocardial sarcoidosis, although rare, may be manifested as heart block, cardiac dysrhythmias, or restrictive cardiomyopathy. Hepatic granulomas and splenomegaly are likely. Fever of unknown etiology is possible. Hypercalcemia is a rare but classic manifestation of sarcoidosis.

Mediastinoscopy is used to provide thoracic lymph node tissue for the diagnosis of sarcoidosis. The diffusion capacity for carbon monoxide across alveolar capillary membranes may be decreased, despite the presence of normal arterial blood gases. Angiotensin-converting enzyme activity is increased in these patients, but the significance of this change is not known. This enzyme is responsible for inactivating bradykinin and converting angiotensin I to angiotensin II. Corticosteroids are frequently used to treat sarcoidosis associated with restrictive lung disease.

Hypersensitivity Pneumonitis

Hypersensitivity pneumonitis is characterized by diffuse interstitial granulomatous reactions in the lungs after the inhalation of dust containing fungi, spores, or animal or vegetable material. Signs and symptoms of hypersensitivity pneumonitis include the onset of dyspnea and cough 4 to 6 hours after inhalation of the antigens, followed by leukocytosis and eosinophilia. Arterial hypoxemia can occur despite hyperventilation. Chest radiographs show multiple pulmonary infiltrates. Repeated episodes of hypersensitivity pneumonitis lead to pulmonary fibrosis.

Eosinophilic Granuloma

Pulmonary fibrosis accompanies the disease process known as eosinophilic granuloma (histiocytosis X). Corticosteroids are beneficial if extensive pulmonary fibrotic changes have not already occurred.

Pulmonary Alveolar Proteinosis

Pulmonary alveolar proteinosis is a disease of unknown etiology characterized by the deposition of lipid-rich proteinaceous material in the alveoli. Dyspnea and arterial hypoxemia are typical clinical manifestations. This process may occur independently or in association with chemotherapy, acquired immunodeficiency syndrome, or inhalation of mineral dusts. Although spontaneous remission may occur, treatment of severe cases consists of whole lung lavage intended to remove alveolar material and improve macrophage function. Lung lavage in a patient with co-existing arterial hypoxemia may even further decrease the level of oxygenation. Airway management during anesthesia for lung lavage includes the placement of a double-lumen endobronchial tube so as to optimize oxygenation during lavage.[12]

Lymphoangiomyomatosis

Lymphoangiomytosis is the benign proliferation of smooth muscle in abdominal and thoracic lymphatics, veins, and bronchioles that occurs in females of reproductive age.[13] Pulmonary function tests show restrictive and obstructive lung disease with a decrease in diffusing capacity. Clinical presentation is as progressive dyspnea, hemoptysis, recurrent pneumothoraces, and ascites. The exclusive female distribution suggests a role for steroid hormone metabolism in the etiology. There is progressive deterioration in pulmonary function, with death generally occurring within 4 years.

CHRONIC EXTRINSIC RESTRICTIVE LUNG DISEASE

Chronic extrinsic restrictive lung disease is most often due to disorders of the thoracic cage that interfere with expansion of the lungs (Table 15-1). The lungs become compressed, and lung volumes are decreased. The work of breathing is increased, owing to abnormal mechanical properties of the chest and increased airway resistance due to decreased lung volumes. Any thoracic deformity will compress pulmonary vasculature and eventually lead to right ventricular dysfunction. Recurrent pulmonary infection resulting from poor cough dynamics may lead to the development of obstructive components of the lung disease.

Pleural Fibrosis

Pleural fibrosis may follow hemothorax, empyema, or surgical pleurodesis for the treatment of recurrent pneumothoraces. Despite obliteration of the pleural space, the functional restrictive lung abnormalities are usually minor. Surgical decortication to remove thick fibrous pleura is technically difficult and is considered only if restrictive lung disease is symptomatic.

Neuromuscular Disorders

Neuromuscular disorders that interfere with the transfer of central nervous system output to skeletal muscles necessary for inspiration and exhalation can result in restrictive lung disease. Acute respiratory failure is a possibility, especially if atelectasis or pneumonia caused by retained secretions owing to an ineffective cough occurs or depressant drugs are administered. The extreme example is cervical spinal cord transection, in which paralysis of abdominal and intercostal muscles precludes a spontaneous cough. Measurement of vital capacity is an important indicator of the total impact of neuromuscular disorders on ventilation.

Bilateral diaphragmatic paralysis is characterized by cephalad movement of the diaphragm, owing to the weight of abdominal contents and the negative intrathoracic pressure created by contraction of the accessory muscles of breathing. As a result, mechanical dysfunction and gas exchange abnormalities similar to those produced by a flail chest may develop. Assumption of the sitting position may produce significant improvement in breathing.

Unilateral diaphragmatic paralysis is most often detected as an asymptomatic radiologic finding. Causes of unilateral diaphragmatic paralysis include compression or destruction of the phrenic nerve by surgery, aneurysmal vessels, or metastatic disease. Reversible paralysis is a complication of cardiac surgery in which the phrenic nerve is transiently injured by cold solutions applied topically to enhance cardioplegia.

Flail Chest

Multiple rib fractures, especially when they occur in a parallel vertical orientation, and separation of a median sternotomy after cardiac surgery may result in loss of chest wall stability, known as flail chest. Stability of the chest wall is necessary for the muscles of inspiration to inflate the lungs. In the presence of flail chest, the underlying lung moves inward as the remainder of the chest expands resulting in decreased tidal volume, arterial hypoxemia, and hypercarbia. Positive-pressure ventilation serves to stabilize the chest wall.

DISORDERS OF THE PLEURA AND MEDIASTINUM

Disorders of the pleura and mediastinum may contribute to mechanical changes that interfere with optimal expansion of the lungs.

Pleural Effusion

Pleural effusion is most often confirmed by a chest radiograph. For example, blunting of the normal sharp costophrenic angle on a lateral chest radiograph indicates the presence of at least 25 to 50 ml of pleural fluid. Larger amounts of fluid produce a characteristic homogeneous opacity that forms a concave meniscus with the chest wall. Ultrasonography and computed tomography are also useful in evaluating a pleural effusion. In patients with congestive heart failure, pleural fluid may collect in the interlobular fissures as an interlobular effusion. Various types of fluid may accumulate in the pleural space, including blood (hemothorax), pus (empyema), lipids (chylothorax), and serous liquid (hydrothorax). All these conditions present with an identical radiographic appearance. Treatment of pleural effusion is thoracentesis. Bloody pleural effusion is common in patients with malignant disease or injuries to the chest. The finding that pleural fluid is blood tinged is not diagnostically useful because 1 to 2 μl of blood added to 1000 ml of pleural fluid results in a serosanguinous appearance.

Pneumothorax

Pneumothorax is the presence of gas within the pleural space owing to disruption of the parietal pleura (external penetrating injury) or visceral pleura (tear in the lung parenchyma). Idiopathic spontaneous pneumothorax occurs most often in males between 20 and 30 years of age. These patients are often tall and slender, and most smoke cigarettes. Recurrent spontaneous pneumothorax is common during the first year after the initial event. Exercise or airline travel do not increase the likelihood of spontaneous pneumothorax.

The most common symptoms of pneumothorax are sudden and severe chest pain accompanied by dyspnea. Distant or absent breath sounds and a chest radiograph confirm the diagnosis. Treatment of pneumothorax is with a chest tube, when large amounts of lung are collapsed. It is acceptable to permit spontaneous resorption of the pneumothorax, when the patient is asymptomatic and the amount of collapsed lung is estimated to be less than about 20%. Spontaneous resorption may be accelerated by the administration of supplemental inspired oxygen, which lowers the partial pressure of nitrogen, favoring the transfer of this gas from the pleural space into the venous circulation. Strict bed rest does not hasten resorption. An air leak from the lung that persists for more than 7 to 10 days may be an indication for surgical intervention. When recurrence is a problem, chemical pleurodesis without a thoracotomy, by instilling tetracycline into the pleural space, may be a consideration.[14]

Tension Pneumothorax

Tension pneumothorax develops when gas enters the pleural space during inspiration and is prevented from escaping during exhalation. The result is a progressive increase in the amount of air trapped under increasing pressure (tension). Tension pneumothorax occurs in less than 2% of patients experiencing an idiopathic spontaneous pneumothorax, but it is a common manifestation of rib fractures or barotrauma in patients requiring mechanical ventilation of the lungs. Dyspnea is severe and arterial hypoxemia and hypotension are likely. Treatment by introduction of a small-bore plastic catheter (catheter over needle) into the second anterior intercostal space may be life-saving.

Mediastinal Mass

Contrast-enhanced computed tomography can distinguish between vascular structures, soft tissue, and calcifications as the causes of mediastinal widening. Lymphomas, thymomas, teratomas, and retrosternal goiters are common causes of anterior mediastinal masses. A large mediastinal tumor may be associated with progressive airway obstruction, loss of lung volume, pulmonary artery or cardiac compression, and superior vena caval obstruction.[15]

Superior Vena Cava Syndrome

Superior vena cava syndrome is a constellation of symptoms that develops in patients with a mediastinal mass, leading to obstruction of venous drainage in the upper thorax.[1] Increased venous pressure leads to (1) dilation of collateral veins in the thorax and neck; (2) edema and cyanosis of the face, neck, and upper chest; (3) edema of the conjunctiva; and (4) evidence of increased intracranial pressure, including headache and altered mental status. Dyspnea is commonly associated with this syndrome. Cancer accounts for nearly all cases of superior vena cava syndrome.

Acute Mediastinitis

Acute mediastinitis usually occurs from bacterial contamination after esophageal perforation. Symptoms include chest pain and fever. Treatment consists of administration of broad-spectrum antibiotics and often surgical drainage.

Pneumomediastinum

Pneumomediastinum may follow tracheostomy and alveolar rupture, although it most often occurs independent of known causes.[16] Spontaneous pneumomediastinum has been observed after the recreational use of cocaine.[17] Symptoms of retrosternal chest pain and dyspnea are typically abrupt in onset and usually follow exaggerated breathing efforts (cough, emesis, Valsalva maneuver). Subcutaneous emphysema may be extensive, including the neck, arms, abdomen, and scrotum. Gas in the mediastinum may decompress into the pleural space, leading to pneumothorax, usually on the left. The diagnosis of pneumomediastinum is established with a chest radiograph. Spontaneous pneumomediastinum resolves without specific therapy although breathing supplemental concentrations of oxygen may accelerate the rate of gas resorption. In adults, only rarely does gas in the mediastinum create sufficient pressure to compress vascular structures; surgical decompression is rarely necessary.

PREOPERATIVE PREPARATION

Preoperative preparation of the patient with restrictive lung disease includes an assessment of the severity of the lung disease and treatment of the reversible components. A preoperative history of dyspnea that limits activity and that can be attributed to restrictive lung disease is an indication for the performance of pulmonary function studies and the measurement of arterial blood gases. The most detailed assessment of flow-resistive properties of the airways is obtained by analysis of flow-volume loops. For example, the patient with restrictive lung disease shows decreased peak flow and a smaller total lung capacity and residual volume, as compared with normal patients[1] (Fig. 15-2). A decrease in the vital capacity from a normal value (about 70 ml·kg^{-1}) to less than 15 ml·kg^{-1}, or the presence of a resting increase in the $PaCO_2$, suggests that these patients are at increased risk of the development of exaggerated pulmonary dysfunction during the postoperative period. Interpretation of pulmonary function tests must consider the dependence of many of these tests on patient effort, as well as the role exerted by co-existing pain. Preoperative preparation also includes eradication of acute pulmonary infection, improvement of sputum clearance, treatment of cardiac dysfunction, exercises to improve strength of those skeletal muscles used in breathing, and training with respiratory therapy techniques that will be used postoperatively.

Preoperative evaluation of the patient with a mediastinal mass includes a chest radiograph, flow-volume loops, computed tomography, and clinical evaluation of evidence of tracheobronchial compression[1] (Fig. 15-2). In general, the size of the mediastinal mass and the degree of tracheal compression can be established by computed tomography. The degree of tracheal compression found on computed tomography is a useful predictor of whether difficulty with the airway during anesthesia may be expected. Flexible fiberoptic bronchoscopy under topical anesthesia is an alternative method for evaluating airway obstruction. Nevertheless, the severity of preoperative pulmonary symptoms may bear no relationship to the degree of respiratory compromise encountered during anesthesia. Indeed, a number of asymptomatic patients have developed unexpected airway obstruction during anesthesia.[1,15,18] For this reason, preoperative radiation should be considered for the patient whose mediastinal tumor is radiation sensitive. In symptomatic patients requiring a diagnostic tissue biopsy, a local anesthetic technique should be considered. Patients may be asymptomatic while awake, yet show the development of airway obstruction during anesthesia; this problem may reflect the effects of the supine position, including a decreased gas volume of the thorax owing to cephalad displacement of the diaphragm and increased central blood volume. Patients with mediastinal masses compressing the pulmonary artery or atria may be relatively asymptomatic while awake, yet life-threatening arterial hypoxemia, hypotension, or cardiac arrest may develop during anesthesia.[19]

MANAGEMENT OF ANESTHESIA

Restrictive lung disease unrelated to the presence of a mediastinal mass does not influence the choice of drugs used for the induction or maintenance of general anesthesia. The need to minimize depression of ventilation that may persist into the postoperative period should be considered in the selection of these drugs. A high index of suspicion for the presence of a pneumothorax and the need to avoid or discontinue nitrous oxide must be maintained. Regional anesthesia can be considered for peripheral operations, but it must be appreciated that sensory levels above T10 can be associated with impairment of respiratory muscle activity necessary for patients with restrictive lung disease to maintain acceptable ventilation. Controlled ventilation of the lungs during the intraoperative period seems a prudent approach to facilitate optimal oxygenation and ventilation. Increased inflation pressures delivered from the ventilator may be necessary to inflate poorly compliant lungs. Mechanical ventilation of the lungs during the postoperative period is often required for those patients with impaired pulmonary function documented preoperatively. Certainly, tracheal tubes should not be removed until patients have met established criteria for extubation (see Chapter 16). Restrictive lung disease contributes to postoperative pulmonary complications, since co-existing decreased lung volumes make it difficult to generate an effective cough for the removal of secretions from the airway.

The method selected for induction of anesthesia and tracheal intubation in the presence of a mediastinal mass depends on the preoperative assessment of the airway. External edema associated with superior vena cava syndrome may be accompanied by similar edema in the mouth and hypopharynx. If edema from venous obstruction is severe, it may be preferable to establish intravenous access in the leg rather than in the arm. Likewise, a central venous or pulmonary artery catheter can be inserted through the femoral vein, if necessary. Monitoring blood pressure through an intra-arterial catheter is common. If the patient must remain in the sitting position to achieve adequate ventilation, the anesthetic induction may proceed from this position using fiberoptic laryngoscopy to secure the airway. Topical airway anesthesia with or without sedation (often midazolam and fentanyl) is useful for fiberoptic laryngoscopy. In the very young patient, an inhalation induction of anesthesia while maintaining spontaneous ventilation may be necessary. Should airway obstruction occur, placing the patient in the lateral or prone position may be life-saving. Spontaneous ventilation and avoidance of the use of muscle relaxants is recommended but not likely to be possible during the maintenance of anesthesia. Acute worsening of superior vena cava syndrome may occur as a result of generous intraoperative fluid replacement. Drug-induced diuresis may decrease tumor volume, but associated decreases in preload in a patient with already comprised venous return may result in unacceptable hypotension. Surgical bleeding is likely to be increased in patients with increased central venous pressure. Postoperatively, reintubation of the trachea may be necessary because of increased airway obstruction owing to tumor swelling as a result of partial resection or biopsy after diagnostic procedures such as mediastinoscopy or bronchoscopy.

DIAGNOSTIC TECHNIQUES

Fiberoptic bronchoscopy has replaced rigid scope bronchoscopy for visualization of the airways and for obtaining samples for culture, cytologic study, and histologic examination. Pneumothorax occurs in 5% to 10% of patients after transbronchial lung biopsies, emphasizing the need for a chest radiograph after this procedure. Likewise, pneumothorax can be anticipated in 10% to 20% of patients after percutaneous needle biopsy of peripheral lung lesions. The principal contraindication to pleural biopsy is a coagulopathy. Pleuroscopy is direct visualization of the pleural surfaces through a fiberoptic scope introduced through an intercostal space into the pleural space. This procedure provides a means of avoiding an exploratory thoracotomy to obtain a biopsy.

Mediastinoscopy is performed through a small transverse incision just above the suprasternal notch during general anesthesia. Blunt dissection along the pretracheal fascia is performed, permitting biopsy of paratracheal lymph nodes to the level of the carina. Complications include pneumothorax, mediastinal hemorrhage, venous air embolism, and injury to the recurrent laryngeal nerve leading to hoarseness and vocal cord paralysis. The mediastinoscope can also exert pressure against the right subclavian artery, causing loss of a distal pulse (erroneous diagnosis of cardiac arrest) or compression of the right carotid artery (postoperative neurologic deficits).

REFERENCES

1. Pullerits J, Holzman R. Anaesthesia for patients with mediastinal masses. Can J Anaesth 1989;36:681–8
2. Bone RC, Jacobs ER. Advances in pharmacologic treatment of acute lung injury and septic shock. In: Stoelting RK, Barash PG, Gallagher TJ, eds. Advances in Anesthesia. Chicago. Year Book Medical Publishers 1986;4:327–45
3. Bernard GR, Luce JM, Sprung CL, et al. High-dose corticosteroids in patients with the adult respiratory distress syndrome. N Engl J Med 1987;317:1565–70
4. Decamp MM, Demling RH. Posttraumatic multisystem organ failure. JAMA 1988;260:530–4
5. Radermacher P, Santak B, Wust HJ, Tarnow J, Falke KJ. Prostacyclin for the treatment of pulmonary hypertension in the adult respiratory distress syndrome: Effects on pulmonary capillary pressure and ventilator-perfusion distributions. Anesthesiology 1990;72:238–44
6. Dudley WR, Marshall BE. Steroid treatment for acid-aspiration pneumonia. Anesthesiology 1974;40:136–41
7. Wynne JW, DeMarco FJ, Hood CI. Physiological effects of corticosteroids in food-stuff aspiration. Arch Surg 1981;116:46–9
8. Braude N, Ludgrove T. Neurogenic pulmonary oedema precipitated by induction of anaesthesia. Br J Anaesth 1989;62:101–3
9. Bartsch P, Maggiorini M, Ritter M, Noti C, Vock P, Oelz O. Prevention of high-altitude pulmonary edema by nifedipine. N Engl J Med 1991;315:1284–9
10. Lang SA, Duncan PG, Shephard DAE, Ha HC. Pulmonary oedema associated with airway obstruction. Can J Anaesth 1990: 37:210–8
11. Willis MH, Harris MM. An unusual airway complication with sarcoidosis. Anesthesiology 1987;66:554–5
12. Spragg RG, Benumof JL, Alfery DD. New method for performance of unilateral lung lavage. Anesthesiology 1982;57:535–8
13. Smith MB, Elwood RJ. Anesthetic management for oophorectomy in a patient with lymphangiomyomatosis. Anesthesiology 1989;70:548–50
14. Krasnik M, Christensen B, Halkier E, et al. Pleurodesis in spontaneous pneumothorax by means of tetracycline: Follow-up evaluation of a method. Scand J Thorac Cardiovasc Surg 1987;21: 181–8
15. John RE, Narang VPS. A boy with an anterior mediastinal mass. Anaesthesia 1988;43:864–6
16. Maunder RJ, Pierson DJ, Hudson LD. Subcutaneous and mediastinal emphysema: Pathophysiology, diagnosis, and management. Arch Intern Med 1984;144:1447–54
17. Shesser R, David C, Edelstine S. Pneumomediastinum and pneumothorax after inhaling alkaloidal cocaine. Ann Emerg Med 1981; 10:213–5
18. deSoto H. Direct laryngoscopy as an aid to relieve airway obstruction in a patient with a mediastinal mass. Anesthesiology 1987;67:116–7
19. Levin H, Bursztein S, Heifetz M. Cardiac arrest in a child with mediastinal mass. Anesth Analg 1985;64:1129–30

16

Acute Respiratory Failure

Respiratory failure is the inability of the lungs to provide adequate arterial oxygenation with or without acceptable elimination of carbon dioxide. A variety of primary or secondary disorders of the airways, lung parenchyma, chest wall, and neural processes involved in breathing may be responsible for the development of respiratory failure, which may be acute, chronic, or acute and superimposed on a chronic disease process.[1,2] There is increasing evidence that fatigue of the muscles of breathing is a principal determinant of acute respiratory failure. Arterial hypoxemia resulting from an intracardiac shunt, anemia, or carbon monoxide poisoning is not considered a cause of acute respiratory failure, since these conditions do not reflect defects in the respiratory system.

DIAGNOSIS

Measurement of arterial blood bases (PaO_2, $PaCO_2$) and pH is mandatory in the diagnosis and management of patients with acute respiratory failure. As a guideline, acute respiratory failure is considered present when the PaO_2 is less than 60 mmHg despite supplemental oxygen. This guideline assumes the absence of a right-to-left intracardiac shunt and is based on the shape of the oxyhemoglobin dissociation curve, in which significant desaturation of hemoglobin in arterial blood (SaO_2) occurs when the PaO_2 declines below about 60 mmHg (see Fig. 24-1). For example, SaO_2 decreases less than 1% when PaO_2 decreases from 100 mmHg to 90 mmHg, while SaO_2 decreases from 88% to 80% when the PaO_2 declines from 55 mmHg to 45 mmHg. The $PaCO_2$ in the presence of acute respiratory failure can be elevated, normal, or decreased, depending on the relationship of alveolar ventilation to the metabolic production of carbon dioxide. A $PaCO_2$ exceeding 50 mmHg, in the absence of respiratory compensation for metabolic alkalosis, is consistent with the diagnosis of acute respiratory failure.

Acute respiratory failure is distinguished from the chronic condition on the basis of the relationship of the $PaCO_2$ to the pH. For example, acute respiratory failure is typically accompanied by an abrupt increase in $PaCO_2$ and by a corresponding decrease in the pH. Conversely, in the presence of chronic respiratory failure, the pHa is usually between 7.35 and 7.45, despite an increased $PaCO_2$. This normal pH reflects compensation, by virtue of renal tubular resorption of bicarbonate.

In addition to arterial hypoxemia, respiratory failure is usually accompanied by a decrease in functional residual capacity (FRC) and lung compliance. There is often bilateral diffuse opacification of the lungs on radiographs of the chest. Pulmonary artery occlusion pressure is usually less than 15 mmHg despite the frequent presence of pulmonary edema (see Chapter 15). Increased pulmonary vascular resistance and pulmonary hypertension are likely to develop when respiratory failure persists. Inhalation of nitric oxide (5 to 80 parts per million) by patients with severe respiratory failure decreases pulmonary artery pressure and improves arterial oxygenation without producing systemic vasodilation.[3]

TREATMENT OF RESPIRATORY FAILURE

Treatment of respiratory failure is directed at initiating specific therapies intended to support pulmonary function until the lungs can recover from the insult responsible for pulmonary dysfunction (Table 16-1). The three principles of management of acute respiratory failure are (1) correction of arterial hypoxemia, (2) removal of excess carbon dioxide, and (3) provision of a patent airway.

Supplemental Oxygen

Correction of arterial hypoxemia begins with providing sufficient supplemental inspired oxygen to maintain the PaO_2 between 60 and 80 mmHg, recognizing that excess oxygen is toxic to the lungs. Supplemental oxygen can be provided to a spontaneously breathing patient, using a nasal cannula, Ven-

Table 16-1. Treatment of Acute Respiratory Failure

Supplemental oxygen	Drug-induced diuresis
Intubation of the trachea	Inotropic support of
Mechanical support of ventilation	cardiac function
Positive end-expiratory pressure	Control of infection
Optimize intravascular fluid volume	Nutritional support

turi mask, a nonrebreathing mask, or a T piece attached to the free end of a tracheal tube. These devices seldom provide an inspired oxygen concentration greater than 50%, emphasizing the value of these methods in correcting the arterial hypoxemia that results from mild to moderate ventilation-to-perfusion abnormalities. When these methods of supplemental oxygen delivery fail to correct arterial hypoxemia, it is necessary to consider a more invasive approach, including intubation of the trachea and mechanical support of ventilation.

Ideally, the inspired concentration of oxygen required to achieve acceptable oxygenation should not exceed 50% for prolonged periods. Administration of more than 50% oxygen for longer than 24 hours may increase the risk of the development of pulmonary oxygen toxicity. For this reason, the use of continuous positive airway pressure (CPAP) or positive end-expiratory pressure (PEEP) is often recommended when the PaO_2 cannot be maintained above 60 mmHg while the patient is breathing less than 50% oxygen. Indeed, in some patients experiencing an acute exacerbation of their lung disease, the delivery of inspiratory positive airway pressure by a tight-fitting face mask may obviate the need for intubation of the trachea and mechanical ventilation of the lungs. Maintenance of PaO_2 above about 80 mmHg is of little benefit, since saturation of hemoglobin with oxygen is nearly 100% at this level.

The notion that administration of oxygen will result in hypoventilation in patients who are dependent on hypoxic drive for breathing seems unfounded. Any increase in $PaCO_2$ that occurs in such patients during supplemental administration of oxygen is more likely to reflect fatigue of breathing muscles, an increase in dead space ventilation, or the Haldane effect. Overall, the risk of supplemental administration of oxygen appears to be overstated and could lead to withholding useful therapy.[2]

Mechanical Ventilation of the Lungs

Intubation of the trachea and mechanical support of ventilation of the lungs should be considered in the presence of (1) a PaO_2 that remains less than 60 mmHg despite an inspired oxygen concentration that exceeds 50%, (2) a $PaCO_2$ that is increasing in association with a decrease in pH, (3) evidence of fatigue of the respiratory muscles, (4) loss of protective upper airway reflexes, and (5) an ineffective cough mechanism.

Intubation of the Trachea

Intubation of the trachea can be performed initially by either the oral or nasal route. Tubes placed in the trachea through the nose tend to provide greater stability with fixation and are better tolerated by the patient. Oral placement of tracheal tubes permits the use of large internal diameter (at least 8-mm) tubes; this procedure facilitates suctioning of secretions from the trachea, as well as the passage of a fiberoptic bronchoscope into the trachea.

It is generally thought that, after about 21 days of supraglottic tracheal intubation, the risk of upper airway complications (laryngostenosis, vocal and paralysis) is sufficiently great to justify recommending a tracheostomy. In addition, a tracheostomy may be preferable to a translaryngeal tube when pulmonary secretions are copious. A serious complication of supraglottic or infraglottic tracheal intubation is tracheal stenosis or tracheomalacia at the site of the mucosal contact with the tube cuff. Minimizing the intracuff pressure (cuff inflated with just enough air to prevent an audible leak of gas during positive pressure ventilation of the lungs) may decrease the risk of ischemic damage to underlying tracheal mucosa.

Positive Airway Pressure

All methods of delivering positive airway pressure in association with mechanical ventilation of the lungs require tracheal intubation. The two basic types of positive-pressure ventilators are (1) volume-cycled, which provides a fixed tidal volume with inflation pressure as the dependent variable; and (2) pressure-cycled, which provides gas flow until a preset pressure is reached, such that tidal volume is the dependent variable. Tidal volume is better maintained with a volume-cycled ventilator during changes in airway resistance or lung compliance, or both. Tidal volume delivered by a pressure-cycled ventilator tends to vary inversely with changes in airway resistance and directly with changes in pulmonary compliance.

When using a volume-cycled ventilator, tidal volume is maintained despite increased inflation pressure that may reflect secretions, active exhalation efforts by the patient, or endobronchial migration of the tube. Similar events in a patient being ventilated with a pressure-cycled machine lead to decreased tidal volume. The disadvantage of a volume-cycled ventilator is the inability of this device to compensate for the development of leaks in the delivery system. For example, a gas leak around the tracheal tube cuff could result in hypoventilation, despite the continued delivery of unchanged ventilatory volumes.

Pressure-cycled ventilators continue to deliver constant inspired volumes in the presence of a leak until a preset time is elapsed or a specific airway pressure is achieved. Overall, a volume-cycled ventilator is most often selected to provide mechanical support of ventilation to patients with acute respiratory failure.

Initial ventilator settings often include a breathing rate of 6 to 10 breaths·min^{-1}, tidal volume of 10 to 15 ml·kg^{-1}, and an inspired concentration of oxygen near 50%. Exhalation is passive and is prolonged by increased resistance to airflow, as in patients with chronic obstructive pulmonary disease or asthma. If the subsequent mechanically delivered breath is initiated before exhalation is complete, there is a risk of air trapping in these patients. In this regard, a slow breathing rate and large tidal volume are most likely to optimize the distribution of ventilation in the presence of regional differences in airway resistance and provide adequate time for exhalation to occur. Subsequent adjustments in the ventilator settings and inspired concentrations of oxygen are based on measurements of arterial blood gases and pH. The goal is to maintain the PaO_2 at 60 to 80 mmHg, the $PaCO_2$ at 35 to 45 mmHg, and the pHa at 7.35 to 7.45.

Sedation (opioids, benzodiazepines) and/or skeletal muscle paralysis (nondepolarizing muscle relaxants) may be utilized to facilitate management of patients during mechanical ventilation of the lungs. There is no evidence, however, that use of drugs in this manner improves outcome. There is evidence that prolonged administration of muscle relaxants (longer than 48 hours) may be associated with persistent weakness, especially in the presence of renal failure and sepsis.[4]

Modes of Ventilation

Modes of positive-pressure mechanical ventilation of the lungs are categorized as controlled, assisted, assisted/controlled, controlled with PEEP, and assisted/controlled employing intermittent mandatory ventilation (IMV) (Fig. 16-1). PEEP is the maintenance of positive airway and intrathoracic pressure during the entire ventilator cycle, with superimposed intermittent inflation of the lungs by cyclic increases in positive pressure. Positive pressure applied during spontaneous breathing is referred to as CPAP. Assisted/controlled modes of ventilation require minimal breathing efforts by the patient and allow the muscles of respiration to be rested. Conversely, IMV exercises inspiratory muscles and decreases mean intrathoracic pressure. High-frequency positive-pressure ventilation (60 to 100 breaths·min^{-1}) has been introduced as an alternative to the more conventional mode of intermittent positive-pressure ventilation.[5] Proposed advantages of this mode of mechanical ventilation include failure of changes in airway resistance or pulmonary compliance to alter tidal volume, and maintenance of low airway pressure, which would appear to decrease the likelihood of barotrauma (pneumothorax) or interference with venous return. Not all reports, however, demonstrate a superiority of high-frequency positive-pressure ventilation over more conventional modes of positive-pressure ventilation.[6]

Positive End-expiratory Pressure

The addition of PEEP to the ventilator cycle is often recommended when the PaO_2 cannot be maintained above 60 mmHg, when breathing 50% oxygen.[1] PEEP is presumed to increase arterial oxygenation, pulmonary compliance, and the FRC, by expanding previously collapsed but perfused alveoli. As a result, ventilation-to-perfusion matching is improved and

the magnitude of the right-to-left intrapulmonary shunting of blood decreased. It is unlikely that PEEP will improve PaO_2 when arterial hypoxemia is due to hypoventilation or is associated with a normal, or even increased, FRC. PEEP does not decrease extravascular lung water or prevent the formation of edema fluid in the lungs. Nevertheless, edema fluid is likely to be distributed to the interstitial lung regions, causing previously flooded alveoli to become ventilated.[7]

Initially, PEEP is added in 2.5- to 5.0-cm H_2O increments, until the PaO_2 is at least 60 mmHg with the patient breathing less than 50% oxygen. The goal is to deliver the amount of PEEP that maximally improves arterial oxygenation, without substantially decreasing the cardiac output. Optimal levels of PEEP, as reflected by maximal oxygen transport (arterial oxygen content times cardiac output), are often associated with the best improvement in pulmonary compliance[8] (Fig. 16-2). Most of these patients show maximal improvement in arterial oxygen transport and pulmonary compliance with levels of PEEP below 15 cm H_2O. Excessive levels of PEEP can decrease PaO_2 by overdistending open alveoli, thereby compressing the capillaries surrounding these alveoli and shunting more blood to collapsed alveoli.

An important adverse effect of PEEP is decreased cardiac output, owing to interference with venous return and a leftward displacement of the ventricular septum, which restricts filling of the left ventricle.[9] It is conceivable that improved PaO_2 produced by PEEP could be offset by decreased tissue blood flow due to decreases in cardiac output. The potential for PEEP to decrease cardiac output is exaggerated in the presence of decreased intravascular fluid volume or normal lungs, or both, permitting maximal transmission of increased airway pressures. Replacement of intravascular fluid volume and administration of a cardiac inotrope may offset the effects of PEEP on venous return and improve myocardial contractility. A pulmonary artery catheter is useful in monitoring the adequacy of intravascular fluid replacement, myocardial contractility, and tissue oxygenation (PvO_2) in patients being treated with PEEP. Measurement of the pulmonary artery occlusion pressure is complicated by transmission of PEEP (intra-alveolar pressure) to the pulmonary capillaries, which is then erroneously interpreted as the pulmonary artery occlusion pressure.

Pneumothorax, pneumomediastinum, and subcutaneous emphysema are examples of pulmonary barotrauma that can be produced by PEEP. Barotrauma is presumed to reflect overdistension and rupture of alveoli owing to PEEP. Abrupt deterioration of the PaO_2 and cardiovascular function during PEEP should arouse suspicion of a tension pneumothorax.

Intravascular Fluid Volume

Maintenance of intravascular fluid volume, as well as optimal water content of the lungs, is important in treating patients exhibiting acute respiratory failure. Excessive accumulation

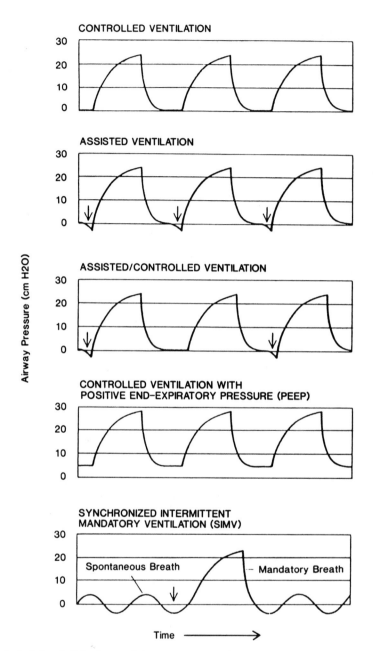

Fig. 16-1. Schematic depiction of tidal volume and airway pressure produced by various modes of ventilation delivered through a tracheal tube. Arrows indicate initiation of a spontaneous breath by the patient that triggers the ventilator to deliver a mechanically assisted breath.

of fluid in the lungs is characteristic of many forms of acute respiratory failure, especially the entity designated adult respiratory distress syndrome (see Chapter 15). Mechanical ventilation of the lungs, particularly in combination with PEEP, may evoke the release of hormones (antidiuretic hormone,

atrial natriuretic hormone) that contribute to fluid retention. Monitors of intravascular fluid volume include measurement of pulmonary artery occlusion pressure, urine output, and body weight. A pulmonary artery occlusion pressure above 15 mmHg or below 15 mmHg may reflect an excessive or an

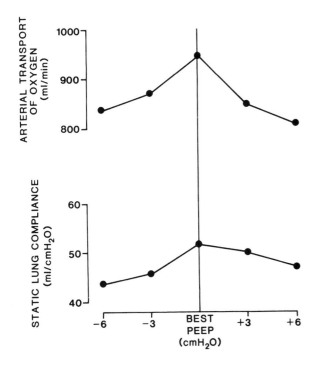

Fig. 16-2. Best positive end-expiratory pressure (PEEP) is defined as that level of PEEP that is associated with maximal arterial oxygenation. (Data from Suter PM, Fairley HB, Isenberg MD. Optimum end-expiratory airway pressure in patients with acute pulmonary failure. N Engl J Med 1975;292:284–9.)

inadequate intravascular fluid volume, respectively. A urine output of 0.5 to 1 ml·kg^{-1}·h^{-1} is consistent with an adequate cardiac output and intravascular fluid volume. Normally, a daily weight loss of 0.2 to 0.4 kg is anticipated in adult patients receiving conventional intravenous fluid therapy. A stable or increasing body weight implies excessive fluid retention. Central venous pressure measurement is probably not a reliable guide for monitoring intravascular fluid volume in patients with acute respiratory failure.

Drug-induced diuresis, using furosemide, is particularly effective in decreasing excessive accumulation of fluid in the lungs. Evidence of the beneficial effects of diuresis includes improved arterial oxygenation and resolution of pulmonary infiltrates on chest radiographs. Diuresis requires careful titration to avoid excessive decreases in the intravascular fluid volume, which could lead to decreased cardiac output, to hypotension, and to tissue oxygen delivery, especially if PEEP is part of the mechanical ventilation mode.

Removal of Secretions

Optimal removal of secretions from the airways is facilitated by adequate systemic hydration and humidification of inspired gases. In addition, chest physiotherapy is important, to en-hance the postural drainage of secretions and to stimulate effective coughing. Tracheal suction with a sterile catheter is useful in stimulating active expiratory efforts and removal of secretions from the airways. Fiberoptic bronchoscopy is indicated for the removal of inspissated secretions that are contributing to atelectasis.

Control of Infection

Control of infection using specific antibiotic therapy based on sputum culture and sensitivity is a valuable adjunct to the management of respiratory failure. The use of prophylactic antibiotics without proven specificity for the infectious organisms, however, is not recommended, since this practice can lead to the overgrowth of resistant bacteria or fungi. Not uncommonly, the earliest evidence of infection in patients with respiratory failure is further deterioration of pulmonary function.

Nutrition

Nutritional support is important, as skeletal muscle weakness can interfere with cessation of mechanical support of ventilation when acute respiratory failure is no longer present.[10] Hypophosphatemia may contribute to skeletal muscle weakness and to poor contractility of the diaphragm that may accompany acute respiratory failure. Increased caloric intake, as associated with hyperalimentation, may increase the metabolic production of carbon dioxide, necessitating an increase in alveolar ventilation that might not be possible without mechanical support of breathing.

The risk of gastrointestinal bleeding is increased in all patients experiencing acute respiratory failure. For this reason, prophylactic administration of antacids or H-2 antagonists, or both, may be instituted, in an attempt to decrease the risk of bleeding.[11]

MONITORING OF TREATMENT

Monitoring the progress of treatment of acute respiratory failure depends on evaluation of pulmonary gas exchange and cardiac function (Table 16-2). A pulmonary artery catheter is useful in making many of these measurements.

Table 16-2. Monitoring of Treatment of Acute Respiratory Failure

Arterial and venous blood gases	Cardiac filling pressures
Arterial pH	Intrapulmonary shunt
Cardiac output	Static compliance

Table 16-3.   Calculation of the Alveolar-to-Arterial Difference for Oxygen (A-aDO$_2$)

$$A\text{-}aDO_2 = P_AO_2 - PaO_2$$

$$P_AO_2 = (P_B - P_{H_2O})F_IO_2 - PaCO_2/0.8$$

Example: Arterial blood gases are PaO$_2$ 100 mmHg breathing 50% oxygen (F$_I$O$_2$ = 0.5) and the PaCO$_2$ is 40 mmHg. The barometric pressure (P$_B$) is 747 mmHg, and the partial pressure of water vapor at 37°C (P$_{H_2O}$) is 47 mmHg. Calculation of the PaO$_2$ and A-aDO$_2$ is as follows:

$$PaO_2 = (747 - 47)0.5 - 40/0.8$$

$$P_AO_2 = 350 - 50$$

$$P_AO_2 = 300 \text{ mmHg}$$

$$A\text{-}aDO_2 = 300 - 100$$

$$A\text{-}aDO_2 = 200 \text{ mmHg}$$

Oxygen Exchange and Arterial Oxygenation

Adequacy of oxygen exchange across the alveolar capillary membrane is reflected by the PaO$_2$. The efficacy of this exchange is paralleled by the difference between the calculated P$_A$O$_2$ and measured PaO$_2$ (Table 16-3). Calculation of the alveolar-to-arterial difference for oxygen (A-aDO$_2$) is useful for evaluating the gas exchange functions of the lung and for distinguishing between the various mechanisms for arterial hypoxemia (Table 16-4). For example, calculation of the A-aDO$_2$ in a patient breathing 100% oxygen provides an estimate of the magnitude of right-to-left intrapulmonary shunting of blood. Conversely, calculation of the A-aDO$_2$ in a patient breathing air reflects ventilation-to-perfusion mismatching, as well as right-to-left intrapulmonary shunting of blood. Normal values for A-aDO$_2$ increase with age (9 mmHg at 20 years and 15 mmHg at 70 years) because of an age-related decrease in PaO$_2$. As a guideline, each 20 mmHg of A-aDO$_2$ measured in a patient breathing oxygen represents venous admixture equivalent to about 1% of the cardiac output. This guideline will underestimate the true magnitude of venous admixture when the SaO$_2$ is less than 100% or when the cardiac output is elevated. An A-aDO$_2$ due to diffusion block of oxygen transfer across the alveolar capillary membrane has not been documented to occur.

A disadvantage of monitoring the A-aDO$_2$ is that the normal range changes with variations in the inspired concentration of oxygen. For this reason, the ratio of arterial-to-alveolar oxygen partial pressure (a/A) may be useful, as this value is less dependent on the inspired oxygen concentration[12] (Table 16-5). For example, a patient with an a/A of 0.5 will have a PaO$_2$ equal to one-half the P$_A$O$_2$, regardless of the inspired concentration of oxygen. An a/A of less than 0.75 suggests that the lungs are not working well as oxygen exchangers.

Significant desaturation of arterial blood occurs only when the PaO$_2$ is less than 60 mmHg, this accounts for the common definition of arterial hypoxemia as a PaO$_2$ of 60 mmHg. Ventilation-to-perfusion mismatching, right-to-left intrapulmonary shunting, and hypoventilation are the key causes of arterial hypoxemia (Table 16-4). Increasing the inspired oxygen concentration is likely to improve the PaO$_2$ in all these conditions, with the exception of a right-to-left intrapulmonary shunt that exceeds 30% of cardiac output.

Compensatory responses to arterial hypoxemia vary enormously among patients. As a guideline, these responses begin with an acute decrease in PaO$_2$ below 60 mmHg; they are also present in chronic hypoxemia when the PaO$_2$ is less than 50 mmHg. Compensatory responses to acute arterial hypoxemia include (1) carotid body-induced increases in alveolar ventilation, (2) regional pulmonary artery vasoconstriction (hypoxic pulmonary vasoconstriction) to divert pulmonary blood flow away from hypoxic alveoli, and (3) increased sympathetic nervous system activity to enhance tissue oxygen delivery by increased cardiac output. When arterial hypoxemia is chronic, increased erythrocyte mass enhances the oxygen-carrying capacity of the blood. Chronic arterial hypoxemia may be associated with somnolence and with decreased renal function.

Table 16-4.   Mechanisms of Arterial Hypoxemia

	PaO$_2$	PaCO$_2$	A-aDO$_2$	Response to Supplemental Oxygen
Low inspired oxygen concentration (altitude)	D	Normal to D	Normal	Improved
Hypoventilation (drug overdose)	D	I	Normal	Improved
Ventilation-to-perfusion mismatching (COPD, pneumonia)	D	Normal to D	I	Improved
Right-to-left shunt (pulmonary edema)	D	Normal to D	I	Poor to none
Diffusion impairment (pulmonary fibrosis)	D	Normal to D	I	Improved

COPD, chronic obstructive pulmonary disease; D, decrease; I, increase.

Table 16-5. Calculation of the Ratio of Arterial-to-Alveolar Oxygen Partial Pressure (a/A)

$$a/A = PaO_2/P_AO_2$$

Example: Arterial blood gases are PaO_2 250 mmHg and $PaCO_2$ 40 mmHg breathing 50% oxygen. The P_B is 747 mmHg and P_{H_2O} is 47 mmHg (see Table 16-3). The calculated P_AO_2 is 300 mmHg (see Table 16-3).

$$a/A = 250/300$$

$$a/A = 0.83 \ (\text{normal} > 0.75)$$

Table 16-7. Calculation of the Dead Space-to-Tidal Volume Ratio

$$V_D/V_T = PaCO_2 - P_ECO_2/PaCO_2$$

Example: The $PaCO_2$ is 40 mmHg and the P_ECO_2 (mixed exhaled partial pressure of carbon dioxide) is 30 mmHg during controlled ventilation of the lungs with isoflurane in oxygen. The calculated V_D/V_T ratio is as follows:

$$V_D/V_T = 40 - 30/40$$

$$V_D/V_T = 10/40$$

$$V_D/V_T = 0.25$$

When the PaO_2 is less than 30 mmHg, compensatory mechanisms fail and cell damage is likely.

Carbon Dioxide Elimination

The adequacy of alveolar ventilation relative to the metabolic production of carbon dioxide is reflected by the $PaCO_2$ (Table 16-6). The efficacy of carbon dioxide transfer across the alveolar capillary membrane is reflected by the dead space ventilation-to-tidal volume ratio (V_D/V_T) (Table 16-7). This ratio depicts areas in the lungs that receive adequate ventilation but inadequate or no pulmonary blood flow. Ventilation to these alveoli is described as "wasted ventilation." Normally, the V_D/V_T is less than 0.3 but may increase to 0.6 or greater when there is an increase in wasted ventilation. An increased V_D/V_T occurs in the presence of acute respiratory failure, decreased cardiac output as due to anesthetic drugs or hypovolemia, and pulmonary embolism.

Hypercarbia is defined as a $PaCO_2$ greater than 45 mmHg. Symptoms of hypercarbia depend on the rate of increase and on the ultimate level of elevation in the $PaCO_2$. Acute increases in the $PaCO_2$ are associated with increased cerebral blood flow and elevated intracranial pressure. Extreme increases in $PaCO_2$ to above 80 mmHg may result in seizures and subsequent central nervous system depression.

Table 16-6. Mechanisms of Hypercarbia

	$PaCO_2$	V_D/V_T	A-aDO_2
Drug overdose	I	Normal	Normal
Restrictive lung disease (kyphoscoliosis)	I	Normal to I	Normal to I
Chronic obstructive pulmonary disease	I	I	I
Neuromuscular disease	I	Normal to I	Normal to I

I, increase; D, decrease.

Mixed Venous Partial Pressure of Oxygen

The mixed venous partial pressure of oxygen ($P\bar{v}O_2$) and the arterial-to-venous difference for oxygen ($CaO_2 - CvO_2$) reflects the overall adequacy of the oxygen transport system (cardiac output) relative to extraction of oxygen by tissues. For example, a decrease in cardiac output that occurs in the presence of unchanged tissue oxygen consumption causes the $P\bar{v}O_2$ to decrease and the $CaO_2 - CvO_2$ to increase. These changes reflect the continued extraction of the same amount of oxygen by the tissues from a decreased tissue blood flow. A $P\bar{v}O_2$ less than 30 mmHg or a $CaO_2 - CvO_2$ greater than 6 ml·dl^{-1} indicates the need to increase cardiac output to facilitate tissue oxygenation. A pulmonary artery catheter permits sampling of mixed venous blood through the distal port for use in measuring the $P\bar{v}O_2$ and in calculating the CvO_2.

Accuracy of Blood Gas Measurements

The recommendation that arterial blood gases should be corrected for differences between the patient's body temperature and the temperature of the measuring electrode (pH-stat management) is based on known temperature-dependent solubility of oxygen and carbon dioxide in blood. For example, placing blood from a patient with a body temperature of less than 37°C into an electrode maintained at 37°C means that more molecules enter the gas phase to be sensed as partial pressure than would be present in vivo at the lower body temperature of the patient. Nevertheless, it has been argued that the $PaCO_2$ and pH measured at an electrode temperature of 37°C (alpha-stat management) reflect the unperturbed acid-base status of the patient, regardless of the body temperature that existed at the time the sample was drawn.[13] If this concept is accepted, it is not necessary to correct measurements of PCO_2 and pH for temperature. Temperature correction of PO_2 measurements remains necessary to assess oxygenation.

Furthermore, calculation of the A-aDO$_2$ requires temperature correction of oxygen and carbon dioxide partial pressure measurements. Nomograms are available to correct arterial blood gas and pH measurements for temperature.

Another consideration in the interpretation of arterial blood gases is consumption of oxygen by leukocytes and platelets that could result in an in vitro reduction of oxygen partial pressures. For this reason, blood samples are placed on ice, especially if the time between obtaining the samples and analysis will exceed 20 minutes.[14] Another source of error is introduced by the presence of air bubbles in blood samples. For example, carbon dioxide can pass along the partial pressure gradient from blood into the air bubble, resulting in a false-low measurement of the PCO$_2$ actually present in the patient. Likewise, oxygen can pass to or from the air bubble, depending on the partial pressure of this gas in the blood, resulting in a false-low or false-high measurement of the PO$_2$ actually present.

Arterial pH

Measurement of pH is necessary to detect acidemia or alkalemia. For example, metabolic acidosis predictably accompanies arterial hypoxemia and inadequate delivery of oxygen to tissues. Furthermore, acidemia due to respiratory or metabolic derangements is associated with cardiac dysrhythmias and with increased pulmonary vascular resistance due to constriction of the pulmonary vasculature.

Alkalemia, as reflected by an increase in the pH, is most often associated with iatrogenic mechanical hyperventilation of the lungs or with drug-induced diuresis leading to loss of chloride and potassium. As with acidemia, the incidence of cardiac dysrhythmias may be increased by metabolic or respiratory alkalosis.[15] The presence of alkalemia in a patient recovering from acute respiratory failure can delay or prevent successful weaning from mechanical support of ventilation because of compensatory hypoventilation by the patient in an attempt to restore total body carbon dioxide stores. The phenomenon known as posthyperventilation hypoxia reflects arterial hypoxemia due to hypoventilation that develops in the absence of administration of supplemental oxygen to a patient in whom previous mechanical hyperventilation of the lungs has led to depletion of carbon dioxide stores.[16]

Cardiac Output

Measurement and maintenance of normal cardiac output are essential in ensuring adequate delivery of oxygen to tissues and evaluating responses to therapeutic interventions during the treatment of respiratory failure. Cardiac output is most frequently measured by a thermodilution technique, using a pulmonary artery catheter.

Cardiac Filling Pressure

Right atrial pressure and pulmonary artery occlusion pressure are measured with a pulmonary artery catheter. Measurement of these cardiac filling pressures combined with the value for cardiac output permits construction of right ventricular and left ventricular function curves for use in guiding fluid administration and drug therapy. In addition, measurement of cardiac filling pressures and the mean pulmonary artery pressure through the pulmonary artery catheter, as well as knowledge of the mean arterial pressure, permit the calculation of the pulmonary and systemic vascular resistance (Table 16-8).

Intrapulmonary Shunt

Right-to-left intrapulmonary shunting of blood occurs when there is perfusion of alveoli that are not ventilated. The net effect is a decreased PaO$_2$, reflecting dilution of oxygen in blood exposed to ventilated alveoli, with blood containing less oxygen coming from unventilated alveoli. Calculation of the shunt fraction provides a reliable assessment of the matching of ventilation to perfusion and serves as a useful estimate of the response to various therapeutic interventions during the treatment of acute respiratory failure (Tables 16-9 and 16-10).

Physiologic shunt normally comprises 2% to 5% of the cardiac output. This degree of right-to-left intrapulmonary shunting reflects the passage of pulmonary arterial blood directly to the left side of the circulation through the bronchial and thebesian veins. It should be appreciated that determina-

Table 16-8. Calculation of Pulmonary Vascular Resistance and Systemic Vascular Resistance

$$PVR = MPAP - PAOP/CO \times 80$$
$$SVR = MAP - CVP/CO \times 80$$

Example: The following cardiovascular measurements are obtained by a pulmonary artery catheter and radial artery catheter: MPAP 15 mmHg; PAOP 8 mmHg; MAP 90 mmHg; CVP 5 mmHg; CO 5 L·min^{-1}. Calculated PVR and SVR is as follows:

$$PVR = 15 - 8/5 \times 80$$
$$PVR = 112 \text{ dyn·s·cm}^{-5} \text{ (normal } 50 - 140 \text{ dyn·s·cm}^{-5})$$
$$SVR = 90 - 5/5 \times 80$$
$$SVR = 1360 \text{ dyn·s·cm}^{-5} \text{ (normal } 900 - 1500 \text{ dyn·s·cm}^{-5})$$

MPAP, mean pulmonary artery pressure; PAOP, pulmonary artery occlusion pressure; MAP, mean arterial pressure; CVP, central venous pressure; CO, cardiac output; PVR, pulmonary vascular resistance; SVR, systemic vascular resistance; 80, factor for conversion to dyn·s·cm^{-5}.

Table 16-9. Calculation of the Intrapulmonary Shunt Fraction

$$Q_s/Q_T = CcO_2 - CaO_2/CcO_2 - CvO_2{}^a$$

$$CaO_2 = (Hb \times 1.39)SaO_2 + PaO_2 \times 0.003$$

$$CcO_2 = \text{same calculation as for } CaO_2$$

$$CvO_2 = \text{same calculation as for } CaO_2$$

Q_s, fraction of pulmonary blood flow not exposed to ventilated alveoli; Q_T, total pulmonary blood flow; CaO_2, oxygen content of arterial blood; CcO_2, oxygent content of pulmonary capillary blood; CvO_2, oxygen content of pulmonary venous blood; Hb, hemoglobin concentration; 1.39 ml oxygen bound by hemoglobin; SaO_2, saturation of hemoglobin with oxygen.

[a] Calculation of the shunt fraction using this equation requires the presence of a pulmonary artery catheter to obtain mixed venous and pulmonary capillary blood samples. Furthermore, the number of calculations makes the equation too complex for routine clinical use. An acceptable alternative equation is shown in Table 16-10.

tion of the shunt fraction in a patient breathing less than 100% oxygen reflects the contribution of ventilation-to-perfusion mismatching, as well as the right-to-left intrapulmonary shunt. Calculation of the shunt fraction from measurements obtained in a patient breathing 100% oxygen eliminates the contribution of ventilation-to-perfusion mismatching.

Static Pulmonary Compliance

Static pulmonary compliance is calculated by dividing the tidal volume by the difference between the plateau airway pressure at end-inspiration and the end-inspiratory pressure.[8] This calculation is a useful indicator of lung volumes and the

Table 16-10. Alternative Method for Calculation of the Intrapulmonary Shunt Fraction

$$Q_s/Q_T = A\text{-}aDO_2 (0.003)/(CaO_2 - CvO2) + A\text{-}aDO_2 (0.003)^a$$

Example: The $A\text{-}aDO_2$ in a patient breathing 100% oxygen is 200 mmHg (see Table 16-3 for calculation). Assuming a $CaO_2 - CvO_2$ difference of 5 ml·dl^{-1} (see Table 16-9, for a precise calculation) the Q_s/Q_T (intrapulmonary shunt fraction) is calculated as follows:

$$Q_s/Q_T = 200 (0.003)/5 + 200 (0.003)$$

$$Q_s/Q_T = 0.6/5.6$$

$$Q_s/Q_T = 0.107 \text{ or } 10.7\% \text{ of total pulmonary blood flow}$$

[a] This equation can be used when patients are breathing 100% oxygen, and the PaO_2 is greater than 150 mmHg so as to ensure maximum saturation of hemoglobin with oxygen. The 0.003 factor in the equation is the solubility coefficient for oxygen in plasma.

optimal level of PEEP for use in treatment of acute respiratory failure.

CESSATION OF MECHANICAL SUPPORT OF VENTILATION

The decision to attempt withdrawal of mechanical support of ventilation (weaning) is guided by measurements of pulmonary function. Ultimately, however, it is often an empirical decision based on clinical and physiologic assessment, as well as trial and error. In reality, the process of weaning occurs in three steps: (1) removal of ventilator support, (2) removal of the tracheal tube, and (3) elimination of the need for supplemental inspired oxygen.

Removal of Ventilator Support

Arbitrary guidelines proposed for indicating the feasibility of discontinuing ventilator support of ventilation include (1) vital capacity greater than 15 ml·kg^{-1}, (2) A-aDO$_2$ less than 350 mmHg while the patient is breathing 100% oxygen, (3) PaO$_2$ greater than 60 mmHg while the patient is breathing less than 50% oxygen, (4) maximal inspiratory pressure greater than minus 20 cm H$_2$O with airway occlusion, (5) maintenance of a normal pH, (6) spontaneous breathing rate less than 20 breaths·min^{-1}, and (7) a V$_D$/V$_T$ less than 0.6.[17] Rapid shallow breathing, as reflected by the ratio of breathing frequency to tidal volume, may be an accurate predictor of the likely success or failure in weaning patients from mechanical ventilation.

Ultimately, the decision to attempt withdrawal of ventilator support is individualized, considering not only the status of pulmonary function but also co-existing abnormalities. For example, the level of consciousness, cardiac function, arterial capacity to carry oxygen (hemoglobin concentration), intravascular fluid volume, electrolyte balance (hypokalemia and phosphate depletion interfere with skeletal muscle strength), and nutritional status must be optimized before attempted removal of mechanical support of ventilation. Likewise, control of infection is important before this step in the weaning process is initiated. The use of sedatives and the presence of bronchospasm or excessive secretions may delay attempts at cessation of mechanical ventilatory support.

T tube or synchronized IMV are two methods commonly employed for initiating removal of mechanical support of ventilation. There is no evidence that one method is preferable. Deterioration of oxygenation after withdrawal of mechanical support of ventilation may reflect progressive alveolar collapse that is responsive to treatment with CPAP rather than reinstitution of mechanical ventilation. A progressive decrease in tidal volume and subsequent increase in the PaCO$_2$ after cessation of mechanical support of ventilation may be a consequence of respiratory muscle fatigue. Events that contribute to respiratory muscle fatigue include disuse atrophy, hypokalemia, phosphate depletion, and increasing mechanical loads imposed by alveolar collapse, airway secretions, or bronchospasm. Elimination and correction of these causes is the best treatment of respiratory muscle fatigue.

T Tube

T tube weaning is initiated by connecting the tube in the patient's trachea to a device (T tube) through which oxygen-enriched and humidified gases are delivered. In addition, CPAP (2.5 to 5 cm H_2O) is often delivered through the T tube to the airway. The use of CPAP minimizes decreases in FRC associated with cessation of positive airway pressure.[18] Initially, patients are allowed to breath spontaneously for 5 to 10 minutes each hour. Tachypnea (greater than 30 breaths·min^{-1}), tachycardia, or deterioration in the level of consciousness during these brief periods of spontaneous ventilation confirms that the weaning attempt has been premature, and mechanical support of ventilation is promptly reinstituted. When pulmonary function has recovered to the extent that weaning from mechanical ventilation is appropriate, it is possible to lengthen the periods of spontaneous ventilation gradually.

Intermittent Mandatory Ventilation

IMV permits the patient to breathe spontaneously between a mechanically delivered tidal volume, using the same inspired concentration of oxygen and PEEP provided by mechanical inflation of the lungs. The mechanical tidal volume can be provided as a nonsynchronous mandatory breath delivered at a preset interval or as a synchronized breath initiated by the patient's spontaneous effort to breath. Cessation of mechanical support of ventilation is initiated by gradually decreasing the number of mechanical breaths delivered each minute. Ideally, the rate of IMV is sequentially decreased as long as the $PaCO_2$ is maintained at a level that results in a pHa of 7.35 to 7.45.

An advantage of IMV is gradual rather than abrupt conversion to spontaneous ventilation. In addition, this mode of ventilation is associated with a low mean airway pressure, which minimizes interference with venous return and decreases the likelihood of pulmonary barotrauma. The presence of spontaneous breathing during IMV also maintains use of muscles of respiration, which should decrease the likelihood of disuse atrophy.

Removal of the Tracheal Tube

Removal of the tracheal tube should be considered if the patient tolerates 2 hours of spontaneous breathing during T tube weaning or when an IMV rate of 1 to 2 breaths·min^{-1} is

tolerated without deterioration of arterial blood gases, mental status, or cardiac function. For example, the PaO_2 should remain above 60 mmHg while breathing less than 50% oxygen. Likewise, the $PaCO_2$ should remain less than 50 mmHg, and the pH should remain above 7.30. Additional important criteria that may be considered before extubation of the trachea include the need for less than 5 cm H_2O PEEP, (2) spontaneous breathing rate less than 30 breaths·min^{-1}, and vital capacity greater than 15 ml·kg^{-1}. These patients should also be alert with active laryngeal reflexes and the ability to generate an effective cough, so as to clear secretions from the airways.

Elimination of the Need for Supplemental Oxygen

Supplemental oxygen is often needed after removal of the secured airway. This need reflects persistence of ventilation-to-perfusion mismatching. Weaning from supplemental oxygen is accomplished by gradual decreases in the inspired concentration of oxygen, as guided by measurement of the PaO_2 and monitoring of the SaO_2 by pulse oximetry.

LUNG TRANSPLANTATION

Single-lung transplantation is a consideration for patients experiencing end-stage respiratory failure especially if the diagnosis is chronic interstitial pulmonary fibrosis.[19] Double-lung transplantation is a more likely selection for patients with chronic obstructive pulmonary disease or cystic fibrosis. Patients with cardiac disease or increased pulmonary vascular resistance owing to cardiac disease are more suited for heart-lung transplantation. Treatment with corticosteroids limits consideration for lung transplantation, in view of the association between this therapy and bronchial dehiscence. Physiologically, patients selected for lung transplantation most often demonstrate a restrictive pattern of lung disease and a large A-aDO$_2$. Mild to moderate degrees of pulmonary hypertension, and possibly some degree of right heart failure, are possible. The ability of the recipient's right ventricle to maintain a sufficient stroke volume in the presence of acute increases in pulmonary vascular resistance produced by clamping the pulmonary artery before pneumonectomy is evaluated preoperatively.

Management of Anesthesia

Management of anesthesia for lung transplantation invokes the principles followed in performing anesthesia for a pneumonectomy. Scrupulous attention to asepsis is important, as these patients are immunosuppressed. Monitors include an intra-arterial and pulmonary artery catheter, pulse oximeter, and capnograph. Pulmonary artery pressure monitoring is especially important in these patients. There are no clear drugs of choice for induction and maintenance of anesthesia and skeletal muscle paralysis. However, drug-induced histamine release would be undesirable, whereas drug-induced bronchodilation would seem useful. Intubation of the trachea is done with a double-lumen endobronchial tube; placement is verified by fiberoptic bronchoscopy. Intraoperative problems may include arterial hypoxemia, especially when one lung anesthesia is initiated, and pulmonary hypertension, when the pulmonary artery is clamped. When arterial hypoxemia accompanies one lung ventilation, a trial of PEEP to the dependent ventilated lung may be considered. Infusion of prostacyclin may be useful for controlling pulmonary hypertension. In extreme cases, support with partial cardiopulmonary bypass may be required. Bronchospasm has been reported after heart-lung transplantation, even though the transplanted lung is denervated.[20] Connection of the donor lung to the recipient is usually in the sequence of pulmonary veins to the recipient's left atrium, anastomosis of the pulmonary artery, and finally bronchial anastomosis, often with an omental wrap. Postoperatively, mechanical support of ventilation is continued until it is appropriate to initiate the weaning process.[21] The principal causes of mortality are bronchial dehiscence or respiratory failure owing to infection or rejection. The denervated donor lung deprives the patient of a normal cough reflex from the lower airways and predisposes to the development of pneumonia. Pulmonary function tests are usually normal, in the absence of rejection.

REFERENCES

1. Bone RC, Jacobs ER. Advances in pharmacologic treatment of acute lung injury and septic shock. In: Stoelting RK, Barash PG, Gallagher TJ, eds. Advances in Anesthesia. Chicago. Year Book Medical Publishers 1986;327–45

2. Schmidt GA, Hall JB. Acute or chronic respiratory failure: Assessment and management of patients with COPD in the emergent setting. JAMA 1989;261:3444–53

3. Rossaint R, Falke KJ, Lopez F, Slama K, Pison U, Zapol WM. Inhaled nitric oxide for the adult respiratory distress syndrome. N Engl J Med 1993;328:399–405

4. Segredo V, Caldwell JE, Matthay MA, Gruenke LD, Miller RD. Persistent paralysis in critically ill patients after long-term administration of vecuronium. N Engl J Med 1992;327:524–8

5. O'Rourke PP, Crone RK. High-frequency ventilation. A new approach to respiratory support. JAMA 1983;250:2845–7

6. Bishop MJ, Benson MS, Sato P, Pierson DJ. Comparison of high-frequency jet ventilation with conventional mechanical ventilation for bronchopleural fistula. Anesth Analg 1987;66:833–8

7. Malo J, Ali J, Wood LDH. How does positive end-expiratory pressure reduce intrapulmonary shunt in canine pulmonary edema? J Appl Physiol 1984;57:1002–8

8. Suter PM, Fairley HB, Isenberg MD. Optimum end-expiratory airway pressure in patients with acute pulmonary failure. N Engl J Med 1975;292:284–9

9. Jardin F, Farcot J-C, Boisante L, et al. Influence of positive end-expiratory pressure on left ventricular performance. N Engl J Med 1981;304:387–92

10. Rochester DF. Malnutrition and the respiratory muscles. Clin Chest Med 1986;7:91–5

11. Shuman RB, Shuster DP, Zuckerman GR. Prophylactic therapy for stress ulcer bleeding: A reappraisal. Ann Intern Med 1987; 106:562–7

12. Doyle DJ. Arterial/alveolar oxygen tension ratio: A critical appraisal. Can Anaesth Soc J 1986;33:471–4

13. Ream AK, Reitz BA, Silverberg G. Temperature correction of PCO_2 and pH in estimating acid-base status: An example of the emperor's new clothes? Anesthesiology 1982;56:41–4

14. Nanju AA, Whitlow KJ. Is it necessary to transport arterial blood samples on ice for pH and gas analysis? Can Anaesth Soc J 1984; 31:568–71

15. Lawson NW, Butler GH, Ray CT. Alkalosis and cardiac arrhythmias. Anesth Analg 1973;52:951–64

16. Sullivan SF, Patterson RW. Posthyperventilation hypoxia: Theoretical considerations in man. Anesthesiology 1968;29:981–6

17. Yang KL, Tobin MJ. A prospective study of indexes predicting the outcome of trials of weaning from mechanical ventilation. N Engl J Med 1991;324:1445–50

18. Brochard L, Isabey D, Piquet J, et al. Reversal of acute exacerbations of chronic obstructive lung disease by inspiratory assistance with a face mask. N Engl J Med 1990;323:1523–30

19. Conacher ID. Isolated lung transplantation: A review of problems and guide to anaesthesia. Br J Anaesth 1988;61:468–74

20. Casella ES, Humphrey LS. Bronchospasm after cardiopulmonary bypass in a heart-lung transplant recipient. Anesthesiology 1988; 69:135–8

21. Smiley RM, Navedo AT, Kirby T, Schulman LL. Postoperative independent lung ventilation in a single-lung transplant patient. Anesthesiology 1991;74:1144–8

17
Diseases of the Nervous System

Perhaps in no other area of anesthesia is the selection of drugs, technique of ventilation of the lungs, and choice of monitors more important than in the care of the patient with a disease involving the central nervous system. In addition, concepts of cerebral protection and resuscitation assume unique importance in these patients.

INTRACRANIAL TUMORS

Intracranial (brain) tumors may be classified as primary tumors (those arising from the brain and its coverings) or metastatic tumors[1] (Table 17-1). Astrocytoma and medulloblastoma are the most common primary brain tumors in children, whereas the most common brain tumors in adults are meningioma, glioblastoma, pituitary adenoma, and metastatic tumor. An astrocytoma typically begins as a slow-growing tumor in a cerebral hemisphere, while a medulloblastoma most often arises in the cerebellum. Meningioma is the most common benign brain tumor, accounting for about 15% of all primary brain tumors. A defect in chromosome 22 is present in many affected patients. Evidence of a hormonal component is the enhanced meningioma growth during pregnancy. This tumor arises from arachnoidal cells, is slow growing, and may infiltrate the skull, with resultant evidence of osteoblastic activity on the skull radiograph. Glioblastoma is a highly malignant and infiltrative intracranial tumor that most often arises in a cerebral hemisphere. The classification of a pituitary adenoma as chromophobe, basophilic, and eosinophilic is based on the staining properties of granules present in cells of the tumor. Nearly 80% of pituitary adenomas are classified as chromophobe. These tumors rarely secrete hormones; rather, they produce panhypopituitarism by virtue of expansion and compression of normal anterior pituitary tissue. In addition, suprasellar extension of this adenoma characteristically produces bitemporal hemianopia, owing to compression of the optic chiasm. A chromophobe adenoma may be part of an inherited syndrome, characterized by multiple endocrine neoplasia (see Chapter 22). A metastatic intracranial tumor is most often from a primary site in the lung or breast. Malignant melanoma, hypernephroma, and carcinoma of the colon are also likely to spread to the brain. A metastatic brain tumor is the likely diagnosis when diagnostic tests indicate the presence of more than one lesion. An acoustic neuroma is a benign tumor that grows from the nerve sheath of the vestibular (cranial nerve VIII) nerve. Initial manifestations of an acoustic neuroma are progressive unilateral sensorineural hearing loss and vertigo, followed by facial palsy and numbness due to compression of the facial nerve as the tumor fills the internal auditory meatus.

Diagnosis

In addition to the classic symptoms and findings on neurologic examination, the presence of an intracranial tumor can be substantiated by specific diagnostic imaging techniques. In this regard, computed tomography with contrast enhancement and magnetic resonance imaging have revolutionized the capability of imaging techniques in identifying brain tumors. Positron emission tomography and single photo emission computed tomography permit imaging not only of structures, but also of some of the functional characteristics of the brain, including blood flow and the concentrations and locations of specific neurotransmitters. Technetium brain scanning and pneumoencephalography are no longer considered useful in the diagnosis of a brain tumor.[1] A vascular mass can be distinguished from a brain tumor on magnetic resonance imaging angiography. Magnetic resonance imaging with contrast agents improves the visualization of certain intracranial tumors (meningiomas, acoustic neuromas) that are not well seen with

181

Table 17-1. Classification of Brain Tumors

Primary Brain Tumor	Histologically Malignant
Histologically Benign	Glioblastoma
Meningioma	Medulloblastoma
Pituitary adenoma	**Metastatic Brain Tumor**
Astrocytoma	
Acoustic neuroma	

computed tomography or that may be inconspicuous in enhanced magnetic resonance imaging. Patients with claustrophobia and those with implanted metal devices (cardiac pacemakers, mechanical heart valves, intracranial metal clips) are not candidates for magnetic resonance imaging.

Treatment

Surgery is part of the initial management of virtually all brain tumors, as it quickly establishes the diagnosis and relieves symptoms due to a space-occupying intracranial mass. The development of the operating microscope, the fusion of the imaging system with the resection technique, and the intraoperative monitoring of sensory evoked responses have combined to improve the effectiveness of tumor resection. Intraoperative monitoring of brain stem auditory evoked responses for the resection of an acoustic neuroma, visual evoked responses for parasellar tumors, and somatosensory evoked responses for parenchymal and brain stem lesions may be useful in guiding the surgical resection. Intraoperative ultrasonography can establish the location of a brain tumor for biopsy or resection. Surgery of the areas of the cortex controlling speech and motor function may be performed under local anesthesia with the use of stereotactic and stimulation techniques to provide precise tumor resection. Laser resection of a brain tumor permits the vaporization of tumor without manipulation of the brain. For a benign tumor, complete resection may be curative, whereas extensive resection of a malignant tumor is likely to prolong survival.

Radiation therapy is particularly useful in the management of a malignant brain tumor. An increase in the neurologic deficit during radiation treatment is probably due to cerebral edema, which usually responds to treatment with a corticosteroid. Cardiorespiratory arrest has been reported after radiation of a brain stem tumor.[2] Brachytherapy is the stereotactic implantation of radiation sources in a tumor for 4 to 6 days. This form of treatment is most useful in prolonging the survival of the patient with a glioblastoma. Radiation therapy is avoided in children younger than 2 years of age because of its long-term effects, which include developmental delay and panhypopituitarism. Chemotherapy, often combination therapy, is the initial treatment for many malignant brain tumors in children. Monoclonal antibody techniques may become useful in the future development of tumor-specific antibodies.

Signs and Symptoms

The major mechanism for the production of signs and symptoms by an intracranial tumor is increased intracranial pressure (ICP). Symptoms of increased ICP include headache, nausea and vomiting, mental changes, and disturbances of consciousness. During the early stages of intracranial hypertension, it is common for symptoms to be most prominent during the early morning hours. The patient will be awakened by a dull headache, followed by spontaneous vomiting. Symptoms will then subside until the next morning. Presumably, increases in the $PaCO_2$ and the associated cerebral vasodilation that accompanies sleep produce an increase in intracranial contents that exceeds the limits of compensation and ICP increases (Fig. 17-1). Progressive increases in ICP eventually result in unexplained fatigue and drowsiness. Papilledema is often accompanied by visual disturbances. A seizure occurring for the first time in an adult, without an apparent cause, should be presumed to be a brain tumor and investigated with computed tomography or magnetic resonance imaging, or both. Systemic blood pressure may be increased, in an attempt to maintain cerebral perfusion pressure in the presence of intracranial hypertension. As the blood pressure increases, there is a corresponding decrease in heart rate, due to reflex activation of the carotid sinus by hypertension. Local tissue destruction by tumor infiltration or compression leads to symptoms determined by the area of the brain involved. For example, mental and behavioral changes may be prominent in a patient with an intracranial tumor in the frontal cortex. Cerebral edema surrounding an expanding intracranial tumor, particularly one with a rapid growth rate, occurs frequently. The edema may contribute to the loss of neurologic function, giving the false impression that the tumor is large and highly destructive. The presence of edema around an intracranial tumor is thought to result from increased permeability of the tumor capillaries, permitting the penetration of protein and fluid into adjacent normal brain tissue. This abnormal permeability is the basis for the lucency of tissues on computed tomography.

An intracranial tumor may result in displacement of the brain, as well as compression of neural tissues at distant sites. The most common example is a supratentorial tumor that leads to herniation of the uncus of the temporal lobe through the incisura of the tentorium. The oculomotor nerve becomes compressed at the tentorial notch, resulting in a dilated, unreactive homolateral pupil. Apnea and unconsciousness follow, if the midbrain is compressed. Compression of the posterior cerebral artery against the edge of the tentorium may lead to infarction of the occipital lobe and contralateral hemianopia. Compression of the cerebral peduncle produces contralateral hemiplegia. A posterior fossa tumor leads to obstruction of the normal flow of cerebrospinal fluid (CSF), and the resulting

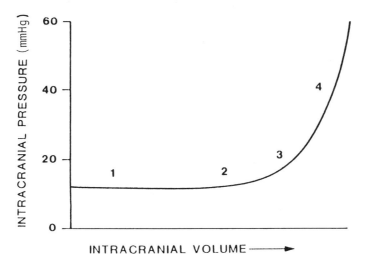

Fig. 17-1. A pressure-volume compliance curve depicts the impact of increasing intracranial volume on intracranial pressure (ICP). As intracranial volume increases from point 1 to 2, ICP does not increase, since cerebrospinal fluid is shifted from the cranium into the spinal subarachnoid space. A patient with an intracranial tumor, but between points 1 and 2 on the curve, is unlikely to manifest symptoms of increased ICP. A patient on the rising portion of the curve (point 3) can no longer compensate for an increase in intracranial volume; ICP begins to increase and is likely to be associated with clinical symptoms. An additional increase in intracranial volume at this point (point 3), as produced by increased cerebral blood flow during anesthesia, can precipitate an abrupt increase in ICP (point 4).

increase in ICP predisposes to herniation of the cerebellar tonsils through the foramen magnum, manifested as a decreased level of consciousness and slow breathing rate.

Management of Anesthesia

Management of anesthesia for the removal of an intracranial tumor requires an understanding of the pressure-volume compliance relationships of the brain, the methods available to monitor and decrease ICP, and the determinants of cerebral blood flow (CBF). The goals of perioperative anesthesia management are often based on keeping the ICP within a normal range and the recognition that autoregulation of CBF may be impaired.

Pressure-Volume Compliance Curve

The pressure-volume compliance curve reflects changes produced by an expanding intracranial tumor (Fig. 17-1). The curve plots the change in ICP that accompanies the alteration in intracranial volume produced by the tumor. As the tumor gradually enlarges, CSF in the cranium is shifted into the spinal subarachnoid space, preventing an increase in ICP above its normal value of about 15 mmHg. In addition, increased absorption of CSF attenuates any increase in pressure produced by an expanding tumor. At this stage, there are minimal clinical

symptoms suggestive of an intracranial tumor. Eventually, a point is reached on the pressure-volume compliance curve at which even a small increase in intracranial volume produced by the expanding tumor results in a marked increase in the ICP. At this point on the pressure-volume compliance curve, anesthetic drugs and techniques that affect cerebral blood volume can adversely and abruptly increase the ICP.

This marked increase in ICP can interfere with the delivery of adequate blood flow to the brain. For example, cerebral perfusion pressure is determined by the difference between mean arterial pressure and right atrial pressure. When ICP is higher than right atrial pressure, the cerebral perfusion pressure is determined by the difference between mean arterial pressure and ICP. If cerebral perfusion pressure is substantially decreased in response to increased ICP, the blood pressure shows a compensatory increase, in an attempt to restore perfusion pressure and thus maintain CBF. Ultimately, this compensatory mechanism fails, producing cerebral ischemia.

Monitoring Intracranial Pressure

ICP can be monitored continuously by a catheter placed through a burr hole into a cerebral ventricle or by a transducer (Richmond bolt) placed on the surface of the brain. A normal ICP wave is pulsatile and varies with the cardiac impulse and breathing. The mean ICP should remain below 15 mmHg. The importance of monitoring ICP in the patient with a space-

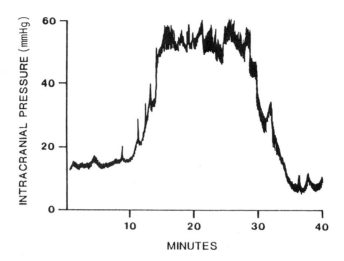

Fig. 17-2. Schematic diagram of a plateau wave. The increased intracranial pressure (ICP) typically occurs abruptly, from normal or near-normal ICP. A plateau wave persists for 10 to 20 minutes, followed by a rapid decrease in the ICP, often to a level below that present before the onset of the plateau wave.

occupying intracranial tumor is emphasized by the observation that an alteration in ICP may not be accompanied by a change in the neurologic examination or in the vital signs. Furthermore, the first evidence of a hazardous increase in ICP in an unresponsive patient may be sudden bilateral pupillary dilation, associated with herniation of the brain stem through the foramen magnum. Delay in the initiation of treatment to reduce ICP until these signs appear may be unrewarding, as irreversible brain damage is likely.

Plateau Wave

An abrupt increase in ICP observed during continuous monitoring is known as a plateau wave (Fig. 17-2). Characteristically, the ICP increases from normal or a near-normal level to as high as 100 mmHg during a plateau wave. During this increase, the patient often becomes overtly symptomatic, and spontaneous hyperventilation can occur. Typically, a plateau wave lasts 10 to 20 minutes, after which ICP rapidly decreases to a level below that present before onset of the waves. The mechanism for this sudden increase is unknown, although an abrupt increase in intracranial blood volume may be responsible. This increased blood volume eventually initiates a decrease in CSF volume, leading to a subsequent decrease in ICP.

Events that can be identified as initiating causes of a plateau wave include anxiety, painful stimulation, and the induction of anesthesia. Indeed, in a normal patient, anxiety and painful stimulation can elicit a substantial increase in oxygen uptake and CBF. In the presence of an intracranial tumor, this increase can lead to an abrupt increase in ICP. Therefore, nox-

ious stimuli should be avoided in the patient with an intracranial tumor, regardless of the level of consciousness. Hence, the liberal use of analgesics to avoid pain, even in the unresponsive patient, is indicated. Obviously, support of ventilation to avoid hypercarbia secondary to drug-induced depression of ventilation will be necessary, especially when an opioid is used. Likewise, it is crucial to establish a depth of anesthesia sufficient to block the pressor response to laryngoscopy or noxious surgical stimulation.

Methods to Decrease Intracranial Pressure

Methods to decrease ICP include posture, hyperventilation of the lungs, CSF drainage, and administration of hyperosmotic drugs, diuretics, corticosteroids, and barbiturates. It is not possible to identify reliably the level of ICP that can interfere with regional CBF in an individual patient. Therefore, a frequent recommendation is to treat any sustained elevation of ICP that exceeds 20 mmHg. Treatment may be indicated when ICP is less than 20 mmHg, if the appearance of an occasional plateau wave suggests low intracranial compliance.

Posture

Posture is important in ensuring optimal venous drainage from the brain. For example, elevation of the head to about 30 degrees will encourage venous outflow from the brain and lower the ICP. Extreme flexion or rotation of the head can obstruct the jugular veins and restrict venous outflow from the brain. The head-down position is to be avoided, as this position can markedly increase ICP.

Hyperventilation

Hyperventilation of the lungs is an effective and rapid method of lowering ICP. In an adult, the recommendation is to maintain the $PaCO_2$ between 25 and 30 mmHg. Extreme hyperventilation of the lungs can theoretically reduce CBF to the point of cerebral ischemia. Nevertheless, there is no evidence that cerebral ischemia occurs when the $PaCO_2$ is above 20 mmHg. Nevertheless, since no additional beneficial therapeutic effect is demonstrable by lowering $PaCO_2$ to an extremely low level, it seems reasonable to strive to achieve a level of 25 to 30 mmHg when treating an elevation of ICP. The duration of the efficacy of hyperventilation of the lungs in decreasing ICP is unknown. In volunteers, however, the effect of hyperventilation wanes with time, and CBF returns to normal after about 6 hours.[3]

In children, it may be appropriate to initiate more aggressive hyperventilation of the lungs than is recommended for adults, so as to maintain the $PaCO_2$ between 20 and 25 mmHg. Presumably, the increased therapeutic benefit of this lower $PaCO_2$ reflects the relatively high CBF blood flow that may be present in children, particularly in the presence of acute head injury. Also, in contrast to adults, there is a suggestion that hyperventilation of the lungs in children is associated with a sustained decrease in CBF beyond 6 hours.

Cerebrospinal Fluid Drainage

CSF drainage from either the lateral cerebral ventricles or the lumbar subarachnoid space is an effective method of reducing intracranial volume and ICP. Lumbar drainage in a patient with increased ICP is not recommended, since herniation of the cerebellum through the foramen magnum might occur. Therefore, lumbar drainage is generally reserved for cases in which surgical exposure may be difficult, such as the patient undergoing an operation on the pituitary gland or surgical removal of an intracranial aneurysm.

Hyperosmotic Drugs

Hyperosmotic drugs, such as mannitol and urea, are important and effective methods of reducing ICP. These drugs produce a transient increase in the osmolarity of plasma, which acts to draw water from tissues, including the brain. The purpose of therapy with a hyperosmotic drug is not to dehydrate the patient, but rather to draw fluid from the brain, along an osmotic gradient. As such, it is an error not to replace some of the intravascular fluid lost through the kidneys (see the section, Fluid Therapy). Failure to replace intravascular fluid volume can result in hypotension and can jeopardize maintenance

of an adequate cerebral perfusion pressure. Likewise, urinary loss of electrolytes, particularly potassium, may require careful monitoring and replacement. Moreover, an intact blood-brain barrier is necessary, so that mannitol or urea can exert maximum beneficial effects on brain size. If the blood-brain barrier is disrupted, these drugs may cross into the brain, causing cerebral edema and an increase in brain size. The brain eventually adapts to a sustained elevation in plasma osmolarity, such that chronic use of a hyperosmotic drug is likely to become less effective.

Mannitol is administered in a dose of 0.25 to 1.0 $g \cdot kg^{-1}$ IV over 15 to 30 minutes. There is little difference in ICP-lowering effects with this dose range, but a higher dose may last longer.[4] A smaller dose requires less volume for administration and avoids the risk of serum hyperosmolarity. This dose range of mannitol permits removal of an estimated 100 ml of water from the brain. After administration, a decrease in ICP is seen within 30 minutes, and the maximum effect occurs within 1 to 2 hours. Urine output can reach 1 to 2 L within 1 hour after initiating the administration of mannitol. Appropriate infusion of crystalloid and colloid solution is often necessary to prevent adverse changes in the plasma concentration of electrolytes and intravascular fluid volume due to the brisk diuresis. Conversely, mannitol can initially increase intravascular fluid volume, emphasizing the need to monitor carefully those patients who have limited cardiac reserve. Mannitol also has direct vascular vasodilating properties that can contribute to increased cerebral blood volume and ICP. The duration of the hyperosmotic effect of mannitol is about 6 hours. Mannitol is not associated with a high incidence of rebound increases in ICP after this time. Furthermore, the incidence of venous thrombosis after the administration of mannitol is low.

Urea is administered in a dose of 1 to 1.5 $g \cdot kg^{-1}$ IV over 15 to 30 minutes. Rebound increases in ICP occur after 3 to 7 hours and last about 12 hours, before once beginning to decline slowly. Rebound hypertension reflects the penetration of urea molecules into the brain and the subsequent passage of water along a concentration gradient. Another disadvantage of urea is a high incidence of venous thrombosis and the possibility of tissue necrosis, should extravasation of the urea occur.

Diuretics

Diuretics, particularly furosemide and ethacrynic acid, have been used in an attempt to promote decreases in ICP. A diuretic is particularly useful when there is evidence of increased intravascular fluid volume and pulmonary edema. In this instance, the promotion of diuresis and systemic dehydration can improve arterial oxygenation, with a concomitant decreases in ICP.

Furosemide (1 $mg \cdot kg^{-1}$ IV) administered to a patient with normal ICP, who is undergoing craniotomy for treatment of an intracranial tumor or aneurysm, is more effective in de-

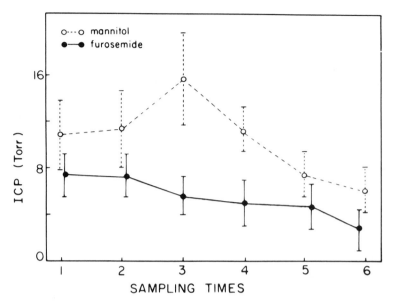

Fig. 17-3. Intracranial pressure (ICP) (mean ± SE) was measured before (sampling times 1 and 2) and after (sampling times 3 to 6) the rapid injection of mannitol (1 g·kg^{-1} IV) or furosemide (1 mg·kg^{-1} IV) to 20 adult patients scheduled for removal of an intracranial tumor. ICP was increased at the onset of mannitol-induced diuresis (3). By contrast, ICP was decreased at all measurement times after administration of furosemide. (From Cottrell JE, Robustelli A, Post K, Turndorf H. Furosemide- and mannitol-induced changes in intracranial pressure and serum osmolarity and electrolytes. Anesthesiology 1977;47:28–30, with permission.)

creasing ICP than is mannitol (1 g·kg^{-1} IV)[5] (Fig. 17-3). Furosemide does not significantly alter either plasma osmolarity or the concentration of potassium. Conversely, mannitol increases plasma osmolarity, and the plasma concentration of potassium is decreased. On the basis of these observations, it has been recommended that furosemide replace mannitol for the treatment of the patient with increased ICP, particularly if the blood-brain barrier is altered or if the water content of the lungs is increased.[5]

Corticosteroids

Corticosteroids are effective in lowering increased ICP due to the development of localized cerebral edema around an intracranial tumor. The drugs most frequently used for this purpose are dexamethasone or methylprednisolone. The mechanism for the beneficial effect of corticosteroids is unknown but may involve stabilization of capillary membranes or reductions in the production of CSF, or both. The patient with a metastatic intracranial tumor and glioblastoma responds best to corticosteroids. Improved neurologic status and the disappearance of signs of increased ICP, such as headache or nausea and vomiting, frequently occur within 12 to 36 hours after initiating treatment with a corticosteroid. The incidence of

pulmonary infection or gastrointestinal hemorrhage has not been shown to be increased by the short-term use of a corticosteroid.

Barbiturates

Administration of barbiturates in high doses is particularly effective in treating increased ICP that develops after an acute head injury. This approach is especially useful when other, more traditional, methods of treatment have failed (see the section, Head Injury).

Determinants of Cerebral Blood Flow

Determinants of CBF include (1) PaCO$_2$, (2) PaO$_2$, (3) arterial blood pressure and autoregulation, (4) venous blood pressure, and (5) anesthetic drugs and techniques. Cerebral blood vessels receive innervation from the autonomic nervous system, but the impact of this innervation on CBF is minimal. For example, it is estimated that neurogenic control can alter CBF by only 5% to 10%.[6] Furthermore, stellate ganglion block does not significantly increase CBF.

PaCO₂

Variations in $PaCO_2$ produce corresponding changes in CBF (Fig. 17-4). As a guideline, CBF (normal is about 50 ml·100 $g^{-1}·min^{-1}$) increases 1 ml·100 $g^{-1}·min^{-1}$ for each 1-mmHg increase in $PaCO_2$ above 40 mmHg. A similar decrease in CBF occurs during hypocarbia, such that CBF is decreased about 50% when $PaCO_2$ is 20 mmHg. The impact of $PaCO_2$ on CBF is mediated by pH variations in the CSF around the walls of arterioles. A decreased pH causes intense cerebral vasodilation, and an increased pH causes vasoconstriction. A corresponding change in resistance to blood flow exerts a predictable effect on CBF.

The ability of hypocapnia to decrease CBF and ICP is the basis for modern neuroanesthesia. Concern that cerebral hypoxia due to vasoconstriction can occur when $PaCO_2$ is lowered below 20 mmHg has not been substantiated.[2] Nevertheless, because there is no evidence of an increased therapeutic benefit at an extremely low $PaCO_2$, it seems reasonable to recommend maintaining $PaCO_2$ between 25 and 30 mmHg during anesthesia for removal of an intracranial tumor. The long-term value of hypocapnia in decreasing ICP is offset by the return of CSF pH to normal, permitting an increase in CBF despite a persistent decrease in $PaCO_2$.[3] This adaptive change, which reflects active transport of bicarbonate ions into or from the CSF, requires about 6 hours before the pH returns to normal.

The influence of carbon dioxide on local CBF may be altered by acidosis, which often surrounds an intracranial tumor. For example, acid metabolites from a tumor diffuse into adjacent tissues, causing maximal vasodilation and increased blood flow around the tumor. These vessels have lost their responsiveness to carbon dioxide, and vasomotor paralysis is present. Increased blood flow in the area of an intracranial tumor has been termed *luxury perfusion*.[6] When $PaCO_2$ is allowed to increase, blood flow is shunted away from the tumor. This response reflects the vasodilation of normal vessels but no change in the vessels that have already been maximally dilated; thus, the pressure gradient for blood flow tends to be reversed. This phenomenon has been termed the *intracerebral steal syndrome*. Conversely, hypocapnia constricts normal vessels, whereas those manifesting vasomotor paralysis are not altered; the result is a change in the pressure gradient that flavors flow to acidotic areas surrounding the tumor. This response is referred to as the inverse steal, or Robin Hood phenomenon. The relative importance of these phenomena is unknown, but it is likely that their occurrence is rare. In the absence of regional CBF measurements, it is not known whether an individual patient will respond physiologically or

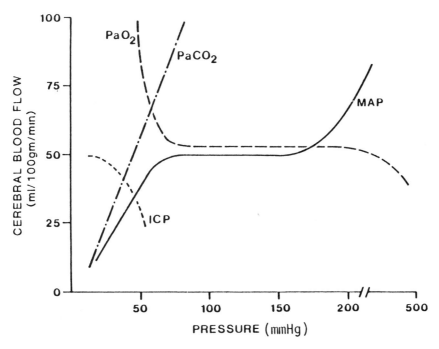

Fig. 17-4. Schematic depiction of the impact of intracranial pressure (ICP), PaO_2, $PaCO_2$, and mean arterial pressure (MAP) on cerebral blood flow.

paradoxically to an alteration in $PaCO_2$. Therefore, the logic of treating focal cerebral ischemia with deliberate hypoventilation or hyperventilation of the lungs is questionable. The prudent approach would be to maintain a normal or moderately decreased $PaCO_2$ when a cerebral steal response is a consideration. If decreased ICP is the goal, the recommendation is to maintain $PaCO_2$ at 25 to 30 mmHg. Inhaled anesthetics do not alter the responsiveness of the cerebral circulation to changes in $PaCO_2$.

PaO_2

Decreased PaO_2 does not lead to significantly increased CBF, until a threshold value of about 50 mmHg is reached (Fig. 17-4). Below this threshold, there is abrupt cerebral vasodilation, and CBF increases. Furthermore, the combination of arterial hypoxemia and hypercarbia exerts a synergistic effect, with an increase in CBF that exceeds the increase that would be produced by either factor alone.[7]

Arterial Blood Pressure and Autoregulation

The ability of the brain to maintain CBF at a constant level, despite a change in mean arterial pressure, is known as autoregulation (Fig. 17-4). Autoregulation is an active vascular response, characterized by arterial constriction when the distending blood pressure is increased, and arterial dilation in response to a decrease in the blood pressure. The upper and lower limits of mean arterial pressure with maintenance of autoregulation have been defined. For example, in a normotensive patient, the lower limit of mean arterial pressure associated with autoregulation is about 60 mmHg. Below this threshold, CBF decreases and becomes directly related to mean arterial pressure. Indeed, at mean arterial pressures of 40 to 55 mmHg, symptoms of cerebral ischemia may appear, in the form of nausea, dizziness, and slow cerebration. Autoregulation of CBF also has an upper limit, above which flow becomes directly proportional to the mean arterial pressure. This upper limit of autoregulation in a normotensive patient is a mean arterial pressure of about 150 mmHg. Above this threshold, CBF increases, causing overdistension of the walls of the cerebral blood vessels. As a result, fluid is forced across vessel walls into the brain tissue, producing cerebral edema.[8]

Autoregulation of CBF is altered in the presence of chronic hypertension. Specifically, the autoregulation curve is displaced to the right, such that a higher mean arterial pressure is tolerated before CBF becomes pressure dependent. However, the adaptation of cerebral vessels to increased blood pressure requires 1 to 2 months. Indeed, acute hypertension, as seen in the child with glomerulonephritis or in the patient with pregnancy-induced hypertension, often produces signs of central nervous system dysfunction at levels of mean arterial pressure tolerated by patients who are chronically hypertensive. Likewise, an acute hypertensive episode associated with

stimulation of laryngoscopy or surgery may cause a breakthrough of autoregulation. The lower limit of autoregulation is also shifted upward in the chronically hypertensive patient, such that acute decreases in blood pressure are not tolerated to the same low level as in normotensive patients. After gradual decreases in blood pressure occur using antihypertensive therapy, however, the tolerance of the brain to hypotension may improve, as the autoregulation curve shifts back toward its original position.[8]

Autoregulation of CBF may be lost or impaired in a variety of conditions, including the presence of an intracranial tumor or head trauma and the administration of a volatile anesthetic. The loss of autoregulation in the blood vessels surrounding an intracranial tumor reflects acidosis leading to maximum vasodilation, such that blood flow becomes pressure dependent.

In animals, autoregulation of CBF in response to changes in blood pressure is retained during the administration of 1 MAC isoflurane but not halothane[9] (Fig. 17-5). The loss of autoregulation during administration of halothane is possibly responsible for the greater brain swelling seen in animals anesthetized with this drug as compared with isoflurane.

Venous Blood Pressure

Venous blood pressure is usually low in the supine or standing position, such that mean arterial pressure is the predominant determinant of cerebral perfusion pressure. An increase in CBF can increase the pressure in cerebral veins, due to the rigid bony orifices surrounding the venous exits from the cranium. Furthermore, the rigidity of dural layers surrounding the intracranial venous sinuses may result in increased venous pressure when CBF is increased. An increase in central venous pressure is directly transmitted to the intracranial veins. The impact of increased central venous pressure on cerebral perfusion pressure and ICP must be appreciated when considering the use of positive airway pressure during intracranial surgery or in a patient with increased ICP. Indeed, the use of positive end-expiratory pressure may produce adverse increases in ICP and thus decrease cerebral perfusion pressure in the patient with an intracranial tumor.[4,10] Elevated venous pressure can also contribute to increased bleeding during intracranial surgery.

Anesthetic Drugs

Volatile anesthetics administered during normocapnia in a concentration above 0.6 MAC are potent cerebral vasodilators that produce dose-dependent increases in CBF[11] (Fig. 17-6). These drug-induced increases in CBF are greatest with halothane, intermediate with enflurane and desflurane, and least for isoflurane, occurring despite a concomitant decrease in cerebral metabolic oxygen requirements. Ketamine is also a potent cerebral vasodilator. Normally, the tendency of ICP to increase in response to an increase in CBF is prevented by the displacement of CSF from the cranium. In the patient with an intracranial tumor, however, this compensatory mecha-

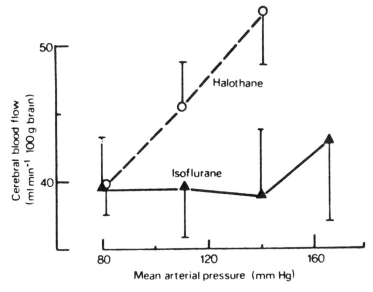

Fig. 17-5. In animals, autoregulation of cerebral blood flow in response to changes in mean arterial pressure is preserved in the presence of 1 MAC isoflurane, but not halothane. (From Eger EI. Pharmacology of isoflurane. Br J Anaesth 1984;56:71S–99S, with permission.)

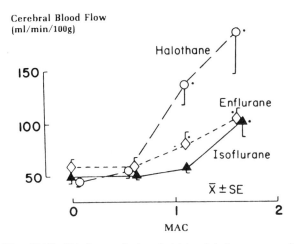

Fig. 17-6. Volatile anesthetics administered during normocapnia to produce a MAC of greater than 0.6 become cerebral vasodilators and produce dose-dependent increases in cerebral blood flow (halothane > enflurane > isoflurane). *$P < 0.05$ versus awake value. (From Eger EI. Isoflurane (Forane). A Compendium and Reference. Madison, WI. Anaquest, A Division of BOC, 1986;1–160, with permission.)

nism may fail, such that a drug-induced increase in CBF may produce an abrupt increase of ICP. In contrast to volatile anesthetics and ketamine, barbiturates and opioids are classified as cerebral vasoconstrictors. Drugs that produce cerebral vasoconstriction predictably decrease CBF and ICP.

The introduction of halothane into the inhaled gases, simultaneously with the initiation of mechanical hyperventilation of the lungs sufficient to decrease $PaCO_2$ to about 25 mmHg, does not reliably prevent a drug-induced increase in ICP in the patient who has an intracranial tumor.[12] Conversely, establishing hypocarbia for about 10 minutes before adding halothane to the inhaled gases prevents an increase in ICP. Enflurane, like halothane, can cause an abrupt increase in ICP in a patient with an intracranial tumor; hypocarbia produced simultaneously with the introduction of this anesthetic does not always protect against an increase in CBF. In contrast to the other volatile anesthetics, the institution of hyperventilation of the lungs, simultaneous to the introduction of isoflurane into the inhaled gases, prevents the increased ICP that can accompany the administration of this drug at normocarbia to a patient with an intracranial tumor. Isoflurane produces a decrease in cerebral metabolic oxygen requirements that exceed those produced by an equivalent MAC of halothane. The greater decrease in cerebral metabolic oxygen requirements produced by isoflurane may explain why CBF increases are minimal below 1.1 MAC[11] (Fig. 17-6). For example, decreased cerebral metabolism means that less carbon dioxide

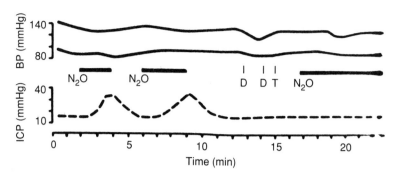

Fig. 17-7. Administration of 70% nitrous oxide to a patient with the abrupt onset of coma due to an unknown cause resulted in an increase in intracranial pressure (ICP). Administration of diazepam (D) or thiopental (T) before introduction of nitrous oxide prevented the nitrous oxide-induced increase in ICP. (From Phirman JR, Shapiro HM. Modification of nitrous oxide-induced intracranial hypertension by prior induction of anesthesia. Anesthesiology 1977;46:150–1, with permission.)

is produced, thus opposing the cerebral vasodilating effects of isoflurane. It is conceivable that isoflurane might produce greater than expected increases in CBF when administered to a patient with co-existing drug or disease-induced depression of CBF. In hypocapnic patients with supratentorial mass lesions, 1 MAC desflurane, but not isoflurane, produces modest increases in ICP.[13]

In contrast to volatile anesthetics, nitrous oxide has less of an effect on CBF, perhaps reflecting restriction of its dose to less than 1 MAC. For this reason, nitrous oxide is unlikely to increase ICP in the patient with an intracranial tumor, maintained at normocarbia. Nevertheless, there is evidence that nitrous oxide is a cerebral vasodilator that, in an occasional vulnerable patient, may increase ICP[14] (Fig. 17-7). Nitrous oxide in contrast to volatile anesthetics does not interfere with autoregulation of CBF. The administration of nitrous oxide during a craniotomy and after closure of the dura may contrib-

ute to the development of a tension pneumocephalus. Tension pneumocephalus reflects the entrance of nitrous oxide into the subdural air cavities.

Barbiturates, such as thiopental, are potent cerebral vasoconstrictors capable of decreasing CBF with an associated decrease in a previously elevated ICP. The decrease in CBF produced by a barbiturate is even greater if hypocarbia is present as well. Prior administration of thiopental can attenuate a ketamine-induced increase in CBF and ICP.[15] Nevertheless, the effect of thiopental on ICP in the presence of ketamine is probably not sufficiently predictable to justify the use of ketamine in a patient with an intracranial tumor. Opioids, like barbiturates, are considered cerebral vasoconstrictors, assuming that opioid-induced ventilatory depression is not permitted to manifest as an increase in $PaCO_2$. In humans, maintained at normocarbia, CBF is unchanged or decreased in the presence of fentanyl or sufentanil[16] (Fig. 17-8).

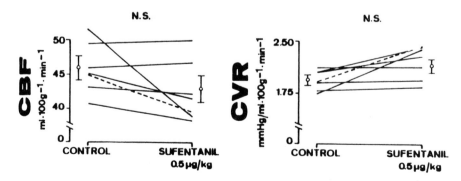

Fig. 17-8. Intravenous administration of sufentanil does not significantly alter cerebral blood flow (CBF) or cerebrovascular resistance (CVR) compared with control values. (From Mayer N, Weinstable C, Podreka I, Spiss CK. Sufentanil does not increase cerebral blood flow in healthy human volunteers. Anesthesiology 1990;73:240–3, with permission.)

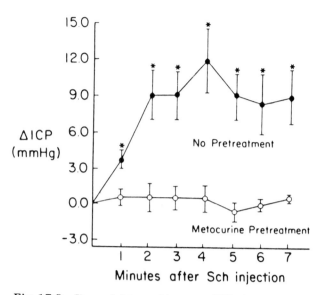

Fig. 17-9. Changes in intracranial pressure (ICP) after administration of succinylcholine (Sch) (1 mg·kg^{-1} IV) with or without prior treatment. Mean ± SE. (From Stirt JA, Grosslight KR, Bedford RF, Vollmer D. Defasciculation with metocurine prevents succinylcholine-induced increases in intracranial pressure. Anesthesiology 1987;67: 50–3, with permission.)

The administration of atracurium or vecuronium to a patient undergoing resection of an intracranial tumor does not result in increased ICP.[17,18] This finding suggests that atracurium may be selected for the production of skeletal muscle paralysis during a neurosurgical operation, despite its potential for evoking histamine release. Histamine release could produce cerebral vasodilation with an associated increase in CBF and ICP. Succinylcholine, administered to a patient with an intracranial tumor, may cause a modest, usually transient, increase in ICP[19] (Fig. 17-9). This response could reflect histamine release or increased venous pressure, or both, due to elevated intra-abdominal and intrathoracic pressure in response to skeletal muscle contractions. Indeed, the prevention of succinylcholine-induced skeletal muscle fasciculations by prior administration of a nondepolarizing muscle relaxant prevents the increase in ICP associated with this drug[19] (Fig. 17-9).

Preoperative Evaluation

Preoperative evaluation of the patient with an intracranial tumor is directed toward establishing the presence or absence of increased ICP. Symptoms of increased ICP include nausea and vomiting, altered level of consciousness, mydriasis and decreased reactivity of the pupils to light, papilledema, bradycardia, hypertension, and disturbances of breathing. Evidence of a midline shift of the brain (greater than 0.5 cm) on computed tomography also suggests the presence of increased ICP.

Preoperative Medication

Preoperative medication that produces sedation or ventilatory depression should be avoided in the patient with an intracranial tumor. The patient with intracranial pathology may be extremely sensitive to the central nervous system depressant effects of drugs such as opioids. Opioid-induced hypoventilation can lead to increased CBF and a consequent increase in ICP. It is difficult to distinguish nausea and vomiting that occurs after administration of preoperative medication from that due to a progressive increase in ICP. Likewise, drug-induced sedation can mask alterations in the level of consciousness that accompany intracranial hypertension. Considering all the potential adverse effects of preoperative medication, it is an inescapable conclusion that pharmacologic premedication should be used sparingly, if at all, in the patient with an intracranial tumor. Certainly no preoperative depressant drugs should be administered to a patient with a depressed level of consciousness. In the alert adult patient with an intracranial tumor, oral administration of diazepam (5 to 10 mg) can provide anxiety relief without introducing the hazard of ventilatory depression. The decision to administer an anticholinergic drug or H-2 receptor antagonist is not influenced by the presence or absence of increased ICP.

Induction of Anesthesia

Induction of anesthesia must be achieved with a drug that produces rapid and reliable anesthesia with a minimal effect on CBF. This goal is often achieved with the injection of thiopental (4 to 6 mg·kg^{-1} IV), preceded by preoxygenation and perhaps voluntary spontaneous hyperventilation. The reduced CBF and increased perfusion-to-metabolism ratio make thiopental a useful induction drug in the presence of increased ICP. Benzodiazepines, etomidate, and propofol also reduce CBF and, in this regard, would be acceptable drugs for the induction of anesthesia. Administration of thiopental is followed by two to three times the ED$_{95}$ dose of vecuronium, atracurium, or pancuronium. Administration of succinylcholine may be associated with a modest and transient increase in ICP[19] (Fig. 17-9). Mechanical hyperventilation of the lungs is instituted after the administration of the muscle relaxant with the goal of decreasing PaCO$_2$ to between 25 to 30 mmHg.

Intubation of the trachea by direct laryngoscopy is carried out when intense skeletal muscle paralysis is confirmed by the absence of an evoked response to the peripheral nerve stimulator. Administration of an additional dose of thiopental or a potent short-acting opioid before the initiation of direct laryngoscopy may reduce the pressor response to this painful stimulus. Likewise, lidocaine (1.5 mg·kg^{-1} IV), administered about 1 minute before beginning direct laryngoscopy, may be

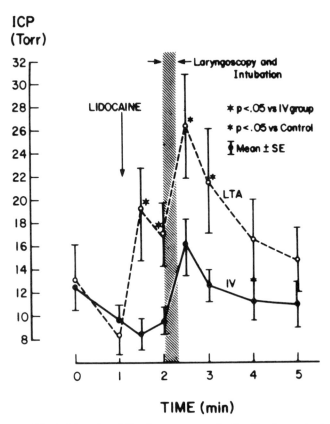

Fig. 17-10. The intravenous (IV) administration of lidocaine was more effective than laryngotracheal administration (LTA) of lidocaine in preventing an increase in intracranial pressure (ICP) during laryngoscopy and tracheal intubation of patients with known intracranial tumors. (From Hamill JF, Bedford RF, Weaver DC, Colohan AR. Lidocaine before endotracheal intubation: Intravenous or laryngotracheal? Anesthesiology 1981;55:578–81, with permission.)

effective in attenuating increased blood pressure and ICP, which may accompany intubation of the trachea[20] (Fig. 17-10). Laryngotracheal lidocaine does not seem to be as effective as intravenous lidocaine in reducing the magnitude of these responses. An abrupt increase in blood pressure in the absence of autoregulation in the area of pathology may be accompanied by cerebral edema and by an undesirable increase in blood flow and ICP. Hypotension should also be avoided, as brain ischemia can occur with decreased cerebral perfusion and autoregulation that is not intact. Any reaction during placement of the tube in the trachea due to inadequate skeletal muscle relaxation can further increase ICP by virtue of an elevation in venous pressure. Likewise, any reaction to movement of the tube after it is placed in the trachea must be prevented, emphasizing the need to maintain skeletal muscle paralysis beyond the period of laryngoscopy. An adequate depth of anesthesia, as well as complete skeletal muscle paralysis, is necessary, since perception of noxious stimulation can abruptly increase the cerebral oxygen requirements and CBF.

After intubation of the trachea, the lungs are ventilated at a rate and tidal volume predicted to maintain PaCO$_2$ between 25 and 30 mmHg. Positive end-expiratory pressure is not recommended, as it could impair cerebral venous drainage and increase ICP.

Maintenance of Anesthesia

Maintenance of anesthesia is often achieved with nitrous oxide plus intravenous supplementation with an opioid or barbiturate, or both. Fentanyl or a similar opioid is an attractive selection, as these drugs are unlikely to alter ICP adversely. Some would question the wisdom of using nitrous oxide in a situation in which the likelihood of air embolism is great, as with an operation performed with the patient in the sitting position. Nevertheless, the incidence or severity of venous air embolism is not influenced by the inclusion of nitrous oxide in the inhaled gases delivered to patients in the sitting position.[21] Volatile anesthetics are administered with caution because of their potential to increase CBF and to interfere with autoregulation. Nevertheless, a low concentration of a volatile drug (less than 0.6 MAC) may be useful in preventing or treating increased blood pressure related to noxious surgical stimulation. In addition to lowering blood pressure, the administration of a volatile anesthetic increases the depth of anesthesia and reduces the likelihood that painful stimulation might increase CBF. The use of a volatile anesthetic requires modest hyperventilation of the lungs to maintain a $PaCO_2$ of 25 to 30 mmHg. The minimal effects of isoflurane on CBF compared with other volatile anesthetics, plus the acceptability of initiating hyperventilation of the lungs simultaneously with introduction of this drug, make isoflurane a useful volatile anesthetic in the patient undergoing an intracranial operation. The use of a peripheral vasodilating drug, such as nitroprusside, or of nitroglycerin may increase CBF and ICP despite a simultaneous reduction in systemic blood pressure. Therefore, the selection of a peripheral vasodilator to treat intraoperative hypertension may be questionable in the patient with increased ICP.

Spontaneous movement by the patient must be avoided during an intracranial operation. Such movement can result in a disastrous increase in ICP, excessive bleeding into the operative site, and bulging of the brain into the wound, making surgical exposure difficult. Therefore, in addition to an adequate depth of anesthesia, skeletal muscle paralysis is often maintained during intracranial surgery.

Fluid Therapy

The selection of an inappropriate fluid solution or infusion of excessive amounts of crystalloid solutions can adversely influence ICP in the patient with an intracranial tumor. Glucose-in-water solutions are not recommended, as they are rapidly and equally distributed throughout total body water. If the concentration of glucose in blood decreases more rapidly than brain glucose, brain water becomes relatively hyperosmolar, and the brain tissues accumulate water, leading to cerebral edema. Furthermore, metabolism of glucose in the brain leaves free water in excess. A hypertonic salt solution, such as 5% glucose in lactated Ringer's solution, is an appropriate fluid selection. This solution will initially tend to reduce brain water by increasing the osmolarity of plasma. Regardless of the crystalloid solution selected, any solution administered in large amounts can increase brain water and elevate ICP in the patient with an intracranial tumor. Therefore, the rate of fluid infusion probably should not exceed 1 to 3 ml·kg^{-1}·h^{-1} during the perioperative period. Intravascular fluid volume depletion due to blood loss during surgery should be corrected with packed red blood cells, whole blood, or a colloid solution, and not with a large volume of balanced salt solution.

Monitoring

Continuous monitoring of blood pressure with a catheter in a peripheral artery is useful for the rapid detection of an excessive increase or decrease in cerebral perfusion pressure. Cap-

nography is helpful in guiding the desired degree of hyperventilation and in serving as a monitor for the detection of venous air embolism (see the section, Venous Air Embolism). A continuous monitor of intracranial pressure is of obvious value, but this monitor cannot be considered as routine during surgery in every patient with an intracranial tumor. Nasopharyngeal or esophageal temperature should be monitored, as unexpected alterations in body temperature can occur. A catheter inserted into the bladder is mandatory, if diuresis is to be produced during the intraoperative period.

Placement of a catheter in the right atrium is helpful in guiding the rate of intravenous fluid infusion. Furthermore, this catheter may be important in aspirating air from the heart, should venous air embolism occur (see the section, Venous Air Embolism). The position of the catheter can be confirmed by (1) a chest radiograph; (2) the configuration of the P wave on the electrocardiogram (ECG), with the saline-filled catheter acting as a unipolar lead; or (3) the transduced venous pressure waveform. The impracticality of obtaining a chest radiograph in the operating room and the electroshock hazard of recording the ECG from a saline-filled catheter are disadvantages to these approaches. Therefore, observation of the phasic pressure waveform recorded from the catheter seems an acceptable criterion for confirming its central venous location. An additional approach is to advance the catheter until a right ventricular pressure waveform is observed and then to withdraw the catheter until the pressure trace becomes atrial. In view of the decrease in mortality from venous air embolism provided by the aspiration of air from a right atrial catheter, it would seem prudent to consider placement of a catheter into the right atrium, whenever venous air embolism is judged to be a likely occurrence during surgery. An extension of this recommendation would be the placement of a pulmonary artery catheter as an alternative.[22]

A peripheral nerve stimulator is helpful in monitoring the persistence of skeletal muscle paralysis. If paresis or paralysis of an upper extremity is associated with an intracranial tumor, it is important to appreciate the presence of resistance (decreased sensitivity) to the effects of nondepolarizing muscle relaxants in the paretic extremity, as compared with the normal extremity[23] (Fig. 17-11). Therefore, monitoring skeletal muscle paralysis with the leads of the peripheral nerve stimulator placed on the paretic arm may be misleading. For example, the evoked response may be erroneously interpreted as inadequate skeletal muscle paralysis. Likewise, at the conclusion of surgery, the same response could be assumed to reflect recovery from the effect of the muscle relaxant when substantial neuromuscular blockade persists. Resistance of the muscles of a paralyzed or paretic extremity to muscle relaxants may reflect the proliferation of acetylcholine-responsive extrajunctional cholinergic receptor sites that can occur within 48 to 72 hours after denervation (see the section, Chronic Spinal Cord Transection).

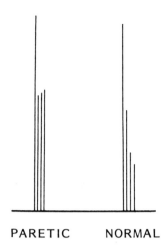

PARETIC   NORMAL

Fig. 17-11. The greater train-of-four ratio recorded from the paretic extremity (0.6) compared with the normal arm (0.3) reflects resistance of the paretic arm to the effects of nondepolarizing muscle relaxants. (From Moorthy SS, Hilgenberg JC. Resistance to nondepolarizing muscle relaxants in paretic upper extremities of patients with residual hemiplegia. Anesth Analg 1980;59:624–7, with permission.)

Monitoring for venous air embolism with a Doppler transducer is often used in the patient undergoing an intracranial operation. The transducer is placed to the right of the sternum, between the third and sixth intercostal spaces. Correct positioning is verified by rapid injection of 5 to 10 ml of crystalloid solution into the right atrial catheter. Turbulence created by this injection of fluid creates a signal (roaring sound) similar to that caused by air. Amounts of air as small as 0.25 ml can be detected by the transducer. Air is detected as a change in the signal from the transducer because the air-blood interface is a much better acoustical reflector than erythrocytes alone. In addition, audible sounds from the transducer may provide early warning of changes in cardiac rate or rhythm.

Monitoring of the ECG is necessary to detect cardiac dysrhythmias related to the presence of an intracranial tumor or from surgical stimulation of vital medullary centers. Indeed, abnormalities on the ECG can indicate an intracranial tumor, presumed to reflect the increased activity of the sympathetic nervous system attributable to increased ICP. More important, alterations in cardiac rate or rhythm may reflect surgical retraction or manipulation of the brain stem or cranial nerves. Indeed, the cardiovascular centers, respiratory control areas, and nuclei of the lower cranial nerves lie in close proximity in the brain stem. Manipulation of the brain stem may produce hypertension and bradycardia or hypotension and tachycardia. Cardiac dysrhythmias range from acute sinus dysrhythmias to ventricular premature beats or ventricular tachycardia.

Position

Craniotomy for the removal of a supratentorial tumor is usually performed with the patient supine and the head elevated 10 to 15 degrees, to facilitate venous drainage from the brain. Excessive flexion or rotation of the head should be avoided, as these positions can impair jugular vein patency and impede venous outflow.

The sitting position is often used for exploration of the posterior cranial fossa, which may be necessary to resect an intracranial tumor, clip an aneurysm, decompress a cranial nerve, or implant electrodes for cerebellar stimulation. Advantages of the sitting position include excellent surgical exposure and facilitation of venous CSF drainage, so as to minimize blood loss and elevation of the ICP. These advantages are offset by reductions in blood pressure and cardiac output produced by this posture and by the potential hazard of venous air embolism. For these reasons, the lateral or prone position may be selected as an alternative. If the sitting position is used, it is mandatory to maintain a high index of suspicion for venous air embolism (see the section, Venous Air Embolism). A serious postoperative complication after posterior fossa craniotomy is apnea due to hematoma formation. Cranial nerve injuries involving innervation to the pharynx and larynx make these patients vulnerable to aspiration.

Venous Air Embolism

Venous air embolism is a potential hazard, whenever the operative site is above the level of the heart, such that the pressure in the veins is subatmospheric. Although this complication is most often associated with neurosurgical procedures, venous air embolism can also occur during operations involving the neck, thorax, abdomen, and pelvis and during open heart procedures, repair of liver and vena cava lacerations, total hip replacement, and vaginal delivery associated with placenta previa. Patients undergoing intracranial surgery are at an increased risk not only because the operative site is usually above the level of the heart, but also because the veins may not collapse, due to attachments to bone or dura. Indeed, the cut edge of bone constituting the skull is a common site for the entry of air into veins held open by bone.

Pathophysiology

The precise mechanism by which venous air embolism leads to cardiovascular collapse is undetermined. Presumably, when air enters the right ventricle, interference with blood flow into the pulmonary artery occurs. Pulmonary edema and reflex bronchoconstriction may result from the movement of air into the pulmonary circulation. Death is usually secondary to acute cor pulmonale and cardiovascular collapse, as well as to arterial hypoxemia from obstruction to right ventricular ejection into the pulmonary artery.

Air can probably pass through pulmonary vessels in small

amounts, to reach the coronary and cerebral circulations; large quantities of air can travel directly to the systemic circulation through a right-to-left intracardiac shunt, as provided by a patent foramen ovale. Indeed, the use of the sitting position inherently predisposes neurosurgical patients to paradoxical air embolism, since the normal interatrial pressure gradient frequently becomes reversed in this position.[24] When the likelihood of venous air embolism is increased, it is useful, but not mandatory, to place a right atrial catheter before beginning surgery (see the section, Monitoring). Death due to paradoxical air embolism results from obstruction of the coronary arteries by air, leading to myocardial ischemia and ventricular fibrillation. Neurologic damage follows air embolism to the brain.

Detection

Early detection of venous air embolism is essential to successful treatment of this complication. A Doppler transducer placed over the right heart is the most sensitive indicator of intracardiac air.[25] Indeed, the small amount of air detected by the transducer is often not clinically significant. In this regard, the transducer does not provide information as to the volume of air that has entered the venous circulation. A sudden decrease in the end-tidal PCO_2 may reflect increased dead space due to continued ventilation of alveoli that are no longer perfused because of obstruction of their vascular supply by air. An increase in right atrial and pulmonary artery pressure reflects acute cor pulmonale and correlates with an abrupt decrease in the end-tidal PCO_2. Although these changes are less sensitive indicators for the presence of air than the Doppler transducer, they reflect the size of the venous air embolism.[25] An increased end-tidal nitrogen concentration, as during continuous mass spectrometry monitoring, may also reflect venous air embolism. Changes in end-tidal nitrogen concentration often precede decreased end-tidal PCO_2 or increased pulmonary artery pressure.[26] During controlled ventilation of the lungs, sudden attempts by the patient to initiate a spontaneous breath (gasp reflex) may be the first indication of the occurrence of venous air embolism. Hypotension, tachycardia, cardiac dysrhythmias, and cyanosis are late signs of venous air embolism. Certainly the detection of the characteristic "millwheel" murmur through the esophageal stethoscope is a late sign of catastrophic venous air embolism.

Treatment

A change in the signal from the Doppler transducer should alert the surgeon to identify and occlude the site of venous air entry by irrigation of the operative site with fluid and by the application of occlusive material to all bone edges. Aspiration of air should be attempted through the right atrial catheter. The ideal location of the right atrial catheter tip is controversial, but evidence suggests that a superior vena cava location

(junction of the superior vena cava with the right atrium) is preferable, as it appears to provide the most rapid aspiration of air.[27] Right atrial multiorifice catheters permit aspiration of a larger amount of air than do single orifice catheters. Because of its small lumen size and slow speed of blood return, a pulmonary artery catheter is not uniquely useful in aspirating air, but it may provide additional evidence that venous embolism has occurred, by virtue of the increased pulmonary artery pressure. Nitrous oxide is promptly discontinued to avoid increasing the size of the venous air bubbles[28] (Fig. 17-12). Indeed, elimination of nitrous oxide from the inhaled gases after the detection of venous air embolism often results in a decrease in pulmonary artery pressure. At the same time that oxygen is substituted for nitrous oxide, it may be helpful to apply positive end-expiratory pressure, in order to increase venous pressure. Despite the logic of this maneuver, the prophylactic use of positive end-expiratory pressure has not been found to be of value in the prevention of venous air embolism. The notion has been raised that positive end-expiratory pressure increases right atrial pressure more than left atrial pressure, predisposing the patient with a probe-patent foramen ovale to paradoxical air embolism. Nevertheless, a level of positive end-expiratory pressure up to 10 cm H_2O probably does not alter the interatrial pressure difference in a sitting neurosurgical patient, and therefore does not increase the

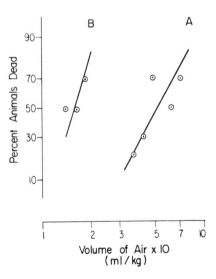

Fig. 17-12. The calculated volume of air necessary to produce death in 50% of animals was greater during the administration of halothane alone (A) compared with halothane–nitrous oxide (B). Presumably, the rapid passage of nitrous oxide into air bubbles, with resultant expansion of the air bubbles, was responsible for the increased lethal effects of venous air embolism in the presence of nitrous oxide. (From Munson ES, Merrick HC. Effect of nitrous oxide on venous air embolism. Anesthesiology 1966;27:783–7, with permission.)

risk of paradoxical air embolism in these patients.[29] Extreme hypotension may require the support of perfusion pressure with a sympathomimetic agent. Likewise, a marked reduction in cardiac output may require infusion of a beta agonist such as dopamine or dobutamine. Bronchospasm is treated with a beta-2 agonist, either by aerosol (metered dose inhaler) or the intravenous route. The traditional admonition to place the patient in the lateral position with the right chest uppermost is rarely possible or safe during an intracranial operation. It is likely that valuable time, better spent aspirating air and supporting circulation, could be lost attempting to attain this position.

After the successful treatment of venous air embolism, the surgical procedure can be resumed. However, the decision to reinstitute administration of nitrous oxide must be individualized. If it is decided not to use nitrous oxide, maintenance of an adequate depth of anesthesia will probably require the administration of a volatile anesthetic. If nitrous oxide is added again to the inhaled gases, it is possible that residual air in the circulation could again produce symptoms. Indeed, increased pulmonary artery pressure after resumption of breathing nitrous oxide should be viewed as evidence that residual air persists despite the apparent successful treatment of venous air embolism.[22] Transfer of a patient to a hyperbaric chamber in an attempt to reduce the size of air bubbles and improve blood flow in the brain is likely to be helpful only if the transfer can be accomplished within 8 hours.

Postoperative Management

Ideally, the effects of anesthetics and muscle relaxants are dissipated or pharmacologically reversed at the conclusion of surgery. This facilitates monitoring of neurologic status and recognition of any adverse effects of the surgery. It is important to prevent any reaction to the tube in the trachea as the patient is allowed to awaken. Lidocaine (0.5 to 1.5 mg·kg^{-1} IV) may be used to attenuate the initial response to the continued presence of the tube in the trachea as the patient awakens. It must be appreciated, however, that this local anesthetic can produce central nervous system depression and reduce the activity of protective upper airway reflexes. If the patient was alert preoperatively, it may be reasonable to place a nasal airway during anesthesia and remove the tracheal tube at the conclusion of surgery, to avoid potentially adverse reactions to the tube. Conversely, if consciousness was depressed preoperatively, it may be best to delay extubation of the trachea, until it can be confirmed that airway reflexes are present and spontaneous ventilation is sufficient to prevent accumulation of carbon dioxide. A decrease in body temperature during anesthesia and surgery to less than 34°C must be considered a possible cause of slow postoperative awakening. It may be inappropriate to remove the tracheal tube in the presence of hypothermia, regardless of the preoperative mental status.

CEREBROVASCULAR DISEASE

Cerebrovascular disease can be manifested as a (1) transient ischemic attack (TIA), with temporary impairment of cerebral function; (2) minor stroke, with recovery to a normal or a near-normal state possible; and (3) major stroke, often resulting in severe, permanent disability or death. Stroke is the third leading cause of death in the United States. Only heart disease and cancer exceed stroke as causes of mortality. The major risk factors for the development of cerebrovascular disease are diabetes mellitus and hypertension. Indeed, effective treatment of hypertension has reduced mortality due to stroke.

Transient Ischemic Attack

TIA is a temporary and focal episode of neurologic dysfunction that develops suddenly and lasts a few minutes to several hours, but never more than 24 hours. The diagnosis of TIA is confirmed by spontaneous recovery within 24 hours, absence of residual neurologic symptoms, and a normal computed tomography brain scan. The peak age for the development of a TIA is during the seventh decade. Such attacks may occur as often as several times daily. Left untreated, about one-third of patients will suffer a minor or major stroke within 5 years.

The causes of a TIA are presumed to be thromboembolism of fibrin-platelet aggregates or atheromatous debris from an atherosclerotic plaque in an extracranial blood vessel. The transient nature of the attack is explained by the rapid fragmentation and dissolution of the microemboli. Disease of the carotid artery or vertebrobasilar arterial system is most often responsible for a TIA (Fig. 17-13). TIAs after spinal anesthesia have been attributed to focal cerebral ischemia produced by anesthetic-induced alterations in CBF in a susceptible patient (co-existing cerebrovascular disease), even in the absence of systemic hypotension.[30] It is important to distinguish neurologic dysfunction due to disease of the carotid artery from that due to vertebrobasilar arterial disease, as the prognosis and treatment are different.

Carotid Artery Disease

The bifurcation of the common carotid artery is a frequent site of atheromatous disease. Disease located in the carotid artery is suggested by complaints of transient ipsilateral monocular visual loss, often associated with a contralateral paresis or sensory disturbance. Transient visual loss (amaurosis fugax) is due to retinal ischemia secondary to the passage of emboli into the ophthalmic artery. The passage of microemboli into the ophthalmic artery is predictable, as this artery is the first branch of the internal carotid artery. Indeed, fundoscopy during the period of blindness can indicate emboli in the retinal arterial system.

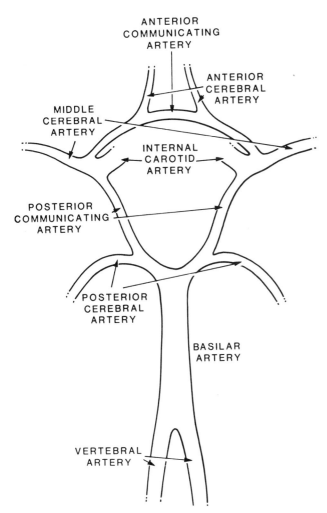

Fig. 17-13. Schematic diagram of the cerebral circulation and circle of Willis. The cerebral blood supply is from the vertebral arteries (arising from the subclavian arteries) and the internal carotid arteries (arising from the common carotid arteries).

of cerebrovascular accident in these patients. There is no evidence that the incidence of postoperative stroke is increased in those patients who undergo non-neurologic surgery.[31] The absence of a bruit does not rule out the presence of significant stenosis of the carotid artery. For example, a bruit may disappear when the degree of stenosis is so severe that blood flow is minimal. Certainly, the absence of a palpable carotid artery pulse in the neck suggests severe occlusive disease. Radionuclide angiography can be used to detect carotid artery disease.

Vertebrobasilar Arterial Disease

Vertebrobasilar arterial disease manifests symptoms referable to ischemia of the posterior portions of the brain, including the occipital lobes and brain stem. Bilateral disturbance of vision results from inadequate blood flow through the posterior cerebral arteries that supply the visual cortex. Visual symptoms range from blurring to total blindness. Diplopia is a common complaint. Attacks of vertigo, ataxia, and nausea and vomiting suggest circulatory disturbances, either in the labyrinth of the inner ear or in the vestibular nuclei of the medulla. Other symptoms of brain stem ischemia include dysarthria, dysphagia, perioral numbness, and weakness or paresthesias of all four limbs. A sudden loss of postural tone in the legs, with consciousness maintained, is characteristic of basilar artery disease. Typically, the patient falls abruptly to the ground, often to a kneeling position. Attempts to arise at once serve to distinguish this event from syncope due to third-degree atrioventricular heart block.

An episode of transient global amnesia is most likely related to vertebrobasilar arterial disease. Characteristically, the patient displays an abrupt onset of memory loss and confusion. During the attack, the patient experiences retrograde amnesia, but self-identity is usually preserved. The attack subsides after several minutes to hours and is ultimately associated with amnesia, permanent only for the period of the ischemic episode. It is presumed that insufficient blood flow to portions of the temporal lobes or thalamus supplied by the posterior cerebral arteries is responsible.

In contrast to the patient with carotid artery occlusive disease, the patient with vertebrobasilar arterial insufficiency is more likely to describe a relationship between symptoms and abrupt changes in posture. Orthostatic hypotension or a low blood pressure for the age of the patient is often present. In addition, the vertebral arteries may be compressed by osteoarthritis of the cervical spine and by movements of the head, particularly hyperextension. Occasionally, vertebrobasilar arterial insufficiency is associated with a bruit over the subclavian artery; a radiograph of the cervical spine may show calcification of the vertebral arteries.

A neurologic examination performed after the patient has experienced a TIA is likely to be normal, as changes are usually mild and their evolution complete within a few seconds. The patient may describe tingling, numbness, or clumsiness of an extremity, as well as momentary difficulty in mentation or in verbal expression, if the dominant cerebral hemisphere is involved. Disturbance of consciousness is rare.

Auscultation may demonstrate a bruit over the common carotid artery in the neck. Indeed, asymptomatic cervical bruits occur in 4% of the population older than 40 years of age, but the risk of myocardial infarction is greater than that

Medical Treatment

Medical treatment of a TIA is preferred in the patient with vertebrobasilar arterial disease or multiple vascular lesions. Medical management consists of long-term administration of an antiplatelet aggregating drug or coumarin anticoagulant. Evidence of the effectiveness of an oral anticoagulant as protection against stroke is not as well defined as it is for aspirin. Nevertheless, warfarin may be selected for medical management of females in whom TIAs develop or of males who do not tolerate aspirin. Spontaneous hemorrhage is the major hazard of oral anticoagulant therapy. Treatment with an oral anticoagulant should be continued for 6 to 12 months after a TIA, as this is the period of greatest risk of stroke. If symptoms are produced by extension or rotation of the head, a cervical collar may be helpful.

Surgical Treatment

Surgical treatment of a patient with an occlusive lesion of greater than 80% in the carotid artery and a history of repeated TIAs is the performance of a carotid endarterectomy. For example, about 75% of patients have an obstructive lesion at a surgically accessible site, most commonly at the bifurcation of the common carotid artery. The presence of an ulcerated atherosclerotic plaque is also an indication for carotid endarterectomy. Approximately 80% of patients improve or become asymptomatic after carotid endarterectomy. Compared with medically treated patients, performance of a carotid endarterectomy increases stroke-free survival. Carotid endarterectomy is not likely to be considered in a patient with an acute stroke or with a stroke in progress because of the greater than 50% incidence of postoperative hemorrhagic infarction. Prophylactic carotid endarterectomy for the patient with asymptomatic carotid disease before cardiac surgery is probably unnecessary.[32]

Management of Anesthesia

The goal during management of anesthesia for carotid endarterectomy surgery is to maintain cerebral perfusion pressure and CBF. The most critical period is the time of surgical occlusion of the common carotid artery. In the vast majority of patients, this occlusion is tolerated by the use of collateral channels provided by the circle of Willis (Fig. 17-13). For example, occlusion of one carotid artery is tolerated because of collateral circulation through the contralateral carotid artery or the vertebral arteries. Other important arterial collaterals are available through the external carotid artery by means of the ophthalmic artery or occipital artery to the distal internal carotid artery. Nevertheless, in some patients, CBF may be inadequate during occlusion of the carotid artery, which is necessary for performance of the endarterectomy.

Preoperative Evaluation

In addition to the neurologic evaluation, these patients should be carefully examined for cardiovascular and renal disease. Predictably, a patient with cerebrovascular occlusive disease will have occlusive disease in other arteries as well. Indeed, ischemic heart disease is a major cause of morbidity and mortality after carotid endarterectomy. Chronic hypertension is a common finding. It is important to establish the range of normal blood pressure in these patients preoperatively, to provide a rational guideline for the range of blood pressure maintenance during surgery. The effects of changes in head position on cerebral function should be ascertained, since extreme head rotation, flexion, or extension in the patient with co-existing vertebral artery disease could lead to angulation and compression of the artery. Recognition of this response preoperatively allows hazardous head positions (especially hyperextension) to be avoided when patients are unconscious during general anesthesia, particularly during direct laryngoscopy for intubation of the trachea. Palpation of the carotid artery is not recommended, as this maneuver could displace fragments of the occlusive lesion, causing a cerebral embolism.

Choice of Anesthesia

Carotid endarterectomy surgery can be performed with regional or general anesthesia. Morbidity and mortality after carotid endarterectomy are similar, whether surgery is performed with regional or general anesthesia.[33]

Regional Anesthesia

During surgery for an occluded carotid artery, it is a distinct advantage to be able to monitor the patient's cerebral function by voice contact. This is possible with cervical plexus anesthesia produced by the injection of a local anesthetic (lidocaine or bupivacaine) at the transverse processes of C3-C4 (deep cervical plexus block), followed by infiltration of a local anesthetic along the posterior inferior border of the sternocleidomastoid muscle (superficial cervical plexus block). Nevertheless, stroke still can occur postoperatively, despite the apparent maintenance of normal cerebral function during regional anesthesia.[34] A disadvantage of regional anesthesia includes a more pronounced cardiovascular response to manipulation in the area of the carotid sinus than occurs with general anesthesia. Furthermore, any cerebral protective effect produced by a drug used for general anesthesia is lost.

General Anesthesia

General anesthesia is acceptably produced by intravenous injection of a barbiturate, benzodiazepine, etomidate, or propofol, followed by the administration of nitrous oxide in combination with a volatile drug or opioid, for maintenance of anesthesia. There is no difference in CBF and cerebral metabolic oxygen requirements in patients anesthetized with nitrous oxide plus isoflurane or sufentanil and undergoing carotid endarterectomy.[35,36] Skeletal muscle paralysis is often produced to permit a decrease in the depth of anesthesia in response to hypotension, without introducing the possibility of unwanted patient movement. Although differences among volatile anesthetics as regards neurologic outcome after carotid endarterectomy are not detectable, there are data suggesting that isoflurane may offer some brain protection, if a volatile anesthetic is selected[34] (Fig. 17-14). Nevertheless, thiopental probably remains the appropriate drug to select under specific circumstances when pharmacologic brain protection is indicated.

Regardless of the drugs selected for anesthesia, the goal is to maintain arterial blood pressure within the normal range for a specific patient. Prolonged and excessive decreases in blood pressure may jeopardize cerebral perfusion pressure and the adequacy of CBF through collateral channels. When decreased blood pressure below the patient's normal range fails to respond to a decrease in the concentration of anesthetic drugs, it may be necessary to return the blood pressure to a normal level (not above) by a continuous infusion of a sympathomimetic drug, such as phenylephrine. Nevertheless, the combination of deep anesthesia with a volatile anesthetic plus phenylephrine to maintain an acceptable blood pressure is more likely to produce evidence of myocardial ischemia than is the same blood pressure but in the presence only of light anesthesia.[37] Presumably, the increased myocardial wall stress produced by phenylephrine is responsible for the evidence of myocardial ischemia. Indeed, the incidence of postoperative myocardial infarction is increased in patients with ischemic

heart disease in whom intraoperative blood pressure is artificially elevated with a sympathomimetic drug. A hazard of uncontrolled hypertension during surgery is cerebral edema, particularly in diseased areas of the brain with altered ability to autoregulate CBF.

Despite the universal concern that hypotension can lead to stroke, there is a lack of evidence to support this notion and some evidence to suggest that a decrease in blood pressure is not the precipitating factor in the genesis of stroke.[38] The questionable role of hypotension in the production of stroke should not be interpreted as a reason to permit blood pressure to remain below a normal level during anesthesia, particularly when the carotid artery is being clamped. It should also be recognized, however, that a transient decrease in blood pressure during the intraoperative period cannot be automatically incriminated as the only etiology, when a postoperative neurologic deficit is manifested.

Surgical manipulation in the area of the carotid sinus during mobilization of the carotid artery may be interpreted as stretch by afferent nerve endings in this area, leading to reflex bradycardia and hypotension (see the section, Carotid Sinus Syndrome). Conversely, during carotid artery occlusion, decreased pressure within the isolated portion of the artery could initiate sympathetic nervous system activity through the carotid sinus, causing tachycardia and hypertension. These intraoperative effects can be modified by an intravenous injection of atropine or by local infiltration of the area of the carotid sinus with 3 to 5 ml of 1% lidocaine, so as to block afferent activity from the baroreceptor.

Current evidence suggests that barbiturates may prolong

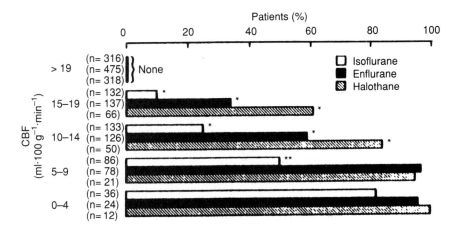

Fig. 17-14. Incidence of EEG ischemic changes within 3 minutes of carotid artery occlusion at different levels of cerebral blood flow (CBF) in patients (%) undergoing carotid endarterectomy in the presence of a volatile anesthetic. Isoflurane appeared to provide a protective effect to the brain although outcome was not different between the anesthetic groups. *Significantly different from each other; **significantly different from the other two. (From Michenfelder JD, Sundt TM, Fode N, Sharbrough FW. Isoflurane when compared to enflurane and halothane decreases the frequency of cerebral ischemia during carotid endarterectomy. Anesthesiology 1987;67:336–40, with permission.)

the tolerance of the brain to focal ischemia as may be produced by clamping the carotid artery during carotid endarterectomy (see the section, Cerebral Protection and Resuscitation). In this regard, it may be reasonable to administer thiopental (4 to 6 mg·kg^{-1} IV) immediately before clamping the carotid artery. Nevertheless, there are no specific data to indicate that a barbiturate used in this manner reduces morbidity after carotid endarterectomy.[39]

Ventilation of the lungs during carotid endarterectomy is with a tidal volume and breathing rate that maintains the PaCO$_2$ at about 35 mmHg. Manipulation of the PaCO$_2$ in an attempt to increase CBF by vasodilation or to produce the inverse steal phenomenon is not recommended. Such manipulation can produce paradoxical and unpredictable cerebrovascular responses in individual patients and cannot be relied on to protect the brain. Monitors during general anesthesia often include continuous recording of blood pressure by a catheter placed in a peripheral artery and capnography, to guide the degree of ventilation required to maintain the PaCO$_2$ within the desired range. In view of the likely presence of ischemic heart disease in many of these patients, it would seem prudent to monitor an appropriate ECG lead for myocardial ischemia.

Adequacy of Cerebral Blood Flow

The goal of monitoring for adequacy of CBF during carotid endarterectomy is to detect the patient whose cerebral collateral circulation is inadequate to prevent cerebral ischemia during occlusion of the carotid artery (Table 17-2). Ideally, this information should identify the patient who requires an intraluminal shunt across the surgically clamped carotid artery. Although some surgeons routinely insert a shunt regardless of data obtained from cerebral perfusion monitors, it must be appreciated that a brief period of carotid occlusion will still be necessary during placement of the shunt. Furthermore, the shunt can interfere with surgical exposure and, in some instances, may induce cerebral embolization. Occlusion of blood flow through the right vertebral artery can occur if inflation of the balloon on the one end of the shunt occludes the innominate artery. Neurologic deficits have been shown to occur,

Table 17-2. Methods to Monitor the Adequacy of Cerebral Blood Flow

Electroencephalogram
   Conventional 16 leads
   Compressed spectral array analysis
   Density-modulated spectral array analysis
   Cerebral function monitor
Somatosensory evoked potentials
Stump pressure
Regional cerebral blood flow
Oculoplethysmography

even when shunts are routinely used. This may reflect inevitable cerebral ischemia during insertion of a shunt, embolization from the carotid artery, or spontaneous distal thrombosis as part of the natural course of the disease.

Electroencephalogram

The electroencephalogram (EEG), using 16 leads, is a reliable method for diagnosing regional cerebral ischemia. Reading and interpretation, however, are still too complex to make the EEG a routine monitor. Furthermore, the EEG will be influenced not only by cerebral ischemia, but also by inhaled anesthetics, body temperature, and the PaCO$_2$. An alternative to recording the conventional EEG is the compressed spectral array or density-modulated spectral array analysis, which provides a three-dimensional pictorial representation of the EEG, compressed with respect to time. Using this form of display, it is possible to compress the continuous recording of the EEG for 1 hour onto a single sheet of paper. This compression facilitates the display of trends. The cerebral function monitor provides a compressed recording of the EEG that is estimated to be equivalent to the integrated microvoltage from a single channel.[40] As a result, this monitor may not be sufficiently discriminating for detection of regional cerebral ischemic changes that can occur in the brain during carotid endarterectomy.

Somatosensory Evoked Potentials

Analysis of cortical somatosensory evoked potentials (SSEPs) in response to a specific extrinsic stimulus can be performed to determine neuronal function, as well as intactness of sensory pathways[41] (Fig. 17-15). SSEPs monitor only sensory function; indeed, there have been reports of disruption of motor function without any change in SSEPs. As with the multiple lead EEG, recording and interpretation of SSEPs remains complex. Inhaled anesthetics produce dose-related depression in the amplitude and an increase in the latency of SSEPs and visual and auditory evoked potentials.[42] Although less than with volatile anesthetics, opioids produce depressant effects on SSEPs with a low-dose continuous infusion of fentanyl, producing less depression than with intermittent injections.[43] Acute hyperventilation of the lungs does not significantly alter the amplitude or latency of SSEP.[44]

Stump Pressure

Stump pressure is the direct measurement of blood pressure in the internal carotid artery distal to the surgical clamp. Therefore, stump pressure reflects the transmitted pressure through the circle of Willis (Fig. 17-13). Stump pressure is determined on the basis of the adequacy of the collateral circulation, cerebral perfusion pressure, and cerebrovascular resistance. The latter is increased by barbiturates and hypocarbia; decreases occur in response to volatile drugs and hypercarbia. Variations in cerebrovascular resistance influence the inter-

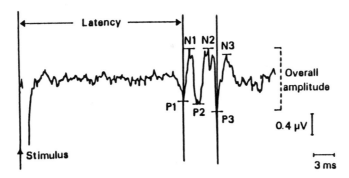

Fig. 17-15. Typical somatosensory evoked potential consisting of three positive peaks (P1, P2, P3) and three negative peaks (N1, N2, N3). A need for change in the surgical technique is indicated by a 50% or greater decrease in amplitude (calculated from the bottom of the lowest positive peak to the top of the highest negative peak) or by complete loss of one or more negative peaks. (From Loghnan BA, Hall GM. Spinal cord monitoring 1989. Br J Anaesth 1989;63:587–94, with permission.)

pretation of stump pressure and its correlation with CBF.[45] For example, an adequate stump pressure during regional anesthesia or an anesthetic technique using nitrous oxide and an opioid is probably higher than that required during administration of a volatile anesthetic. This speculation is based on the predictable presence of a higher cerebrovascular resistance in an awake patient or in a patient receiving nitrous oxide and an opioid, as compared with the lower resistance associated with a volatile anesthetic. Furthermore, the administration of a barbiturate just before clamping of the carotid artery will most likely increase stump pressure, by virtue of the cerebral vasoconstriction induced by the barbiturate. Nevertheless, the available data suggest that a stump pressure greater than 60 mmHg provides adequate perfusion of normal areas of the brain during general anesthesia, regardless of the drugs administered[45] (Fig. 17-16). This observation implies that an

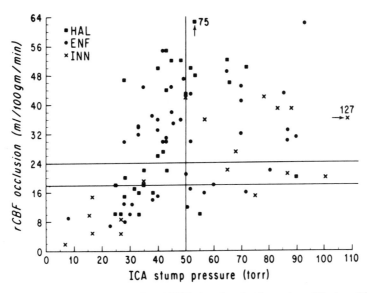

Fig. 17-16. Scattergram of regional cerebral blood flow (rCBF) plotted against internal carotid artery (ICA) stump pressure in patients anesthetized with nitrous oxide plus halothane (HAL), enflurane (ENF), or Innovar (INV). A stump pressure greater than 60 mmHg was associated with a rCBF greater than 18 ml·100 g^{-1}·min^{-1}, in most patients. (From McKay RD, Sundt TM, Michenfelder JD, et al. Internal carotid endarterectomy: Modification by halothane, enflurane, and Innovar. Anesthesiology 1976; 45:390–9, with permission.)

intraluminal shunt should probably be used when stump pressure is less than 60 mmHg. Despite its drawbacks, stump pressure measurement has the advantages of being simple and readily available in most operating rooms.

Regional Cerebral Blood Flow

Measurement of regional cerebral blood flow by the use of an isotope-washout technique, alone or in combination with the EEG, is a useful method for monitoring the adequacy of CBF. It is commonly recommended that regional CBF be maintained above $18 \text{ ml} \cdot 100 \text{ g}^{-1} \cdot \text{min}^{-1}$. This technique remains too complex for routine clinical use.

Oculoplethysmography

Oculoplethysmography assesses supraorbital arterial blood flow as a reflection of the adequacy of blood flow through the intraluminal shunt placed at surgery. A delay in the ocular pulse signifies inadequate flow through the shunt and may alert the surgeon to the need for adjusting its position.

Postoperative Problems

Postoperative problems that follow a carotid endarterectomy include lability of systolic blood pressure, airway compression due to hematoma formation at the operative site, loss of carotid body function, myocardial infarction, and stroke.[46-49]

Hypertension is frequently observed during the immediate postoperative period, occurring most commonly in the patient with co-existing hypertension.[48] Blood pressure is often increased maximally 2 to 3 hours after surgery and may persist for 24 hours. Blood pressure must be lowered to a normal range, to avoid the hazards of cerebral edema and myocardial ischemia. Indeed, the incidence of neurologic deficits is increased threefold in patients who become hypertensive postoperatively. Continuous infusion of nitroprusside is an acceptable treatment with which to lower blood pressure acutely. When hypertension persists, longer-acting drugs, such as labetalol or hydralazine, should be considered. The mechanism for hypertension is unknown, but it may reflect increased intravascular fluid volume, altered activity of the carotid sinus, or loss of carotid sinus function due to denervation during surgery. Likewise, hypotension can be explained on the basis of increased afferent nerve activity perceived by a carotid sinus previously shielded by an atheromatous plaque. Treatment of hypotension is with a vasopressor such as phenylephrine, infusion of fluid, and infiltration of the carotid sinus with a local anesthetic.

The incidence of stroke after carotid endarterectomy is about 5%, most often reflecting cerebral embolism or hemorrhagic infarction. Angiography may be necessary to exclude cerebral thrombosis at the operative site. Preoperative risk factors (transient ischemic attacks, occlusion of the contralateral internal carotid artery, plaque extension beyond surgical access, ischemic heart disease, hypertension) are the best predictors of subsequent carotid endarterectomy-related stroke.[49] The severity of postoperative stroke is not influenced by intraoperative events, including cross-clamp time, shunt placement, and intravenous administration of glucose-containing solutions.

Destruction of the nerve supply to the carotid body, like that to the carotid sinus, is also likely during carotid endarterectomy surgery.[47] Unilateral loss of carotid body function is unlikely to alter the ability of the patient to increase ventilation, in response to a decrease in PaO_2. The ventilatory response to hypoxia, however, is lost in the patient who has undergone a bilateral carotid endarterectomy. Should arterial hypoxemia occur, this patient would be less able to compensate with an increase in alveolar ventilation, as compared with a patient who has intact carotid body function.

Damage to the peripheral nerves may occur during exposure of the carotid artery. For example, trauma to the facial nerve may be manifested as unilateral perioral weakness, whereas hypoglossal nerve damage results in weakness of the tongue. Persistent hoarseness during the postoperative period may reflect surgical trauma to the recurrent laryngeal nerve.

Stroke

Stroke is a heterogeneous collection of different disorders that affect the vasculature of the brain.[50] The two major subdivisions of stroke are hemorrhage and ischemia. Hemorrhage can be further subdivided into subarachnoid hemorrhage and intracerebral hemorrhage. In subarachnoid hemorrhage, blood surrounds the brain, usually from a sudden rupture of a congenital arterial aneurysm. In intracerebral hemorrhage, blood escapes directly into the brain parenchyma, most often from rupture of a small penetrating artery damaged by hypertension. Ischemia is characterized as a focal region of the brain deprived of needed blood supply, owing to systemic hypoperfusion, embolism, or thrombosis. Each of the subtypes of stroke is characterized by common features requiring different strategies for diagnostic evaluation and treatment[50] (Table 17-3).

Localized neurologic dysfunction manifested initially during the immediate postoperative period in a previously normal patient most likely reflects intraoperative thromboembolism, cerebral ischemia, or hemorrhage.[32] Neurologic dysfunction that occurs after cardiopulmonary bypass is most likely due to air emboli, which are especially apt to occur when a cardiac chamber is opened to perform cardiac valve replacement. Computed tomography, review of the history for possible predisposing causes (TIA, atrial fibrillation, bruit over the carotid artery, intraoperative course), and consultation with an appropriate specialist are indicated when a new neurologic deficit occurs postoperatively. Computed tomography is the most

Table 17-3. Characteristics of Stroke Subtypes

	Subarachnoid Hemorrhage	Intracerebral Hemorrhage	Systemic Hypoperfusion	Embolism	Thrombosis

Risk factors	Often absent
	Hypertension
	Coagulopathy
	Drugs
	Trauma
		Hypertension
		Coagulopathy
		Drugs
		Trauma
			Hypotension
			Hemorrhage
			Cardiac arrest
				Smoking
				Ischemic heart disease
				Peripheral vascular
				  disease
				Diabetes mellitus
				White male
					Smoking
					Ischemic heart disease
					Peripheral vascular
					  disease
					Diabetes mellitus
					White male

Onset	Sudden, often during exertion	Gradually progressive	Parallels risk factors	Sudden	Often preceded by a TIA Progressive
Signs and symptoms	Headache Vomiting Transient loss of consciousness	Headache Vomiting Decreased level of consciousness Seizures	Pallor Diaphoresis Hypotension	Headache	Headache
Imaging	CT: hyperdensity (white) MRI	CT: focal hyperdensity (white) MRI	CT: low density (black) MRI	CT: low density (black) MRI	CT: low density (black) MRI

CT, computed tomography; MRI, magnetic resonance imaging.
(Data from Caplan LR. Diagnosis and treatment of ischemic stroke. JAMA 1991;266:2413–8.)

reliable technique for differentiating between cerebral hemorrhage and infarction, but magnetic resonance imaging is more sensitive in detecting acute cerebral infarction. The EEG is not useful in the initial diagnosis of an acute localized neurologic dysfunction.

Cerebral Thrombosis

Cerebral thrombosis may be manifested as neurologic dysfunction that progresses over several minutes to hours. The dysfunction may be either minor and transient or severe and irreversible. Nearly 50% of patients who experience a stroke have had one or more previous TIAs. Commonly, thrombotic events occur during sleep, presumably reflecting decreased blood pressure and CBF that are likely to occur at this time. The symptoms of cerebral thrombosis depend on which cerebral vessel has become occluded by thrombus. In most cases, the middle cerebral artery, or a branch of this artery, is occluded. When the main trunk is occluded, infarction of a large portion of the cerebral hemisphere will result, producing symptoms of hemiplegia, homonymous hemianopsia, and, if the dominant hemisphere is involved, an expressive and receptive aphasia. Thrombosis of the anterior cerebral artery characteristically produces a more profound degree of impairment in the leg than in the face and arm. Vertebrobasilar arterial thrombosis is suggested by ipsilateral cranial nerve palsy combined with contralateral hemiplegia. Infarction of the medulla produces ipsilateral paralysis of the tongue and contralateral paralysis of the limbs; the face is spared.

Cerebral thrombosis is most likely to develop in a patient who has extensive atherosclerosis associated with essential hypertension or diabetes mellitus. Indeed, the treatment of essential hypertension with antihypertensive drugs has greatly reduced the incidence of stroke. Other causes of cerebral thrombosis include (1) hypotension, as can follow a myocardial infarction; (2) inflammatory diseases of blood vessels, as associated with temporal arteritis, polyarteritis nodosa, and systemic lupus erythematosus; and (3) hematologic disorders, including polycythemia, thrombotic thrombocytopenic purpura, and sickle cell anemia. The use of oral contraceptive drugs has been alleged to be associated with an increased incidence of cerebral thrombosis.

Treatment of cerebral thrombosis may include an attempt to arrest propagation of the thrombus. Therefore, if the CSF is clear, these patients may receive heparin initially, followed by chronic anticoagulation with warfarin. Aspirin therapy is an alternative to an oral anticoagulant.

Cerebral Embolism

Cerebral embolism is most commonly from the heart, in the presence of mitral valve disease with atrial fibrillation, a prosthetic heart valve, or subacute bacterial endocarditis. Occasionally, cerebral embolism represents fat, tumor cells, or air. Unlike cerebral thrombosis, the symptoms of cerebral embolism have an abrupt onset. Headache on the affected side is common. Neurologic deficits will depend on the vessel that is occluded. Emboli are responsible for most ischemic events that occur in the distribution of the carotid arteries, whereas thrombosis is likely to include the vertebrobasilar vessels (Fig. 17-13). The diagnosis of cerebral embolism, although suggested by the abruptness of the onset, is definitive only if a stroke occurs in a patient with valvular heart disease, with or without atrial fibrillation, or if there are emboli elsewhere in the body. Echocardiography may be useful in determining the source of emboli. Treatment of cerebral embolism in the acute phase is the same as for a cerebral thrombosis. Long-term administration of an anticoagulant is helpful in preventing a recurrent cerebral embolism.

INTRACRANIAL HEMORRHAGE

Intracranial hemorrhage accounts for about 10% of all strokes that occur in the United States.[51] The most common cause is rupture of a small arteriole or aneurysm in association with chronic hypertension. Intracranial aneurysms result from a congenital weakness in the media of cerebral arteries, which can rupture, leading to subarachnoid hemorrhage at any age, although most often in the fourth through sixth decades. Congenital intracranial aneurysms may be single or multiple. About 50% occur in the middle cerebral artery. Approximately 30% of congenital aneurysms are present in the region in which the anterior communicating artery joins the anterior cerebral arteries. The key factor predisposing to rupture of a congenital intracranial aneurysm is size. An intracranial aneurysm greater than 10 mm in diameter is associated with a high incidence of spontaneous rupture. Hypertension is also thought to predispose to an increased incidence of rupture, but this has not been confirmed. Neither age, sex, nor number and location of intracranial aneurysms influences the incidence of rupture. Mycotic aneurysms are caused by weakening of the arterial wall around a septic embolus from the heart. Intracranial hemorrhage can also be due to an arteriovenous malformation. Systemic anticoagulation with heparin or warfarin is associated with an increased likelihood of intracranial hemorrhage.

Signs and Symptoms

Signs and symptoms of intracranial hemorrhage reflect the site of hemorrhage and the development of increased ICP. Rupture of an intracranial aneurysm results in a hematoma that displaces the brain structures. For example, a hemorrhage deep in a cerebral hemisphere results in flaccid hemiplegia, hemianesthesia, and hemianopia. Vomiting and a sudden violent headache are common. Hypertension is often present. Fever and leukocytosis reflect meningeal irritation from blood. Cerebral vasospasm occurs in most patients who have sustained a subarachnoid hemorrhage and, depending on its severity, may be accompanied by cerebral ischemia[52,53] (Fig. 17-17). If vasospasm occurs in the vessels supplying the hypothalamus, the resulting ischemia may lead to stimulation of the heart through sympathetic nervous system pathways, result-

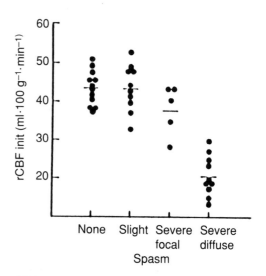

Fig. 17-17. Relationship between mean initial regional cerebral blood flow (rCBF init) and degree of vasospasm in patients experiencing a recent subarachnoid hemorrhage. (From Voldby B, Enevoldsen EM, Jensen FT. Regional CBF, intraventricular pressure, and cerebral metabolism in patients with ruptured intracranial aneurysms. J Neurosurg 1985;62:48–58, with permission.)

ing in the appearance of Q waves, deep inverted T waves, prolonged Q-T intervals, and ST elevation on the ECG. It is important to recognize that when these abnormalities are seen on the ECG after subarachnoid hemorrhage, they most likely reflect a neurologic mechanism, and not myocardial damage.[54,55] Nimodipine, a calcium entry blocker, reduces the incidence of cerebral vasospasm and associated ischemia after subarachnoid hemorrhage.[56] Coma and decerebrate rigidity may result from increased ICP. Cerebellar hemorrhage leads to unsteadiness of gait, nuchal rigidity, and peripheral facial weakness. Mortality may exceed 50% during the first month after rupture of a congenital intracranial aneurysm.[56] Another 30% of patients will experience a repeat episode of intracranial hemorrhage during this period.

In contrast to the rapid onset of neurologic dysfunction associated with hemorrhage due to rupture of an intracranial aneurysm, leakage of blood from a low-pressure arteriovenous malformation does not always produce an abrupt onset of symptoms. In fact, a patient may experience repeated bouts of intracranial hemorrhage from the arteriovenous malformation, with little permanent neurologic deficit.

Diagnosis

Computed tomography and cerebral angiography are performed to establish the diagnosis of intracranial hemorrhage. Hemorrhage but not dysfunction due to transient ischemia appears as a hyperdense area on computed tomography. Several hours to days after an ischemic event that leads to irreversible damage, lucent areas will be visible on computed tomography. When hemorrhage has been extensive, the CSF is usually bloody and under increased pressure. Lumbar puncture, if performed, should be accomplished using a small needle because of the risk of herniation after withdrawal of fluid. Xanthochromia develops in the spinal fluid within 4 hours, distinguishing subarachnoid hemorrhage from a traumatic tap. The presence of known increased ICP is a reason not to perform a lumbar puncture.

Treatment

Immediate management of the patient with intracranial hemorrhage is directed toward the reduction of increased ICP. The prognosis associated with massive intracranial hemorrhage is grave, with nearly 80% of patients dying during the acute illness. There is considerable controversy regarding the management of patients who have experienced intracranial hemorrhage due to rupture of a congenital aneurysm. For example, high doses of aminocaproic acid may be effective in decreasing the incidence of repeat hemorrhage. Other investigators, however, do not find this protective effect. Furthermore, aminocaproic acid may increase the incidence of venous thromboembolism and aggravate vasospasm associated with intracranial hemorrhage. Cerebral vasospasm may be reduced by treatment with the calcium entry blocker, nimodipine.[56] Although early operative intervention after rupture of a congenital intracranial aneurysm has traditionally been deemed hazardous, other evidence suggests that prompt surgical treatment is no more dangerous than the natural course of the disease. Likewise, there is no consensus on the management of the patient with a congenital intracranial aneurysm that has not ruptured. Nevertheless, it is likely that surgical intervention will be planned when the diameter of an intact aneurysm is shown to exceed 7 mm.

Management of Anesthesia

The goal during the management of anesthesia for resection of a congenital intracranial aneurysm is to prevent dangerous elevations in systemic blood pressure and to facilitate surgical exposure and vascular control of the aneurysm by producing controlled hypotension.

Preoperative Evaluation

Preoperative evaluation of a patient with a congenital intracranial aneurysm must assess mental status and estimate ICP. Sedation before induction of anesthesia is desirable, to reduce apprehension, but it must be titrated to prevent hypoventilation and any associated increase in CBF. Oral or intramuscular administration of a benzodiazepine, combined with intramuscular scopolamine, produces desirable sedation and relief of anxiety, without introducing significant cardiopulmonary depression. Prophylactic administration of nimodipine before

surgery for clipping of an intracranial aneurysm does not influence the anesthetic requirements or dose of nitroprusside required to maintain controlled hypotension.[53]

Induction of Anesthesia

Induction of anesthesia is often achieved with an intravenous injection of a barbiturate, benzodiazepine, etomidate, or propofol, followed by a muscle relaxant to facilitate control of ventilation and subsequent intubation of the trachea. The use of succinylcholine may be influenced by the report of exaggerated potassium release after administration of this drug to patients undergoing general anesthesia for repair of a previously ruptured cerebral aneurysm.[57] It is important to prevent an excessive, prolonged elevation in blood pressure that predictably occurs in response to direct laryngoscopy and to intubation of the trachea. The pressor response to intubation of the trachea is minimized by establishing an adequate depth of anesthesia with a volatile anesthetic or opioid, or both, before initiation of direct laryngoscopy. It is important to limit the duration of laryngoscopy to as short a period as possible (ideally less than 15 seconds). The administration of lidocaine (1 to 2 mg·kg^{-1} IV), about 1 minute before intubation of the trachea, may attenuate the pressure response and blunt the increase in ICP that may accompany direct laryngoscopy[20,58] (Fig. 17-10). If the blood pressure increases despite these precautions, it may be useful to administer nitroprusside (1 to 2 μg·kg^{-1} IV) as a rapid injection.[59]

Maintenance of Anesthesia

Acceptable maintenance of anesthesia is achieved with nitrous oxide and a volatile anesthetic. Potent volatile drugs are useful in preventing and treating excessive increases in blood pressure that can occur in response to surgical stimulation. A volatile anesthetic is also likely to decrease the dose of vasodilator necessary for the production of controlled hypotension. Furthermore, unchanged CBF and decreased cerebral metabolic oxygen requirements during the administration of isoflurane indicate that the global cerebral oxygen supply-demand balance is favorably altered in patients anesthetized with this anesthetic.[60] Management of ventilation, fluid therapy, the use of monitors, and treatment of increased ICP are similar to that described for patients undergoing removal of intracranial tumors.

Controlled Hypotension

Surgical exposure and control of an intracranial aneurysm are facilitated by the production of controlled hypotension. Continuous intravenous delivery of nitroprusside, using a calibrated infusion pump, is most often used to achieve the desired level of decrease in blood pressure. In the presence of adequate anesthesia, as provided by a volatile anesthetic, the dose of nitroprusside seldom exceeds 3 μg·kg^{-1}·min^{-1}. Propranolol or esmolol can be used to slow the heart rate, if reflex tachycardia that accompanies the decrease in blood pressure offsets the hypotensive effect of nitroprusside. The maximum acceptable infusion rate of nitroprusside is 8 to 10 $\mu g \cdot kg^{-1} \cdot min^{-1}$, not to exceed 1.5 mg·kg^{-1} for a 1- to 3-hour administration.[61] If the dose of nitroprusside approaches this infusion rate, it is important to monitor arterial pH, at intervals of about 1 hour. The appearance of metabolic acidosis in a patient receiving a high dose of nitroprusside suggests the development of cyanide toxicity; infusion of the drug should be promptly discontinued.

Alternative drugs to nitroprusside for producing controlled hypotension are trimethaphan, nitroglycerin, and labetalol. Trimethaphan is both a ganglionic blocker and a peripheral vasodilator. Although trimethaphan provides excellent minute-to-minute control of blood pressure, its use for neuroanesthesia is limited because this drug produces mydriasis, which interferes with the evaluation of neurologic status. Perhaps more important is the observation in animals that trimethaphan decreases CBF more than cerebral metabolic oxygen requirements; thus, trimethaphan decreases the brain oxygen reserve while producing controlled hypotension.[62] Furthermore, tachyphylaxis commonly develops to the blood pressure-lowering effects of trimethaphan. Nitroglycerin acts predominantly on capacitance vessels, to decrease the blood pressure by decreasing venous return. As such, decreased blood pressure produced by nitroglycerin may be more dependent on intravascular fluid volume, as compared with nitroprusside. In addition, nitroglycerin is less potent than nitroprusside in decreasing blood pressure.[63] Labetalol is a mixed alpha and beta antagonist that promptly decreases blood pressure when administered intravenously, making it a potentially useful drug in the production of controlled hypotension.

Decreased PaO$_2$ as reflected by pulse oximetry often accompanies the production of drug-induced controlled hypotension. Drugs used to produce controlled hypotension also act as cerebral vasodilators. As a result, CBF and ICP can increase, despite decreases in systemic blood pressure. This increase in ICP has been documented with nitroprusside and can be attenuated by inducing hyperventilation of the lungs before administration of the drug.[21] In view of this effect, it might be prudent to withhold administration of a vasodilating drug until after the dura is opened.

The estimated safe level of controlled hypotension can be calculated on the basis of predicted CBF, limits of autoregulation of CBF, and PaCO$_2$. For example, in a normotensive awake patient (mean arterial pressure 90 mmHg), CBF is about 50 ml·100 g^{-1}·min^{-1}. Evidence of cerebral ischemia on the EEG is not shown when CBF remains above 25 ml·100 g^{-1}·min^{-1}.[64] Assuming that CBF decreases linearly below a perfusion pressure of 60 mmHg, blood flow to the brain would be decreased to 25 ml·100 g^{-1}·min^{-1}, when cerebral perfusion pressure corresponds to a mean arterial pressure of about 45 mmHg—provided the central venous pressure is 10 mmHg

(cerebral perfusion pressure equals mean arterial pressure minus central venous pressure). CBF is also decreased about 1 ml for each 1-mmHg decrease in PaCO$_2$. Therefore, it is probably important to maintain the PaCO$_2$ at about 35 mmHg during controlled hypotension. On the basis of these concepts, safe cerebral perfusion pressure during controlled hypotension would be produced by a mean arterial pressure of about 50 mmHg. This mean arterial blood pressure corresponds to a systolic blood pressure of about 60 to 70 mmHg. It should also be appreciated that a patient will safely tolerate a mean arterial pressure of less than 50 mmHg for a short period, as may be needed to place a clip on an intracranial aneurysm. Tolerance to a low perfusion pressure is also improved by the zero ICP present when the dura is open. Conversely, hypotension produced by hemorrhage is not as well tolerated as a similar decrease in blood pressure produced by a vasodilating agent. Presumably, the development of cerebral ischemia during hemorrhagic hypotension reflects sympathetic nervous system discharge, leading to increased cerebral metabolic oxygen requirements. As a result, evidence of cerebral ischemia during hemorrhage is likely to develop at a blood pressure and CBF that would be considered safe when produced by a vasodilating agent, but in the absence of sympathetic nervous system stimulation.

When controlled hypotension is considered in a hypertensive patient, it is important to appreciate the likely rightward shift of the curve for autoregulation of CBF. The lower limit of 60 mmHg assumed for autoregulation in a normotensive patient (mean arterial pressure 90 mmHg) should be adjusted upward by an equal amount for each 1 mmHg that the mean arterial pressure exceeds 90 mmHg. Therefore, the lower limit of autoregulation would be 85 mmHg in a chronically hypertensive patient, with a mean arterial pressure of 115 mmHg. This lower limit of autoregulation value should be used instead of 60 mmHg in calculating the safe level of controlled hypotension.

An alternative to these calculations as a guideline for the safe level of controlled hypotension is to decrease mean arterial pressure no more than 30 to 40 mmHg below the normal awake level. This guideline assumes a central venous pressure of 10 mmHg or less and a PaCO$_2$ of about 35 mmHg.

The need for accurate monitoring of blood pressure entails strict attention to accurate calibration of the transducer used to measure arterial pressure and to proper positioning of the transducer relative to the heart level. Accuracy of systolic blood pressure measured from a catheter placed in a peripheral artery of the upper extremity can be confirmed by inflating an encircling cuff placed proximal to the artery, until no blood flow is present. Slow deflation of the occlusive cuff is permitted, until the first sign of pulsatile blood flow is detected from the peripheral artery. When this "reflow" occurs, the pressure on the mercury manometer represents true systolic blood pressure. Confirmation by this method is known as the return-to-flow technique. This confirmation is helpful, since a false-high reading of systolic blood pressure from the intra-arterial catheter could lead to an unrecognized and potentially ischemic levels of cerebral perfusion pressure during controlled hypotension. Equally important in confirming the accuracy of the blood pressure recorded from the arterial catheter is proper positioning of the arterial pressure transducer. As a guideline, blood pressure decreases about 0.7 mmHg for each centimeter that the head is above the level of the heart. Therefore, recording the mean arterial pressure from a transducer placed at heart level would not accurately reflect the perfusion pressure at the brain, if the head were elevated above the heart level. For example, when the head is elevated 20 cm above heart level, cerebral perfusion pressure will be about 14 mmHg less than the mean arterial pressure present at heart level. If controlled hypotension were produced to a mean arterial pressure of 50 mmHg, as recorded from a transducer at heart level, the actual perfusion pressure at the brain would be about 36 mmHg. A useful approach during controlled hypotension is to place the transducer at the same height as the circle of Willis. From a practical standpoint, an arterial pressure transducer placed at the level of the external auditory canal will reflect mean arterial pressure at the circle of Willis.

ACUTE HEAD TRAUMA

Acute head trauma most often follows a motor vehicle accident and is the leading cause of death in persons less than 24 years of age. It is frequently associated with other injuries, including cervical spine injury and thoracoabdominal trauma. Initial management of head injury includes immobilization of the cervical spine, establishment of a patent upper airway, and protection of the lungs from the aspiration of gastric contents. The most useful diagnostic procedure, in terms of simplicity and rapidity, is computed tomography, which should be performed as soon as possible. In this regard, computed tomography has greatly facilitated the identification of an epidural or subdural hematoma. The Glasgow Coma Scale provides a reproducible method for assessing the seriousness of brain injury (less than 8 points is severe injury) and for following the patient's neurologic status (Table 17-4). Patients with a scale score less than 8 points are by definition in coma and about 50% of these patients die or remain in a vegetative state. The age of the patient and type of injury are important determinants of outcome in patients with low scores. For example, a patient with an acute subdural hematoma has a poorer prognosis than that of a patient with a diffuse contusion injury. Mortality in children with a severe head injury is lower than in adults.

Table 17-4. Glasgow Coma Scale

Response	Score
Eye Opening	
Spontaneous	4
To speech	3
To pain	2
Nil	1
Best Motor Response	
Obeys	6
Localizes	5
Withdraws (flexion)	4
Abnormal flexion	3
Extensor response	2
Nil	1
Verbal Response	
Oriented	5
Confused conversation	4
Inappropriate words	3
Incomprehensible sounds	2
Nil	1

Epidural Hematoma

Epidural hematoma results from arterial bleeding into the space between the skull and dura. The cause is usually rupture of a meningeal artery associated with a skull fracture. Classically, the patient experiences loss of consciousness in association with the head injury, followed by regained consciousness and a variable lucid period. Hemiparesis, mydriasis, and bradycardia reflecting uncal herniation and brain stem compression develop suddenly within a few hours after injury. If an epidural hematoma is suspected on computed tomography, the treatment is prompt placement of burr holes at the site of the skull fracture.

Subdural Hematoma

Subdural hematoma results from a lacerated or torn bridging vein that bleeds into the space between the dura and the arachnoid. The CSF, which is subarachnoid, remains clear. Symptoms characteristically evolve gradually over several days because the hematoma results from slow venous bleeding. The most common cause is head trauma, which may be considered so minor that the responsible event has been forgotten by the patient. Trivial head injury leading to a subdural hematoma is particularly likely in an elderly patient. Occasionally, a subdural hematoma is spontaneous, as in a patient on hemodialysis or being treated with an anticoagulant.

Headache is a universal complaint of the patient with a subdural hematoma. Drowsiness and obtundation are characteristic findings, but these changes may fluctuate in magnitude from hour to hour. Lateralizing neurologic signs, manifesting as hemiparesis, hemianopsia, and language disturbances, eventually occur. An elderly patient may have an unexplained progressive dementia. The diagnosis of subdural hematoma is confirmed by computed tomography. Conservative medical management may be acceptable for the patient whose condition has stabilized. Nevertheless, the most frequent treatment is surgical evacuation of the clot, as the prognosis is poor if coma develops.

DEGENERATIVE DISEASES OF THE NERVOUS SYSTEM

Degenerative diseases of the nervous system may reflect defects in the development of the neural tube, which might not result in symptoms until adulthood. Often, a hereditary pattern is responsible for these disorders. Pathologic processes may be diffuse or may involve only those neurons that are anatomically and functionally related.

Aqueductal Stenosis

Aqueductal stenosis is caused by congenital narrowing of the cerebral aqueduct that connects the third and fourth ventricles. Obstructive hydrocephalus can develop in infancy, when the narrowing is severe. Lesser degrees of obstruction result in a slowly progressive hydrocephalus, which may not be evident until adulthood. The symptoms of aqueductal stenosis are the same as those seen with increased ICP. A seizure disorder is present in about one-third of these patients. Computed tomography confirms the presence of obstructive hydrocephalus. Aqueductal stenosis sufficient to produce signs of hydrocephalus, and increased ICP is treated by ventricular shunting. Management of anesthesia for the creation of a ventricular shunt must consider the likely presence of increased ICP in these patients.

Arnold-Chiari Malformation

The Arnold-Chiari malformation consists of the downward displacement of the tonsillar portion of the cerebellum and caudal portion of the medulla through the foramen magnum into the upper cervical spinal canal. Cerebellar herniation results in the formation of arachnoidal adhesions, leading to obstruction of the flow of CSF from the fourth ventricle. This obstruction can lead to hydrocephalus and increased ICP. In addition, there is progressive entrapment of cranial nerves, as well as torsion of the brain stem.

Signs and Symptoms

Signs and symptoms of the Arnold-Chiari malformation appear at any age. The most common complaint is an occipital headache, often extending into the shoulders and arms, with a corresponding cutaneous dysesthesia. Pain is aggravated by coughing or movement of the head. Visual disturbances, intermittent vertigo, and ataxia are prominent symptoms. Signs of syringomyelia are present in about 50% of patients with this disorder.

Treatment

Treatment of the Arnold-Chiari malformation consists of surgical decompression by freeing adhesions and enlarging the foramen magnum. Management of anesthesia must consider the possibility of an associated increase in ICP.

Syringomyelia

Syringomyelia is a chronic, slowly progressive degeneration of the spinal cord, leading to cavitation. Presumably, this degeneration reflects an abnormality of embryologic development associated with obstruction to the outflow of CSF from the fourth ventricle. The pressure of the CSF is directed into the central canal of the spinal cord, which eventually leads to cyst formation.

Signs and Symptoms

Signs and symptoms of syringomyelia usually begin in the third or fourth decades of life. Early complaints are those of dissociated sensory impairment in the upper extremities, reflecting destruction of crossing fibers that convey the sensation of pain and temperature. As cavitation of the spinal cord progresses, destruction of lower motor neurons ensues, with the development of skeletal muscle weakness and wasting, with areflexia. Thoracic scoliosis may result from weakness of paravertebral muscles. Extension of the cavitation process cephalad into the medulla results in syringobulbia, characterized by paralysis of the palate, tongue, and vocal cords and loss of sensation over the face. Magnetic resonance imaging is the preferred diagnostic procedure.

Treatment

No known treatment is effective in arresting the progressive degeneration of the spinal cord or medulla. Surgical procedures designed to restore the normal flow of CSF or to plug the central cavity have not been predictably effective.

Management of Anesthesia

Management of anesthesia in a patient with syringomyelia or syringobulbia should consider the neurologic deficits associated with this disease. Thoracic scoliosis can contribute to ventilation-to-perfusion mismatching. The presence of lower motor neuron disease, leading to skeletal muscle wasting, suggests the possibility that hyperkalemia could develop after the administration of succinylcholine.[65] Likewise, co-existing skeletal muscle weakness could be associated with an exaggerated response to nondepolarizing muscle relaxants. Body temperature is often monitored, as thermal regulation may be impaired. The selection of drugs for induction and maintenance of anesthesia is not influenced by the disease. The possible presence of decreased or absent protective airway reflexes should be considered when contemplating removal of the tracheal tube during the postoperative period.

Amyotrophic Lateral Sclerosis

Amyotrophic lateral sclerosis (ALS) is a degenerative disease of the motor cells throughout the central nervous system and spinal cord that most commonly afflicts males between 40 and 60 years of age. Limitation of the degenerative process to the motor cortex is designated primary lateral sclerosis; limitation to the brain stem nuclei is known as pseudobulbar palsy. Werdnig-Hoffmann disease resembles ALS, except that manifestations of this disease occur during the first 3 years of life. Although the cause of ALS is unknown, occasionally a genetic pattern is shown. The possibility of a viral etiology has also been proposed.

Signs and Symptoms
Signs and symptoms of ALS reflect upper and lower motor neuron dysfunction. Frequent initial manifestations include atrophy, weakness, and fasciculations of skeletal muscles, often beginning in the intrinsic muscles of the hand. With time, atrophy and weakness involve most of the skeletal muscles, including those of the tongue, pharynx, larynx, and chest. Early symptoms of bulbar involvement include fasciculations of the tongue, as well as dysphagia leading to pulmonary aspiration. For reasons that are unclear, the ocular muscles are spared. Evidence of autonomic nervous system dysfunction in these patients manifests as orthostatic hypotension and resting tachycardia. An inability to control emotional responses is characteristic. Complaints of cramping and aching sensations, particularly in the lower extremities, are common. Carcinoma of the lung has been associated with ALS. The plasma creatine kinase concentration is normal, distinguishing this disease from chronic polymyositis. ALS has no known treatment, and death is likely within 6 years after the onset of clinical symptoms.

Management of Anesthesia
The patient with a lower motor neuron disease such as ALS is vulnerable to hyperkalemia after administration of succinylcholine.[65] Furthermore, these patients may show prolonged responses to nondepolarizing muscle relaxants. Indeed, changes of ALS, as displayed on the electromyogram, resemble those of myasthenia gravis. Bulbar involvement with dysfunction of pharyngeal muscles may predispose to pulmonary aspiration. There is no evidence that a specific anesthetic drug

or combination of drugs is best for administration to a patient with this disease. Epidural anesthesia has been successfully administered to patients with ALS.[66]

Friedreich's Ataxia

Friedreich's ataxia is an autosomal recessive inherited condition, characterized by degeneration of the spinocerebellar and pyramidal tracts. Cardiomyopathy is present in 10% to 50% of cases. Kyphoscoliosis, producing a steady deterioration of pulmonary function, is present in nearly 80% of affected patients. Ataxia is the typical presenting symptom. Dysarthria, nystagmus, skeletal muscle weakness and spasticity, and diabetes mellitus may be present. Friedreich's ataxia is usually fatal by early adulthood, often due to cardiac failure.

Management of anesthesia for Friedreich's ataxia is as described for ALS. In addition, the potential for exaggerated negative inotropic effects of anesthetic drugs in the presence of cardiomyopathy should be considered. Although experience is limited, the response to muscle relaxants seems normal.[67] Kyphoscoliosis may make epidural anesthesia technically difficult, whereas spinal anesthesia has been successfully used.[68] The likelihood of postoperative ventilatory failure may be increased, especially in the presence of kyphoscoliosis.

Paralysis Agitans

Paralysis agitans (Parkinson's disease) is an adult-onset degenerative disease of the central nervous system (extrapyramidal system), characterized by the loss of dopaminergic fibers normally present in the basal ganglia of the brain. As a result of the degeneration of these fibers, the levels of dopamine are depleted in the basal ganglia. Dopamine is presumed to be a neurotransmitter, which acts by inhibiting the rate of firing of neurons that control the extrapyramidal motor system. Depletion of dopamine results in diminished inhibition of the extrapyramidal motor system and an unopposed action of acetylcholine.

Although the cause of paralysis agitans is generally unknown, the disease has been observed to develop after encephalitis, intoxication with carbon monoxide, and chronic ingestion of antipsychotic drugs. Males between 40 and 60 years of age are most often afflicted.

Signs and Symptoms
The classic signs and symptoms of paralysis agitans are decreased spontaneous movements, rigidity of the extremities, facial immobility, a shuffling gait, and a rhythmic resting tremor. These symptoms reflect diminished inhibition of the activity of the extrapyramidal motor system due to depletion of dopamine from the basal ganglia. Skeletal muscle rigidity first appears in proximal muscles of the neck. The earliest manifestation can be loss of associated arm swing when walk-

ing and the absence of head rotation when turning. Facial immobility is characterized by infrequent blinking and by a paucity of emotional responses. Tremor is characterized as rhythmic, alternating flexion and extension of the thumb and digits at a rate of four to five movements per second. These movements are often described as a pill-rolling tremor. The tremor is prominent in the resting limb but disappears briefly during the course of a movement, which distinguishes it from an essential or familial tremor. Seborrhea, oily skin, pupillary abnormalities, diaphragmatic spasms, and oculogyric crises are frequent. Dementia and depression are often noted.

Treatment

The treatment of paralysis agitans is designed to increase the concentration of dopamine in the basal ganglia or to decrease the neuronal effects of acetylcholine. The drugs most often used to achieve these goals are levodopa, anticholinergics, and antihistamines.

Levodopa

Exogenous administration of dopamine will not increase the concentration of this inhibitory neurotransmitter in the basal ganglia, since dopamine cannot readily cross the blood-brain barrier. However, the immediate precursor of dopamine, levodopa, does cross the blood-brain barrier and is then converted to dopamine in the central nervous system by a decarboxylase enzyme. Therefore, the oral administration of levodopa (4 to 6 g·d^{-1}) can be used to increase the central nervous system concentration of dopamine. The decarboxylating enzyme responsible for the conversion of levodopa to dopamine in the central nervous system is also present in the systemic circulation and other tissues. As a result, administration of levodopa results in total body increases in the concentration of dopamine. Furthermore, conversion of levodopa to dopamine in the systemic circulation limits the amount of drug available for transfer to the central nervous system. For this reason, levodopa is often combined with a drug that inhibits the activity of decarboxylase enzyme in the systemic circulation. Indeed, the combination of levodopa with such an enzyme inhibitor, carbidopa, often permits a 75% reduction in the dose of levodopa, with an associated decrease in the dose-related adverse side effects of this drug.

The adverse side effects of levodopa are seen in the cardiovascular, gastrointestinal, and central nervous systems. Increased levels of dopamine, converted from levodopa, can increase myocardial contractility and heart rate, predisposing to cardiac irritability. Norepinephrine stores in the heart may become depleted by the chronic administration of levodopa. Dopamine is known to increase renal blood flow, glomerular filtration rate, and excretion of sodium. Renin release is also reduced during levodopa therapy. As a result of these renal effects of dopamine, it is likely that intravascular fluid volume

will be decreased, and the activity of the renin-angiotension-aldosterone system will be reduced. Therefore, orthostatic hypotension is a common finding in patients chronically treated with levodopa. Another mechanism for orthostatic hypotension is decreased production of norepinephrine in sympathetic nervous system nerve endings due to the negative feedback inhibition by a high concentration of dopamine on the synthesis of catecholamines. In addition, dopamine replaces norepinephrine at many sites and, because of its weaker pressor actions, is less able to support blood pressure. Gastrointestinal side effects of levodopa therapy include nausea and vomiting, most likely reflecting stimulation of the chemoreceptor trigger zone by dopamine. Central nervous system effects of chronic levodopa therapy are most often manifested as psychiatric symptoms, including agitation, confusion, depression, and overt psychosis. The most serious problem is the appearance of dyskinesis, which develops in about 80% of patients after a year or more of treatment with levodopa.

Anticholinergic and Antihistaminic Drugs

Anticholinergic drugs may be the initial selection for therapy when symptoms of paralysis agitans are mild. Antihistaminic drugs are also useful for the control of mild symptoms of extrapyramidal motor system overactivity, particularly as produced by phenothiazines or butyrophenones.

Management of Anesthesia

Management of anesthesia in the patient with paralysis agitans is based on an understanding of the treatment of this disease and of the associated potential adverse drug effects. Levodopa therapy should be continued during the perioperative period, including the usual morning dose on the day of surgery. The elimination half-time of levodopa, and of the dopamine it produces, is short, so that interruption of therapy for more than 6 to 12 hours can result in an abrupt loss of therapeutic benefit derived from this drug. Indeed, the abrupt withdrawal of levodopa can lead to skeletal muscle rigidity that interferes with the maintenance of adequate ventilation.[69]

The possibility of orthostatic hypotension, cardiac dysrhythmias, and even hypertension must be kept in mind during the administration of anesthesia to a patient being treated with levodopa. The selection of drugs to be administered in the preoperative medication and for the production of anesthesia must consider the ability of phenothiazines and butyrophenones to antagonize the effects of dopamine in the basal ganglia. Therefore, droperidol, as present in Innovar, would not be a likely selection in the patient being treated with levodopa. An acute dystonic reaction after the administration of alfentanil has been speculated to reflect an opioid-induced decrease in central dopaminergic transmission.[70] The use of ketamine may be questionable because of the possible provocation of exaggerated sympathetic nervous system responses. Nevertheless, ketamine has been used successfully in patients treated with levodopa.[69] Cardiac dysrhythmias may be more likely to occur when halothane is selected, although this speculation has not been documented. The presence of decreased intravascular fluid volume may be manifested by a decrease in blood pressure during the induction of anesthesia, requiring aggressive administration of crystalloid or colloid solutions. The choice of muscle relaxants does not seem to be influenced by the presence of paralysis agitans. The single report of a patient in whom hyperkalemia developed after the intravenous administration of succinylcholine has not been confirmed by others to be a risk in these patients.[71] Continuation of levodopa therapy during the postoperative period is as important as maintaining treatment up to the induction of anesthesia.

Hallervorden-Spatz Disease

Hallervorden-Spatz disease is a rare autosomal recessive disorder of the basal ganglia. It follows a slowly progressive course from its onset in late childhood to death in about 10 years. No specific laboratory tests are diagnostic for this condition, and no effective treatment is known. Dementia and dystonia with torticollis, as well as scoliosis, are commonly present. Dystonic posturing is likely to disappear with the induction of anesthesia, although skeletal muscle contractures and bony changes may accompany the chronic forms of the disease, leading to immobility of the temporomandibular joint and cervical spine, even in the presence of deep general anesthesia or neuromuscular blockade.

Management of Anesthesia

Management of anesthesia must consider the possibility of being unable to position the patient optimally for intubation of the trachea, after induction of anesthesia.[72] Noxious stimulation, as produced by attempted awake intubation of the trachea, can intensify dystonia. For these reasons, induction of anesthesia may be preferably achieved by inhalation and maintenance of spontaneous ventilation. Administration of succinylcholine is questionable, since skeletal muscle wasting and diffuse axonal changes in the brain, which may involve the upper motor neurons, could accentuate the release of potassium. Any required skeletal muscle relaxation is probably best provided by an increased concentration of a volatile anesthetic or a nondepolarizing muscle relaxant. Emergence from anesthesia will be predictably accompanied by return of dystonic posturing.

Huntington's Chorea

Huntington's chorea is a premature degenerative disease of the central nervous system, characterized by marked atrophy of the caudate nucleus and, to a lesser degree, of the putamen and globus pallidus.[73] Biochemical abnormalities include defi-

ciencies in the basal ganglia of acetylcholine and its synthesizing enzyme choline acetyltransferase and gamma aminobutyric acid. A selective loss of gamma aminobutyric acid may reduce inhibition of the dopamine nigrostriatal system. This disease is transmitted as an autosomal dominant trait, but its delayed appearance until 35 to 40 years of age interferes with effective genetic counseling.

Signs and Symptoms

Manifestations of Huntington's chorea consist of progressive dementia combined with choreoathetosis. Chorea is usually considered the first sign of Huntington's chorea, although behavioral changes (depression, dementia) may precede the onset of involuntary movement by several years. Involvement of the pharyngeal muscles makes these patients susceptible to pulmonary aspiration. The disease progresses over several years, and accompanying mental depression makes suicide a prominent cause of death. The duration of Huntington's chorea from onset to the patient's death averages 17 years.

Treatment

Treatment of Huntington's chorea is symptomatic and is directed at reducing choreiform movements. Haloperidol or chlorpromazine is used to control the chorea and emotional lability associated with this disease. The most useful therapy for the control of involuntary movements is with drugs that interfere with the neurotransmitter effects of dopamine. As such, butyrophenones and phenothiazines may be helpful in the management of these patients. Diazepam and lithium have also been tried, with varying success.

Management of Anesthesia

Experience with the management of anesthesia in Huntington's chorea patients is too limited to propose specific drugs or techniques. Nitrous oxide combined with an opioid and droperidol would seem a useful approach, in view of the potential antagonism of dopamine by droperidol. Nevertheless, the use of nitrous oxide and a volatile anesthetic is also acceptable. Delayed awakening and generalized tonic spasms were observed after the administration of thiopental to a single patient.[74] The importance of this observation, if any, remains unclear. Decreased plasma cholinesterase activity, with prolonged responses to succinylcholine, have been reported.[75] Likewise, it has been suggested that these patients may be sensitive to the effects of nondepolarizing muscle relaxants.[76]

Preoperative and postoperative sedation with a butyrophenone or phenothiazine may be helpful in controlling choreiform movements. The increased likelihood of pulmonary aspiration must be considered if pharyngeal muscles are involved.

Spasmodic Torticollis

Spasmodic torticollis is thought to result from disturbances of basal ganglia function. The most frequent mode of presentation is spasmodic contraction of nuchal muscles, which may progress to involvement of the limb and girdle muscles. Hypertrophy of the sternocleidomastoid muscle may be present. Spasm may involve the muscles of the vertebral column, leading to lordosis and scoliosis and impaired ventilation. Treatment is not particularly effective, but a bilateral anterior rhizotomy at C1 and C3, with a subarachnoid section of the spinal accessory nerve, may be attempted. This operation may cause postoperative paralysis of the diaphragm, resulting in respiratory distress. No known problems are related to the selection of anesthetic drugs, but spasm of nuchal muscles can interfere with maintenance of a patent upper airway before institution of skeletal muscle paralysis. Furthermore, awake intubation of the trachea may be necessary, if chronic skeletal muscle spasm has led to fixation of the cervical vertebrae. The sudden appearance of torticollis after the induction of general anesthesia with fentanyl, thiopental, and isoflurane was described in a patient treated chronically with chlorpromazine.[77] The administration of diphenhydramine (25 to 50 mg IV) produces dramatic reversal of drug-induced torticollis.

Shy-Drager Syndrome

Shy-Drager syndrome is characterized by autonomic nervous system dysfunction in association with widespread parenchymatous degeneration in the central nervous system and spinal cord. Although the primary defect is loss of neuronal cells, an element of sympathetic nervous system dysfunction can result from the depletion of norepinephrine from peripheral efferent nerve endings. Idiopathic orthostatic hypotension, rather than Shy-Drager syndrome, is considered to be present when autonomic nervous system dysfunction occurs in the absence of central nervous system degeneration.

Signs and Symptoms

Signs and symptoms of Shy-Drager syndrome are related to dysfunction of the autonomic nervous system, as manifested by orthostatic hypotension, urinary retention, bowel dysfunction, diminished sweating, and sexual impotence. Postural hypotension is often severe enough to produce syncope. The plasma concentration of norepinephrine fails to show a normal increase after standing or exercise. Sweating may be absent, pupillary reflexes sluggish, and control of breathing abnormal. Further evidence of autonomic nervous system dysfunction is failure of baroreceptor reflexes to produce an increase in heart rate or vasoconstriction in response to hypotension. Symptoms of paralysis agitans often develop in these patients.

Treatment

Treatment of orthostatic hypotension is symptomatic and includes head-up body tilt at night, elastic stockings, high-sodium diet to expand the intravascular fluid volume, and administration of an alpha agonist.[78] Death usually occurs within 8

years of diagnosis, most often due to cerebral ischemia from prolonged hypotension. Theoretically, orthostatic hypotension can be lessened by treatment with a selective alpha-2 antagonist, such as yohimbine, which would facilitate continued release of norepinephrine from postganglionic nerve endings. Levodopa is administered to reduce the symptoms of paralysis agitans.

Management of Anesthesia

Management of anesthesia is based on understanding the impact of reduced autonomic nervous system activity on the cardiovascular responses to such events as changes in body position, positive airway pressure, and acute blood loss, as well as on the effects produced by the administration of negative inotropic anesthetic agents. Preoperative evaluation may elicit such signs of autonomic nervous system dysfunction as orthostatic hypotension and the absence of beat-to-beat variability in heart rate assoicated with deep breathing. Despite the obvious vulnerability of these patients to events likely to occur during the perioperative period, clinical experience has shown that most patients tolerate general anesthesia without undue risk.[79] The key to management of these patients is continuous monitoring of blood pressure and prompt correction of hypotension by the infusion of crystalloid or colloid solutions. Continuous measurement of arterial blood pressure and cardiac filling pressures is useful in guiding the rate of intravenous fluid infusion. If a vasopressor is needed, it should be appreciated that these patients can exhibit exaggerated responses to drugs that act by provoking the release of norepinephrine. Presumably, this excessive response reflects denervation hypersensitivity. An appropriate selection to treat hypotension pharmacologically would be a direct-acting drug such as phenylephrine. Even the dose of phenylephrine should be initially reduced, until the response of each individual patient can be confirmed. A continuous infusion of phenylephrine (0.5 to 1.5 $\mu g \cdot kg^{-1} \cdot min^{-1}$ IV) has been used to maintain blood pressure in affected patients during general anesthesia.[78] The risk of hypotension after the administration of spinal or epidural anesthesia detracts from the use of these techniques in affected patients. Excessive decreases in cardiac output, due to myocardial depression from a volatile anesthetic, can result in exaggerated hypotension. This is because compensatory responses such as vasoconstriction or tachycardia are unlikely, in view of absent carotid sinus activity. Likewise, positive-pressure ventilation of the lungs or acute blood loss are not readily compensated for by increased sympathetic nervous system activity. Bradycardia, which contributes to hypotension, is best treated with atropine. Signs of the depth of anesthesia may be less apparent in these patients because of a decreased response of the sympathetic nervous system to noxious stimulation. Induction of anesthesia with diazepam and fentanyl, in addition to pancuronium for skeletal muscle paralysis, has been described in these patients, followed by maintenance of anesthesia with a low dose of a volatile anesthetic, combined with nitrous oxide.[79] Administration of a muscle relaxant with minimal to absent effects on circulation would also seem a useful alternative to pancuronium. Thiopental, as used for the induction of anesthesia, might provoke an exaggerated decrease in blood pressure if the rate of administration is rapid or if the intravascular fluid volume is decreased. Conversely, the possibility of an accentuated blood pressure increase after administration of ketamine should be considered.

Familial Dysautonomia

Familial dysautonomia (Riley-Day syndrome) is a rare inherited disorder of the central nervous system, found almost exclusively in children of Eastern European Jewish ancestry (see Chapter 32).

Congenital Insensitivity to Pain

Congenital insensitivity to pain with anhidrosis is a rare hereditary disorder that leads to self-mutilation and defective thermoregulation. The plasma concentration of catecholamines may be decreased, and autonomic nervous system dysfunction may be present. Skeletal muscle weakness and joint laxity are characteristic. Management of anesthesia includes preoperative medication to relieve apprehension in a patient who is often mentally retarded, monitoring of body temperature, and avoidance of joint extension.[80] The use of an anticholinergic drug is questionable, considering the presence of anhidrosis, as well as potential autonomic nervous system dysfunction. Indeed, hypertension and tachycardia has been described after the intravenous administration of scopolamine.[81]

Progressive Blindness

Degenerative diseases of the central nervous system limited to the optic nerve and retina include Leber's optic atrophy, retinitis pigmentosa, and the Kearns-Sayer syndrome.

Leber's Optic Atrophy

Leber's optic atrophy is characterized by degeneration of the retina and atrophy of the optic nerve, culminating in blindness. Transmission of this disease is as a sex-linked autosomal recessive trait. Since the defect responsible for optic atrophy is most likely related to an abnormality of cyanide metabolism, these patients should probably not receive nitroprusside.

Retinitis Pigmentosa

Retinitis pigmentosa describes a genetically and clinically heterogeneous group of inherited retinopathies characterized by degeneration of the retina. These debilitating disorders collec-

tively represent the most frequent forms of human visual handicap, with an estimated prevalence of about 1 in 3000. Mutations responsible for retinitis pigmentosa occur in genes responsible for encoding transmembranes proteins of the rod photoreceptor outer disc. Examination of the retina shows areas of pigmentation, particularly in the peripheral regions. Vision is lost from the periphery of the retina toward the center, until total blindness develops.

Kearns-Sayer Syndrome

Kearns-Sayer syndrome is characterized by retinitis pigmentosa associated with progressive external ophthalmoplegia, typically manifested before 20 years of age. Cardiac conduction abnormalities, ranging from bundle branch block to third-degree atrioventricular heart block, are common in these patients. Third-degree atrioventricular heart block can occur abruptly, leading to death before an artificial cardiac pacemaker can be inserted. Generalized degeneration of the central nervous system has been observed. This finding, as well as the often elevated concentration of protein in the CSF, suggests a viral etiology for this disease.

Although Kearns-Sayer syndrome is extremely rare, one could conceivably encounter a patient requiring surgery for a procedure other than insertion of an artificial cardiac pacemaker. Management of anesthesia requires a high index of suspicion and prior preparation to treat third-degree atrioventricular heart block, if this cardiac conduction abnormality occurs during the perioperative period. This preparation includes prompt availability of isoproterenol for infusion as a chemical cardiac pacemaker, to maintain an adequate heart rate until artificial cardiac pacing can be established. Experience is too limited to recommended specific drugs for the induction and maintenance of anesthesia. Apparently, the response to succinylcholine and nondepolarizing muscle relaxants is not altered, suggesting that this disease does not involve the neuromuscular junction.[82]

Alzheimer's Disease

Alzheimer's disease is responsible for about 60% of cases of severe dementia in the United States.[83] The incidence of this disease is about 10% for patients between 75 and 85 years of age, increasing to 20% for patients who are older than 85 years of age. About one-half of all nursing home beds are occupied by patients with Alzheimer's disease. A diagnosis of probable Alzheimer's disease is made when the dementing illness is characterized by insidious onset, progressive worsening of memory, and a normal level of consciousness. Computed tomography typically shows ventricular dilation and marked cortical atrophy. Positron emission tomography may demonstrate areas of decreased blood flow. The definitive diagnosis of Alzheimer's disease can be made only after examination of brain tissue. In this regard, proteins or protein fragments are found to have precipitated as amyloid and fibrillar aggregates. Cholinergic neurons in the brain may be selectively destroyed early in the course of the illness; the activity of choline acetyltransferase, which catalyzes the synthesis of acetylcholine, is decreased as much as 90%. Nevertheless, centrally active anticholinesterase drugs have not been predictably effective in these patients. Ergoloids are the most commonly prescribed drugs for the patient with Alzheimer's disease. Mental depression and anxiety generally accompany the symptoms of cognitive decline. Treatment of mental depression is with either a heterocylic antidepressant or a monoamine oxidase inhibitor. Tricyclic antidepressants with anticholinergic effects are avoided. The average duration of the disease is 6 to 10 years, with death commonly due to total debilitation or infection.

Signs and Symptoms

Dementia in an adult is characterized by intellectual deterioration severe enough to interfere with occupational or social performance. Cognitive changes include disturbances not only in memory, but also in other cognitive areas, such as language use, the ability to learn necessary skills, to think abstractly, and to make judgments. Initially, retention of new information is impaired, followed by global dementia. Social avoidance and anxiety are common. Irritability, agitation, and physical aggression toward family members may develop. Seizures are not likely to occur.

Management of Anesthesia

Management of anesthesia is based on an understanding of the pathophysiology of Alzheimer's disease. The major problem during the perioperative period is dealing with a patient who is unable to comprehend the environment or to cooperate with those responsible for providing medical care. Sedative drugs, as might be used in preoperative medication, should rarely be administered to these patients, as further mental confusion could result. A centrally acting anticholinergic drug should probably not be included in the preoperative medication, whereas reversal of nondepolarizing neuromuscular blockade might logically include glycopyrrolate, rather than atropine. Maintenance of anesthesia can be acceptably achieved with an inhaled or injected drug. A possible advantage of an inhaled drug would be a more predictable return to the level of preoperative mental function after surgery. Possible drug interactions based on co-existing treatment with a centrally acting anticholinesterase drug should be considered.

Creutzfeldt-Jakob Disease

Creutzfeldt-Jakob disease (subacute spongiform encephalopathy) is a rare, noninflammatory disease of the central nervous system caused by transmissible slow infectious pathogens known as prions. Prions differ from viruses in that they lack RNA and DNA and fail to produce any detectable immune reaction. Inactivation of the causative agent is reliably achieved by steam, ethylene oxide sterilization, as well as sodium hypochlorite. The incubation period is measured in months or years. The patient with this disease exhibits progressive presenile dementia, with death usually occurring within 6 months of onset. It would seem prudent to avoid contact with body fluids and to label clearly specimens of a patient undergoing a brain biopsy for the diagnosis of an unknown central nervous system disease. Instruments used for surgery in these patients should be carefully sterilized to avoid transmission of the disease with subsequent use of the instruments. Indeed, the disease has manifested in two patients 2.3 and 2.5 years after stereotactic EEG exploration with silver electrodes sterilized in alcohol and formaldehyde but previously implanted in an infected patient. Contact with infected tissue and blood is best prevented by the use of gloves and gowns. Accidental percutaneous exposure to infected tissue or blood should be followed by thorough cleansing of the wound with iodine or sodium hypochlorite. Overall, this disease is only remotely contagious, and there seems no justification for hospital personnel to exercise other than usual precautions in the care of these patients, including the administration of anesthesia.[84]

Leigh Syndrome

Leigh syndrome (subacute necrotizing encephalomyelopathy) is a chronic neurologic disease that is usually diagnosed before 4 years of age.[85] Symmetric lesions are generally found in the brain stem and lateral walls of the third ventricle, explaining the common clinical features, which include hypotonia, ataxia, breathing difficulties, propensity to aspiration, altered temperature regulation, and seizures. The syndrome is progressive and is marked by remissions and acute exacerbations, which may develop after surgery.

The most likely enzyme abnormality is a defect in the activation of pyruvate dehydrogenase. Indeed, an increased blood lactate and pyruvate concentration is frequently present. In this regard, crystalloid solutions containing lactate are avoided to minimize any iatrogenic contribution to co-existing lactic acidosis. Likewise, iatrogenic respiratory alkalosis due to intraoperative hyperventilation of the lungs could result in inhibition of pyruvate carboxylase and accentuation of lactic acidosis. Experience in management of anesthesia of these patients is too limited to permit specific recommendations for drug selection.

Rett Syndrome

Rett syndrome is a progressive neurologic disease manifested exclusively in females as dementia, autistic behavior, stereotyped hand movements, and an abnormality of breathing control that results in frequent episodes of apnea and arterial hypoxemia. In the chronic phase, there is diffuse and progressive muscle wasting; survival beyond 30 years of age is unlikely. Among severely retarded females, the incidence of this syndrome may be as high as 25%. In view of skeletal muscle weakness and wasting, the likelihood of pulmonary aspiration, release of excessive amounts of potassium after administration of succinylcholine, and the need for mechanical support of ventilation are considerations in the management of anesthesia.[86] Vasomotor disturbances and unexpected hypothermia may occur during anesthesia.

Sotos Syndrome

Sotos syndrome (cerebral gigantism) is the association of mental retardation and macrocephaly. This syndrome is inherited as an autosomal dominant trait. Rapid skeletal growth may account for the high incidence of scoliosis in these patients and the likely need for corrective spinal surgery. Considerations in the management of anesthesia include the anatomic characteristics of the facies that may make management of the airway difficult, as well as severe mental retardation that impairs the ability of these patients to cooperate. In this regard, aggressive behavior may contraindicate the use of a "wakeup test" during corrective spinal surgery for correction of scoliosis, emphasizing the potential value of SSEP monitoring.[88] Selection of drugs for maintenance of anesthesia may be influenced by the decision to use SSEP monitoring and the likely impact of anesthetic drugs on interpretation of this monitor.

Menkes Syndrome

Menkes syndrome is an X-linked recessive disorder of copper absorption and metabolism. Defective processing of copper results in abnormalities of many enzymes, manifesting as dysfunction of multiple organ systems. Onset is generally within the first 2 months of life with progressive cerebral degeneration; death usually occurs by 3 years of age due to intractable seizures or pneumonia. Affected children often require anesthetic care during diagnostic procedures such as magnetic resonance imaging. The major anesthetic implications of this syndrome are related to the disease's effects on the central nervous system.[88] Seizures often require multiple anticonvulsant drugs for control. Preoperative measurement of plasma anticonvulsant concentrations with adjustments to ensure therapeutic levels may be indicated. Progressive central nervous system deterioration may be accompanied by gastroesophageal reflux, poor pharyngeal muscle control, and recurrent aspiration. Defective collagen formation similar to Ehler-Danlos syndrome may be associated with perioperative hemorrhage. Experience is too limited to recommend specific anesthetic drugs. The choice of muscle relaxants is likely to exclude succinylcholine, although there is no evidence to support this practice.

Table 17-5. Clinical Characteristics of Leukodystrophies

Disease	Clinical Characteristics
Pelizaeus-Merzbacher	Onset in infancy Progressive central nervous system deterioration
Metachromatic leukodystrophy	Most common leukodystrophy Onset at 1–2 years of age Bouts of fever and abdominal pain Gallbladder dysfunction
Krabbe's disease (globoid cell leukodystrophy)	Onset at 4–6 months of age
Adrenoleukodystrophy (subanophilic cerebral sclerosis)	Onset at 5–10 years of age Hypoadrenalism
Canavan's disease	Onset at 2–4 months of age Increased plasma membrane permeability to water and cations Macrocephaly without evidence of hydrocephalus
Alexander's disease	Onset in first year of life

Leukodystrophies

Leukodystrophies are represented by a group of genetically determined progressive degenerative diseases of cerebral white matter that reflect defective formation of myelin[89] (Table 17-5). Typically, these diseases present during the first year of life with skeletal muscle spasticity, arrest of motor development, and gait disturbances. Because of their progressive nature, afflicted children often require anesthesia during diagnostic imaging procedures or surgical procedures intended to correct the sequelae of their disease. Relevant anesthetic concerns include a high likelihood of seizure disorders, gastroesophageal reflux with the risk of aspiration, and airway complications related to poor pharyngeal muscle control and copious oral secretions. Intraoperative doses of intravenous anesthetic drugs and muscle relaxants may need to be increased due to the increased hepatic enzyme function seen in patients being treated chronically with anticonvulsants. In view of the upper motor neuron disease characteristic of these disorders, it may be prudent to avoid the administration of succinylcholine. Adrenal involvement with this disease may necessitate the administration of supplemental corticosteroids.

Multiple Sclerosis

Multiple sclerosis is an acquired disease of the central nervous system, characterized by random and multiple sites of demyelination of corticospinal tract neurons in the brain and spinal cord.[89] Neuropathologic changes consist of loss of the myelin covering the axons in the form of demyelinative plaques. The disease does not affect the peripheral nervous system. Multiple sclerosis is a disease of young adults; the onset of symptoms before 15 years or after 40 years of age is rare.

Etiology

The relationship between geographic latitude and the risk of the development of multiple sclerosis is striking. For example, the incidence is high (75 to 150 per 100,000 population) in the northern temperate zone in North America and Europe and in the southern portions of New Zealand and Australia. The incidence of multiple sclerosis is low near the equator. Studies of migrant populations have disclosed that factors determining susceptibility are acquired before 15 years of age. In addition, the incidence of multiple sclerosis is greater among urban dwellers and affluent socioeconomic groups. Evidence for the role of genetic factors is demonstrated by the 12- to 15-fold increase of the disease among first-degree relatives. In addition, a high percentage of patients share common histocompatibility antigens. For example, 60% of patients share the antigen designated HLA-DW2, whereas only 18% of patients without the disease have this antigen. These features of multiple sclerosis lend support to theories of a viral etiology. Conceivably, a viral infection initiates an altered immune reaction against myelin in a genetically susceptible person. Indeed, several viruses can cause demyelination of the central nervous system in animals, but to date none has been shown to be causative for multiple sclerosis in humans.

Signs and Symptoms

Manifestations of multiple sclerosis reflect sites of demyelination in the central nervous system and spinal cord. For example, disease of the optic nerve causes visual disturbances; involvement of the cerebellum leads to gait disturbances; and lesions of the spinal cord cause limb paresthesias and weakness, as well as urinary incontinence and sexual impotence. Ascending spastic paresis of the skeletal muscles is often prominent. Optic neuritis is characterized by diminished visual acuity and defective pupillary reaction to light. Demyelination of the pathways in the brain stem that coordinate eye movement causes paresis of the medial rectus muscle on lateral conjugate gaze. Nystagmus is seen in the abducting eye. Intramedullary disease of the cervical cord is suggested by an electrical sensation, which runs down the back into the legs in response to flexion of the neck (Lhermitte sign). Typically, symptoms develop over the course of a few days, remain stable for a few weeks, and then improve. Since remyelination in the central nervous system probably does not occur, remission of symptoms most likely results from the correction of transient chemical and physiologic disturbances that have interfered with nerve conduction, in the absence of complete demyelination. There is an increased incidence of seizure disorders in patients with multiple sclerosis.

The course of multiple sclerosis is characterized by exacerbation and remission of symptoms at unpredictable intervals over a period of several years. Residual symptoms eventually persist during remission, leading to severe disability from visual failure, incoordination, spastic weakness, and urinary incontinence. Nevertheless, the disease in some patients remains benign, with infrequent mild episodes of demyelination, followed by prolonged, and occasionally permanent, remission. The onset of multiple sclerosis after 35 years of age is most likely to be associated with a slow progression.

Diagnosis

The diagnosis of multiple sclerosis must be made on clinical grounds, as there are no specific laboratory tests.[90] Visual, brainstem-, auditory-, and SSEP responses can be used to demonstrate slowing of nerve conduction due to demyelination in specific areas of the central nervous system. Computed tomography and magnetic resonance imaging may demonstrate demyelinative plaques. Immersion of patients in water at a temperature of 40°C may produce new symptoms or the recurrence of previously experienced symptoms.[90] The mechanism by which immersion in hot water provokes symptoms of multiple sclerosis is unknown, but it is likely that elevated temperature causes complete blocking of conduction in demyelinated nerves. Indeed, raising the body temperature 0.5°C in animals with experimentally produced demyelination can produce complete conduction blockade. One of the most widely used diagnostic tests for multiple sclerosis is examination of the CSF. Approximately 70% of patients with multiple sclerosis have elevations of immunoglobulin G proteins in the CSF. This elevation of CSF protein is not specific for multiple sclerosis, as similar changes occur with infections, connective tissue diseases, encephalopathies, and neurosyphilis. Another test using CSF is measurement of myeline basic protein by radioimmunoassay. Elevation in the concentration of this protein indicates destruction of myelin.

Treatment

No treatment is curative for multiple sclerosis. Treatment with adrenocorticotropic hormone or with corticosteroids will shorten the duration of an acute attack, but there is no evidence that these drugs influence the ultimate progression of the disease. Nonspecific measures include avoidance of excessive fatigue, emotional stress, and marked changes in environmental temperature. Stress as produced by surgery is unwise, and elective surgical procedures are rarely performed. Pregnancy appears to introduce no special risk. Drugs used in the treatment of skeletal muscle spasticity associated with multiple sclerosis include diazepam, dantrolene, and baclofen. Hepatic function should be monitored in the patient treated with dantrolene, as this drug can lead to liver damage. Painful dysesthesias, tonic seizures, and attacks of paroxysmal dysarthria and ataxia are best treated with carbamazepine. Immunosuppressive therapy has been provided with azathioprine and cyclophosphamide, but data to support the efficacy of this treatment are lacking. Plasmapheresis may produce a beneficial response in some patients.

Management of Anesthesia

Management of anesthesia in the patient with multiple sclerosis must consider the impact of surgical stress on the natural progression of the disease. For example, regardless of the anesthetic technique or drugs selected for use during the perioperative period, it is likely that symptoms of multiple sclerosis will be exacerbated during the postoperative period. In this regard, any increase in body temperature that follows surgery may be more likely than drugs to be responsible for exacerbation of multiple sclerosis during the postoperative period. Furthermore, the unpredictable cycle of exacerbation and remission of this disease could lead to the incorrect association of changing manifestations with drugs or events present during the perioperative period. Certainly, the changing neurologic picture in the patient with multiple sclerosis must be appreciated when considering the selection of regional anesthesia. Indeed, spinal anesthesia has been implicated in postoperative exacerbations of multiple sclerosis, whereas exacerbation of the disease after epidural anesthesia or peripheral nerve blocks has not been described.[91] For this reason, epidural anesthesia has been used in parturients with multiple sclerosis.[92] The mechanism by which spinal anesthesia may exacerbate multiple sclerosis is unknown but could reflect local anesthetic neurotoxicity. In this regard, the lack of a protective nerve sheath around the spinal cord and the associated demyelination of multiple sclerosis may render the spinal cord more susceptible to potential neurotoxic effects of local anesthetics. Epidural anesthesia may be less of a risk than spinal anesthesia because the concentration of local anesthetic in the white matter of the spinal cord is three to four times lower after epidural, as compared with spinal, administration.

General anesthesia is most often chosen. There are no unique interactions between multiple sclerosis and the drugs used to provide general anesthesia. There is no evidence to support recommendations for selection of a specific inhaled or injected anesthetic. The selection of a muscle relaxant should consider the possibility of exaggerated release of potassium after administration of succinylcholine to these patients. A prolonged response to a muscle relaxant would be consistent with co-existing weakness (myasthenia-like) and decreased skeletal muscle mass. Conversely, resistance to the effects of nondepolarizing muscle relaxants has been observed, perhaps reflecting proliferation of extrajunctional cholinergic receptors characteristic of upper motor neuron lesions.[93] Supplementation with a corticosteroid may be indicated when using these drugs in chronic treatment. Efforts must be made during the perioperative period to recognize and prevent even modest increases in body temperature (greater than 1°C), as this change might lead to deterioration of nerve tissue at the sites of demyelination. Neurologic evaluation during the postoperative period may be useful in detecting any new symptoms of multiple sclerosis.

Optic Neuritis

Optic neuritis represents a demyelinating disease of the central nervous system that is limited to the optic nerve. Eventually, about 50% of these patients show evidence of multiple sclerosis. Evaluation of patients with optic neuritis includes examination of the CSF and determination of histocompatibility antigens. Visual loss is the most prominent symptom, although visual acuity generally returns with time. Intravenous administration of methylprednisolone followed by oral prednisone may speed the recovery of visual acuity.[94]

Transverse Myelitis

Transverse myelitis is an inflammation of the spinal cord that can follow a viral infection or radiation treatment. Multiple sclerosis may be initially manifested as transverse myelitis. The cause of transverse myelitis, however, is most often unknown. The onset of this disease process is characterized by a rapid ascending weakness of the legs associated with bladder paralysis and a sensory level to the thoracic region. The entire progression of symptoms can occur over a period of hours, with permanent sequelae likely. When transverse myelitis is preceded or followed by bilateral optic neuritis, the diagnosis is one of Devic's disease or neuromyelitis optica.

Stiff-Man Syndrome

Stiff-man syndrome is a rare central nervous system disease characterized by the onset, in a previously normal adult, of continuous skeletal muscle rigidity and painful spasms resembling tetanus. Unlike tetanus, however, trismus does not accompany stiff-man syndrome. Skeletal muscle rigidity may interfere with adequate ventilation; when severe, it has resulted in disruption of the muscles, fracture of the long bones, and bending of internal orthopaedic appliances. Electromyography reveals continuous motor unit activity in the affected skeletal muscles indistinguishable from voluntary contraction. The congenital form of stiff-man syndrome, known as stiff-baby syndrome, is inherited as an autosomal dominant trait. There is evidence that adults with stiff-man syndrome have developed an antibody against the enzyme glutamic acid decarboxylase, which is responsible for the synthesis of the inhibitory neurotransmitter, gamma aminobutyric acid.[95] Antibody formation against a specific enzyme (antigen) could be the result of an infectious process, while the resulting loss of central inhibition provided by gamma aminobutyric acid could be the mechanism of stiff-man syndrome.[95]

NEUROPATHIES

Neuropathies may involve cranial or peripheral nerves (Table 17-6). Interruption of the axon leads to degeneration of its distal segment (wallerian degeneration). Failure of nerve impulse transmission results, producing paresis and trophic

Table 17-6.   Classification of Neuropathies

Cranial Mononeuropathies
Idiopathic facial paralysis (Bell's palsy)
Trigeminal neuralgia (tic douloureux)
Glossopharyngeal neuralgia
Vestibular neuronitis
Metastatic cancer

Peripheral Entrapment Neuropathies
Carpal tunnel syndrome
Ulnar nerve palsy
Brachial plexus palsy
Radial nerve palsy
Meralgia paresthetica
Femoral nerve palsy
Peroneal nerve palsy

Peripheral Metabolic Neuropathies
Alcohol
Vitamin B_{12} deficiency
Diabetes mellitus
Hypothyroidism
Uremia
Porphyria

Systemic Disease-Related Peripheral Neuropathies
Cancer
Sarcoidosis
Collagen vascular disease
Acute idiopathic polyneuritis (Guillain-Barré syndrome)

Toxic Peripheral Polyneuropathies
Drugs
  Sulindac
  Amiodarone
  Hydralazine
  Nitrous oxide
  Disulfiram
  Phenytoin
  Isoniazid
  Cisplatin
  Vincristine
Industrial agents
Insecticides
Heavy metals

Peripheral Hereditary Neuropathies
Peroneal muscular atrophy (Charcot-Marie-Tooth disease)
Refsum's disease
Möbius syndrome

Table 17-7.   Questions to Determine the Etiology of a Peripheral Neuropathy

1. Is the disturbance a mononeuropathy or a mononeuropathy multiplex (asymmetric involvement of more than one nerve)? If the answer is yes, the etiology is most likely local entrapment, compression, traction, or ischemia.
2. Is the disturbance a symmetric polyneuropathy? If the answer is yes, the etiology is most likely metabolic, systemic, or toxic (see Table 17-6).
3. Is the neuropathy primarily motor (acute idiopathic polyneuritis, porphyria)?
4. Is the neuropathy primarily sensory (vitamin deficiency)?
5. Is there a family history of neuropathy (see Table 17-6)?

changes in the corresponding skeletal muscle. Degeneration of Schwann cells, which provide myelination of axons, leads to segmental demyelination; the result is slowing of nerve conduction. Segmental demyelination produces paresis but no trophic changes in the corresponding skeletal muscle. The application of nerve conduction velocity and electromyographic techniques has aided in the diagnosis and classification of peripheral neuropathies as either predominantly axonal or demyelinating disorders.

Characteristic features of a peripheral neuropathy include distal skeletal muscle weakness and wasting, stocking glove sensory loss, and loss of tendon reflexes. Conduction velocity studies and electromyography are helpful diagnostic aids. Specific questions during the initial clinical examination can aid in the search for an etiology of the peripheral neuropathy (Table 17-7). The patient with a co-existing ulnar nerve lesion may describe tingling in the fingers innervated by this nerve, when asked to flex the arm to its fullest extent. Recovery from peripheral neuropathy is slow, often taking 3 to 12 months; unfortunately, during this time, the patient may experience pain and disability.

Postoperative Neuropathy

Peripheral nerve injury, and resulting neuropathy, is a significant source of anesthesia-related liability claims.[96] Brachial plexus injury, particularly that involving the ulnar nerve, is common after median sternotomy and cardiopulmonary bypass.[96–101] Damage to the brachial plexus in association with median sternotomy may be due to penetration of the plexus by a fractured first rib, especially with wide sternal separation.[99] Peripheral neuropathy after cardiopulmonary bypass is unrelated to internal mammary artery dissection or internal jugular vein catheterization.[99,100] Perioperative brachial plexus injury is estimated to have a frequency of 0.02% among patients undergoing noncardiac surgery under general anesthesia.[97] The traditional explanation, when a postoperative neuropathy occurs, is a position-related compression or traction to the involved nerve(s).[97] In this regard, it is often assumed that proper positioning and padding during anesthesia and surgery will decrease the risk of peripheral nerve injury. Nevertheless, there is compelling evidence that upper extremity nerve injury, exhibited initially during the postoperative period, may occur despite appropriate padding and independent of the arm position (abducted or at the side, pronated or supinated) during surgery[96–101] (see the sections, Ulnar Nerve Palsy and Brachial Plexus Palsy).

Idiopathic Facial Paralysis

Idiopathic facial paralysis (Bell's palsy) is characterized by the rapid onset of motor weakness or paralysis of all the facial muscles innervated by the facial nerve. Often the onset is first noted on arising in the morning and looking into a mirror. Additional symptoms can include the loss of taste sensation over the anterior two-thirds of the tongue, as well as hyperacusis and diminished salivation and lacrimation. The absence of cutaneous sensory loss emphasizes that the facial nerve is a motor nerve. The cause of idiopathic facial paralysis is presumed to be inflammation and edema of the facial nerve, most often in the facial canal of the temporal bone. A viral inflammatory mechanism (perhaps herpes simplex virus) may be the cause. Indeed, the onset of this neuropathy is often preceded by a viral prodrome.

Spontaneous recovery usually occurs over about 12 weeks. If no recovery occurs within 16 to 20 weeks, the disease is probably not idiopathic facial paralysis. Prednisone (1 $mg \cdot kg^{-1} \cdot d^{-1}$ orally, for 5 to 10 days), depending on the degree of facial nerve paralysis, dramatically relieves pain and reduces the number of patients experiencing complete denervation of the facial nerve. The eye should be covered, to protect the cornea. Surgical decompression of the facial nerve may be required for persistent or severe cases of idiopathic facial paralysis or for facial paralysis secondary to trauma. Trauma to the facial nerve can reflect stretch injury produced by excessive traction on the angle of the mandible during maintenance of the upper airway in an unconscious patient.[102] Uveoparotid fever (Heerfordt syndrome) is a variant of sarcoidosis, characterized by bilateral anterior uveitis, parotitis, and mild pyrexia, as well as the presence of facial nerve paralysis in 50% to 70% of patients. Facial nerve paralysis associated with uveoparotid fever appearing during the postoperative period may be erroneously attributed to mechanical pressure over the nerve during general anesthesia.[103]

Facial nerve palsy associated with the placement of an extradural blood patch for the treatment of a spinal headache has been described.[104] A sudden increase in ICP caused by the blood patch is speculated to have transiently compromised the blood supply to the facial nerve.

Trigeminal Neuralgia

Trigeminal neuralgia (tic douloureux) is characterized by the sudden onset of brief but intense unilateral facial pain triggered by local sensory stimuli to the affected side of the face.[105] The second and third divisions of the trigeminal nerve are usually involved. Trigeminal neuralgia is most often seen in patients older than 50 years of age. The appearance of this neuralgia at an earlier age should arouse suspicion of multiple sclerosis. Indeed, about 2% of patients with multiple sclerosis also experience trigeminal neuralgia. This finding is consistent with histologic evidence of degeneration or absence of myelin along the trigeminal nerve of patients with trigeminal neuralgia. The etiology of these changes is unknown, but proposed mechanisms include viral infections and vascular compression of the nerve.

Treatment

Medical treatment of trigeminal neuralgia is with an anticonvulsant drug such as carbamazepine. The rationale for the use of this drug is based on the analogy of paroxysmal neuronal discharges in epilepsy and the possibility that similar discharges may produce the sudden attacks of pain characteristic of trigeminal neuralgia. Surgical treatment consists of selective radiofrequency destruction of trigeminal nerve fibers, transection of the sensory root of the trigeminal nerve, and microsurgical decompression of the trigeminal nerve.

Management of Anesthesia

There are no special considerations for the management of anesthesia in the patient with trigeminal neuralgia. The patient undergoing surgical therapy of trigeminal neuralgia, however, may experience a dramatic, life-threatening increase in blood pressure during radiofrequency destruction of nerve fibers, requiring treatment with nitroprusside.[105] The potential effects of anticonvulsant drug therapy on hepatic microsomal enzymatic activity should be remembered when selecting drugs, particularly enflurane or halothane. In addition, carbamazepine can cause altered hepatic function, leukopenia, and thrombocytopenia, emphasizing the importance of evaluating these systems preoperatively in patients receiving this drug.

Glossopharyngeal Neuralgia

Glossopharyngeal neuralgia is characterized by attacks of intense pain in the throat, neck, tongue, and ear. Swallowing chewing, coughing, or talking can trigger the pain. This neuralgia can also be associated with severe bradycardia and syncope, presumably reflecting activation of the motor nucleus of the vagus nerve. Hypotension, seizures due to cerebral ischemia, and even cardiac arrest can occur in some patients.

Diagnosis

Glossopharyngeal neuralgia is usually idiopathic but has been described in patients with cerebellopontine angle vascular anomalies and tumors, vertebral and carotid artery occlusive disease, arachnoiditis, and extracranial tumors arising in the area of the pharynx, larynx, and tonsils. The presence of glossopharyngeal neuralgia is supported by the occurrence of pain in the distribution of the glossopharyngeal nerve; the presence of a site in the oropharynx, which reproduces the symptoms, when stimulated; and the relief of pain by topical anesthesia of the oropharynx.

In the absence of pain, cardiac symptoms associated with glossopharyngeal neuralgia may be confused with sick sinus syndrome or carotid sinus syndrome. Sick sinus syndrome can be ruled out by the absence of characteristic changes on the ECG. The failure of carotid sinus massage to produce cardiac symptoms rules out the presence of carotid sinus hypersensitivity. Glossopharyngeal nerve block is useful in differentiating glossopharyngeal neuralgia from atypical trigeminal neuralgia. This block does not differentiate glossopharyngeal neuralgia from the carotid sinus syndrome, since afferent pathways of both syndromes are mediated by the glossopharyngeal nerve. Topical anesthesia of the oropharynx blocks receptors in the trigger area responsible for initiating glossopharyngeal neuralgia, distinguishing this response from the carotid sinus syndrome.

Treatment

Treatment of glossopharyngeal neuralgia associated with cardiac symptoms should be aggressive, as affected patients are vulnerable to sudden death. Cardiovascular symptoms are treated with atropine, isoproterenol, and/or an artificial cardiac pacemaker. The pain associated with this syndrome is managed by chronic administration of an anticonvulsant drug, such as phenytoin or carbamazepine. Topical anesthesia of the pharyngeal or oral mucosa, or a glossopharyngeal nerve block, effectively relieves pain, but only for the duration of the effect of the local anesthetic. Prevention of cardiovascular symptoms and provision of predictable pain relief are achieved by the intracranial section of the glossopharyngeal nerve and the upper two roots of the vagus nerve. Although permanent pain relief after repeated glossopharyngeal nerve blocks is possible, this neuralgia is sufficiently life-threatening to justify intracranial transection of nerves in the patient who is unresponsive to medical therapy.

Management of Anesthesia

Preoperative evaluation of the patient with glossopharyngeal neuralgia is directed at assessing the intravascular fluid volume and cardiac status.[106] A significant deficit of intravascular fluid volume may be present, as these patients avoid oral intake and its associated pharyngeal stimulation in attempts to prevent triggering painful attacks. Furthermore, drooling and loss of saliva can contribute to loss of intravascular fluid volume. A preoperative history of syncope or documented bradycardia, concurrent with the presence of neuralgia, introduces the consideration for prompt ability to provide noninvasive transcutaneous pacing or actual placement of a prophylactic transvenous artificial cardiac pacemaker before the induction of anesthesia. Continuous monitoring of the ECG and of arterial blood pressure through a catheter in a peripheral artery is useful. Topical anesthesia of the oropharynx with lidocaine is helpful in preventing bradycardia and hypotension, which may occur in response to triggering of this syndrome during direct laryngoscopy and intubation of the trachea. Furthermore, intravenous administration of atropine or glycopyrrolate just before laryngoscopy is recommended.[106]

Cardiovascular changes in response to surgical manipulation and intracranial section of cranial nerve roots should be expected. For example, bradycardia and hypotension are likely during manipulation of the vagus nerve. An anticholinergic drug must be promptly available to treat this vagal-mediated response. Hypertension, tachycardia, and ventricular premature beats can occur after transection of the glossopharyngeal nerve and the upper two roots of the vagus nerve. These events may reflect the sudden loss of sensory input from the carotid sinus. Hypertension is usually transient but may persist in some patients into the postoperative period. Persistence of hypertension is due to increased sympathetic nervous system activity. Administration of hydralazine during the postoperative period is effective in treating hypertension. Experience is too limited to permit a recommendation for a specific anesthetic drug or muscle relaxant. Thiopental, nitrous oxide, halothane, succinylcholine, and pancuronium have been administered to these patients without adverse or unusual responses.[106] The possibility of the development of vocal cord paralysis after transection of the vagus nerve should be considered, if airway obstruction occurs after tracheal extubation.

Vestibular Neuronitis

Vestibular neuronitis is characterized by vertigo, vomiting, and gait disturbances. These symptoms are thought to reflect irritation of the vestibular portion of the eighth cranial nerve. The absence of hearing loss distinguishes vestibular neuronitis from endolymphatic hydrops (Menière's disease). Vestibular neuronitis is a benign condition, for which no specific treatment is necessary.

Metastatic Cancer

Cranial nerve palsy can reflect compression or infiltration by leukemia or lymphomas. Metastatic disease from the breast or lung may invade the trigeminal nerve, causing numbness of the chin or cheek. Similar invasion of the hypoglossal nerve produces atrophy of the tongue.

Möbius Syndrome

Möbius syndrome is a rare congenital dysplasia of the cranial nerves. The spinal accessory and facial nerves are most often affected, resulting in esotropia or partial facial paralysis. Occasionally, involvement of other cranial nerves is manifested as difficulties in mastication, swallowing, and coughing, often leading to aspiration and recurrent pneumonia.

Carpal Tunnel Syndrome

Carpal tunnel syndrome is the most frequent of the entrapment neuropathies. The median nerve is compressed, and perhaps rendered ischemic, in the confined space between the carpal bones and the flexor retinaculum of the wrist. Resulting symptoms include pain and paresthesias in the thumb, index, and middle fingers, often with nocturnal exacerbation. Neurologic signs include sensory loss in the distribution of the median nerve[107] (Fig. 17-18) and weakness and atrophy of the adductor pollicis brevis in the thenar eminence. Tinel sign is the provocation of pain by percussion over the median nerve at the wrist.

Carpal tunnel syndrome occurs most often in females aged 30 to 50 years, often in association with pregnancy. The incidence is increased in patients with acromegaly, hypothyroid-

ism, multiple myeloma, or amyloidosis. Bilateral carpal tunnel syndrome is not uncommon. The diagnosis of this syndrome is by demonstration of a conduction delay in the median nerve at the wrist. Surgical decompression is the recommended treatment, when conservative measures, such as immobilization and local injection of corticosteroid, are not effective.

Ulnar Nerve Palsy

The ulnar nerve is vulnerable to trauma and external compression at the condylar groove of the fully flexed elbow. Severe or recurrent injury can lead to local fibrosis and entrapment of the ulnar nerve, manifested as weakness, atrophy, and sensory loss in the ulnar field of the hand[107] (Fig. 17-18). Nerve conduction studies reveal localized conduction blockade at the elbow. Surgical transposition of the nerve in the condylar groove of the elbow may be necessary.

Ulnar nerve injury is the most common postoperative peripheral neuropathy; the etiology is often not apparent[96-101] (see the section, Postoperative Neuropathy). Symptoms of ulnar nerve palsy that have previously been mild or even unrecognized by the patient may become more obvious and disabling during the postoperative period. Furthermore, the appearance of this neuropathy may be spontaneous without any relationship to anesthesia and surgery. The appearance of a postoperative ulnar nerve neuropathy in some patients is delayed, manifesting 2 to 30 days postoperatively.[96] This delayed appearance suggests that some ulnar nerve injuries may occur during the postoperative period, rather than during anesthesia and surgery. Electromyographic studies are indicated for any patient who complains of a sensory or motor deficit. In cases of injury to the ulnar nerve at operation, active denervation potentials should not appear until approximately 3 weeks after the event and should be confined to the neuromuscular pathway of the ulnar nerve. If active denervation potentials occur at an earlier date, the factor responsible for the sensory disturbance or skeletal muscle weakness was co-existing and was not the result of an injury at operation. Electromyography is also useful in following the progression of the lesion.

The male predominance of perioperative ulnar nerve injury suggests an anatomic predisposition (perhaps the depth of the condylar groove at the elbow) associated with the male body habitus. The ulnar nerve is probably more susceptible to external compression in the cubital tunnel either when the elbow is fully flexed or when the hand is pronated, or both[99] (Fig. 17-19). Nevertheless, even with the routine utilization of preventive measures (elbow padding, forearm in supination, avoidance of prolonged elbow flexion, loose application of the blood pressure cuff), some patients who have subclinical entrapment of the ulnar nerve in the cubital tunnel may become symptomatic after a surgical procedure.[98] A patient in whom a postoperative ulnar nerve neuropathy develops will invariably

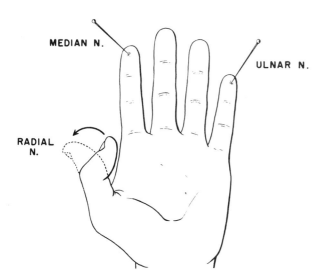

Fig. 17-18. Schematic diagram for the rapid identification of peripheral nerve injury to the upper extremity. Injury to the musculocutaneous nerve results in loss of biceps function and inability to flex the forearm; injury to the axillary nerve results in loss of deltoid function and inability to abduct the arm. (From McAlpine FS, Seckel BR. Complications of positioning. The peripheral nervous system. In: Martin JT, ed. Positioning in Anesthesia and Surgery. Philadelphia. WB Saunders 1987;303–28, with permission.)

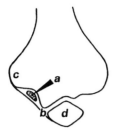

Fig. 17-19. Schematic depiction of the relationship of the ulnar nerve (a) to the arcuate ligament (b) that extends from the medial epicondyle of the humerus (c) to the olecranon of the ulna (d) at the elbow, forming the roof of the cubital tunnel. Pronation of the forearm rotates the cubital tunnel, such that both the medial epicondyle and olecranon rest on the same flat surface, increasing the possibility of ulnar nerve compression in the cubital tunnel. Likewise, flexion of the elbow tenses the arcuate ligament and decreases the size of the cubital tunnel. (From Wadsworth TG. The cubital tunnel and the external compression syndrome. Anesth Analg 1974;53:303–8, with permission.)

display an abnormality of nerve conduction testing, in both the affected and contralateral arm.[97] This finding implies that a co-existing lesion of the ulnar nerve is common, if not universal. Nevertheless, the unexpected clinical appearance during the postoperative period may erroneously suggest a new disturbance.

Brachial Plexus Palsy

The development of localized weakness of one or both arms, after a virus-like infection, may signal the onset of brachial plexus palsy. Initially, patients describe pain across the shoulder and into the upper arm. Pain subsides over a period of a few days, but weakness or paralysis is then exhibited. The muscles of the shoulder girdle, particularly the deltoid muscle, are most often affected. Sensory loss is usually not prominent. There is no specific treatment. Complete recovery can be expected, although this may take 1 to 2 years. Nerve conduction velocity studies confirm the diagnosis and avoid unnecessary myelography.

The brachial plexus is especially vulnerable to trauma during thoracic surgery, owing to its long superficial course in the axilla between two points of fixation: the vertebrae above and the axillary fascia below (see the section, Postoperative Neuropathy). Stretching is the principal perioperative cause of damage to the brachial plexus, with compression having only a secondary role.

Radial Nerve Palsy

Radial nerve palsy due to compression of the radial nerve is manifested as wrist drop and paralysis of the extensor muscles of the fingers[107] (Fig. 17-18). The mechanical effects of differential pressure exerted at the distal edge of the inflatable cuff of an automated blood pressure monitor may be a rare cause of injury to the radial nerve.[108] Placing the blood pressure cuff higher on the arm, away from the elbow and the most superficial portion of the radial nerve, may decrease the likelihood of this rare type of injury.

Long Thoracic Nerve Palsy

Long thoracic nerve palsy is characterized by paralysis of the serratus anterior muscle and "winging" of the scapula. The appearance of this palsy following an obstetric delivery or a surgical procedure unrelated to the anatomic area of the nerve presents a diagnostic dilemma. Consideration of the etiology of a postoperative long thoracic nerve palsy must include a coincidental infectious neuropathy as an alternative to any assertion that a preventable injury occurred during anesthesia.[109]

Meralgia Paresthetica

Entrapment of the lateral femoral cutaneous nerve as it passes under the inguinal ligament can cause burning pain over the anterolateral aspect of the thigh. Hypalgesia and hypesthesia are present in the involved area. Obesity and tight belts can contribute to its development. Relief of pain can be obtained by weight loss, removal of mechanical pressure produced by clothing, and block of the lateral femoral cutaneous nerve with a local anesthetic.

Femoral Neuropathy

Disturbed function of the femoral nerve is characterized by sensory deficits over the anterior aspect of the thigh, as well as motor weakness, most apparent in the quadriceps muscles (difficulty climbing stairs). A reduced or absent knee jerk is the most reliable objective sign of femoral neuropathy. Diabetes mellitus is present in most patients in whom femoral neuropathy develops.[110] Hip flexion produced by the lithotomy position (vaginal hysterectomy) and pressure on the greater psoas muscle by the retractor blades (abdominal hysterectomy) have been associated with femoral neuropathy.[110]

Peroneal Nerve Palsy

Peroneal nerve palsy reflects compression of the common peroneal nerve at the level of the head of the fibula. Improper positioning in the lithotomy position or prolonged periods with the legs crossed may be responsible for damage to this nerve. Manifestations are footdrop and sensory loss over the dorsum of the foot[107] (Fig. 17-20).

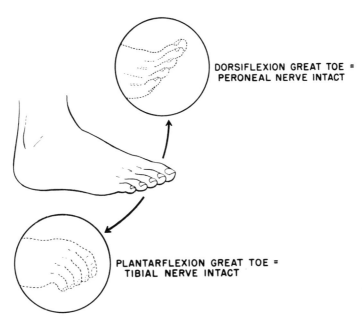

DORSIFLEXION GREAT TOE =
PERONEAL NERVE INTACT

PLANTARFLEXION GREAT TOE =
TIBIAL NERVE INTACT

Fig. 17-20. Schematic diagram for the rapid identification of peripheral nerve injury of the lower extremity. Injury to the femoral nerve results in loss of quadriceps function. (From McAlpine FS, Seckel BR. Complication of positioning. The peripheral nervous system. In: Martin JT, ed. Positioning in Anesthesia and Surgery. Philadelphia. WB Saunders 1987;303–28, with permission.)

Fabella Syndrome

Peroneal nerve palsy may be due to compression of the common peroneal nerve by a sesamoid bone (fabella) embedded in the tendinous portion of the gastrocnemius muscle.[111] This bone is present in about 12% of patients. A fabella should be considered one of the causes of peroneal nerve palsy, especially after a lengthy operation in the supine position, in which a leg strap is applied tightly above the knees. Fabella syndrome, in addition to skeletal muscle weakness and sensory changes, is accompanied by local tenderness and pain in the area of the fabella, intensified by full extension of the knees.

Alcoholic Neuropathy

Polyneuropathy of chronic alcoholism is nearly always associated with a nutritional deficiency. Presumably, a vitamin deficiency is a contributing factor in the pathogenesis of alcoholic neuropathy. Symptoms characteristically begin in the lower extremities, with pain and numbness in the feet. Weakness and tenderness of the intrinsic muscles of the feet, absent Achilles tendon reflexes, and hypalgesia in a stocking distribution are the early findings. Restoration of a proper diet, abstinence from alcohol, and multivitamin therapy promote a slow, but predictable, resolution of the neuropathy.

Vitamin B$_{12}$ Deficiency

The earliest neurologic symptoms of vitamin B$_{12}$ deficiency resemble the neuropathy typically seen in the patient who uses alcohol in excess. Paresthesias in the legs, with a sensory loss in a stocking distribution and absent Achilles tendon reflexes, are characteristic findings. Similar neurologic findings have been reported in dentists who are chronically exposed to nitrous oxide.[112] This is of concern, since nitrous oxide is known to inactivate certain vitamin B$_{12}$-dependent enzymes, which could lead to a deficiency of this essential vitamin (see Chapter 29).

Diabetes Mellitus

It is estimated that more than 1 million Americans suffer from diabetic peripheral neuropathy, with the greatest incidence in those with long-standing disease. Strictness of the control of the blood glucose concentration does not appear to influence the development of a peripheral neuropathy. The electromyogram may show evidence of denervation, and nerve conduction velocity is likely to be slowed.

The most common neuropathy is a distal, symmetric, and predominantly sensory disturbance. The principal manifestations are unpleasant tingling, numbness, burning and aching in the lower extremities, skeletal muscle weakness, and distal sensory loss. Discomfort is particularly prominent at night and is often relieved by walking. Symptoms often progress and may extend to the upper extremities. Impotence, urinary retention, and postural hypotension are common and reflect autonomic nervous system dysfunction.

Diabetic neuropathy may be characterized by the rapid development of pain and skeletal muscle weakness confined to the distribution of one or two nerves in the leg, most often the femoral or sciatic nerve, or both. The neuropathy may affect first one leg and than the other. Occasionally, an isolated sciatic neuropathy suggests the diagnosis of a herniated intervertebral disc. Sciatic neuropathy in a patient with diabetes mellitus is not associated with pain in response to straight-leg raising, serving to distinguish this peripheral neuropathy from lumbar disc disease. Spontaneous and complete recovery usually occurs, but the rate of return of normal nerve function is unpredictable.

Hypothyroidism

A distal sensory neuropathy may be one of the first signs of myxedema. Delayed relaxation of tendon reflexes, especially the Achilles tendon reflex, is characteristic.

Uremia

A distal polyneuropathy with sensory and motor components often occurs in the extremities of patients with chronic renal failure. Symptoms tend to be more prominent in the legs than in the arms. Presumably, metabolic abnormalities are responsible for axonal degeneration and segmental demyelination, which accompany this neuropathy. Slowing of nerve conduction has been correlated with an elevated plasma concentration of parathormone and myoinositol, which is a component of myelin. Improved nerve conduction velocity often occurs within a few days after renal transplantation. Hemodialysis does not appear to be equally effective in reversing the polyneuropathy.

Porphyria

The neuropathy associated with porphyria is distinctive in that it is predominantly motor. Cranial nerves and respiratory muscles may be involved by the neuropathic process.

Cancer

Peripheral sensory or motor neuropathies, or both, occur in patients with a variety of malignancies, especially those involving the lung, ovary, and breast. Polyneuropathy that develops in older patients should always arouse suspicion of undiagnosed cancer. Myasthenic syndrome (Eaton-Lambert syndrome) is characteristically observed in patients with carcinoma of the lung. This syndrome, however, is an abnormality of the neuromuscular junction, rather than of the nerves.

Sarcoidosis

Polyneuropathy is a frequent finding in the patient with sarcoidosis. Facial nerve paralysis on one or both sides may result from involvement of this nerve in the parotid gland.

Collagen Vascular Disease

Collagen vascular disease is commonly associated with peripheral neuropathies. The most common conditions are systemic lupus erythematosus, polyarteritis nodosa, rheumatoid arthritis, and scleroderma. The detection of multiple mononeuropathies suggests vasculitis of nerve trunks and should stimulate a search for the presence of a collagen vascular disease.

Acute Idiopathic Polyneuritis

Acute idiopathic polyneuritis (Guillain-Barré syndrome) is characterized by a sudden onset of weakness or paralysis typically exhibited in the legs, spreading cephalad over the next few days to involve skeletal muscles of the arms, trunk, and head. With the virtual elimination of poliomyelitis, this syndrome has become the most common cause of acute generalized paralysis, with an annual incidence of 0.75 to 2 cases per 100,000 population.[112] Bulbar involvement is most frequently manifested as bilateral facial paralysis. Difficulty in swallowing due to pharyngeal muscle weakness and impaired ventilation due to intercostal muscle paralysis are the most serious symptoms. Because of lower motor neuron involvement, paralysis is flaccid, and corresponding tendon reflexes are diminished. Sensory disturbances occur as paresthesias, most prominently in the distal part of the extremities and generally preceding the onset of paralysis. Pain often exists in the form of headache, backache, or tenderness of skeletal muscles to deep pressure.

Autonomic nervous system dysfunction is a prominent finding in the patient with acute idiopathic polyneuritis. Wide fluctuations in blood pressure, sudden profuse diaphoresis, peripheral vasoconstriction, resting tachycardia, and cardiac conduction abnormalities on the ECG reflect alterations in the level of autonomic nervous system activity. Orthostatic hypotension may be so severe that elevating the head on a pillow leads to syncope. Thromboembolism occurs with increased frequency. Sudden death is associated with this disease, most likely due to autonomic nervous system dysfunction. A rare complication is increased ICP.

Complete spontaneous recovery from acute idiopathic polyneuritis can occur within a few weeks, when segmental demyelination is the predominant pathologic change. Axonal degeneration, however, as shown by electromyography, may result in slow recovery over several months, with some degree of permanent weakness remaining. Mortality from this syndrome is 3% to 8%, from largely avoidable complications, such as sepsis, adult respiratory distress syndrome, pulmonary emboli, or, in rare cases, unexplained cardiac arrest, perhaps related to autonomic nervous system dysfunction.

Diagnosis

The diagnosis of acute idiopathic polyneuritis is based on typical clinical findings[112] (Table 17-8). The diagnosis is supported by the finding of an increased concentration of protein in the CSF, although cell counts remain normal. Support of a viral etiology is the observation that this syndrome develops after a respiratory or gastrointestinal infection in about one-half of cases.

Treatment

Treatment of acute idiopathic polyneuritis is mainly symptomatic. Vital capacity should be monitored; when it is less than 15 ml·kg^{-1}, the need to support ventilation of the lungs must be considered. Measurement of arterial blood gases will help guide the adequacy of ventilation. Pharyngeal muscle weakness, even in the absence of ventilatory failure, may necessitate the placement of a cuffed tube in the trachea, so as to protect the lungs from aspiration of secretions and gastric fluid. Autonomic nervous system dysfunction may require treatment of hypertension or hypotension. Corticosteroids are not considered useful therapy for this disorder. Plasma exchange or infusion of gamma globulin may be of some benefit.

Management of Anesthesia

Altered function of the autonomic nervous system and the presence of lower motor neuron lesions are the two key considerations for management of anesthesia in the patient with acute idiopathic polyneuritis. Compensatory cardiovascular responses may be absent, resulting in profound hypotension in response to changes in posture, blood loss, or positive airway pressure. Conversely, noxious stimulation, as during laryngoscopy, could be manifested as an exaggerated increase in blood pressure, reflecting the labile activity of the autonomic nervous system in these patients. In view of these unpredictable changes in blood pressure, it would seem prudent to monitor blood pressure continuously with a catheter in a peripheral artery. An exaggerated response to indirect-acting vasopressors should be considered when selecting a drug, rather than intravenous infusion of fluid, to treat hypotension.

Succinylcholine should not be administered, since the possibility of excessive potassium release exists in the presence of lower motor neuron lesions.[65] A nondepolarizing muscle relaxant with minimal circulatory effects would seem a better selection than pancuronium. Even if spontaneous ventilation is present preoperatively, it is likely that depression from anesthetic drugs will necessitate mechanical ventilation of the lungs during surgery. Certainly, continued support of ventilation is likely to be necessary during the postoperative period.

Peroneal Muscular Atrophy

Peroneal muscular atrophy (Charcot-Marie-Tooth disease) is a rare degenerative disease of the peripheral nervous system, transmitted as an autosomal dominant trait. The hallmark of the disease is peroneal muscle atrophy. High pedal arches and talipes (clubfeet) are common, and pes cavus may be present. Onset is typically in the second decade of life, making this disease the most common cause of chronic peripheral neuropathy in childhood. Later, mild distal sensory impairment develops, and eventually the process spreads to involve the upper extremities. Pregnancy may be associated with an exacerbation of this disease. Incapacitation is rare, and death usually occurs from other causes.

Management of Anesthesia

Management of anesthesia in patients with peroneal muscular atrophy introduces concerns regarding responses to muscle relaxants, susceptibility to malignant hyperthermia, and the likelihood of development of postoperative ventilatory failure. Although experience is limited, succinylcholine and nondepolarizing muscle relaxants have been administered to these patients without adverse effects.[113,114] Likewise, the incidence of malignant hyperthermia or postoperative pulmonary complications does not appear to be increased.[113,114] Regional anesthetic techniques may be avoided because of the co-existing neurologic dysfunction.

Refsum's Disease

Refsum's disease is a multisystem disorder manifested by polyneuropathy, ichythyosis, deafness, retinitis pigmentosa, cardiomyopathy, and cerebellar ataxia. The metabolic defect

---

Table 17-8. Diagnostic Criteria for Acute Idiopathic Polyneuritis

Features Required for Diagnosis
  Progressive bilateral weakness in legs and arms
  Areflexia

Features Strongly Supporting the Diagnosis
  Progression of symptoms over several days
  Symmetry of symptoms
  Mild sensory symptoms or signs (sensory level makes diagnosis doubtful)
  Cranial nerve involvement (especially bilateral facial muscle weakness)
  Spontaneous recovery beginning 2–4 weeks after progression ceases
  Autonomic nervous system dysfunction
  Absence of fever at onset
  Increased concentration of protein in the cerebrospinal fluid

responsible for this disease reflects a failure to oxidize phytic acid, a fatty acid that subsequently accumulates in excessive concentrations. Transmission of Refsum's disease is an autosomal recessive trait.

SPINAL CORD TRANSECTION

Spinal cord transection is the description of damage to the spinal cord manifested as paralysis of the lower extremities (paraplegia) or all the extremities (quadriplegia). Anatomically, the spinal cord is not divided, but the effect physiologically is the same as if it were. Spinal cord transection above the level of C2–C4 is incompatible with survival, as innervation to the diaphragm is likely to be destroyed.

The most common cause of spinal cord transection is the trauma associated with a motor vehicle or diving accident, resulting in fracture dislocation of cervical vertebrae. It is estimated that cervical spine injury occurs in 1.5% to 3% of all major trauma victims. The trauma patient's neck must be promptly immobilized, preferably with a rigid collar. Cervical vertebral injury can occur without cord damage because the spinal canal is widest in the cervical region. Two-thirds of all trauma patients have multiple injuries that can interfere with cervical spine evaluation, which is ideally accomplished with computed tomography or magnetic resonance imaging. Nevertheless, routine computed tomography or magnetic resonance imaging is not practical, considering the risk of transporting a potentially unstable patient. For this reason, standard radiographic views of the cervical spinal are often relied on. In an alert patient, the absence of neck pain or tenderness virtually eliminates the presence of cervical spine injury.[115]

Occasionally, rheumatoid arthritis of the spine leads to spontaneous dislocation of the C1 vertebra on the C2 vertebra, producing progressive quadriparesis. These patients can suddenly become quadriplegic. Treatment of cervical fracture dislocation entails immediate immobilization and traction as provided by a halo-thoracic brace. The most frequent nontraumatic cause of spinal cord transection is multiple sclerosis. In addition, infections or vascular and developmental disorders may be responsible for permanent damage to the spinal cord.

Pathophysiology

Spinal cord transection initially produces flaccid paralysis, with total absence of sensation below the level of injury. In addition, there is loss of temperature regulation and of spinal cord reflexes below the level of injury. Decreased systemic blood pressure and bradycardia are common findings. Abnormalities on the ECG are frequent during the acute phase of spinal cord transection and include ventricular premature beats and ST-T wave changes suggestive of myocardial ischemia. This initial phase, occurring after acute transection of

the spinal cord is known as spinal shock and typically lasts 1 to 3 weeks. During this period, the major cause of morbidity and mortality is impaired alveolar ventilation, combined with an inability to protect the airway and to clear bronchial secretions. Aspiration of gastric fluid or contents, as well as pneumonia and pulmonary embolism, are constant threats during spinal shock.

Several weeks after acute transection of the spinal cord, the spinal cord reflexes gradually return, and patients enter a chronic stage, characterized by overactivity of the sympathetic nervous system and involuntary skeletal muscle spasms. Sequelae of this chronic stage, which jeopardize the patient's well-being, include impaired alveolar ventilation; cardiovascular instability manifested as autonomic hyperreflexia; chronic pulmonary or genitourinary tract infections, or both; anemia; and altered thermoregulation.

Mental depression and pain are very real problems after spinal cord injury. Root pain is localized at or near the level of the transection. Visceral pain is produced by distension of the bladder or bowel. Phantom body pain can occur in areas of complete sensory loss. As a result of mental depression or the presence of pain, or both, these patients may be ingesting drugs, which must be considered when planning management of anesthesia.

Pulmonary System

Spontaneous ventilation is impossible if the level of spinal cord transection results in paralysis of the diaphragm. A transection between the level of C2–C4 may result in apnea due to denervation of the diaphragm. When function of the diaphragm is intact, tidal volume is likely to remain adequate. Nevertheless, the ability to cough and clear secretions from the airway is often impaired because of decreased expiratory reserve volume. Indeed, acute transection of the spinal cord at the cervical level is accompanied by a marked decrease in vital capacity. Furthermore, arterial hypoxemia is a consistent early finding during the period after cervical spinal cord injury. Tracheobronchial suctioning has been associated with bradycardia and cardiac arrest in these patients, emphasizing the importance of establishing optimal arterial oxygenation before undertaking this maneuver.

Autonomic Hyperreflexia

Autonomic hyperreflexia is a disorder that appears after resolution of spinal shock and in association with return of the spinal cord reflexes.[116] This reflex response can be initiated by cutaneous or visceral stimulation below the level of spinal cord transection. Distension of a hollow viscus, such as the bladder or rectum, is a common stimulus. The incidence of autonomic hyperreflexia depends on the level of spinal cord transection. For example, about 85% of patients with spinal cord transections above T6 will exhibit this reflex; it is unlikely

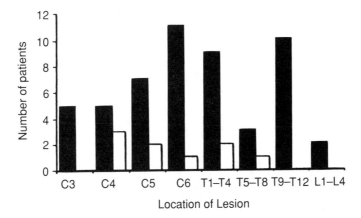

Fig. 17-21. Autonomic hyperreflexia (AHR) did not occur in any patient undergoing extracorporeal shock-wave lithotripsy (ESWL) and a spinal cord transection below T9. Shaded bars, lesions (n = 52); open bars, AHR (n = 9). (From Stowe DF, Bernstein JS, Madsen KE, McDonald DJ, Ebert TJ. Autonomic hyperreflexia in spinal cord injured patients during extracorporeal shock wave lithotripsy. Anesth Analg 1989;68:788–91, with permission.)

to be associated with a transection below T10. Surgery, however, is a particularly potent stimulus to the development of autonomic hyperreflexia, and even patients with no previous history of this response may be at risk during operative procedures. Patients with spinal cord transection undergoing extracorporeal shock wave lithotripsy may experience autonomic hyperreflexia even in the presence of general or spinal anesthesia[116] (Fig. 17-21).

Mechanism

Stimulation below the level of spinal cord transection initiates afferent impulses that enter the spinal cord below that level (Fig. 17-22). These impulses elicit reflex sympathetic activity over the splanchnic outflow tract. In neurologically intact patients, this outflow is modulated by inhibitory impulses from higher centers in the central nervous system. In the presence of spinal cord transection, however, this outflow is isolated

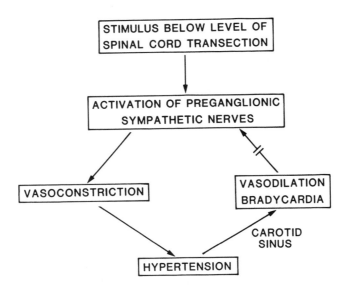

Fig. 17-22. Schematic diagram of the sequence of events associated with clinical manifestations of autonomic hyperreflexia. Because the impulses that produce vasodilation cannot reach the neurologically isolated portion of the spinal cord, vasoconstriction and hypertension persist.

from inhibitory impulses, such that generalized vasoconstriction persists below the level of injury. Vasoconstriction results in an increase of blood pressure, which is then perceived by the carotid sinus. Subsequent activation of the carotid sinus results in decreased efferent sympathetic nervous system activity from the central nervous system, manifested as a predominance of parasympathetic nervous system activity at the heart and peripheral vasculature. This predominance, however, cannot be produced below the level of spinal cord transection, as this part of the body remains neurologically isolated. Therefore, vasoconstriction persists below the level of spinal cord transection. If the level of spinal cord transection is above the level of splanchnic outflow (T4–T6), vasodilation in the neurologically intact portion of the body is insufficient to offset the effects of vasoconstriction, as reflected by persistent hypertension.

Signs and Symptoms

Hypertension and bradycardia are the hallmarks of autonomic hyperreflexia.[116] Stimulation of the carotid sinus from hypertension is manifested as bradycardia and cutaneous vasodilation above the level of spinal cord transection. Hypertension persists, since vasodilation cannot occur below the level of injury. Nasal stuffiness reflects vasodilation. The patient may complain of headache and blurred vision as manifestations of severe hypertension. A precipitous increase in blood pressure can lead to cerebral, retinal, or subarachnoid hemorrhage, as well as increased operative blood loss. Loss of consciousness and seizures can occur. Cardiac dysrhythmias are also present in most of these patients. Pulmonary edema reflects acute left ventricular failure, due to increased afterload produced by elevations in blood pressure.

Treatment

Treatment of autonomic hyperreflexia consists of ganglionic blocking drugs (trimethaphan, pentolinium), alpha-adrenergic antagonists (phentolamine, phenoxybenzamine), direct-acting vasodilators (nitroprusside), and general or regional anesthesia.[117] Drugs that lower blood pressure by a central action alone are not predictably effective.

Although the most practical approach to lowering blood pressure in an awake patient would seem to be with an intravenous infusion of nitroprusside, clinical experience with the use of nitroprusside for this purpose has not been reported. Intravenous phentolamine has been recommended, but large doses may be required, emphasizing that the hypertension of autonomic hyperreflexia is not due to increased circulating levels of catecholamines. Institution of epidural anesthesia has been reported to be effective for the treatment of autonomic hyperreflexia provoked by uterine contractions.[118] In this same patient, an attempt to control blood pressure with nitroprusside was not successful. Epidural administration of meperidine has been used during labor to control hyperreflexia.[119]

Genitourinary Tract System

Renal failure is the leading cause of death in the patient with chronic spinal cord transection. Chronic urinary tract infections and immobilization predispose to the development of renal calculi. Amyloidosis of the kidney can be manifested as proteinuria, leading to a decrease in the concentration of albumin in the plasma.

Musculoskeletal System

Prolonged immobility leads to osteoporosis, skeletal muscle atrophy, and the development of decubitus ulcers. Pathologic fractures can occur when moving these patients. Pressure points should be well protected and padded, to minimize the likelihood of trauma to the skin and the development of decubitus ulcers.

Management of Anesthesia

Management of anesthesia in the patient with transection of the spinal cord is largely determined by the duration of the injury.[116] Regardless of the duration of spinal cord transection, the institution of preoperative hydration is helpful in preventing hypotension during the induction and maintenance of anesthesia.

Acute Spinal Cord Transection

The patient with acute spinal cord transection may require special precautions in the management of the airway. It is important to recognize that undertaking any airway maneuver results in some movement of the cervical spine. Topical anesthesia and placement of the tube into the trachea, using a fiberoptic laryngoscope, is an alternative to rapid-sequence induction of anesthesia with an intravenous anesthetic and muscle relaxant. In an alert patient, the absence of neck pain or tenderness virtually excludes the possibility of cervical spine injury or the likelihood of neurologic damage during tracheal intubation. When the cervical spine is unstable or when there is a high index of suspicion for the presence of cervical spine injury, it is important to proceed carefully, as extension of the head (as during direct laryngoscopy for intubation of the trachea) could further damage the spinal cord. Nevertheless, there is no evidence of increased neurologic morbidity after elective or emergency oral tracheal intubation of the anesthetized or awake patient who has an unstable cervical spine.[113,120,121] Even manual-in-line stabilization to reduce cervical vertebrae movement during tracheal intubation has been discouraged, for fear that application of cervical traction may result in dislocation in the unstable neck.[112] Although the muscles in the neck exert some stabilizing force, their contribution toward clinical stability of the cervical spine has not been determined.[123] All factors considered, airway management in the presence of cervical spine injury should be dictated by common sense, and not by a dogmatic approach. Certainly, clinical experience in the management of these patients supports the safety of a variety of techniques.[120]

The absence of compensatory responses of the sympathetic nervous system makes these patients particularly likely to show extreme decreases in blood pressure, in response to an acute change in body posture, blood loss, or positive airway pressure. Liberal intravenous infusion of a crystalloid solution may be necessary to fill the vascular space, which has been abruptly increased by vasodilation. Likewise, blood loss should be replaced promptly in these patients. Breathing is best managed by mechanical ventilation of the lungs, as abdominal and intercostal muscle paralysis, combined with general anesthesia, mitigates against maintenance of adequate spontaneous ventilation. Hypothermia should be guarded against, as these patients tend to become poikilothermic below the level of spinal cord transection. Anesthesia is maintained with drugs that will ensure central nervous system sedation and facilitate tolerance of the endotracheal tube. Nitrous oxide combined with a volatile or injected drug is satisfactory for this purpose. Pulse oximetry is useful in guiding the delivered concentration of oxygen, keeping in mind that arterial hypoxemia is a frequent finding after acute spinal cord transection.

The need for a muscle relaxant will be dictated by the operative site and the level of spinal cord transection. If a muscle relaxant is necessary, the sympathomimetic effect of pancuronium makes this drug an attractive choice. Succinylcholine is unlikely to provoke an excessive release of potassium during the first few hours after acute spinal cord transection. Nevertheless, it would seem reasonable to avoid the use of this drug, except for the rare instances in which the rapid onset of short-duration skeletal-muscle paralysis is mandatory.

Chronic Spinal Cord Transection

The critical objective during management of anesthesia for the patient with chronic transection of the spinal cord is prevention of autonomic hyperreflexia. Surgery is an intense stimulus for its development, emphasizing that patients who have a negative history for this reflex response are vulnerable to its occurrence during operation. General anesthesia, which includes volatile drugs, is effective in preventing this response.[114] Epidural and spinal anesthesia are also effective, but it may be technically difficult to perform these procedures in the patient with spinal cord injury. Furthermore, control of the level of anesthesia is not easy to attain. Nevertheless, spinal anesthesia seems particularly effective in preventing autonomic hyperreflexia.[117] Conversely, epidural anesthesia has been reported to be ineffective occasionally in preventing hypertension during urologic endoscopic procedures in patients with spinal cord injury.[123] This problem might be predictable, as epidural anesthesia does not always provide adequate sacral anesthesia. Block of afferent pathways with a topical local anesthetic applied to the urethra, as for a cystoscopic procedure, is often ineffective in preventing autonomic hyperreflexia, since this form of anesthesia does not block the bladder muscle proprioceptors, which are stimulated by bladder distension. Regardless of the technique selected for anesthesia, a drug such as nitroprusside must be readily available to treat precipitous hypertension. Nitroprusside administered as a rapid injection (1 to 2 $\mu g \cdot kg^{-1}$ IV) is an effective method of treating sudden hypertension.[59] Persistence of hypertension will require a continuous intravenous infusion of nitroprusside. It is also important to appreciate that autonomic hyperreflexia may be manifested postoperatively, when the effects of the anesthetic begin to dissipate.

When general anesthesia is selected, administration of a muscle relaxant may be necessary to facilitate intubation of the trachea and to prevent reflex skeletal muscle spasms in response to surgical stimulation. A nondepolarizing muscle relaxant is used for this purpose, since succinylcholine is likely to provoke the release of potassium, particularly within the first 6 months of spinal cord injury.[124] Indeed, there is evidence that increased release of potassium after administration of succinylcholine can begin to occur within 4 days of denervation injury[125] (Fig. 17-23). Peak release of potassium after administration of succinylcholine occurs when the injury is about 14 days old. Cardiac arrest due to succinylcholine-induced hyperkalemia, however, has been observed as early as 7 days after spinal cord transection.[125] Furthermore, the magnitude of potassium release does not seem to be dose dependent, as evidenced by the development of hyperkalemia after intravenous administration of 20 mg of succinylcholine to a paraplegic adult patient.[126] In addition, prior administration of a nonparalyzing dose of a nondepolarizing muscle relaxant does not reliably attenuate the release of potassium in response to succinylcholine.

Excess release of potassium presumably reflects proliferation of the extrajunctional cholinergic receptors that are responsive to acetylcholine (Fig. 17-24). These receptor sites may develop within 48 to 72 hours of denervation, providing an increased number of sites at which potassium exchange can occur during succinylcholine-induced depolarization.[127] All factors considered, it would seem reasonable to avoid the use of succinylcholine in patients with transection of the spinal cord that is more than 24 hours old. The duration of susceptibility to the hyperkalemic effects of succinylcholine is unknown, but the risk is probably reduced after 3 to 6 months. Nevertheless, the presence of resistance to the effects of a nondepolarizing muscle relaxant in a patient 463 days after a burn injury suggests the persistence of the same extrajunctional receptors presumed to be responsible for succinylcholine-induced

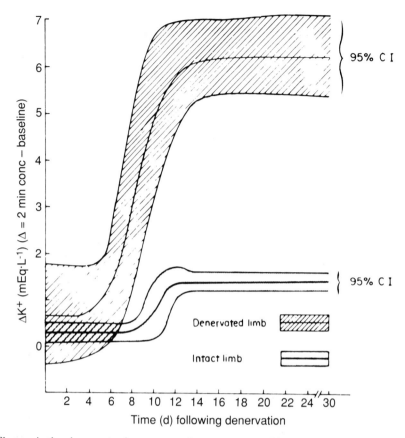

Fig. 17-23. Changes in the plasma potassium concentration were measured in the venous effluent blood from a denervated intact limb of anesthetized animals 2 minutes after the administration of succinylcholine (2 mg·kg⁻¹ IV) over 1 minute. The half-peak increase in plasma potassium concentration occurred 8.4 days after denervation, and the peak increase was present 14 days after denervation. An increase in the plasma potassium concentration was evident as early as 4 days after denervation. (From John DA, Tobey RE, Homer LD, Rice CL. Onset of succinylcholine-induced hyperkalemia following denervation. Anesthesiology 1976; 45:294–9, with permission.)

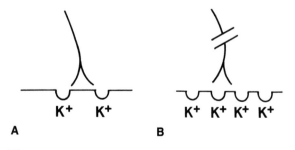

Fig. 17-24. Schematic diagram of the neuromuscular junction (**A**) before and (**B**) after denervation. Denervation is associated with a proliferation of extrajunctional cholinergic receptors that participate in the exchange of potassium in response to depolarization induced by acetylcholine. As a result, prolonged depolarization of the neuromuscular junction, as produced by succinylcholine, leads to hyperkalemia.

hyperkalemia.[128] If this is true, patients could remain at risk of the hyperkalemic effects of succinylcholine far beyond the speculated 3- to 6-month period after spinal cord transection.

CEREBRAL PROTECTION AND RESUSCITATION

Cardiac arrest, stroke, and head injury are the events most likely to require attempts directed toward cerebral protection and resuscitation.

Cardiac Arrest

The early doctrine that 4 to 6 minutes of global cerebral ischemia produced by cardiac arrest results in irreversible brain injury is no longer tenable.[129] The evidence suggests that central nervous system neurons can tolerate 20 to 60 minutes of complete anoxia without always sustaining irreversible injury. Furthermore, events that follow cerebral ischemia may be more likely than the initial insult to produce permanent brain damage. For example, profound cerebral hypoperfusion (cerebral blood flow often less than 10% of normal) with areas of no reflow may occur 15 to 90 minutes after resuscitation from circulatory arrest. This massive and progressive increase in cerebral small vessel resistance may reduce blood flow below levels sufficient to maintain neuronal viability. Regardless of the time from cardiac arrest to initiation of cardiopulmonary resuscitation, more than 6 minutes of closed chest massage is associated with increased neurologic morbidity.[129]

Historically, management of the patient who fails to awaken after cardiac arrest has included hypothermia, hyperventilation of the lungs, and large doses of corticosteroids. Enthusiasm for hypothermia has waned because of the absence of convincing data that this complex procedure induced after cardiac arrest is beneficial. Nevertheless, recent animal data suggest that even a mild decrease of body temperature (2° to 3°C) present at the time of arterial hypoxemia may contribute to cerebral protection.[130] Certainly hypothermia is the only method available to depress cellular oxygen requirements below that needed for normal cellular function. Hyperventilation of the lungs, in the absence of increased ICP, has not been shown to improve outcome after cardiac arrest and, like hypothermia, cannot be routinely recommended. Therapy with corticosteroids remains a common intervention, but the value of these drugs is also controversial. Perhaps a low risk-to-benefit ratio has contributed to their continued use. Administration of calcium during and after cardiopulmonary resuscitation may be questionable in view of the possible role of neuronal calcium overload in small vessel vasoconstriction and postresuscitation cerebral hypoperfusion.[129] In this regard, calcium antagonists may find a role in prevention or attenuation of postresuscitation cerebral hypoperfusion.[129] Hypertonic saline may be a preferred solution in the resuscitation of patients experiencing hemorrhagic shock associated with increased ICP.[131]

Barbiturates

The use of barbiturates in brain protection after an ischemic insult is based on the ability of these drugs to produce dose-related decreases in cerebral metabolic oxygen requirements until maximum reductions of about 50% are achieved. This maximum reduction corresponds to an isoelectric EEG and is evidence that additional doses of barbiturates are not necessary. This drug-induced decrease in oxygen requirements reflects depression of mentation, and not a decrease in oxygen needed to maintain cellular viability. From this evidence, it can be predicted that barbiturate protection will occur only if the ischemic insult does not interfere with basal cellular metabolism, as evidenced by the continued presence of electrical activity on the EEG.[132] During cardiac arrest (global ischemia), the EEG becomes flat within 20 to 30 seconds, and subsequent administration of a barbiturate would not be expected to improve neurologic outcome. Indeed, administration of thiopental (30 mg·kg^{-1} IV), as a single injection to comatose survivors of cardiac arrest, does not increase survival or improve neurologic outcome.[133] Likewise, controlled animal studies fail to demonstrate improved neurologic outcomes when administration of thiopental precedes or follows global cerebral ischemia.[134,135] In contrast to global ischemia, incomplete ischemia with maintenance of electrical activity on the EEG is likely to be associated with improved neurologic outcome when a barbiturate is administered to produce metabolic suppression. Consistent with this concept is the observation that neuropsychiatric complications after cardiopulmonary bypass, presumably due to embolism, clear more rapidly in patients treated prospectively with thiopental (average dose 39.5 mg·kg^{-1} IV) to maintain EEG silence.[136] Other patients at risk of incomplete cerebral ischemia who might benefit from prior barbiturate-induced EEG silence include those scheduled for carotid endarterectomy or for resection of a thoracic aneurysm. In view of these data from patient and animal studies, it does not seem appropriate to recommend administration of a barbiturate to a patient who has been resuscitated from a cardiac arrest.

Postanoxic Encephalopathy

Neurologic sequelae after an episode of acute cerebral hypoxia range from mild psychiatric disturbances to an irreversible vegetative state. Cortical blindness is a potential complication. The presence of coma after successful cardiopulmonary resuscitation is a grave prognostic sign. The prognosis for acceptable neurologic recovery is about 1% for patients who remain comatose 24 hours after resuscitation from a cardiac arrest with the absence of two of three reflexes (pupillary, corneal, oculovestibular).

Brain Death

The need to define and confirm irreversible brain damage that occurs after successful cardiopulmonary resuscitation is apparent. The diagnosis of brain death in the very young is difficult, as the resistance of the immature brain to the damaging effects of arterial hypoxemia is well documented. In the absence of hypothermia (body temperature above 32°C), coupled with the elimination of a depressant drug overdose as the cause of coma, the criteria for establishment of brain death in an adult are as follows[137]:

1. *Coma (absent cerebral responsivity)* due to a known structural or metabolic insult that has persisted for 12 hours (coma due to an overdose of depressant drug must be ruled out by history and appropriate laboratory studies)

2. *Vital brain stem function absent,* as reflected by fixed and unreactive pupils, absent oculocephalic reflexes, no ocular responses to ice water irrigation of the ears, and no spontaneous ventilation, despite normal to elevated $PaCO_2$ (spinal reflex activity does not preclude the diagnosis of brain death)

3. *Cortical function absent,* as reflected by an isoelectric EEG at maximum gain for 60 minutes (again, this assumes that a depressant drug overdose is not present)

4. *Absence of cerebral circulation,* or a clinical defect of cerebral circulation, as determined by angiography, even in the presence of a depressant drug overdose

Recording for SSEPs is useful in monitoring the comatose patient and predicting neurologic outcome. Measurement of SSEPs may also be useful in confirming brain death.

Stroke

Stroke models in laboratory animals have been shown to benefit from the administration of barbiturates before or after initiation of the stroke.[137] Nevertheless, lesions resulting from the abrupt occlusion of a single cerebral vessel in an otherwise healthy animal cannot be equated to that encountered in the elderly patient with co-existing cerebrovascular disease. On the basis of current animal data, production of barbiturate coma in stroke patients cannot be recommended. More important is the recognition from animal models that the brain does not immediately infarct after occlusion of a single major vessel; rather, irreversible damage may not occur for as long as 2 to 3 hours.

Head Injury

The greatest success in cerebral protection and resuscitation has been in patients who sustain a head injury. In contrast to patients who suffer cardiac arrest or stroke, these patients are often young, and co-existing cerebrovascular disease is minimal or absent. Routine monitoring of ICP is useful in guiding the management of these patients. Administration of hyperosmotic drugs and corticosteroids and the institution of mechanical hyperventilation of the lungs to produce a $PaCO_2$ between 25 to 30 mmHg are standard interventions to decrease ICP.

Barbiturates

Administration of a barbiturate is recommended when ICP remains elevated despite traditional therapy. This recommendation is based on the predictable ability of these drugs to decrease ICP, presumably by decreasing CBF and cerebral blood volume secondary to cerebrovascular vasoconstriction. In addition, a drug-induced decrease in neuronal metabolism can lead to even further decreases in cerebral blood volume, by decreasing CBF in response to metabolic autoregulation.

The goal of barbiturate therapy is to maintain ICP at less than 20 mmHg without the occurrence of plateau waves. An effective regimen is the administration of an initial dose of pentobarbital (3 to 5 $mg \cdot kg^{-1}$ IV), followed by a continuous rate of infusion to maintain the blood concentration of the barbiturate at 3 to 6 $mg \cdot dl^{-1}$.[138,139] An alternative to measuring the blood concentration of pentobarbital every 12 to 24 hours is to adjust the infusion rate to maintain an isoelectric EEG, which confirms the presence of maximum drug-induced depression of cerebral metabolic requirements for oxygen. Barbiturates also decrease the dose of mannitol necessary to keep the ICP below 20 mmHg. This reduction in dose decreases the likelihood of plasma hyperosmolarity and electrolyte disturbances secondary to diuresis. Discontinuation of the barbiturate infusion can be considered when the ICP has remained within a normal range for 48 hours.

One of the hazards of barbiturate therapy, as used to lower ICP, is hypotension, which can jeopardize the maintenance of an adequate cerebral perfusion pressure. Hypotension is particularly likely in elderly patients and in the presence of decreased intravascular fluid volume. In patients, a dose of thiopental or methohexital sufficient to produce an isoelectric EEG produces peripheral vasodilation and myocardial depression.[140,141] In animals, thiopental is more likely than pentobarbital to produce hypotension and ventricular fibrillation when administered in doses sufficient to cause electrical silence in the brain.[142] Inotropic support of cardiac output may be necessary in some patients being treated with barbiturates.

Failure of a barbiturate to lower ICP is a grave prognostic sign. Even when barbiturates are effective, the overall morbidity and mortality in a head trauma patient have not been shown to be improved by the use of these drugs, as compared with patients treated aggressively with diuretics, corticosteroids, and hyperventilation.[142] Likewise, there is no evidence that high-dose dexamethasone is useful in improving the long-term outcome of the patient with severe head injury.

EPILEPSY

Chronic recurrent epilepsy (seizure disorder) affects about 0.5% to 1% of the population. It is estimated that 2% to 5% of the population will experience a nonfebrile seizure at some point during their lifetime.[144] Idiopathic seizure disorders usually begin in childhood, whereas the onset of epilepsy in an adult should arouse suspicion of focal brain disease, such as an intracranial tumor, head trauma, or infection. Withdrawal from alcohol or other addicting drugs may also be a cause of seizures in an adult. The EEG is the most important diagnostic test, although a normal tracing does not exclude the possibility

Table 17-9.   Classification of Adult Seizure Disorders

Type	Clinical Features	Effective Drugs	Half-time (h)	Therapeutic Blood Level ($\mu g \cdot ml^{-1}$)
Partial (focal)				
Simple partial	Focal motor or sensory disturbances (jacksonian epilepsy); consciousness not impaired	Valproic acid	12	50–100
		Carbamazepine	12	4–10
		Phenytoin	24	10–20
Complex partial	Bizarre behavior and impaired consciousness; auras prominent	As for simple partial seizures		
Generalized				
Absence	Brief loss of consciousness, staring; little or no motor activity	Valproic acid Ethosuximide	55	50–100
Myoclonic	Isolated clonic jerks, often evoked by a sensory stimulus	Valproic acid		
Continual				
Status epilepticus	Continual seizure activity	Diazepam Phenytoin Carbamazepine Valproic acid		

of epilepsy. Magnetic resonance imaging is superior to computed tomography in detecting a focal intracranial lesion such as atrophy. Examination of the CSF is indicated if infection is a possible cause of seizures. Seizures are categorized as (1) those arising in part of one cerebral hemisphere accompanied by focal EEG abnormalities, and (2) those with clinical and EEG manifestations that indicate essentially simultaneous involvement of all or large parts of both cerebral hemispheres from the beginning[145] (Table 17-9).

Pathophysiology

Epilepsy is not a disease, but rather a symptom of a disorder of neuronal dysfunction. A seizure results from the excessive discharge of an aggregate of neurons that depolarize in synchronous fashion. A focal area of neuronal hyperexcitability in the cerebral cortex may remain localized, if there is a surrounding field in which the neurons are hyperpolarized and inexcitable. Conversely, hyperactive neurons may impinge on the adjoining cerebral cortex, recruiting more neurons and generating sufficient energy to spread by anatomic connections to the thalamus and brain stem. In such instances, massive synchronous discharges appear, resulting in generalized seizures. The concept that generalized seizures can result from localized areas in the cerebral cortex is the basis for using the initial symptomatology, or aura, as a clue to the location of the focal discharge. For example, generalized seizures after an aura of an ill-defined odor indicates focal lesions in the temporal lobe.

Treatment

Treatment of chronic epilepsy is ideally with a single drug, determined principally by the classification of the seizure disorder. Nonsedating drugs are preferable to sedating drugs, such as phenobarbital (Table 17-9). Valproic acid may be the preferable drug in the initial treatment of most forms of epilepsy.[146] Only after failure of single-drug therapy is combination therapy likely to be considered. Monitoring the blood level of the anticonvulsant has become common, although the clinical response is the most important observation.

The need to treat a patient after a single seizure is controversial. The likelihood of a recurrent seizure is about 50% during the first 3 years, with the greatest incidence during the first 6 months. For this reason, there may be some logic in treating for 6 months after an initial seizure. Conversely, most agree that gradual withdrawal of anticonvulsant therapy is a consideration, when seizure activity has been controlled for a sustained period, often 2 years.[147] There is an increased risk of congenital malformation in the infant of a mother who conceives during anticonvulsant drug therapy.[148] Furthermore, an anticonvulsant drug that produces enzyme induction can decrease the efficacy of an oral contraceptive by increasing its metabolism.

A surgical procedure such as cortical resection and transection of the anterior portion of the corpus collosum may be considered in the patient who is resistant to control with anticonvulsant therapy. The use of positron emission tomography to measure brain glucose metabolism may be helpful in preoperative localization of the epileptogenic focus.

Grand Mal Seizure

Grand mal seizure is a generalized, continuous seizure (status epilepticus). It is a medical emergency, as adequate ventilation and oxygenation are not possible, and death is inevitable if treatment is not provided. The first priority of treatment is establishment of a patent upper airway and administration of oxygen. Seizure activity is suppressed by administration of diazepam (2 mg·min^{-1} IV), until seizures stop, or to a total of 20 mg.[149] To prevent recurrence of seizure activity as the effect of diazepam wanes, it is recommended that an infusion of phenytoin (50 mg·min^{-1} IV) to a total of 18 mg·kg^{-1}, be initiated simultaneously with administration of the benzodiazepine. Intravenous administration of lorazepam with its associated long duration of action, may be a useful alternative to diazepam for the initial treatment of a grand mal seizure. Phenytoin may be a better choice than diazepam for the management of continuous seizure activity associated with head trauma or global cerebral ischemia, as drug-induced alterations of consciousness would be undesirable. In an extreme situation, general anesthesia using halothane or isoflurane and a skeletal muscle relaxant to provide neuromuscular blockade and facilitate ventilation of the lungs is necessary to control seizure activity. Treatment with only a skeletal muscle relaxant is questionable, as continuous firing of neurons (more than 60 minutes) can result in cell damage despite adequate cerebral oxygenation.[149]

Management of Anesthesia

Management of anesthesia in the patient with a seizure disorder must include consideration of the impact of anticonvulsant drugs on organ function, coagulation, and response to anesthetic drugs. Known adverse effects of these drugs should be evaluated with appropriate preoperative tests. Coexisting sedation produced by an anticonvulsant drug may have an additive effect with the anesthetic, whereas drug-induced enzyme induction could alter responses to other drugs or even contribute to organ toxicity associated with administration of halothane or enflurane.

The selection of drugs used for induction and maintenance of anesthesia should include consideration of the effects of these drugs on central nervous system electrical activity. For example, methohexital can activate epileptic foci and has been recommended as a method of delineating these foci in patients undergoing surgical treatment of epilepsy.[150] The ability of ketamine to elicit seizure activity in patients with known seizure disorders, as well as in patients with no known central nervous system disease, has not been a consistent observation.[151] Concurrent use of ketamine with other drugs, such as aminophylline, can result in lowering of the seizure threshold for both drugs.[152] Seizures and opisthotonos have been observed after propofol anesthesia, suggesting caution in the administration of this drug to patients with known seizure disorders.[153] In selecting a muscle relaxant, the central ner-

vous system-stimulating effects of laudanosine, a metabolite of atracurium, may merit consideration.

Most inhaled anesthetics, including nitrous oxide, have been reported to produce seizure activity.[154] The presence of halogen atoms is an important determinant of the convulsant properties of volatile anesthetics, with fluorine incriminated as epileptogenic. Nevertheless, seizure activity is very rare after administration of halothane and has not been shown to occur in response to the administration of isoflurane.[154] Conversely, enflurane predictably produces spike and wave activity on the EEG, which can be accompanied by visible skeletal muscle twitching. These changes occur in normal patients, as well as in those with known co-existing seizure disorders. The likelihood of seizure activity is greatest when the inhaled concentration of enflurane is above 2.5% and when hypocarbia (less than 25 mmHg) is present. Seizure activity on the EEG, however, has been observed in normal children who have inhaled concentrations of enflurane as low as 1%.[154] Auditory stimulation can also elicit seizure activity during the administration of enflurane. Although adverse effects on the brain are not produced by this seizure activity, the wisdom of administering an epileptogenic anesthetic to a patient with a seizure disorder remains doubtful. Conceivably, enflurane could be used to facilitate identification of seizure foci in patients undergoing diagnostic procedures.

In view of the availability of drugs that do not lower the seizure threshold, it would seem reasonable to avoid administration of potentially epileptogenic drugs to the patient with epilepsy. In this regard, thiobarbiturates, opioids, and benzodiazepines do not lower the seizure threshold or predispose to seizure activity. Halothane, isoflurane, or desflurane would seem good choices when a volatile anesthetic that does not produce seizure activity in the central nervous system is desired. Regardless of the drugs used for anesthesia, it is important to maintain treatment with the pre-established anticonvulsant drug throughout the perioperative period.

SYNCOPE

Syncope is a sudden transient loss of consciousness with concurrent loss of postural tone followed by spontaneous recovery. This disorder must be differentiated from seizures and other states of altered consciousness such as dizziness, vertigo, and narcolepsy. It is estimated that syncope accounts for 1% to 6% of hospital admissions and 3% of emergency department visits. The most common causes of syncope are vasovagal reactions, orthostatic hypotension, drug-induced, and cardiac disease (obstruction to left ventricular outflow, bradydysrhythmias, tachydysrhythmias).[155]

TOURETTE SYNDROME

Tourette syndrome is a complex neuropsychiatric disorder of lifelong duration, with onset during childhood.[156] Symptoms begin as an attention deficit disorder, progressing to spasmodic repetitious movements, which may be confused with seizures. Intelligence is usually above average, but nonspecific abnormalities are present on the EEG in about one-half of cases. Some patients exhibit coprolalia (profane vocalizations) and echolalia (repetitious speech).

Drugs administered in an attempt to provide symptomatic relief of Tourette syndrome include haloperidol, clonidine, and pimozide. Side effects associated with drug therapy include extrapyramidal symptoms (haloperidol), sedation and reduced anesthetic requirements (clonidine), and cardiac dysrhythmias secondary to prolongation of the Q-T interval (pimozide) on the ECG. Sudden unexpected deaths in patients treated with high doses of pimozide (greater than 0.3 mg·kg^{-1}) have been attributed to cardiac dysrhythmias. There are no unique features of this syndrome that influence the selection of anesthetic drugs or muscle relaxants.

HEADACHE

Headache is one of the most common symptoms described by patients. In most cases, the cause of a headache is benign, and no treatment is required. Occasionally, headache is a symptom of central nervous system disease. Perioperative caffeine withdrawal syndrome may be manifested as postoperative headache in susceptible patients.[157]

Migraine Headache

Migraine headache is a disorder of youth, occurring most often in females between 20 and 35 years of age.[158] A family history of migraine headache is present in about 60% of patients, and the incidence of hypertension, stroke, and ischemic heart disease is increased. The onset of migraine headache in middle age or its accentuation by maneuvers that increase ICP (coughing, bending over) suggests a focal intracranial tumor.

Signs and Symptoms

Signs and symptoms of migraine headache commonly begin in childhood (abdominal pain, vertigo, motion sickness), but the actual headache may not be experienced until later. Classic migraine headache begins with prodroma characterized by neurologic symptoms suggestive of cerebral ischemia. Visual blurring and tingling paresthesias of the face and arms are frequent. After about 30 minutes, these symptoms wane, followed by an intense (pounding) unilateral headache. Nausea and vomiting may occur. Typically, the headache subsides in about 6 hours.

Common migraine headache differs from classic migraine headache in that the prodromal signs are absent and the headache is often protracted and may be present on awakening. A small number of patients manifest symptoms (vertigo, diplopia, ataxia) characterized as basilar artery migraine. Ophthalmic migraine is characterized by headache and ocular paralysis

(ptosis due to oculomotor nerve involvement), presumably reflecting compression of the cranial nerve by an edematous carotid or basilar artery. The traditional explanation for migraine headache is initial vasoconstriction causing the prodromal phase of brain ischemia, followed by secondary extracranial vasodilation manifesting as headache. Nevertheless, there is no evidence of an initial decrease in CBF to support this hypothesis. A more likely explanation of the initiating event seems to be a neuronal change characterized by a spreading inhibition of the cortical neurons. Abnormal serotoninergic transmission may be involved in the development of migraine headache. Indeed, migraine headache can be precipitated by drugs that release serotonin.[158]

Treatment

Treatment of migraine headache is most often with ergonovine or methysergide. These drugs are not recommended for the parturient or in the presence of co-existing hypertension. Chronic treatment with methysergide has been associated with pleuropulmonary fibrosis, thickening of heart valves, and retroperitoneal fibrosis. Sumatriptan, a selective agonist of a subpopulation of serotonin receptors (type 1D), is effective for the treatment of migraine and cluster headache.[159] Other drugs that are sometimes helpful in the treatment of migraine headache include verapamil, propranolol, timolol, prednisone, cyproheptadine, and amitriptyline.

Management of Anesthesia

Management of anesthesia for the patient with a history of migraine headache should consider the possible adverse interactions of anesthetic drugs with ergot preparations. Specifically, administration of a vasopressor to the patient treated with these drugs might produce an exaggerated increase in blood pressure. There are no known unique hazards of anesthetic drugs when administered to these patients.

Cluster Headache

Cluster headache (histamine cephalgia, atypical facial neuralgia) is a vasodilating headache that typically awakens the patient at night as excruciating unilateral pain, often involving the temple or malar region. Maximum intensity is reached in 20 to 30 minutes, followed by the disappearance of symptoms over the next 1 to 2 hours. Visual disturbances or paresthesias typical of migraine are absent, but ptosis and miosis may occur. Attacks occur in a cluster, followed by long symptom-free intervals. Middle-aged males are most often affected.

Treatment

Treatment of cluster headache is usually more difficult than treatment of migraine headache. It includes prophylaxis with ergonovine or methysergide. Intranasal administration of lidocaine on the same side as the pain may relieve cluster headache, perhaps by anesthetizing nerves in the sphenopalatine fossa. Even nasal inhalation of oxygen by virtue of its vasoconstrictive effects may be helpful in some refractory cases. Other drugs reported to be useful in the treatment of cluster headache include sumatriptan, lithium, indomethacin, and prednisone.

Increased Intracranial Pressure

Headache can be the initial manifestation of increased ICP due to an intracranial tumor, abscess, or hematoma. Commonly, this headache occurs in the early morning, often awakening the patient. Presumably, this timing reflects decreased alveolar ventilation during physiologic sleep, leading to an increase in the $PaCO_2$ and a corresponding increase in CBF. Spontaneous vomiting may accompany the headache. Headache may also be provoked by coughing, which leads to increased ICP by impeding venous outflow from the brain.

Benign Intracranial Hypertension

Benign intracranial hypertension (pseudotumor cerebri) is defined as a syndrome characterized by (1) increased ICP above 20 mmHg, (2) normal composition of CSF, (3) normal level of consciousness, and (4) absence of a focal intracranial lesion.[160] Computed tomography indicates a normal or even small ventricular system. Headache and bilateral visual disturbances typically occur in an obese female with menstrual irregularities. Symptoms of benign intracranial hypertension may be exaggerated during pregnancy. This syndrome may also occur after withdrawal of corticosteroids or after initiation of therapy for hypothyroidism. In most patients, no identifiable cause of the increased ICP is found. The condition is self-limited, and the prognosis is excellent.

Treatment

Treatment of benign intracranial hypertension includes lumbar puncture to remove 20 to 40 ml of CSF, administration of acetazolamide to decrease formation of CSF, and dexamethasone to decrease cerebral edema. The principal indication for treatment is loss of visual acuity. Initial treatment is often repeated lumbar puncture to remove CSF with a large needle, which also facilitates measurement of CSF pressure (ICP). Furthermore, continued leakage of CSF through the dural puncture site may be therapeutic. Lumbar puncture would not be safe in a patient with increased ICP secondary to a space-occupying lesion. In such a patient, lumbar puncture could lead to herniation of the cerebellar tonsils and pressure on the medulla oblongata. In the patient with benign intracranial hypertension, the presence of uniform swelling of the brain plus the normal position of the cerebellar tonsils prevents herniation and compression of the brain stem. Chronic administration of acetazolamide can result in acidemia, presumably reflecting inhibition of hydrogen ion secretion by renal tubules. Surgical therapy, most often a lumboperitoneal shunt, is indicated only after medical therapy has failed and vision shows deterioration.

Management of Anesthesia

Management of anesthesia in the patient with benign intracranial hypertension who is undergoing a lumboperitoneal shunt incorporates the same principles outlined for removal of an intracranial tumor. In the parturient, spinal anesthesia may be beneficial, since continued leakage of CSF is welcomed.[160] When a lumboperitoneal shunt is present, a skull radiograph is helpful to localize the area of entry into the subarachnoid space before performance of a lumbar puncture. Furthermore, there is a theoretical possibility that an injection of a local anesthetic into the subarachnoid space could escape into the peritoneal cavity, resulting in inadequate anesthesia. Therefore, general anesthesia may be a more logical choice in the presence of a lumboperitoneal shunt.

HERNIATION OF AN INTERVERTEBRAL DISC

The intervertebral disc is composed of a compressible nucleus pulposus surrounded by a fibrocartilaginous anulus fibrosis. The disc acts as a shock absorber between vertebral bodies. Trauma or degenerative changes lead to changes in the intervertebral disc. Nerve root compression results when the nucleus pulposus protrudes through the posterolateral aspect of the annulus fibrosis. Occasionally, central protrusion of the disc may occur. If protrusion is into the cervical or thoracic region, there will be signs of spinal cord compression; signs of cauda equina compression occur if protrusion is into the lumbar region. Low back pain ranks second only to upper respiratory tract disease as a reason for office visits to physicians.[161] An estimated 70% of adults experience low back pain at some time. Among chronic conditions, low back pain is the most common cause of limitation of activity in patients younger than 45 years of age. Cancer (primary or metastatic) is the most common systemic disease affecting the spine, although it accounts for less than 1% of all episodes of low back pain.

Cervical Disc Disease

Lateral protrusion of a cervical disc usually occurs at the C5-C6 or C6-C7 intervertebral space. Protrusion can be secondary to trauma or occur spontaneously. Pain starting in the neck that radiates to the shoulder and down the outer aspect of the arm into the thumb is characteristic of a C5-C6 disc protrusion. The biceps reflex is reduced, and the biceps muscle is weak. Pain in the scapula, triceps region, and the middle and index fingers reflects protrusion at the C6-C7 intervertebral space. Symptoms are commonly aggravated by coughing. The same symptoms can be due to osteophytes that compress nerve roots in the intervertebral foramina. Initial treatment of cervical disc protrusion is with traction. Surgical decompression is necessary if symptoms do not abate with conservative treatment.

Cervical Spondylosis

Cervical spondylosis is a common disorder that leads to osteophyte formation and degenerative disc disease. There is narrowing of the spinal canal and compression of the spinal cord by transverse osteophytes, in addition to nerve root compression by bony spurs in the intervertebral foramina. Spinal cord dysfunction may also reflect ischemic infarction secondary to bony compression of the spinal arteries. Symptoms typically develop insidiously after 50 years of age. Neck pain and radicular pain in the arm and shoulders are accompanied by sensory loss and skeletal muscle wasting. Later sensory and motor signs appear in the legs, producing an unsteady gait. Sphincter disturbances are uncommon. A radiograph of the spine often demonstrates osteoarthritic changes, but these changes correlate poorly with neurologic symptoms. Surgery may be necessary to arrest progression of the symptoms.

Lumbar Disc Disease

The most common site for lumbar disc protrusion is the L4-L5 and L5-S1 intervertebral space. Both sites produce low back pain, which radiates down the posterior and lateral aspects of the thigh and calf (sciatica). Sensory loss and skeletal muscle weakness correspond to compression of the L5 or S1 nerve root. A history of trauma is usually associated with sudden back pain that signals protrusion. This trauma may be trivial in nature, however. Pain is aggravated by coughing or stretching of the sciatic nerve, as produced by straight-leg raising. These mechanical signs help distinguish protrusion from peripheral nerve disorders, as may accompany diabetes mellitus, which are not accompanied by such signs. The finding of a herniated disc in an asymptomatic patient indicates that the results of imaging studies (computed tomography, magnetic resonance imaging) might be misleading. In such cases, valid decision making requires correlation with the history and physical examination.[161,162]

Initial treatment of lumbar disc protrusion consists of absolute bed rest and the use of centrally acting muscle relaxants such as diazepam. In the patient without neuromotor deficits, the clinical outcome is similar, with 2 days of bed rest, as compared with longer periods.[163] When neurologic symptoms do not abate with bed rest, surgery (laminectomy or microdisectomy) should be considered. An alternative to surgery may be the placement of a corticosteroid in the epidural space.[164] Corticosteroids may reduce the inflammation and edema produced by compression of the nerve roots. Although not documented in human studies, the placement of a large dose of

triamcinolone into the epidural spaces of dogs has demonstrated evidence of reduced responsiveness of the pituitary-adrenal axis for up to 4 weeks.[165]

SLEEP DISORDERS

It is estimated that one in four adults in the United States suffers from insomnia or the belief they obtain too little sleep. Excessive sleepiness is a less frequent complaint; most of these patients have narcolepsy. Sleep apnea is a rare form of sleep disorder. Even less frequent are Kleine-Levin syndrome (hypersomnia with excessive eating) and pickwickian syndrome (hypersomnia, hypoventilation, and obesity).

Insomnia

Insomnia is the most common sleep disorder, being more prevalent in females and the elderly.[166,167] About 10% to 15% of patients with chronic insomnia have an underlying problem of substance abuse, especially alcohol. Common causes of transient insomnia include grief, hospitalization, and pain. Pharmacologically induced insomnia may be due to stimulants such as caffeine or nicotine. Air travel across time zones (jet lag) is often associated with insomnia. The most common sleep-related forms of neuromuscular dysfunction affecting the elderly include restless leg syndrome (strong urge to move legs interferes with going to sleep) and nocturnal myoclonus (periodic leg movements during sleep cause repeated awakening).[167]

Sleeping pills do not cure insomnia, but they may provide symptomatic relief. Benzodiazepines, because of their efficacy and safety (death from overdose is unlikely and addiction potential is low), are the drugs of choice for the treatment of insomnia. An estimated 0.3% of the adult population have taken drugs to produce sleep on a nightly basis for a year.[166] A long-acting benzodiazepine such as flurazepam is more likely to produce a sedative effect the next day, whereas a short-acting drug such as triazolam may be associated with rebound insomnia and anterograde amnesia. Antidepressant drugs with sedative effects (amitriptyline, doxepine, trazodone) may be administered in a low dose at bedtime for treatment of insomnia.

Narcolepsy

Narcolepsy is a distinct neurologic disorder characterized by an uncontrollable urge to sleep and by abnormalities of rapid eye movement sleep.[168] Abnormalities of monoaminergic and cholinergic functioning in the brain are likely to be present. Cataplexy, the sudden loss of postural tone leading to collapse, can accompany narcolepsy. Methylphenidate and dextroamphetamine are used as stimulants to prevent narcolepsy, whereas a tricyclic antidepressant is considered the primary treatment for cataplexy.

Sleep Apnea Syndrome

Sleep apnea syndrome (cessation of airflow at the mouth for longer than 10 seconds) can reflect (1) loss of central nervous system drive to maintain ventilation, (2) mechanical upper airway obstruction, or (3) combinations of both.[169,170] Absence of neural drive to ventilation when voluntary control of breathing is diminished by sleep (central alveolar hypoventilation syndrome, Ondine's curse) is characterized by cessation of breathing movements and airflow, most likely reflecting a defect in the function of the medullary ventilatory center. Conversely, obstructive sleep apnea is due to an abnormal relaxation of the genioglossus muscle that normally pulls the tongue forward and relaxation of the pharyngeal muscles. This change may reflect decreased neural input to these muscles from the brain stem. Normally, subatmospheric pressure in the airway generated by contraction of the diaphragm is opposed by contraction of the pharyngeal muscles. Obstructive sleep apnea occurs when the balance between these two forces is disturbed.

Signs and Symptoms

Signs and symptoms of sleep apnea syndrome reflect the chronic effects of intermittent apnea in these patients (Table 17-10). Breathing effort is persistent, but the movement of air is absent, owing to upper airway obstruction. Intense snoring accompanies obstructive sleep apnea. The prevalence of multiple apneic episodes increases with age and may be exacerbated by the use of depressant drugs such as alcohol.[167] Multiple episodes of arterial hypoxemia (blood oxygen saturation less than 80%), hypercarbia, repeated awakening from sleep, morning headaches, and daytime sedation are present. Repeated bouts of acidosis and hypoxemia are presumed responsible for the cardiac dysrhythmias, pulmonary hypertension, and cor pulmonale that may occur in these patients. A subset of patients with sleep apnea syndrome who are morbidly obese

Table 17-10. Signs and Symptoms of Sleep Apnea Syndrome

Signs	Symptoms
Obesity	Insomnia
Hypertension	Intense snoring
Hypoxemia	Thrashing during sleep
Hypercarbia	Morning headache
Polycythemia	Daytime somnolence
Cor pulmonale	Intellectual deterioration

and hypersomnolent and who experience cor pulmonale are designated as having pickwickian syndrome.

Treatment

Treatment of obstructive sleep apnea may include correction of nasal problems associated with increased nasal airway resistance (septal deviation, nasal polyps, adenoid hypertrophy). In overweight patients, weight loss is associated with improved status, presumably reflecting increased airway size with the disappearance of excess fat deposits from the base of the tongue and along the walls of the hypopharynx. The avoidance of alcohol and of sedatives before sleep is intended to increase upper airway muscle tone during sleep. Continuous positive nasal airway pressure (5 to 20 cm H_2O) delivered to the upper airway by a tight-fitting mask designed to fit over the nose acts to provide an artificial splint to the upper airway. The traditional surgical treatment of obstructive sleep apnea is tracheostomy, designed to bypass the obstruction. Alternatively, uvulopalatopharyngoplasty, designed to widen the posterior pharynx by excision of the uvula and redundant oropharyngeal tissues, may be effective in relieving obstructive symptoms that accompany sleep. Treatment of central alveolar hypoventilation may include a respiratory stimulant, such as acetazolamide, and electrophrenic pacing. Phrenic nerve damage is a significant complication of electrophrenic pacing.

Management of Anesthesia

Management of anesthesia in the patient with a history of sleep apnea syndrome must consider the likely exquisite sensitivity to drugs that depress ventilation.[171] Furthermore, since anesthetics may depress upper airway muscle activity, special attention to the possibility of airway obstruction with induction of anesthesia in the patient with a history of obstructive sleep apnea is important, whereas the history of central alveolar hypoventilation may increase the likelihood of unexpected postoperative apnea.[169] In this regard, prolonged mechanical support of ventilation may be required, especially in the patient with central alveolar hypoventilation syndrome. Postoperative pain relief poses an additional risk, and neuraxial opioids have been recommended to minimize the systemic effects of these drugs on ventilation.[171,172] Emergence from anesthesia after a uvulopalatopharyngoplasty may be associated with upper airway obstruction, emphasizing the need to delay tracheal extubation until full return of consciousness is evident.[173]

ABNORMAL PATTERNS OF VENTILATION

Irregular breathing patterns may reflect an abnormality of an specific site in the central nervous system (Table 17-11). Ataxic (Biot's) breathing is characterized by a completely ran-

Table 17-11. Abnormal Patterns of Ventilation

	Pattern	Site of Lesion
Ataxic (Biot's breathing)	Unpredictable sequence of breaths varying in rate and tidal volume	Medulla
Apneustic breathing	Repetitive gasps with prolonged pauses at full inspiration	Pons
Cheyne-Stokes breathing	Cyclic crescendo-decrescendo tidal volume pattern interrupted by apnea	Cerebral hemispheres Congestive heart failure
Central neurogenic hyperventilation	Hypocarbia	Cerebral thrombosis or embolism
Posthyperventilation apnea	Awake apnea following moderate decreases in the $PaCO_2$	Frontal lobes

dom pattern of tidal volumes that results from disruption of medullary neural pathways by trauma, hemorrhage, or extrinsic compression. Mechanical ventilation of the lungs may be necessary if apnea is a problem. Apnea may occur in response to sedatives or opioids. A lesion in the pons may result in apneustic breathing characterized by a prolonged end-inspiratory pause maintained for as long as 30 seconds. Occlusion of the basilar artery leading to pontine infarction is a common cause of apneustic breathing. Cheyne-Stokes breathing is characterized by breaths of progressively increasing, and then decreasing, volume (crescendo-decrescendo pattern), followed by periods of apnea lasting 15 to 20 seconds. Arterial blood gases typically also fluctuate in a cyclic pattern. This pattern of breathing may reflect brain damage (cerebral hemispheres or basal ganglia) due to arterial hypoxemia or may accompany congestive heart failure. In the presence of congestive heart failure, the delay in circulation time from the pulmonary capillaries to the carotid bodies is presumed responsible for Cheyne-Stokes breathing. Central neurogenic hyperventilation is most often due to an acute neurologic insult as associated with a cerebral thrombosis or cerebral embolism. Hyperventilation is spontaneous and may be so severe that the $PaCO_2$ is decreased to less than 20 mmHg. Posthyperventilation apnea occurs in the patient with frontal lobe disease after a sequence of five deep breaths that lower the $PaCO_2$ by about 10 mmHg. Breathing in such cases resumes when apnea is of sufficient duration to return the $PaCO_2$ to the level present before hyperventilation. In a normal patient, the same sequence of voluntary deep breaths does not produce apnea despite a similar decrease in $PaCO_2$, reflecting the presence of a voluntary drive to breathe.

ACUTE MOUNTAIN SICKNESS

Acute mountain sickness is characterized by headache, fatigue, and anorexia, most likely due to cerebral edema that accompanies rapid ascent to altitude. Symptoms are rare below 2440 m and common above 3660 m. The onset of acute mountain sickness may not occur until 8 to 24 hours after ascent; symptoms usually subside within 2 to 4 days. Severe cases of cerebral edema may be accompanied by ataxia, obtundation, and coma. Computed tomography of the brain indicates cerebral edema. Cerebral edema is probably caused by increased CBF (vasogenic edema), as well as cellular swelling related to hypoxia (cytotoxic edema). Prompt descent and oxygen therapy are the principal treatment. Dexamethasone and acetazolamide may be recommended. Furosemide is avoided, since diuresis may result in orthostatic hypotension.

EPISTAXIS

The arteries that supply the nasal chamber and that give rise to epistaxis are the terminal branches of the internal carotid artery (ethmoidal arteries) and external carotid artery (sphenopalatine artery). Epistaxis originating from the anterior nasal chamber (most often from a blood vessel in the mucous membrane of the nasal septum) often stops spontaneously or as the result of conservative measures, such as external application of pressure or cold. Spontaneous bleeding from the posterior aspects of the nasal chamber is likely to be arterial and associated with hypertension. In some instances, blood loss may be extensive, with accompanying hypotension. Treatment of posterior nasal hemorrhage usually requires sedation and placement of a postnasal pack. In an emergency, a Foley catheter serves as an effective postnasal pack. The tip of this catheter should be covered with antibiotic ointment before being inserted into the nostril; the balloon is filled with saline, rather than air, to prevent loss of pressure and gradual collapse.

Any posterior pack that effectively blocks the postnasal space will also block normal pathways for drainage of secretions, predisposing the patient to acute sinusitis. Obstruction of the eustachian tube orifice may result in acute otitis media. For these reasons, systemic antibiotics are routinely administered to these patients. Obstruction of the nasal airway may also result in arterial hypoxemia, particularly in an elderly debilitated patient.

Surgical ligation of a bleeding site, especially from the ethmoidal area, may be required when packing fails to control epistaxis. Angiography is occasionally used to delineate hemorrhage from the ethmoidal or sphenopalatine arteries. The anterior ethmoidal artery is ligated through an incision along the side of the nose. The sphenopalatine artery is approached surgically by opening the maxillary sinus and ligating the artery in the pterygopalatine fissure.

ENDOLYMPHATIC HYDROPS

Endolympathic hydrops (Menière's disease) is a disorder of the membranous labyrinth of the inner ear, characterized by the triad of hearing loss, tinnitus, and vertigo. This disease occurs most commonly between 30 and 60 years of age; in most patients, the etiology is unknown. Endolymphatic hydrops should be distinguished from other causes of vertigo, which include acoustic neuroma, vestibular neuronitis, hypoglycemia, and hypothyroidism. The pathognomonic feature of endolymphatic hydrops is distension of the endolymphatic system of the inner ear. Treatment of Menière's disease is surgical, if bed rest and sedation with benzodiazepines are not

effective. Surgical therapy is a labyrinthectomy or transection of the vestibular nerve, requiring a craniotomy.

MIDDLE EAR COMPLICATIONS RELATED TO THE USE OF NITROUS OXIDE

The middle ear is an air-filled cavity bounded by the tympanic membrane and the inner ear (Fig. 17-25). During the administration of nitrous oxide, middle ear pressure may increase. This increase reflects the passage of nitrous oxide into the noncompliant confines of the middle ear. Under normal conditions, this pressure buildup in the middle ear is passively vented through the eustachian tubes into the nasopharynx. Narrowing of the eustachian tubes by acute inflammation or the presence of scar tissue, as is likely after an adenoidectomy, impairs the ability of the middle ear to vent passively any pressure increase produced by nitrous oxide. Excessive middle ear pressure could jeopardize the integrity of the tympanic membrane. The presence of bright red blood in the external auditory canal, as evidence of membrane rupture, has been described during the administration of nitrous oxide, even in the absence of middle ear disease.[174,175] Disruption of previous middle ear reconstructive surgery has also been observed when nitrous oxide is administered at a later date for operative procedures not involving the ear.[176] A manifestation of this disruption is recurrence of hearing loss in the previ-

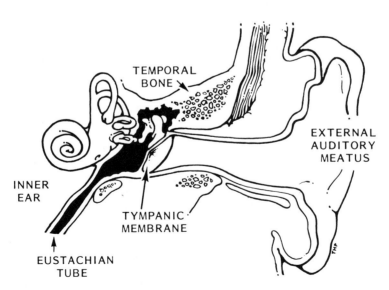

Fig. 17-25. The middle ear is an air-filled cavity bounded by the tympanic membrane and inner ear. Diffusion of nitrous oxide into this cavity can increase the middle ear pressure, particularly when passive venting of the pressure into the nasopharynx is impaired because of obstruction of the eustachian tube.

ously diseased ear, on awakening from anesthesia. Administration of nitrous oxide during tympanoplasty may result in displacement of a freshly placed graft, reflecting the presence of air bubbles containing nitrous oxide in the middle ear. Postoperative nausea and vomiting could also be due to increased middle ear pressure that persists after administration of nitrous oxide.

Absorption of nitrous oxide after discontinuation of the administration of this drug can also exert deleterious effects on the middle ear. For example, rapid resorption of nitrous oxide can result in negative pressure in the middle ear, causing rupture of the tympanic membrane. Transient hearing impairment after administration of nitrous oxide to a previously normal patient most likely reflects negative pressure in the middle ear.[177] Serous otitis can also be a manifestation of this negative pressure.

Potential adverse effects of nitrous oxide on the middle ear raise questions as to the wisdom of administering this drug to a patient with narrowing of the eustachian tubes due to acute inflammation or scarring. Likewise, a preoperative history of previous middle ear surgery introduces concern. Nevertheless, it is undeniable that many patients with a history of middle ear surgery have received nitrous oxide on subsequent occasions, without detectable detrimental effects on hearing.

GLAUCOMA

Glaucoma is characterized by increased intraocular pressure. Left untreated, blindness results, due to interference with blood flow to the retina and compression of the optic disc. Increased intraocular pressure is caused by obstruction to the outflow of aqueous humor from the anterior chamber of the eye into the venous circulation. Normal intraocular pressure is 10 to 20 mmHg; a value of greater than 25 mmHg is considered pathologic.

There are two types of glaucoma: open-angle and angle-closure. Open-angle glaucoma is the most common form, manifesting as a slowly progressive bilateral disorder. An estimated 12% to 30% of blindness in the United States is due to open-angle glaucoma. Angle-closure glaucoma is less frequent but can be precipitated acutely by mydriasis in a susceptible person.

Treatment

Treatment of glaucoma consists of the use of drugs designed to lower intraocular pressure by decreasing the resistance to outflow of aqueous humor or by reducing the rate of formation of aqueous humor. Miosis decreases resistance by contracting the ciliary muscle, which stretches the trabecular meshwork in the anterior chamber of the eye. Open-angle glaucoma can often be controlled with medical management; angle-closure glaucoma will ultimately require surgery.

Parasympathomimetics

Pilocarpine is a short-acting parasympathomimetic drug that produces miosis. Topical administration of this drug three to four times a day often provides adequate control of intraocular pressure. Carbachol is a parasympathomimetic drug that can be substituted, if intolerance to pilocarpine develops or if a slightly stronger or longer-acting drug is needed. Echothiophate is a long-acting parasympathomimetic miotic drug. An adverse effect of this drug is inhibition of plasma cholinesterase activity, which persists for about 4 weeks after echothiophate eyedrops are discontinued. A potential undesirable effect produced by the chronic use of topical miotic drugs is the formation of cataracts.

Epinephrine

Topical administration of epinephrine reduces intraocular pressure by decreasing the resistance of outflow of aqueous humor from the anterior chamber of the eye into the venous circulation. In addition, epinephrine is likely to reduce the formation of aqueous humor. Epinephrine is variably effective and can produce systemic sympathomimetic symptoms. Furthermore, the use of topical epinephrine is associated with local allergic reactions in about 20% of patients.

Carbon Anhydrase Inhibitors

Oral administration of carbonic anhydrase inhibitors, such as acetazolamide, lowers intraocular pressure, presumably by decreasing the formation of aqueous humor.

Beta Antagonist Drugs

Oral or topical administration of beta antagonist drugs lowers intraocular pressure. The topical route is preferred because of a lower incidence of systemic side effects. The ability of these drugs to lower intraocular pressure seems to involve a decrease in the formation of aqueous humor, rather than an increase in outflow.

Propranolol lowers intraocular pressure, but its local anesthetic effect, when applied topically, is undesirable. Timolol is a long-acting, nonselective, beta-adrenergic antagonist drug, without significant local anesthetic effects when applied topically to the cornea. After topical application of a single dose of timolol (1 drop of a 0.25% solution), intraocular pressure begins to decrease within 20 minutes, with the effect persisting even after 24 hours.[178] Timolol does not alter the diameter of the pupil or its reactivity to light. Timolol is absorbed into the systemic circulation after topical application, producing side effects related to blockade of cardiac and noncardiac beta receptors. Indeed, bradycardia and hypotension, which are refractory to atropine treatment, have been observed during anesthesia in patients being treated with topical timolol.[179] In addition, systemic absorption of timolol can result in the appearance of bronchospasm. Lethargy and fatigue are central nervous system effects of topical timolol and other beta antagonist drugs.

Management of Anesthesia

Management of anesthesia for the patient with glaucoma includes maintenance of miosis by the continuation of parasympathomimetic therapy throughout the perioperative period. For example, the topical application of pilocarpine would be appropriate on the morning of surgery. This practice decreases the likelihood of an attack of acute angle-closure glaucoma.

The inclusion of an anticholinergic drug in the preoperative medication is acceptable, since the amount of drug reaching the eye is too little to dilate the pupil.[180] Furthermore, the use of an anticholinergic drug in combination with an anticholinesterase drug to reverse a nondepolarizing muscle relaxant is acceptable. For example, it is estimated that the administration of atropine (2 mg IV) will result in the delivery of only 0.004 mg to the eye. Despite these assurances, it would seem reasonable to limit use of an anticholinergic drug in patients with glaucoma. Indeed, scopolamine (0.4 mg IM) produces a significant increase in the diameter of the pupils in healthy subjects and, therefore, may not be an appropriate drug to administer to patients with glaucoma.[181] By contrast, the same dose of atropine does not alter the size of the pupils. Although not evaluated, glycopyrrolate, administered systemically, would predictably also have minimal effects on the diameter of the pupils. Administration of an anticholinergic drug in combination with drugs that produce miosis (opioids, anticholinesterases) may prevent dilating effects on the pupils normally produced by the anticholinergic drug.

Another important goal during the administration of anesthesia to the patient with glaucoma is prevention of an increase in intraocular pressure. Succinylcholine-induced increases in intraocular pressure are maximal 2 to 4 minutes after administration of the muscle relaxant, returning to baseline values after about 6 minutes.[180] These increases in intraocular pressure are not reliably obscured by any method, including prevention of skeletal muscle fasciculations by prior administration of a nondepolarizing muscle relaxant.[182] The implications of this drug-induced increase in intraocular pressure in a patient with glaucoma are unknown. Presumably, a patient with adequate medical control of glaucoma would not be jeopardized by a transient elevation of intraocular pressure produced by succinylcholine. Other events that increase intraocular pressure are hypercarbia and increased central venous pressure. The effect of ketamine on intraocular pressure is unclear, as reports are contradictory.[183] Intraocular pressure is lowered

by hypocarbia and decreased central venous pressure, as produced by drug-induced osmotic diuresis, opioids, and volatile anesthetic drugs. The fluctuations in arterial pressure and skeletal muscle paralysis produced by a nondepolarizing muscle relaxant exert only minor influences on intraocular pressure, although pancuronium may produce a decrease in this pressure.[182]

Interactions of drugs administered during anesthesia with those used to treat glaucoma must be considered. The rare patient being treated with echothiophate is at risk of prolonged paralysis after administration of succinylcholine. If succinylcholine is administered, the initial dose should be reduced to 0.1 mg·kg^{-1} IV; the responses should be observed, using a peripheral nerve stimulator. Bradycardia and exaggerated hypotension have been attributed to beta blockade produced by chronic topical administration of timolol.[179]

Postoperatively, the patient with glaucoma should be observed for dilated pupils that are irregular and asymmetric—signaling an acute attack of angle-closure glaucoma. The patient with such an attack is also likely to complain of pain in and around the eye, as well as a loss of vision. By contrast, the patient with a corneal abrasion will complain of pain only in the eye.

CATARACT EXTRACTION

Cataract extraction may be performed using a retrobulbar block or under general anesthesia. A risk of retrobulbar block is the passage of local anesthetic along the optic nerve sheath into the subarachnoid space, leading to apnea. In this regard, increased resistance encountered during injection of local anesthetic in performance of a retrobulbar block may reflect incorrect position of the needle in the optic nerve sheath, rather than proper placement in the retrobulbar adipose tissue.[184]

The patient who requires general anesthesia for cataract extraction is likely to be elderly, with one or more co-existing medical diseases. General anesthesia must ensure immobility of the patient, as sudden movement or an attempt to cough when the eye is open could result in extrusion of vitreous and permanent ocular damage. An adequate depth of anesthesia, with or without skeletal muscle paralysis, is essential. Although succinylcholine increases intraocular pressure, this elevation is transient. Nevertheless, the use of an intermediate- or short-acting nondepolarizing muscle relaxant may serve as a useful alternative. Modest hyperventilation of the lungs to produce hypocarbia and a 10- to 15-degree head-up tilt to promote venous drainage will likely decrease intraocular pressure during intraocular surgery. It is important to minimize the possibility of stimulation due to the endotracheal tube at the conclusion of surgery. In this regard, tracheal extubation may be considered before airway depression from the anesthetic drug was waned. If the tube is left in the trachea as the patient awakens, it may be helpful to administer lidocaine (0.5 to 1.5 mg·kg^{-1} IV), in an attempt to attenuate the tracheal reflex response to the presence of the tube.

It is helpful to minimize the incidence of vomiting during the postoperative period. In this regard, the use of an opioid in the preanesthetic medication is often avoided. Routine aspiration of the stomach with an orally inserted tube at the conclusion of general anesthesia serves not only to remove gastric fluid, but also to decrease gastric distension that could contribute to postoperative nausea and vomiting. A number of antiemetic drugs have been recommended, with questionable efficacy. In a well-controlled study, however, administration of droperidol (1.25 mg IV), 5 minutes before the conclusion of general anesthesia, was effective in reducing the incidence of postoperative emesis.[185]

OCULAR TRAUMA

Ocular trauma characterized by a penetrating eye injury requires prompt surgical treatment, if the eye is to be salvaged. Management of anesthesia is often complicated by the recent ingestion of food by the patient. Therefore, protection of the airway must be balanced against the hazard of producing an increase in intraocular pressure and the potential extrusion of intraocular contents. The obvious controversy relates to the use of succinylcholine to facilitate intubation of the trachea. The rapid onset of skeletal muscle paralysis provided by this drug is useful for prompt placement of a cuffed tube in the trachea. Against the selection of succinylcholine is the predictable increase in intraocular pressure, even when fasciculations are prevented. Despite the controversy associated with the use of succinylcholine, no published case reports describe a loss of intraocular contents attributable to this drug. An alternative to succinylcholine is the administration of large doses (0.15 mg·kg^{-1}) of pancuronium, which is alleged to produce rapid onset of skeletal muscle paralysis without the hazard of increased intraocular pressure.[186] The disadvantage of using pancuronium is a prolonged duration of action for what may be a short operation. In this regard, a large dose (two to three times ED$_{95}$) of an intermediate- or short-acting muscle relaxant may be a useful alternative. Regardless of the muscle relaxant selection, it is mandatory to confirm the presence of skeletal muscle paralysis with the use of a peripheral nerve stimulator, before initiating direct laryngoscopy for intubation of the trachea. Premature placement of the tube in the trachea will provoke movement of the patient and defeat all attempts designed to minimize an increase in intraocular pressure. Maintenance of anesthesia is acceptably accomplished with inhaled or injected drugs. Timing of the removal of the cuffed tube from the trachea at the end of surgery is influenced by the likely presence or absence of gastric contents.

GLOMUS JUGULARE TUMORS

Glomus jugulare tumors (chemodectomas) arise from the glomus body at the dome of the jugular bulb.[187] These tumors are typically slow growing and benign, although they have a propensity for local invasion.

Signs and Symptoms

Symptoms produced by a glomus jugulare tumor are related to its vascularity, principally from the external carotid artery and its invasion of surrounding structures. Because of its vascularity, a bruit may be heard over these tumors. Unilateral pulsatile tinnitus is often the patient's initial complaint. Hearing loss results, as tumor extension limits the mobility of the eardrum or ossicles. Cranial nerve involvement may be manifested as dysphagia, recurrent aspiration, upper airway obstruction, and difficulty handling secretions. Invasion of the posterior fossa may obstruct the aqueduct of Sylvius, causing hydrocephalus. It is common for a glomus jugulare tumor to invade the internal jugular vein; finger-like projections may extend to the right atrium. A mass in the neck occurs when the glomus jugulare tumor extends inferiorly and laterally. Occasionally, the glomus jugulare tumor secretes norepinephrine, producing symptoms that mimic pheochromocytoma.

Treatment

Surgical excision, often preceded by radiotherapy or embolization to diminish vascularity, is the treatment for a glomus jugulare tumor. Preoperative evaluation may include arteriography to evaluate the location and blood supply to the tumor, venography to detect extension into the internal jugular vein, and computed tomography for evidence of intracranial extension. Examination of cranial nerve function is important to evaluate the risk of aspiration. Evidence of increased ICP is sought when obstructive hydrocephalus is suspected.

Management of Anesthesia

Management of anesthesia is influenced by the potential for massive and rapid blood loss and likely prolonged (often 8 hours or more) operative time. Invasive arterial and venous pressure monitoring is indicated; urine output is followed after placement of a Foley catheter. An internal jugular vein involved by tumor should not be cannulated for placement of a right atrial or pulmonary artery catheter. Hypothermia is likely, especially with prolonged surgery, emphasizing the usefulness of warming inhaled gases and infused fluids. Drugs and techniques designed to control ICP may be necessary. Controlled hypotension minimizes blood loss and may facilitate surgical excision of the tumor. Venous air embolism is a hazard, particularly if the internal jugular vein is opened for removal of tumor. It is also a hazard if excision of tumor that has invaded temporal bone results in the exposure of veins, which cannot collapse because of bony attachments. As a precaution, mechanical ventilation of the lungs may be useful; the addition of skeletal muscle paralysis minimizes the possibility of a gasp reflex. Appropriate monitors for detection of venous air embolism are indicated when venous air embolism is considered a hazard (see the section, Venous Air Embolism). Sudden unexplained cardiovascular collapse and death during resection of these tumors may reflect the presence of venous air embolism or tumor emboli. If the surgeon finds it necessary to identify the facial nerve, avoidance of profound skeletal muscle paralysis or temporary pharmacologically induced antagonism of the neuromuscular blockade may be required. The choice of anesthetic drugs is not uniquely influenced by the presence of a glomus jugulare tumor, although the potential adverse effects of nitrous oxide should be recognized if venous air embolism occurs.

CAROTID SINUS SYNDROME

Carotid sinus syndrome is an uncommon entity caused by exaggeration of normal activity of the baroreceptors in response to mechanical stimulation. For example, stimulation of the carotid sinus by external massage, which in normal patients produces slight decreases in heart rate and blood pressure, can produce syncope in affected patients. There is a high incidence of associated vascular disease in these patients. Indeed, carotid sinus syndrome is a known complication of carotid endarterectomy.

Two distinct types of cardiovascular response may be noted with carotid sinus hypersensitivity. In about 80% of affected patients, a cardioinhibitory reflex is mediated by the vagus nerve, resulting in profound bradycardia. In about 10% of patients, a vasodepressor reflex is mediated by inhibition of sympathetic nervous system vasomotor tone, with resultant decreases in systemic vascular resistance and profound hypotension. The remaining 10% of patients exhibit components of both reflexes.

Treatment of carotid sinus syndrome may consist of administration of drugs, placement of a permanent demand artificial cardiac pacemaker, or ablation of the carotid sinus. Use of anticholinergic drugs and vasopressors is limited by side effects and is rarely effective in patients with vasodepressor or mixed forms of carotid sinus hypersensitivity. Since most patients have the cardioinhibitory type of carotid sinus syndrome, implantation of an artificial cardiac pacemaker is the usual initial treatment. In patients in whom the vasodepressor reflex response is refractory to cardiac pacing, ablation of the carotid sinus may be attempted. Glossopharyngeal nerve block may be an alternative therapy in patients who are refractory to artificial cardiac pacing or drug therapy.[188]

Management of anesthesia is often complicated by hypotension, bradycardia, and cardiac dysrhythmias.[188] Infiltration of lidocaine around the carotid sinus before dissection usually improves hemodynamic stability but may also interfere with determination of the completeness of surgical denervation. Such drugs as atropine, isoproterenol, and epinephrine should be readily available.

NEUROFIBROMATOSIS

Neurofibromatosis is due to an autosomal dominant mutation that is not limited to racial or ethnic origin. Both sexes are affected with equal frequency and severity. Expressivity is variable, but penetrance of the trait is virtually 100%. Manifestations are classified as classic (von Recklinghausen's disease), acoustic, and segmental neurofibromatosis. It is estimated that neurofibromatosis affects 80,000 people in the United States.

Signs and Symptoms

The diversity of clinical features of neurofibromatosis emphasizes the protean nature of this disease (Table 17-12). One feature common to all patients, however, is progression of the disease with time.

Café-au-lait spots are present in more than 99% of patients with neurofibromatosis. Six or more spots larger than 1.5 cm in diameter are considered diagnostic. Café-au-lait spots are usually present at birth and continue to increase in number and size during the first decade of life. Café-au-lait spots vary in size from 1 mm to more than 15 cm. The distribution of spots is random, except for disproportionately small numbers on the face. Other than an adverse cosmetic effect, café-au-lait spots pose no threat to health.

Table 17-12. Manifestations of Neurofibromatosis

Café au lait spots	Kyphoscoliosis
Neurofibromas	Short stature
Cutaneous	Cancer
Neural	Endocrine dysfunction
Vascular	Learning disability
Intracranial tumor	Seizures
Spinal cord tumor	Congenital heart
Pseudarthrosis	disease
	Pulmonic stenosis

Neurofibromas virtually always involve the skin, but they can also occur in the deeper peripheral nerves and nerve roots and in or on viscera or blood vessels innervated by the autonomic nervous system. They may be nodular and discrete or diffuse, with extensive interdigitation with surrounding tissue. Although neurofibromas are histologically benign, functional compromise and cosmetic disfigurement may result. Compromise of the airway may occur when neurofibromas develop in the laryngeal, cervical, or mediastinal regions. Neurofibromas may be highly vascular. Pregnancy or puberty can lead to increases in the number and size of neurofibromas.

Intracranial tumors occur in 5% to 10% of patients with neurofibromatosis, accounting for a major portion of the morbidity and mortality associated with this disease. Computed tomography to rule out the presence of an intracranial tumor is indicated when the diagnosis of neurofibromatosis is considered. The bilateral presence of an acoustic neuroma in a patient with café-au-lait spots establishes the diagnosis of acoustic neurofibromatosis.

Congenital pseudarthrosis is commonly due to neurofibromatosis. The tibia is involved most often; the radius is the second most frequent site. Ordinarily, only a single site is involved in any one patient. The severity of pseudoarthrosis ranges from an asymptomatic radiologic presentation to the need for amputation. Kyphoscoliosis occurs in about 2% of patients afflicted with neurofibromatosis. The cervical and thoracic vertebrae are most frequently involved. Paravertebral neurofibromas are often present, but their role, if any, in the development of kyphoscoliosis is not defined. Left untreated, this manifestation progresses, leading to cardiorespiratory and neurologic compromise. Short stature is a recognized feature of neurofibromatosis.

There is an increased incidence of cancer in patients with neurofibromatosis. Clearly associated cancers include neurofibrosarcomas, malignant schwannomas, Wilms tumor, rhabdomyosarcoma, and leukemia. Other cancers, including neuroblastomas, medullary thyroid carcinomas, and pancreatic adenocarcinoma, are less clearly associated with neurofibromatosis.

It is a misconception that neurofibromatosis entails diffuse endocrine dysfunction. Associated endocrine disorders, however, include pheochromocytoma, disturbances in reaching puberty, medullary thyroid carcinoma, and hyperparathyroidism. Pheochromocytoma occurs with a frequency of probably less than 1% and is virtually unknown in children with neurofibromatosis.

Intellectual impairment occurs in about 40% of patients with neurofibromatosis. Mental retardation is less frequent than is impairment classified as a learning disability. The intellectual handicap is usually apparent by school age and does not progress with time. Major and minor motor seizures are known complications of neurofibromatosis. Seizures may be idiopathic or may reflect the presence of intracranial tumors.

Treatment

Treatment of neurofibromatosis consists of symptomatic drug therapy (antihistamines for pruritus, anticonvulsants) and appropriately timed surgery. Surgical removal of cutaneous neurofibromas is reserved for those that are particularly disfiguring or functionally compromising. Progressive kyphoscoliosis is best treated with surgical stabilization. Surgery is indicated for symptoms due to nervous system involvement by neurofibromas or to associated endocrine dysfunction.

Management of Anesthesia

Management of anesthesia for the patient with neurofibromatosis must include consideration of the multiple clinical features of this disease.[189] Although rare, the possible presence of pheochromocytoma should be considered in the preoperative evaluation. Signs of increased ICP may reflect the presence of an expanding intracranial tumor. Airway patency may be jeopardized by an expanding laryngeal neurofibroma.[190] Patients with neurofibromatosis and scoliosis are also likely to have cervical spine defects that can influence positioning for an operative procedure. There are no known unique considerations for the selection of inhaled or injected anesthetic drugs. Responses to muscle relaxants must be monitored carefully, since these patients have been reported to be both sensitive and resistant to succinylcholine and sensitive to nondepolarizing muscle relaxants.[191] Selection of regional anesthesia must recognize the possible future development of neurofibromas involving the spinal cord.

REFERENCES

1. Black P McL. Brain tumors. N Engl J Med 1991;324:1471–6; 1555–65
2. Brose WG, Samuels SI, Steinberg GK. Cardiorespiratory arrest following initiation of cranial irradiation for treatment of a brain stem-tumor. Anesthesiology 1989;71:450–1
3. Raichle ME, Posner JB, Plum F. Cerebral blood flow during and after hyperventilation. Arch Neurol 1970;23:394–403
4. Marsh ML, Marshall LF, Shapiro HM. Neurosurgical intensive care. Anesthesiology 1977;47:149–63
5. Cottrell JE, Robustelli A, Post K, Turndorf H. Furosemide- and mannitol-induced changes in intracranial pressure and serum osmolality and electrolytes. Anesthesiology 1977;47:28–30
6. Lassen NA, Christensen MS. Physiology of cerebral blood flow. Br J Anaesth 1976;48:719–34
7. Cohen PJ, Alexander SC, Smith TC, et al. Effects of hypoxia and normocarbia on cerebral blood flow and metabolism in man. J Appl Physiol 1967;23:183–9
8. Strandgaard S. Autoregulation of cerebral blood flow in hypertensive patients: The modifying influence of prolonged antihypertensive treatment on the tolerance to acute drug-induced hypotension. Circulation 1976;53:720–7

9. Eger EI. Pharmacology of isoflurane. Br J Anaesth 1984;56: 71S–99S

10. Aidinis S, Lafferty J, Shapiro H. Intracranial responses to PEEP. Anesthesiology 1976;45:275–86

11. Eger EI. Isoflurane (Forane). A Compendium and Reference. Madison, WI. Anaquest, A Division of BOC 1986;1–160

12. Adams RW, Gronert GA, Sundt TM, Michenfelder JD. Halothane, hypocapnia, and cerebrospinal fluid pressure in neurosurgery. Anesthesiology 1972;37:510–7

13. Muzzi DA, LoSasso TJ, Dietz NM, Faust RJ, Cucchiara RF, Milde LN. The effect of desflurane and isoflurane on cerebrospinal fluid pressure in humans with supratentorial mass lesions. Anesthesiology 1992;76:720–4

14. Phirman JR, Shapiro HM. Modification of nitrous oxide-induced intracranial hypertension by prior induction of anesthesia. Anesthesiology 1977;46:150–1

15. Wyte SR, Shapiro HM, Turner P, Harris AB. Ketamine-induced intracranial hypertension. Anesthesiology 1972;36:174–6

16. Mayer N, Weinstabl C, Podreka I, Spiss CK. Sufentanil does not increase cerebral blood flow in healthy human volunteers. Anesthesiology 1990;73:240–3

17. Rosa G, Orfei P, Sanfilippo M, et al. The effects of atracurium besylate (Tracrium) on intracranial pressure and cerebral perfusion pressure. Anesth Analg 1986;65:381–4

18. Rosa G, Sanfilippo M, Vilardi V, et al. Effects of vecuronium bromide on intracranial pressure and cerebral perfusion pressure. Br J Anaesth 1986;58:437–40

19. Stirt JA, Grosslight KR, Bedford RF, Vollmer D. "Defasciculations" with metocurine prevents succinylcholine-induced increases in intracranial pressure. Anesthesiology 1987;67:50–3

20. Hamill JF, Bedford RF, Weaver DC, Colohan AR. Lidocaine before endotracheal intubation: Intravenous or laryngotracheal? Anesthesiology 1981;55:578–81

21. Losasso TJ, Black S, Muzzi DA, Michenfelder JD, Cucchiara RF. Fifty percent nitrous oxide does not increase the risk of venous air embolism in neurosurgical patients operated upon in the sitting position. Anesthesiology 1992;77:21–30

22. Marshall WK, Bedford RF. Use of a pulmonary-artery catheter for detection and treatment of venous air embolism: A prospective study in man. Anesthesiology 1980;52:131–4

23. Moorthy SS, Hilgenberg JC. Resistance to nondepolarizing muscle relaxants in paretic upper extremities of patients with residual hemiplegia. Anesth Analg 1980;59:624–7

24. Perkins-Pearson NAK, Marshall WK, Bedford RF. Atrial pressures in the seated position. Implications for paradoxical air embolism. Anesthesiology 1982;57:493–7

25. English JB, Westenshown D, Hodges MR, Stanley TH. Comparison of venous air embolism monitoring methods in supine dogs. Anesthesiology 1978;48:425–9

26. Matjasko J, Petrozza P, Mackenzie CF. Sensitivity of end-tidal nitrogen in venous air embolism detection in dogs. Anesthesiology 1985;63:418–25

27. Bunegin L, Albin MS, Helsel PE, et al. Positioning the right atrial catheter: A model for reappraisal. Anesthesiology 1981; 55:343–8

28. Munson ES, Merrick HC. Effect of nitrous oxide on venous air embolism. Anesthesiology 1966;27:783–7

29. Zasslow MA, Pearl RG, Larson CP, Silverberg G, Shuer LF. PEEP does not affect atrial-right pressure difference in neurosurgical patients. Anesthesiology 1988;68:760–3

30. Chung RA, Goodwin AM. Transient ischaemic attack after spinal anaesthesia. Br J Anaesth 1991;67:635–7

31. Chambers BR, Norris JW. Outcome in patients with asymptomatic neck bruits. N Engl J Med 1986;315:860–5

32. Wong DHW. Perioperative stroke. Part II. Cardiac surgery and cardiogenic embolic stroke. Can J Anaesth 1991;38:471–88

33. Anderson CA, Rich NM, Collins GJ, et al. Carotid endarterectomy: Regional versus general anesthesia. Ann Surg 1980;46: 323–7

34. Michenfelder JD, Sundt TM, Fode N, Charbrough FW. Isoflurane when compared to enflurane and halothane decreases the frequency of cerebral ishcemia during carotid endarterectomy. Anesthesiology 1987;67:336–40

35. Young WL, Prohovnik I, Correll JW, et al. A comparison of the cerebral hemodynamic effects of sufentanil and isoflurane in humans undergoing carotid endarterectomy. Anesthesiology 1989;71:863–9

36. Carlsson C, Smith DS, Keykhah MM, Englebach I, Harp JHR. The effects of high-dose fentanyl on cerebral circulation and metabolism in rats. Anesthesiology 1982;57:375–80

37. Smith JS, Roizen MF, Cahalan MK, et al. Does anesthetic technique make a difference? Augmentation of systolic blood pressure during carotid endarterectomy: Effects of phenylephrine versus light anesthesia and of isoflurane versus halothane on the incidence of myocardial ischemia. Anesthesiology 1988;69: 846–53

38. Torvik A, Skullerud K. How often are brain infarcts caused by hypotensive episodes? Stroke 1976;7:255–7

39. Keats AS. Anesthesia for carotid endarterectomy. Cleve Clin Q 1981;48:68–71

40. Cucchiara RF, Sharbrough FW, Messick JM, Tinker JH. An electroencephalographic filter-processor as an indicator of cerebral ischemia during carotid endarterectomy. Anesthesiology 1979;51:77–9

41. Loughman BA, Hall GM. Spinal cord monitoring 1989. Br J Anaesth 1989;63:587–94

42. Peterson DI, Drummond JC, Todd MM. Effects of halothane, enflurane, isoflurane, and nitrous oxide on somatosensory evoked potentials in humans. Anesthesiology 1986;65:35–40

43. Pathak KS, Brown RH, Cascorbi HF, Nash CL. Effects of fentanyl and morphine on intraoperative somatosensory cortical-evoked potentials. Anesth Analg 1984;63:833–7

44. Schubert A, Drummond JC. The effect of acute hypocapnia on human median nerve somatosensory evoked responses. Anesth Analg 1986;65:240–4

45. McKay RD, Sundt TM, Michenfelder JD, et al. Internal carotid artery stump pressure and cerebral blood flow during carotid endarterectomy: Modification by halothane, enflurane and Innovar. Anesthesiology 1976;45:390–9

46. Riles TS, Kopelman I, Imparato AM. Myocardial infarction following carotid endarterectomy: A review of 683 operations. Surgery 1979;85:249–52

47. Wade JG, Larson CP, Hickey RF, et al. Effect of carotid endarterectomy on carotid chemoreceptor and baroreceptor function in man. N Engl J Med 1970;282:823–9

48. Asiddao CB, Donegan JH, Whitesell RC, Kalbfleisch JH. Factors

associated with perioperative complications during carotid endarterectomy. Anesth Analg 1982;61:631–7

49. Sieber FE, Toung TJ, Diringer MN, Wang H, Long DM. Preoperative risks predict neurological outcome of carotid endarterectomy related stroke. Neurosurgery 1992;30:847–54

50. Caplan LR. Diagnosis and treatment of ischemic stroke. JAMA 1991;266:2413–8

51. EC/IC Bypass Study Group. Failure of extracranial-intracranial arterial bypass to reduce the risk of ischemic stroke: Results of an international randomized trail. N Engl J Med 1985;313:1191–1200

52. Voldby B, Enevoldsen EM, Jensen FT. Regional CBF, intraventricular pressure, and cerebral metabolism in patients with ruptured intracranial aneurysms. J Neurosurg 1985;62:48–58

53. Archer DP, Shaw DA, Leblanc RL, Trammer BI. Haemodynamic considerations in the management of patients with subarachnoid hemorrhage. Can J Anaesth 1991;38:454–70

54. White JC, Parker SD, Rogers MC. Preanesthetic evaluation of a patient with pathologic Q waves following subarachnoid hemorrhage. Anesthesiology 1985;62:351–4

55. Davies KR, Gelb AW, Manninen PH, Boughner DR, Bisnaire D. Cardiac function in aneurysmal subarachnoid hemorrhage: A study of electrocardiographic and echocardiographic abnormalities. Br J Anaesth 1991;67:58–63

56. Allen GS, Ahn HS, Preziosi TJ, et al. Cerebral arterial spasm—a controlled trial of nimodipine in patients with subarachnoid hemorrhage. N Engl J Med 1983;308:619–24

57. Iwatsuki N, Kuroda N, Amaha K, Iwatsuki K. Succinylcholine-induced hyperkalemia in patients with ruptured central aneurysms. Anesthesiology 1980;53:64–7

58. Stoelting RK. Circulatory changes during direct laryngoscopy and tracheal intubation: Influence of duration of laryngoscopy with or without prior lidocaine. Anesthesiology 1977;47:381–3

59. Stoelting RK. Attenuation of blood pressure response to laryngoscopy and tracheal intubation with sodium nitroprusside. Anesth Analg 1979;58:116–9

60. Newman B, Gelb AW, Lam AM. The effect of isoflurane-induced hypotension on cerebral blood flow and cerebral metabolic rate for oxygen in humans. Anesthesiology 1986;58:1–10

61. Michenfelder JD, Tinker JH. Cyanide toxicity and thiosulfate protection during chronic administration of sodium nitroprusside in the dog: Correlation with a human case. Anesthesiology 1977;47:441–8

62. Sivarajan M, Amory DW, McKenzie SM. Regional blood flows during induced hypotension produced by nitroprusside or trimethaphan in the Rhesus monkey. Anesth Analg 1985;64:759–66

63. Fahmy NR. Nitroglycerin as a hypotensive drug during general anesthesia. Anesthesiology 1978;49:17–20

64. Sundt TM, Sharbrough FW, Anderson RE, Michenfelder JD. Cerebral blood flow measurements and electroencephalograms during carotid endarterectomy. J Neurosurg 1974;41:310–20

65. Rosenbaum KJ, Neigh JL, Stobel GE. Sensitivity to nondepolarizing muscle relaxants in amyotrophic lateral sclerosis: Report of two cases. Anesthesiology 1971;35:38–41

66. Kochi T, Oka T, Mizuguchi T. Epidural anesthesia for patients with amyotrophic lateral sclerosis. Anesth Analg 1989;68:410–2

67. Bird TM, Strunin L. Hypotensive anesthesia for a patient with

68. Kubal K, Pasricha SK, Bhargava M. Spinal anesthesia in a patient with Friedreich's ataxia. Anesth Analg 1991;72:257–8

69. Hetherington A, Rosenblatt RM. Ketamine and paralysis agitans. (Letter.) Anesthesiology 1980;52:527

70. Mets B. Acute dystonia after alfentanil in untreated Parkinson's disease. Anesth Analg 1991;72:557–8

71. Muzzi DA, Black S, Cucchiara RF. The lack of effect of succinylcholine on serum potassium in patients with Parkinson's disease. Anesthesiology 1989;71:322

72. Roy RC, McLain S, Wise A, Shaffner LD. Anesthetic management of a patient with Hallervorden-Spatz disease. Anesthesiology 1983;58:382–4

73. Martin JB, Gusella JF. Huntington's disease. Pathogenesis and management. N Engl J Med 1986;315:1267–76

74. Davies DD. Abnormal response to anesthesia in a case of Huntington's chorea. Br J Anaesth 1966;38:490–1

75. Propert DN. Pseudocholinesterase activity and phenotypes in mentally ill patients. Br J Psychiatry 1979;134:477–81

76. Lamont AMS. Brief report: Anaesthesia and Huntington's chorea. Anaesth Intensive Care 1979;7:189–90

77. Stemp LI, Taswell C. Spastic torticollis during general anesthesia: Case report and review of receptor mechanisms. Anesthesiology 1991;75:365–6

78. Osborne PJ, Lee LW. Idiopathic orthostatic hypotension, midodrine, and anaesthesia. Can J Anaesth 1991;38:499–501

79. Malan MD, Crago RR. Anaesthetic considerations in idiopathic orthostatic hypotension and the Shy-Drager syndrome. Can Anaesth Soc J 1979;26:322–7

80. Mitaka C, Tsunoda Y, Kikawa Y, et al. Anesthetic management of congenital insensitivity to pain with anhydrosis. Anesthesiology 1985;63:328–9

81. Kashtan HI, Heyneker TJ, Morell RC. Atypical response to scopolamine in a patient with type IV hereditary sensory and autonomic neuropathy. Anesthesiology 1992;76:140–2

82. D'Ambra MN, Dedrick D, Savarese JJ. Kearns-Sayer syndrome and pancuronium-succinylcholine-induced neuromuscular blockade. Anesthesiology 1979;51:343–5

83. Katzman R. Alzheimer's disease. N Engl J Med 1983;314:964–73

84. deMoulin GC, Hedley-Whyte J. Hospital-associated viral infection and the anesthesiologist. Anesthesiology 1983;59:51–65

85. Ward DS. Anesthesia for a child with Leigh's syndrome. Anesthesiology 1981;55:90–1

86. Maguire D, Bachman C. Anaesthesia and Rett syndrome: A case report. Can J Anaesth 1989;36:478–81

87. Suresh D. Posterior spinal fusion in Sotos' syndrome. Br J Anaesth 1991;66:728–32

88. Tobias JD. Anaesthetic considerations in the child with Menkes' syndrome. Can J Anaesth 1992;39:712–5

89. Tobias JD. Anaesthetic considerations for the child with leukodystrophy. Can J Anaesth 1992;39:394–7

90. Hart RG, Sherman DG. The diagnosis of multiple sclerosis. JAMA 1982;247:498–503

91. Crawford JS, James FM, Nolte H, et al. Regional anaesthesia for patients with chronic neurological disease and similar conditions. Anaesthesia 1981;365:821–8

Freidreich's ataxia and cardiomyopathy. Anesthesiology 1984;60:377–80

92. Warren TM, Datta S, Ostheimer GW. Lumbar epidural anesthesia in a patient with multiple sclerosis. Anesth Analg 1982;61:1022–3

93. Brett RS, Schmidt JH, Gage JS, et al. Measurement of acetylcholine receptor concentration in skeletal muscle from a patient with multiple sclerosis and resistance to atracurium. Anesthesiology 1987;66:837–9

94. Beck RW, Cleary PA, Anderson MM, et al. A randomized, controlled trial of corticosteroids in the treatment of acute optic neuritis. N Engl J Med 1992;326:581–8

95. Layzer RB. Stiff-man syndrome—an autoimmune disease? N Engl J Med 1988;318:1060–3

96. Kroll DA, Caplan RA, Posner K, Ward RJ, Cheney FW. Nerve injury associated with anesthesia. Anesthesiology 1990;73:202–7

97. Dawson DM, Krarup C. Perioperative nerve lesions. Arch Neurol 1989;46:1355–60

98. Alvine FG, Schurrer ME. Postoperative ulnar-nerve palsy. J Bone Joint Surg 1987;69A:255–9

99. Wadsworth TG. The cubital tunnel and the external compression syndrome. Anesth Analg 1974;53:303–8

100. Roy RC, Stafford MA, Charlton JE. Nerve injury and musculoskeletal complaints after cardiac surgery: Influence of internal mammary artery dissection and left arm position. Anesth Analg 1988;67:277–9

101. Seyfer AE, Grammer NY, Goubumill GP, Provost JM, Chandry U. Upper extremity neuropathies after cardiac surgery. J Hand Surg 1985;10A:16–9

102. Nightingale PJ, Longreen A. Iatrogenic facial nerve paresis. Anesthesiology 1982;37:322–3

103. Vaghadia H. Facial paresis after general anesthesia. Report of an unusual case: Heerfordt's syndrome. Anesthesiology 1986;64:513–4

104. Lowe DM, McCullough AM. 7th Nerve palsy after extradural blood patch. Br J Anaesth 1990;65:721–2

105. Sweet WH. The treatment of trigeminal neuralgia (tic douloureux). N Engl J Med 1986;315:174–7

106. Rao NL, Drupin BR. Glossopharyngeal neuralgia with syncope-anesthetic considerations. Anesthesiology 1981;54:426–8

107. McAlpine FS, Seckel BR. Complications of positioning. The peripheral nervous system. In: Martin JT, ed. Positioning in Anesthesia and Surgery. Philadelphia. WB Saunders 1987;303–28

108. Bickler PE, Schapera A, Baintain CR. Acute radial nerve injury from use of an automatic blood pressure monitor. Anesthesiology 1990;73:186–8

109. Martin JT. Postoperative isolated dysfunction of the long thoracic nerve: A rare entity of uncertain etiology. Anesth Analg 1989;69:614–9

110. Schreiner EJ, Lipson SF, Bromage PR, Camporesi EM. Neurological complications following general anaesthesia. Anaesthesia 1983;38:226–9

111. Kubota Y, Toyoda Y, Kubota H, et al. Common peroneal nerve palsy associated with the fabella syndrome. Anesthesiology 1986;65:552–3

112. Ropper AH. The Guillain-Barré syndrome. N Engl J Med 1992;326:1130–6

113. Greenberg RS, Parker SD. Anesthetic management for the child with Charcot-Marie-Tooth disease. Anesth Analg 1992;74:305–7

114. Antognini JF. Anaesthesia for Charcot-Marie-Tooth disease: A review of 86 cases. Can J Anaesth 1992;39:398–400

115. Hastings RH, Marks JD. Airway management for trauma patients with potential cervical spine injuries. Anesth Analg 1991;73:471–82

116. Stowe DF, Bernstein JS, Madsen KE, McDonald DJ, Ebert TJ. Autonomic hyperreflexia in spinal cord injured patients during extracorporeal shock wave lithotripsy. Anesth Analg 1989;68:788–91

117. Lambert DH, Deane RS, Mazuzan JE. Anesthesia and the control of blood pressure in patients with spinal cord injury. Anesth Analg 1982;61:344–8

118. Ravindran RS, Cummins DF, Smith IE. Experience with the use of nitroprusside and subsequent epidural analgesia in a pregnant quadriplegic patient. Anesth Analg 1981;60:1–3

119. Baraka A. Epidural meperidine for control of autonomic hyperreflexia in a paraplegic parturient. Anesthesiology 1985;62:688–90

120. Suderman VS, Crosby ET, Lui A. Elective oral tracheal intubation in cervical spine-injured adults. Can J Anaesth 1991;38:785–9

121. Meschino A, Devitt JH, Kock J-P, Schwartz ML. The safety of awake tracheal intubation in cervical spine injury. Can J Anaesth 1992;39:114–7

122. Turner LM. Cervical spine immobilization with axial traction: A practice to be discouraged. J Emerg Med 1989;7:385–6

123. Crosby ET, Lui A. The adult cervical spine: Implications for airway management. Can J Anaesth 1990;37:77–93

124. Gronert GA, Theye RA. Pathophysiology of hyperkalemia induced by succinylcholine. Anesthesiology 1975;43:89–99

125. John DA, Tobey RE, Homer LD, Rice CL. Onset of succinylcholine-induced hyperkalemia following denervation. Anesthesiology 1976;45:294–9

126. Tobey RE. Paraplegia, succinylcholine, and cardiac arrest. Anesthesiology 1970;32:359–64

127. Shayevitz JR, Matteo RS. Decreased sensitivity to metocurine in patients with upper motor-neuron disease. Anesth Analg 1985;64:767–72

128. Martyn JAJ, Matteo RS, Szyfelbein SK, Kaplan RF. Unprecedented resistance to neuromuscular blocking effects of metrocurine with persistence and complete recovery in a burned patient. Anesth Analg 1982;61:614–7

129. White BC, Weigentstein JG, Winegar CD. Brain ischemic anoxia. Mechanisms of injury. JAMA 1984;251:1586–90

130. Berntman L, Welsh FA, Harp JR. Cerebral protective effect of low-grade hypothermia. Anesthesiology 1981;55:495–8

131. Prough DS, Whitley JM, Taylor CL, Deal DD, DeWitt DS. Regional cerebral blood flow following resuscitation from hemorrhagic shock with hypertonic saline. Influence of a subdural mass. Anesthesiology 1991;75:319–27

132. Michenfelder JD. A valid demonstration of barbiturate-induced brain protection in man—at last. Anesthesiology 1986;64:140–2

133. Brain Resuscitation Clinical Trial I Study Group. Randomized clinical study of thiopental loading in comatose survivors of cardiac arrest. N Engl J Med 1986;314:397–403

134. Todd MM, Chadwick HS, Shapiro HM, et al. The neurologic effects of thiopental therapy following experimental cardiac arrest in cats. Anesthesiology 1982;57:76–86

135. Gisvold SE, Safar P, Hendrick HHL, et al. Thiopental treatment after global brain ischemia in pigtailed monkeys. Anesthesiology 1984;60:88–96

136. Nussmeier NA, Arlund C, Slogoff S. Neuropsychiatric complications after cardiopulmonary bypass: Cerebral protection by a barbiturate. Anesethesiology 1986;64:165–70

137. Plum F, Posner JB. The Diagnosis of Stupor and Coma. Philadelphia. FA Davis 1972;286

138. Smith AL. Barbiturate protection in cerebral hypoxia. Anesthesiology 1977;47:285–93

139. Rockoff MA, Marshall LF, Shapiro HM. High dose barbiturate therapy in humans: A clinical review of 60 patients. Ann Neurol 1979;6:194–9

140. Todd MM, Drummond JC, Sang H. The hemodynamic consequences of high-dose methohexital anesthesia in humans. Anesthesiology 1984;61:495–501

141. Todd MM, Drummond JC, Sang H. The hemodynamic consequences of high-dose thiopental anesthesia. Anesth Analg 1985; 64:681–7

142. Roesch C, Haselby KA, Paradise RP, et al. Comparison of cardiovascular effects of thiopental and pentobarbital at equivalent levels of CNS depression. Anesth Analg 1983;62:749–53

143. Ward JD, Becker DP, Miller DJ, et al. Failure of prophylactic barbiturate coma in the treatment of severe head trauma. J Neurosurg 1985;62:383–8

144. Sander JWAS, Shorvon SD. Incidence and prevalence studies in epilepsy and their methodological problems: A review. J Neurol Neurosurg Psychiatry 1987;50:829–39

145. Scheuer ML, Pedley TA. The evaluation and treatment of seizures. N Engl J Med 1990;323:1468–74

146. Browne TR. Valproic acid. N Engl J Med 1980;302:661–6

147. Callaghan N, Garrett A, Goggin T. Withdrawal of anticonvulsant drugs in patients free of seizures for two years: A prospective study. N Engl J Med 1988;318:942–6

148. Schmidt D. Adverse Effects of Antiepileptic Drugs. New York. Raven Press 1982

149. Delgado-Escueta AV, Wasterlain C, Treiman DM, Porter RJ. Current concepts in neurology. Management of status epilepticus. N Engl J Med 1982;306:1337–40

150. Ford EW, Morrell F, Whisler WW. Methohexital anesthesia in the surgical treatment of uncontrollable epilepsy. Anesth Analg 1982;61:997–1001

151. Celesia GG, Chen R-C, Bamforth BJ. Effects of ketamine in epilepsy. Neurology 1975;25:169–72

152. Hirshman CA, Krieger W, Littlejohn G, et al. Ketamine-aminophylline-induced decrease in seizure threshold. Anesthesiology 1982;56:464–7

153. DeFriez CB, Wong HC. Seizures and opisthotonos after propofol anesthesia. Anesth Analg 1992;75:630–2

154. Steen PA, Michenfelder JD. Neurotoxicity of anesthetics. Anesthesiology 1979;50:437–53

155. Kapoor WN. Evaluation and the management of the patient with syncope. JAMA 1992;268:2553–60

156. Morrison JE, Lockhart CH. Tourette syndrome: Anesthetic implications. Anesth Analg 1986;65:200–2

157. Fennelly M, Galletly DC, Purdie GI. Is caffeine withdrawal the mechanism of postoperative headache? Anesth Analg 1991;72:446–53

158. Gilman S. Advances in neurology. N Engl J Med 1992;326:1608–16

159. Raskin NH. Serotonin receptors and headache. N Engl J Med 1991;325:353–4

160. Abouleish E, Ali V, Tang RA. Benign intracranial hypertension and anesthesia for cesarean section. Anesthesiology 1985;63:705–7

161. Deyo RA, Ranville J, Kent DL. What can the history and physical examination tell us about low back pain? JAMA 1992;268:760–5

162. Boden SD, Davis DO, Dina TS, Patronas NJ, Wiesel SW. Abnormal magnetic resonance scans of the lumbar spine in asymptomatic subjects. J Bone Joint Surg 1990;72:403–8

163. Deyo RA, Diehl AK, Rosenthal M. How many days of bed rest for acute low back pain? N Engl J Med 1986;315:1064–70

164. Abram SE. Subarachnoid corticosteroid injection following inadequate response to epidural steroids for sciatica. Anesth Analg 1978;57:313–5

165. Gorski DW, Rao TLK, Glisson SN, et al. Epidural triamcinolone and adrenal response to hypoglycemic stress in dogs. Anesthesiology 1982;57:364–66

166. Gillin JC, Byerley WF. The diagnosis and management of insomnia. N Engl J Med 1990;322:239–48

167. Prinz PN, Vitiello MV, Raskind MA, Thorpy MJ. Geriatrics: Sleeping disorders and aging. N Engl J Med 1990;323:520–6

168. Aldrech MS. Narcolepsy. N Engl J Med 1990;323:389–94

169. Kuna ST, Sant'Ambrogio G. Pathophysiology of upper airway closure during sleep. JAMA 1991;266:1384–9

170. Hoffstein V, Zamel N. Sleep apnea and the upper airway. Br J Anaesth 1990;65:139–50

171. Wiesel S, Fox GS. Anaesthesia for a patient with central alveolar hypoventilation syndrome (Ondine's curse). Can J Anaesth 1990;37:122–6

172. Pellecchia DJ, Bretz KA, Barnette RE. Postoperative pain control by means of epidural narcotics in a patient with obstructive sleep apnea. Anesth Analg 1987;66:280–2

173. Gabrielczyk MR. Acute airway obstruction after uvulopalatopharyngoplasty for obstructive sleep apnea syndrome. Anesthesiology 1988;69:941–3

174. Owens WD, Gustave F, Sclaroff A. Tympanic membrane rupture with nitrous oxide anesthesia. Anesth Analg 1978;57:283–6

175. White PF. Spontaneous rupture of the tympanic membrane occurring in the absence of middle ear disease. Anesthesiology 1983;59:368–9

176. Man A, Segal S. Ear injury caused by elevated intratympanic pressure during general anaesthesia. Acta Anaesth Scand 1980; 24:224–6

177. Perreault L, Normandin N, Plamondon L, et al. Tympanic membrane rupture after anesthesia with nitrous oxide. Anesthesiology 1982;57:325–6

178. Kosman ME. Timolol in the treatment of open angle glaucoma. JAMA 1979;241:2301–3

179. Mishra P, Calvey TN, Williams NE, Murray GR. Intraoperative bradycardia and hypotension associated with timolol and pilocarpine eye drops. Br J Anaesth 1983;55:897–9

180. Cunningham AJ. Intraocular pressure—physiology and implications for anaesthetic management. Can Anaesth Soc J 1986;33:195–208

181. Garde JF, Aston R, Endler GC, Sison OS. Racial mydriatic response to belladonna premedication. Anesth Analg 1978;57:572–6

182. Meyers EF, Krupin T, Johnson M, Zink H. Failure of nondepolarizing neuromuscular blockers to inhibit succinylcholine-induced increased intraocular pressure, a controlled study. Anesthesiology 1978;48:149–51

183. Ausinsch B, Rayburn RL, Munson ES, Levy NS. Ketamine and intraocular pressure in children. Anesth Analg 1976;55:773–5

184. Wang BC, Bogart B, Hillman DE, Turndorf H. Subarachnoid injection—a potential complication of retrobulbar block. Anesthesiology 1989;71:845–7

185. Kortilla K, Kauste A, Auvinen J. Comparison of domperidone, droperidol, and metoclopramide in the prevention and treatment of nausea and vomiting after balanced general anesthesia. Anesth Analg 1979;58:396–400

186. Brown EM, Krishnaprasad S, Similer BG. Pancuronium for rapid induction technique for tracheal intubation. Can Anaesth Soc J 1972;26:489–91

187. Ghani GA, Sung Y-F, Per-Lee JH. Glomus jugulare tumors—origin, pathology, and anesthetic considerations. Anesth Analg 1983;62:686–91

188. Kodama K, Seo N, Murayama T, Yoshizawa Y, Terasako K, Yaginuma T. Glossopharyngeal nerve block for carotid sinus syndrome. Anesth Analg 1992;75:1036–7

189. Krishna G. Neurofibromatosis, renal hypertension, and cardiac dysrhythmias. Anesth Analg 1975;54:542–5

190. Yamashita M, Matsuki A, Oyama R. Anaesthetic considerations in von Recklinghausen's disease (multiple neurofibromatosis). Anaesthetist 1977;26:177–8

191. Baraka A. Myasthenia response to muscle relaxants in von Recklinghausen's disease. Br J Anaesth 1974;46:701–3

18

Diseases of the Liver and Biliary Tract

Diseases of the liver and biliary tract can be categorized as parenchymal liver disease (acute and chronic hepatitis, cirrhosis of the liver) and cholestasis with or without obstruction of the extrahepatic biliary pathway. Management of anesthesia in these patients requires an understanding of the physiologic functions of the liver. In addition, the impact of anesthesia and surgery on hepatic blood flow has important implications for the management of anesthesia. Liver function tests are useful in detecting unsuspected co-existing liver disease. Furthermore, these tests are helpful in establishing the diagnosis when postoperative liver dysfunction occurs.

PHYSIOLOGIC FUNCTIONS OF THE LIVER

The liver is the largest gland in the body, weighing about 1500 g and representing 2% of adult body weight. Hepatocytes represent about 80% of the cell mass of the liver. These cells perform diverse and complex functions (Table 18-1 and Fig. 18-1).

Metabolic Function

The main function of the liver in carbohydrate metabolism is the storage of glycogen. In this regard, the liver plays an important role in maintaining normal blood glucose levels. The breakdown of glycogen (glycogenolysis) releases glucose back into the systemic circulation, to maintain a normal blood glucose concentration, especially during periods of fasting, as before elective surgery. It must be remembered that the liver can store only about 75 g of glycogen. This amount of glycogen can be depleted by 24 to 48 hours of starvation. External sources of glucose become important in the prevention of

hypoglycemia during the perioperative period, when glycogen stores are depleted owing to poor preoperative nutrition or co-existing liver disease. Specific functions of the liver in fat metabolism consist of beta oxidation of fatty acids and the formation of lipoproteins. Fatty liver infiltration as may accompany a variety of diseases (obesity, malnutrition) usually reflects excess accumulation of triglycerides in the liver. The most important function of the liver in protein metabolism consists of deamination of amino acids, formation of urea for the removal of ammonia, and the formation of plasma proteins. All proteins, except gamma globulins and antihemophiliac factor, are produced by the rough endoplasmic reticulum of the liver. Protein synthesis is important in drug binding, coagulation, and hydrolysis of drugs with ester linkages.

The liver normally produces 10 to 15 g of albumin daily, which is sufficient to maintain the plasma albumin concentration in the range of 3.5 to 5.5 $g \cdot dl^{-1}$. Liver disease can be associated with decreased albumin production, resulting in decreased colloid osmotic pressure of the plasma and fewer protein sites available for drug binding. As a result, unbound pharmacologically active fractions of drugs, such as thiopental, increase, causing unexpected drug sensitivities[1] (Fig. 18-2). Increased drug sensitivities owing to decreased protein binding are most likely to occur when plasma albumin concentrations are less than 2.5 $g \cdot dl^{-1}$. Acute hepatic dysfunction is not likely to be associated with hypoalbuminemia, since the elimination half-time of albumin from plasma is 14 to 21 days.

Clotting abnormalities must be suspected in patients with liver disease, since hepatocytes are responsible for synthesis of most clotting factors including prothrombin, fibrinogen, and factors V, VII, IX, and X. The adequacy of clotting factor levels is evaluated by measuring the prothrombin time and partial thromboplastin time. Liver function must be dramatically decreased before impaired coagulation manifests, since many of the coagulation factors require only 20% to 30% of

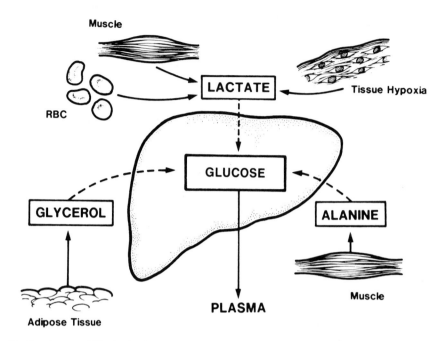

Fig. 18-1. The liver is responsible for the formation and release of glucose into the systemic circulation. Lactate, glycerol, and alanine from peripheral sites can enter the liver for conversion to glucose by the process of gluconeogenesis. Metabolic acidosis can occur when severe hepatic dysfunction interferes with the ability of the liver to clear lactate from the systemic circulation. Glucose is stored in the liver as glycogen. Glycogenolysis provides glucose for release into plasma, to maintain a normal blood glucose concentration.

their normal concentrations to prevent bleeding. Nevertheless, plasma half-times of hepatic-produced clotting factors are relatively brief (hours), and acute liver dysfunction may be associated with clotting abnormalities.

Liver disease associated with splenomegaly can alter the normal coagulation mechanism by platelet trapping in the spleen. Another factor predisposing to a bleeding diathesis is failure of a diseased liver to clear plasma activators of the fibrinolytic system, leading to an enhancement of fibrinolysis. Decreased prothrombin production may reflect severe hepatocellular disease or impaired vitamin K absorption owing to

Table 18-1. Physiologic Functions of the Liver

Glucose homeostasis
Fat metabolism
Protein synthesis
   Drug binding
   Coagulation
   Hydrolysis of ester linkages
Drug and hormone metabolism
Bilirubin formation and excretion

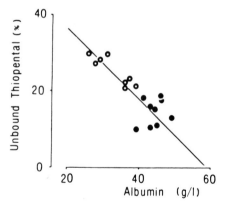

Fig. 18-2. The pharmacologically active unbound fraction of thiopental in the plasma parallels the albumin concentration in patients with cirrhosis of the liver (open symbols) and those with normal hepatic function (solid symbols). A decreased plasma albumin concentration in patients with cirrhosis results in an increased unbound plasma concentration of thiopental. (From Pandele G, Chaux F, Salvadori C, et al. Thiopental pharmacokinetics in patients with cirrhosis. Anesthesiology 1983;59:123–6, with permission.)

biliary obstruction and absence of bile salts. Parenteral vitamin K restores prothrombin production when decreases are due to biliary obstruction, but it may not be effective if hepatocellular disease is severe.

Plasma cholinesterase (pseudocholinesterase) is a protein produced in the liver, which is responsible for the hydrolysis of drugs with ester linkages, such as succinylcholine and certain local anesthetics. Severe liver disease may decrease cholinesterase production to the extent that the duration of apnea after the administration of succinylcholine is prolonged.[2] The prolonged effects of succinylcholine (greater than 30 minutes), however, are unlikely from liver disease alone, and atypical plasma cholinesterase enzyme must be suspected. Acute liver failure is unlikely to be associated with a slowed rate of succinylcholine hydrolysis because the plasma half-time for cholinesterase is about 14 days.

Drug Metabolism

The conversion of lipid-soluble drugs to more water-soluble and less pharmacologically active products is under the control of microsomal enzymes present in the smooth endoplasmic reticulum of hepatocytes. The hepatic elimination of a drug by metabolism is determined principally by hepatic blood flow and microsomal enzymatic activity. Hepatic clearance of drugs from the plasma that have a high hepatic extraction ratio is greatly influenced by hepatic blood flow, whereas drugs with low hepatic extraction ratios are more influenced by changes in microsomal enzymatic activity and protein binding. Chronic liver disease may interfere with the metabolism of drugs by virtue of decreased numbers of enzyme-containing hepatocytes or decreased hepatic blood flow, or both (see the section, Hepatic Blood Flow). Conversely, cirrhosis of the liver may be associated with accelerated drug metabolism and the resulting resistance to the pharmacologic effects of drugs. This response may reflect enzyme induction, owing to exposure of a decreased number of hepatocytes to drugs for metabolism.

HEPATIC BLOOD FLOW

The liver receives a dual afferent blood supply from the hepatic artery and vein (Fig. 18-3). Total hepatic blood flow is approximately 1450 ml·min^{-1}, or about 30% of the cardiac output. Of this amount, the portal vein provides 75% of the total flow, but only 50% to 55% of the hepatic oxygen supply, because this blood is partially deoxygenated before it reaches the liver. The hepatic artery provides only 25% of total hepatic blood flow but supplies 45% to 50% of the hepatic oxygen requirements. Hepatic artery blood flow is autoregulated such

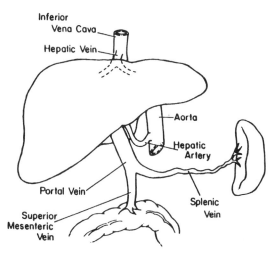

Fig. 18-3. Schematic depiction of the dual afferent blood supply to the liver provided by the portal vein and hepatic artery.

that a decrease in portal vein blood flow is accompanied by an increase in hepatic artery blood flow. Isoflurane preserves the ability of hepatic artery blood flow to increase when portal vein blood flow decreases, whereas halothane preserves this autoregulation to a limited extent, and only when used in doses (1 MAC or less) that do not decrease blood pressure greater than about 20%[3] (Fig. 18-4). As a result, hepatic oxygen delivery is better maintained in the presence of isoflurane than during administration of halothane. Surgical stimulation may further decrease hepatic blood flow independent of the anesthetic drug administered. The largest decreases in hepatic blood flow occur during intra-abdominal operations, presumably because of mechanical interference to blood flow related to retraction in the operative area, as well as the local release of vasoconstricting substances.

Fibrotic constriction characteristic of hepatic cirrhosis can increase resistance to portal vein blood flow, as evidenced by portal venous pressures of 20 to 30 mmHg. Ascites occurs when increased portal venous pressure causes transudation of protein-rich fluid through the outer surface of the liver capsule into the abdominal cavity.

LIVER FUNCTION TESTS

The ability to interpret liver function tests is useful in appreciating the presence of liver disease preoperatively and to facilitate the differential diagnosis of postoperative liver dysfunction. It is important to remember that liver function tests are rarely specific. Furthermore, in view of the enormous

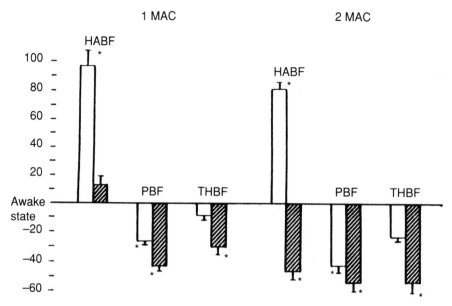

Fig. 18-4. Changes in hepatic blood flow in the presence of 1 MAC and 2 MAC isoflurane (open bars) or halothane (hatched bars) administered to dogs. HABF, hepatic artery blood flow; PBF, portal vein blood flow; THBF, total hepatic blood flow. *$P<0.05$ isoflurane versus halothane at comparable doses. (From Gelman S, Fowler KC, Smith LR. Liver circulation and function during isoflurane and halothane anesthesia. Anesthesiology 1984;61:726–30, with permission.)

reserve of the liver, considerable hepatic damage may be present before liver function tests are altered. Indeed, cirrhosis of the liver may produce little change in liver function, and only when some additional insult (surgery) produces further deterioration does the underlying liver disease become obvious. In adult patients scheduled for elective operations, routine performance of liver function tests demonstrates unsuspected evidence of liver disease in about 1 of every 700 otherwise asymptomatic patients.[4,5]

Postoperatively, the magnitude of liver dysfunction, as reflected by liver function tests, is exaggerated by operations close to the liver[6] (Fig. 18-5). The specific anesthetic drug does not influence the magnitude of postoperative liver dysfunction, as reflected by liver function tests[6] (Fig. 18-5). In animals rendered cirrhotic, the administration of a volatile anesthetic (halothane) produces greater derangement of liver function tests than that observed in noncirrhotic animals[7] (Fig. 18-6).

Bilirubin

Jaundice is likely to be present when the plasma bilirubin concentration exceeds 3 mg·dl^{-1} (normal plasma concentration 0.3 to 1.1 mg·dl^{-1}). Protein-bound (indirect-reacting or unconjugated) bilirubin cannot be excreted by the kidneys, whereas conjugated (direct-reacting) bilirubin may appear in

the urine. Increased plasma concentrations of unconjugated bilirubin are likely to accompany hemolysis of erythrocytes. Increased plasma concentrations of conjugated bilirubin reflect an impaired ability to secrete bilirubin into the biliary tract (cholestasis) due either to hepatocellular disease or to biliary tract obstruction, as produced by tumor or stones. Often, there is no correlation between the plasma level of bilirubin and severity of liver disease.

Transaminase Enzymes

Hepatocytes contain large amounts of transaminase enzymes (aspartate aminotransferase [AST], formerly SGOT; alanine aminotransferase [ALT], formerly SGPT), such that acute hepatocellular damage, as may occur in response to arterial hypoxemia, drugs, or viruses, will cause these enzymes to spill into the circulation. Other tissues, including the heart, lungs, and skeletal muscles, also contain transaminase enzymes. Therefore, measurement of plasma transaminase concentrations may not be specific for liver damage. Indeed, postoperative increases in plasma transaminase concentrations may reflect skeletal muscle damage from intramuscular injections administered preoperatively or damage to skeletal muscles during surgery. Nevertheless, marked increases of plasma transaminase concentrations (three times normal) during the postoperative period suggest acute hepatocellular

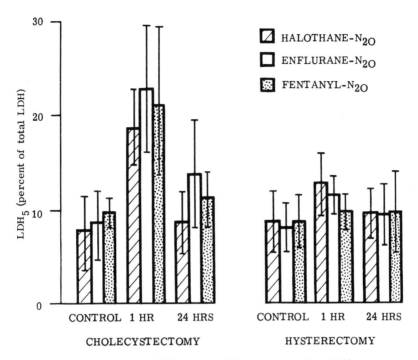

Fig. 18-5. Lactate dehydrogenase isoenzyme 5 (LDH_5, mean $\pm$ SD) was measured 1 and 24 hours postoperatively in patients undergoing cholecystectomy or hysterectomy. These data suggest that the site of operation, and not the drugs used for anesthesia, is responsible for postoperative increases in the plasma concentration of LDH_5. (From Viegas OJ, Stoelting RK. LDH_5 changes after cholecystectomy or hysterectomy in patients receiving halothane, enflurane or fentanyl. Anesthesiology 1979;51:556–8, with permission.)

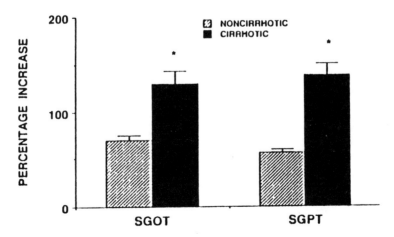

Fig. 18-6. Increase (mean $\pm$ SE) in the plasma concentration of SGOT and SGPT in noncirrhotic and cirrhotic rats after 1.05% halothane for 3 hours. *$P<0.05$ cirrhotic compared with noncirrhotic rats. (From Baden JM, Serra M, Fujinaga M, Mazze RI. Halothane metabolism in cirrhotic rats. Anesthesiology 1987;67:600–4, with permission.)

damage. The magnitude of plasma transaminase enzyme elevation typically parallels the severity of hepatocellular damage. Acute biliary tract obstruction as due to cholelithiasis may also cause increased plasma transaminase concentrations. Initially, increased transaminase concentrations decrease as hepatocellular recovery occurs or, on rare occasions, as a reflection of continued hepatocellular damage such that too few hepatocytes remain to serve as a source of enzymes.

Alkaline Phosphatase

Alkaline phosphatase enzyme is present in bile duct cells such that even slight degrees of biliary obstruction result in increases (three times normal) in plasma concentrations of this enzyme. Therefore, this test helps differentiate between hepatic dysfunction due to biliary obstruction and that due to hepatocellular damage. Despite the predominant presence of this enzyme in bile duct cells, it is well recognized that increases in plasma alkaline phosphatase concentrations may also accompany hepatocellular disease. As with transaminase enzymes, there are also extrahepatic stores of alkaline phosphatase, particularly in bone.

Albumin

The liver is the sole site of synthesis of albumin. Hepatocellular damage predictably results in decreased plasma albumin concentrations (normal plasma concentration 3.5 to 5.5 $g \cdot dl^{-1}$). Plasma albumin concentrations of less than 2.5 $g \cdot dl^{-1}$ may signify significant liver disease or loss of protein into ascitic fluid. Altered responses to drugs owing to decreased protein binding are more likely when plasma albumin concentrations are less than 2.5 $g \cdot dl^{-1}$. The plasma half-time for albumin is 14 to 21 days, emphasizing that acute liver dysfunction will not be reflected by decreased plasma albumin levels. Albumin-to-globulin ratios have little significance as a measure of hepatic function, since immunoglobulin production does not take place in the liver.

DIFFERENTIAL DIAGNOSIS OF POSTOPERATIVE HEPATIC DYSFUNCTION

When postoperative hepatic dysfunction occurs, a predetermined approach, including serial liver function tests and a search for extrahepatic causes of hepatic dysfunction, facilitates the differential diagnosis. The causes of hepatic dysfunction, most often manifested as jaundice, can be categorized as prehepatic, intrahepatic or hepatocellular, and as posthepatic or cholestatic, on the basis of repeated measurements of the plasma concentrations of bilirubin, transaminase enzymes, and alkaline phosphatase (Table 18-2).

The causes of postoperative hepatic dysfunction are most likely multifactorial and difficult to confirm, because few pathognomonic features are unique to specific etiologies. Furthermore, liver function often returns to normal without specific treatment. Maintenance of hepatic oxygen delivery relative to demand during exposure to anesthetics is important, since hepatocyte hypoxia is likely to be important in the etiology of postoperative hepatic dysfunction. When postoperative hepatic dysfunction occurs, the following steps should be taken in search of a cause before assuming, without supporting evidence, that anesthetic drugs are the responsible hepatotoxins:

1. Review all drugs administered, as every drug, regardless of how innocuous it may seem, must be considered as a potential cause of hepatocyte damage. Administration of catecholamines or sympathomimetics may evoke splanchnic vasoconstriction sufficient to interfere with an adequate hepatic blood flow.
2. Check for sources of sepsis. The development of jaundice is common in patients with severe infection.
3. Evaluate bilirubin load. A 500-ml transfusion of fresh whole blood contains 250 mg of bilirubin. This bilirubin load increases as the age of transfused blood increases. Patients with normal hepatic function can receive large amounts of blood without appreciable increases in bilirubin concentrations. This response can be different in patients with co-existing hepatic disease.
4. Rule out occult hematomas. Resorption of large hematomas may produce hyperbilirubinemia for several days. Furthermore, patients with Gilbert syndrome have limited ability to conjugate bilirubin, and even small increases in bilirubin load may lead to jaundice (see the section, Gilbert Syndrome).
5. Rule out hemolysis. Decreases in the hematocrit or increases in the reticulocyte count may reflect the hemolysis of erythrocytes.
6. Review perioperative records. Evidence of hypotension, arterial hypoxemia, hypoventilation, and hypovolemia must be considered as possible etiologic factors in postoperative hepatic dysfunction.
7. Consider extrahepatic abnormalities. Extraheptic causes of hepatic dysfunction include congestive heart failure, respiratory failure, pulmonary embolism, and renal insufficiency.
8. A phenomenon designated benign postoperative intrahepatic cholestasis has been described in association with extensive and prolonged surgery, especially if complicated by hypotension, arterial hypoxemia, and massive blood transfusion[8] (see the section, Benign Postoperative Intrahepatic Cholestasis).

Table 18-2. Liver Function Tests and Differential Diagnosis

Hepatic Dysfunction	Bilirubin	Transaminase Enzymes	Alkaline Phosphatase	Causes
Prehepatic	Increased unconjugated fraction	Normal	Normal	Hemolysis Hematoma resorption Bilirubin overload from whole blood
Intrahepatic (hepatocellular)	Increased conjugated fraction	Markedly increased	Normal to slightly increased	Viral Drugs Sepsis Hypoxemia Cirrhosis
Posthepatic (cholestatic)	Increased conjugated fraction	Normal to slightly increased	Markedly increased	Stones Sepsis

ACUTE HEPATITIS

Acute hepatitis is an inflammatory disease of hepatocytes, most often due to a viral infection or ingestion of a toxic drug. Rarely, acute hepatitis, characterized by fatty liver infiltration, is associated with pregnancy. Other causes of acute hepatitis include sepsis and congestive heart failure.

Viral Hepatitis

The most frequent organisms responsible for viral hepatitis are type A virus (infectious or short incubation hepatitis), type B virus (serum or long incubation hepatitis), and type C virus (non-A, non-B hepatitis) (Table 18-3). In the United States,

it is estimated that more than 300,000 persons acquire hepatitis B annually, with overt jaundice developing in only 25% of these patients.[9] Viral hepatitis due to infection with type D virus, Epstein-Barr virus, or cytomegalovirus is less common. Many cases of viral hepatitis are unrecognized because they remain subclinical or anicteric. It is likely that a number of patients undergo elective operations while in the asympatomatic prodromal phase of viral hepatitis.

Signs and Symptoms

The onset of viral hepatitis may be gradual or sudden. The symptoms are variable, but most often include dark urine, fatigue, and anorexia (Table 18-4). Dehydration may result from repeated vomiting; low-grade fever is common. The liver

Table 18-3. Characteristic Features of Viral Hepatitis

	Type A	Type B	Type C	Type D
Transmission	Fecal-oral, contaminated shellfish	Percutaneous, venereal	Percutaneous	Percutaneous
Incubation period (d)	20–37	60–110	35–70	60–110
Results of serum antigen and antibody tests	IgM early and IgG during convalescence	HBsAg and anti-HBc early and persist in carriers	Anti-HVC in 6 months	Anti-HVD late and may be short-lived
Immunity	45% have antibodies	5–15% have anti-HBs	Unknown	Protected if immune to type B
Course	Does not progress to chronic liver disease	Chronic liver disease develops in 1–10%	Chronic liver disease develops in >50%	Co-exists with type B
Prevention	Pooled gamma globulin	Hepatitis B vaccine, hepatitis B immunoglobulin	Unknown	Unknown
Mortality	≤0.2%	0.3–1.5%	Unknown	2–20%

HBcAg, hepatitis B core antigen; HBsAg, hepatitis B surface antigen; HVC, HVD, herpes virus types C and D; IgG, IgM, immunoglobulins G and M.

Table 18-4. Incidence of Symptoms
in Acute Viral Hepatitis

Symptom	Patients (%)
Dark urine	94
Fatigue	91
Anorexia	90
Nausea	87
Fever	76
Emesis	71
Headache	70
Abdominal discomfort	65
Light-colored stools	52
Pruritus	42

is often enlarged and tender. Asterixis, peripheral edema, or ascites implies unusually severe disease and a poor prognosis. Clinical and histologic features may not distinguish viral hepatitis from that resulting from other causes.

Laboratory Tests

Most patients have mild anemia and a lymphocytosis. Aminotransferase concentrations increase 7 to 14 days before the onset of jaundice and begin to decrease shortly after jaundice appears. The degree of aminotransferase increase does not necessarily parallel disease severity. If increased, gamma globulin concentrations suggest chronic, rather than acute, hepatitis. Severe acute hepatitis may be associated with decreased plasma albumin concentrations and prolonged prothrombin time as evidence of impaired protein synthesis functions of the liver.

Radioimmunoassay for hepatitis B surface antigen (HBsAg) is performed promptly, as this antigen appears in the plasma of all patients with hepatitis B early in the course of the disease. The appearance of immunoglobulin M (IgM) antibody to hepatitis A virus provides evidence of hepatitis A. An enzyme-linked immunosorbent assay for antibody to hepatitis C virus is used for screening blood products for contamination with this virus. Antibody to hepatitis C virus is usually detectable within 3 months after infection with the virus.

Clinical Course

Viral hepatitis typically produces symptoms for 1 to 2 weeks before the onset of dark urine and jaundice. As jaundice intensifies, appetite begins to return and malaise decreases. Aminotransferase concentrations usually begin to decrease just before peak jaundice occurs and decrease rapidly thereafter. Plasma bilirubin concentrations increase for 10 to 14 days and then decrease for 2 to 4 weeks, paralleling an improved sense of well-being in the patient. Usually, the clinical course is un-

eventful, and liver function returns to normal. Nevertheless, in some patients, symptoms persist and hepatic coma may develop.

Treatment

Treatment is often symptomatic, as it is unlikely that any therapy alters the course of the disease. A high-calorie diet is encouraged, but nausea and vomiting may be so severe that hospitalization and intravenous fluid and electrolyte replacement are necessary. Abstention from alcohol is advised during the acute phase of the disease, although alcohol has not been shown to have an adverse effect on the prognosis. Vitamin K is indicated if the prothrombin time is prolonged. Corticosteroids have not been shown to influence the course of the disease.[10] In extreme cases, liver transplantation may be considered.[11]

Epidemiology

Special features permit differentiation of the various forms of hepatitis (Table 18-3).

Hepatitis A

Hepatitis A virus is a 27-nm particle and a member of the picornavirus family. The virus is shed for 14 to 21 days before the onset of jaundice. Patients are unlikely to be infectious more than 21 days after the illness has begun. Hepatitis A is highly contagious, being transmitted by food that has been contaminated by the feces-soiled hands of infected persons. Ingestion of sewage-contaminated shellfish has led to epidemics of hepatitis A. Viremia is present from 1 to 25 days before the onset of symptoms, but transmission by blood is rare.

IgM antibody to hepatitis A is detectable at the onset of clinical illness and usually disappears within 60 to 120 days.[12] Immunoglobulin G (IgG) antibody reaches a high titer during convalescence, persists indefinitely, and confers immunity. Indeed, about 50% of the adult population has a high concentration of plasma antibody to hepatitis A virus.[13]

Pooled gamma globulin administered intramuscularly after exposure to the virus decreases the clinical occurrence of hepatitis A severalfold. Administration more than 2 weeks after exposure is not protective. Pooled gamma globulin should be given to all persons who share a household or hospital room with a hepatitis A patient.

The prognosis of patients in whom type A hepatitis develops is good, with symptoms disappearing and plasma transaminase concentrations decreasing within 3 to 4 weeks. Chronic liver disease does not develop, and a chronic carrier state does not occur.

Hepatitis B

Hepatitis B virus (also termed the Dane particle) consists of a 28-nm central core surrounded by a protein cover, creating a total diameter of 42 nm. Transmission is usually by parenteral routes, such as blood transfusion or percutaneous innoculation. Nonparenteral routes (oral to oral and sexual) can also be responsible. The incubation period for hepatitis B is 4 to 24 weeks. The prevalence of antibodies to HBsAg varies among subpopulations ranging from 5% in middle-class whites to 48% among homosexual males. This antibody confers immunity to hepatitis B.

Detection of Hepatitis B Viral Infection

A number of tests are available for the diagnosis of hepatitis B. The HBsAg is detectable in the serum of infected persons as early as 1 to 2 weeks after parenteral injection of virus and may persist for months. If HBsAg remains in the serum of an infected individual for 6 months after an episode of acute hepatitis B, it is likely to persist indefinitely. The presence of HBsAg in the blood indicates infectivity. Another core antigen (HBcAg), when present, indicates the presence of hepatitis B virus in the blood and a high risk of infectivity.

Persistence of HBsAg for longer than 6 months in the absence of antibodies indicates that the patient is a chronic carrier and potentially infective to others. Approximately 1 in every 200 adults in the United States is classified as a chronic carrier on this basis. These patients do not appear to be susceptible to reactivation of the virus, when subjected to anesthesia and operation. Furthermore, HBsAg is rarely present in the plasma of patients, with unexplained jaundice during the postoperative period. Chronic active hepatitis develops in an unknown percentage of chronic carriers of HBsAg, often progressing to cirrhosis of the liver with esophageal varices and ascites. Primary hepatocellular carcinoma is also more likely to develop in chronic carriers.

The antibody (anti-HBs) to HBsAg typically appears in the blood 2 to 4 months after an attack of hepatitis B and usually when HBsAg is no longer detectable. Antibody to core antigen (anti-HBc) appears promptly in the blood of infected individuals and persists indefinitely serving as a marker for prior or chronic hepatitis B infection. Immunity to hepatitis B infection is confirmed by the presence of anti-HBs or anti-HBc antibodies.

Prophylaxis

Hepatitis B vaccine produced by recombinant DNA techniques is highly effective in inducing antibodies to hepatitis B virus and thus preventing hepatitis B. Vaccination is recommended for high-risk groups, including health care workers with frequent exposures to blood products. Indeed, personnel who administer anesthesia are about 5 times more likely than the general population to show serologic evidence of prior hepatitis B infection.[14,15] Unfortunately, immunosuppressed patients show a poor antibody response to vaccination. After successful vaccination, titers of antibody to HBsAg begin to decline; in 5 years, 20% to 30% of these patients lack protec-

tive levels.[16] These patients will respond to a booster dose of vaccine, although the need has not been confirmed. The vaccine is useless in hepatitis B virus carriers, and it is unnecessary for those already immune (blood contains antibodies) to hepatitis B; however, the vaccine has no detrimental effects in these groups.

Avoiding exposure to high-risk patients (hemodialysis, immunosuppressed, homosexuals, intravenous drug abusers) is unreliable prophylaxis, considering infective patients who are asymptomatic and unrecognized. Proper techniques for all patients includes wearing gloves by those involved in patient care, using disposable equipment, and labeling blood specimens as possibly coming from patients with hepatitis. Hepatitis B virus can survive on contaminated surfaces at room temperature for prolonged periods. In this regard, heating to 60°C for 4 hours, heat or steam sterilization, or 2% glutaraldehyde destroys the hepatitis virus. Pooled gamma globulin contains low titers of anti-HBs, emphasizing the need to administer hepatitis B immunoglobulin and vaccine to an unprotected health care worker who has been exposed to a contact source known to be HBsAg positive.

Hepatitis C

Hepatitis C virus is responsible for most, if not all, cases of post-transfusion hepatitis. Chronic liver disease develops in more than one-half of patients with post-transfusion hepatitis C.[17] The antibody to hepatitis C virus is present in 0.5% of blood donors with normal aminotransferase concentrations and in 44% of blood donors with increased aminotransferase levels. Presumably, persons who are positive for antibodies to hepatitis C virus carry the viral infection. The presence of circulating antibodies is used to screen blood donors, although seroconversion may be delayed for 3 months or longer after infection, or it may not occur at all.[18,19] The value of pooled gamma globulin in prophylaxis against hepatitis C is not documented.

Hepatitis D

Hepatitis D virus (delta agent) requires the presence of hepatitis B viral infection for its expression.[20] When anti-HVD is present in the plasma, markers for hepatitis B such as HBcAg are usually absent. Successful vaccination against hepatitis B will prevent hepatitis D infection.

Other Viruses

Epstein-Barr virus and cytomegalovirus are infrequent causes of acute hepatitis in adults.

Epstein-Barr Hepatitis

Epstein-Barr virus is a herpes virus that usually produces mild hepatitis associated with nausea and vomiting, modest increases of plasma aminotransferase concentrations, and jaundice in some patients. In most instances, the hepatitis is part of the clinical syndrome of infectious mononucleosis. Rarely, hepatic dysfunction is severe and fatal, especially in immunocompromised patients.[21] An increase in the titer of specific fluorescent antibodies to Epstein-Barr virus confirms the diagnosis.

Cytomegalovirus Hepatitis

Cytomegalovirus is a herpes virus that is present in most adults, as evidenced by serum complement-fixation reactivity. The most severe outcome of infection with this virus is damage to the immature central nervous system in neonates. Liver involvement is usually mild and does not progress to chronic liver disease.

DRUG-INDUCED HEPATITIS

Several classes of drugs, including but not limited to antibiotics, antihypertensives, anticonvulsants, analgesics, tranquilizers, and anesthetics, are occasionally associated with hepatic dysfunction that may be indistinguishable histologically from viral hepatitis. These idiosyncratic drug reactions are rare, unpredictable, and not dose dependent. Clinical signs of liver dysfunction usually occur 2 to 6 weeks after the initiation of drug therapy but can be seen as early as the first day or as late as 6 months. Treatment consists of the early recognition of alterations in liver function and discontinuation of the responsible drug. Nevertheless, in some patients, the disease may progress despite withdrawal of the drug.

Anesthetic Drugs

All anesthetic drugs studied in the hypoxic rat model, which includes enzyme induction, may produce centrilobular necrosis, but the incidence is greatest with halothane, followed in order by fentanyl and nitrous oxide[22] (Fig. 18-7). It is likely that inadequate hepatocyte oxygenation (oxygen supply relative to demand) is the principal mechanism responsible for hepatic dysfunction that follows anesthesia and surgery. Any anesthetic that either decreases alveolar ventilation or reduces hepatic blood flow, or both, could interfere with adequate hepatocyte oxygenation. Co-existing liver disease, such as cirrhosis, may be associated with marginal hepatocyte oxygenation, which would be further jeopardized by the depressant effects of anesthetics or hepatic blood flow or arterial oxygenation, or both. Hypothermia that decreases hepatic oxygen demand may protect the liver from drug-induced events that decrease hepatic oxygen delivery.

Halothane

Halothane is speculated to produce two types of hepatotoxicity. The first is a mild self-limited postoperative hepatotoxicity characterized by transient increases in aminotransferase con-

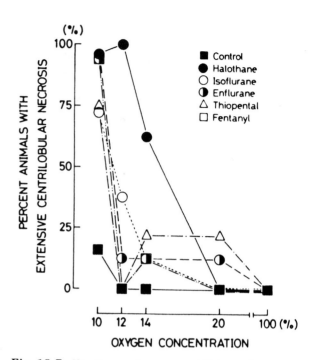

Fig. 18-7. Hepatic necrosis was present 24 hours after exposure to 10% oxygen for 2 hours in nearly all animals receiving an inhaled or injected anesthetic. When the oxygen concentration was increased to 12% or greater, halothane was the only anesthetic associated with hepatic necrosis in more than 50% of animals. (From Shingu K, Eger EI, Johnson BH, et al. Effect of oxygen concentration on anesthetic-induced hepatic injury in rats. Anesth Analg 1983;62:146–50, with permission.)

centrations. The less frequent and more severe from of hepatotoxicity (halothane hepatitis) occurs between 1 in 22,000 and 1 in 35,000 administrations of halothane and may lead to hepatic necrosis and death.[23,24] It is likely that the more common self-limited form of hepatic dysfunction after administration of halothane is a nonspecific drug effect owing to changes in hepatic blood flow that impair hepatocyte oxygenation. Conversely, the more rare but life-threatening form of hepatic dysfunction characterized as halothane hepatitis is most likely an immune-mediated hepatotoxicity.

Halothane Hepatitis

Clinical manifestations of halothane hepatitis that suggest an immune-mediated response include eosinophilia, fever, rash, arthralgia, and prior exposure to halothane. More important, the plasma of many patients with a clinical diagnosis of halothane hepatitis has been found to contain specific antibodies that react with halothane-induced liver antigens (neoantigens), whereas the plasma of patients with other forms of hepatitis does not contain antibodies of this specificity.[25] These neoantigens are formed by the covalent interaction of the reactive oxidative trifluoroacetyl halide metabolite of halothane with hepatic microsomal proteins. This acetylation of liver proteins in effect changes these proteins from self to nonself (neoantigens), resulting in the formation of antibodies against this now foreign protein. It is presumed that the subsequent antigen-antibody interaction is responsible for the liver injury associated with halothane hepatitis. The possibility of a genetic susceptibility factor is suggested by case reports of halothane hepatitis in closely related females of Spanish American origin.[26]

Several observations suggest that reductive metabolism is not the primary mechanism in halothane hepatitis. For example, neither enflurane nor isoflurane undergoes reductive metabolism, yet both drugs produce centrilobular necrosis in the hypoxic rat model. Furthermore, metabolites produced by reductive metabolism of halothane do not themselves produce hepatotoxicity. Furthermore, fasting does not alter metabolism; rather, it enhances hepatotoxicity produced by volatile anesthetics.

Halothane hepatitis, in the absence of documentation of the existence of antibodies, is a diagnosis of exclusion based on the elimination of other possible causes as likely explanations (see the section, Extrahepatic Causes of Hepatic Dysfunction). Undoubtedly, halothane has been wrongly incriminated in many patients when a more detailed investigation would have exonerated the anesthetic. Nevertheless, most cases of alleged halothane hepatitis have occurred in middle-aged obese females, especially with repeat administration of halothane within 4 weeks of a previous halothane anesthetic. Sensitivity to halothane may persist for prolonged periods, as suggested by the development of fatal halothane hepatitis with documented antibodies in a patient 28 years after the initial exposure to halothane.[27] Typically, hepatic dysfunction is manifested as fever and increased aminotransferase concentrations within the first 7 days postoperatively, or sooner, if a repeated halothane anesthetic is involved. Halothane should not be administered to patients who have experienced postoperative hepatic dysfunction for unknown reasons after previous operations that included administration of halothane. Pediatric patients seem less likely than adults to develop halothane hepatitis, even with repeated short interval exposures, although alleged cases have been described.[28]

Enflurane and Isoflurane

Mild self-limited postoperative hepatic dysfunction associated with enflurane or isoflurane most likely reflects anesthetic-induced alterations in hepatic oxygen delivery relative to demand that result in inadequate hepatocyte oxygenation. More disturbing, however, is the realization that an oxidative halide metabolite of both anesthetics is capable of acetylating the same liver proteins rendered antigenic by the trifluoroacetyl halide metabolite of halothane.[29] As a result, acetylated liver proteins capable of evoking an antibody response could occur after exposure to halothane, enflurane, or isoflurane. Furthermore, because of the cross-sensitivity between halogenated anesthetics, changing them in patients requiring multiple exposures will not necessarily reduce the risk of anesthetic-induced liver injury in susceptible patients. Considering the magnitude of metabolism of these volatile drugs, however, it is predictable that the incidence of anesthetic-induced hepatitis attributable to an immune-mediated mechanism would be greatest after administration of halothane, intermediate with enflurane, and lowest with isoflurane. Indeed, based on the estimated use of enflurane and isoflurane, the alleged incidence of hepatic dysfunction produced by these anesthetics, as indicated by the number of published reports, is less than the spontaneous attack rate of viral hepatitis.[30] Nevertheless, the development of an enzyme-linked immunosorbent assay for the detection of antibodies evoked by acetylation of liver proteins would be useful in establishing any rare cases of sensitization due to prior exposure to halothane; presumably, these patients would be at increased risk of subsequent exposure to enflurane or isoflurane.[31] Hepatic injury after administration of desflurane seems unlikely considering the nearly nonexistent metabolism of this drug.

CHRONIC HEPATITIS

Chronic hepatitis is categorized as chronic active hepatitis or chronic persistent hepatitis based on clinical features and interpretation of a liver biopsy[32] (Table 18-5). Chronic hepatitis does not occur with hepatitis A but does occur in 1% to 10% of acute hepatitis B infections and in 10% to 40% of patients with hepatitis C infections[33] (Table 18-3). Drug-induced (methyldopa, iproniazid, aspirin, dantrolene) chronic hepatitis usually resolves when the causative agent is discon-

Table 18-5. Differentiating Features in Chronic Hepatitis

Feature	Chronic Active Hepatitis	Chronic Persistent Hepatitis
Jaundice	Common	Rare
Aminotransferases	Markedly increased	Mildly increased
Bilirubin	Increased	Normal
Gamma globulin	Increased	Normal
Prothrombin time	Prolonged	Normal
Albumin	Decreased	Normal
HBsAg (incidence)	10–20%	10–20%

tinued.[34] In some patients with chronic hepatitis, there may be circulating antibodies to liver-specific membrane antigens, suggesting an autoimmune process. A genetic predisposition to the development of chronic active hepatitis is suggested by the frequency of specific histocompatability antigens.[35] There is no evidence that patients with chronic hepatitis need to restrict their activity, alter their diet, or avoid an evening cocktail. Potentially, hepatotoxic drugs should be avoided and drugs metabolized in the liver carefully titrated to effect. Chronic hepatitis B predisposes the infected person to the development of primary hepatocellular carcinoma.[36]

Chronic Active Hepatitis

Chronic active hepatitis is the most serious form of chronic hepatitis, ultimately leading to widespread destruction of hepatocytes, to cirrhosis, and to hepatic failure. Death is usually due to gastrointestinal varices or hepatoma. Esophageal varices, ascites, or hepatic encephalopathy are infrequent.

Patients with chronic active hepatitis who are HBsAg negative may be treated with corticosteroids, usually 15 to 20 mg·d^{-1}. Azathroprine may be added to corticosteroids. Although this treatment increases the 5-year survival from less than 50% to more than 85%, severe complications, including diabetes mellitus, hypertension, cataracts, and osteoporosis with vertebral collapse, develop in more than one-half of patients treated with corticosteroids for longer than 18 months. Azathioprine may cause bone marrow depression.

Patients with chronic active hepatitis often experience marked fatigue; jaundice is common. Extrahepatic manifestations are likely and include arthritis, neuropathy, myocarditis, glomerulonephritis, thrombocytopenia, and truncal obesity. Serum aminotransferase levels are invariably increased, and sudden increases may herald an exacerbation of the disease. Plasma albumin concentrations may be decreased and the prothrombin time prolonged. A positive lupus erythematosus cell preparation is present in 10% to 20% of patients.

Chronic Persistent Hepatitis

Chronic persistent hepatitis is a benign nonprogressive inflammatory disease largely confined to portal areas. Aminotransferase concentrations may remain elevated for years despite the benign course of the disease. Nutritional support, avoidance of potential hepatotoxins, and continued observation is the accepted treatment. Chronic active hepatitis develops in about 10% of these patients, for whom corticosteroid therapy becomes a consideration.

CIRRHOSIS OF THE LIVER

Cirrhosis of the liver is a sequela of a variety of chronic diseases characterized by scarring of the liver parenchyma. In the United States, the most common cause of cirrhosis is excessive intake of alcohol. Regardless of the etiology, the decreased hepatic blood flow resulting from increased intrahepatic resistance to flow through the portal vein (portal hypertension) reflects the fibrotic process associated with cirrhosis. This increased resistance leads to a decrease in the proportion of hepatic blood flow delivered through the portal vein and to an increase in the contribution to total hepatic blood flow from the hepatic artery. Therefore, decreases in systemic perfusion pressure or arterial oxygenation, as may occur during the perioperative period, are more likely to jeopardize the adequacy of hepatic blood flow and the delivery of oxygen to the liver in patients with cirrhosis, as compared with normal patients. Despite these predictable changes, liver function tests are usually normal or only slightly deranged. Often, only when additional insults, such as anesthesia and surgery, are imposed is cirrhosis indicated by the changes in liver function tests. Percutaneous liver biopsy is often the only procedure that can unequivocally establish the presence of cirrhosis. Esophagoscopy is the most useful procedure to establish the presence of esophageal varices.

Types of Cirrhosis

Alcoholic Hepatitis

Alcoholic hepatitis is directly attributable to chronic ingestion of large amounts of alcohol. It is estimated that about 10% of those who consume the equivalent of 80 g of alcohol daily for 10 to 15 years will show the development of cirrhosis of the liver. Concomitant malnutrition is common, but not necessary, for the development of cirrhosis. As alcoholic cirrhosis progresses, the patient loses skeletal muscle mass in the face, neck, shoulders, and arms. Weight loss is often offset by the accumulation of ascitic fluid. Hepatomegaly is almost invariably present, and splenomegaly is common. Palmar erythema appears, and spider angiomas are common over the face, back, chest, and arms. Subcutaneous bleeding often occurs as a result of both vitamin deficiencies and decreased coagulation factors. Gynecomastia and esophageal varices are usually present. Aminotransferases are increased, prothrombin time prolonged, and plasma albumin concentration is likely to be decreased. The only established treatment for patients with alcoholic liver disease is absention from alcohol. Treatment with corticosteroids, prophylthiouracil, or colchicine has not been documented to be efficacious.[37]

Postnecrotic Cirrhosis

Postnecrotic cirrhosis is characterized by a shrunken liver containing regenerating nodules. The most common cause of this form of cirrhosis is chronic active hepatitis, although the etiology in many patients is unknown (cryptogenic hepatitis). The distinguishing clinical features of postnecrotic cirrhosis are its predominance in females and increased plasma concentrations of gamma globulin. The disease often progresses insidiously, with the usual cause of death being gastrointestinal bleeding or hepatic failure. Primary liver cell carcinoma occurs in 10% to 15% of these patients. Treatment is supportive and symptomatic, although corticosteroids may be administered when the disease is associated with chronic active hepatitis.

Primary Biliary Cirrhosis

Primary biliary cirrhosis occurs most often in females between 30 and 50 years of age, typically manifested initially as fatigue and pruritus. Jaundice may not develop until 5 to 10 years after the onset of pruritus. Osteoporosis is common, manifested as bone pain, multiple fractures, and vertebral collapse. An autoimmune mechanism is suggested by the presence of autoantibodies in most patients. Alkaline phosphatase is markedly elevated, and prothrombin time may be prolonged. A moderate number of patients with primary biliary cirrhosis have concomitant disease, such as renal tubular acidosis, hypothyroidism, scleroderma, CREST syndrome, or Sjögren syndrome. Corticosteroids, azathioprine, penicillamine, and colchicine have been suggested as therapy. Exacerbation of osteoporosis may accompany administration of corticosteroids.

Hemochromatosis

Hemochromatosis develops when large amounts of iron are deposited in hepatocytes, leading to hepatic scarring, cirrhosis, and portal hypertension. This disease is inherited as an autosomal recessive defect, most often afflicting males 40 to 60 years of age. Iron deposits in the pancreas lead to the development of diabetes mellitus in about 50% of patients, whereas cardiac iron deposits are responsible for congestive heart failure and cardiac dysrhythmias in about 15% of patients. Primary liver cell carcinoma occurs in 15% to 20% of patients.

The diagnosis of hemochromatosis can be established only by liver biopsy, as an increased plasma iron or ferritin concentration is also possible with other forms of hepatitis. Mild increases in the aminotransferase concentrations and alkaline phosphate concentrations are likely, but jaundice is unusual. Plasma albumin concentrations and prothrombin time remain normal until late in the course of the disease. Treatment of hemochromatosis is removal of excess iron by periodic phlebotomies. If patients are identified before the development of cirrhosis and total body iron depletion is successful, life expectancy approaches normal.

Wilson's Disease

Wilson's disease (hepatolenticular degeneration) is an autosomal recessive disorder characterized by accumulation of copper in tissues, as a result of defective biliary excretion of this metal. Neurologic or hepatic dysfunction is usually manifested by 15 years of age. Hepatic damage is reflected by jaundice,

ascites, and hemorrhage from esophageal varices. Neurologic symptoms include tremors, skeletal muscle rigidity, and personality changes. Associated hemolytic anemia is a clue to the diagnosis. The pathognomonic finding of Wilson's disease is the Kayser-Fleischer ring, a thin, brown crescent of pigmentation at the periphery of the cornea. Distinguishing laboratory findings are decreased or absent plasma ceruloplasmin concentrations (a copper-binding globulin) and increased urinary copper excretion.

Treatment of Wilson's disease is with the administration of penicillamine, a chelating drug that binds copper and that promotes its urinary excretion. This drug is associated with nausea and may produce leukopenia and thrombocytopenia. In a small number of patients, the nephrotic syndrome develops. Pyridoxine is administered weekly, to offset the pyridoxine antagonist effects of pencillamine.

Alpha-1-Antitrypsin Globulin Deficiency

Alpha-1-antitrypsin globulin deficiency is associated with progressive hepatic cirrhosis in adults. Pulmonary emphysema is also typically present. Genetic variants have been found, reflecting the existence of more than 25 different alleles for the gene that controls production of alpha-1-antitrypsin. Measurement of plasma alpha-1-antitrypsin concentrations confirms the diagnosis.

Jejunoileal Bypass

Increased hepatic fat accumulation occurs in many patients during the period of rapid weight loss after jejunoileal bypass surgery. In a small number of patients, progressive liver disease develops that is indistinguishable from alcoholic cirrhosis. The cause of this syndrome is not known. The only effective treatment of this complication is reanastomosis of the bowel.

Complications of Cirrhosis

Hepatic and extrahepatic complications of hepatic cirrhosis, especially alcoholic cirrhosis, develop predictably in patients afflicted with progressive disease (Table 18-6). Acute hepatic

Table 18-6. Complications of Hepatic Cirrhosis

Portal vein hypertension	Hepatorenal syndrome
Varices	Hypoglycemia
Ascites	Duodenal ulcer
Hyperdynamic circulation	Gallstones
Cardiomyopathy	Impaired immune defense
Anemia	Hepatic encephalopathy
Coagulopathy	Hepatic cancer
Arterial hypoxemia	

failure is characterized by the increased expression of these complications.

Portal Vein Hypertension

Typically, portal vein hypertension does not develop until several years after the first attack of alcoholic hepatitis, followed by progressive scarring of the liver. The resulting elevated resistance to blood flow through the portal vein system, combined with hypoalbuminemia and increased secretion of antidiuretic hormone, contributes to the development of ascites. The most striking finding on physical examination is the presence of hepatomegaly with or without splenomegaly and ascites.

Varices

Gastroesophageal varices are massively dilated submucosal veins, permitting the passage of splanchnic venous blood from the high-pressure portal system to the low-pressure azygous and hemiazygous thoracic veins. It is important to recognize that not all patients with cirrhosis of the liver acquire esophageal varices, and not all patients with varices will bleed from their varices. However, when it does occur, variceal hemorrhage is usually from the distal esophagus or proximal stomach and often is hemodynamically significant.

Treatment

Treatment of active variceal bleeding includes the administration of whole blood to maintain the hematocrit close to 30%.[38] In patients with coagulopathy due to hypoprothrombinemia or thrombocytopenia, fresh frozen plasma or platelets, or both, are necessary. In the presence of significant hemorrhage, especially in patients with hepatic encephalopathy, intubation of the trachea may be performed to prevent pulmonary aspiration and facilitate endoscopic evaluation of the bleeding site. Balloon tamponade provided by a Sengstaken-Blakemore tube placed through the nose or mouth will stop bleeding in more than 90% of cases. Placement of this tube is often preceded by tracheal intubation and by subsequent insertion of a nasogastric tube above the balloon, to prevent the accumulation of blood and mucus. Sclerotherapy, the injection of a sclerosing substance into esophageal varices by an endoscope during general anesthesia, is effective in the immediate control of variceal bleeding.[39] Respiratory distress may occur 24 to 48 hours after sclerotherapy. Percutaneous transhepatic obliteration of varices also controls acute variceal hemorrhage in most patients, although recurrent bleeding is likely.

Intra-arterial injection of vasopressin may temporarily control variceal bleeding but does not improve overall survival and its administration requires specialized angiographic expertise. Vasopressin administered intravenously as a continuous infusion does not seem to be effective.[40] Propranolol produces a sustained decrease in portal venous pressure, but the efficacy

of this treatment in preventing bleeding from esophageal varices is not a consistent finding.[41]

Recurrent or continued bleeding may indicate a need for a portosystemic shunt. This operation has a mortality of about 40% when performed as an emergency, whereas mortality is substantially less when esophageal bleeding is controlled and the operation is performed electively. Portosystemic shunts may not prolong survival, but they do prevent subsequent variceal bleeding. The principal postoperative complication is hepatic encephalopathy and hepatic failure. The incidence of this complication may be less with a distal splenorenal (Warren) shunt and gastroesophageal devascularization that decompresses esophageal varices while maintaining mesenteric blood flow to the liver.[42] In the future, decompression of the portal venous system in the patient with variceal hemorrhage may be accomplished with the creation of a percutaneous transjugular intrahepatic portosystemic shunt, by means of an expandable stent placed between the hepatic and portal veins.[43]

Ascites

Ascites is a common sequela of many forms of cirrhosis, manifested as a fluid wave of the abdomen on physical examination or as a right-sided pleural effusion. Factors that contribute to ascites are portal vein hypertension, hypoalbuminemia, and increased secretion of antidiuretic hormone. Initial therapy for ascites often includes administration of spironolactone. The maximum diuresis of ascitic fluid should not exceed 1000 $ml \cdot d^{-1}$ (daily weight loss of 0.5 to 1 kg), as a more rapid diuresis can lead to undesirable degrees of hypovolemia, electrolyte abnormalities, and encephalopathy. Ascites that fails to respond to diuretic therapy may be treated by placement of a LeVeen shunt that routes ascitic fluid subcutaneously from the peritoneal cavity to the internal jugular vein through a one-way valve. Complications of shunt placement include peritonitis and disseminated intravascular coagulation. Paracentesis is rarely recommended as a chronic treatment, although paracentesis may still have a place in the initial treatment of patients with the recent onset of ascites.[44]

Circulation

A hyperdynamic circulation characterized by increased cardiac output is often present in patients with hepatic cirrhosis. This increased cardiac output has been attributed to vasodilating substances, such as glucagon, to increased intravascular fluid volume, to decreased viscosity of blood secondary to anemia, and to arteriovenous communications, especially in the lungs. Conversely, cardiomyopathy manifested as congestive heart failure can occur in patients with alcoholic cirrhosis. Megaloblastic anemia is frequent and is probably due to antagonism of folate by alcohol, rather than to dietary deficiencies. Thrombocytopenia is likely; accumulation of fibrin degradation products may reflect the presence of disseminated intravascular coagulation or the inability of the diseased liver to clear these substances from the circulation.

Arterial Hypoxemia

Despite the frequent presence of hyperventilation due to accumulation of ammonia, PaO_2 values of 60 to 70 mmHg are common in patients with cirrhosis of the liver. A possible explanation for unanticiapted low PaO_2 values is impaired movement of the diaphragm, owing to accumulation of ascitic fluid. In addition, right-to-left intrapulmonary shunts may develop in the presence of portal vein hypertension, leading to arterial hypoxemia. Likewise, many patients with hepatic cirrhosis smoke, and chronic obstructive airway disease is likely. Arterial hypoxemia may reflect pneumonia, a frequent occurrence in alcoholic patients. Vulnerability to the development of pneumonia may reflect the ability of alcohol to inhibit the phagocytic activity normally present in the lungs. As a result, bacteria inhaled into the respiratory tract are more likely to lead to pneumonia. Indeed, most lung abscesses are found in chronic alcoholic patients. Also, regurgitation of gastric contents is made more likely by alcohol-induced decreases in lower esophageal sphincter tone.

Hepatorenal Syndrome

See Chapter 20 for a discussion of hepatorenal syndrome.

Hypoglycemia

Hypoglycemia is a constant threat in patients with hepatic cirrhosis, especially in those who abuse alcohol. This may reflect glycogen depletion owing to malnourishment plus alcohol-induced glycogenolysis and to interference with glucogenogenesis. The liver is responsible for clearing lactic acid from the circulation and subsequently converting lactate to glucose by gluconeogenesis. Severe hepatic cirrhosis may impair its function, contributing not only to hypoglycemia but to the development of metabolic acidosis as well.

Duodenal Ulcer

Duodenal ulcer disease is more common in patients with hepatic cirrhosis. Bleeding from a duodenal ulcer, like that from varices, contributes to anemia and presents an increased ammonia load to the gastrointestinal tract, which may aggravate hepatic encephalopathy. Gastrointestinal bleeding owing to duodenal ulcer is differentiated from variceal bleeding with upper gastrointestinal endoscopy.

Gallstones

The incidence of gallstones is increased in patients with hepatic cirrhosis, presumably reflecting chronic increases in the bilirubin load caused by persistent hemolytic anemia and sple-nomegaly. The presence of gallstones complicates the differential diagnosis, if jaundice occurs.

Impaired Immune Defense

Alcohol ingestion suppresses immune defense mechanisms, rendering alcoholic patients vulnerable to bacterial and viral infections, tuberculosis, and the development of cancer.[45] In this regard, the patient using alcohol in excess, either episodically or on a regular basis, should be viewed as immunocompromised. Spontaneous bacterial peritonitis develops in nearly 10% of patients with ascites and hepatic cirrhosis owing to alcohol, perhaps reflecting bacteria that enter the portal venous system through the portosystemic collaterals, bypassing the major reticuloendothelial system in the liver. Fever, abdominal pain, and absent bowel sounds may herald the onset of this complication. Despite aggressive antibiotic therapy, the mortality in patients in whom spontaneous bacterial peritonitis develops is about 50%.

Hepatic Encephalopathy

Metabolic encephalopathy may be due to several different mechanisms (Table 18-7). Hepatic encephalopathy is characterized by mental obtundation, asterixis, and fetor hepaticus, which are thought to occur because nitrogenous waste products, specifically ammonia, have direct access to the systemic circulation due to portosystemic shunting.[46] Normally, the ammonia produced in the gastrointestinal tract by the bacteria-induced deamination of amino acids is converted in the liver to urea. Asterixis is most easily elicited by asking the patient to hold the arm horizontally with the hands extended. The flapping motion caused by intermittent loss of extensor tone is a hallmark of hepatic encephalopathy, although asterixis may also develop in patients with uremia or severe pulmonary disease. Slowing or flattening of waves on the electroencephalogram verifies the presence of hepatic encephalopathy. Cerebral edema and increased intracranial pressure often accompany hepatic encephalopathy and are the most likely causes of death.

Treatment of hepatic encephalopathy includes the elimination of exogenous sources of ammonia by restriction of dietary protein intake and control of gastrointestinal bleeding. Oral neomycin is poorly absorbed from the gastrointestinal tract; by decreasing the bacterial population, it will reduce thea-

Table 18-7. Mechanisms of Metabolic Encephalopathy

Toxic metabolic products (hepatic and/or renal failure)
Substrate deficiency (glucose, oxygen)
Acid-base disorders
Altered plasma osmolarity (<260 mOsm·L^{-1} or >325 mOsm·L^{-1})
Electrolyte imbalance

mount of urea converted to ammonia by bacterial ureases. Lactulose may be effective in decreasing concentrations of ammonia, by virtue of its ability to decrease the pH of fluid in the colon, causing the conversion of ammonia to ammonium, which is poorly absorbed and thus excreted in the feces.

MANAGEMENT OF ANESTHESIA IN THE PATIENT WITH HEPATIC CIRRHOSIS

It is estimated that 5% to 10% of all patients with cirrhosis of the liver undergo surgery during the last 2 years of life. Postoperative morbidity is increased, especially with respect to poor wound healing, bleeding, infection, and deterioration of hepatic function, including encephalopathy. Preoperative criteria may correlate with the surgical risk and the postoperative outcome of patients with cirrhosis of the liver undergoing major surgery[47] (Table 18-8).

Acute Hepatic Failure

Only surgery designed to correct a life-threatening situation should be considered in patients with acute hepatic failure. Preoperative correction of coagulation abnormalities with fresh frozen plasma may be indicated. Depressant or sedative drugs are not required. Nitrous oxide may be sufficient to provide analgesia and total amnesia in these critically ill patients. An injection of anesthetic may produce prolonged effects in the absence of normal rates of hepatic metabolism. Muscle relaxants are appropriate in providing operative exposure and facilitating the management of ventilation. The choice of muscle relaxants must consider the impact of decreased hepatic function, and often associated renal dysfunction, on the clearance of these drugs from the plasma. Since the plasma half-time of cholinesterase is 14 days, it is unlikely that acute liver failure will be associated with prolonged responses to succinylcholine.

Table 18-8. Prediction of Surgical Risk Based on Preoperative Evaluation

	Minimal	Modest	Marked
Bilirubin (mg·dl^{-1})	<2	2–3	>3
Albumin (g·dl^{-1})	>3.5	3–3.5	<3
Prothrombin time (seconds prolonged)	1–4	4–6	>6
Encephalopathy	None	Moderate	Severe
Nutrition	Excellent	Good	Poor
Ascites	None	Moderate	Marked

(Data from Strunin I. Preoperative assessment of the patient with liver dysfunction. Br J Anaesth 1978;50:25–34.)

Provision of exogenous glucose is important, and, in long operations, plasma glucose measurements to confirm the absence of hypoglycemia are prudent. Blood should be warmed and administered at as slow a rate as practical to minimize the likelihood of citrate intoxication. The use of fresh whole blood optimizes delivery of coagulation factors and minimizes the ammonia load. Monitoring of arterial blood gases, pH, and electrolytes is helpful, as these patients are vulnerable to the development of arterial hypoxemia, metabolic acidosis, and decreased potassium, calcium, and magnesium concentrations. Hypotension and its potential adverse effects on hepatic blood flow and hepatocyte oxygenation must be appreciated. Urine output is maintained with intravenous infusion of crystalloid or colloid solutions and, if necessary, by the administration of mannitol. Invasive monitoring, including a systemic arterial and pulmonary artery catheter, is helpful in guiding perioperative management. These patients are vulnerable to infections, emphasizing the importance of aseptic techniques during the insertion of intravascular catheters. Institution of neomycin or lactulose therapy during the preoperative period will decrease the ammonia load and help prevent the development of hepatic encephalopathy.

Sober Alcoholic Patient

Management of anesthesia in the sober patient with alcohol-induced cirrhosis of the liver is based on an understanding of the pathophysiologic changes associated with chronic liver disease (Table 18-6). The optimal anesthetic drug choice or technique in the presence of liver disease is unknown. It is important to remember, however, that a constant feature of chronic liver disease is decreased hepatic blood flow owing to increased resistance to flow through the portal vein. As a result, hepatic blood flow and hepatocyte oxygenation are more dependent on hepatic artery blood flow than in normal patients. Hepatic artery blood flow and PaO_2 may be impaired by intraoperative events associated with decreases in blood pressure or arterial oxygenation, or both. Among the volatile anesthetics, isoflurane may be associated with the best maintenance of hepatic blood flow, and thus hepatocyte oxygenation[3] (Fig. 18-3). It is probably prudent to limit the dose of isoflurane (limit decrease in blood pressure to about 20% of awake values) by combining the volatile drug with nitrous oxide or an opioid. Injected anesthetic agents may serve as valuable adjuncts to nitrous oxide with or without volatile anesthetics, but it must be appreciated that cumulative drug effects are likely if liver disease is severe enough to slow metabolism[1] (Fig. 18-2). Regardless of the drugs selected for anesthesia, postoperative liver dysfunction is likely to be exaggerated in patients with chronic liver disease, presumably owing to the detrimental nonspecific effects of anesthetic drugs and to stress-induced activation of the sympathetic nervous system on hepatocyte oxygenation. Regional anesthesia is useful in patients with advanced liver disease, assuming that coagulation status is acceptable.

The cardiac depressant effects of volatile anesthetics may be enhanced in patients with alcohol-induced cardiomyopathy. There may be decreased responsiveness to catecholamines, manifested as decreased tolerance to blood loss. Likewise, decreased protein binding of injected anesthetics in the presence of hypoalbuminemia owing to liver disease could theoretically increase the pharmacologic effects of these drugs. Disulfiram inhibits dopamine beta oxidase enzyme, necessary for the conversion of dopamine to norepinephrine, consistent with the observation of hypotension during anesthesia in patients treated with this drug.[48] Sedation and inhibition of other drug-metabolizing enzymes that result in potentiation of drugs such as diazepam may accompany disulfiram administration. The selection of regional anesthesia may be influenced by occasional patients treated with disulfiram in whom polyneuropathy develops.

It is a clinical impression that sober alcoholic patients display resistance (cross-tolerance) to other central nervous system depressant drugs, such as volatile anesthetics and barbitu-

rates. Indeed, animal studies have shown that chronic alcohol abuse increases anesthetic requirements (MAC) for halothane and isoflurane[49,50] (Fig. 18-8). The most likely explanation is cellular tolerance. Alcohol may produce enzyme induction, but increased metabolism will not alter the brain partial pressure required to produce anesthesia; nevertheless, the amount of drug delivered to achieve this partial pressure might be increased by enzyme induction. Surprisingly, thiopental dose requirements have not been shown to be increased in the sober alcoholic patient[51] (Fig. 18-9).

Muscle Relaxants

The role of the liver in the clearance of muscle relaxants must be considered when selecting these drugs for administration to patients with cirrhosis of the liver. Succinylcholine is acceptable, although severe liver disease may decrease plasma cholinesterase activity sufficiently to produce a modestly prolonged duration of action of this drug. The increased volume

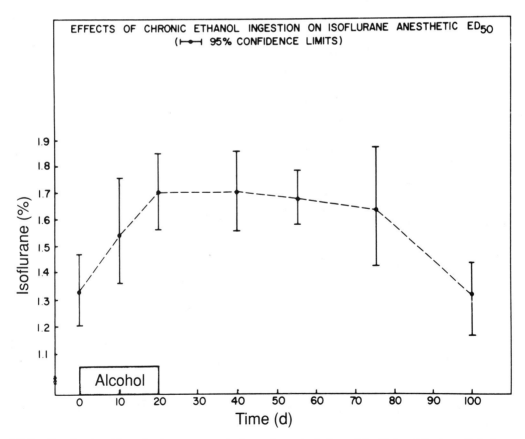

Fig. 18-8. Chronic ethanol ingestion increases anesthetic requirements during and for 55 days following unlimited access to alcohol. (From Johnstone RE, Kulp RA, Smith TC. Effects of acute and chronic ethanol administration on isoflurane requirement in mice. Anesth Analg 1975;54:277–81, with permission.)

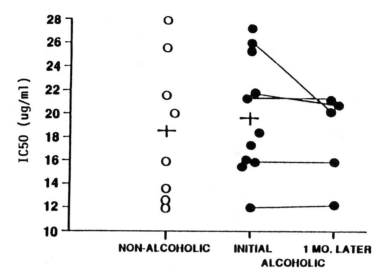

Fig. 18-9. The plasma concentration of thiopental needed to achieve one-half of the maximal decrease of the spectral edge on the electroencephalogram (IC50) was similar in nonalcoholic and alcoholic patients. The mean value is indicated by a plus (+) sign. Individual alcoholic patients studied a second time are indicated by a connecting line. (From Swerdlow BN, Holley FO, Maitre PO, Stanski DR. Chronic alcohol intake does not change thiopental anesthetic requirement, pharmacokinetics, or pharmacodynamics. Anesthesiology 1990;72:455–61, with permission.)

of distribution that accompanies cirrhosis may result in the need for larger initial doses of nondepolarizing muscle relaxants to produce the required plasma concentration, but the resulting neuromuscular blockade may be prolonged if these drugs depend on hepatic clearance mechanisms. Indeed, the elimination half-time of pancuronium is prolonged, owing to decreased hepatic clearance of this drug in patients with cirrhosis.[52] Hepatic dysfunction does not alter the elimination half-time of atracurium.[53,54] The elimination half-time of vecuronium in the presence of hepatic dysfunction or biliary tract obstruction is not increased until the dose exceeds 0.1 mg·kg^{-1}, consistent with the dependence of this drug on hepatic clearance mechanisms[53,55,66] (Fig. 18-10). Altered protein binding of muscle relaxants in patients with hepatic cirrhosis is probably insignificant as a mechanism of altered responses in these patients. All factors considered, intermediate-acting muscle relaxants, especially atracurium, would seem to be attractive selections for producing skeletal muscle paralysis in patients with severe liver disease.

Monitoring

Monitoring of intraoperative arterial blood gases, pH, and urine output, as well as provision of exogenous glucose, are important principles. Arterial hypoxemia may be exaggerated intraoperatively if drugs used for anesthesia produce vasodilation of co-existing portosystemic and intrapulmonary shunts.[57] Intravenous infusion of glucose during the perioperative pe-

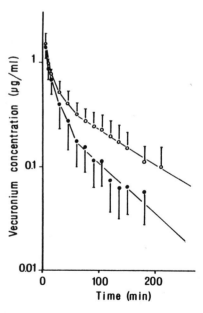

Fig. 18-10. Disappearance of vecuronium from the plasma of patients with cirrhosis of the liver (open circles) and control patients (solid circles), after a single bolus dose of 0.2 mg·kg^{-1} IV. (From Lebrault C, Berger JL, D'Hollander AA, Gomeni R, Henzel D, Duvaldestin P. Pharmacokinetics and pharmacodynamics of vecuronium (ORG NC45) in patients with cirrhosis. Anesthesiology 1985;62:601–5, with permission.)

riod is important, not only to prevent hypoglycemia, but also to decrease the likelihood of deposition of potentially harmful lipid-soluble metabolic products of volatile anesthetics in hepatocytes. Repeated blood glucose determinations may be helpful, especially during prolonged surgical procedures. Intraoperative maintenance of urine output, particularly in patients with co-existing jaundice, is important in decreasing the likelihood of postoperative renal failure. Mannitol may be necessary to establish diuresis. A small dose of dopamine may be beneficial, owing to drug-induced improvement in renal blood flow and an anti-aldosterone effect.

The need for invasive intraoperative monitoring is determined by the extent and urgency of the surgery. Management of anesthesia for surgical creation of a portocaval shunt includes monitoring of systemic arterial and cardiac filling pressures. A practical point is the avoidance of unnecessary esophageal instrumentation in the patient with known esophageal varices.

Intoxicated Alcoholic Patient

In contrast to the chronic but sober alcoholic, the acutely intoxicated patient requires less anesthetic, since there is an additive depressant effect between alcohol and anesthetics. The acutely intoxicated patient is also ill equipped to withstand stress and blood loss. Furthermore, alcohol tends to decrease the tolerance of the brain to hypoxia. Intoxicated patients may be more vulnerable to regurgitation of gastric contents, as alcohol slows gastric emptying and decreases tone of the lower esophageal sphincter. Surgical bleeding may reflect alcohol-induced interference with platelet aggregation. Alcohol, even in moderate doses, causes increased plasma concentrations of catecholamines, most likely reflecting inhibition of neurotransmitter uptake back into the presynaptic nerve endings. It is unknown whether the development of intraoperative cardiac dysrhythmias is influenced by this phenomenon.

IDIOPATHIC HYPERBILIRUBINEMIA

Hyperbilirubinemia may occur in the absence of hemolysis or overt hepatobiliary disease. Unconjugated hyperbilirubinemia will be present if there are defects before the conjugation steps in hepatocytes. These conjugation steps render bilirubin water soluble and are under the control of the hepatic enzyme, glucuronyl transferase. If the defect in transport occurs after conjugation, conjugated bilirubin will reenter the circulation to produce a conjugated hyperbilirubinemia.

Gilbert Syndrome

The most common example of idiopathic hyperbilirubinemia (present in varying degrees in 5% to 10% of the population) is Gilbert syndrome, inherited as an autosomal dominant trait with variable penetrance. The primary defect is decreased bilirubin uptake by hepatocytes, resulting in increases of the plasma concentrations of unconjugated bilirubin. Plasma bilirubin concentrations seldom exceed 5 mg·dl^{-1}.

Crigler-Najjar Syndrome

Crigler-Najjar syndrome is a rare form of severe unconjugated hyperbilirubinemia, owing to decreased or absent glucuronyl transferase enzyme. Children who lack this enzyme are jaundiced at birth; kernicterus develops with plasma bilirubin concentrations close to 30 mg·dl^{-1}. These children seldom survive to adulthood. When some enzymatic activity is present, plasma bilirubin concentrations average 15 mg·dl^{-1}, and jaundice is less severe. In these less severely afflicted patients, chronic phenobarbital therapy may decrease jaundice by stimulating enzymatic activity of glucuronyl transferase. Alternatively, plasmapheresis and phototherapy represent temporary treatments. Liver transplantation is the only permanent therapy available.

In the anesthetic management of children with this syndrome, bilirubin phototherapy lights should be available.[58] Fasting should be minimized because this stress is known to increase the plasma concentration of bilirubin. Morphine is metabolized by a different glucuronyl transferase enzyme system from that deficient in Crigler-Najjar syndrome. For this reason, morphine can be safely administered to these patients. Barbiturates, inhaled anesthetics, and muscle relaxants are acceptable selections in these patients.

Dubin-Johnson Syndrome

Dubin-Johnson syndrome is due to a decreased ability to transport organic ions from hepatocytes into the biliary system, resulting in conjugated hyperbilirubinemia. Inheritance of this syndrome is autosomal recessive.

Benign Postoperative Intrahepatic Cholestasis

Benign postoperative intrahepatic cholestasis may occur when surgery is prolonged, especially if complicated by hypotension, arterial hypoxemia, and the need for blood transfusions.[8] Patients who experience these responses are often elderly. Jaundice, in association with conjugated hyperbilirubinemia, is usually apparent within 24 to 48 hours and may persist for 2 to 4 weeks. Liver function tests other than the plasma bilirubin concentration are usually normal or only slightly deranged. The prognosis depends on the underlying surgical or medical condition.

ORTHOTOPIC LIVER TRANSPLANTATION

Orthotopic liver transplantation is the only curative therapy for a patient in hepatic failure. Hepatoma, biliary tract tumors, and genetically determined metabolic disturbances may also be treated with liver transplantation. Preoperative disturbances include arterial hypoxemia, anemia, thrombocytopenia, disseminated intravascular coagulation, hypokalemia, hypocalcemia, congestive heart failure, and encephalopathy.[59] The urgent nature of the operation and the severity of the hepatic dysfunction often limit the time available to optimize these disturbances before proceeding with surgery. An awareness of the association between portal hypertension and primary pulmonary hypertension is important, as these patients may be asymptomatic.[60] Only cadaver livers are used, but perfusion techniques permit procurement from long distances.

Management of Anesthesia

Management of anesthesia for liver transplantation includes invasive monitoring of arterial pressure and cardiac filling pressures, as well as placement of large-bore intravenous catheters to optimize volume replacement.[59] The radial artery is preferred over infradiaphragmatic sites because the abdominal aorta is occasionally cross-clamped during hepatic arterial anastomosis. Clamping of the suprahepatic inferior vena cava dictates placement of venous access catheters above the diaphragm. Massive blood and fluid requirements require the use of cell-saver devices. Calcium administration is often required to treat citrate-induced hypocalcemia and myocardial depression. Decreased venous return when the inferior vena cava is clamped may require the use of cardiac inotropes (dopamine) or sympathomimetics. Venovenous bypass to decompress venous congestion when the inferior vena cava is clamped may be considered. Hypothermia must be guarded against by warming inhaled gases and infused fluids.

Hypotension may accompany unclamping of the inferior vena cava, perhaps reflecting washout of negative inotropic or vasodilating factors from the previously ischemic tissues, which may occur even when venovenous bypass is used. Multiple types of coagulopathies can occur (thrombocytopenia, decreased levels of coagulation factors, fibrinolysis) requiring complex monitoring (thrombelastography) and appropriate blood component therapy. Metabolic acidosis during surgery is predictable; when combined with electrolyte disturbances and hypothermia, it may lead to cardiac dysrhythmias. Life-threatening hyperkalemia may accompany unclamping of previously clamped vessels or escape of potassium-rich perfusate from the newly transplanted liver. Blood glucose concentrations are monitored, as both hypoglycemia and hyperglycemia are potential problems. Maintenance of urine output is important, and oliguria may reflect co-existing renal dysfunction or hypovolemia.

Ketamine is a useful drug for the induction of anesthesia. Prolongation of the action of succinylcholine administered to facilitate intubation of the trachea is not a clinical problem because of the duration of surgery and the utilization of multiple blood transfusions, which are likely to contain cholinesterase enzyme. Maintenance of anesthesia is often with isoflurane with or without opioids. Large doses of opioids are not recommended, in view of the role of the liver in the clearance of these drugs. Co-existing pulmonary hypertension may require vasodilator therapy, although the risk of systemic hypotension may limit the full benefit of these drugs (hydralazine, nifedipine, nitroprusside) on the pulmonary vasculature.[60] Nitrous oxide is usually not administered because of possible bowel distension and the risk of air embolism at the time of revascularization of the liver, reflecting the presence of air previously trapped in the liver. The presence of co-existing portosystemic shunts may also increase the risk, should air embolism occur. Indeed, venous air embolism can occur during hepatic resection in supine patients, even in the absence of an open large vein, presumably reflecting entrainment of air through small hepatic veins open to the atmosphere.[61] Hepatic and renal routes of elimination must be considered in the selection of muscle relaxants during maintenance of anesthesia. Because of its independence from renal or hepatic clearance mechanisms, atracurium is a useful selection in these patients.[62] By contrast, the principal metabolite of atracurium, laudanosine, is dependent on hepatic clearance and may accumulate during the anhepatic phase of liver transplantation.[63] It is likely that mechanical support of ventilation will be required during the early postoperative period.

Complications

Early postoperative deaths may be caused by thrombosis of graft vessels, cholangitis, and air embolism, including systemic arterial air emboli through pulmonary arteriovenous shunts. Rejection is signaled by abnormalities in liver function tests and must be distinguished from mechanical factors, infections (viral hepatitis, cytomegalovirus), and effects of hepatotoxic drugs, including cyclosporine. Central nervous system toxicity, manifested as confusion, seizures, and coma, has been attributed to the administration of cyclosporine. Because cyclosporine is metabolized exclusively in the liver, frequent monitoring of blood levels is required during periods of changing hepatic function.

DISEASES OF THE BILIARY TRACT

An estimated 15 to 20 million adults in the United States have biliary tract disease, displayed by the presence of gallstones.[64] Gallstones may be present in 10% of males and in 20% of females between 55 and 65 years of age. The causes of gallstone formation are most likely related to abnormalities in the physicochemical aspects of the various components of bile. Approximately 90% of gallstones are radiolucent, composed primarily of hydrophobic cholesterol molecules. The remaining gallstones are usually radiopaque and are typically composed of calcium bilirubinate. These types of gallstones develop most often in patients with cirrhosis of the liver or hemolytic anemia. Diseases of the biliary tract may present as acute cholecystitis or as chronic cholelithiasis and cholecystitis.

Acute Cholecystitis

Acute cholecystitis is almost always due to obstruction of the cystic duct by gallstones. The cardinal symptom of acute cholecystitis is the abrupt onset of severe midepigastric pain (biliary colic) that extends into the right upper abdomen. This pain is typically accentuated by inspiration (Murphy sign). Localized tenderness may indicate perforation with peritonitis. Ileus may be present. Body temperature is usually elevated, and there is often a mild leukocytosis. Plasma bilirubin, alkaline phosphatase, and amylase concentrations are frequently increased. Jaundice is present when the cystic duct is completely obstructed by gallstones. Myocardial infarction is distinguished from acute cholecystitis on the basis of the electrocardiogram and measurement of plasma aminotransferases specific for cardiac muscle. Cholescintigraphy (intravenous injection of a labeled material selectively excreted by the gallbladder) or ultrasonography is used to confirm the clinical diagnosis of acute cholecystitis and the presence of gallstones. The differential diagnosis of acute cholecytstitis includes diseases characterized by severe epigastric pain and transient liver function abnormalities (Table 18-9).

Table 18-9. Differential Diagnosis of Acute Cholecystitis

Acute viral hepatitis
Alcoholic hepatitis
Penetrating peptic ulcer
Appendicitis
Pyelonephritis
Right lower lobe pneumonia
Pancreatitis
Myocardial infarction

The initial management of patients with acute cholecystitis consists of gastric suction, and of intravenous fluid and volume replacement, especially if vomiting has been prominent. Even though opioids can cause spasm of the choledochoduodenal sphincter, it is often necessary to administer these drugs to relieve the intense pain produced by acute cholecystitis. The presence of free air in the abdomen or of peritonitis suggests perforation of the gallbladder, necessitating emergency laparotomy.

Chronic Cholelithiasis and Choledocholithiasis

In patients who experience repeated attacks of acute cholecystitis, a fibrotic gallbladder eventually develops that is incapable of contracting to expel bile. Acute common bile duct obstruction by a gallstone produces symptoms similar to those described for acute cholecystitis. Ultrasonography and computed tomography may identify a dilated common bile duct and biliary tree. Direct visualization of the biliary tree may be accomplished by percutaneous transhepatic cholangiography.

Chronic cholangitis is inflammation of the hepatic biliary tree, which develops most often in patients with recurrent obstruction of the common bile duct. Fatigue, intermittent chills and fever, and weight loss are common complaints in these patients.

Elimination of Gallstones

Elimination of gallstones should be accompanied by the relief of symptoms and should prevent the development of more serious complications, such as cholecystitis, cholangitis, obstructive jaundice, and pancreatitis. Gallstones composed of cholesterol may be susceptible to dissolution with oral administration of chenodiol (chenodeoxycholic acid). Ursodoxycholic acid may be more effective than chenodiol. Infusion of methyl terbutyl ether through a transhepatic catheter placed directly into the gallbladder may be effective in dissolving gallstones. Overflow of this drug into the duodenum can result in intestinal irritation, hemolysis, or the onset of unconsciousness. Litholytic therapy is limited to selected patients and may require months to be effective. Furthermore, gallstones may recur in these patients.[64] Extracorporeal shock-wave lithotripsy, often in conjunction with oral litholytic treatment, may be effective in some patients. Historically, cholecystectomy through a subcostal incision has been used reliably to cure gallbladder disease and eliminate the risk of recurrent stones. Common bile duct exploration and removal of the impacted stone at the time of cholecystectomy constitutes the treatment of choice for choledocholithiasis. A T tube is left in the common bile duct through which cholangiography is performed to confirm the absence of common bile duct stones. In the absence of abdominal adhesions, an alternative to open cholecystectomy is laparoscopic laser cholecystectomy.[64,65] Postoperatively, patients undergoing this procedure experience only modest discomfort as the incision is small, are often able to eat the evening of surgery, and frequently leave the hospital the next day.

Management of Anesthesia

Treatment of gallbladder disease by open or laparoscopic cholecystectomy is most often performed with general anesthesia supplemented with muscle relaxants. Complete biliary tract obstruction could interfere with the clearance of muscle relaxants, such as vecuronium and pancuronium, which depend on this route for elimination.[66] Regional anesthesia is an unlikely selection, since the necessary sensory level would be extensive and surgical retraction around the diaphragm could interfere with adequate spontaneous ventilation.

Anesthetic considerations for laparoscopic cholecystectomy are similar to those for other laparoscopic procedures.[67] Insufflation of the abdominal cavity (pneumoperitoneum) with carbon dioxide introduced through a needle placed by a supraumbilical incision results in increased intra-abdominal pressure

that may interfere with the adequacy of spontaneous ventilation and venous return. During laparoscopic cholecystectomy, placement of the patient in the reverse Trendelenburg position favors movement of abdominal contents away from the operative site and may improve ventilation. This position may further interfere with venous return, however, emphasizing the need to maintain intravascular fluid volume. Mechanical ventilation of the lungs is recommended to ensure adequate ventilation in the presence of increased intra-abdominal pressure and to offset the effects of systemic absorption of carbon dioxide used in the creation of the pneumoperitoneum. High intra-abdominal pressure may increase the risk of passive reflux of gastric contents. Clearly, tracheal intubation with a cuffed tube will minimize the risk of pulmonary aspiration, should reflux occur. Venous carbon dioxide embolism may be responsible for cardiovascular collapse in the operating room or during the immediate postoperative period.[68] Because of the need to monitor ventilation, the chance of carbon dioxide embolism, and the risk of cardiac dysrhythmias owing to hypercarbia, capnography monitoring seems prudent. Intraoperative decompression of the stomach with a nasogastric or orogastric

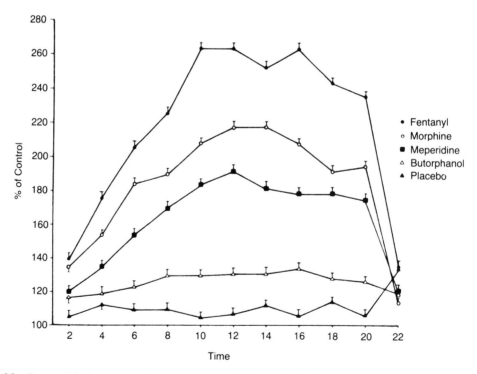

Fig. 18-11. Common bile duct pressure (percentage of control) increased after intravenous administration of an agonist opioid, but not after injection of an opioid antagonist, naloxone (placebo). Butorphanol, an opioid agonist-antagonist produced only a modest increase in common bile duct pressure. (From Radnay PA, Duncalf D, Navakovic M, Lesser ML. Common bile duct pressure changes after fentanyl, morphine, meperidine, butorphanol, and naloxone. Anesth Analg 1984;63:441–4, with permission.)

tube may decrease the risk of visceral puncture at needle insertion for production of the pneumoperitoneum, subsequently improving laparoscopic visualization and facilitating retraction of right upper quadrant structures. As with all laparoscopic procedures, careful observation for accidental injury to abdominal structures is important. The loss of hemostasis or injury to the hepatic artery or liver may require prompt intervention with an open laparotomy. There is no evidence that nitrous oxide (70%) expands bowel gas or interferes with surgical working conditions during laparoscopic cholecystectomy.[69]

The co-existing presence of liver disease may influence the selection of volatile anesthetics. Nevertheless, there is no evidence that hepatic dysfunction is uniquely deranged after elective cholecystectomy performed with general anesthesia that included a volatile anesthetic[6] (Fig. 18-5). The use of opioids for anesthesia in patients undergoing open cholecystectomy and common bile duct exploration is controversial based on the known ability of these drugs to cause spasm of the choledochoduodenal sphincter (sphincter of Oddi) and subsequent choledochol hypertension[70–72] (Fig. 18-11). Opioid-induced spasm of the choledochoduodenal sphincter may impair passage of contrast medium into the duodenum, erroneously suggesting the need for a sphincteroplasty or the presence of common duct stones. Despite these concerns, opioids have been used in many instances without adverse effects, emphasizing that not all patients respond to opioids with choledochoduodenal sphincter spasm. Indeed, it has been suggested that the incidence of opioid-induced sphincter spasm during open cholecystectomy is so low (less than about 3%) that this response should not influence the selection of these drugs.[73] Furthermore, should opioid-induced sphincter spasm occur, it is possible to antagonize this effect with the intravenous administration of naloxone (which may also antagonize desirable analgesic effects) or glucagon.[71,74] Glucagon predictably produces hyperglycemia and, in awake patients, is likely to be associated with vomiting. It should be remembered that intraoperative manipulation of the biliary duct system with probes and the use of cold or irritating solutions (radiopaque dyes) may produce spasm of the choledochoduodenal sphincter, which is independent of drugs used to produce anesthesia.

Emergency surgery for acute cholecystitis or common bile duct obstruction associated with vomiting may necessitate volume and electrolyte replacement. Many of these patients will have ileus and should be considered at increased risk of pulmonary aspiration of gastric contents.

Postoperative pain is intense after cholecystectomy. In this regard, patient-controlled analgesia or neuraxial opioids contribute to patient comfort and early ambulation, which helps decrease the likelihood of pulmonary complications.

REFERENCES

1. Pandele G, Chaux F, Salvadori C, et al. Thiopental pharmacokinetics in patients with cirrhosis. Anesthesiology 1983;59:123–6
2. Foldes FF, Swerdlow M, Lipschitz E, et al. Comparison of the respiratory effects of suxamethonium and suxethonium in man. Anesthesiology 1956;17:559–68
3. Gelman S, Fowler KC, Smith LR. Liver circulation and function during isoflurane and halothane anesthesia. Anesthesiology 1984;61:726–30
4. Schemel WH. Unexpected hepatic dysfunction found by multiple laboratory screening. Anesth Analg 1976;55:810–2
5. Wataneeyawech M, Kelly KA. Hepatic diseases unsuspected before surgery. NY State J Med 1975;75:1278–81
6. Viegas OJ, Stoelting RK. LDH5 changes after cholecystectomy or hysterectomy in patients receiving halothane, enflurane, or fentanyl. Anesthesiology 1979;51:556–8
7. Baden JM, Serra M, Fujinaga M, Mazze RI. Halothane metabolism in cirrhotic rats. Anesthesiology 1987;67:660–4
8. LaMont JT, Isselbacher KJ. Postoperative jaundice. N Engl J Med 1973;288:305–7
9. Recommendations for the Immunization Practices Advisory Committee (ACIP): Update on hepatitis B prevention. MMWR 1987;36:353–7
10. Ware AJ, Cuthbert JA, Shorey J, et al. A prospective trial of steroid therapy in severe viral hepatitis. Gastroenterology 1981;80:219–26
11. Edmond JC, Aran PP, Whitington PF, et al. Liver transplantation in the management of fulminant hepatic failure. Gastroenterology 1989;96:1583–9
12. Kao HW, Ashcaval M, Redeker AG. The persistence of hepatitis A IgM antibody after acute clinical hepatitis A. Hepatology 1984;4:933–9
13. Szmuness W, Dienstag JL, Purcell RH, et al. Distribution of antibody to hepatitis A antigen in urban adult populations. N Engl J Med 1976;295:755–82
14. Oxman MN. Hepatitis B vaccination of high-risk hospital personnel. Anesthesiology 1984;60:1–3
15. Berry AJ, Isaacson IJ, Hunt D, Kane M. The prevalence of hepatitis B markers in anesthesia personnel. Anesthesiology 1984;60:6–9
16. Wainwright RE, McMahon BJ, Bulkow LR, et al. Duration of immunogenicity and efficacy of hepatitis B vaccine in a Yupik Eskimo population. JAMA 1989;261:2362–8
17. Alter M, Margolis HS, Krawczynski K, et al. The natural history of community-acquired hepatitis C in the United States. New Engl J Med 1992;327:1899–905
18. Esteban JI, Gonzalez A, Hernandez JM, et al. Evalaution of antibodies to hepatitis C virus in a study of transfusion associated hepatitis. N Engl J Med 1990;323:1107–12
19. Aach RD, Stevens CE, Hollinger FB, et al. Hepatitis C virus infection in post-transfusion hepatitis. N Engl J Med 1991;325:1325–9
20. Hoofnagle JH. Type D (delta) hepatitis. JAMA 1989;261:1321–6
21. Markin RS, Linder J, Juerlein K, et al. Hepatitis in fatal infectious mononucleosis. Gastroenterology 1987;93:1210–6

22. Shingu K, Eger EI, Johnson EH, et al. Effect of oxygen concentration, hyperthermia, and choice of vendor on anesthetic-induced hepatic injury in rats. Anesth Analg 1983;62:146–50

23. Summary of the national halothane study. JAMA 1966;197:775–88

24. Mushin WW, Rosen M, Jones EV. Post-halothane jaundice in relation to previous administration of halothane. Br Med J 1971;3:18–22

25. Hubbard AK, Roth TP, Gandolfi AJ, Brown BR, Webster NR, Nunn JF. Halothane hepatitis patients generate an antibody response toward a covalently bound metabolite of halothane. Anesthesiology 1988;68:791–6

26. Hoft RH, Bunker JP, Goodman HI, Gregory PB. Halothane hepatitis in three pairs of closely related women. N Engl J Med 1981;304:1023–4

27. Martin JL, Dubbink DA, Plevak DJ, et al. Halothane hepatitis 28 years after primary exposure. Anesth Analg 1992;74:605–8

28. Lewis RB, Blair M. Halothane hepatitis in a young child. Br J Anaesth 1982;54:349–52

29. Christ DD, Kenna JG, Kammerer W, Satoh H, Pohl LR. Enflurane metabolism produces covalently bound liver adducts recognized by antibodies from patients with halothane hepatitis. Anesthesiology 1988;69:833–8

30. Brown BR, Gandolfi AJ. Adverse effects of volatile anaesthetics. Br J Anaesth 1987;59:14–23

31. Martin JL, Kenna JG, Pohl LR. Antibody assays for the detection of patients sensitized to halothane. Anesth Analg 1990;70:154–9

32. Boyer JL. Chronic hepatitis: A perspective on classification and determinants of prognosis. Gastroenterology 1976;70:1161–71

33. Rakela J, Redeker AG. Chronic liver disease after acute non-A, non-B viral hepatitis. Gastroenterology 1979;77:1200–4

34. Kaplowitz N, Aw TY, Simon FR, et al. Drug-induced hepatotoxicity. Ann Intern Med 1986;104:826–38

35. Robertson DA, Zhant SL, Guy EC, et al. Persistent measles viral genome in autoimmune chronic active hepatitis. Lancet 1987;2:9–10

36. Shafritz DA, Shouval D, Sherman HI, et al. Integration of hepatitis B virus DNA into the genome of liver cells in chronic liver disease and hepatocellular carcinoma: Studies in percutaneous liver biopsies and postmortem tissue specimens. N Engl J Med 1981;305:1067–78

37. Boyer JL, Ransohoff DF. Is colchicine effective therapy for cirrhosis? N Engl J Med 1988;318:1751–2

38. Cello JP, Crass RA, Grendell JH, Trunkey DD. Management of the patient with hemorrhaging esophageal varices. JAMA 1986;256:1480–4

39. Westaby D, Macdougall BRD, Williams R. Improved survival following injection sclerotherapy for esophageal varices: Final analysis of a controlled trial. Hepatology 1985;5:827–32

40. Fogel MR, Krauer CM, Andres LL, et al. Continuous intravenous vasopressin in active upper gastrointestinal bleeding: A placebo controlled trial. Ann Intern Med 1982;96:565–71

41. LeBrec D, Poynard T, Bernuau J, et al. A randomized controlled study of propranolol for prevention of recurrent gastrointestinal bleeding in patients with cirrhosis: A final report. Hepatology 1984;4:355–61

42. Langer B, Taylor BR, Mackenzie DR, et al. Further report of a prospective randomized trial comparing distal splenorenal shunt with end-to-side portacaval shunt: An analysis of encephalopathy, survival, and quality of life. Gastroenterology 1985;88:424–32

43. Zemel G, Katzen BT, Becker GJ, Benenati JF, Sallee DS. Percutaneous transjugular portosystemic shunt. JAMA 1991;266:390–3

44. Quintero E, Gines P, Arroyo V, et al. Paracentesis versus diuretics in the treatment of cirrhotics with tense ascites. Lancet 1985;1:611–3

45. MacGregor RR. Alcohol and immune defense. JAMA 1986;256:1474–9

46. Fraser CL, Arieff AI. Hepatic encephalopathy. N Engl J Med 1985;313:865–72

47. Strunin L. Preoperative assessment of the patient with liver dysfunction. Br J Anaesth 1978;50:25–34

48. Diaz JH, Hill GE. Hypotension with anesthesia in disulfiram-treated patients. (Letter.) Anesthesiology 1979;51:366–8

49. Han YH. Why do chronic alcoholics require more anesthesia? Anesthesiology 1969;30:341–2

50. Johnston RE, Kulp RA, Smith TC. Effects of acute and chronic ethanol administration on isoflurane requirement in mice. Anesth Analg 1975;54:277–81

51. Swerdlow BN, Holley FO, Maitre PO, Stanski DR. Chronic alcohol intake does not change thiopental anesthetic requirement, pharmacokinetics, or pharmacodynamics. Anesthesiology 1990;72:455–61

52. Duvaldestin P, Agoston S, Henzel D, et al. Pancuronium pharmacokinetics in patients with liver cirrhosis. Br J Anaesth 1978;50:1131–6

53. Bell CF, Hunter JM, Jones RS, Utting JE. Use of atracurium and vecuronium in patients with oesophageal varices. Br J Anaesth 1985;57:160–8

54. Parker CJR, Hunter JM. Pharmacokinetics of atracurium and laudanosine in patients with hepatic cirrhosis. Br J Anaesth 1989;62:177–83

55. Arden JR, Lynam DP, Castagnoli KP, Canfell PC, Cannol JC, Miller RD. Vecuronium in alcoholic liver disease: A pharmacokinetic and pharmadocynamic analysis. Anesthesiology 1988;68:771–6

56. Lebrault C, Berger JL, D'Hollander AA, Gomeni R, Henzel D, Duvaldestin P. Pharmacokinetics and pharmacodynamics of vecuronium (ORG NC45) in patients with cirrhosis. Anesthesiology 1985;62:601–5

57. Kaplan JA, Bitner RL, Dripps RD. Hypoxia, hyperdynamic circulation, and the hazards of general anesthesia in patients with hepatic cirrhosis. Anesthesiology 1971;35:427–31

58. Prager MC, Johnson KL, Ascher NL, Roberts JP. Anesthetic care of patients with Crigler-Najjar syndrome. Anesth Analg 1992;74:162–4

59. Carmichael FJ, Lindop MJ, Farman JV. Anesthesia for hepatic transplantation: Cardiovascular and metabolic alterations and their management. Anesth Analg 1985;64:108–16

60. Cheng EY, Woehlck HJ. Pulmonary artery hypertension complicating anesthesia for liver transplantation. Anesthesiology 1992;77:389–92

61. Hatano Y, Murakawa M, Segawa H, Nishida Y, Mori K. Venous air embolism during hepatic resection. Anesthesiology 1990;73:1282–5

62. O'Kelly B, Jayais P, Veroli P, Lhuissier C, Ecoffey C. Dose

requirements of vecuronium, pancuronium, and atracurium during orthotopic liver transplantation. Anesth Analg 1991;73:794–8

63. Pittett J-F, Tassonyi E, Schopfer C, et al. Plasma concentrations of laudanosine, but not of atracurium, are increased during the anhepatic phase of orthotopic liver transplantation in pigs. Anesthesiology 1990;72:145–52

64. Way LW. Changing therapy for gallstone disease. N Engl J Med 1990;323:1273–4

65. Wolfe BM, Gardiner B, Frey CF. Laparoscopic cholecystectomy: A remarkable development. JAMA 1991;265:1573–4

66. Westra P, Vermeer GA, deLange AR, et al. Hepatic and renal disposition of pancuronium and gallamine in patients with extrahepatic cholestasis. Br J Anaesth 1981;53:331–8

67. Marco PA, Yeo CJ, Rock P. Anesthesia for the patient undergoing laparoscopic cholecystectomy. Anesthesiology 1990;73:1268–70

68. Clark CC, Weeks DB, Gusdon JP. Venous carbon dioxide embolism during laparoscopy. Anesth Analg 1977;56:650–2

69. Taylor E, Feinstein R, White PF, Soper N. Anesthesia for laparoscopic cholecystectomy. Is nitrous oxide contraindicated? Anesthesiology 1992;76:541–3

70. Murphy P, Saleman J, Roseman DL. Narcotic anesthetic drugs. Arch Surg 1980;115:710–1

71. Radnay PA, Duncalf D, Novakovic M, Lesser ML. Common bile duct pressure changes after fentanyl, morphine, meperidine, butorphanol, and naloxone. Anesth Analg 1984;63:441–4

72. McCammon RL, Viegas OJ, Stoelting RK, Dryden GE. Naloxone reversal of choledochoduodenal sphincter spasm associated with narcotic administration. Anesthesiology 1978;48:437

73. Jones RM, Detmer M, Hill AB, Bjoraker DE. Incidence of choledochoduodenal sphincter spasm during fentanyl-supplemented anesthesia. Anesth Analg 1981;60:638–40

74. Jones RM, Fiddian-Gree R, Knight PR. Narcotic-induced choledochoduodenal sphincter spasm reversed by glucagon. Anesth Analg 1980;59:946–7

19

Diseases of the Gastrointestinal System

The principal function of the gastrointestinal tract is to provide the body with a continual supply of water, nutrients, and electrolytes. Each section of the gastrointestinal tract is adapted for specific functions, such as passage of food in the esophagus, storage of food in the stomach, and digestion and absorption of nutrients in the small intestine and proximal colon.

ESOPHAGEAL DISEASES

Dysphagia is the classic symptom produced at some stage in all disorders of the esophagus. Barium contrast examination is recommended in patients with dysphagia. After the barium contrast study, esophagoscopy permits direct viewing of the esophagus, as well as recovery of biopsy and cytology specimens.

Diffuse Esophageal Spasm

Diffuse esophageal spasm occurs most often in elderly patients. It is most likely due to an alteration in the innervation of the esophagus by the autonomic nervous system. Pain produced by esophageal spasm may mimic angina pectoris. Indeed, some patients respond favorably to nitroglycerin. Nifedipine and isosorbide, which decrease lower esophageal sphincter (LES) pressure, may also relieve pain produced by esophageal spasm.[1]

Chronic Peptic Esophagitis

Chronic peptic esophagitis is caused by reflux of acidic gastric fluid into the esophagus, producing retrosternal discomfort (heartburn) relieved by oral administration of antacids. Reflux esophagitis is a common clinical problem, with more than one-third of healthy adults experiencing the symptoms of heartburn at least once a month.[2] Normally, the LES exerts a relatively high resting pressure in the terminal 1 to 2 cm of the esophagus; this pressure tends to protect against spontaneous gastroesophageal reflux. The underlying defect leading to esophagitis seems to be a decrease in the resting tone of the LES. Indeed, patients with reflux esophagitis have decreased LES pressures (average 13 mmHg versus 29 mmHg in normal patients).[3]

Treatment of reflux esophagitis is initially with oral antacids and avoidance of substances (fat, chocolate, alcohol, nicotine) that decrease LES pressure. Cimetidine or an equivalent drug may promote healing in these patients. Persistent and severe symptoms may be relieved by a surgical procedure designed to create a valve mechanism, by wrapping a gastric pouch around the distal esophagus (Nissen fundoplication). Alternatively, an antrectomy with Roux-en-Y duodenal diversion or placement of a C-shaped plastic prosthesis (Angelchick valve) around the distal esophagus may be beneficial. Patients with chronic esophagitis are at risk of the development of a stricture at the distal esophagus, requiring treatment with tapered dilators.

Management of Anesthesia

Preoperative evaluation of the patient with chronic peptic esophagitis logically involves the exclusion of pneumonia, as may be evident on a chest radiograph. The decision to include an anticholinergic drug in the preoperative medication must be weighed against the known ability of these drugs to decrease LES tone.[4] Theoretically, an anticholinergic drug, by decreasing LES pressure, could increase the likelihood of silent regurgitation and the possibility of pulmonary aspiration. This potential adverse effect of anticholinergic drugs has not been documented. Furthermore, a decrease in the pH of esophageal fluid as evidence of gastric fluid reflux during general anesthesia is unlikely in the absence of upper airway obstruction or patient movement in response to the presence of a tracheal tube.[5,6] In this regard, the incidence of postoperative symptoms attributable to pulmonary aspiration is impressively minimal when adult and pediatric patients undergo elective operations.[7-9] For these reasons, it does not seem justifiable to avoid an anticholinergic drug in the preoperative medication solely because a patient is known to experience reflux esophagitis. Likewise, routine use of metoclopramide or an H-2 receptor antagonist, or both, in the preoperative medication of these patients cannot be supported by the available data. Succinylcholine increases LES pressure, but barrier pressure (LES pressure minus gastric pressure) is unchanged since fasciculations are associated with an increase in gastric pressure.[10]

Hiatus Hernia

Hiatus hernia is a protrusion of a portion of the stomach through the hiatus of the diaphragm and into the thoracic cavity. The sliding type of hiatus hernia, formed by movement of the upper stomach through an enlarged hiatus, can be identified in about 30% of patients undergoing an upper gastrointestinal radiographic examination. Because hiatus hernia and peptic esophagitis frequently co-exist by chance, they have been erroneously considered to have a cause-and-effect relationship. Based on the assumption that the hiatus hernia predisposes to the development of peptic esophagitis, surgical repair of the hernia may be recommended. Nevertheless, most patients with hiatus hernia do not have symptoms of reflux esophagitis, emphasizing the importance of the integrity of the LES. Oral antacids or therapy with H-2 antagonists is not necessary for patients with hiatus hernia in the absence of symptoms of reflux esophagitis.

Achalasia

Achalasia is a syndrome of aperistalsis and hypertonia of the LES. The esophagus consequently becomes progressively dilated. The cause of achalasia is unknown, but the syndrome is usually associated with a decrease in the number, or complete absence, of the neurons in the myenteric plexus of the esophageal muscle layers. Nifedipine administered sublingually decreases or eliminates symptoms of dysphagia in most patients with achalasia.[1]

Collagen Vascular Disease

Scleroderma, dermatomyositis, and polymyositis may involve the esophagus, manifested as slowed distal movement of food through the esophagus and decreased LES pressure that predisposes the patient to reflux esophagitis. Dysphagia is not seen early, presumably because decreased LES pres-

sure permits emptying of the esophagus by gravity. Eventually, chronic reflux of acidic gastric fluid produces a stricture in most patients.

Esophagitis Due to Drugs

Tablets often remain in the esophagus for 5 minutes or longer when swallowed with a small volume of liquid (about 15 ml).[11] Preferably, tablets are swallowed with at least 100 ml of water, with the patient remaining upright for at least 90 seconds, to ensure that the drug passes promptly into the stomach. Unless this precaution is taken, drugs such as aspirin may produce irritation of the esophageal mucosa.

Esophagitis and Stricture Due to Caustic Chemicals

Esophageal damage occurs in nearly all patients who ingest liquid caustic materials, especially when they contain alkali. The mouth and pharynx should be examined for oral burns. Diagnostic endoscopy is indicated for evaluation of esophageal or gastric mucosal damage.

Esophageal Infections

Esophageal infections owing to *Candida albicans* is a problem in immunosuppressed patients, typically developing several weeks after organ transplantation. Symptoms include dysphagia and retrosternal pain. Esophagoscopy is necessary for documentation of inflammation.

Esophageal Diverticula

Esophageal diverticula are classified according to their location as Zenker's diverticulum (upper esophagus), traction diverticulum (midesophageal), and epiphrenic diverticulum (near the LES). Regurgitation of previously ingested food from a Zenker's diverticulum may predispose patients to pulmonary aspiration, even in the absence of recent food intake. Surgical excision of this diverticulum may be performed in two stages, with an initial mobilization of the pouch, followed by complete excision after granulation tissue has formed.

Carcinoma of the Esophagus

For a discussion of carcinoma of the esophagus, see Chapter 28.

PEPTIC ULCER DISEASE

Peptic ulcer disease refers to an ulceration of the mucous membrane of the esophagus, stomach, or duodenum caused by hydrochloric acid and pepsin in the gastric fluid. Vagal stimulation causes cells in the antrum of the stomach to release gastrin, which enters the circulation. Gastrin subsequently causes the parietal cells in the body of the stomach to secrete hydrochloric acid. Hydrochloric acid secretion is also stimulated by histamine-mediated activation of H-2 receptors.

Duodenal Ulcer Disease

The development of a chronic ulcer in the duodenum just beyond the pylorus constitutes peptic ulcer disease of the duodenum. Because the clinical syndrome and response to treatment are similar for ulcers occurring in the distal antrum of the stomach and pylorus, these are also considered to be duodenal. The highest incidence of chronic duodenal ulceration is found in males aged 45 to 65 years and in females older than 55 years. The disease is about twice as common in males as in females, and is three times more common in first-degree relatives of patients with known ulcer disease.

The causes of duodenal ulcer disease are unknown, but affected patients have about twice the normal number of parietal cells. Contrary to popular belief, drugs such as indomethacin, corticosteroids, and alcohol do not predispose to the development of peptic ulcer disease. Aspirin on a regular basis in doses of 1.2 to 2.4 g·d^{-1} probably predisposes to peptic ulcer disease. Emotional stress has been implicated in the development of peptic ulcer disease, but there is little evidence to support this association.[3] The incidence of duodenal ulcer disease seems to be increased in patients with chronic obstructive airway disease, rheumatoid arthritis, cirrhosis of the liver, and hyperparathyroidism. Critically ill patients may be at increased risk of the development of peptic ulcer disease with bleeding. In this regard, administration of antacids or H-2 receptor antagonists, or both, to maintain a gastric fluid pH of greater than 3.5 has been recommended.

Signs and Symptoms

The typical complaint of duodenal ulcer disease is aching pain in the midepigastrum that may awaken the patient and is relieved by food or antacids. Vomiting is unlikely, and weight gain may reflect increased ingestion of food for pain relief. Serum electrolytes and liver function tests are usually normal, whereas anemia may reflect chronic hemorrhage.

Complications of duodenal ulcer disease are unusual. When they do develop, they typically include bleeding, gastrointestinal obstruction owing to edema, or fibrosis in the area of the liver, and perforation into the peritoneal cavity or pancreas. Gastric outlet obstruction is suggested by a retained gastric fluid volume of greater than 300 ml, present 30 minutes after oral ingestion of 750 ml of saline.

Treatment

Dietary therapy, consisting of a bland diet and ingestion of multiple small meals, has not been shown to accelerate ulcer healing. Milk is a poor antacid and may actually stimulate the

secretion of hydrochloric acid. Oral antacids are the mainstay of duodenal ulcer therapy, with H-2 receptor antagonists, sucralfate, and anticholinergics serving as alternative therapies. Peptic ulcers heal more slowly in smokers than in nonsmokers. Surgical therapy may ultimately be necessary in some patients.

Antacids

Antacids produce a beneficial effect on peptic ulcer healing equivalent to H-2 antagonists.[12] Potential complications of antacid therapy are acid rebound, milk-alkali syndrome, and phosphorus depletion. Acid rebound is the increase in gastric acid secretion that may occur after neutralization produced by calcium-containing antacids. Milk-alkali syndrome is characterized by hypercalcemia, increased blood urea nitrogen, and alkalosis that may occur in patients taking calcium-containing antacids and ingesting large amounts (about 1 L) of milk daily. In the acute stage of milk-alkali syndrome, skeletal muscle weakness and polyuria may occur. Phosphorus depletion can occur in patients who ingest large doses of aluminum-containing antacids, as this drug binds phosphate in the intestinal lumen, preventing absorption. Acute phosphorous depletion can produce anorexia, skeletal muscle weakness, and fatigue, whereas osteoporosis and pathologic fractures may accompany chronic phosphorus depletion.

H-2 Receptor Antagonists

H-2 receptor antagonists (cimetidine, ranitidine, famotidine) block hydrochloric acid secretion in the stomach and are as effective as antacids in promoting the healing of duodenal ulcers.[13] The side effects of H-2 antagonists may have important anesthetic implications (Table 19-1). In this regard, famotidine may be less likely to alter the hepatic microsomal P-450 system and prolong the elimination half-times of concomitantly administered drugs.

Sucralfate

Sucralfate is an aluminum salt of sulfated sucrose that adheres to ulcers to promote healing. In addition, sucralfate appears to increase the gastric mucus layer. Clinical trials demonstrate

Table 19-1. Side Effects of H-2 Antagonists

Decreased hepatic blood flow
Inhibition of P-450 enzyme system
Mental confusion
Leukopenia and thrombocytopenia
Interstitial nephritis
Hepatitis
Polymyositis
Bradycardia and hypotension
Gynecomastia

that sucralfate is as effective as antacids or H-2 antagonists for accelerating duodenal ulcer healing and is devoid of significant side effects.

Anticholinergics

Anticholinergic drug therapy for duodenal ulcer disease is based on the fact that these drugs competitively inhibit the actions of acetylcholine on acid-secreting cells in the stomach. The value of this therapy is limited, as the effective dose is likely to produce unacceptable side effects, such as blurring of vision and urinary retention. Anticholinergic drugs do seem to augment and prolong the inhibitory effects of H-2 antagonists on gastric acid secretion. Pirenzepine is an anticholinergic that selectively inhibits gastric acid secretion without producing side effects.

Surgery

Surgical treatment of peptic ulcer disease is used less than previously, reflecting the effectiveness of medical therapy. Treatment of gastric outlet obstruction consists of continuous nasogastric suction to remove hydrochloric acid and to permit edema to subside. When gastric outlet obstruction is the result of scarring it is usually unresponsive to nasogastric suction; a surgical procedure such as pyloroplasty (a drainage procedure) plus vagotomy is the preferred treatment. Patients who have persistent recurrent peptic ulcer disease may benefit from an antrectomy with a Billroth I or II anastomosis.[14] Patients subjected to gastric surgical procedures are at risk of the development of the dumping syndrome, manifested as nausea, skeletal muscle weakness, and diaphoresis within 15 to 60 minutes after meals. Treatment of a perforated peptic ulcer is laparotomy and sealing of the perforation, most often with a piece of omentum. Posterior perforation of an ulcer into the pancreas producing acute pancreatitis is usually treated with antacids and nasogastric suction.

Gastrinoma

Gastrinoma is a neoplasm that usually develops in the pancreas or duodenum. This tumor secretes gastrin, which stimulates parietal cells to secrete enormous amounts of hydrochloric acid. Zollinger-Ellison syndrome is present when a gastrinoma causes intractable pain and ulcers. Abdominal pain and diarrhea are common presenting complaints. Other endocrine neoplasias (insulinoma, pituitary adenoma, parathyroid adenoma, thyroid adenoma) occur in about one-fourth of patients with a gastrinoma. This association is known as multiple endocrine neoplasia type I (MEN I).

Treatment of gastrinoma is surgical excision, as antacids are not effective. Often multiple adenomas or metastases are present. H-2 antagonists may be useful when surgical cure is not possible. Alternatively, omeprazole, a proton pump inhibitor, may be useful.

Management of Anesthesia

Management of anesthesia for surgical excision of a gastrinoma must consider gastric hypersecretion and the likelihood of a large gastric fluid volume at the time of induction of anesthesia. Esophageal reflux is common in these patients despite the ability of gastrin to increase LES tone. Depletion of intravascular fluid volume and electrolyte imbalance (hypokalemia and metabolic alkalosis) may accompany profuse watery diarrhea. Associated endocrine abnormalities (MEN I) could also influence management of anesthesia in these patients.

Gastric Ulcer

Gastric ulcers, in contrast to more common duodenal ulcers, are associated with normal gastric acid secretion, or even hypochlorhydria. A change in mucosal resistance most likely predisposes to the development of a gastric ulcer. Weight loss is common, owing to the associated pain and anorexia. Malignant degeneration of a benign gastric ulcer accounts for less than 3% of gastric carcinomas. If medical therapy does not promote healing of the gastric ulcer within 3 months, surgical excision of the ulcer, with or without vagotomy, and pyloroplasty is a consideration.

IRRITABLE BOWEL SYNDROME

Patients with irritable bowel syndrome (spastic or mucous colitis) often complain of generalized bowel discomfort, usually confined to the left lower quadrant. There may be constipation, but more commonly the frequency of stools is increased, and the feces are covered with mucus. Many patients have associated symptoms of vasomotor instability, including tachycardia, hyperventilation, fatigue, diaphoresis, and headaches. Air trapped in the splenic flexure may produce pain in the left shoulder, radiating down the left arm. This latter symptom is the reason for the occasional designation of this disease as the splenic flexure syndrome. Despite the frequent occurrence of irritable bowel syndrome, there is no known etiologic agent or structural or biochemical defect. The syndrome appears to be an intense intra-abdominal response to emotional tension.

INFLAMMATORY BOWEL DISEASE

Ulcerative colitis and Crohn's disease represent types of inflammatory bowel disease that have different manifestations, prognosis, and treatment[15] (Table 19-2).

Ulcerative Colitis

Ulcerative colitis is an inflammatory disease of the colonic mucosa that primarily affects the rectum and distal colon. The cause of the disease is unknown, and remissions followed by exacerbations are common. There is a definite clustering of the disease within certain ethnic groups; it is most common among those of Jewish origin. Females, usually between the ages of 25 and 45 years, are affected most often. Most patients have mild disease characterized by intermittent diarrhea and cramping abdominal pain. Fatigue, low-grade fever, and weight loss occur during exacerbations.

Severe ulcerative colitis is associated with complications classified as colonic and extracolonic (Table 19-3). Toxic megacolon is manifested as the sudden onset of fever, tachycardia, dehydration, and dilation of the colon. Intestinal perforation is associated with rebound pain, except when high doses of corticosteroids mask the symptoms. Apparently because of the presence of chronic inflammation produced by ulcerative colitis, patients are at increased risk of the development of carcinoma of the colon. Elective colectomy is considered when epithelial dysplasia is discovered during colonoscopic surveillance, especially when the duration of the disease exceeds 8 years. Arthritis tends to be restricted to large joints and is most often present when the colitis is clinically active. Patients with ulcerative colitis have an increased incidence of ankylosing spondylitis. Liver disease is manifested most often as fatty liver infiltration or pericholangitis with jaundice and increased plasma alkaline phosphatase.

Table 19-3. Complications Associated With Ulcerative Colitis

Complication	Incidence (%)
Colonic	
Toxic megacolon	1–3
Intestinal perforation	3
Carcinoma of the colon	2.5–30
Hemorrhage	4
Stricture	10
Extracolonic	
Erythema nodosum	3
Iritis	5–10
Ankylosing arthritis	5–10
Fatty liver infiltration	40
Pericholangitis	30–50
Cirrhosis of the liver	3

Treatment

Initial treatment of ulcerative colitis is with antidiarrheal drugs and sulfasalazine. Treatment with systemic corticosteroids is reserved for patients with persistent symptomatic disease. Abrupt exacerbations may require hospitalization to replace electrolytes and intravascular fluid volume. The only curative treatment is proctocolectomy with ileostomy. About 25% of patients with ulcerative colitis undergo this procedure during the first 5 years of the disease.

Crohn's Disease

Crohn's disease is characterized by ileal and colonic involvement (granulomatous ileocolitis) in about 50% of patients, whereas the remainder are equally divided between those with disease restricted to the small intestine (regional enteritis) and those with disease confined to the colon. The cause of Crohn's disease is unknown; the peak incidence is at about 30 years of age.

There is chronic inflammation of all layers of the bowel, often leading to the development of fistulas between the diseased intestinal loops and adjacent structures. Rectal fissures, rectocutaneous fistulas, or perirectal abscesses occur in as many as 50% of patients. Extracolonic complications include arthritis and iritis. Renal stones and gallstones containing calcium oxalate are common, especially if the distal ileum is involved, reflecting increased colonic absorption of oxalate. Anemia is likely and may be due to chronic hemorrhage, iron deficiency, vitamin B_{12} deficiency, or folate deficiency. Decreased plasma albumin concentrations reflect protein loss through diseased bowel mucosa. Distinction from ulcerative

Table 19-2. Comparative Features of Ulcerative Colitis and Crohn's Disease

Feature	Ulcerative Colitis	Crohn's Disease
Acute toxicity	Common	Rare
Stools	Bloody, watery	Watery
Perirectal involvement	Occurs in 10–20%, but usually self-limiting	Rectocutaneous fistulas in 50%
Extracolonic complications	Common	Common
Carcinoma of colon	5% after 10 years	1%, but unrelated to extent or duration of the disease
Treatment	Proctocolectomy is curative	Recurrence likely despite surgical resection

colitis is important, since Crohn's disease is infrequently associated with cancer, and recurrence after surgical resection is common (20% to 80% within 5 years).

Treatment

Treatment of Crohn's disease is similar to that of ulcerative colitis, including systemic corticosteroids. Corticosteroids produce a prompt remission but must be continued chronically to maintain an asymptomatic state. Other potentially useful drugs include sulfasalazine, metronidazole, and azathioprine. Hyperalimentation may be indicated if weight loss and malnutrition are prominent. An estimated 60% of patients will require surgery because of drug failure or the development of complications such as intra-abdominal fistulas.

Pseudomembranous Enterocolitis

Pseudomembranous enterocolitis is attributable to unknown causes although it is often associated with antibiotic therapy (especially clindamycin and lincomycin), bowel obstruction, uremia, congestive heart failure, and intestinal ischemia. Clinical manifestations include fever, watery diarrhea,

dehydration, hypotension, cardiac dysrhythmias, skeletal muscle weakness, intestinal ileus, and metabolic acidosis.

Management of Anesthesia

Surgical treatment of inflammatory bowel disease most often involves the resection of varying lengths and portions of the gastrointestinal tract. Management of anesthesia requires preoperative evaluation of intravascular fluid volume and electrolyte status, and assessment of both colonic and extracolonic complications (anemia, arthritis, liver disease) that may be associated with the inflammatory bowel process (Table 19-3). Underlying liver disease may influence the choice of volatile anesthetics and muscle relaxants. In the presence of bowel distension, the administration of nitrous oxide may be limited or avoided. The need to provide additional corticosteroids during the perioperative period is introduced when these drugs have been used as part of the medical therapy. Adverse effects associated with hyperalimentation must be appreciated (see Chapter 23). Although the reversal of nondepolarizing muscle relaxants with an anticholinesterase drug will increase gastrointestinal intraluminal pressure, there is no evidence this results in a risk of colon suture line dehiscence[16–18] (Fig. 19-1).

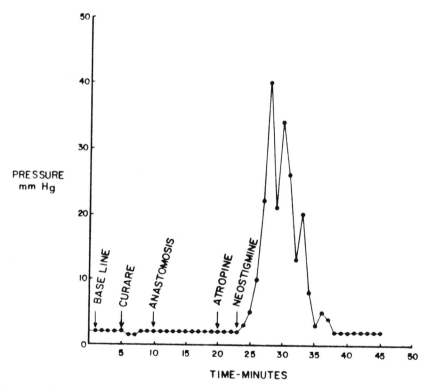

Fig. 19-1. Intraluminal colonic pressure was measured in a single anesthetized dog after division of the colon and a standard two-layer anastomosis. There was no evidence that the neostigmine-induced increase in intracolonic pressure caused disruption of the freshly completed bowel anastomosis. (From Yellin YE, Newman J, Donovan AJ. Neostigmine-induced hyperperistalsis. Effects on security of colonic anastomoses. Arch Surg 1973;106:779–81, with permission.)

CARCINOID TUMORS

Carcinoid tumors arise from enterochromaffin tissues and are typically found in the gastrointestinal tract. Indeed, carcinoid tumors are the most common neoplasms of the small intestine, with the highest incidence in the appendix, where these tumors can mimic acute appendicitis. On occasion, carcinoid tumors arise in the bronchi, where they are histologically indistinguishable from undifferentiated small cell carcinomas. Rarely, carcinoid tumors arise from the ovaries. The diagnosis of carcinoid tumor is supported by increased urinary excretion of 5-hydroxyindoleacetic acid, the degradation product of serotonin.

Carcinoid Syndrome

Carcinoid syndrome is present when vasoactive substances (serotonin, kallikreins, histamine) released from cells of carcinoid tumors result in clinical symptoms[19] (Table 19-4). Kallikreins are important because they activate a plasma factor (kininogen) that subsequently produces a group of polypeptides (kinins) that includes bradykinin. Normally, release of vasoactive substances produces minimal if any symptoms, as the liver is able to inactivate these substances effectively before they reach the systemic circulation. Manifestations of the carcinoid syndrome occur when the output of vasoactive substances overwhelms the ability of the liver to inactivate these substances. Hepatic metastases are usually present when manifestations of carcinoid syndrome develop. Indeed, the presence of metastatic carcinoid cells in the liver may permit direct access of these vasoactive substances to the circulation. Overall, carcinoid syndrome develops in about 5% of patients with carcinoid tumor.[20]

Carcinoid tumors in the bronchi or ovaries may produce symptoms of the carcinoid syndrome earlier than similar tumors located in the jejunum or ileum because pulmonary or ovarian tumors do not drain into the portal venous system. As a result, vasoactive substances are not inactivated in the liver. Carcinoid tumors in the appendix have never been reported to produce the carcinoid syndrome.

Table 19-4. Signs and Symptoms of the Carcinoid Syndrome

Bronchoconstriction-asthma
Tricuspid regurgitation and/or pulmonic stenosis
Premature atrial beats and supraventricular tachydysrhythmias
Episodic cutaneous flushing or cyanosis
Venous telangiectasia
Chronic abdominal pain and diarrhea
Hepatomegaly
Hyperglycemia
Decreased plasma albumin concentrations

Signs and Symptoms

Bronchoconstriction in a patient with a carcinoid tumor reflects the release of vasoactive substances capable of producing constriction of airway smooth muscle (Table 19-4). Tricuspid regurgitation or pulmonic stenosis represents the type of right-sided valvular heart lesion that can result from valve cusp distortion produced by metastases from a carcinoid tumor. The valves on the left side of the heart are spared, which may reflect the ability of pulmonary parenchymal cells to inactivate vasoactive substances. Patients with carcinoid syndrome have an increased incidence of atrial premature beats and supraventricular tachydysrhythmias.

Episodic cutaneous flushing initially involves the face and neck; with increasing intensity and duration, it may spread to involve the trunk and upper extremities. During cutaneous flushing, arterial blood pressure is usually decreased, and cardiac output is likely to be decreased. Bradykinin is a potent vasodilator that seems the most likely cause of cutaneous flushing. Chronic intermittent abdominal pain and diarrhea are most likely due to release of serotonin by carcinoid tumor cells. Hepatomegaly may reflect extensive hepatic metastases from carcinoid tumors. Mild hyperglycemia and decreased plasma albumin concentrations may be present in patients with carcinoid tumors. Hyperglycemia most likely reflects the ability of serotonin to mimic the metabolic effects of epinephrine and to stimulate glycogenolysis and gluconeogenesis. Hypoalbuminemia may reflect the diversion of tryptophan from the production of protein to synthesis of serotonin. Normally, less than 2% of dietary tryptophan is used in the synthesis of serotonin, but up to 60% of this amino acid can be used for this purpose by tumor cells in patients with carcinoid tumors.

Management of Anesthesia

Carcinoid tumors and their manifestations have important implications for the management of anesthesia. Patients with carcinoid syndrome may present in the operating room for primary resection of the carcinoid tumor or for removal of hepatic metastases. On occasion, these patients may require replacement of a heart valve. Preoperative preparation of these patients with a drug(s) that blocks effects of vasoactive substances secreted by the carcinoid tumor cells is recommended. In this regard, pretreatment with octreotide, a synthetic somatostatin analogue, is useful in inhibiting ectopic hormone release.[21-23] The recommended dose of octreotide is 50 μg IV and 50 μg subcutaneously, prior to manipulation of the tumor. Somatostatin is a growth hormone release inhibitory hormone that is known to inhibit the release of several gastrointestinal hormones and of vasoactive substances from carcinoid tumors. The use of somatostatin or an analogue has rendered administration of antihistamine drugs and antiserotonin drugs (cyproheptadine, ketanserin) superfluous.[21] The therapeutic effects of somatostatin are limited because of its short

(2- to 3-minute) half-time, when administered intravenously. Intraoperative carcinoid crises (hypotension, bronchospasm) most often associated with manipulation of the tumor have also been effectively treated with somatostatin or an analogue.[21,24]

No specific anesthetic drugs or techniques have proved superior in patients with carcinoid tumors.[25] Since hypotension may stimulate the release of vasoactive substances from tumor cells, it is important to consider the potential adverse effects of deep anesthesia or the effects of peripheral sympathetic nervous system blockade, as produced by regional anesthetic techniques. In this regard, preoperative hydration may be prudent. Although not popularized, regional anesthesia seems an acceptable alternative to general anesthesia in these patients, especially for peripheral tissue operative procedures.[23] Drugs such as ketamine, which may activate the sympathetic nervous system, are unlikely selections, since catecholamines are known to activate kallikreins. Likewise, drug-induced histamine release should be avoided, if possible. Increased central nervous system levels of serotonin are associated with sedation, suggesting that anesthetic requirements might be decreased in these patients.

DISEASES OF THE PANCREAS

Acute Pancreatitis

Conditions that predispose to acute pancreatitis include excessive alcohol ingestion, gallstones, blunt abdominal trauma, and a penetrating peptic ulcer. Pancreatic cellular injury is common after cardiopulmonary bypass and may be associated with the intraoperative administration of large doses of calcium.[26] Acute pancreatitis is manifested by an elevated plasma amylase concentration in a patient experiencing intense midepigastric pain. Bilirubin and alkaline phosphatase concentrations may be increased, owing to compression of the common bile duct by the edematous head of the pancreas or by a stone in the common bile duct. Intestinal ileus is common. Hypotension and hypovolemia are related to exudation of plasma into the pancreatic area. Acute renal failure may occur if hypotension is prolonged. Hypocalcemia may develop, and patients should be observed for signs of tetany. Hemorrhagic pancreatitis may result in diabetic coma. Breathing may be painful in the presence of a pleural effusion and pleuritis. The differential diagnosis of acute pancreatitis includes acute cholecystitis, acute myocardial infarction, and pneumonia. Ultrasonography and computed tomography may demonstrate an enlarged edematous pancreas. Treatment of acute pancreatitis consists of nasogastric suction, fluid and electrolyte repletion, and opioids for analgesia. Surgical therapy may be attempted if pancreatitis is caused by duct obstruction produced by stones or an adenoma. Hypoglycemia may be a risk after surgery of the pancreas.

Chronic Pancreatitis

Chronic pancreatitis characteristically presents in emaciated males who are chronic alcoholics. Predisposing conditions in addition to alcoholism include severe biliary tract disease and blunt abdominal trauma that may have occurred many years earlier. Plasma amylase concentrations are often normal during recurrent episodes of chronic pancreatitis. Jaundice occurs in about 10% of patients. Maldigestion of fat and protein supervenes when about 80% of the pancreas is destroyed. Mild diabetes mellitus is common, and fatty liver filtration is likely to be present.

Pancreatic Cancer

For a discussion of pancreatic cancer, see Chapter 28.

GASTROINTESTINAL BLEEDING

Gastrointestinal bleeding is most often from a duodenal ulcer or is a manifestation of gastritis (Table 19-5). Endoscopy is useful in identifying the site of gastrointestinal bleeding. Specific sites of bleeding are also suggested by the history. For example, epigastric pain that precedes passage of black stools suggests peptic ulcer disease. Lower abdominal pain, fever, and bloody diarrhea are common in the presence of diverticulosis. The passage of bright red blood through a nasogastric tube suggests bleeding esophageal varices or a Mallory-Weiss tear at the esophagogastric junction. Patients in intensive care units are at increased risk of gastroduodenal bleeding because of the stress of their acute illness.

Most acute gastrointestinal bleeding is self-limited, ceasing within 24 to 48 hours in 80% or more of patients treated with conservative medical management. Laser photocoagulation may be useful in controlling hemorrhage in some patients. When upper gastrointestinal bleeding is rapid and severe, the

Table 19-5.   Causes of Upper Gastrointestinal Bleeding

Cause	Incidence (%)
Duodenal ulcer	27
Gastritis	23
Varices	14
Esophagitis	13
Gastric ulcer	8
Mallory-Weiss tear	7
Bowel infarction	3
Idiopathic	5

blood urea nitrogen concentration may exceed 40 mg·dl^{-1} because of the absorbed nitrogen load from blood in the small intestine. Colonic bleeding does not usually cause an increase in the blood urea nitrogen concentration. Hypotension associated with massive gastrointestinal hemorrhage may result in myocardial infarction, renal failure, and hepatic centrilobular necrosis.

DISEASES PRODUCING MALABSORPTION AND MALDIGESTION

Malabsorption denotes altered food absorption owing to a defect in the mucosa of the small intestine or in a resection of the small intestine, whereas maldigestion is caused by deficiencies of pancreatobiliary secretions (Table 19-6). There are important differences between diseases that produce malabsorption or maldigestion (Table 19-7). Weight loss, vitamin deficiencies, anemia, and hypoalbuminemia (protein loss through damaged intestinal mucosa) are more likely with malabsorption, while steatorrhea is the hallmark of maldigestion. Hypocalcemia and hypomagnesemia may result in tetany and mental confusion in patients with disease of the small intestine. In severe malabsorption, vitamin K deficiency may prolong the prothrombin time to the extent that ecchymoses develop.

Celiac Sprue

Celiac sprue is characterized by weight loss, fatigue, and megaloblastic anemia owing to folic acid deficiency. This disease is often associated with short stature (150 cm) in females. Therapy is directed at removal of glutein (wheat, barley, oats, beer, whiskey) from the diet. The most important complications of celiac sprue are the development of ulcerations and

Table 19-6. Diseases Associated With Malabsorption or Maldigestion

Malabsorption (Small Intestine Defects)	Maldigestion (Pancreatic Defects)
Celiac sprue	Chronic pancreatitis
Tropical sprue	Bile salt deficiency syndrome
Diabetes mellitus	Postgastrectomy steatorrhea
Resection of the ileum	
Ischemia of the small intestine	
Radiation enteritis	
Regional enteritis	
Amyloidosis	
Systemic mastocytosis	
Acquired immunodeficiency syndrome	

Table 19-7. Differences Between Malabsorption (Small Intestine Disease) and Maldigestion (Pancreatic Disease)

	Malabsorption	Maldigestion
Weight loss	Marked	Mild to absent
Vitamin deficiency (A, B, E, K, B$_{12}$)	Common	Rare
Anemia	Common (usually megaloblastic)	Rare (unless associated with alcoholism)
Hypoalbuminemia	Common	Rare
Hypomagnesemia	Common	Rare
Steatorrhea	Moderate ($<$35 g·d^{-1})	Marked (40–80 g·d^{-1})

small intestine malignancies. Prednisone may be administered for the treatment of ulcerations, although surgery is often necessary.

Tropical Sprue

Tropical sprue is characterized by fatigue, weight loss, and severe megaloblastic anemia (hematocrit less than 25%). Folic acid therapy is effective in most patients; in the remainder, the addition of an antibiotic (ampicillin) is effective.

Diabetes Mellitus

Autonomic nervous system neuropathy causing stasis in the small intestine develops in a significant number of patients with diabetes mellitus. Watery diarrhea is prominent and malabsorption occurs in some patients, presumably as a result of bacterial overgrowth. In this regard, broad-spectrum antibiotics may be effective.

Resection of the Ileum

Extensive jejunal resection results in only mild malabsorption because of compensation by the ileum. By contrast, ileal resection is often followed by severe nutritional problems because the jejunum cannot readily adapt to the loss of ileum, particularly to the loss of the specialized sites for bile salt and vitamin B$_{12}$ absorption. Extensive resection of the small intestine may be associated with profuse diarrhea, as malabsorption of solutes causes an excessive osmotic load. There is an increased incidence of cholelithiasis and nephrolithiasis in these patients.

Ischemia of the Small Intestine

Atherosclerosis of blood vessels supplying the small intestine is manifested as severe abdominal pain after a meal. Malabsorption is usually not severe; nevertheless, weight loss is common, as patients avoid eating to escape postprandial discomfort. With acute ischemia, abdominal signs suggesting peritonitis may be present. Emergency surgery may be required if bowel necrosis is suspected, whereas arterial bypass graft surgery may be considered in stable patients. Ischemic heart disease or cerebralvascular disease, or both, is often present in those patients with atherosclerosis involving the small intestinal vessels.

Radiation Enteritis

Radiation enteritis after treatment of intra-abdominal cancer has become a relatively common cause of malabsorption. Acute radiation enteritis occurs within a few days after therapy, manifested as acute watery diarrhea. Corticosteroids may be necessary in the management of these patients.

DIVERTICULOSIS AND DIVERTICULITIS

Diverticulosis is characterized by multiple outpouchings of the colonic mucosa, most often located in the sigmoid colon. These outpouchings are demonstrable in about 50% of patients older than 60 years of age, who are undergoing barium enema. The pathogenesis of diverticulosis has not been clearly defined, although it may be linked to an increase in intracolonic pressure or to a structural weakness in the colonic submucosa, or both. The relationship between diverticulosis and irritable bowel syndrome has not been clearly established.

The incidence of diverticular bleeding is infrequent (less than 2% of afflicted patients) but, when it does occur, it can be massive. Nevertheless, the bleeding generally stops spontaneously, with rebleeding unlikely. Segmental colectomy is considered either when bleeding does not cease spontaneously or when it recurs.

Diverticulitis develops in only about 1% of patients who have diverticulosis. Clinical manifestations include cramping, lower abdominal pain, fever attributable to bacteremia, and profuse diarrhea that may result in hypovolemia and hypokalemia. In some patients, colonic obstruction or perforation occurs, and ileus may develop because of inflammation of the overlying peritoneum. A barium-contrast abdominal radiograph and computed tomography can be useful in identifying an inflammatory mass. Diverticulitis of the right colon or cecum often necessitates exploratory surgery because of the difficulty in differentiating this condition from acute appendicitis.

Appendicitis

Acute appendicitis occurs in about 7% of the U.S. population, with the highest incidence in those aged 10 to 30 years. Clinical manifestations of acute appendicitis are likely to be related to the stage of the disease and the location of the appendix. Initially, when inflammation is limited to the interior lining of the appendix, the perception of pain is vague and is often referred to the epigastric or periumbilical area. Within 12 to 24 hours, the inflammation spreads to the surface and involves the parietal peritoneum, producing pain that is more localized and accentuated by contraction of the abdominal muscles, for example, by coughing. Physical examination at this time produces rebound tenderness. If the appendix is in a location that does not lead to involvement of the parietal peritoneum, or when the involvement of the parietal peritoneum occurs late (a true retrocecal location), pain remains vague and poorly localized. Patients with retrocecal appendicitis are often diagnosed late in the course of the disease, and the incidence of rupture in these patients is high. Overall, the likelihood of appendiceal perforation increases rapidly about 72 hours after the onset of symptoms. Patients being treated with corticosteroids are at increased risk of perforation, since these drugs mask the initial symptoms of acute appendicitis. Peritonitis resulting from a ruptured or gangrenous appendix may be life-threatening and may be associated with subsequent adhesions and intestinal obstruction.

There is no specific test for the laboratory diagnosis of acute appendicitis. It is debatable whether the white blood count and differential count are useful, as perforation has been observed in the absence of leukocytosis. Furthermore, leukocytosis is common in patients who have conditions that mimic appendicitis but that do not require an operation. Fever is not a more useful indication than blood counts, as some patients remain afebrile. An abdominal radiograph demonstrating a fecalith in the right lower quadrant or air in the lumen of the appendix suggests acute appendicitis, but these are rare findings. Ultrasonography may be useful when the diagnosis of acute appendicitis is uncertain.[27] Appendectomy is the accepted treatment for acute appendicitis.

Differential Diagnosis

Several gynecologic conditions, including acute salpingitis, tubal pregnancy, ruptured ovarian cyst, and ovarian torsion, closely mimic acute appendicitis. A pregnancy test may be useful in evaluating some of these conditions. Mesenteric adenitis mimics acute appendicitis, although lymphocytosis may be suggestive of adenitis. Perforated duodenal ulcers may leak down the right lumbar gutter and present as right lower quadrant peritonitis. Inflammatory bowel disease also mimics acute appendicitis.

GASTROINTESTINAL POLYPS

Polypoid lesions of the gastrointestinal tract are common. Adenomas are the most important because of their association with malignant disease. Colonic polyps are the most prevalent and important, as they are considered premalignant. More than 95% of colonic polyps can be removed endoscopically, but larger or sessile lesions may require surgery. Segmental colon resection may be necessary when the adenoma contains invasive carcinoma.

Familial Polyposis Coli

Familial polyposis coli is inherited as an autosomal dominant trait, with multiple polyps usually appearing by 10 years of age. Left untreated, the incidence of malignant degeneration is nearly 100%. Surgical therapy is usually total colectomy with a permanent ileostomy. Gardner syndrome is characterized by familial polyposis plus multiple osteomas, cutaneous tumors, and abnormal dentition. Turcot's syndrome is multiple colonic polyps and tumors of the central nervous system. Peutz-Jeghers syndrome is manifested as melanotic spots on the lips and on the dorsum of the fingers and toes, as well as by colonic polyps that are not premalignant. The usual presentation of this syndrome is cramping abdominal pain in children, owing to intussusception.

REFERENCES

1. Richter JE, Dalton CB, Buice RG, et al. Nifedipine: A potent inhibitor of contractions in the body of the human esophagus: Studies in healthy volunteers and patients with the nutcracker esophagus. Gastroenterology 1985;89:549–55
2. Nebel OT, Fornes MF, Castell DO. Symptomatic gastroesophageal reflux: Incidence and precipitating factor. Dig Dis Sci 1976; 21:953–60
3. Feldman M, Walker P, Green JL, et al. Life events, stress and psychosocial factors in men with peptic ulcer disease. Gastroenterology 1986;91:1370–8
4. Brock-Utne JG, Welman RS, Dimopoulos GE, et al. The effect of glycopyrrolate (Robinal) on the lower esophageal sphincter. Can Anaesth Soc J 1978;25:144–6
5. Hardy J-F, Lepage Y, Bonneville-Chouinard N. Occurrence of gastroesophageal reflux on induction of anaesthesia does not correlate with the volume of gastric contents. Can J Anaesth 1990; 37:502–8
6. Illing L, Duncan PG, Yip R. Gastroesophageal reflux during anaesthesia. Can J Anaesth 1992;39:466–70
7. Tiret L, Nwoche Y, Hatton F, Desmonts JM, Vour'h G. Complications related to anaesthesia in infants and children: A prospective survey of 40,240 anaesthetics. Br J Anaesth 1988;61:263–9
8. Olsson GL, Hallen B, Hambraeus-Jonzon K. Aspiration during anaesthesia. A computer-aided study of 185,358 anaesthetics. Acta Anaesthesiol Scand 1986;30:84–92
9. Cote CJ. NPO after midnight for children—a reappraisal. Anesthesiology 1990;72:589–92
10. Smith G, Dalling R, Williams TIR. Gastroesophageal pressure gradient changes produced by induction of anaesthesia and suxamethonium. Br J Anaesth 1978;50:1137–42
11. Evans KT, Robert GM. Where do all tablets go? Lancet 1976;2: 1237–8
12. Faizallah R, DeHaan HA, Krasner N, et al. Is there a place in the United Kingdom for intensive antacid treatment for chronic peptic ulceration? Br Med J 1984;289:869–73
13. Bianchi-Porro G, Dicenta C, Cook T, et al. Review of an extensive worldwide study of a new H2-receptor antagonist, famotidine, as compared to ranitidine in the treatment of acute duodenal ulcer. J Clin Gastroenterology 1987;2:14–19
14. Strom M, Bodemar G, Lindhagen J, et al. Cimetidine or parietal-cell vagotomy in patients with juxtapyloric ulcers. Lancet 1984; 2:894–6
15. Podolsky DK. Inflammatory bowel disease. N Engl J Med 1991; 325:928–37
16. Yellin AE, Newman J, Conovan AJ. Neostigmine-induced hyperperistalsis. Effects on security of colonic anastomoses. Arch Surg 1973;106:779–81
17. Aitkenhead AR. Anaesthesia and bowel surgery. Br J Anaesth 1984;56:95–101
18. Hunter AR. Colorectal surgery for cancer: The anaesthetist's contribution? Br J Anaesth 1986;58:825–6
19. Oates JA. The carcinoid syndrome. N Engl J Med 1986;315: 702–4
20. Weidner FA, Ziter FMH. Cardinoid tumors of the gastrointestinal tract. JAMA 1981;245:1153–5
21. Parris WCV, Oates JA, Kambam J, Shmerling R, Sawyers JF. Pretreatment with somatostatin in the anaesthetic management of a patient with carcinoid syndrome. Can J Anaesth 1988;35: 413–6
22. Watson JT, Badner NH, Ali MJ. The prophylactic use of octreotide in a patient with ovarian carcinoid anal valvular heart disease. Can J Anaesth 1990;37:798–800
23. Monteith K, Roaseg OP. Epidural anaesthesia for transurethral resection of the prostate in a patient with carcinoid syndrome. Can J Anaesth 1990;37:349–52
24. Marsh MH, Martin JK, Kvols LK, et al. Carcinoid crisis during anesthesia: Successful treatment with somatostatin analogue. Anesthesiology 1987;66:89–91
25. Mason RA, Steans PA. Carcinoid syndrome: Its relevance to the anaesthetist. Anaesthesia 1976;31:228–42
26. Castillo CF-D, Harringer W, Warshaw AL, et al. Risk factors for pancreatic cellular injury after cardiopulmonary bypass. N Engl J Med 1991;325:382–7
27. Schwerk WB, Wichtrup B, Rathmund M, et al. Ultrasonography in the diagnosis of acute appendicitis: A prospective study. Gastroenterology 1989;97:630–7

20
Renal Disease

The principal function of the kidneys is to maintain a constant extracellular environment by regulating the excretion of fluid and electrolytes. Co-existing renal disease, which often presents in elderly patients, can predispose to perioperative morbidity and mortality.[1] Furthermore, the possibility of impaired renal function during the intraoperative and postoperative periods should be considered in otherwise healthy patients undergoing major operations.

FUNCTIONAL ANATOMY OF THE KIDNEYS

The functional unit of the kidneys is the nephron, which consists of the glomerulus and the renal tubule (Fig. 20-1). The glomerulus is a network of capillaries originating from an afferent arteriole. These capillaries are surrounded by the dilated blind end of the nephron, known as Bowman's capsule. The renal tubule consists of the proximal convoluted tubule, the loop of Henle, and the distal convoluted tubule. The distal ends of several distal convoluted tubules join to form the collecting tubules, which subsequently drain into the renal pelvis.

The proximal convoluted tubule is a direct continuation of Bowman's capsule. About 65% of the filtered sodium, chloride, and water is resorbed from the proximal convoluted tubules back into peritubular capillaries. Glucose is actively resorbed from the proximal convoluted tubules back into peritubular capillaries against a concentration gradient. When blood glucose concentrations exceed about 180 mg·dl^{-1}, the resorption threshold is exceeded, and glucose appears in the urine. Most of the filtered potassium is resorbed back into the peritubular capillaries from the proximal convoluted tubules. In addition, potassium is secreted by distal convoluted tubules into the peritubular capillaries. Resorption of calcium into peritubular capillaries from the proximal convoluted tubules is enhanced by parathyroid hormone. The loops of Henle are a continuation of the proximal convoluted tubules; this portion of the renal tubule is responsible for the formation of hypertonic fluid, by the countercurrent mechanism. Sodium, chloride, and water can be resorbed from the distal renal tubules, principally under the influence of aldosterone. Antidiuretic hormone (ADH) increases the permeability of distal convoluted tubules and collecting tubules, such that water is resorbed back into the peritubular capillaries and a small volume of highly concentrated urine enters the renal pelvis. The secretion of hydrogen ions by the renal tubular cells of distal convoluted tubules facilitates the elimination of acid metabolites, which result from normal dietary intake. Indeed, metabolic acidosis is a predictable feature of renal failure.

Endocrine Functions

In addition to serving as target organs for various hormones (parathyroid hormone, aldosterone, ADH), the kidneys are involved in both the metabolism and secretion of regulatory substances. For example, insulin is metabolized by the kidneys, which may explain the occasional improvement in glucose tolerance that occurs in diabetic patients in whom renal failure develops. Renin is a proteolytic enzyme secreted into the circulation by specialized smooth muscle cells of renal arterioles and segments of distal convoluted tubules known as the macula densa. Together, these specialized areas are designated the juxtaglomerular apparatus. Renin acts in the plasma on alpha-2-globulins synthesized in the liver (angiotensinogen), to form angiotensin I. Angiotensin I is then split by angiotensin-converting enzyme in the lungs, to form angiotensin II. Angiotensin II is a potent renal artery vasoconstrictor (decreases glomerular filtration rate and renal blood flow) that stimulates the release of aldosterone from the adrenal cortex. Prostaglandins are produced in the renal medulla and act as vasodilators (attenuate vasoconstriction produced by sympathetic nervous system activity and angiotensin II) or vasoconstrictors. Optimal effects of ADH may also be dependent on prostaglandins.

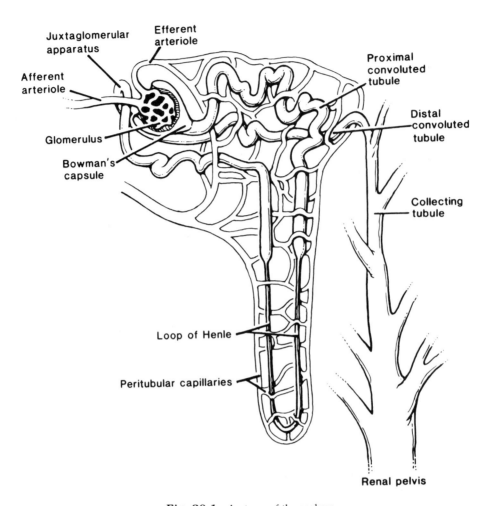

Fig. 20-1. Anatomy of the nephron.

Glomerular Filtration Rate

Despite relatively low filtration pressure (hydrostatic pressure minus plasma oncotic pressure), the glomerular capillaries are able to filter about 125 ml·min^{-1}, which is considered the normal glomerular filtration rate (GFR). About 90% of the fluid resulting from glomerular filtration is resorbed from the renal tubules back into the peritubular capillaries. Decreased perfusion pressure reduces hydrostatic pressure in the glomerular capillaries, and outward filtration is predictably decreased. Hemorrhage or dehydration can increase plasma oncotic pressure, resulting in decreased filtration pressure.

Renal Blood Flow

The kidneys represent about 0.5% of total body weight but receive 20% to 25% of the resting cardiac output. About two-thirds of the renal blood flow is to the renal cortex. Renal blood flow is autoregulated, remaining constant between a mean arterial pressure ranging from about 60 to 160 mmHg. By virtue of maintaining renal blood flow, the glomerular capillary hydrostatic pressure, and thus GFR, remain unchanged despite alterations in perfusion pressure over the range of autoregulation. Renal blood flow becomes pressure dependent outside the range of mean arterial pressure associated with autoregulation. Likewise, sympathetic nervous system stimulation produces renal artery vasoconstriction and decreased renal blood flow and GFR, despite maintenance of perfusion pressure within the range associated with autoregulation. Furthermore, any decrease in renal blood flow will initiate renin release, which, along with the release of catecholamines, can further decrease renal blood flow as well as alter distribution of blood flow in the kidneys. Prostaglandins may produce vasodilation, offsetting, to some extent, the renal artery vasoconstriction that results from release of renin.

TESTS FOR EVALUATION OF RENAL FUNCTION

Baseline renal function is defined by standard laboratory tests that evaluate GFR and renal tubular function (Table 20-1). GFR is the most frequently evaluated index of renal function. Although it is a useful tactic to consider glomerular function and renal tubular function separately when evaluating renal function, most diseases affecting the kidneys interfere with both. For example, anything that decreases GFR will compromise renal tubular function as well. This is predictable, since renal tubular cells are dependent on glomerular filtration for the delivery of fluid for selective absorption (water, sodium, glucose) or secretion (hydrogen, potassium).

It must be appreciated that most renal function tests are insensitive measurements, and significant renal disease can be present despite normal laboratory values. Indeed, at least one-half of normal renal function may be lost before tests of GFR show abnormal findings. Furthermore, clinical evidence of renal failure becomes evident only after more than 75% of nephrons are nonfunctional. Trends are more useful than isolated measurements in evaluating renal function.

Blood Urea Nitrogen

Blood urea nitrogen (BUN) varies inversely with GFR in patients ingesting a normal diet. Nevertheless, the BUN concentration is not a sensitive index of GFR because urea clearance also depends on the production rate and renal tubular resorption rate of urea. As a result, BUN can be abnormal despite a normal GFR. For example, the production rate of urea is increased by a high-protein diet or by gastrointestinal bleeding (hemoglobin is digested, as is blood in ingested meat). Other causes of increased BUN, despite a normal GFR, include increased catabolism during a febrile illness and enhanced resorption of urea from the renal tubules, owing to the slow movement of fluid through the renal tubules. Slow renal tubular flow allows more time for the action of ADH. Congestive heart failure is the most common cause of increased BUN, presumably reflecting the increased resorption of urea, owing to the slow rate of fluid flow through the renal

tubules. Likewise, increased BUN observed during dehydration or fluid deprivation most likely reflects increased urea resorption back into peritubular capillaries. When slow movement of fluid through the renal tubules is responsible for increased BUN, the plasma creatinine concentration remains normal.

BUN can remain normal in the presence of a low-protein diet (starvation, hemodialysis patients) despite marked decreases in GFR. Conversely, low levels of BUN can reflect an excess of total body water content. Despite these extraneous influences, a BUN above 50 mg·dl^{-1} almost always reflects a decreased GFR.

Plasma Creatinine

Plasma creatinine is a specific indicator of GFR, independent of protein metabolism or the rate of fluid flow through renal tubules. When skeletal muscle mass is constant (the source of creatinine), the plasma concentration of creatinine is dependent on GFR, as this material is not resorbed by the renal tubules. As GFR declines with advancing age, creatinine production also decreases because of decreasing skeletal muscle mass. Consequently, in an elderly patient, the plasma creatinine concentration may remain within normal limits, even though GFR decreases with aging. Indeed, a modest increase in the plasma creatinine concentration in an elderly patient should suggest significant renal disease. Likewise, in patients with chronic renal failure, measured plasma creatinine concentrations may not accurately reflect the GFR because of decreased production in the presence of reduced skeletal muscle mass. In general, however, a 50% increase in the plasma creatinine concentration reflects a corresponding decrease in GFR.

An important clinical consideration is the speed with which the plasma creatinine concentration increases after an abrupt change in GFR. The rate of change in the plasma creatinine concentration depends on the relationship between total body water and GFR. As a general rule, about 17 hours is required for equilibration to occur. Even at the maximal rate of increase in the absence of concurrent dilution, at least 8 hours is required for the plasma creatinine concentration to increase from a normal level to that suggestive of acute renal failure. Furthermore, with the total absence of renal function, the plasma creatinine concentration eventually plateaus, apparently as a result of nonrenal (gastrointestinal) excretion or inhibition of the production of creatinine.[2]

Creatinine Clearance

Creatinine clearance is the most reliable clinical estimate of GFR, independent of patient age and of whether a steady state is present. The principal disadvantage of this test is the need for accurate urine collections over a specified period of time.

Table 20-1.   Tests Used for Evaluation of Renal Function

Glomerular Filtration Rate	Renal Tubular Function
Blood urea nitrogen (10–20 mg·dl^{-1})	Urine specific gravity (1.003–1.030)
Plasma creatinine (0.7–1.5 mg·dl^{-1})	Urine osmolarity (38–1400 mOsm·L^{-1})
Creatinine clearance (110–150 ml·min^{-1})	

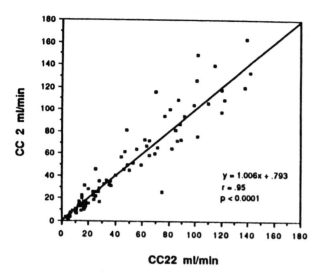

Fig. 20-2. Correlation between the 2-hour (CC 2) and 22-hour (CC 22) creatinine clearance. (From Sladen RN, Endo E, Harrison T. Two-hour versus 22-hour creatinine clearance in critically ill patients. Anesthesiology 1987;67:1013–6, with permission.)

Collection over 24 hours, however, may not be necessary, in view of accurate measurements obtained with a 2-hour collection period[3] (Fig. 20-2).

Moderate renal dysfunction is present when creatinine clearance values are less than 25 ml·min⁻¹. In these patients, the doses of drugs that depend on renal excretion, such as long-acting nondepolarizing muscle relaxants, should be decreased, and electrolyte and water replacement must be carefully monitored. Patients with a creatinine clearance of less than 10 ml·min⁻¹ can be considered anephric and will require hemodialysis for water and electrolyte hemostasis.

Urine Concentrating Ability

Renal tubular dysfunction is manifested as polyuria and dehydration and the demonstration that the kidneys do not produce appropriately concentrated urine in the presence of an adequate physiologic stimulus for the release of ADH. In the absence of diuretic therapy or glycosuria, a urinary specific gravity above 1.018 after an overnight fast makes impaired ability of renal tubules to concentrate urine an unlikely diagnosis.[4] Conversely, if urine osmolarity does not increase significantly above the osmolarity of plasma (at least 300 mOsm·L⁻¹) after standard periods of water deprivation, an impaired ability of renal tubules to concentrate urine is likely.

Exogenous ADH (vasopressin) may be administered after confirmation that urine osmolarity does not increase appropriately, in response to a physiologic stimulus such as overnight fasting. If urine osmolarity increases in response to vasopressin, the diagnosis of diabetes insipidus is established. If the administration of vasopressin does not increase the osmolarity of urine, it is likely that the renal tubules are unresponsive to ADH and that water is not undergoing resorption back into the peritubular capillaries. This renal tubular unresponsiveness to ADH is known as nephrogenic diabetes insipidus. Fluoride nephrotoxicity, as occurs after administration of such drugs as methoxyflurane, and rarely, enflurance, is an example of drug-induced nephrogenic diabetes insipidus.[5,6] Other causes of nephrogenic diabetes insipidus include the action of lithium, amphotericin B, and osmotic diuretics and the effects of hypercalcemia and hypokalemia.

Sodium Excretion

Urinary excretion of greater than 40 mEq·L⁻¹ sodium suggests a decreased ability of renal tubules to resorb sodium, as may accompany acute renal failure, owing to acute tubular necrosis of acute renal failure. Urine osmolarity is likely to be less than 350 mOsm·L⁻¹. Conversely, the decreased renal blood flow that accompanies hypovolemia-induced secretion of ADH results in resorption of sodium from the renal tubules. As a result, urinary sodium excretion is usually less than 15 mEq·L⁻¹, and urinary osmolarity may exceed 500 mOsm·L⁻¹.

Proteinuria

Proteinuria is associated with almost every pathologic process that afflicts the kidneys. It may also occur in the absence of renal dysfunction (exercise, fever, orthostatic, congestive heart failure). Severe proteinuria (greater than 3 g·d⁻¹) usually reflects significant underlying glomerular disease. Microalbuminuria is the earliest sign of diabetic nephropathy. The systemic effect of proteinuria is evaluated by measuring the plasma albumin concentration.

Hematuria

Hematuria can be caused by bleeding anywhere between the glomerulus and urethra. Microhematuria may be benign (focal nephritis) or may reflect glomerulonephritis, renal calculi, or cancer of the genitourinary tract. Sickle cell disease is a consideration in black patients who exhibit hematuria. Joggers may experience hematuria, presumably as a result of trauma to the urinary tract. In the absence of proteinuria or erythrocyte (RBC) casts, glomerular disease as a cause of hematuria is unlikely. Intravenous urography (pyelogram) or cystoscopy may be indicated to determine the site of bleeding.

Urine Sediment

Examination of the centrifuged sediment of a fresh urine specimen provides information similar to that provided by a renal biopsy. For example, RBC casts are virtually diagnostic of glomerulonephritis or vasculitis, whereas free RBCs can originate anywhere in the genitourinary tract, including trauma to the urethra produced by the placement of a bladder catheter. The finding of epithelial cell casts in a patient with acute renal failure is suggestive of acute tubular necrosis.

Urine Volume

Urine volume may not reflect the severity of renal dysfunction, as even patients with advanced renal failure may maintain normal or even increased urine output. Measurement of urine volume is chiefly used for the patient in whom anuria develops (less than 50 ml·d^{-1} of urine), most likely due to shock (hypotension and renal vasoconstriction) or to urinary tract obstruction. In rare instances, bilateral vascular occlusion, as caused by a dissecting aortic aneurysm, may be responsible for anuria. Prerenal disease and acute tubular necrosis, the most common causes of acute renal failure, are likely to be associated with oliguiria, but not with anuria.

Additional Diagnostic Studies

Intravenous urography is the basic method for evaluating gross renal structure. Exposure to radiocontrast dyes may result in signs of acute renal failure, especially in patients with co-existing renal disease (plasma creatinine above 2 mg·dl^{-1}). Characteristically, oliguria appears within 24 hours after the radiologic procedure and lasts several days, with recovery over the next 7 to 14 days. A few patients with unusually severe co-existing renal disease have experienced irreversible renal damage. In the absence of co-existing renal dysfunction, nephrotoxicity owing to contrast material is negligible.[7]

Ultrasound is a useful diagnostic technique for determining kidney size and the presence of renal masses. Residual urine volume exceeding 100 ml can be detected by ultrasound. Computed tomography provides information similar to that of ultrasound and is a useful alternative when ultrasound is inconclusive. Magnetic resonance imaging has advantages over ultrasound and computed tomography in evaluating renal anatomy, although calcifications are not demonstrated by this technique. Radionuclide imaging depends on renal uptake of isotopes, which may be altered in patients with renal failure, urinary tract obstruction, and dehydration.

Renal Biopsy

Renal biopsy may be performed in the patient with unexplained proteinuria, hematuria, or renal insufficiency. Contraidications to renal biopsy include the presence of a single kidney, coagulation abnormalities, uncontrolled hypertension, and the patient who is unable to cooperate by voluntary breathholding during the procedure.

EFFECTS OF ANESTHETIC DRUGS ON RENAL FUNCTION

Anesthetic drugs are predictably associated with decreased GFR, renal blood flow, and urine output. Inhaled anesthetic drugs most likely depress renal function by producing decreased cardiac output and blood pressure. During the administration of halothane, and presumably other volatile anesthetics as well, decreased GFR and renal blood flow is attenuated by preoperative hydration and the administration of a low concentration of anesthetic, which is more likely to maintain blood pressure at a near normal level[8] (Table 20-2). There is no evidence that volatile anesthetics interfere with the normal autoregulation of GFR or renal blood flow[9] (Fig. 20-3). Isoflurane-induced deliberate hypotension does not further decrease GFR or renal blood flow, as compared with values measured during anesthesia and normotension.[10] When alterations in renal hemodynamics occur during regional anesthesia, the most likely explanation is a sustained decreased in perfusion pressure.

Decreased urine output during anesthesia suggests the release of ADH. Nevertheless, plasma ADH concentration does not change during halothane or high-dose morphine anesthesia in the absence of surgical stimulation[11] (Fig. 20-4). Surgical stimulation, however, results in a significant increase in the circulating concentration of ADH. Hydration before the induction of anesthesia attenuates the increase in plasma ADH concentration produced by surgical stimulation. Positive-pressure ventilation of the lungs may result in increased atrial pressures, leading to the decreased release of atrial natriuretic factor, perhaps accounting in part for the antidiuretic and antinatriuretic effect of positive end-expiratory pressure.[12]

Suggestions that anesthetic drugs increase renin release have not been confirmed in animals, although increases do occur during halothane or enflurane anesthesia in the presence

Table 20-2. Impact of Inspired Concentration of Halothane and Preoperative Hydration on Renal Function

Inspired Halothane Concentration (%)	Preoperative Hydration	Decrease from Control (%)	
		Renal Blood Flow	Glomerular Filtration Rate
0.5–1.0	No	61	48
	Yes	12	8
1.2–3.0	No	69	58
	Yes	47	40

(Data from Barry KG, Mazze RI, Schwartz FD. Prevention of surgical oliguria and renal hemodynamic suppression by sustained hydration. N Engl J Med 1964;270:1371–7.)

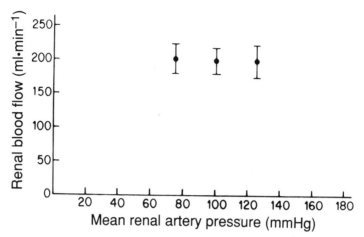

Fig. 20-3. Renal blood flow in dogs (mean ± SE) was similar at a mean arterial pressure of 75 mmHg, 100 mmHg, and 125 mmHg, in the presence of 0.9% end-exhaled halothane. These observations suggest that autoregulation of renal blood flow is not altered by halothane anesthesia. (From Bastron RD, Perkins FM, Payne JL. Autoregulation of renal blood flow during halothane anesthesia. Anesthesiology 1977;46:142–4, with permission.)

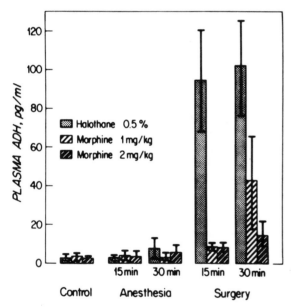

Fig. 20-4. Plasma antidiuretic hormone (ADH) concentrations (mean ± SE) in adult patients were not altered from control measurements during anesthesia with nitrous oxide (50%) plus halothane or morphine. Thiopental was also administered to patients who subsequently received halothane. Surgical stimulation increased plasma ADH levels with the largest increase occurring in those patients receiving halothane. (From Philbin DM, Coggins CH. Plasma antidiuretic hormone levels in cardiac surgical patients during morphine and halothane anesthesia. Anesthesiology 1978;49:95–8, with permission.)

of sodium depletion.[13] This finding suggests that preoperative hydration is important in determining the intraoperative release of renin. Increases in circulating renin levels produced by surgical stimulation are indeed attenuated by hydration.

Direct Nephrotoxicity

In a sense, all anesthetics are direct nephrotoxins, as they produce generalized depression of measurable renal function. This depression of renal function is transient, however, and is usually clinically insignificant.

Delayed nephrotoxicity secondary to fluoride resulting from metabolism of methoxyflurane and possibly enflurane may occur[5,14–16] (Table 20-3). Metabolism of sevoflurane to fluoride resembles enflurane. Typically renal failure due to fluoride nephrotoxicity is characterized by an inability to concentrate urine. Polyuria leads to dehydration, hypernatremia, and increased plasma osmolarity. Defluorination of halothane and

Table 20-3. Plasma Fluoride Concentrations in Nonobese Adults

	Dose (MAC hours)	Maximum Plasma Fluoride ($\mu M \cdot L^{-1}$)	Time of Maximum Increase (Hours Postanesthesia)
Methoxyflurane	2.5	61	24
Enflurane	2.5	22	4
Isoflurane	4.5	4.4	6
Halothane	4.5	No change	—

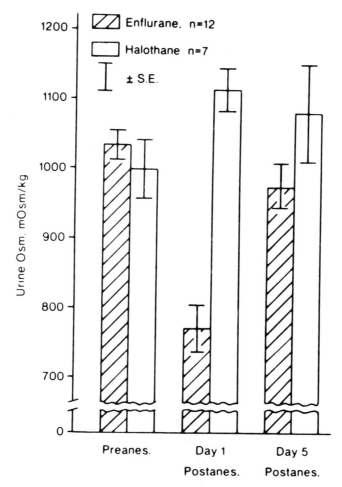

Fig. 20-5. The ability to concentrate urine (maximum urine osmolarity) in response to exogenous vasopressin was measured in volunteers without renal disease before anesthesia (Preanes.) and 1 day and 5 days after anesthesia (Postanes.) with enflurane (9.6 MAC hours) or halothane (13.7 MAC hours). The ability to concentrate urine in response to vasopressin was decreased on day 1 after enflurane anesthesia, but not after halothane anesthesia. By day 5 after anesthesia, mean values for enflurane patients had returned to preanesthetic levels. (From Mazze RI, Calverley RK, Smith NT. Inorganic fluoride nephrotoxicity: Prolonged enflurane and halothane anesthesia in volunteers. Anesthesiology 1977;46:265–71, with permission.)

isoflurane is insufficient to lead to plasma fluoride levels capable of producing nephrotoxicity[5,8,9,25] (Table 20-3). The metabolism of enflurane to fluoride, although much less than with methoxyflurane, is potentially great enough to produce nephrotoxicity, particularly after prolonged administration (1 MAC for 9.6 hours), as reflected by decreased urine concentrating ability when plasma fluoride levels averaged 15 $\mu M \cdot L^{-1}$ (Fig. 20-5).[17] This finding suggests that potentially nephrotoxic levels of plasma fluoride may be substantially less than the speculated level of 50 $\mu M \cdot L^{-1}$. By contrast, shorter anesthetic exposures (1 MAC for 2.7 hours) indicate no difference between enflurane or halothane with respect to urine concentrating ability or intraoperative changes in GFR, renal blood flow, or urine output[14] (Fig. 20-6).

The use of enflurane or sevoflurane in patients vulnerable to the development of postoperative renal dysfunction may be questioned. This concern is based on the realization that excretion of fluoride depends on GFR. Therefore, it is likely that patients with decreased GFR will maintain elevated circulating levels of fluoride for longer periods of time than will normal patients. Nephrotoxicity depends on the duration of the exposure of renal tubules of fluoride, as well as on the levels of plasma fluoride. Therefore, it is possible that patients with decreased GFR are at increased risk in the presence of plasma fluoride concentrations that are usually considered nontoxic (below 50 $\mu M \cdot L^{-1}$). Indeed, postoperative renal dysfunction has been reported after administration of enflurane to a patient with co-existing renal disease.[6] Nevertheless,

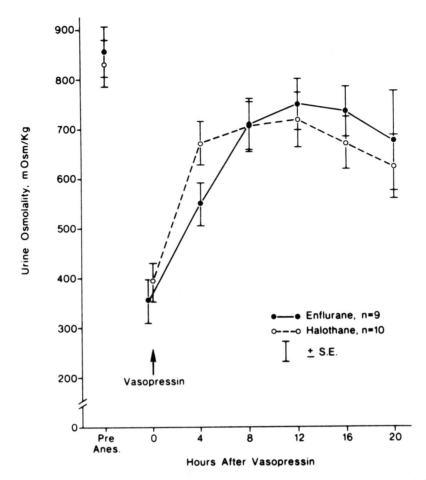

Fig. 20-6. The ability to concentrate urine after administration of exogenous vasopressin was similar in surgical patients without renal disease after anesthesia with enflurane (2.7 MAC hours) or halothane (4.9 MAC hours). (From Cousins MJ, Greenstein LR, Hitt BA, Mazze RI. Metabolism and renal effects of enflurane in man. Anesthesiology 1976;44:44–53, with permission.)

a large series of patients with chronic renal disease (plasma creatinine concentrations 1.5 to 3.0 mg·dl^{-1}), undergoing elective operations with halothane or enflurane, manifested evidence of improved renal function postoperatively.[18] Furthermore, peak plasma fluoride concentrations (19 μmol·L^{-1}), as well as the rate of disappearance of fluoride from the circulation, was similar to that in patients without renal disease. Presumably, storage of fluoride in bone offsets the effect of the reduced GFR on fluoride clearance from the plasma, thereby preventing sustained exposure of renal tubules to this potential nephrotoxin. On the basis of these observations, it is not possible to justify a recommendation to avoid the routine administration of enflurane for nonrenal surgery to patients with co-existing renal dysfunction. It is unden-

iable, however, that the differential diagnosis of postoperative renal dysfunction may be unnecessarily complicated if enflurane or sevoflurane, rather than equally acceptable alternative drugs, is administered to a patient with co-existing renal disease or to a patient undergoing an operation associated with a high incidence of postoperative renal dysfunction. In this regard, minimal to nonexistent metabolism of isoflurane, halothane, and desflurane to fluoride suggests that renal dysfunction is unlikely from nephrotoxic metabolites after administration of these drugs.

Obese patients have been shown to have higher plasma fluoride concentrations after the administration of methoxyflurane or enflurane, as compared with nonobese patients.[19,20] Nevertheless, the incidence of renal dysfunction has not been reported to increase after administration of these drugs to obese patients. Likewise, enzyme induction produced by the administration of phenobarbital does not significantly increase defluorination of enflurane. Isoniazid administration has been shown to increase defluorination of enflurane.

CHRONIC RENAL FAILURE

Despite different causes (diabetic nephropathy, chronic glomerulonephritis, pyelonephritis) the common denominator present in patients in whom chronic renal failure develops is progressive and irreversible loss of functioning nephrons with an associated decrease in GFR. Renal reserve is decreased, but patients remain asymptomatic when at least 40% of the nephrons continue to function. Renal insufficiency is present when only 10% to 40% of nephrons are functioning. These patients are compensated, but there is no renal reserve; as a result, excess catabolic loads or toxic substances (aminoglycosides, potassium load from hemolysis) can exacerbate renal insufficiency. The loss of greater than 90% of functioning nephrons results in uremia (urine in the blood) and the need for dialytic treatment. No single toxin reproduces the uremic syndrome, although BUN is a useful clinical indicator of the severity of the syndrome. By contrast, plasma creatinine concentration, although a good measure of GFR, correlates poorly with manifestations of the uremic syndrome.

Characteristic Changes

Rational management of anesthesia in patients with chronic renal failure requires an understanding of those changes characteristic of chronic renal failure (Table 20-4).

Anemia

Anemia (hemoglobin 5 to 8 g·dl^{-1}) is a well-recognized complication of chronic renal failure; it may be the cause of many of the symptoms associated with the uremic syndrome, including chronic fatigue. Decreased renal production of erythropoietin is responsible for this anemia. Administration of recombinant human erythropoietin can correct the anemia of end-stage chronic renal failure, improving the patient's ability to function and virtually eliminating the need for blood transfusions designed to increase the oxygen-carrying capacity of the patient's blood.[21] Eryuthropoietin is administered until a hematocrit of 30% to 33% is achieved. A side effect of treatment with erythropoietin is the development of hypertension or exacerbation of co-existing hypertension.

Table 20-4.   Changes Characteristic of Chronic Renal Failure

Chronic Anemia
    Increased cardiac output
    Oxyhemoglobin dissociation curve shifted to the right

Pruritus

Coagulopathies
    Platelet dysfunction
    Systemic heparinization

Altered Hydration and Electrolyte Balance
    Unpredictable intravascular fluid volume
    Hyperkalemia
    Hypermagnesemia
    Hypocalcemia

Metabolic Acidosis

Systemic Hypertension
    Congestive heart failure
    Attenuated sympathetic nervous system activity due to therapy
        with antihypertensive drugs

Increased Susceptibility to Infection
    Decreased activity of phagocytes
    Immunosuppressant drugs

Pruritus

Pruritus occurs in most patients with end-stage renal disease. Administration of erythropoietin lowers the plasma concentration of histamine and may decrease the intensity of pruritus.

Coagulopathies

Patients with chronic renal failure exhibit a bleeding tendency despite a normal prothrombin time, plasma thromboplastin time, and platelet count.[22] The screening test best correlated with a bleeding tendency is the bleeding time. Recognized hemostatic abnormalities in these patients include the release of defective von Willebrand factor. Although bleeding from the gastrointestinal tract is the most frequent manifestation of uremic bleeding, epistaxis, hemorrhagic pericarditis, and subdural hematoma may occur as well.

Treatment of uremic bleeding may include the administration of desmopressin or cryoprecipitate, especially when surgery is planned. For example, infusion of desmopressin, a nonvasoconstricting analogue of vasopressin (0.3 to 0.4 mg·kg^{-1} IV over 30 minutes), decreases the prolonged bleeding time, producing a peak effect in 1 to 4 hours and lasting 4 to 8 hours. A more prolonged beneficial coagulation response (14 days) is produced by estrogen therapy. Treatment of anemia with erythropoietin shortens bleeding time in these patients. Indeed, there is evidence that bleeding time is shortened in the uremic patient with a hematocrit greater than 26%.[23] Dialysis has not consistently improved coagulation in patients with uremic bleeding.

Hyperkalemia

Hyperkalemia is the most serious electrolyte abnormality in patients with chronic renal failure. Changes on the electrocardiogram (peaked T waves, followed by prolongation of the P-R interval and the QRS complex, and ultimately heart block or ventricular fibrillation) remain the best guide to the need for treatment of hyperkalemia. Because of the potential dangers of hyperkalemia, elective surgery is commonly recommended against, unless the plasma potassium concentration is less than 5.5 mEq·L^{-1}. Even when hemodialysis has been performed within the previous 6 to 8 hours, it is useful to measure the plasma potassium concentration before induction of anesthesia, as hyperkalemia can occur both rapidly and unexpectedly. If surgery cannot be delayed, the plasma potassium concentration can be decreased promptly by deliberate hyperventilation of the lungs (decrease about 0.5 mEq·L^{-1} for every 10-mmHg decrease in PaCO$_2$) and intravenous administration of glucose with insulin (see Chapter 21). Intravenous administration of calcium is effective in restoring normal cardiac conduction in the presence of hyperkalemia.

Hypocalcemia

Hypocalcemia occurs in patients with chronic renal failure when the GFR declines to the level of the development of hyperphosphatemia, leading to a reciprocal change in the plasma calcium concentration. Hypocalcemia stimulates the release of parathyroid hormone and subsequent bone resorption (renal osteodystrophy), making patients vulnerable to pathologic fractures as during positioning for anesthesia and surgery. Skeletal radiographs show demineralization as evidence of hyperparathyroid bone disease. Hypocalcemia is further aggravated by diminished renal production of the active form of vitamin D, resulting in decreased gastrointestinal absorption of calcium. If hypocalcemia persists despite medical management, a surgical subtotal parathyroidectomy may be necessary. Dementia and bone disease may reflect aluminum toxicity, either from aluminum in the dialysate fluid or from aluminum salts in antacids administered to prevent hyperphosphatemia.

Hypermagnesemia

Hypermagnesemia may accompany chronic renal failure, especially if magnesium-containing antacids are being used. Central nervous system depression owing to excessive magnesium concentrations can lead to coma, hypotension, and hypoventilation. Potentiation of depolarizing and nondepolarizing muscle relaxants may accompany increased plasma concentrations of magnesium.[24] Plasma sodium concentrations are usually normal in patients with chronic renal disease because the osmoreceptor mechanism is functioning; thirst prevents hypernatremia.

Metabolic Acidosis

The kidneys normally excrete 50 to 100 mEq of hydrogen ions every day, reflecting metabolism of dietary protein. Chronic metabolic acidosis (pH less than 7.3) stimulates compensatory hyperventilation and depresses neuromuscular responsiveness. Hemodialysis is effective in restoring the arterial pH to near-normal values. In patients requiring emergency surgery, intravenous administration of sodium bicarbonate may be considered if acidosis is severe (pH less than 7.15). Care should be taken to avoid correcting the acidosis too rapidly, especially if hypocalcemia is present. In this regard, metabolic acidosis protects against the effects of hypocalcemia; left unopposed, these effects could precipitate seizures.

Hypertension

Hypertension afflicts more than 80% of patients with end-stage renal disease and is the most significant risk factor for the development of congestive heart failure, myocardial infarction, and stroke, in these patients. Congestive heart failure can be aggravated by the arteriovenous fistula used for hemodialysis. Intravascular volume expansion and activation of the renin-angiotensin-aldosterone system are the most likely explanations for hypertension. In this regard, blood pressure control can often be achieved by hemodialysis and the removal of excess fluid. In patients with increased renin levels, even vigorous dialysis may not be effective, necessitating the use of increasing doses of antihypertensive agents. Medical control of hypertension with angiotensin-converting enzyme inhibitors or calcium entry blockers has replaced bilateral nephrectomy for the management of patients with refractory hypertension and elevated plasma renin concentrations.

Pericardial Disease

Pericardial disease in patients with chronic renal failure is manifested as pericardial effusion with or without cardiac tamponade. The diagnosis of pericardial effusion is made by cardiac ultrasonography. Treatment consists of hemodialysis or pericardiocentesis, if the cardiac effusion is hemodynamically significant. The beneficial response evoked by renal dialysis suggests that a circulating toxin may be important in producing uremic pericarditis. Acute pericardial tamponade is the principal life-threatening complication of uremic pericarditis.

Nervous System Abnormalities

Abnormalities of the central nervous system and the peripheral nervous system may accompany renal failure. Encephalopathy may be manifested as mental depression or sedation that progresses to coma. Seizures may accompany uremia or reflect cerebral edema from acute hypertension. A distal symmetric mixed motor and sensory polyneuropathy (median and common peroneal nerves most often) may develop. Autonomic nervous system dysfunction commonly accompanies uremia and may contribute to attenuated compensatory responses to changes in blood volume or positive-pressure ventilation of the lungs. Hemodialysis may be effective in reversing both uremic encephalopathy and uremic neuropathy.

Infection

The most serious problem facing patients with chronic renal failure is infection. Indeed, the most common cause of death in patients with renal failure is sepsis, often originating from a pulmonary infection. Strict attention to asepsis is important when placing vascular catheters and endotracheal tubes in these patients.

The increased incidence of viral hepatitis in patients with chronic renal disease most likely reflects the frequent use of blood products. Approximately one-third of patients with chronic renal failure who become infected with hepatitis virus become chronic carriers.

Management of Anesthesia

Precise quantitation of the GFR is not usually necessary for managing patients with renal disease.[25] The most important observation in these patients is an assessment of whether the disease is stable, progressing, or improving. This information is most simply obtained by monitoring the plasma concentration of creatinine.

Preoperative Evaluation

The preoperative evaluation of a patient with chronic renal failure includes consideration of concomitant drug therapy and evaluation of those changes considered characteristic of chronic renal failure (Table 20-4). Estimates of blood volume status may be made by comparison of body weight both before and after hemodialysis, consideration of vital signs (orthostatic hypotension, heart rate), and measurement of atrial filling pressure. Diabetes mellitus is often present in these patients. Insulin replacement regimens may require attention. Signs of digitalis toxicity should be sought in treated patients, emphasizing the role of renal clearance of this and other drugs. Antihypertensive drug therapy is usually continued. Preoperative medication must be individualized, remembering that these patients may exhibit uremia-induced slowing of gastric emptying as well as unexpected sensitivity to central nervous system depressant drugs. In addition to patients with known pre-

Table 20-5.   Patients at Risk of Perioperative Renal Failure

Co-existing renal disease
Hypovolemia
Cirrhosis of the liver
Biliary tract obstruction
Sepsis
Multiple organ system trauma
Congestive heart failure
Abdominal aneurysm resection
Cardiopulmonary bypass
Advanced age

operative renal dysfunction, it is important to recognize others at high risk of perioperative renal failure, even in the absence of co-existing renal disease[1] (Table 20-5). Preservation of renal function intraoperatively depends on maintaining an adequate intravascular fluid volume and minimizing cardiovascular depression.

Induction of Anesthesia

Induction of anesthesia and intubation of the trachea can be safely accomplished with intravenous drugs (propofol, etomidate, barbiturates, midazolam) plus succinylcholine. An alternative to succinylcholine, if the possibility of increased gastric fluid volume does not mandate the rapid onset of skeletal muscle paralysis, would be an intermediate- or short-acting muscle relaxant that does not depend on renal clearance mechanisms. Logic would suggest slow injection of the induction drug, to minimize the likelihood of drug-induced decreases in blood pressure. Regardless of blood volume status, these patients often respond to induction of anesthesia as if they were hypovolemic. The likelihood of hypotension during induction of anesthesia may be increased if sympathetic nervous system function is attenuated by antihypertensive drugs or uremia. Attenuated sympathetic nervous system activity impairs compensatory peripheral vasoconstriction; thus, small decreases in blood volume, institution of positive-pressure ventilation of the lungs, abrupt changes in body position, or drug-induced myocardial depression can result in an exaggerated decrease in blood pressure.

Exaggerated central nervous system effects of anesthetic induction drugs may reflect uremia-induced disruption of the blood-brain barrier. Furthermore, decreased protein binding of drugs may result in the availability of more unbound drug to act at receptor sites. Indeed, the amount of pharmacologically active unbound thiopental in plasma is increased in patients with chronic renal failure.

Potassium release after administration of succinylcholine is not exaggerated in patients with chronic renal failure, although there is a theoretical concern that those with extensive uremic neuropathies might be at increased risk. Likewise, caution is indicated when the preoperative plasma potassium concentration is in a high-normal range, since this finding combined with maximum drug-induced potassium release (0.5 to 1.0 mEq·L^{-1}) could result in dangerous hyperkalemia. It is important to recognize that a small dose of nondepolarizing muscle relaxant administered before the injection of succinylcholine (pretreatment) does not reliably attenuate the succinylcholine-induced release of potassium.[26]

Maintenance of Anesthesia

In patients with chronic renal disease who are not dependent on hemodialysis, or in patients vulnerable to renal dysfunction because of advanced age or the need for major abdominal vascular surgery, the maintenance of anesthesia is often achieved with nitrous oxide combined with isoflurane, halothane, desflurane, or a short-acting opioid. Enflurane and sevoflurane may be avoided because of concerns for the potential adverse effects of fluoride on the diseased kidneys (see the section, Direct Nephrotoxicity).

A potent volatile anesthetic is useful in controlling intraoperative hypertension and reducing the dose of muscle relaxant needed for adequate surgical relaxation. The high incidence of associated liver disease in patients with chronic renal disease should be considered, however, when selecting these drugs, particularly halothane. Furthermore, excessive depression of cardiac output is a potential hazard of volatile anesthetics. Reductions in tissue blood flow must be minimized in the presence of anemia, to avoid jeopardizing oxygen delivery to the tissues. Opioids decrease the likelihood of cardiovascular depression and avoid the concern of liver toxicity. Nevertheless, opioids are not reliably effective in controlling intraoperative blood pressure elevations. Furthermore, prolonged sedation and depression of ventilation from small doses of an opioid have been described in anephric patients.[27] Conceivably, pharmacologically active metabolites of opioids accumulate in the circulation and in the cerebrospinal fluid, when renal function is absent.

When hypertension does not respond to an adjustment in the depth of anesthesia, it may be appropriate to administer a vasodilator, such as hydralazine or nitroprusside. Cyanide from the breakdown of nitroprusside is unlikely to cause toxicity in these patients. Indeed, animal data have demonstrated resistance to the development of cyanide toxicity, in the absence of renal function.[28] The most likely explanation for this resistance is decreased renal excretion of thiosulfate. Thiosulfate serves as an endogenous sulfur donor and facilitates conversion of cyanide to thiocyanate.

Ventilation of the lungs during general anesthesia should be designed to maintain normocapnia and minimize the effects of positive intrathoracic pressure on cardiac output. Hypoventilation with resulting respiratory acidosis is undesirable, as decreases in arterial pH can result in the transfer of potassium from cells into the circulation, accentuating hyperkalemia. Conversely, respiratory alkalosis from hyperventilation of the lungs shifts the oxyhemoglobin dissociation curve to the left and reduces oxygen availability to the tissues. This change may be particularly undesirable in patients with anemia. Changes in cardiac output produced by positive-pressure ventilation of the lungs can be minimized by using a slow breathing rate, to permit sufficient time for venous return during pauses between mechanical breaths.

Maintenance of anesthesia in patients requiring chronic hemodialysis is often achieved with nitrous oxide combined with isoflurane, enflurane, or desflurane. These drugs provide sufficient potency to reduce excessive increases in blood pressure due to surgical stimulation and also decrease the dose of nondepolarizing muscle relaxants needed to produce skeletal muscle relaxation. Furthermore, the use of isoflurane, enflurane, or desflurane in the presence of co-existing liver disease is less controversial than the use of halothane. Excessive plasma fluoride elevations do not occur in anephric patients receiving enflurane, since storage of fluoride in bone can offset the lack of its renal excretion.[29]

Regional Anesthesia

Brachial plexus block is useful for the placement of a vascular shunt necessary for chronic hemodialysis. In addition to providing analgesia, this form of regional anesthesia also abolishes vasospasm and provides optimal surgical conditions by producing maximal vascular vasodilation. The suggestion that duration of brachial plexus anesthesia is shortened in patients with chronic renal failure has not been confirmed in controlled studies.[30–32] Adequacy of coagulation should be considered and the presence of uremic neuropathies excluded before regional anesthesia is performed in these patients. Co-existing metabolic acidosis may decrease the seizure threshold for local anesthetics.

Muscle Relaxants

Renal disease slows the clearance of long-acting nondepolarizing muscle relaxants from the plasma. For this reason, prolonged responses are predictable, if the usual doses of these drugs are administered to these patients. By contrast, the impact of renal failure on the duration of action of atracurium and mivacurium is predictably absent, even with large doses of these drugs[33] (Fig. 20-7). The clearance of vecuronium from the plasma is slowed in patients with chronic renal failure, and the duration of action may be less predictable than in patients receiving atracurium[33] (Fig. 20-7). It is estimated that about 30% of an administered dose of vecuronium appears in the urine as unchanged drug during the first 24 hours.[34] Plasma concentrations of laudanosine after the administration

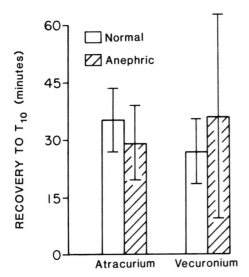

Fig. 20-7. Time to recovery of twitch response to 10% of control (T_{10}) (Mean $\pm$ SE) after rapid administration of atracurium (0.5 mg·kg^{-1} IV) or vecuronium (0.1 mg·kg^{-1} IV) to normal or anephric patients during nitrous oxide–fentanyl–thiopental anesthesia. Absence of renal function did not prolong the duration of action of either muscle relaxant, although variability in response was greatest in anephric patients receiving vecuronium. (From Hunter JM, Jones RS, Utting JE. Comparison of vecuronium, atracurium and tubocurarine in normal patients and in patients with no renal function. Br J Anaesth 1984;56:941–50, with permission.)

of atracurium are higher, and the elimination half-time is prolonged in patients with renal failure as compared with normal patients.[35,36] There is evidence of resistance to the effects of vecuronium (slower onset, high plasma concentration of drug at 25% recovery) in patients with chronic renal failure compared with patients with normal renal function.[34] A similar, but less prominent, degree of tolerance may also occur after administration of atracurium to patients in renal failure.[33] Overall, atracurium or mivacurium would seem to be the most useful nondepolarizing muscle relaxants for administration to patients with severe renal disease.

Renal excretion accounts for about 50% of the clearance of neostigmine and about 75% of the elimination of edrophonium and pyridostigmine. As a result, the elimination half-time of these drugs is greatly prolonged by renal failure[37] (Fig. 20-8). Therefore, recurarization is unlikely, because plasma clearance of anticholinesterase drugs will be delayed for as long as, if not longer than, the nondepolarizing muscle relaxants. When skeletal muscle weakness persists or recurs postoperatively, other causes of recurarization, such as inadequate initial antagonism of neuromuscular blockade, respiratory acidosis, elec-trolyte derangements, or drug-induced effects, as from antibiotics, must be considered.

Fluid Management and Urine Output

Patients with severe renal dysfunction but not requiring hemodialysis, as well as those patients without renal disease undergoing operations associated with a high incidence of postoperative renal failure may benefit from preoperative hydration with administration of 10 to 20 ml·kg^{-1} IV of a balanced salt solution[1] (Table 20-2). Indeed, most patients come to the operating room with a contracted extracellular fluid volume unless corrective measures are taken. Lactated Ringer's solution (4 mEq·L^{-1} of potassium) or other potassium-containing fluids should not be administered to anuric patients. Administration of 3 to 5 ml·kg^{-1}·h^{-1} IV of a balanced salt solution is often recommended to maintain a urine output greater than 0.5 ml·kg^{-1}·h^{-1}. In general, when urine output is less than 0.5 ml·kg^{-1}·h^{-1}, GFR can be assumed to be decreased. Often, a small dose of furosemide (5 mg IV) will increase urine output, if oliguria is due to ADH release, but not if it is due to hypovolemia and decreased renal blood flow. Rapid infusion of a balanced salt solution (500 ml IV) should increase urine output in the presence of hypovolemia. Stimulation of urine output with an osmotic (mannitol) or tubular (furosemide) diuretic in the absence of adequate intravascular fluid volume replacement is discouraged. Indeed, the most likely reason for oliguria is an inadequate circulating fluid volume, which can only be further compromised by drug-induced diuresis. Furthermore, although the administration of mannitol or furosemide will predictably increase urine output, there is no evidence of corresponding improvements in GFR.[38] Likewise, intraoperative urine output has not been shown to be predictive of postoperative renal insufficiency after abdominal vascular surgery (see Fig. 10-3).

If fluid replacement is not effective in restoring urine output, the diagnosis of congestive heart failure may be considered. Dopamine (0.5 to 3 μg·kg^{-1}·min^{-1} IV) increases renal blood flow and subsequent urine output by stimulating renal dopaminergic receptors. Higher doses of dopamine (3 to 10 μg·kg^{-1}·min^{-1} IV) stimulate beta receptors, making this drug useful in treating oliguria caused by congestive heart failure. It is helpful, but not always possible, to confirm the diagnosis of congestive heart failure and a beneficial response to drugs with measurements obtained from a pulmonary artery catheter. Another consideration in the differential diagnosis of oliguria is mechanical obstruction of the urinary catheter or pooling of urine in the dome of the bladder, in response to the head-down position.

Patients dependent on hemodialysis require special attention, with respect to perioperative fluid management. Absence

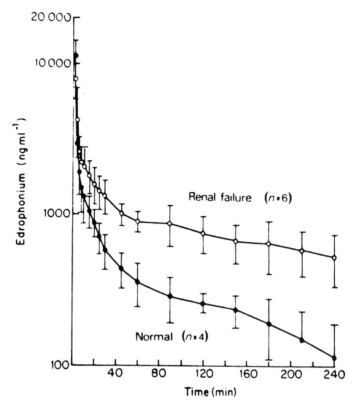

Fig. 20-8. The plasma concentration of edrophonium declines more slowly in patients with renal failure than in normal patients. Delayed clearance of edrophonium, and other anticholinesterase drugs, parallels the delayed clearance of nondepolarizing muscle relaxants. (From Morris RB, Cronnelly R, Miller RD, et al. Pharmacokinetics of edrophonium in anephric and renal transplant patients. Br J Anaesth 1981;53:1311–3, with permission.)

of renal function narrows the margin of safety between insufficient and excessive fluid administration to these patients. Noninvasive operations require replacement of only insensible water losses, with 5% glucose in water (5 to 10 ml·kg^{-1} IV). The small amount of urine output can be replaced with 0.45% sodium chloride. Thoracic or abdominal surgery can be associated with a loss of significant intravascular fluid volume to the interstitial spaces. This loss is often replaced with balanced salt solutions or with a 5% albumin solution (Plasmanate). Blood transfusion may be considered if oxygen-carrying capacity must be increased or blood loss is excessive.

Monitoring

Minor surgical procedures can be monitored by noninvasive methods. Permanent vascular shunts should be protected. Their patency may be monitored with a Doppler sensor to confirm continued patency during the operative procedure.

Continuous monitoring of intra-arterial blood pressure is helpful when major operative procedures are being performed. A femoral or dorsalis pedis artery is often used, since patients may require the availability of arteries in the upper extremity for placement of vascular shunts. Intravenous fluid replacement is guided by central venous pressure measurements and urine output. A pulmonary artery catheter can be useful if the interpretation of central venous measurements is questionable, as in the presence of co-existing chronic obstructive airway disease or left ventricular dysfunction. Furthermore, measurement of thermodilution cardiac outputs and calculation of systemic vascular resistance can be helpful in guiding doses of anesthetic drugs and recognizing the need for inotropic drugs, such as dopamine. Strict asepsis is mandatory for the placement of intravascular catheters, such as those for measurement of blood pressure or pulmonary artery occlusion pressure.

Postoperative Management

Diagnosis of recurarization should be considered in an anephric patient who shows signs of skeletal muscle weakness during the postoperative period. A weak hand grip or inability to maintain head lift and improvement after the administration of edrophonium (5 to 10 mg IV) confirms the diagnosis.

Hypertension is a common problem during the postoperative period. Hemodialysis is a useful treatment, if hypervolemia is the cause. Vasodilators (nitroprusside, hydralazine, labetalol) are helpful until excess fluid can be removed by hemodialysis.

Caution is indicated in the use of parenteral opioids for postoperative analgesia, in view of the report describing exaggerated central nervous system depression, as well as hypoventilation, after even small doses of opioids.[27] Administration of naloxone may be necessary if depression of ventilation is severe. Continuous monitoring of the electrocardiogram is helpful in the detection of cardiac dysrhythmias, as may be related to hyperkalemia. Continuation of supplemental oxygen into the postoperative period is a consideration, especially if anemia is present.

PERIOPERATIVE OLIGURIA

Acute perioperative oliguria (less than 0.5 ml·kg^{-1}·h^{-1}) must be treated promptly, as prolonged perioperative oliguria can lead to acute renal failure, with a mortality exceeding 50%.[1,39] Perioperative renal failure accounts for approximately one-half of the cases in the United States requiring acute hemodialysis. The causes of perioperative oliguria can be categorized as prerenal, renal, and postrenal (Table 20-6). Postrenal obstuction or bilateral renal artery occlusion is uncommon, diagnosed by the presence of anuria. Thus, the usual differential diagnosis distinguishes between prerenal (undamaged renal tubules conserve sodium in an attempt to restore intravascular fluid volume) and renal (damaged renal

Table 20-6. Causes of Perioperative Oliguria

Prerenal (Decreased Renal Blood Flow)
 Hypovolemia
 Decreased cardiac output

Renal (Acute Tubular Necrosis)
 Renal ischemia due to prerenal causes
 Nephrotoxic drugs
 Release of hemoglobin or myoglobin

Postrenal
 Bilateral ureteral obstruction
 Extravasation due to bladder rupture

Table 20-7. Differential Diagnosis of Perioperative Oliguria

	Prerenal	Renal
Urinary sodium (mEq·L^{-1})	<40	>40
Urine osmolarity (mOsm·L^{-1})	>400	250–300
Urine osmolarity/plasma osmolarity	>1.8	<1.1

tubules limited in ability to conserve sodium) causes (Table 20-7). Prior administration of a diuretic increases urine sodium excretion and decreases urine osmolarity, making it difficult to confirm the diagnosis of acute renal tubular dysfunction. The most common cause of acute renal failure is prolonged (30- to 60-minute) renal hypoperfusion, most often owing to hypovolemia. The key strategy in decreasing the likelihood of oliguria progressing to acute renal failure is to limit the duration and magnitude of renal hypoperfusion. Urine output is a commonly observed variable in diagnosing acute renal failure, although this variable may remain normal or even elevated despite dramatic renal dysfunction, especially if diuretics have been administered.

The pathophysiology of acute oliguric renal failure is unclear and may vary among patients. The term acute vasomotor nephropathy is applied to patients in whom blood flow to the renal cortex and glomeruli is greatly decreased. Another term, acute tubular necrosis, emphasizes the concept that glomerular filtration continues, but the renal tubules are necrotic. Another mechanism of acute oliguric renal failure is obstruction of renal tubules by cellular debris or edema of tubular cells. In the absence of a precise understanding of the mechanism of acute oliguric renal failure, it is difficult to evaluate the advantages of proposed therapies, such as the administration of osmotic or loop diuretics.

Treatment

Aggressive and early treatment of perioperative oliguria is most important for those patients at increased risk of the development of acute renal failure[1] (Table 20-5). Transient oliguria during an elective operation in a young patient without co-existing renal disease does not require the same aggressive treatment used for oliguria in an elderly patient with co-existing renal disease (Prough DS: personal communication) (Fig. 20-9). Oliguria in patients considered at risk of the development of acute renal failure is treated initially with rapid intravenous infusion of 500 ml of a balanced salt solution. Administration of a diuretic at this point could evoke further detrimental effects on renal blood flow if drug-induced diuresis accentuated co-existing hypovolemia. Furthermore, furosemide shows no evidence of benefit in preventing renal failure in at-risk pa-

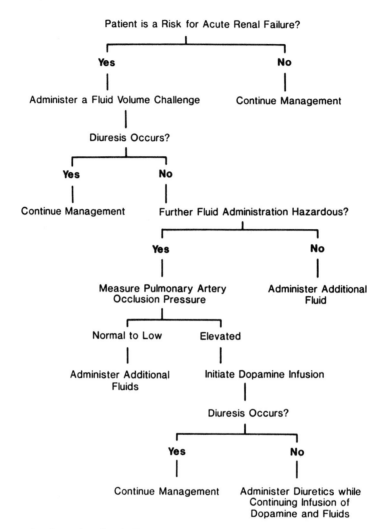

Fig. 20-9. Treatment of perioperative oliguria (Data from Prough DS, Bowman Gray School of Medicine, personal communication.)

tients.[1] Brisk diuresis in response to a fluid challenge suggests hypovolemia as the cause of oliguria. When this fluid challenge does not produce a therapeutic response, additional fluids may be infused with or without monitoring of atrial filling pressures, depending on whether patients are at risk of the development of cardiac dysfunction. When patients are at risk of the development of cardiac dysfunction, and left atrial filling pressure is normal, or below normal, treatment with additional intravenous fluids is acceptable. In the presence of an elevated left atrial filling pressure, the possibility of oliguria and decreased renal blood flow owing to low cardiac output (congestive heart failure) should be considered. In this situation, infusion of do-

pamine (most often 3 to 10 $\mu g \cdot kg^{-1} \cdot min^{-1}$ IV) provides useful therapy. Failure of dopamine to improve urine output may be an indication to administer a diuretic such as mannitol (0.5 to 1 $g \cdot kg^{-1}$ IV) with or without furosemide (1 to 3 $mg \cdot kg^{-1}$ IV). Combinations of dopamine and furosemide may facilitate the conversion of oliguric to nonoliguric renal failure, which is easier to manage but is not associated with a decrease in mortality.[1] Likewise, dopamine has not been shown to improve outcome in critically ill patients with decreased renal function. Hemodialysis is often recommended when the BUN exceeds 100 $mg \cdot dl^{-1}$, or when there is severe fluid overload, metabolic acidosis, or hyperkalemia.

PRIMARY DISEASES OF THE KIDNEYS

A number of pathologic processes can primarily involve the kidneys or occur in association with dysfunction of other organ systems. A knowledge of the associated pathology and characteristics of the renal disease is important in planning management of these patients during the perioperative period.

Glomerulonephritis

Glomerulonephritis is the most common cause of end-stage renal failure in adults. Acute glomerulonephritis is usually due to deposition of antigen-antibody complexes in the glomeruli. The source of antigens may be either exogenous (poststreptococcal infection) or endogenous (collagen diseases). Clinical manifestations of glomerular diseases (acute nephritic syndrome, nephrotic syndrome, interstitial nephritis) include hematuria, proteinuria, hypertension, edema, and an increased plasma creatinine concentration. RBC casts are suggestive of glomerular disease, rather than of nonglomerular disease, such as nephrolithiasis or prostatic disease. Proteinuria reflects an increase in glomerular permeability. Most glomerular diseases are diagnosed by renal biopsy.

Acute Nephritic Syndrome
Poststreptococcal glomerulonephritis, most commonly after infection with group A beta-hemolytic streptococci, is the classic entity associated with the acute nephritic syndrome. The disease occurs most often in children, manifesting as hematuria and RBC casts, 1 to 3 weeks after a streptococcal infection. Proteinuria and hypertension are often present. Antimicrobial therapy with penicillin does not appear to prevent the production of antibody to the glomerular basement membrane that leads to cellular proliferation.

Goodpasture Syndrome
Goodpasture syndrome is a combination of pulmonary hemorrhage and glomerulonephritis, occurring most often in young males. Antibodies account for renal lesions and also apparently react with similar antigens in the lungs, producing alveolitis, which results in hemoptysis. Typically, hemoptysis precedes clinical evidence of renal disease. The prognosis is poor, with no known effective therapy to prevent progression to renal failure, usually within 1 year of diagnosis.

Nephrotic Syndrome
Patients with nephrotic syndrome typically present with proteinuria (greater than 3 $g \cdot d^{-1}$), hypoalbuminemia, hypercholesterolemia, and thromboembolic episodes. The marked hypoalbuminemia and resulting decrease in plasma oncotic pressure lead to edema, ascites, pleural effusion, and hypovolemia. It is likely that persistent hypercholesterolemia increases the risk of atherosclerosis. The increased incidence of arterial and venous thromboemboli, particularly deep vein and renal vein thrombosis, most likely reflects a hypercoagulable state. Renal vein thrombosis is often asymptomatic; it is recognized when the patient is evaluated for a pulmonary embolus.

Causes of the nephrotic syndrome are diverse, with renal biopsy the standard diagnostic approach. Administration of corticosteroids, usually prednisone, is often effective in producing a remission. Chemotherapeutic drugs such as cyclophosphamide or chlorambucil and the immunosuppressant cyclosporine are alternatives to corticosteroid therapy. Even without treatment, most adult patients undergo spontaneous remission. Renal failure is rare.

Interstitial Nephritis
Interstitial nephritis has been observed as an allergic reaction to drugs, including sulfonamides, allopurinol, phenytoin, and diuretics. Patients exhibit decreased urine concentrating ability, proteinuria, and hypertension. Corticosteroid therapy may be beneficial.

Hereditary nephritis (Alport syndrome) is often accompanied by hearing loss and ocular abnormalities. Males are afflicted most often, with the disease culminating in hypertension and renal failure. Drug therapy has not proved successful, although lowering the intraglomerular pressure with an angiotensin-converting enzyme inhibitor may offer some protection.

Polycystic Renal Disease

Polycystic renal disease is inherited as an autosomal dominant trait. The disease typically progresses slowly, until renal failure occurs in middle age. Mild hypertension and proteinuria are common. Decreased urine concentrating ability develops early in the course of the disease. Cysts may also be present in the liver and in the central nervous system, as intracranial aneurysms. Hemodialysis or renal transplantation will eventually be necessary in most patients.

Fanconi Syndrome

Fanconi syndrome results from inherited or acquired disturbances of proximal renal tubular function, causing hyperaminoaciduria, glycosuria, and hyperphosphaturia. There is renal loss of substances normally conserved by proximal renal tubules, including potassium, bicarbonate, and water. Symptoms of Fanconi syndrome reflect the abnormality of the renal tubules and include polyuria, polydipsia, metabolic acidosis due to loss of bicarbonate, and skeletal muscle weakness related to hypokalemia. Dwarfism with osteomalacia, reflecting loss of phosphate, is prominent in these patients. Indeed, presentation as vitamin D-resistant rickets is frequent. Management of anesthesia must include the appreciation of fluid and electrolyte disorders characteristic of this syndrome and the recognition that left ventricular cardiac failure secondary to uremia is often present in the final stages.[40]

Bartter Syndrome

Bartter syndrome is characterized by renal juxtaglomerular apparatus hyperplasia, with an elevated plasma concentration of renin, angiotensin II, and aldosterone. Hypokalemic hypochloremic metabolic alkalosis develops; there is also decreased vascular reactivity to the vasopressor actions of angiotensin II and norepinephrine. Despite these changes, patients with Bartter syndrome are characteristically normotensive. A cardinal feature of this syndrome is overproduction of prostaglandins.

Treatment of Bartter syndrome consists of oral supplements to replace sodium and potassium losses. Administration of spironolactone, an aldosterone antagonist, acts to preserve total body potassium. Propranolol has been used to decrease release of renin from the kidneys. Inhibition of prostaglandin synthesis is accomplished with drugs such as aspirin or indomethacin. Blocking the conversion of angiotensin I to angiotensin II with captopril may be helpful. Surgical removal of the adrenal glands in an effort to control hyperaldosteronism has not proved effective.

Management of Anesthesia

Management of anesthesia for the patient with Bartter syndrome is influenced by the status of renal function and the intravascular fluid volume.[41] For example, the selection of enflurane or sevoflurane may not be wise if there is preoperative evidence of renal dysfunction. Patients treated with spironolactone and propranolol may be hypovolemic but may fail to exhibit chronotropic responses because of beta-blockade. A brisk diuresis with associated loss of potassium may occur during the perioperative period, requiring careful monitoring of acid-base and electrolyte status. Because of the tendency toward hypokalemic metabolic alkalosis, it is important to avoid hyperventilation of the lungs. It is conceivable, although undocumented, that diminished reactivity of blood vessels to catecholamines could be associated with the exaggerated decreases in blood pressure produced by anesthetic drugs. Medications used to treat these patients should be continued throughout the perioperative period, even if it is necessary to administer oral medications through a nasogastric tube.

Renal Hypertension

Renal disease is the most frequent cause of secondary hypertension. Accelerated or malignant hypertension is likely to be associated with renal disease. Furthermore, the appearance of hypertension in a young patient suggests the diagnosis of renal, rather than essential, hypertension. Hypertension due to renal dysfunction reflects either parenchymal disease of the kidneys or renovascular disease.

Chronic pyelonephritis and glomerulonephritis are parenchymal diseases often associated with hypertension, particularly in younger patients. Less common forms of renal parenchymal disease that can cause hypertension include diabetic nephropathy, cystic disease of the kidneys, and renal amyloidosis. Renovascular disease is characterized by atherosclerosis; it accounts for only a small percentage of patients with hypertension. However, the sudden onset of a marked elevation in blood pressure or the presence of hypertension before the age of 30 years should arouse suspicion of renovascular disease. A bruit may be audible on auscultation of the abdomen over the areas of the kidneys. This type of hypertension does not respond well to antihypertensive drugs.

The mechanism for the production of hypertension in the presence of renal disease is not established. Stimulation of the renin-angiotensin-aldosterone system is a possible, but unproven, mechanism. Alternatively, the kidneys may function to some extent as antihypertensive organs, possibly producing substances with vasodepressor activity. Regardless of the mechanism, the treatment of hypertension due to renal parenchymal disease is usually with antihypertensive drugs, including beta-adrenergic antagonist drugs, which inhibit the release of renin from the kidneys. Treatment of hypertension due to renovascular disease is with renal artery endarterectomy or nephrectomy.

Uric Acid Nephropathy

Acute uric acid nephropathy is distinct from gout. It occurs when uric acid crystals are precipitated in the renal collecting tubules or ureters, producing acute oliguric renal failure. This precipitation occurs when the uric acid concentration reaches a saturation point in acidic urine. This condition is particularly likely to occur when uric acid production is greatly increased, as in patients with myeloproliferative disorders being treated with chemotherapeutic drugs for cancer. These patients are particularly vulnerable to uric acid nephropathy if they have good renal function and urine concentrating ability and then become dehydrated or acidotic because of reduced caloric intake.

Hepatorenal Syndrome

Acute oliguria manifested in the patient with decompensated cirrhosis of the liver is designated hepatorenal syndrome. Indeed, cirrhosis of the liver is associated with decreased GFR and renal blood flow preceding overt renal dysfunction by several weeks. The typical patient is deeply jaundiced and moribund; ascites, hypoalbuminemia, and hypoprothrombinemia are present. In these patients, renal failure may reflect hypovolemia, owing to vigorous attempts to treat ascites. Treatment is directed at intravascular fluid volume replacement, remembering that saline and albumin may aggravate ascites. Therefore, whole blood or packed RBCs may be a more appropriate form of volume replacement. A peritoneal to venous shunt for the treatment of ascites may also be associated with improvement in renal function. In some patients, a circulating toxin may be responsible for extreme renal vasoconstriction and renal failure. Nevertheless, hemodialysis has not been reliable for eliminating suspected hepatic toxins.

There is an increased incidence of postoperative renal failure in patients with obstructive jaundice who undergo surgery. The cause of renal failure in these patients is unclear, but preoperative administration of mannitol appears to provide some protection.

NEPHROLITHIASIS

Although the pathogenesis of renal stones in poorly understood, several predisposing factors are recognized for the five major types of stones[42] (Table 20-8). Most stones are composed of calcium oxalate; the causes of hypercalcemia (hyperparathyroidism, sarcoidosis, malignant disease, idiopathic) must be sought in these patients. Urinary tract infection with urea-splitting organisms that produce ammonia favors the formation of magnesium ammonium phosphate stones. Formation of uric acid stones is favored by a persistently acid urine (pH less than 6.0) that decreases the solubility of uric acid. About 50% of patients with uric acid stones have gout.

Stones in the renal pelvis are typically painless, unless they are complicated by infection or obstruction. By contrast, renal stones passing down the ureter can produce intense flank pain, often radiating to the groin, associated with nausea and vomiting, and mimicking an acute surgical abdomen. Hematuria is common during ureteral passage of a stone, whereas ureteral obstruction may lead to signs and symptoms of renal failure.

Treatment

Treatment depends on identification of the composition of the stone and correction of predisposing factors, such as hyperparathyroidism, urinary tract infection, or gout. High fluid intake sufficient to maintain daily urine output at 2 to 3 L is often part of therapy. Extracorporeal shock-wave lithotripsy is a noninvasive treatment of renal stones that produces destruction of stones by shock waves. As an alternative to percutaneous nephrolithotomy, this approach has advantages of low morbidity and short hospital stay. Contraindications to extracorporeal shock-wave lithotripsy include pregnancy, morbid obesity, aortic aneurysm, and coagulopathy. The presence of an artificial cardiac pacemaker does not prohibit treatment with lithotripsy.[43,44]

Management of Anesthesia

Patients undergoing extracorporeal shock-wave lithotripsy experience pain at the flank entry site, necessitating anesthesia. Various anesthetic techniques (general, spinal, epidural, intercostal block with local infiltration, intravenous sedation with drugs such as midazolam, alfentanil, and ketamine) have been used successfully, and no one technique can be considered superior.[43–48] Regardless of the technique selected, immobilization is important. Any movement can displace the stone from the predetermined focus site, leading to unnecessary trauma to adjacent tissues, as well as incomplete dissolution of the stone. Indeed, the lungs, being air-filled sacs, present a different acoustic impedance to shock waves; they may also be injured by shock waves. In this regard, shock-wave-induced pulmonary contusion and hemoptysis have resulted in life-threatening arterial hypoxemia.[50] Even spontaneous or mechanical ventilation of the lungs with associated movement of the diaphragm causes stones to move as much as 30 mm along a vertical axis. For this reason, high-frequency jet ventilation has been used in an attempt to keep the stone stationary.[45] Complications of jet ventilation (air trapping, broncho-

Table 20-8. Composition and Characteristics of Renal Stones

Type of Stone	Incidence (%)	Radiographic Appearance	Etiology
Calcium oxalate	65	Opaque	Primary hyperparathyroidism Idiopathic hypercalciuria Hyperoxaluria Hypercuricosuria
Magnesium ammonium phosphate (struvite)	20	Opaque	Alkaline urine (usually due to chronic bacterial infection)
Calcium phosphate	7.5	Opaque	Renal tubular, acidosis
Uric acid	5	Lucent	Acid urine, gout Hyperuricosuria
Cystine	1.5	Opaque	Cystinuria

spasm, hypoventilation, inaccurate delivery of anesthetic gases) detract from the popularity of this mode of ventilation. Alternatively, mechanical ventilation of the lungs using a slow breathing rate ensures a long expiratory pause, during which the stone is stationary. A sensory level to T6 is recommended when epidural or spinal anesthesia is selected, keeping in mind that sympathetic nervous system blockade may be more pronounced with a spinal anesthetic.

Patients undergoing extracorporeal shock-wave lithotripsy are placed in a semireclining position into a hydraulically operated chair-like support system and then submerged in water from the clavicles down, in a large immersion tub. The head-up position during anesthesia can be associated with peripheral pooling of blood. This effect is usually offset, however, by immersion in water, which increases hydrostatic pressure on the abdomen and thorax such that venous return, cardiac output, and blood pressure are maintained. In patients with limited cardiac reserve, rapid immersion and displacement of blood into the central circulation by virtue of increased hydrostatic pressure may result in acute congestive heart failure. Likewise, hydrostatic forces on the thorax result in decreased chest wall compliance, vital capacity, and functional residual capacity. These changes may produce or aggravate ventilation-to-perfusion mismatches. Diuresis, natriuresis, and kaliuresis may follow immersion, perhaps reflecting suppression of ADH release. The water in the immersion tube must be kept warm to avoid hypothermia. Catheter insertion sites, as for epidural anesthesia, must be protected with water-impermeable dressings. The use of electrical equipment in contact with the water bath could introduce a significant electrical safety hazard, if the grounding system fails. The need for positioning in the chair introduces the need for extra-long anesthesia delivery tubing and cords for monitors. A unique problem is sudden exaggerated peripheral vasodilation and hypotension, when the patient is removed from the bath. Fluid replacement during lithotripsy is calculated to result in a urine output that facilitates passage of the disintegrated stones. Ear plugs may be used to decrease the noise intensity.

Cardiac dysrhythmias may occur during delivery of shock waves, although they are usually self-limited and rarely require treatment with lidocaine. To minimize the risk of initiating cardiac dysrhythmias, shock waves are triggered by the R wave of the electrocardiogram and delivered to the kidney during the absolute refractory period. Lithotripsy has been performed in patients with artificial cardiac pacemakers including an automatic implantable cardioverter defibrillator without incident.[43,44]

Postoperative pain is minimal, and most patients do not require opioids. Future lithotripters may not require the use of a water bath. Furthermore, the shock waves generated may be less painful, eliminating the need for anesthesia.

BENIGN PROSTATIC HYPERTROPHY

Benign prostatic hypertrophy (BPH) affects an estimated 15 million American males, typically developing after 50 years of age and manifested initially as frequency, nocturia, and a feeling of incomplete emptying. Obstruction to urine flow may result in urinary retention and renal failure. Because patients are often elderly, they are likely to have co-existing medical problems, especially cardiopulmonary disorders.

Medical management of BPH may be initiated with a drug that selectively inhibits the conversion of testosterone to dihydrotestosterone, which is necessary for growth of the prostate gland. As a result, the prostate gland decreases in size, serving to decrease the urinary obstruction. Nevertheless, definitive treatment of BPH requires transurethral resection of the prostate (TURP). Indeed, TURP is the most common surgical procedure performed in males older than 50 years of age. The surgical procedure is accompanied by absorption of nonelectrolyte irrigating fluids used to distend the bladder and wash away blood and prostatic tissue. This intravascular absorption of fluid may be sufficient to produce cardiovascular and central nervous system manifestations, known as the TURP syndrome[51] (Table 20-9). Intravascular absorption of large amounts of electrolyte-free fluid leads to dilutional hyponatremia; symptoms are most likely to develop if the serum sodium concentration is abruptly decreased below 120 $mEq \cdot L^{-1}$ (Table 20-10). Glycine, the most commonly used irrigating solution, has an osmolarity of 288 $mOsm \cdot L^{-1}$. Thus, its absorption may be associated with a near-normal plasma osmolarity despite profound hyponatremia. Transient visual disturbances have been observed, presumably reflecting the function of glycine as an inhibitory neurotransmitter at the retina.[52–54] Metabolism of glycine to ammonia has been associated with postoperative somnolence.

The amount of irrigating fluid absorbed into the patient's circulation is determined by a number of factors[51] (Table 20-11). Ideally, the duration of the resection is limited to less than 60 minutes and the hydrostatic pressure of the irrigating fluid should not exceed 70 cm H_2O. It is estimated that 10 to

Table 20-9.   Manifestations of the TURP Syndrome

Cardiovascular	Central Nervous System
Hypertension	Restlessness
Increased central venous pressure	Confusion
	Nausea
Bradycardia	Visual disturbances
Myocardial ischemia	Seizures
Shock	Coma

Table 20-10. Manifestations of Acute Hyponatremia

Serum Sodium ($mEq \cdot L^{-1}$)	Electrocardiogram	Central Nervous System
120	Possible widening of QRS	Restless Confusion
115	Widened QRS Elevated ST segment	Nausea Somnolence
110	Ventricular tachycardia Ventricular fibrillation	Seizures Coma

30 ml of irrigating fluid is absorbed into the patient's circulation for every minute of operating time, although volumes exceeding 1200 ml have been absorbed in 75 to 120 minutes. Prompt detection of excessive intravascular fluid absorption can be facilitated by the use of an ethanol-tagged irrigating solution and by measurement of the ethanol concentration in the patient's exhaled breath[55–57] (Fig. 20-10).

Management of Anesthesia

Spinal anesthesia has been recommended for TURP, because an awake patient may demonstrate central nervous system signs of excessive intravascular absorption of irrigating fluid (Table 20-9). Furthermore, accidental perforation of the bladder may be recognized by referred pain to the shoulder, reflecting subdiaphragmatic irritation by irrigating fluid in the peritoneal activity. At least a T10 sensory level is desirable for TURP. The inclusion of morphine (0.1 to 0.2 mg) with the local anesthetic solution injected into the subarachnoid space provides prolonged postoperative analgesia.[58] General anesthesia may mask signs of excessive intravascular absorption of irrigating fluid; nevertheless, it may be a more desirable approach in the patient who is unable to cooperate.

Intraoperative monitoring of the plasma sodium concentration, osmolarity, and hematocrit may be useful in detecting excessive hemodilution due to intravascular absorption of irrigating fluid. Increased central venous pressure and blood pressure is likely to accompany this acute hypervolemia. When hyponatremia is suggestive of excessive hemodilution (plasma sodium concentration less than 120 $mEq \cdot L^{-1}$), administration of mannitol or furosemide may be indicated.[59] On rare occasions, hypertonic saline may be required to treat hyponatremia. Assessment of blood loss during TURP is difficult because dilution of blood with irrigating fluids and the usual hemodynamic responses to blood loss (tachycardia and hypotension) are unreliable. Bleeding is estimated to be about 15 $ml \cdot g^{-1}$ of resected tissue.

Table 20-11. Factors Influencing Absorption of Irrigation Fluid

Hydrostatic pressure produced by irrigation fluid
Number and size of open venous sinuses
Peripheral venous pressure
Duration of surgery

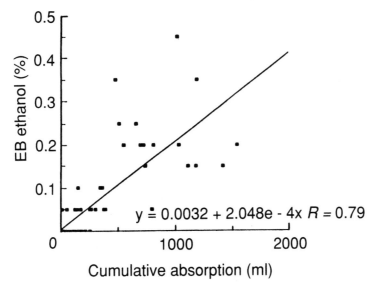

Fig. 20-10. Ethanol concentration in the exhaled gases (EB ethanol) parallels the cumulative absorption of irrigating fluid. (From Hulten J, Sarma VJ, Hjertberg H, Palmquist B. Monitoring of irrigating fluid absorption during transurethral prostatectomy. A study in anaesthetized patients using a 1% ethanol tag solution. Anaesthesia 1991;46:349–53, with permission.)

RENAL TRANSPLANTATION

Candidates for renal transplantation are selected from patients with end-stage renal disease who are on an established program of chronic hemodialysis. In adults, the most common causes of end-stage renal disease are diabetes mellitus, glomerulonephritis, polycystic kidney disease, and hypertension. Despite concerns about the recurrence of disease in the donor kidney, this has generally been only slowly progressive. The kidney must be removed from the donor and transplanted into the recipient promptly, to minimize the potential for ischemic damage to the organ. Kidneys from cadaver donors can be preserved by perfusion at low temperatures for 24 to 36 hours. Attempts are made to match human leukocyte antigens (HLA), as well as ABO blood groups, between donors and recipients. Paradoxically, the presence of certain common or shared HLA in blood administered to a potential transplant recipient has been observed to induce tolerance to donor antigens and thus improve allograft survival.[60] The donor kidney is placed in the lower abdomen and receives its vascular supply from the iliac vessels. The ureter is anastomosed directly to the bladder. Immunosuppressive therapy is instituted during the perioperative period.

Management of Anesthesia

Management of anesthesia for renal transplantation invokes the same principles as detailed for chronic renal failure patients: hemodialysis before surgery to optimize coagulation and hydration and to improve electrolyte and acid-base balance. Many of these patients are diabetics, emphasizing the need to monitor the blood glucose concentration during the perioperative period. In addition, strict asepsis must be adhered to during placement of intravascular catheters and intubation of the trachea.

Both regional and general anesthesia have been successfully used during renal transplantation. Advantages of regional anesthesia include elimination of the need for intubation of the trachea in an immunosuppressed patient, as well as the need for muscle relaxants. These advantages are negated, however, if regional anesthesia must be extensively supplemented with injected or inhaled drugs. Furthermore, blockade of the peripheral sympathetic nervous system, as produced by regional anesthesia, can complicate the control of blood pressure, especially considering the unpredictable intravascular fluid volume status of these patients. The use of regional anesthesia, particularly epidural anesthesia, is controversial in the presence of abnormal coagulation. For these reasons, general anesthesia is often the preferred approach for the management of patients undergoing renal transplantation.

When general anesthesia is selected, a useful approach is administration of nitrous oxide combined with a volatile drug

or short-acting opioid. The use of a volatile anesthetic may have a potential disadvantage, however. For example, administration of enflurane or sevoflurane is questionable, since elimination of fluoride depends on the GFR, which is often decreased in the early period after renal transplantation. In addition, the likely presence of liver disease in patients undergoing chronic hemodialysis, and the frequent occurrence of hepatic dysfunction after renal transplantation, must be remembered when considering the use of halothane. Furthermore, decreased cardiac output due to negative inotropic effects of volatile drugs must be minimized, to avoid jeopardizing the adequacy of tissue oxygen delivery, especially if anemia is present. All factors considered, the skeletal muscle relaxant effects of isoflurane and desflurane, plus their minimal metabolism, make these volatile anesthetics an attractive choice. Disadvantages of opioids used during anesthesia for renal transplantation are their lack of skeletal muscle relaxant effects and that excessive elevations in blood pressure cannot be reliably prevented or treated with these drugs.

The choice of muscle relaxants must take into account the principal route of elimination of these drugs, which most often is renal clearance. Furthermore, renal function may be unpredictable after transplantation. In this regard, atracurium or mivacurium, which are largely independent of renal function for their clearance, are logical selections. A newly transplanted but functioning kidney is able to clear muscle relaxants, as well as anticholinesterase drugs, used in their reversal at the same rate as normal patients.[61]

Fluid management includes intravenous replacement of intravascular fluid volume lost due to surgical trauma. In addition, intravenous fluids are necessary to optimize intravascular fluid volume and thereby maintain renal blood flow to the newly transplanted kidney. Potassium-containing intravenous fluid solutions should be used with caution in these patients. The anuric patient typically requires about 8 $ml \cdot kg^{-1} \cdot d^{-1}$ to replace insensible water loss. Humidification of inhaled gases during surgery reduces this requirement of maintenance fluid. Replacement of this insensible water loss, as well as fluid translocated due to surgical trauma, is often with a 5% glucose solution with 0.45% sodium chloride, to minimize sodium load until renal function is established after renal transplantation. Oxygen delivery to the tissues can be improved by the administration of erythrocytes. In the absence of cardiopulmonary disease, monitoring central venous pressure is a useful guide to the optimal rate of intravenous fluid infusion. Optimal hydration during the intraoperative period improves early function of the transplanted kidney.[62]

Diuretics are often administered to facilitate urine formation by the newly transplanted kidney. In this regard, an osmotic diuretic such as mannitol will facilitate urine output and reduce excess tissue and intravascular fluid. Unlike loop diuretics (furosemide or ethacrynic acid), mannitol does not depend on renal tubular concentrating mechanisms to produce diuresis.

Cardiac arrest has been described after completion of the artery anastomosis to the transplanted kidney.[63] This event occurred with the release of the occlusion clamp and most likely reflected sudden hyperkalemia, due to establishment of blood flow to the transplanted kidney and washout of the potassium-containing solution used to preserve the kidney before transplantation. In addition, if clamping of the external iliac artery is necessary during the renal artery anastomosis, potassium can be released into the circulation from the ischemic limb after removal of the clamp. Unclamping may also be followed by hypotension due to the abrupt addition of up to 300 ml to the capacity of the intravascular fluid space, as well as the release of vasodilating chemicals from previously ischemic tissues. When it does occur, this hypotension is often treated with intravenous infusion of fluids.

Complications

Acute immunologic rejection of the newly transplanted kidney can occur. This rejection is manifested in the vasculature of the transplanted kidney. It can be so rapid that inadequate circulation is evident almost immediately after the blood supply to the kidneys is established. The only treatment for this acute rejection reaction is removal of the transplanted kidney, especially if the rejection process is accompanied by disseminated intravascular coagulation. Postoperative hematoma may arise in the graft, causing vascular or ureteral obstruction.

Delayed signs of graft rejection usually include fever, local tenderness, and deterioration of urine output. Treatment with high doses of corticosteroids and antilymphocyte globulin may be helpful. The acute tubular necrosis that occurs in the transplanted kidney secondary to prolonged ischemia usually responds to hemodialysis. Cyclosporine toxicity may also cause acute renal failure. Ultrasonography and needle biopsy are performed to differentiate between the possible causes of kidney malfunction.

Opportunistic infections owing to chronic immunosuppression are common after renal transplantation. Hepatitis B was a frequent problem until the availability of a vaccine decreased the infection rate to less than 5%. Long-term survival is unsatisfactory in renal transplant patients who are immunosuppressed and who also carry hepatitis B surface antigen. The frequency of cancer is 30 to 100 times greater in transplant recipients than in the general population, presumably reflecting the loss of protective effects due to immunosuppression. Large cell lymphoma is a well-recognized complication of transplantation, occurring almost exclusively in patients with evidence of Epstein-Barr virus infection.

REFERENCES

1. Byrick RJ, Rose DK. Pathophysiology and prevention of acute renal failure: The role of the anaesthetist. Can J Anaesth 1990; 37:457–67

2. Mitch WE, Collier VU, Walser M. Creatinine metabolism in chronic renal failure. Clin Sci 1980;58:327–33

3. Sladen RN, Endo E, Harrison T. Two-hour versus 22-hour creatinine clearance in critically ill patients. Anesthesiology 1987;67: 1013–6

4. Curtis JR, Donovan BA. Assessment of renal concentrating ability. Br Med J 1979;1:304–5

5. Cousins MJ, Mazze RI. Methoxyflurane nephrotoxicity—a study of dose response in man. JAMA 1973;225:1611–6

6. Loehning RW, Mazze RI. Possible nephrotoxicity from enflurane in a patient with severe renal disease. Anesthesiology 1974;40: 203–5

7. Parfrey PS, Griffiths SM, Barrett BJ, et al. Contrast material-induced renal failure in patients with diabetes mellitus, renal insufficiency, or both. A prospective controlled study. N Engl J Med 1989;320:143–9

8. Barry KG, Mazze RI, Schwartz FD. Prevention of surgical oliguria and renal hemodynamic suppression by sustained hydration. N Engl J Med 1964;270:1371–7

9. Bastron RD, Perkins FM, Pyne JL. Autoregulation of renal blood flow during halothane anesthesia. Anesthesiology 1977;46:142–4

10. Lessard MR, Trepanier CA. Renal function and hemodynamics during prolonged isoflurane-induced hypotension in humans. Anesthesiology 1991;74:860–5

11. Philbin DM, Coggins CH. Plasma antidiuretic hormone levels in cardiac surgical patients during morphine and halothane anesthesia. Anesthesiology 1978;49:95–8

12. Kharasch ED, Yeo K-T, Kenny MA, Buffington CW. Atrial natriuretic factor may mediate the renal effects of PEEP ventilation. Anesthesiology 1988;69:862–9

13. Miller ED, Ackerly JA, Peach MJ. Blood pressure support during general anesthesia in a renin-dependent state in the rat. Anesthesiology 1978;48:404–8

14. Cousins MJ, Greenstein LR, Hitt BA, Mazze RI. Metabolism and renal effects of enflurane in man. Anesthesiology 1976;44:44–53

15. Mazze RI, Cousins MJ, Barr GA. Renal effects and metabolism of isoflurane in man. Anesthesiology 1974;40:536–42

16. Creasser C, Stoelting RK. Serum inorganic fluoride concentrations during and after halothane, fluroxene and methoxyflurane anesthesia in man. Anesthesiology 1973;39:537–40

17. Mazze RI, Calverley RK, Smith NT. Inorganic fluoride nephrotoxicity: Prolonged enflurane and halothane anesthesia in volunteers. Anesthesiology 1977;46:265–71

18. Mazze RI, Sievenpiper TS, Stevenson J. Renal effects of enflurane and halothane in patients with abnormal renal function. Anesthesiology 1984;60:161–3

19. Young SR, Stoelting RK, Peterson C, Madura JA. Anesthetic biotransformation and renal function in obese patients during and after methoxyflurane or halothane anesthesia. Anesthesiology 1975;42:451–7

20. Bentley JB, Vaughn RW, Miller MS, et al. Serum inorganic fluoride levels in obese patients during enflurane anesthesia. Anesth Analg 1979;58:409–12

21. Eschbach JW, Kelley MR, Haley NR, et al. Treatment of the anemia of progressive renal failure with recombinant human erythropoietin. N Engl J Med 1989;321:158–66

22. Carvalho AC. Bleeding in uremia. A clinical challenge. N Engl J Med 1983;308:38–46

23. Fernandez F, Goudable C, Sie P, et al. Low haematocrit and prolonged bleeding time in uraemic patients: Effect of red cell transfusions. Br J Haematol 1985;59:139–43

24. Ghoneim MM, Long JP. The interaction between magnesium and other neuromuscular blocking agents. Anesthesiology 1970;32:23–7

25. Weir PH, Chung FF. Anaesthesia for patients with chronic renal disease. Can Anaesth Soc J 1984;31:468–80

26. Gronert GA, Lambert EH, Theye RA. The response of denervated skeletal muscle to succinylcholine. Anesthesiology 1973;39:13–22

27. Don HF, Dieppa RA, Taylor P. Narcotic analgesics in anuric patients. Anesthesiology 1975;42:745–7

28. Tinker JH, Michenfelder JD. Increased resistance to nitroprusside-induced cyanide toxicity in anuric dogs. Anesthesiology 1980;52:40–7

29. Carter R, Heerdt M, Acchiardo S. Fluoride kinetics after enflurane anesthesia in healthy and anephric patients and in patients with poor renal function. Clin Pharmacol Ther 1977;20:565–70

30. Bromage PR, Gertel M. Brachial plexus anesthesia in chronic renal failure. Anesthesiology 1972;36:488–93

31. McEllistrem RF, Schell J, O'Malley KO, O'Toole DO, Cunningham AJ. Interscalene brachial plexus blockade with lidocaine in chronic renal failure—a pharmacokinetic study. Can J Anaesth 1989;36:59–63

32. Beauregard L, Martin R, Tetrault JP. Brachial plexus block and chronic renal failure. Can J Anaesth 1987;34:S118

33. Hunter JM, Jones RS, Utting JE. Comparison of vecuronium, atracurium and tubocurarine in normal patients and in patients with no renal function. Br J Anaesth 1984;56:941–50

34. Bencini AF, Scaf AHF, Sohn YJ, et al. Disposition and urinary excretion of vecuronium bromide in anesthetized patients with normal renal function or renal failure. Anesth Analg 1986;65:245–51

35. Fahey MR, Rupp SM, Canfell C, et al. Effect of renal function on laudanosine excretion in man. Br J Anaesth 1985;57:1049–51

36. Parker CJR, Jones JE, Hunter JM. Disposition of infusions of atracurium and its metabolite, laudanosine, in patients in renal and respiratory failure in an ITU. Br J Anaesth 1988;61:531–40

37. Morris RB, Cronnelly R, Miller RD, et al. Pharmacokinetics of edrophonium in anephric and renal transplant patients. Br J Anaesth 1981;53:1311–3

38. Paul MD, Mazer CD, Byrick RJ, Rose DK, Goldstein MB. Influence of mannitol and dopamine on renal function during elective infrarenal aortic clamping in man. Am J Nephrol 1986;6:427–34

39. Tilney NL, Lazarus JM. Acute renal failure in surgical patients. Surg Clin North Am 1983;63:357–77

40. Joel M, Rosales JK. Fanconi syndrome and anesthesia. Anesthesiology 1981;55:455–6

41. Nishikawa T, Dohi S. Baroreflex function in a patient with Bartter's syndrome. Can Anaesth Soc J 1985;32:646–50

42. Coe FL, Parks JH, Asplin JR. The pathogenesis and treatment of kidney stones. N Engl J Med 1992;327:1141–52

43. Celentano WJ, Jahr JS, Nossaman BD. Extracorporeal shock wave lithotripsy in a patient with a pacemaker. Anesth Analg 1992;74:770–2

44. Long AL, Venditti FJ. Lithotripsy in a patient with an automatic implantable cardioverter defibrillator. Anesthesiology 1991;74:937–8

45. Perel A, Hoffman B, Podeh D, Davidson DJT. High frequency positive pressure ventilation during general anesthesia for extracorporeal shock wave lithotripsy. Anesth Analg 1986;65:1231–4

46. Berger JJ, Boysen PG, Gravenstein JS, et al. Failure of high frequency jet ventilation to ventilate patients adequately during extracorporeal shock-wave lithotripsy. Anesth Analg 1987;66:262–3

47. Duvall JO, Griffith DP. Epidural anesthesia for extracorporeal shock wave lithotripsy. Anesth Analg 1985;64:544–6

48. Monk TG, Boure B, White PF, Meretyk S, Clayman RV. Comparison of intravenous sedative-analgesic techniques for outpatient immersion lithotripsy. Anesth Analg 1991;72:616–21

49. Monk TG, Rater JM, White PF. Comparison of alfentanil and ketamine infusions in combination with midazolam for outpatient lithotripsy. Anesthesiology 1991;74:1023–8

50. Malhotra V, Rosen RJ, Slepian RL. Life-threatening hypoxemia after lithotripsy in an adult due to shock-wave-induced pulmonary contusion. Anesthesiology 1991;75:529–31

51. Jensen V. The TURP syndrome. Can J Anaesth 1991;38:90–7

52. Roesch RP, Stoelting RK, Lingeman JE, et al. Ammonia toxicity resulting from glycine absorption during a transurethral resection of the prostate. Anesthesiology 1983;58:577–9

53. Ovassaian A, Joshi CW, Brunner EA. Visual disturbance: An unusual symptom of transurethral prostatic resection reaction. Anesthesiology 1982;57:332–4

54. Wang JM-L, Creel DJ, Wong KC. Transurethral resection of the prostate, serum glycine levels, and ocular evoked potentials. Anesthesiology 1989;70:36–41

55. Hulten J, Samra VJ, Hyertberg H, Palmquist B. Monitoring of irrigating fluid absorption during transurethral prostatectomy. A study in anaesthetized patients using a 1% ethanol tag solution. Anaesthesia 1991;46:349–53

56. Hahn RG. Ethanol monitoring of irrigating fluid absorption in transurethral prostatic surgery. Anesthesiology 1988;68:867–73

57. Hahn R, Mjoberg M. Immediate detection of irrigant absorption during transurethral prostatectomy: Case report. Can J Anaesth 1989;36:86–8

58. Kirson LE, Goldman JM, Slover RB. Low-dose intrathecal morphine for postoperative pain control in patients undergoing transurethral resection of the prostate. Anesthesiology 1989;71:192–5

59. Crowley K, Clarkson K, Hannon V, McShane A, Kelly DG. Diuretics after transurethral prostatectomy: A double-blind controlled trial comparing furosemide and mannitol. Br J Anaesth 1990;65:337–41

60. vanTwuyver, Mooijaart RJD, tenBerge IJM, et al. Pretransplantation blood transfusion revisited. N Engl J Med 1991;325:1210–3

61. Cronnelly R, Stanski DR, Miller RD, Sheiner LB. Pyridostigmine kinetics with and without renal function. Clin Pharmacol Ther 1980;28:78–81

62. Carlier M, Squifflet JP. Maximal hydration during anesthesia increases pulmonary artery pressure and improves function of human renal transplants. Transplantation 1982;34:701–4

63. Hirshman CA, Leon D, Edelstein G, et al. Risk of hyperkalemia in recipients of kidneys preserved with an intracellular electrolyte solution. Anesth Analg 1980;59:283–6

21

Water, Electrolyte, and Acid-Base Disturbances

Alterations of water and electrolyte content and distribution, as well as acid-base disturbances, can produce multiple organ system dysfunction during the perioperative period. For example, impairment of central nervous system, cardiac, and neuromuscular function is likely in the presence of water, electrolyte (sodium, potassium, calcium, magnesium), and acid-base disturbances. Furthermore, those disorders often accompany events associated with the perioperative period (Table 21-1). Management of patients with water and electrolyte disorders requires an understanding of the distribution of water and electrolytes and the electrophysiology of cells. Often the manifestations of water and electrolyte disturbances are related more to the rate of change and less to the absolute change.

DISTRIBUTION OF BODY WATER

Total body water content is greatest at birth, representing about 70% of the body weight in kilograms (Fig. 21-1). With increasing age, total body water content decreases, constituting about 60% of the body weight of an average adult male and 50% of the body weight of an adult female. This difference is attributable to the greater fat content of females. Since fat is essentially anhydrous, it contributes to body weight without a proportionate increase in the volume of total body water. Constant total body water content is important for the viability of cells. Indeed, water is the medium in which all metabolic reactions occur. Furthermore, all nutrients and solutes of the body are dissolved or suspended in water.

Total body water content is categorized as intracellular fluid or extracellular fluid, according to the location of water relative to cell membranes (Fig. 21-2). Intracellular fluid represents about 55% of the total body water content; the remaining water is distributed as extracellular fluid. Extracellular fluid is further divided into interstitial and intravascular (plasma) fluid on the basis of the location of water relative to capillary membranes. The water content of these fluid spaces is calculated in Table 21-2.

The body's main priority is to maintain intravascular fluid volume. Acute reductions in this volume, as occur with fluid deprivation during the preoperative period, blood loss, or surgical trauma that results in tissue edema ("third-space loss"), elicit the release of antidiuretic hormone (ADH), renin, and possibly atrial natriuretic factor. These substances subsequently result in responses at renal tubules that lead to the restoration of intravascular fluid volume. Furthermore, interstitial fluid is in dynamic equilibrium with intravascular fluid, serving as an available reservoir from which water and electrolytes can be mobilized into the circulation. Conversely, interstitial fluid spaces can accept water and electrolytes, if these substances are present in excess amounts in the intravascular fluid spaces. Peripheral edema is a manifestation of excess amounts of water in the interstitial fluid spaces.

The pressure necessary to prevent movement of solvent (water) to another fluid space is designated the osmotic pressure. Indeed, osmotic pressure is the principal determinant of the distribution of water among the three major compartments. Sodium is the most important cation for determining plasma osmolarity. In this regard, plasma osmolarity can be predicted clinically by doubling the plasma sodium concentration (Table 21-3). Low plasma osmolarity (below 285 $mOsm \cdot L^{-1}$) means a high concentration of water; a high osmolarity (above 295 $mOsm \cdot L^{-1}$) means a low concentration.

Intravenous solutions administered to patients are considered isotonic, hypotonic, or hypertonic, according to their effective osmotic pressures relative to plasma. Normal saline and 5% glucose in water have an osmolarity similar to that of

Table 21-1.   Etiology of Water, Electrolyte, and Acid-
Base Disturbances During the Perioperative Period

Disease States
  Endocrinopathies
  Nephropathies
  Gastroenteropathies

Drug Therapy
  Diuretics
  Corticosteroids

Nasogastric Suction

Surgery
  Transurethral resection of the prostate
  Translocation of fluid due to tissue trauma
  Resection of portions of the gastrointestinal tract

Management of Anesthesia
  Intravenous fluid administration
  Alveolar ventilation
  Hypothermia

Table 21-2.   Calculation of Total Body Water Content
and Distribution in a 70-kg Adult

	Male	Female
Total body water	42 L $(70 \times 0.6)^a$	35 L $(70 \times 0.5)^a$
Total intracellular water	23 L $(42 \times 0.55)^b$	19 L $(35 \times 0.55)^b$
Total extracellular water	19 L (42×0.45)	16 L (35×0.45)

[a] Total body water content constitutes 60% of the body weight (kg) of an adult male and 50% of the body weight of an adult female.

[b] Intracellular water represents about 55% of the total body water content.

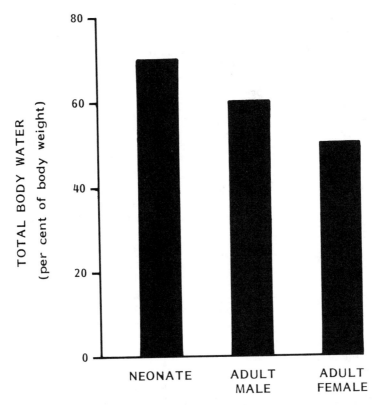

Fig. 21-1. Total body water represents about 70% of the body weight (kg) of a neonate, 60% of an adult male, and 50% of an adult female. Anhydrous fat contributes disproportionately to the body weight of an adult female, explaining the decreased amount of body water relative to body weight.

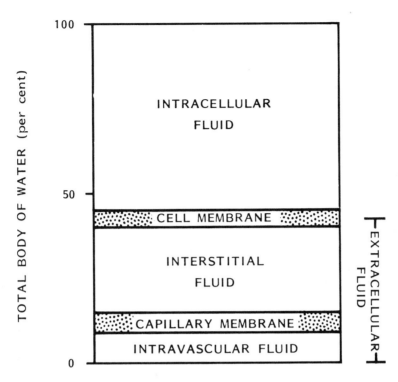

Fig. 21-2. Total body water is designated as intracellular or extracellular fluid, depending on the location of water relative to the cell membrane. Water in the extracellular compartment is further subdivided as interstitial or intravascular (plasma) fluid, depending on its location relative to the capillary membrane. About 55% of total body water is intracellular, 37% interstitial, and the remaining 8% intravascular.

body fluids. Therefore, these fluids are classified as isotonic solutions. It is important to understand, however, that the metabolism and cellular uptake of glucose present in 5% glucose in water result in hypotonic solutions. The resulting free water can distribute itself among all fluid compartments, with less than 10% remaining intravascular. Lactated Ringer's solution, containing 5% glucose, is initially hypertonic (about 527 $mOsm·L^{-1}$), but the hypertonicity diminishes as glucose is metabolized and taken up by cells.

The intravascular pressure produced by the heart results in a hydrostatic pressure gradient of approximately 20 mmHg across capillary membranes. If this pressure gradient is not counterbalanced, it tends to force intravascular water into the interstitial fluid compartment. Indeed, were it not for large protein molecules (principally albumin), which cannot freely cross capillary membranes, there would be a continuous loss of intravascular fluid volume. The concentrations of these proteins are just sufficient to balance the hydrostatic pressure difference of about 20 mmHg that exists between the intravascular and interstitial fluid compartments. The osmotic effect produced by the proteins maintains the circulating plasma volume. This osmotic effect is called the colloid osmotic pressure, or oncotic pressure. An important way to increase circulating plasma volume is to infuse albumin, which draws water from the interstitial into the intravascular fluid space.

Table 21-3.   Calculation of Plasma Osmolarity

Plasma osmolarity = 2 (plasma sodium concentration)
$$+ \frac{BUN}{2.8} + \frac{glucose}{18}$$

Normal plasma osmolarity is 285–295 $mOsm·L^{-1}$. In the presence of a normal blood urea nitrogen concentration (BUN, 10–20 $mg·dl^{-1}$) and blood glucose concentration (60–100 $mg·dl^{-1}$), plasma osmolarity can be predicted as twice the plasma sodium concentration. As BUN or blood glucose concentrations increase, a greater impact is exerted by these substances on plasma osmolarity.

DISTRIBUTION OF ELECTROLYTES

The distribution and concentration of electrolytes differ greatly among the fluid compartments for body water (Table 21-4). The major cation in intravascular fluid is sodium, as well

Table 21-4. Approximate Composition of Extracellular and Intracellular Fluid (mEq·L^{-1})^a

	Extracellular		Intracellular
	Intravascular	Interstitial	
Sodium	140	145	10
Potassium	5	4	150
Calcium	5	2.5	<1
Magnesium	2	1.5	40
Chloride	103	115	4
Bicarbonate	28	30	10

^{a} Total anion concentration consists of phosphates, sulfates, organic acids, and negatively charged sites on proteins.

as small amounts of potassium, calcium, and magnesium. By contrast, the major cation in intracellular fluid is potassium. The net effect is a concentration of total cation that is essentially equal throughout body water. These positive charges are balanced by anions such as chloride, bicarbonate, phosphate, and the negatively charged sites on proteins.

Sodium is unique in that changes in the concentration of this ion in extracellular fluid are usually due to changes in the volume of solvent (water), and not to changes in the total body content of sodium. Therefore, a change in the plasma sodium concentration must be interpreted with respect to total body water content. Indeed, an acute change in the plasma sodium concentration usually reflects an alteration in total body water content, and not sodium content.

Plasma potassium concentrations are easily measured, but only about 2% (80 mEq) of total body potassium content is present in the extracellular fluid. Skeletal muscles are the major storage site of potassium.

ELECTROPHYSIOLOGY OF CELLS

The electrophysiology of excitable cells is dependent on the intracellular and extracellular concentrations of sodium, potassium, and calcium. An essential characteristic of excitable cells is their ability to maintain concentration gradients for sodium and potassium across their membranes. This unequal distribution of ions (excess potassium inside and sodium outside cells) produces an electrochemical difference across cell membranes, with the interior of cells negative relative to the exterior (Fig. 21-3). At rest, the interior of cells is about -90 mV with respect to the outside of cells. The negative electrical potential of cell interiors is designated the resting membrane potential. The arrival of an appropriate stimulus (electrical,

chemical, mechanical) results in altered permeability of cell membranes, such that sodium enters and potassium leaves the cells. The net effect of this change is a decrease in the electrical potential difference (the resting membrane potential becomes less negative) across the cell membrane. When the difference across cell membranes is about -70 mV, a sudden additional influx of sodium reverses the electrical charge across the cell membranes, producing an action potential.

The electrophysiology of cells, and the resulting action potential, are altered by changes in the concentrations of electrolytes (Fig. 21-3). Potassium gradients across cell membranes are the key determinants of resting membrane potentials. An increase in the extracellular concentration of potassium results in a less negative resting membrane potential that is closer to the threshold potential. Conversely, a reduction in the extracellular concentration of potassium makes the resting membrane potential more negative. Excitability of cells is partly related to the distance between the resting membrane potential and the threshold potential. Since hyperkalemia brings the resting membrane potential closer to the threshold potential, a smaller impulse is required to elicit an action potential. Therefore, the excitability of cells is considered to be increased. The effects of potassium on the rate of spontaneous depolarization and conduction velocity of neural impulses must also be considered when predicting effects of changes in the concentration of this electrolyte on the excitability of cells. For example, a decrease in the plasma potassium concentration increases the rate of spontaneous depolarization, while a high concentration of extracellular potassium slows the conduction velocity of neural impulses. All factors considered, it is difficult to predict reliably the effects of changes in the plasma concentration of potassium on the excitability of cells. Sodium is also necessary for the cellular depolarization and generation of an action potential. Indeed, the amplitude of the action potential is decreased in the presence of hyponatremia. Calcium is also an ion necessary for the maintenance of threshold potentials.

TOTAL BODY WATER EXCESS

The hallmark of total body water excess is a plasma sodium concentration below 135 mEq·L^{-1}, in the presence of a normal or increased intravascular fluid volume. Because the kidneys have an extraordinary ability to excrete increased amounts of water, patients with excess body water are also likely to have impaired renal function. The ability of the kidneys to excrete excess body water is impaired, for example, in patients with congestive heart failure, nephrosis, or cirrhosis of the liver. Peripheral edema is a manifestation of excess body water that accompanies these disease processes.

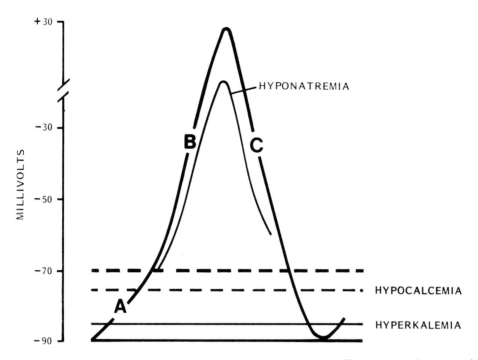

Fig. 21-3. Schematic diagram of the action potential of an automatic (pacemaker) cell. The resting membrane potential (bottom line) is normally -90 mV. Continuous movement of sodium and potassium across the cell membrane results in spontaneous depolarization (A) until the threshold potential (top dashed line) is reached at about -70 mV. When the threshold potential is reached, there is a sudden increase in the permeability of the cell membrane to sodium, and rapid depolarization (B) leads to the production of an action potential. After propagation of the action potential, permeability of the cell membrane is restored, sodium is pumped out of the cell, and repolarization occurs (C). Disturbances of electrolyte concentrations alter the electrophysiology of the cell. For example, hyponatremia decreases the amplitude of the action potential. Hyperkalemia results in a less negative resting membrane potential. Hypocalcemia results in a more negative threshold potential.

Excess body water can also be due to inappropriate secretion of ADH, but edema does not occur (see the section, Inappropriate Secretion of Antidiuretic Hormone). Intravascular absorption of large volumes of water, as during transurethral resection of the prostate, can result in iatrogenic water intoxication (see Chapter 20). Regardless of the etiology, an excess of body water results in a decrease of the plasma sodium concentration and in a decrease in plasma osmolarity.

Signs and Symptoms

Signs and symptoms of total body water excess depend on the absolute plasma sodium concentration and the rate of its decline. Plasma osmolarity and hematocrit are predictably decreased when excess body water is present. Other evidence of excess body water is arterial hypertension, increased central venous pressure, and pulmonary edema. When water retention is sufficient to decrease the plasma sodium concentration below 120 mEq·L^{-1}, it is likely that central nervous system signs ranging from confusion to drowsiness will be

manifested. Further declines to less than 110 mEq·L^{-1} can produce seizures and coma. These central nervous system abnormalities most likely reflect cerebral edema and increased intracranial pressure. Cardiac dysrhythmias, including ventricular fibrillation, can occur when the plasma sodium concentration decreases below 100 mEq·L^{-1}.

Treatment

Emergency treatment of excess body water consists of reducing the water content of the brain by administering hypertonic saline, mannitol, or furosemide. As a rough guide, 1 ml of 5% saline will increase the sodium concentration of 1 liter of a body water by 1 mEq. For example, to increase the plasma sodium concentration from 130 mEq·L^{-1} to 140 mEq·L^{-1} in a 70-kg adult male (predicted total body water content 42 L) would require about 420 ml of 5% saline (1 ml × 10 mEq × 42 L). The rate of sodium administration varies from 30 minutes to several hours, depending on the urgency of the situation and should stop, once seizures cease or cardiac dysrhythmias are corrected. In contrast to saline, mannitol not only removes water from cells but also results in an osmotic diuresis. Both saline and mannitol will initially expand the extracellular fluid volume.

Inappropriate Secretion of Antidiuretic Hormone

Inappropriate secretion of ADH results in water retention, low output of a highly concentrated urine, and dilutional hyponatremia. In addition, urinary excretion of sodium is increased, further lowering the plasma sodium concentration. Despite this excess sodium loss, hypovolemia does not occur, since the concomitant retention of water has expanded the intravascular fluid volume. Secretion of ADH is considered to be inappropriate, since there is no physiologic stimulus present to stimulate elaboration of this hormone.

Inappropriate secretion of ADH has been described after a number of events (Table 21-5). The possible occurrence of this response in the postoperative period should be appreciated. For example, a consistent metabolic response to surgery is the release of ADH for up to 96 hours postoperatively.[1,2] Indeed, acute hyponatremia is the most common acute biochemical change found after surgery. The most likely mechanism for this hyponatremia is acute expansion of intravascular fluid volume secondary to hormone-induced resorption of water by renal tubules. This excess hormone release (aldosterone as well) may be an exaggerated response to decreases in intravascular fluid volume that often occurs during invasive operations (Fig. 21-4). Abrupt reductions in the plasma concentrations of sodium (especially below 110 mEq·L^{-1}) can lead to cerebral edema and seizures. Indeed, intravenous administration of sodium deficient solutions to oliguric postoperative patients has led to hyponatremia, seizures, and permanent brain damage.[3]

Inappropriate elevated urinary sodium concentrations and osmolarity in the presence of hyponatremia and decreased plasma osmolarity (less than 280 mOsm·L^{-1}) is virtually diagnostic of inappropriate ADH secretion. Treatment is initially with reductions in water intake to 500 ml·d^{-1}. Establishment of a negative water balance leads to a spontaneous decrease of ADH release and often is the only treatment necessary in postoperative patients in whom the abnormality of ADH secretion is transient. Demeclocycline may be administered to antagonize the effects of ADH on renal tubules. Restriction of fluid intake and administration of demeclocycline, however, are not immediately effective for management of patients manifesting acute neurologic symptoms due to hyponatremia. In these patients, intravenous infusion of hypertonic saline solutions sufficient to elevate the plasma concentration of sodium 0.5 mEq·L^{-1}·h^{-1} is a useful guideline. Overly rapid correction of symptomatic hyponatremia has been associated with a fatal neurologic disorder known as central pontine myelinolysis.[3–5]

Management of Anesthesia

Management of anesthesia must consider the likely presence of renal, cardiac, or liver disease as an etiology for excess body water. Decreased excitability of cells due to the low plasma sodium concentration could result in poor cardiac contractility and in increased sensitivity to nondepolarizing muscle relaxants. This former possibility should be considered when hypotension occurs, particularly during administration of anesthetics with known negative inotropic effects. Likewise, the dose of muscle relaxants should be titrated, observing responses evoked by a peripheral nerve stimulator.

TOTAL BODY WATER DEFICIT

The hallmark of total body water deficit is a plasma sodium concentration above 145 mEq·L^{-1}. Pure water deficit is rare, as most conditions leading to water loss are accompanied by loss of electrolytes. Causes of pure water loss include deficiencies or absence of ADH (diabetes insipidus) or resistance of renal tubules to the effects of this hormone. For example, pure water loss due to renal tubular unresponsiveness to ADH can accompany hypercalcemia, hypokalemia, and chronic nephritis. Pure water deficit can also occur in elderly or confused patients who do not respond to the sensation of thirst. Prolonged mechanical ventilation of the lungs with unhumidified gases can also lead to substantial water loss.

Table 21-5. Factors Associated With Inappropriate Secretion of Antidiuretic Hormone

Postoperative period

Positive-pressure ventilation of the lungs

Endocrine disorders
  Adrenocortical insufficiency
  Anterior pituitary damage

Carcinoma of the lung

Central nervous system dysfunction
  Infection
  Hemorrhage
  Trauma

Drugs
  Chlorpropamide
  Opioids
  Diuretics
  Antimetabolites

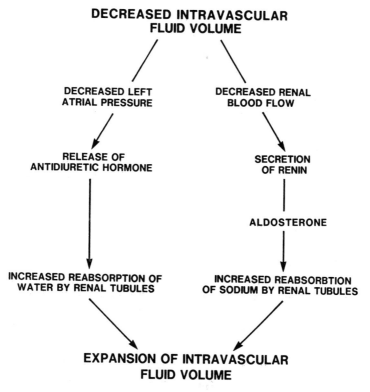

**DECREASED INTRAVASCULAR
FLUID VOLUME**

**DECREASED LEFT
ATRIAL PRESSURE**

**DECREASED RENAL
BLOOD FLOW**

**RELEASE OF
ANTIDIURETIC HORMONE**

**SECRETION
OF RENIN**

ALDOSTERONE

**INCREASED REABSORPTION OF
WATER BY RENAL TUBULES**

**INCREASED REABSORBTION
OF SODIUM BY RENAL TUBULES**

**EXPANSION OF INTRAVASCULAR
FLUID VOLUME**

Fig. 21-4. An acute decrease in intravascular fluid volume elicits changes designed to expand the intravascular fluid volume.

Signs and Symptoms

Clinical manifestations of a total body water deficit reflect loss of water from all fluid compartments. For example, mucous membranes are dry, and skin turgor is reduced. When dehydration is severe, blood pressure, venous pressure, and urine output are decreased, and heart rate is increased. Orthostatic hypotension is often present. Peripheral cyanosis reflects a sluggish peripheral circulation, with marked desaturation of the venous blood. Central nervous system dysfunction (drowsiness, coma) can occur. Because both intracellular and extracellular fluid volumes are reduced, the hematocrit will probably not increase. Blood urea nitrogen and serum creatinine concentrations will increase, as hypovolemia leads to decreased blood pressure and cardiac output, causing a reduced renal blood flow and glomerular filtration rate. If the kidneys are responding normally, the urine concentrating system will be functioning at its maximum level resulting in a urine with a high osmolarity (above 800 mOsm·L^{-1}) and specific gravity (above 1.030). Peripheral edema is absent, emphasizing that a decrease in total body water content is responsible for the increased plasma sodium concentration.

Treatment

Treatment of a total body water deficit consists of administering free water on the basis of a measured reduction in body weight or, more commonly, the magnitude of elevation of the plasma sodium concentration. An acceptable approach is administration of 5% glucose in water, with the volume and rate of administration guided by changes in blood pressure, central venous pressure, urine output, and repeated determinations of the plasma sodium concentration. It should be appreciated that the brain does not necessarily shrink to the same extent that total body water diminishes, particularly if dehydration is gradual. Thus, if correction of the body water deficit is too rapid, the brain can take up excessive water, leading to the development of cerebral edema. To avoid brain damage from too rapid correction, it is recommended that hypernatremia be gradually corrected at a maximum rate of 0.5 mEq·L^{-1}·h^{-1}.[3–5]

Management of Anesthesia

Induction and maintenance of anesthesia in the presence of a decreased intravascular fluid volume due to a total body water deficit is likely to be accompanied by a decrease in blood pressure. Specifically, peripheral vasodilation, produced by opioids, barbiturates, or volatile anesthetic drugs, can unmask hypovolemia. Ketamine is less likely to decrease blood pressure when intravascular fluid volume is reduced. Positive-pressure ventilation of the lungs and blood loss are likely to produce exaggerated blood pressure decreases in these patients.

A contracted intravascular fluid volume also results in decreased volume of distribution for drugs such as nondepolarizing muscle relaxants, which are limited in their distribution primarily to the extracellular fluid. Conceivably, these patients could have an increased sensitivity to muscle relaxants. Measurements of cardiac filling pressures and urine output are helpful in guiding the volume and rate of intravenous fluid administration.

SODIUM EXCESS

Total body excess of sodium is reflected by a plasma sodium concentration that exceeds 145 mEq·L^{-1}. The kidneys closely regulate total body sodium content, such that excess accumulation of sodium is almost impossible, unless there is impaired renal function. For example, impairment of sodium excretion by the kidneys often occurs in patients with congestive heart failure, nephrotic syndrome, and cirrhosis of the liver with ascites. Increased resorption of sodium by renal tubules is a classic response to excess aldosterone secretion by the adrenal cortex. Indeed, in patients with primary aldosteronism, hypernatremia predominates, with little evidence of expansion of the interstitial fluid volume. It must be remembered, however, that the most common cause of hypernatremia is not an excess of total body sodium, but rather a total body water deficit.

Signs and Symptoms

Peripheral edema is the hallmark of increased total body sodium content. Interstitial fluid spaces, however, can be expanded by as much as 5 L in normal adults, before edema is detectable. Other features of total body sodium excess include ascites, pleural effusion, and an expanded intravascular fluid volume manifested as hypertension.

Treatment

Treatment of excess total body sodium consists of facilitated excretion of sodium through the kidneys. This is accomplished by the administration of diuretics that prevent resorption of sodium by the renal tubules. In this regard, furosemide may be administered to treat edema owing to congestive heart failure, whereas edema due to cirrhosis of the liver is treated with spironolactone.

Management of Anesthesia

Other than the recognition of an increased intravascular fluid volume, there are no specific recommendations regarding management of anesthesia. Although the volume of distribution for parenteral drugs is increased, clinical responses produced by these drugs do not seem to be altered predictably. In animals, abrupt increases in sodium concentrations of cerebrospinal fluid and accompanying hyperosmolarity are associated with increased anesthetic requirements for halothane[6] (Fig. 21-5).

SODIUM DEFICIT

Total body deficit of sodium is reflected by a plasma sodium concentration below 135 mEq·L^{-1}. Excessive loss of sodium can result from vomiting, diarrhea, diaphoresis, third-degree burns, and administration of thiazide diuretics. As with total body sodium excess, it is important to remember that the most common cause of hyponatremia is not a deficiency of total body sodium, but rather a total body water excess.

Signs and Symptoms

The total body deficit of sodium is evidenced by decreased intravascular fluid volume and cardiac output. Conversely, hyponatremia due to total body water excess is associated with an increased intravascular fluid volume. Manifestations of reduced intravascular fluid volume include decreased blood pressure, venous pressure, and glomerular filtration rate, as well as an increased heart rate. The hematocrit is typically increased, reflecting a reduction in intravascular fluid volume without concomitant loss of erythrocytes.

A reduction of interstitial fluid volume in association with a total body deficit of sodium is reflected by a decrease in skin turgor. Because the amount of underlying fat can also affect the elasticity of the skin, a useful site to look for decreased skin turgor is the forehead. Loss of skin elasticity in the extremities cannot be distinguished from poor skin turgor accompanying the aging process.

Treatment

Treatment of a total body deficit of sodium is difficult because there is usually an accompanying loss of body water. An approximation of the sodium deficit, however, can be calculated from the plasma sodium concentration and the predicted total body water content (Table 21-6). Despite the substantial calculated deficits of total body sodium, the use of hypertonic saline is usually reserved for symptomatic hyponatremia, which is most likely to be present when the plasma sodium concentration is below 110 mEq·L^{-1}.

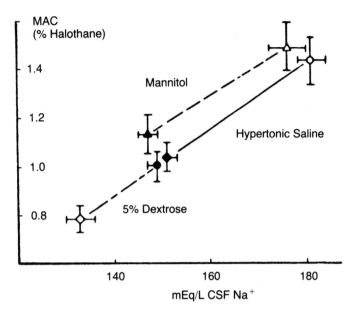

Fig. 21-5. Halothane MAC in animals parallels changes in the sodium concentration (Na^+) and osmolarity of cerebrospinal fluid (CSF) produced by the infusion of mannitol, hypertonic saline, or 5% dextrose in water. (From Tanifuji Y, Eger EI. Brain sodium, potassium and osmolarity: Effects on anesthetic requirement. Anesth Analg 1978;57:404–10, with permission.)

Management of Anesthesia

Considerations for management of anesthesia in the presence of a total body deficit of sodium are similar to those outlined for patients with total body water deficits. In animals, abrupt decreases in sodium concentrations of cerebrospinal fluid and accompanying hypo-osmolarity are associated with decreased anesthetic requirements for halothane[6] (Fig. 21-5).

HYPERKALEMIA

Hyperkalemia (plasma potassium concentration above 5.5 $mEq \cdot L^{-1}$) can be due to an increased total body potassium content or to an alteration in distribution of potassium between intracellular and extracellular sites (Table 21-7).

Table 21-6.   Calculation of Total Body Sodium Deficit

Sodium deficit = 140 − plasma sodium concentration   × total body water (weight in kg × 0.6)

Example: The predicted sodium deficit in an 80-kg male with a plasma sodium concentration of 120 $mEq \cdot L^{-1}$ would be calculated as follows:
        = (140 − 120) × (80 × 0.6)
        = 20 × 48
        = 960 mEq

Increased Total Body Potassium Content

Increased total body potassium content occurs when the kidneys are unable to excrete sufficient potassium to maintain the plasma potassium concentration below 5.5 $mEq \cdot L^{-1}$.

Table 21-7.   Causes of Hyperkalemia

Increased Total Body Potassium Content
    Acute oliguric renal failure
    Chronic renal disease
    Hypoaldosteronism
    Drugs that impair potassium excretion
        Triamterene
        Spironolactone
        Nonsteroidal anti-inflammatory drugs
    Drugs that inhibit the renin-angiotensin-aldosterone system
        Beta antagonists
        Angiotensin-converting enzyme inhibitors

Altered Distribution of Potassium Between Intracellular and Extracellular Sites
    Succinylcholine
    Respiratory or metabolic acidosis
    Hemolysis
    Lysis of cells due to chemotherapy
    Iatrogenic bolus

Pseudohyperkalemia

Acute oliguric renal failure is the classic cause of hyperkalemia. By contrast, patients with chronic renal disease do not usually develop hyperkalemia until the glomerular filtration rate decreases to less than 15 ml·min^{-1}. Patients with severe renal disease, but not requiring hemodialysis, may be vulnerable to hyperkalemia if they are challenged with potassium loads. This potential hazard must be considered when penicillin (1.7 mEq of potassium for every 1 million units of penicillin) or banked whole blood (about 1 mEq of potassium L^{-1}·d^{-1} of storage) is administered to patients with chronic renal disease. Hypoaldosteronism favors potassium retention such that hyperkalemia can result. Likewise, diuretics such as spironolactone and triamterene, which act as aldosterone antagonists, can interfere with renal elimination of potassium.

Altered Distribution of Potassium

Altered distribution of potassium between intracellular and extracellular sites can result in hyperkalemia, even in the absence of changes in total body content of potassium. For example, the release of intracellular potassium and subsequent hyperkalemia after succinylcholine administration to patients with burns, spinal cord transection, or muscle trauma is well recognized. Respiratory or metabolic acidosis favors passage of potassium from intracellular to extracellular locations. Specifically, a 0.1-unit decrease in arterial pH (pHa), as produced by a 10-mmHg increase of the $PaCO_2$, can increase plasma potassium concentrations by about 0.5 mEq·L^{-1} (Fig. 21-6).[7] Increased plasma potassium concentrations can result from tumor lysis and release of intracellular constituents, including potassium. This response is most likely to occur in patients receiving cancer chemotherapeutic drugs for the treatment of leukemia or lymphoma. Iatrogenic hyperkalemia has been attributed to poor mixing of potassium chloride added to plastic fluid containers, resulting in intravenous delivery of the added potassium chloride to patients as a bolus.[8] The likelihood of inadequate mixing is minimal when potassium chloride is added with plastic containers held in the inverted position, with the injection port uppermost.

Signs and Symptoms

The adverse effects of hyperkalemia are likely to accompany an acute increase in the plasma potassium concentration. By contrast, chronic hyperkalemia is more likely to be associated with normalization of gradients between extracellular and intracellular concentrations of potassium and return of the resting membrane potentials of excitable cells to near normal.

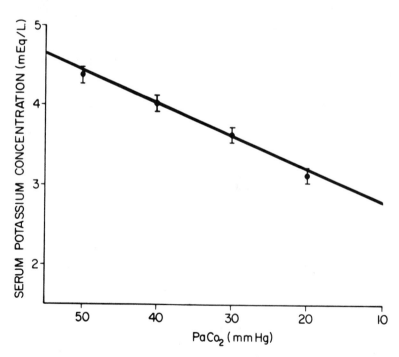

Fig. 21-6. The serum potassium concentration (mean ± SE) is directly related to $PaCO_2$. A 10-mmHg change in $PaCO_2$ results in a corresponding change in the plasma potassium concentration of about 0.5 mEq·L^{-1}. (From Edwards R, Winnie AP, Ramamurthy S. Acute hypocapneic hypokalemia: An iatrogenic anesthetic complication. Anesth Analg 1977;56:786–92, with permission.)

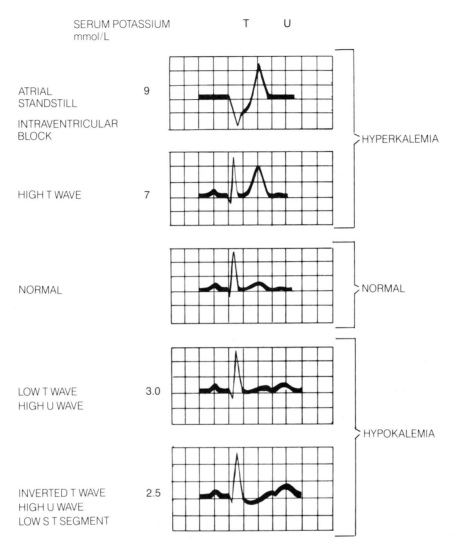

Fig. 21-7. Manifestations on the electrocardiogram of changes in the plasma potassium concentration. (From Goudsouzian NG, Karamanian A. The electrocardiogram. In: Physiology for the Anesthesiologist. E. Norwalk, CT. Appleton-Century-Crofts, 1977; 37, with permission.)

Indeed, patients with chronic elevations of potassium are often asymptomatic, supporting the greater importance of appropriate potassium gradients across cell membranes rather than the absolute plasma concentrations of potassium.

The most detrimental effect of hyperkalemia is on the cardiac conduction system. Characteristic changes produced on the electrocardiogram (ECG) by hyperkalemia are prolongation of the P-R interval progressing to loss of the P wave, widening of the QRS complex, and peaking of the T wave[9] (Fig. 21-7). Ventricular tachycardia and ventricular fibrillation may occur, although the most likely event in the presence of hyperkalemia is cardiac standstill in diastole. The electrocardiographic changes of hyperkalemia may be difficult to distinguish from idioventricular rhythm or acute myocardial infarction.

Appearance of abnormalities on the ECG depends on the absolute level of plasma potassium, as well as on the rapidity with which the plasma concentration increases. Cardiac conduction abnormalities are frequently present when the plasma potassium concentration exceeds $7.0 \text{ mEq} \cdot \text{L}^{-1}$. Nevertheless, these changes can be manifested at even lower plasma concentrations, if the increase has been acute. Peaking of T waves, although diagnostic, occurs in less than 25% of patients with hyperkalemia.

Hyperkalemia decreases the intracellular to extracellular potassium ratio, compromising neuromuscular function. Presumably, this is the explanation for the common presence of skeletal muscle weakness in these patients.

Treatment

Immediate treatment is indicated in the presence of electrocardiographic signs of hyperkalemia or in the presence of a plasma potassium concentration that exceeds 6.5 mEq·L^{-1} (Table 21-8). Initial treatment of hyperkalemia is directed at antagonizing the adverse effects of potassium on the heart (intravenous calcium) and facilitating the movement of potassium from the plasma into cells (intravenous glucose, insulin, and bicarbonate and hyperventilation of the lungs). Insulin is administered to ensure that glucose enters cells and carries potassium with it. Because these measures only temporarily control hyperkalemia, efforts to facilitate potassium excretion (ion exchange resins) may be instituted simultaneously. Dialysis is instituted if these measures are not promptly effective. If the plasma potassium concentration is less than 6.5 mEq·L^{-1} and there are no indications of cardiac toxicity on the ECG, the treatment of hyperkalemia may be conservative, directed at correction of the underlying problem.

Management of Anesthesia

A common recommendation is that the plasma potassium concentration should be below 5.5 mEq·L^{-1} before subjecting patients to elective operations that require an anesthetic. If this is not possible, it is important to adjust the anesthetic technique so as to recognize adverse effects of hyperkalemia intraoperatively and to minimize the likelihood of any additional increase in the plasma potassium concentration. Specifically, it is important to monitor the ECG continuously to detect adverse cardiac effects produced by hyperkalemia. Ventilation of the lungs must be managed in a way that ensures the absence of carbon dioxide accumulation, which would lead to respiratory acidosis and the transfer of potassium from intracellular to extracellular sites. Metabolic acidosis due to unrecognized arterial hypoxemia or to excessive depths of anesthesia would also contribute to an extracellular distribution of potassium. Mild hyperventilation of the lungs during the intraoperative period would seem logical, since a 10-mmHg decrease in the PaCO$_2$ reduces the plasma potassium concentration by about 0.5 mEq·L^{-1} (Fig. 21-6).[7] These goals are facilitated by measuring arterial blood gases and pH.

Responses to muscle relaxants must also be considered when hyperkalemia is present. The plasma potassium concentration increases by about 0.3 to 0.5 mEq·L^{-1}, after administration of 1 to 2 mg·kg^{-1} of succinylcholine.[10] The implications of a 0.5-mEq·L^{-1} increase must be considered when co-existing plasma potassium concentrations are elevated. Since there is no effective way to prevent release of potassium after administration of succinylcholine (including pretreatment with a subparalyzing dose of nondepolarizing muscle relaxant), it may be prudent to avoid administration of this drug to patients with elevated plasma potassium concentrations. Nevertheless, the institution of hyperventilation before the injection of succinylcholine may provide some degree of protection. Responses to nondepolarizing muscle relaxants in the presence of hyperkalemia are unclear. Presence of skeletal muscle weakness preoperatively would suggest the possibility of decreased muscle relaxant requirements intraoperatively. Evidence from an animal study suggests that dose requirements for pancuronium are directly related to the plasma potassium concentration[11] (Fig. 21-8). A useful approach would seem to be titration of muscle relaxants until desired effects are obtained, as evidenced by monitoring with a peripheral nerve stimulator.

Perioperative intravenous fluids must be selected with the realization that most solutions contain potassium. Lactated Ringer's solution contains 4 mEq·L^{-1}, Normosol-R 5 mEq·L^{-1}, and Normosol-M 13 mEq·L^{-1} of potassium. Drugs such as calcium and glucose-insulin must be readily available to treat intraoperative manifestations of hyperkalemia. Unlike alterations in plasma concentrations of sodium, hyperkalemia

Table 21-8. Treatment of Hyperkalemia

	Dose	Mechanism	Onset	Duration
Calcium gluconate	10–20 ml of a 10% solution IV	Direct antagonism	Rapid	15–30 min
Sodium bicarbonate	50–100 mEq IV	Shift intracellular	15–30 min	3–6 h
Glucose and insulin	25–50 g with 10–20 units IV	Shift intracellular	15–30 min	3–6 h
Hyperventilation	PaCO$_2$ 25–30 mmHg	Shift intracellular	Rapid	
Kayexelate		Remove	1–3 h	
Peritoneal dialysis		Remove	1–3 h	
Hemodialysis		Remove	Rapid	

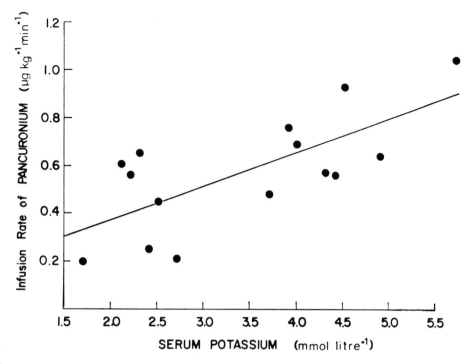

Fig. 21-8. The relationship between the infusion rate of pancuronium necessary to maintain 90% twitch depression and the plasma potassium concentration is depicted by means of an animal model. (From Miller RD, Roderick LL. Diuretic-induced hypokae-lemia, pancuronium neuromuscular blockade and its antagonism by neostigmine. Br J Anaesth 1978;50:541–4, with permission.)

is not associated with alterations in requirements for volatile anesthetics.[6]

PSEUDOHYPERKALEMIA

Pseudohyperkalemia (benign or spurious hyperkalemia) is characterized by an increased serum concentration of potassium (as high as 7 mEq·L^{-1}) due to the in vitro release of intracellular stores of this ion from leukocytes and platelets during the clotting or separation process.[12] This abnormal in vitro leakage of potassium may reflect an inherited trait and usually occurs only in a patient with a very high leukocyte or platelet count.[13] Clinically, pseudohyperkalemia is distinguished from hyperkalemia by measuring both the plasma and serum concentration of potassium. In pseudohyperkalemia, only the serum concentration of potassium is increased while the plasma level is normal. These patients are asymptomatic and lack detectable adrenal or renal abnormalities. Failure to recognize this syndrome could lead to hypokalemia if aggressive pharmacologic attempts are instituted to lower the plasma potassium concentration. Other causes of spurious hyperka-

lemia include hemolysis of the blood sample used to measure the plasma potassium concentration and perhaps the practice of repeatedly clenching and unclenching the fist during venipuncture[14] (Fig. 21-9). Confirmation of the presence of pseudohyperkalemia preoperatively removes the concerns typically expressed for management of anesthesia in the presence of hyperkalemia.

HYPOKALEMIA

Hypokalemia (plasma potassium concentration below 3.5 mEq·L^{-1}) can be due to decreased total body potassium content or to an alteration in distribution of potassium between intracellular and extracellular sites (Table 21-9). Chronic hypokalemia is likely to be associated with decreased total body content of potassium, as well as a reduction in the plasma concentration of this ion. By contrast, acute hypokalemia is usually due to intracellular translocation of potassium, without a change in total body content.

Clinically, the only practical means of assessing hypokalemia is by measuring the plasma concentration of potassium.

Table 21-9.   Causes of Hypokalemia

Decreased Total Body Postassium Content

    Gastrointestinal loss
        Vomiting-diarrhea
        Nasogastric suction
        Villous adenoma of the colon
    Renal loss
        Osmotic or tubular diuretics
        Hyperglycemia
        Aldosteronism
        Excess endogenous or exogenous cortisol
        Surgical trauma
    Insufficient oral intake

Altered Distribution of Potassium Between Intracellular and Extracellular Sites

    Respiratory or metabolic alkalosis
    Glucose and insulin
    Familial periodic paralysis
    Beta-2 agonist stimulation
    Hypercalcemia
    Hypomagnesemia

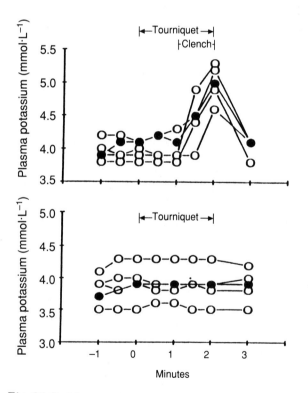

Fig. 21-9. Measurement of the plasma concentration of potassium in a venous blood sample drawn while the subject is clenching the fist results in an increase in the concentration of this ion compared with that present when only a tourniquet is used. (From Don BR, Sebastian A, Cheitlin M, Christiansen M, Schambelan M. Pseudohyperkalemia caused by fist clenching during phlebotomy. N Engl J Med 1990;322:1290–3, with permission.)

Nevertheless, it is important to remember that 98% of total body potassium is intracellular and thus not measured by plasma determinations (Table 21-4). Furthermore, as extracellular potassium is lost, intracellular potassium crosses cell membranes along a concentration gradient, in an attempt to restore extracellular fluid concentrations and thus maintain the normal ratio of intracellular to extracellular potassium. Indeed, enormous potassium deficits can be present despite only a small decrease in the plasma potassium concentration. For example, it is estimated that a chronic decrease of 1 mEq·L^{-1} in the plasma potassium concentration can reflect a total body deficit of 600 to 800 mEq of potassium.

Decreased Total Body Potassium Content

Decreased total body potassium content is most often due to increased chronic loss of this ion through the gastrointestinal tract or the kidneys. Gastrointestinal losses of potassium responsible for hypokalemia include vomiting, diarrhea, laxative abuse, nasogastric suction, and villous adenomas of the colon. Renal losses of potassium occur in response to osmotic and tubular diuretics, hyperglycemia, and excess secretion of aldosterone or cortisol. Hypokalemia accompanying administration of many diuretics is usually self-limited. For example, the plasma potassium concentration rarely decreases to less than 3 mEq·L^{-1} and may spontaneously reverse during continued therapy.[15] The significance of diuretic-induced hypokalemia is controversial, although there is general agreement that normokalemia should be maintained in patients being treated with digitalis. Trauma as produced by surgery results in loss of potassium (50 mEq·d^{-1} for the first 2 days postoperatively) through the kidneys. Inadequate oral intake of potassium is an uncommon cause of hypokalemia, unless the patient's only source of nutrition is potassium-free parenteral fluids.

Differentiating hypokalemia due to gastrointestinal versus renal losses is facilitated by measuring the concentration of potassium in the urine. If the gastrointestinal tract is the source of loss, the kidneys will respond by reducing urinary excretion of potassium to less than 10 mEq·L^{-1}. Conversely, if the kidneys are the source, urine potassium content is likely to exceed 40 mEq·L^{-1}.

Altered Distribution of Potassium

Hypokalemia without changes in total body potassium content occurs when potassium is acutely shifted from the extracellular fluid into cells to replace hydrogen ions, which have left cells to offset an increased pHa. For example, the plasma potassium concentration decreases approximately 0.5 mEq·L^{-1} for every 10-mmHg reduction in the PaCO$_2$ (Fig. 21-6).[7] Hyperventilation of the lungs during anesthesia is the most frequent cause of acute hypokalemia due to changes in the distribution of potassium between the cells and extracellular fluid. Another cause of acute hypokalemia attributable to this mechanism is glucose-insulin infusions that drive potassium into cells without altering the total body content of potassium. Likewise, rapid correction of hyperglycemia with the administration of insulin can abruptly promote potassium entry into cells and produce hypokalemia. The hypokalemic form of familial periodic paralysis is also characterized by abrupt intracellular shifts of potassium from the intravascular fluid space (see Chapter 26).

The sympathetic nervous system modulates distribution of potassium between intracellular and extracellular sites. In this regard, it has been observed that the plasma potassium concentration measured in a sample obtained immediately before the induction of anesthesia is frequently lower (0.28 to 0.8 mEq·L^{-1}) than that measured in a sample obtained 1 to 3 days preoperatively[16,17] (Fig. 21-10). The most likely explanation for this finding is stress-induced catecholamine release during the immediate preoperative period leading to a beta-2 mediated translocation of potassium into intracellular sites[18] (Fig. 21-11). Indeed, pretreatment of patients with a nonselective beta antagonist such as propranolol negates this discrepancy between the timing of potassium samples, presumably by blocking the beta-2 agonist effects of epinephrine[16,18,19] (Fig. 21-12). Atenolol, which is a selective beta-1 antagonist, does not reliably prevent the observed decrease in plasma potassium concentrations measured immediately before induction of anesthesia[16] (Fig. 21-12). The possible presence of acute stress-induced hypokalemia should be considered when interpreting the plasma potassium concentration, as measured during the immediate preoperative period. Hypokalemia is also a hazard of treating bronchial asthma or premature labor with a beta-2 agonist.[19,20]

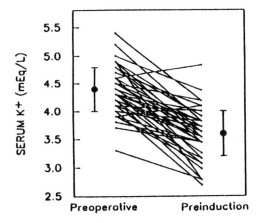

Fig. 21-10. Individual and mean ($\pm$SE) preoperative (measured 1 to 3 days before surgery) and preinduction plasma potassium concentrations measured in adult patients. (From Kharasch ED, Bowdle A. Hypokalemia before induction of anesthesia and prevention by β_2 adrenoceptor antagonism. Anesth Analg 1991;72:216–20, with permission.)

Signs and Symptoms

Neuromuscular function depends on the electrical potential difference across cell membranes, which is largely determined by the ratio of intracellular to extracellular potassium concentration. In potassium deficiency, the extracellular potassium concentration usually decreases more than the intracellular concentration, thereby altering this ratio. This ratio change is presumably at least partially responsible for skeletal muscle weakness, intestinal ileus, and abnormalities of cardiac electrical conduction that may accompany hypokalemia. Skeletal muscle weakness is most prominent in the legs and rarely affects muscles innervated by cranial nerves. The kidneys respond to potassium deficiency with a decrease in concentrating ability, often resulting in polyuria. Metabolic alkalosis is common, and extreme potassium deficiency may result in hypoventilation.

Acute hypokalemia, as produced by hyperventilation of the lungs, is unlikely to produce significant alterations in cardiac contractility or conduction. By contrast, intracellular depletion of potassium, as is likely with chronic hypokalemia, is associated with poor myocardial contractility. Furthermore, abrupt additional decreases in the plasma potassium concentration in the presence of co-existing chronic hypokalemia are more likely to produce cardiac conduction and rhythm abnormalities than is the same degree of hypokalemia produced acutely but in the absence of co-existing chronic total body potassium depletion. It is speculated that sudden decreases in the plasma potassium concentration exert more profound effects on electrochemical gradients for potassium in chronically hypokalemic patients. Orthostatic hypotension in the presence of hypokalemia may reflect autonomic nervous system dysfunction.

Changes on the ECG produced by hypokalemia characteristically reflect impaired cardiac conduction[9] (Fig. 21-7). Initially, a U wave appears immediately after the T wave and, if erroneously considered part of the T wave, results in calculation of a falsely prolonged Q-T interval. As hypokalemia becomes more severe, the P-R interval is prolonged, the ST segment is depressed, the T wave is inverted, and a prominent U wave is present. There is increased automaticity of the atria and ventricles, reflecting the more rapid rate of spontaneous depolarization, which occurs in the presence of hypokalemia. Ventricular fibrillation is a common terminal dysrhythmia in the presence of hypokalemia. Despite the commonly described characteristic changes on the ECG produced by hypokalemia, the extent to which these changes correlate with the plasma potassium concentration or total body potassium deficit is controversial.

Treatment

Treatment of hypokalemia depends on whether the decreased plasma potassium concentration is associated with normal or decreased total body potassium content. When total

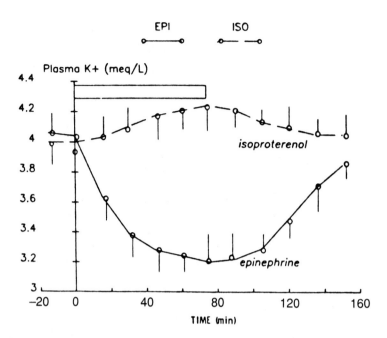

Fig. 21-11. Beta-2 agonist effects of epinephrine (EPI) are responsible for intracellular movement of potassium and an associated decrease in the plasma potassium concentration. Plasma potassium concentrations return slowly to the control level after discontinuation of the epinephrine infusion. (From Brown MJ, Brown DC, Murphy MB. Hypokalemia from beta-2 receptor stimulation by circulating epinephrine. N Engl J Med 1983;309:1414–9, with permission.)

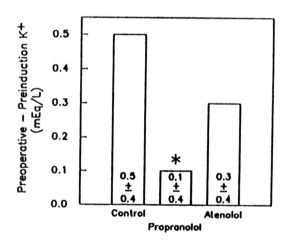

Fig. 21-12. The discrepancy between the preoperative (measured 1 to 3 days before surgery) and preinduction plasma potassium concentration is attenuated more by propranolol (mixed beta-1 and beta-2 antagonist effects) than by the selective beta-1 antagonist, atenolol. (From Kharasch ED, Bowdle TA. Hypokalemia before induction of anesthesia and prevention by β_2 adrenoceptor antagonism. Anesth Analg 1991;72:216–20, with permission.)

body potassium content is normal, as with acute hypokalemia, treatment begins with correction of the underlying cause, such as excessive intraoperative hyperventilation of the lungs.

Chronic hypokalemia associated with decreased total body potassium content is treated with supplemental potassium chloride. Chloride is important, since hypochloremic metabolic alkalosis is frequently associated with hypokalemia. Despite the common practice of administering supplemental potassium chloride, there is evidence that such therapy may be both ineffective and unnecessary.[21,22] For example, about 50% of patients with diuretic-induced hypokalemia fail to attain a normal plasma concentration of potassium despite potassium supplementation. Indeed, in many treated patients, most of the ingested supplemental potassium is excreted in the urine despite persistence of hypokalemia.

It must be appreciated that chronic hypokalemia is often associated with a total body potassium deficit exceeding 500 mEq or even 1000 mEq. This finding emphasizes that potassium content cannot be totally corrected within the 12 to 24 hours preceding elective surgery. Nevertheless, an infusion of potassium chloride ($0.2 \text{ mEq·kg}^{-1}\text{·h}^{-1}$ IV) during the few hours preceding surgery has been suggested to be beneficial, even in severely depleted patients.[23] The explanation is not clear, but it is possible that even small amounts of potassium are helpful in normalizing the electrophysiology of cells. Continuous monitoring of the ECG during intravenous administration of potassium is important. Repeat plasma potassium measurements every 12 to 24 hours should be used to guide continued replacement and rates of infusion. When digitalis toxicity is suspected, potassium chloride can be administered in 0.5- to 1-mEq intravenous boluses every 3 to 5 minutes, until the ECG reverts to normal. A practical point is to administer the potassium in a glucose-free solution; hyperglycemia would favor potassium entrance into cells, which could further exaggerate the degree of hypokalemia.

Management of Anesthesia

The advisability of proceeding with elective surgery in the presence of chronic plasma potassium concentrations below 3.5 mEq·L^{-1} is controversial.[24] It is suggested that chronically hypokalemic patients are at increased risk of the development of cardiac dysrhythmias intraoperatively, particularly if plasma potassium concentrations are less than 3 mEq·L^{-1}. Nevertheless, it is impossible to confirm or defend arbitrary plasma potassium concentrations acceptable for elective surgery. Indeed, the incidence of intraoperative cardiac dysrhythmias is not increased in asymptomatic patients with chronic hypokalemia (2.6 to 3.5 mEq·L^{-1}) undergoing elective operations.[17,25] It is not possible to support the practice of routine preoperative potassium repletion in otherwise asymptomatic patients (with or without cardiovascular disease) solely on the basis of the determination of the preoperative plasma potassium concentration.[17] It must be emphasized that adverse effects of hypokalemia are most likely when acute decreases in the plasma potassium concentration are superimposed on co-existing chronic hypokalemia.

It would seem logical to repeat the plasma potassium measurement and obtain an ECG for evaluation of cardiac rhythm before the induction of anesthesia in a patient considered at risk of hypokalemia. In this regard, it is important to recognize that the plasma potassium concentration measured just before induction of anesthesia is often lower than the value measured 24 hours earlier[16,17] (Fig. 21-10) (see the section, Altered Distribution of Potassium). During surgery, intravenous fluids should be selected to avoid glucose loads, as hyperglycemia could contribute to hypokalemia. The addition of 10 to 20 mEq of potassium chloride to every liter of intravenous fluid maintenance can be considered, but this approach must be weighed against the hazards of too rapid administration, should infusion rates be inadvertently increased during the intraoperative period. The use of exogenous epinephrine should be discouraged, as beta-2 agonist stimulation may shift potassium intracellularly and exaggerate co-existing hypokalemia[18] (Fig. 21-11). Furthermore, the potassium-depleted heart may be vulnerable to the arrhythmogenic effects of catecholamines, digitalis, and calcium. Excessive hyperventilation of the lungs must be avoided. Capnography and measurement of arterial blood gases and pHa are helpful in confirming the proper management of ventilation.

The potential for prolonged responses to nondepolarizing muscle relaxants must be anticipated. A prudent approach is to reduce the initial muscle relaxant dose 30% to 50%. Administration of subsequent doses should be based on responses shown by a peripheral nerve stimulator. Nevertheless, chronic hypokalemia is likely to be associated with a normal ratio of intracellular to extracellular potassium such that responses to muscle relaxants are not altered.

No specific anesthetic drugs or techniques appear to be superior for administration to patients with hypokalemia. Nevertheless, it should be recalled that chronic hypokalemia has been associated with reduced myocardial contractility and postural hypotension. Therefore, patients with chronic hypokalemia might be unusually sensitive to the cardiac depressant effects of volatile anesthetics. Likewise, exaggerated blood pressure reductions in response to positive-pressure ventilation of the lungs or blood loss are likely in the presence of reduced sympathetic nervous system activity. The association of chronic hypokalemia with polyuria must also be remembered in choosing anesthetic drugs metabolized to fluoride. There is evidence that epinephrine included in the local anesthetic solution used to perform an axillary block may result in electrocardiographic evidence of hypokalemia.[19] For this reason, it would seem prudent to avoid the inclusion of epinephrine in local anesthetic solutions administered to patients with co-existing hypokalemia.

It is important to monitor the ECG continuously during the intraoperative and postoperative period for evidence of hypokalemia. The appearance of abnormalities on the ECG related to hypokalemia requires prompt treatment with intravenous infusions of potassium chloride, including consideration of the administration of 0.5- to 1.0-mEq bolus injections, until the ECG reverts to normal.

CALCIUM

Calcium is essential for nerve and skeletal muscle excitability and contractility. Total plasma calcium concentration is maintained at 4.5 to 5.5 mEq·L^{-1} by the actions of parathyroid hormone. The physiologically active form of calcium, however, is the ionized fraction, which normally represents about 45% of the total plasma concentration. The normal plasma ionized calcium concentration is therefore 2.0 to 2.5 mEq·L^{-1}.

Symptoms due to an altered concentration of calcium reflect changes in the plasma level of ionized calcium. This finding emphasizes the need to evaluate disturbances in calcium homeostasis by measurement of the ionized calcium concentration. It must be remembered that the concentration of ionized calcium is dependent on the pHa; for example, acidosis increases the concentration, while alkalosis decreases it. The plasma albumin concentration must also be considered in interpreting the plasma calcium measurement. For example, the total plasma calcium concentration can be reduced in the presence of hypoalbuminemia, but symptoms of hypocalcemia do not occur unless the ionized calcium concentration is reduced as well. Likewise, an elevated plasma albumin concentration is associated with an increased total calcium concentration, but the ionized fraction can be normal.

Hypercalcemia

The most common causes of hypercalcemia (plasma calcium concentration above 5.5 mEq·L^{-1}) are hyperparathyroidism and neoplastic disorders with bone metastasis. Less common causes include pulmonary granulomatous diseases (sarcoidosis), vitamin D intoxication, and immobilization.

Signs and Symptoms

Hypercalcemia produces changes that affect the central nervous system, gastrointestinal tract, kidneys, and heart. Early signs and symptoms include sedation and vomiting. Persistently elevated plasma calcium concentrations (7 to 8 mEq·L^{-1}) can interfere with urine-concentrating ability, and polyuria results. In addition, an increased plasma calcium concentration can contribute to the formation of renal calculi. Oliguric renal failure can occur in advanced cases of hypercalcemia. When the plasma calcium concentration exceeds 8 mEq·L^{-1}, cardiac conduction disturbances, characterized on the ECG as a prolonged P-R interval, wide QRS complex, and shortened Q-T interval occur.

Treatment

The cornerstone of treatment of hypercalcemia is hydration with normal saline (2.5 to 4 L·d^{-1}).[26] Hydration lowers the plasma calcium concentration by dilution, and sodium acts to inhibit the renal resorption of calcium. Diuresis produced with furosemide (80 to 100 mg IV every 1 to 2 hours) minimizes the risk of overhydration and further facilitates renal elimination of calcium. Volume expansion must precede the administration of furosemide because the effect of the drug depends on delivery of calcium to the renal tubules. Thiazide diuretics are not administered for the treatment of hypercalcemia, as these drugs may enhance the renal tubular resorption of calcium. Ambulation is an important aspect of treatment, as it decreases calcium release from bone associated with immobilization.

An elevated plasma calcium concentration secondary to myeloproliferative disorders can be lowered by the administration of the cancer chemotherapeutic drug, plicamycin. Administration of plicamycin (25 μg·kg^{-1} IV) over 4 to 6 hours begins to lower the plasma calcium concentration as early as 12 hours after the administration of the drug; the maximum decrease occurs in 48 to 72 hours. Clearly, this drug is not helpful in the acute management of life-threatening hypercalcemia. Side effects of plicamycin include nausea, hepatotoxicity, nephrotoxicity, and thrombocytopenia.

Management of Anesthesia

The key principle for management of anesthesia in the presence of hypercalcemia is maintenance of hydration and urine output with intravenous fluids containing sodium. Continuous monitoring of the ECG is useful to warn of adverse effects on cardiac conduction produced by an excessive increase in the plasma calcium concentration. The choice of anesthetic drugs should include consideration of the impaired urine-concentrating ability associated with polyuria, which could be confused with anesthetic-induced fluoride nephrotoxicity, during the postoperative period. Theoretically, hyperventilation of the lungs would be undesirable, as respiratory alkalosis lowers the plasma potassium concentration and would leave the actions of calcium unopposed. Nevertheless, by lowering the ionized fraction of calcium, alkalosis could also be beneficial. The response to nondepolarizing muscle relaxants is not well defined, but the preoperative existence of skeletal muscle weakness would suggest decreased dose requirements for these drugs.

Hypocalcemia

The most common cause of hypocalcemia (plasma calcium concentration below 4.5 mEq·L^{-1}) is a decreased plasma albumin concentration. Critically ill patients with low plasma albumin concentrations characteristically have low plasma calcium levels, but plasma ionized calcium measurements may be normal.[27] Conversely, a normal total plasma calcium concentration in the presence of hypoalbuminemia may indicate an increased concentration of ionized calcium. Other causes of hypocalcemia include acute pancreatitis, hypoparathyroidism (especially after thyroid surgery), decreased plasma magnesium concentration (malnutrition, sepsis, aminoglycoside administration), vitamin D deficiencies, and renal failure. Radiographic contrast media contains calcium chelators (edetate and citrate) and may acutely lower the plasma calcium concentration. Hyperventilation of the lungs may result in reductions in the plasma ionized concentration of calcium due to alkalosis-induced increases in calcium binding to proteins. This mechanism can lead to acute ionized hypocalcemia in patients given sodium bicarbonate for control of metabolic acidosis. Increased plasma free fatty acid concentrations, as associated with total parenteral nutrition, may lower the plasma ionized calcium concentration, without altering the total calcium concentration.[27] Hypocalcemia and hyperphosphatemia resulting from the use of hypertonic phosphate enemas (Fleet enema) have been associated with cardiac arrest during induction of anesthesia.[28]

Signs and Symptoms

Hypocalcemia is reflected in the central nervous system, heart, and neuromuscular junction. Numbness and circumoral paresthesias can progress to confusion, and occasionally to seizures. Abrupt decreases in the ionized portion of the plasma calcium concentration are associated with hypotension and with increased left ventricular filling pressures.[29,30] The Q-T interval on the ECG can be prolonged, but this is not a consistent observation; therefore, the Q-T interval is not clinically reliable as a guide to the presence of hypocalcemia. Impaired neuromuscular function in the presence of hypocalcemia probably reflects the decreased presynaptic release of acetylcholine. Indeed, many patients with chronic hypocalcemia complain of skeletal muscle weakness and fatigue. Rapid decreases in the plasma calcium concentration, as can follow a total parathyroidectomy, can produce skeletal muscle spasm, manifested by laryngospasm. Skeletal muscle spasm is most likely to occur when the plasma calcium concentration abruptly decreases below 3.5 mEq·L^{-1}. In anesthetized or critically ill and unresponsive patients, the only evidence of hypocalcemia may be hypotension due to decreased myocardial contractility.[31]

Treatment

The initial management of hypocalcemia entails the correction of any co-existing respiratory or metabolic alkalosis. An intravenous infusion of calcium should be considered when there are symptoms of hypocalcemia (hypotension, tetany) or when the plasma calcium concentration decreases below 3.5 mEq·L^{-1}. Treatment consists mainly of intravenous administration of 10% calcium chloride (1.36 mEq·ml^{-1}) or calcium gluconate (0.45 mEq·ml^{-1}). Equal elemental calcium doses of calcium chloride (2.5 mg·kg^{-1} IV) or calcium gluconate (7.5 mg·kg^{-1} IV) are equivalent in their ability to increase the plasma ionized calcium concentration.[32] Calcium should be administered until the plasma concentration approaches 4 mEq·L^{-1} or the ECG returns to a normal pattern.

Management of Anesthesia

Management of anesthesia is designed to prevent further decreases in the plasma calcium concentration and to recognize and treat adverse effects of hypocalcemia, particularly on the heart. For this reason, it may be important to monitor the plasma ionized calcium concentration in a patient considered to be at risk of hypocalcemia, during the perioperative period. During surgery and anesthesia, it is important to appreciate that respiratory or metabolic alkalosis can rapidly decrease the plasma ionized calcium concentration. This can occur during hyperventilation of the lungs or after intravenous administration of sodium bicarbonate for treatment of metabolic acidosis. The development of life-threatening hypocalcemia during general anesthesia has been observed in patients with renal insufficiency who are undergoing vascular surgery.[31]

The administration of whole blood containing citrate preservative usually does not reduce the plasma calcium concentration because calcium is rapidly mobilized from body stores. The ionized calcium concentration can be decreased, however, with rapid infusions of blood (500 ml every 5 to 10 minutes) or when metabolism or elimination of citrate is limited by hypothermia, cirrhosis of the liver, or renal dysfunction.[33] Although there is no evidence that co-existing hypocalcemia predisposes to citrate intoxication, it would seem prudent to maintain a high index of suspicion, when whole blood is administered.

Continuous monitoring of the ECG to facilitate recognition of changes characteristic of hypocalcemia is important during the perioperative period. Intraoperative hypotension may reflect the exaggerated cardiac depression produced by anesthetic drugs in the presence of a decreased plasma ionized calcium concentration. Measurement of the arterial blood gases, pHa, and plasma calcium (particularly the plasma ionized calcium concentration) is useful in guiding intraoperative management. The importance of the plasma albumin concentration and administration of protein in the intravenous maintenance and replacement fluids considered in the interpretation of the plasma calcium concentration. Administration of colloid solutions is particularly important in the face of loss of intravascular fluid into the tissues due to surgical trauma.

Responses to nondepolarizing muscle relaxants could be potentiated by hypocalcemia. Nevertheless, clinical experience is too limited to confirm this speculation. Theoretically, coagulation abnormalities could also accompany extreme decreases in the plasma concentration of calcium. Postoperatively, it should be appreciated that sudden decreases in the plasma calcium concentration can produce skeletal muscle spasm, including laryngospasm.

MAGNESIUM

Total body magnesium stores are about 2000 mEq. Most of this magnesium is distributed to the intracellular spaces (Table 21-4). Excretion of magnesium is by the gastrointestinal tract and kidneys. In its absence in the diet, the kidneys are able to conserve magnesium, excreting less than 1 mEq·d^{-1}. The most important physiologic effect of magnesium is regulation of the presynaptic release of acetylcholine from nerve endings. The extensive use of magnesium in obstetric practice, as well as its interactions with drugs used during anesthesia, emphasizes the importance of this ion in the management of patients in the perioperative period.[34]

Hypermagnesemia

Hypermagnesemia is present when the plasma magnesium concentration exceeds 2.5 mEq·L^{-1}. The most common causes of hypermagnesemia are iatrogenic, including administration of magnesium sulfate to treat pregnancy-induced hypertension and excessive individual use of antacids or laxatives. Patients with chronic renal dysfunction are at increased risk of the development of hypermagnesemia, since magnesium elimination is dependent on the glomerular filtration rate. Indeed, the plasma magnesium level predictably increases when exogenous magnesium is administered to patients with glomerular filtration rates below 30 ml·min^{-1}.

Signs and Symptoms

Hypermagnesemia can have adverse effects on the central nervous system, heart, and neuromuscular junction. Central nervous system depression is displayed as hyporeflexia plus sedation, which may progress to coma. Cardiac depression may be prominent. Skeletal muscle weakness, presumably reflecting reduced acetylcholine release secondary to increased magnesium levels, can be so severe as to impair ventilation. Indeed, the most common cause of death from hypermagnesemia is cardiac and/or ventilatory arrest.

Treatment

Signs and symptoms of hypermagnesemia can be temporarily reversed with the intravenous administration of calcium. Elimination of magnesium can be facilitated by fluid loading and diuresis, produced by diuretics. The definitive therapy for persistent and life-threatening hypermagnesemia requires either peritoneal dialysis or hemodialysis.

Management of Anesthesia

Acidosis and dehydration must be prevented intraoperatively, as these events lead to increased concentrations of plasma magnesium. Therefore, ventilation of the lungs should be managed to ensure the absence of respiratory acidosis due to hypoventilation. Capnography, arterial blood gases, and pHa determinations are useful in guiding the management of ventilation of the lungs and in ensuring the absence of systemic acidosis. Intravenous fluid maintenance and replacement should be adjusted to maintain urine output. Stimulation of urine output with a diuretic, such as furosemide, may be necessary.

Hypermagnesemia potentiates the action of nondepolarizing and depolarizing muscle relaxants[35] (Fig. 21-13), emphasizing the importance of decreasing the initial doses of muscle relax-ants. Subsequent doses are based on responses observed with a peripheral nerve stimulator.

It is conceivable that cardiac depression produced by anesthetic drugs could be exaggerated in the presence of hypermagnesemia. Furthermore, increased plasma magnesium levels produce peripheral vasodilation, which might be further accentuated by drugs used during anesthesia. These speculations remain undocumented, but it would seem prudent to titrate the doses of anesthetic drugs, maintaining a high index of suspicion for magnesium-anesthetic drug interactions, should hypotension occur.

Hypomagnesemia

Plasma magnesium concentrations below 1.5 mEq·L^{-1} are associated with chronic alcoholism, malabsorption syndromes, hyperalimentation therapy without added magnesium, and protracted vomiting or diarrhea.[34] Hypomagnesemia may be a cause of hypokalemia that is resistant to potassium supplement therapy.[36]

Signs and Symptoms

Signs and symptoms of hypomagnesemia are similar to those observed in patients with hypocalcemia. Indeed, both hypomagnesemia and hypocalcemia frequently present as combined electrolyte disorders. Predictable manifestations of hypomagnesemia include central nervous system irritability reflected by hyperreflexia and seizures, skeletal muscle spasm, and cardiac irritability. Hypomagnesemia can potentiate digitalis-induced cardiac dysrhythmias. Cardiac dysrhythmias attributed to diuretic-induced hypokalemia may in fact be due to hypomagnesemia.[37]

Treatment

Treatment of hypomagnesemia is with magnesium sulfate (1 g IV) administered over 15 to 20 minutes. Blood pressure, heart rate, and patellar reflexes should be monitored. Depression or disappearance of patellar reflexes is an indication to stop magnesium replacement.

Management of Anesthesia

The importance of hypomagnesemia in the management of anesthesia is primarily related to associated disturbances such as alcoholism, malnutrition, and hypovolemia. Conceivably, decreased plasma magnesium concentrations could interfere with the response to muscle relaxants, but this possibility has not been studied.

ACID-BASE DISTURBANCES

Acid-base disturbances are classified as respiratory or metabolic based on the measurement of the arterial hydrogen ion concentration (pHa) and PaCO$_2$ and estimation of the plasma bicarbonate concentration from a nomogram[38,39] (Table 21-10). The first determination is whether the pHa is less than

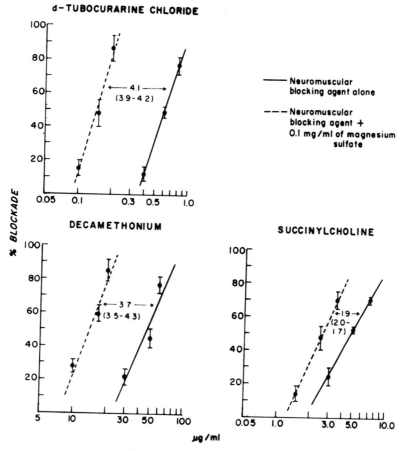

Fig. 21-13. Dose-response curves (mean ±SE) for production of neuromuscular blockade in the presence or absence of magnesium sulfate, using the rat phrenic nerve–diaphragm preparation. Displacement of the dose response curve to the left reflects increased sensitivity to the neuromuscular blocking effects of the muscle relaxant in the presence of magnesium. (From Ghoneim MM, Long JP. The interaction between magnesium and other neuromuscular blocking agents. Anesthesiology 1970;32:23–7, with permission.)

Table 21-10.   Direction of Changes During Acute and Chronic Acid-Base Disturbances

	pHa	PaCO$_2$	HCO$_3$
Respiratory acidosis			
Acute	Moderate decrease	Marked increase	Slight increase
Chronic	Slight decrease	Marked increase	Moderate increase
Respiratory alkalosis			
Acute	Moderate increase	Marked decrease	Slight decrease
Chronic	Slight increase to no change	Marked decrease	Moderate decrease
Metabolic acidosis			
Acute	Moderate to marked decrease	Slight decrease	Marked decrease
Chronic	Slight decrease	Moderate decrease	Marked decrease
Metabolic alkalosis			
Acute	Marked increase	Moderate increase	Marked increase
Chronic	Marked increase	Moderate increase	Marked increase

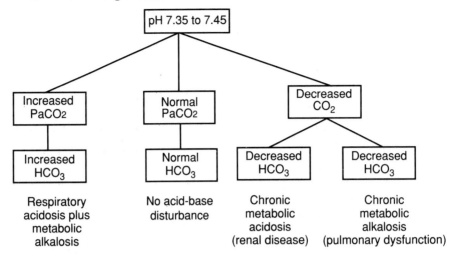

Fig. 21-14. Diagnostic approach to the interpretation of a normal arterial pH based on $PaCO_2$ and HCO_3 (bicarbonate) concentration.

7.35, greater than 7.45, or in between. A normal pHa may reflect the absence of an acid-base disturbance, a chronic disturbance with compensation, or a mixed acid-base disturbance (Fig. 21-14). If the pHa is less than 7.35, the diagnosis is either respiratory acidosis or metabolic acidosis (Fig. 21-15). If the pH is greater than 7.45, the diagnosis is either metabolic alkalosis or respiratory alkalosis, as determined by measurement of the $PaCO_2$ and bicarbonate concentration (Fig. 21-

16). Once the nature of the acid-base disturbance has been established, the search for causes can begin and the appropriate treatment instituted.

When the acid-base disturbance results principally from changes in alveolar ventilation, the designation is respiratory acidosis or alkalosis. By convention, $PaCO_2$ greater than 45 mmHg represents hypoventilation, whereas hyperventilation is present when $PaCO_2$ is less than 35 mmHg. Hypoventilation

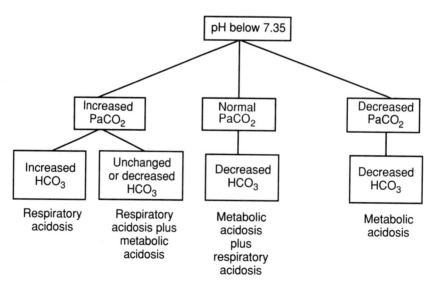

Fig. 21-15. Diagnostic approach to the interpretation of an arterial pH below 7.35 based on $PaCO_2$ and HCO_3 (bicarbonate) concentration.

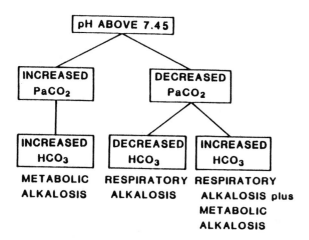

Fig. 21-16. Diagnostic approach to the interpretation of an arterial pH above 7.45 based on the PaCO₂ and HCO₃ (bicarbonate) concentration.

is synonymous with respiratory acidosis, and hyperventilation is synonymous with respiratory alkalosis. Changes in pHa unrelated to a primary alteration in PaCO₂ are designated metabolic acidosis or alkalosis.

The normal pHa is regulated over a narrow range of 7.35 to 7.45. In this regard, a normal pHa depends on maintenance of an optimal 20:1 ratio of the concentration of bicarbonate to the concentration of carbon dioxide (Henderson-Hasselbalch equation) (Table 21-11). Acid-base disturbances characterized by changes in the plasma bicarbonate concentration are predictably accompanied by appropriate compensatory changes in PaCO₂ secondary to alterations in alveolar ventilation. If a 20:1 ratio is maintained, the pHa will remain within the normal range, despite the presence of an acid-base disturbance (Fig. 21-14). For example, respiratory acidosis or alkalosis is compensated for by renal-induced changes in the plasma bicarbon-

Table 21-11. Henderson-Hasselbalch Equation

$$pHa = pK + \log \frac{HCO_3}{0.03 \times PaCO_2}$$

pHa = negative logarithm of the arterial concentration of
    hydrogen ions
pK = 6.1 at 37°C
HCO₃ = concentration of bicarbonate, mEq·L⁻¹
PaCO₂ = mmHg

Substitution of average values for pHa (7.4) and PaCO₂ (40 mmHg) results is a calculated HCO₃ concentration of 24 mEq·L⁻¹. Maintenance of a normal HCO₃ concentration relative to the concentration of carbon dioxide results in an optimal ratio of about 20:1 (24 mEq·L⁻¹ divided by 1.2). This optimal ratio of 20:1 permits maintenance of a relatively normal pHa despite deviations from normal in the HCO₃ concentration.

$$CO_2 + H_2O \rightleftharpoons H_2CO_3 \rightleftharpoons HCO_3^- + H^+$$

Fig. 21-17. Hydration of carbon dioxide results in H₂CO₃ (carbonic acid), which can subsequently dissociate into HCO₃⁻ (bicarbonate) and H⁺ (hydrogen) ions.

ate concentration that begin in 6 to 12 hours and serve to maintain a 20:1 ratio. After a few days, as a result of this renal compensation, pHa in the presence of chronic respiratory acidosis or alkalosis is returned to normal despite persistent alterations in the PaCO₂ (Table 21-10). Acid-base disturbances due to metabolic acidosis or alkalosis are compensated for by ventilation-induced changes in the PaCO₂ that tend to restore the 20:1 ratio and return the pHa toward normal (Table 21-10). In contrast to the renal compensatory mechanisms that restore pHa to normal in the presence of respiratory acidosis or alkalosis, the ventilatory compensatory mechanism only partially corrects the pHa in the presence of metabolic acidosis or alkalosis.

Interpretation of the nomogram-derived estimate of the plasma concentration of bicarbonate as a reflection of acid-base disturbances due to metabolic processes requires an adjustment for the impact of ventilation. For example, an increase in PaCO₂ will lead to the hydration of carbon dioxide to carbonic acid with a subsequent increase in the plasma concentration of bicarbonate (Fig. 21-17). Conversely, lowering PaCO₂ will reverse the direction of this reaction, resulting in a decrease in the plasma concentration of bicarbonate. These changes are nearly linear and permit the use of a guideline for clinical interpretation and adjustment of the estimated plasma bicarbonate concentration (Table 21-12). For example, using this guideline, hypoventilation leading to an acute increase in PaCO₂ to 70 mmHg would result in a normalized plasma bicarbonate concentration of 27 mEq·L⁻¹, assuming a normal value of 24 mEq·L⁻¹.

The principal manifestation of respiratory or metabolic acidosis is depression of the central nervous system. Conversely, the principal manifestation of respiratory or metabolic alkalosis is increased excitability of the peripheral nervous system (tetany) and central nervous system (seizures). Acidosis decreases myocardial contractility, although little clinical

Table 21-12. Impact of Ventilation on Plasma Bicarbonate Concentration

Change in PaCO₂ Equal to 10 mmHg	Change in Bicarbonate Concentration (from 24 mEq·L⁻¹)
Acute increase	Increase 1 mEq·L⁻¹
Chronic increase	Increase 3 mEq·L⁻¹
Acute decrease	Decrease 2 mEq·L⁻¹
Chronic decrease	Decrease 5 mEq·L⁻¹

effect is seen until the pHa decreases below 7.2, perhaps reflecting the effects of catecholamine release in response to acidosis.[40] When the pHa is less than 7.1, cardiac responsiveness to catecholamines decreases, and compensatory inotropic effects are diminished. Detrimental effects of acidosis may be accentuated in those with underlying left ventricular dysfunction or myocardial ischemia or in those in whom sympathetic nervous system activity is impaired, as by beta blockade or general anesthesia. Direct effects of alkalosis on myocardial contractility are less than acidosis. Cardiac dysrhythmias in the presence of alkalosis may be accentuated by hypokalemia. Alkalosis may also produce cerebral and coronary artery vasoconstriction and shift the oxyhemoglobin dissociation curve to the left, thus impairing the release of oxygen from hemoglobin to the tissues.

Respiratory Acidosis

Respiratory acidosis is present when a decrease in alveolar ventilation results in an increase in the $PaCO_2$ sufficient to lower the pHa to less than 7.35. Carbonic acid resulting from dissolved carbon dioxide is considered a respiratory acid. The most likely causes of respiratory acidosis include (1) drug-induced depression of alveolar ventilation, (2) disorders of neuromuscular function, and (3) intrinsic lung disease. Rarely, respiratory acidosis may result from increased metabolic production of carbon dioxide as in patients experiencing malignant hyperthermia or being treated with hyperalimentation solutions.

Respiratory acidosis may be complicated by metabolic acidosis when renal perfusion is decreased to the extent that resorption mechanisms through the kidneys are impaired (Fig. 21-15). For example, cardiac output and renal blood flow may be so decreased in patients with chronic obstructive pulmonary disease and cor pulmonale as to lead to metabolic acidosis.

Treatment of respiratory acidosis is by correction of the disorder responsible for hypoventilation. Mechanical ventilation of the lungs will be necessary when the elevation in $PaCO_2$ is marked. It must be remembered that rapid lowering of a chronically elevated $PaCO_2$ by mechanical hyperventilation will decrease body stores of carbon dioxide more rapidly than the kidneys can produce a corresponding decrease in the plasma concentration of bicarbonate. The resulting metabolic alkalosis can result in neuromuscular irritability and excitation of the central nervous system, exhibited as a seizure. For this reason, it is important to decrease $PaCO_2$ slowly, so as to permit sufficient time for renal tubular elimination of bicarbonate. Metabolic alkalosis may also accompany respiratory acidosis when there are decreased body stores of chloride and potassium. For example, a decrease in the plasma concentration of chloride facilitates renal resorption of bicarbonate, leading to metabolic alkalosis. Hypokalemia stimulates renal tu-

Table 21-13. Causes of Respiratory Alkalosis

Iatrogenic
Decreased barometric pressure
Arterial hypoxemia
Central nervous system injury
Hepatic disease
Pregnancy
Salicylate overdose

bules to excrete hydrogen, which may produce metabolic alkalosis or aggravate a co-existing alkalosis, owing to chloride deficiency. Treatment of metabolic alkalosis associated with these electrolyte disturbances is with the intravenous administration of potassium chloride.

Respiratory Alkalosis

Respiratory alkalosis is present when an increase in alveolar ventilation results in a decrease in the $PaCO_2$ sufficient to increase the pHa to greater than 7.45 (Table 21-13). The most likely cause of acute respiratory alkalosis during the perioperative period is iatrogenic hyperventilation of the lungs, as may occur during general anesthesia. Treatment of respiratory alkalosis is directed at correcting the underlying disorder responsible for alveolar hyperventilation. During anesthesia, this is most often accomplished by adjusting the mechanical ventilator to decrease alveolar ventilation. In addition, dead space can be added to the breathing circuit to increase rebreathing of exhaled gases containing carbon dioxide. In selected patients, it may be appropriate to add carbon dioxide from a metered source to the inspired gases, in an attempt to re-establish a more normal $PaCO_2$. Hypokalemia and hypochloremia that characterize respiratory alkalosis may also require treatment.

Metabolic Acidosis

Metabolic acidosis is characterized by a decrease in the pHa, owing to accumulation of nonvolatile acids, as is likely to accompany major organ dysfunction, especially renal failure (Table 21-14). Decreased cardiac output that results in inade-

Table 21-14. Causes of Metabolic Acidosis

Inadequate tissue oxygenation (lactic acidosis)
Renal failure
Diabetic ketoacidosis
Hepatic failure
Increased skeletal muscle activity
Cyanide poisoning
Carbon monoxide poisoning

Table 21-15. Calculation of the Dose of Sodium Bicarbonate to Treat Metabolic Acidosis

Sodium bicarbonate (mEq)	=	body weight (kg)	×	deviation of plasma bicarbonate concentration from normal	×	extracellular fluid volume as a fraction of body mass (0.2)

Evaluation of an 80-kg patient in hemorrhagic shock reveals the following: pHa, 7.20; $PaCO_2$, 60 mmHg; and bicarbonate, 16 mEq·L^{-1}. The normalized bicarbonate concentration corrected for the increased $PaCO_2$ would be 26 mEq·L^{-1} (see Table 21-12). The calculated dose of sodium bicarbonate to replace the bicarbonate deficit would be 160 mEq (80 kg × 10 mEq·L^{-1} × 0.2). About one-half of this calculated dose of sodium bicarbonate should be administered intravenously, followed by a repeat measurement of the pHa, to evaluate the impact of therapy.

quate tissue oxygenation results in anaerobic metabolism and accumulation of lactic acid.[41] Severe diarrhea and loss of bicarbonate can lead to metabolic acidosis, especially in pediatric patients. Plasma bicarbonate concentrations decrease owing to buffering of nonvolatile acids in the circulation.

Metabolic acidosis is treated by removal of the causes of the accumulation of nonvolatile acids in the circulation. It has been a common practice to treat acute metabolic acidosis with the intravenous administration of sodium bicarbonate, especially if myocardial depression or cardiac dysrhythmias are present. A formula designed to calculate the dose of sodium bicarbonate is based on deviation of the plasma concentration of bicarbonate from normal, the percentage of body mass that consists of extracellular fluid, and the ideal body weight (Table 21-15). A useful approach is to administer about one-half the calculated dose of sodium bicarbonate, followed by a repeat measurement of the pHa to evaluate the impact of treatment. It is important to recognize that sodium bicarbonate administration results in endogenous carbon dioxide production (1 mEq·kg^{-1} IV will produce about 180 ml of carbon dioxide), necessitating an increase in alveolar ventilation to prevent both hypercarbia and a worsening of the already existing acidosis. In this regard, the use of sodium bicarbonate to treat metabolic acidosis has been challenged.[40,42] Indeed, administration of sodium bicarbonate during cardiopulmonary resuscitation is considered less important than alveolar ventilation for the correction of acidosis.

Metabolic Alkalosis

Metabolic alkalosis is characterized by a loss of nonvolatile acids from the extracellular fluid (Table 21-16). For example, prolonged vomiting and nasogastric suction can result in the loss of hydrochloric acid, with subsequent metabolic alkalosis. Diuretics that inhibit resorption of sodium and potassium by the renal tubules lead to hypokalemia and an associated metabolic alkalosis. In the past, overzealous intravenous administration of sodium bicarbonate to treat metabolic acidosis during cardiopulmonary resuscitation has resulted in metabolic alkalosis.

Depletion of intravascular fluid volume is often the most important factor in the maintenance of metabolic alkalosis. Indeed, hypovolemia should be considered in the postoperative patient in whom metabolic alkalosis develops. Since loss of potassium often parallels loss of sodium, hypokalemia is frequently present when hypovolemia complicates metabolic alkalosis. Skeletal muscle weakness also accompanies hypokalemia. Urinary chloride excretion is usually less than 10 mEq·L^{-1} in the presence of metabolic alkalosis associated with depletion of intravascular fluid volume.[43]

Treatment of metabolic alkalosis is directed at resolution of those events responsible for the acid-base derangement, as well as appropriate replacement of electrolytes. On occasion, intravenous infusion of hydrogen in the form of ammonium chloride or 0.1 N hydrochloric acid (no greater than 0.2 mEq·kg^{-1}·h^{-1}) is used to facilitate the return of pHa to near-normal levels. Administration of acid requires insertion of a central venous catheter, as a peripheral injection can cause sclerosis of the vein and hemolysis.

Table 21-16. Causes of Metabolic Alkalosis

Vomiting	Hypovolemia
Nasogastric suction	Hyperaldosteronism
Diuretic therapy	Chloride-wasting diarrhea
Iatrogenic	

REFERENCES

1. Chung H-M, Kluge R, Schrier RW, Anderson RJ. Postoperative hyponatremia: A prospective study. Arch Intern Med 1986;146:333–6
2. Hemmer M, Viquerat CE, Suter PM, Valotton MB. Urinary antidiuretic hormone excretion during mechanical ventilation and weaning in man. Anesthesiology 1980;52:395–400
3. Arieff AI. Hyponatremia, convulsions, respiratory arrest, and permanent brain damage after elective surgery in healthy women. N Engl J Med 1986;314:1529–35
4. Sterns RH, Thomas DJ, Herndon RM. Brain dehydration and

neurologic deterioration after correction of hyponatremia. Kidney Int 1989;35:69–76

5. Ayxis JC, Krothapalli RK, Arieff AI. Treatment of symptomatic hyponatremia and its relation to brain damage: A prospective study. N Engl J Med 1987;317:1190–7

6. Tanifuji Y, Eger EI. Brain sodium, potassium, and osmolality: Effects on anesthetic requirement. Anesth Analg 1978;57:404–10

7. Edwards R, Winnie AP, Ramamurthy S. Acute hypocapneic hypokalemia: An iatrogenic anesthetic complication. Anesth Analg 1977;56:786–92

8. Williams RP. Potassium overdosage: A potential hazard of non-rigid parenteral fluid containers. Br Med J 1973;1:714–5

9. Goudsouzian NG, Karamanian A. The electrocardiogram. In: Physiology for the Anesthesiologist. E. Norwalk, CT. Appleton-Century-Crofts 1977;37

10. Stoelting RK, Peterson C. Adverse effects of increased succinylcholine dose following d-tubocurarine pretreatment. Anesth Analg 1975;54:282–8

11. Miller RD, Roderick LL. Diuretic-induced hypokaelemia, pancuronium neuromuscular blockade and its antagonism by neostigmine. Br J Anaesth 1978;50:541–4

12. Naidu R, Steg NL, MacEwen GD. Hyperkalemia: Benign, hereditary autosomal dominant trait. Anesthesiology 1982;56:226–8

13. Ho AM-H, Woo JCH, Kelton JG, Chiu L. Spurious hyperkaelemia associated with severe thrombocytosis and leukocytosis. Can J Anaesth 1991;38:613–5

14. Don BR, Sebastian A, Cheitlin M, Christiansen M, Schambelan M. Pseudohyperkalemia caused by fist clenching during phlebotomy. N Engl J Med 1990;322:1290–2

15. Sandor FF, Pickens PT, Crallan J. Variations of plasma potassium concentrations during long-term treatment of hypertension with diuretics without potassium supplements. Br Med J 1982;284:711–5

16. Kharasch ED, Bowdle TA. Hypokalemia before induction of anesthesia and prevention by β_2 adrenoceptor antagonism. Anesth Analg 1991;72:216–20

17. Hirsch IA, Tomlinson DL, Slogoff S, Keats AS. The overstated risk of preoperative hypokalemia. Anesth Analg 1988;67:131–6

18. Brown MJ, Brown DC, Murphy MB. Hypokalemia from beta$_2$-receptor stimulation by circulating epinephrine. N Engl J Med 1983;309:1414–9

19. Toyoda Y, Kuboa Y, Kubota H, et al. Prevention of hypokalemia during axillary nerve block with 1% lidocaine and epinephrine 1:100,000. Anesthesiology 1988;69:109–12

20. Hurlbert BJ, Edelman JD, David K. Serum potassium levels during and after terbutaline. Anesth Analg 1981;60:723–5

21. Papademetrious V, Burris J, Kukich S, Freis ED. Effectiveness of potassium chloride or triamterene in thiazide hypokalemia. Arch Intern Med 1985;145:1986–90

22. Papademetrious V, Fletcher R, Khatri IM, Freis ED. Diuretic-induced hypokalemia in uncomplicated systemic hypertension: Effect of plasma potassium correction on cardiac arrhythmias. Am J Cardiol 1983;52:1017–22

23. Wong KC, Wetstone D, Martin WE, et al. Hypokalemia during

anesthesia: The effects of d-tubocurarine, gallamine, succinylcholine, thiopental, and halothane with or without respiratory alkalosis. Anesth Analg 1973;52:522–8

24. Harrington JT, Isner JM, Kassirer JP. Our national obsession with potassium. Am J Med 1982;73:155–9

25. Vitez TS, Soper LE, Wong KC, Soper P. Chronic hypokalemia and intraoperative dysrhythmias. Anesthesiology 1985;63:130–3

26. Bilezikian JP. Management of acute hypercalemia. N Engl J Med 1992;326:1196–1203

27. Zaloga GP, Chernow B. Hypocalcemia in critical illness. JAMA 1986;256:1924–9

28. Reedy JC, Zwiren GT. Enema-induced hypocalcemia and hyperphosphatemia leading to cardiac arrest during induction of anesthesia in an outpatient surgery center. Anesthesiology 1983;59:578–9

29. Denlinger JK, Nahrwold ML. Cardiac failure associated with hypocalcemia. Anesth Analg 1976;55:34–6

30. Scheidegger D, Drop LJ. The relationship between duration of Q-T interval and plasma ionized calcium concentration: Experiments with acute, steady-state (Ca^{++}) changes in the dog. Anesthesiology 1979;51:143–8

31. Prielipp RC, Zaloga GP. Life-threatening hypocalcemia after abdominal aortic aneurysm repair in patients with renal insufficiency. Anesth Analg 1991;73:638–41

32. Cote CJ, Drop LJ, Danniels AL, Hoaglin DC. Calcium chloride versus calcium gluconate: Comparison of ionization and cardiovascular effects in children and dogs. Anesthesiology 1987;66:465–70

33. Denlinger JK, Nahrwold ML, Gibbs PS, Lecky JP. Hypocalcemia during rapid blood transfusion in anesthetized man. Br J Anaesth 1976;48:995–1000

34. James MFM. Clinical use of magnesium infusions in anesthesia. Anesth Analg 1992;74:129–36

35. Ghoneim MM, Long JP. The interaction between magnesium and other neuromuscular blocking agents. Anesthesiology 1970;32:23–7

36. Whang R, Flink EB, Dyckner, et al. Magnesium depletion as a cause of refractory potassium repletion. Arch Intern Med 1985;145:1686–90

37. Harris MNE, Crowther A, Jupp RA, Aps C. Magnesium and coronary revascularization. Br J Anaesth 1988;60:779–83

38. Narins RG, Emmett M. Simple and mixed acid-base disorders: A practical approach. Medicine 1980;59:161–87

39. Siggard-Anderson O. Blood acid base alignment nomogram. Scand J Clin Lab Invest 1963;15:211–7

40. Hindman BJ. Sodium bicarbonate in the treatment of subtypes of acute lactic acidosis: Physiologic considerations. Anesthesiology 1990;72:1064–76

41. Mizock BA. Controversies in lactic acidosis. Implications in critically ill patients. JAMA 1987;258:497–501

42. Graf H, Leach W, Arieff AI. Metabolic effects of sodium bicarbonate in hypoxic lactic acidosis in dogs. Am J Physiol 1985;249:F630–5

43. Sherman RA, Eisinger RP. The use (and misuse) of urinary sodium and chloride measurements. JAMA 1982;247:3121–4

22

Endocrine Disease

Endocrine disease is characterized by the overproduction or underproduction of single or multiple hormones. Alterations in the physiologic responses to stress or to changes in homeostatic mechanisms, or both, reflect the impact of excessive or deficient amounts of these hormones. An endocrine gland disorder may be the primary reason for surgery, or it may coexist in a patient requiring an operation unrelated to endocrine gland dysfunction. The presence of unsuspected endocrine disease may be determined by seeking the answer to specific questions in the patient's preoperative evaluation (Table 22-1).

DIABETES MELLITUS

Diabetes mellitus is a chronic systemic disease characterized by a broad array of abnormalities, the most notable of which is disturbed glucose metabolism, resulting in inappropriate hyperglycemia. Indeed, the diagnosis of diabetes is traditionally based on a blood glucose concentration usually greater than 185 mg·dl^{-1} present 1 hour after a glucose load. It is estimated that 2.4% of the U.S. population, or about 5.5 million persons, are diabetic.[1] In addition, 3.2% of the population with no history of diabetes have glucose intolerance.

Diabetics are divided into two categories (Table 22-2). A patient who depends on exogenous insulin for the prevention of ketoacidosis has insulin-dependent diabetes mellitus (IDDM). IDDM most often develops in childhood or adolescence (before 16 years of age), accounting for its prior designation as juvenile-onset diabetes or type I diabetes. A diabetic patient who does not require exogenous insulin to prevent ketoacidosis has noninsulin-dependent diabetes mellitus (NIDDM). NIDDM most often develops in middle or later life (after 35 years of age), accounting for its prior designation as maturity-onset diabetes or type II diabetes. Although many maturity-onset diabetics may be on insulin therapy, they are usually not prone to ketoacidosis and are classified as having

NIDDM. Nevertheless, NIDDM may progress to the extent that insulin is needed to prevent ketoacidosis. Patients with NIDDM, who are almost all overweight, constitute more than 90% of all diabetics. Obese nondiabetics require two to five times more insulin than do nonobese nondiabetics, emphasizing that obesity may unmask latent diabetes.

The two categories of diabetes are pathologically and genetically distinct entities. IDDM probably results from destruction of pancreatic beta cells by an autoimmune process that may be precipitated by a viral infection. About 15% of patients with IDDM have other autoimmune diseases such as hypothyroidism, Graves' disease, Addison's disease, and myasthenia gravis. The genetic predisposition for the development of IDDM is a reflection of the susceptibility for the development of the disease, rather than of inheritance of the disease. The genes controlling susceptibility to IDDM are present near or within the major histocompatibility complex (HLA) on chromosome 6. NIDDM is characterized by a gradual decline in pancreatic beta cell function and skeletal muscle and hepatic resistance to the effect of insulin, which is further enhanced by obesity. The prevalence of NIDDM increases steadily with age, especially after 45 years, and seems particularly prominent among black females. As with IDDM, there is evidence for a genetic basis of NIDDM. Gestational diabetes is estimated to occur in 2.4% of all pregnancies in the United States. Secondary causes of diabetes are due to diseases that alter hormone levels (Cushing syndrome, pheochromocytoma, acromegaly) or to pancreatic destruction or resection.

Treatment

Treatment of diabetes includes diet, oral hypoglycemic drugs, and exogenous insulin. Of paramount importance is the primary prevention of NIDDM by the avoidance or treatment of obesity. Transplantation of pancreatic tissue may be considered in select patients. The use of cyclosporine to treat recent-onset IDDM is based on the presumption that it is an autoimmune disease.[2]

Table 22-1. Preoperative Evaluation of Endocrine Function

Does urinalysis demonstrate glycosuria?

Are blood pressure and heart rate normal?

Is body weight unchanged?

Is sexual function normal?

Is there a history of medication with drugs relevant to endocrine function?

Table 22-3. Oral Hypoglycemia Drugs

	Relative Potency	Duration of Action (h)
First generation		
Tolbutamine	1	6–10
Acetohexamide	2.5	12–18
Tolazamide	5	16–24
Chlorpropamide	6	24–72
Second generation		
Glyburide	150	18–24
Glipizide	100	16–24

Oral Hypoglycemic Drugs

Oral hypoglycemic drugs are useful when blood glucose control cannot be attained with diet alone (Table 22-3). These drugs require the presence of functional pancreatic beta cells and thus are not effective in patients with IDDM. Likewise, a patient with NIDDM who has required more than 40 units of exogenous insulin will probably not respond to an oral hypoglycemic drug. The most serious drug-induced complication is prolonged hypoglycemia, which is most likely to develop in the patient with renal disease. In this regard, it is useful to remember that tolbutamide is metabolized in the liver, whereas chlorpropamide is entirely dependent on renal excretion. Skin rashes, cholestatic hepatitis, and drug interactions (enhanced effects of barbiturates, thiazides, anticoagulants) may occur.

Exogenous Insulin

A number of types of insulin are available, including pork insulin, beef insulin, and human insulin (Humulin), which was developed through recombinant DNA research (Table 22-4). Advantages of human insulin include a decreased risk of the development of anti-insulin antibodies. Single-peak Lente or NPH insulin (100 units·ml^{-1}; U-100) are the most commonly prescribed intermediate-acting insulin preparations. Some diabetics require only a single injection of Lente insulin before breakfast. Nevertheless, most diabetics require a combination of regular (rapid-acting) and Lente (intermediate-acting) insulin before breakfast and a second injection of Lente before the evening meal or at bedtime. These two separate insulin injections permit simulation of the normal physiologic pattern in which endogenous insulin release occurs after each of three meals. It is important to recognize that rebound hyperglycemia (Somogyi effect) may follow a hypoglycemic reaction; for example, notation of increased glycosuria, as on arising in the morning, may not indicate the need for additional insulin.

Table 22-2. Classification of Diabetes Mellitus

	IDDM	NIDDM
Age of onset (y)	<16	>35
Onset	Abrupt	Gradual
Manifestations	Polyphagia Polydipsia Polyuria	May be asymptomatic
Require exogenous insulin	Yes	Not always
Susceptibility to ketoacidosis	Yes	Not always
Blood glucose concentration	Wide fluctuations	Relatively stable
Nutrition	Thin	Obese
Microangiopathy	Common	Infrequent
Macroangiopathy	Infrequent	Common
Other autoimmune diseases present	Maybe	No

Table 22-4. Classification of Insulin Preparations

	Hours After Subcutaneous Administration (Estimated)		
	Onset	Peak	Duration
Fast-acting			
Regular[a]	0.5–1	2–4	6–8
Semilente	1–3	5–10	16
Intermediate-acting			
Isophane (NPH)[a]	2–4	6–12	18–26
Lente[a]	2–4	6–12	18–26
Long-acting			
Protamine zinc	4–8	14–24	28–36
Ultralente	4–8	14–24	28–36

NPH, neutral (N) solution, protamine (P), with origin in Hagedorn's laboratory (H).

[a] Available as human insulin (Humulin).

Patients treated with protamine-containing insulin preparations, such as NPH or protamine zinc insulin, may be more likely to experience a life-threatening allergic reaction when protamine is administered intravenously to antagonize the effects of heparin.[3] Presumably, low-dose antigenic stimulation from the protamine-containing insulin preparation evokes the production of antibodies to protamine. The use of tight metabolic control (blood glucose 75 to 125 mg·dl^{-1}) to prevent diabetic complications is controversial as its role in preventing microvascular and renal complications and neuropathy is unclear.[4,5]

Insulin Infusion Pump

Insulin infusion pumps that deliver insulin continuously by the intravenous route, based on the blood glucose concentration and in anticipation of meals, are being used more frequently.[6] These battery driven pumps are placed subcutaneously in the abdomen or chest. Complications of infusion pump therapy may include hypoglycemia, ketoacidosis owing to pump failure, and abscess formation at the infusion site.

Pancreas Transplantation

Pancreas transplantation (whole grafts, segmental grafts, or processed islet cells) may offer treatment for the patient with IDDM who has labile plasma blood glucose concentrations and who exhibits progressive microangiopathy.[7] The corrosive effects of pancreatic exocrine secretions are prevented by polymer instillation to produce fibrosis and occlusion of the pancreatic duct. Function of the islet cells is maintained despite fibrosis of the exocrine pancreas. The use of the body and tail of the pancreas with the attached splenic artery and vein simplifies vascular anastomosis to the external iliac vessels in the iliac fossa. Insulin is normally secreted into the portal venous circulation and is thus delivered directly to the liver. By contrast, insulin from a pancreatic transplant is delivered into the systemic venous circulation. Nevertheless, difficulties in glucose homeostasis have not occurred in transplant patients. When islet cells are transplanted, they are infused into either the liver or spleen. Management of anesthesia for pancreas transplantation requires frequent monitoring for hypoglycemia or hyperglycemia and consideration of the impact of immunosuppressant drugs.[7]

Rejection of the transplanted pancreas is a major problem. When a kidney and pancreas from a single donor are transplanted, rejection can be monitored for both organs by surveillance for renal rejection alone. Hyperglycemia is a late sign of rejection, since control of plasma glucose is maintained until about 95% of pancreatic endocrine tissue is destroyed. Vascular thrombosis of graft vessels is another cause of graft rejection. Human leukocyte antigen matching and immunosuppression greatly improve graft survival. Successful transplantation results in return of blood glucose levels to normal within hours. Diabetic nephropathy and diabetic retinopathy are arrested by successful pancreatic transplantation.

Complications

The most serious acute metabolic complication of diabetes is ketoacidosis. Late complications of diabetes may be manifested as macroangiopathy (coronary artery disease, cerebrovascular disease, peripheral vascular disease), microangiopathy (retinopathy, nephropathy) and disorders of the nervous system (autonomic nervous system neuropathy, peripheral neuropathy). Microvascular complications predominate in the patient with IDDM, whereas macrovascular complications are more common in the patient with NIDDM. Macrovascular sequelae, such as premature myocardial infarction, angina pectoris, or peripheral vascular insufficiency, may be the presenting symptoms in an undiagnosed diabetic. Diabetic retinopathy occurs in 80% to 90% of those who have add IDDM for at least 20 years. In young and middle-aged adults in the United States, diabetes is the leading cause of kidney failure requiring dialysis and is the leading cause of blindness.[8] Autonomic nervous system dysfunction may affect more than 15% of diabetics.[9] Perioperative morbidity is increased in diabetics with evidence of autonomic neuropathy.[10] Delayed wound healing and postoperative infection (leukocyte function is not optimal) are more likely to occur in the diabetic. Infection is often the cause of a sudden increase in the insulin requirement.

Ketoacidosis

Hyperglycemia in the presence of metabolic acidosis and a history of diabetes are sufficient to establish the diagnosis of ketoacidosis. The patient with diabetic ketoacidosis often presents with nausea, vomiting, lethargy, and signs of hypovolemia owing to dehydration. Complaints of abdominal pain and the associated presence of leukocytosis may suggest the need for laporatomy. Causes for ketoacidosis are usually poor patient compliance although insulin resistance owing to infection (urinary tract, pneumonia) or silent myocardial infarction may also be the explanation. Inhibition of premature labor utilizing a beta-2 agonist but in the presence of IDDM may abruptly precipitate ketoacidosis, even with the prior subcutaneous administration of insulin.[11]

Initial treatment of ketoacidosis includes repletion of intravascular fluid volume (750 to 1000 ml of saline IV), regular insulin (0.2 units·kg^{-1} IV, followed by 0.1 unit·kg^{-1}·h^{-1} IV), potassium (40 mEq·h^{-1} IV) until the blood glucose concentration begins to decrease, and sodium bicarbonate administered intravenously if the pHa is less than 7.2 and the bicarbonate ion concentration is less than 10 mEq·L^{-1} (see Table 21-15). Even in the presence of hypovolemia, there is usually some urine output because of the osmotic effect of glucose.

Atherosclerosis

Atherosclerosis as a manifestation of macroangiopathy can appear at an early age in the patient with diabetes. Cerebrovascular accident is twice as common, myocardial infarction is 2 to 10 times more frequent, and peripheral vascular disease is 5 to 10 times more frequent in the diabetic than in the nondiabetic.[12] Cardiomyopathy is not an uncommon problem in diabetics.

Microangiopathy

Microangiopathy correlates with the degree and duration of hyperglycemia. Thickened but leaky capillary wall linings primarily affect the eyes and kidneys. In this regard, the diabetic is 25 times more susceptible to partial loss of vision, and the risk of cataracts is 4 to 6 times greater in the diabetic than in the nondiabetic. There is a twofold greater risk of glaucoma in the diabetic. Photocoagulation of leaking vessels with an argon laser may improve visual acuity in the patient with diabetic retinopathy. Vitreous surgery is being used for the treatment of vitreous hemorrhage and of retinal detachment. Renal failure occurs eventually in about one-third of patients with IDDM, reflecting a lesion in the microvasculature of the renal glomerulus. Microalbuminuria is an early sign of the development of diabetic nephropathy. Renal transplantation may be a consideration in the treatment of this diabetic complication.

Autonomic Neuropathy

Autonomic neuropathy reflects dysfunction of the autonomic nervous system as a result of diabetes[13] (Table 22-5). Cardiovascular manifestations of autonomic neuropathy include orthostatic hypotension, resting tachycardia, and decreased or absent beat-to-beat variation of the heart rate during voluntary deep breathing. The basic defect in orthostatic hypotension associated with diabetes is the lack of vasoconstriction, owing to sympathetic nervous system dysfunction. The plasma concentration of norepinephrine increases less when the diabetic with symptoms of orthostatic hypotension assumes the standing position. Cardiac vagal denervation often occurs early and is reflected by the loss of variability in heart rate during deep

breathing. The heart rate response to drugs such as atropine and propranolol is blunted in the diabetic with evidence of autonomic neuropathy compared with the nondiabetic.[14] The shortening of the Q-T interval on the electrocardiogram in association with autonomic neuropathy may result in serious cardiac dysrhythmias. Autonomic neuropathy may interfere with control of breathing and make the patient with diabetes more susceptible to depressant effects of drugs as administered during anesthesia. Unexpected cardiac or respiratory arrest, or both, may occur in the diabetic patient with autonomic neuropathy.[13,15-18] The presence of autonomic neuropathy may prevent the development of angina pectoris and thus obscure the presence of ischemic heart disease.[15] Unexplained hypotension may be due to painless myocardial infarction in the diabetic with autonomic neuropathy. It is not inconceivable that autonomic neuropathy could place the patient at increased risk for sudden death during the perioperative period. Indeed, once autonomic neuropathy develops, the prognosis is poor, with mortality exceeding 50% over a 5-year period.[19] Restoration of normoglycemia, as with a pancreatic transplant, does not reliably reverse manifestations of autonomic neuropathy.

Delayed gastric emptying (gastroparesis) is a manifestation of autonomic neuropathy with obvious risk implications for the diabetic patient during the perioperative period[20] (Fig. 22-1). It is estimated that gastroparesis occurs in 20% to 30% of all

Table 22-5. Manifestations of Diabetic Autonomic Neuropathy

Orthostatic hypotension
Resting tachycardia
Absent variation in heart rate with deep breathing
Gastroparesis
    Vomiting
    Diarrhea
    Abdominal distension
Bladder atony
Impotence
Cardiac dysrhythmias
Altered regulation of breathing
Asymptomatic hypoglycemia
Sudden death syndrome

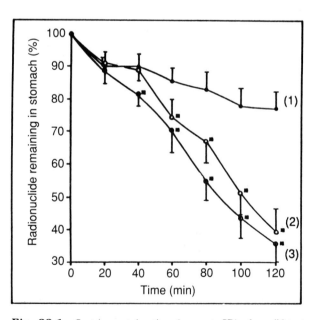

Fig. 22-1. Gastric emptying time (mean ± SD) of a solid test meal in patients with (1) diabetes (line 1), (2) diabetes and receiving metoclopramide (10 mg IV) before the test meal (line 2), and (3) no evidence of diabetes (line 3). (From Wright RA, Clemente R, Wathen R. Diabetic gastroparesis: An abnormality of gastric emptying of solids. Am J Med Sci 1985;289:240–2, with permission.)

diabetic patients, manifested as nausea, vomiting, and abdominal distension. Symptoms may appear early in the disease and occur in patients with IDDM and NIDDM. Metoclopramide improves gastric emptying and decreases symptoms of gastroparesis. Bowel dysfunction, characterized by intermittent diarrhea, and bladder dysfunction may be elicited from the medical history. Impotence is a prominent sign of autonomic neuropathy. Hypoglycemic unawareness (blood glucose concentration often less than 50 mg·dl^{-1}) is characterized by an absence of symptoms. Peripheral sympathetic nervous system denervation results in increased arteriovenous shunting and decreased skin-capillary blood flow, as well as decreased sweating in the extremities. These changes contribute to the development of neuropathic foot problems in the diabetic patient.

Sensory Neuropathy

Sensory neuropathy may be manifested as nocturnal sensory discomfort of the lower extremities. There is an increased incidence of carpal tunnel syndrome in these patients. Segmental demyelinization and vascular occlusion of nutrient arteries, especially to the cranial nerves, as well as the median and ulnar nerves of the forearm, are often involved. Sensory neuropathy and autonomic neuropathy may develop in parallel. In an occasional patient, the discomfort produced by sensory neuropathy requires treatment with an analgesic such as an opioid.

Stiff Joint Syndrome

An estimated 30% to 40% of patients with IDDM show evidence of limited joint mobility, most often initially manifesting in the small joints of the digits and hands.[21] An inability to approximate the palmar surfaces of the interphalangeal joints ("prayer sign") correlates with the presence of the stiff joint syndrome.[22] The atlanto-occipital joint may be involved, contributing to difficulties in laryngoscopy for intubation of the trachea.[22] In addition to joint involvement, the afflicted patient often has rapidly progressive microangiopathy (microalbuminuria, renal failure), nonfamilial short stature, and tight waxy skin. Glycosylation of tissue proteins from chronic hyperglycemia seems to be responsible for this complication.

Glycohemoglobin

The concentration of glycosylated hemoglobin (glycohemoglobin, hemoglobin A_{1c}) is probably the best measure of overall blood glucose control.[23] Increased amounts of glucose exposed to a target protein, such as hemoglobin, leads to increased covalent binding of glucose to the target protein (glycosylation). In this regard, the concentration of glycohemoglobin increases from a normal value of 5% to 7% to as high as 20% in the presence of severe hyperglycemia. The incidence of diabetic retinopathy and nephropathy is increased in the patient with a persistent increase in glycohemoglobin concentration.[5]

Scleredema

Diabetic scleredema is manifested as thickening and hardening of the skin characteristically over the back of the neck, shoulders, and upper back but can involve the hands, arms, and legs. The induration is nonpitting and usually symmetric. It may develop after an acute infection in the patient with poorly controlled diabetes or it may occur without a known cause. In children with diabetes, associated findings may include carpal tunnel syndrome and limited mobility of the finger joints. A report of anterior spinal artery syndrome as a complication of epidural anesthesia in a patient with diabetic scleredema was attributed to a restriction of arterial blood flow to the spinal cord. This problem was caused by a marked increase in epidural pressure, when the large volume of local anesthetic solution was placed into an epidural space containing noncompressible collagen.[24]

Management of Anesthesia

The principal goal in the management of anesthesia for the diabetic patient undergoing elective surgery is to mimic normal metabolism as closely as possible by avoiding hypoglycemia, excessive hyperglycemia, ketoacidosis, and electrolyte disturbances.[25,26] Hypoglycemia is prevented by ensuring an adequate supply of exogenous glucose. Hyperglycemia and associated ketoacidosis, dehydration, and electrolyte abnormalities are prevented by the administration of exogenous insulin. The goal for control of the blood glucose concentration is to maintain a level well above that considered hypoglycemic, but below the level at which the deleterious effects of hyperglycemia (hyperosmolarity, osmotic diuresis, electrolyte disturbances, impaired phagocyte function, impaired wound healing) become evident. In this regard, a recommendation is to maintain the blood glucose concentration at 120 to 180 mg·dl^{-1}.[26] Despite the technical ability to normalize the blood glucose concentration, prospective data comparing surgical outcomes following improved blood glucose control during the perioperative period are not available. Furthermore, there is no consensus on the optimal medical management of the diabetic patient in the perioperative period.[25]

Preoperative Evaluation

It is frequently recommended that the diabetic patient be scheduled for surgery early in the day, if possible. Most agree that the well-controlled, diet-treated NIDDM patient does not require prior hospitalization or any special treatment (including insulin) either before or during surgery. Likewise, the patient with well-controlled IDDM undergoing a brief outpatient surgical procedure may not require any adjustment in the usual subcutaneous insulin regimen. If an oral hypoglycemic drug is being administered, it may be continued until the evening before surgery, remembering that these drugs may produce hypoglycemia several hours (as long as 36 hours with chlorpropamide) after their administration in the absence of caloric intake. Preadmission to the hospital is probably indicated only for the patient with poorly controlled IDDM.

Preoperative evaluation and treatment of hyperglycemia, electrolyte disturbances, and ketoacidosis is important before proceeding with elective surgery. Measurement of the glycohemoglobin concentration is a practical means of estimating the average blood glucose concentration of the previous 1 to 3 weeks. Evidence of ischemic heart disease, cerebrovascular disease, and renal dysfunction should be sought. Indeed, the most common cause of perioperative morbidity in the diabetic patient is ischemic heart disease. The electrocardiogram and a search for proteinuria provide useful information in the IDDM patient. Signs of peripheral neuropathy (which may influence selection of regional anesthesia) and autonomic neuropathy are noted (Table 22-5). The patient with evidence of autonomic nervous system dysfunction may be at increased risk of aspiration on induction of anesthesia and intraoperative cardiovascular lability (hypotension requiring vasopressor therapy)[10] (Fig. 22-2). Evaluation of the IDDM patient for evidence of limited joint mobility is important in predicting possible difficulty in performing direct laryngoscopy for intubation of the trachea. Indeed, an increased incidence of difficult tracheal intubation has been described in patients with long-standing IDDM.[21,22] Furthermore, the common presence of obesity in this patient population may influence the ease of tracheal intubation or performance of regional anesthetic techniques.

Exogenous Insulin

There is a consensus that the IDDM patient undergoing major surgery should be treated with insulin; however, the accepted route of administration (subcutaneous, intravenous) remains unsettled.[26] Furthermore, there is no evidence to confirm that close control of the blood glucose concentration during the relatively brief intraoperative period benefits the diabetic patient. Nevertheless, understanding the metabolic response to surgery and how this response is altered by insulin provides the rationale for administration of insulin during the perioperative period. In this regard, a traditional time-tested approach is the administration of one-fourth to one-half the usual daily intermediate-acting dose of insulin on the morning of surgery. If regular insulin is part of the morning schedule, the intermediate-acting insulin dose may be increased by 0.5 unit for each unit of regular insulin, remembering that the stress of anesthesia increases the need for insulin. It is a common practice to initiate an intravenous infusion of glucose (5 to 10 g·h^{-1}) during the preoperative period, along with the subcutaneous insulin, to minimize the likelihood of hypoglycemia. In addition, the administration of potassium (2 mEq·L^{-1}) is often included with the glucose. An alternative to routine preoperative subcutaneous administration of a partial insulin dose is to withhold

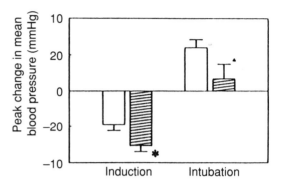

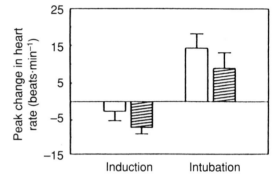

Fig. 22-2. Mean arterial (blood) pressure decreased more ($P < 0.05$) during induction of anesthesia and heart rate increased less ($P < 0.06$) during intubation of the trachea in patients with diabetes mellitus (cross-hatched bars) and preoperative evidence of autonomic nervous system dysfunction compared with nondiabetic patients (open bars). (From Burgos LG, Ebert TJ, Asiddao C, et al. Increased intraoperative cardiovascular morbidity in diabetics with autonomic neuropathy. Anesthesiology 1989;70:591–7, with permission.)

insulin and measure the blood glucose concentration frequently (every hour) during the intraoperative period[27] (Fig. 22-3). On the basis of this measurement, the blood glucose concentration can be maintained at 100 to 200 mg·dl^{-1} during the intraoperative period by the intravenous infusion of additional glucose or regular insulin[27] (Table 22-6).

There is increasing interest in the continuous intravenous infusion of regular insulin to manage the patient with IDDM undergoing any form of surgery.[25,26] The intravenous route of insulin administration circumvents the unpredictable absorption of subcutaneous insulin exaggerated by changes in blood pressure and cutaneous blood flow that might occur during the perioperative period. Although the insulin dose required for optimal control of the blood glucose concentration is unknown, the usual starting dose for the variable rate insulin infusion is 1 unit·h^{-1} (Table 22-7).[25] It is reasonable to initiate the insulin infusion at 0.5 unit·h^{-1} in a patient such as a thin

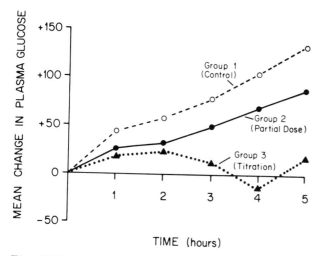

Fig. 22-3. Changes in the plasma glucose concentrations were determined during the intraoperative period in insulin-dependent adult diabetic patients. Group 1 patients received no preoperative insulin or glucose. Group 2 patients received one-fourth to one-half of their usual dose of insulin at 7 AM on the morning of surgery. In addition, glucose (6.25 g·h^{-1} IV) was initiated at the time of insulin administration. Group 3 patients received no insulin or glucose preoperatively but were treated with regular insulin administered intravenously if the measured blood glucose concentration exceeded 200 mg·dl^{-1}. (From Walts LF, Miller J, Davidson MB, Brown J. Perioperative management of diabetes mellitus. Anesthesiology 1981;55:104–9, with permission.)

female who may be more sensitive to insulin. Cardiopulmonary bypass is associated with significant metabolic derangements and insulin resistance owing to hypothermia. As a result, the continuous intravenous infusion rate of insulin may have to be increased to greater than 10 units·h^{-1}, to maintain euglycemia. There does not appear to be general agreement regarding the frequency of monitoring of the blood glucose concentration

Table 22-6.   Intermittent Intravenous Insulin Injection During the Perioperative Period

1. Begin an infusion of glucose (5–10 g·h^{-1} IV) and potassium (2–4 mEq·h^{-1} IV) during the perioperative period
2. Measure the blood glucose concentration every 1–2 hours during surgery and during the early postoperative period
3. Administer regular insulin (5–10 units IV), if the blood glucose concentration is >250 mg·dl^{-1}
4. Increase the rate of intravenous glucose infusion if the blood glucose concentration is <100 mg·dl^{-1}

(Data from Walts LF, Miller J, Davidson MB, Brown J. Perioperative management of diabetes mellitus. Anesthesiology 1981;55: 104–9.)

Table 22-7.   Continuous Intravenous Infusion of Regular Insulin During the Perioperative Period

1. Mix 50 units of regular insulin in 500 ml normal saline (1 unit·h^{-1} = 10 ml·h^{-1})
2. Initiate intravenous infusion at 0.5–1 unit·h^{-1}
3. Measure blood glucose concentration as necessary (usually every hour), and adjust insulin infusion rate accordingly:

<80 mg·dl^{-1}	Turn infusion off for 30 minutes Administer 25 ml of 50% glucose Remeasure blood glucose concentration in 30 minutes
80–120 mg·dl^{-1}	Decrease insulin infusion by 0.3 unit·h^{-1}
120–180 mg·dl^{-1}	No change in insulin infusion rate
180–220 mg·dl^{-1}	Increase insulin infusion by 0.3 unit·h^{-1}
>220 mg·dl^{-1}	Increase insulin infusion by 0.5 unit·h^{-1}

4. Provide sufficient glucose (5–10 g·h^{-1}) and potassium (2–4 mEq·h^{-1})

(Data from Hirsh IB, Magill JB, Cryer PE, White PF. Perioperative management of surgical patients with diabetes mellitus. Anesthesiology 1991;74:346–59.)

although a schedule of glucose checks every 1 to 2 hours in the operating room is often recommended.[27] The use of a blood glucose meter is recommended over visually read capillary glucose estimates for the patient receiving a continuous intravenous infusion of insulin. Estimation of the urine glucose concentration and the use of a sliding scale based on this observation to manage perioperative insulin needs is not optimal, since the sliding scale regimen is based on retrospective hyperglycemia.[25] Furthermore, this approach requires the presence of a bladder catheter in the sedated or anesthetized patient. In view of the potential for infection, a bladder catheter should probably not be placed only to monitor glycosuria in the diabetic patient.

Induction and Maintenance

The choice of drugs for induction and maintenance of anesthesia is less important than monitoring the blood glucose concentration and treatment of potential physiologic derangements associated with diabetes. Rapid and accurate measurement of the blood glucose concentration with a blood glucose meter should be possible in the operating room. The use of a sliding scale based on glycosuria to manage perioperative insulin requirements is not as precise as measurement of the blood glucose concentration. Intubation of the trachea with a cuffed tube seems prudent, in view of the potential for delayed gastric emptying in the patient with autonomic neuropathy. Hyperglycemia during surgery most likely reflects an increase in the plasma concentration of cortisol, growth hormone, and norepinephrine. In addition, volatile anesthetics impair the release of insulin in response to administration of glucose.[28] With respect to glucose intolerance, there is no evidence that maintenance of anesthesia with a specific volatile agent in a diabetic patient is advantageous. Epidural and low spinal anesthesia preserve glucose tolerance, presumably due to inhibition of the epinephrine response to surgery. Large doses of local anesthetic, as administered for brachial plexus block, have been associated with myocardial depression in diabetic patients.[29] The high incidence of peripheral neuropathy is a consideration in choosing a regional anesthetic technique in the diabetic patient. Conversely, there may be an increased risk of nerve injury in the diabetic patient who is rendered unconscious, emphasizing the importance of proper positioning of the extremities.

Episodes of bradycardia and hypotension that develop suddenly and are unresponsive to atropine and ephedrine have been described during maintenance of anesthesia in diabetic patients with preoperative evidence of cardiac autonomic neuropathy (orthostatic hypotension, resting tachycardia).[17,18,29] Prompt intervention with external cardiac massage and intravenous administration of epinephrine may be the only effective therapy.

If a patient is receiving adequate insulin, glucose, and potassium, any additional fluids administered during surgery for treatment of intraoperative blood loss need not contain glucose. Administration of lactated Ringer's solution to a diabetic patient is controversial, since lactate is converted to glucose. For this reason, a higher insulin dose may be required for the diabetic patient receiving lactated Ringer's solution during the perioperative period. Metoclopramide increases gastric motility and may be an effective postoperative antiemetic in the diabetic patient with gastroparesis.

Emergency Surgery

The most common emergency operations performed in the diabetic patient are appendectomy, incision and drainage procedures, and lower extremity amputation for infection. In this situation, it is useful to evaluate the patient's metabolic status (blood glucose concentration, electrolytes, pH, urine ketones) before proceeding with anesthesia. If diabetic ketoacidosis is present, surgery can be delayed while standard treatment of this metabolic emergency is instituted with infusion of fluids, insulin, and potassium. Indeed, treatment of diabetic ketoacidosis may result in the disappearance of abdominal pain and tenderness.[25] Placement of a central venous catheter may be helpful in guiding volume replacement therapy.

Hyperosmolar Hyperglycemic Nonketotic Coma

Hyperosmolar hyperglycemic nonketotic coma (HHNC) has been reported as a postoperative complication of NIDDM.[30] This syndrome is characterized by marked hyperglycemia,

Table 22-8. Hyperosmolar Hyperglycemic Nonketotic Coma

Hyperosmolarity (>330 mOsm·L^{-1})
Hyperglycemia (>600 mg·dl^{-1})
Normal pH
Osmotic diuresis (hypokalemia)
Hypovolemia (hemoconcentration)
Central nervous system dysfunction

plasma hyperosmolarity, profound dehydration, absence of ketoacidosis, and variable mental status changes (Table 22-8). Hyperglycemia and insulin resistance present during cardiopulmonary bypass in patients with NIDDM make this patient population vulnerable to the development of HHNC.[25] Other factors that may precipitate HHNC include sepsis, advanced age, hyperalimentation, and certain surgical procedures, such as pancreatectomy. About two-thirds of patients in whom HHNC develops do not have a history of diabetes and do not require exogenous insulin supplementation after recovery from this syndrome. Treatment of HHNC is directed at the correction of hypovolemia and hyperosmolarity. Insulin treatment is maintained until the blood glucose concentration decreases to about 300 mg·dl^{-1}. Potassium supplementation may be required to replace that lost owing to osmotic diuresis.

INSULINOMA

Insulinoma is an insulin-secreting tumor of pancreatic beta cells manifested as fasting hypoglycemia. A failure of the plasma insulin concentration to decrease as the blood glucose concentration decreases is suggestive of the presence of an insulinoma. Diagnosis of inappropriate secretion of insulin by an islet cell tumor is difficult in the obese patient, since obesity results in insulin resistance and in the need for increased circulating concentrations of this hormone. About 10% of these tumors are malignant, metastasizing to the liver. Streptozotocin has activity against pancreatic beta cells and is used as palliative therapy for inoperable metastatic disease.

The principal challenge during anesthesia for surgical excision of an insulinoma is the maintenance of a normal blood glucose concentration.[31] Profound hypoglycemia can occur, particularly during manipulation of the tumor, whereas marked hyperglycemia can follow successful surgical removal of the tumor. Nevertheless, a hyperglycemic response is both variable and unpredictable, making this observation an unreliable clinical indicator of the completeness of surgical removal of the tumor.[32] An artificial pancreas that continuously analyzes the blood glucose concentration and automatically infuses insulin or glucose has been used for the intraoperative management of these patients.[33] A blood glucose meter is necessary to permit frequent (every 15 minutes) measurement of the blood glucose concentration.[32] Since evidence of hypoglycemia (hypertension, tachycardia, diaphoresis) may be masked during anesthesia, it is probably wise to include glucose in the intravenous fluids administered intraoperatively. The known ability of volatile anesthetics to inhibit insulin release is a theoretical advantage for the maintenance of anesthesia during surgical resection of an insulinoma, remembering that the efficacy of this effect is unproved in these patients.[28,29] The minimum glucose level needed to maintain glucose transport across the blood-brain barrier and into brain cells is undefined. Some patients adapt to blood glucose concentrations as low as 40 $mg \cdot dl^{-1}$, whereas others could experience a hypoglycemic reaction when the blood glucose level is abruptly decreased from 300 $mg \cdot dl^{-1}$ to 100 $mg \cdot dl^{-1}$.

THYROID GLAND DYSFUNCTION

Thyroid gland dysfunction reflects the overproduction or underproduction of either triiodothyronine (T_3) or thyroxine (tetraiodothyronine, T_4), or both. These two physiologically active thyroid gland hormones act on cells through the adenylate cyclase system, producing changes in the speed of biochemical reactions, total body oxygen consumption, and energy (heat) production.

Thyroid Function Tests

Thyroid function tests are used to assess the rate of production of T_3 and T_4 in the detection of hyperthyroidism and hypothyroidism (Table 22-9). In the absence of clinical evidence of thyroid gland dysfunction, routine screening of adults by performance of thyroid function tests is not cost-effective, except possibly for females older than 65 years of age.[34,35] If thyroid gland dysfunction is suspected, the efficient initial approach is to measure the total plasma T_4 level (Table 22-10). The T_4 level most closely reflects the functional state of the thyroid gland, being increased in about 90% of hyperthyroid patients and decreased in about 85% of hypothyroid patients. The resin T_3 uptake (RT_3U) test is used to document changes in the T_4 level not due to thyroid dysfunction (Table 22-10). If measurement of T_4 and RT_3U suggest thyroid gland dysfunction, it is appropriate to measure a total T_3 level (hyperthyroidism) or thyroid stimulating hormone (TSH) level (hypothyroidism). Measurement of the T_3 level may be misleading in a euthyroid patient with cirrhosis of the liver or in a patient with uremia or malnutrition in whom the peripheral conversion of T_4 to T_3 is decreased. The T_3 level is decreased in only about 50% of hypothyroid patients, reflecting the production of more T_3 than T_4 as the thyroid gland fails. An increased TSH level is the most sensitive test for detecting primary hypothyroidism, emphasizing the extreme sensitivity

Table 22-9. Tests of Thyroid Gland Function

Test	Purpose
Total plasma thyroxine (T_4) level	Detects >90% of hyperthyroid patients; influenced by level of T_4-binding globulin (see Table 22-10)
Resin triiodothyronine uptake (RT_3U)	Clarifies whether changes in T_4 level are due to thyroid gland dysfunction or alterations in T_4-binding globulin
Total plasma triiodothyronine (T_3) level	Confirm diagnosis of hyperthyroidism; may be low in absence of hypothyroidism in patients who are cirrhotic, uremic, or malnourished
Thyroid stimulating hormone (TSH) level	Confirms diagnosis of primary hypothyroidism; may be increased before T_4 level is decreased
Thyroid scan	Demonstrates iodide-concentrating capacity of thyroid gland; functioning thyroid gland tissue is rarely malignant
Ultrasonography	Discriminates between cystic (rarely malignant) and solid (may be malignant) nodules
Antibodies to thyroid gland components	Distinguishes Hashimoto's thyroiditis from cancer

of the hypothalamic-pituitary axis to even modest decreases in circulating concentrations of T_3 and T_4. Indeed, the TSH level may be increased before the serum T_4 concentration is decreased. Whether every patient with an increased TSH level is, by definition, hypothyroid, especially if the T_4 and T_3 levels remain normal, is an unsettled question. Secondary hypothyroidism in which the anterior pituitary gland does not secrete TSH is detected by both a decrease in both the T_4 and TSH level.

Hyperthyroidism

Hyperthyroidism is a generic term for all conditions in which body tissues are exposed to increased circulating concentrations (5 to 15 times normal) of T_3 or T_4, or both. Graves' disease or diffuse toxic goiter is the most common form of hyperthyroidism, occurring most often in females between 20 and 40 years of age. An autoimmune pathogenesis for Graves' disease is suggested by the presence of immunoglobulin G autoantibodies such as long-acting thyroid stimulator in the plasma, which mimics the effects of TSH and produces effects for up to 12 hours, compared with 1 hour for normal TSH.

Table 22-10. Differential Diagnosis of Thyroid Gland Dysfunction[a]

Condition	T_4	RT_3U	T_3	TSH
Hyperthyroidism	Increased	Increased	Increased	Normal
Primary hypothyroidism	Decreased	Decreased	Decreased	Increased
Secondary hypothyroidism	Decreased	Decreased	Decreased	Decreased
Pregnancy	Increased	Decreased	Normal	Normal

[a] See Table 22-9 for definitions.

Hyperthyroidism occurs in about 0.2% of parturients and is most often due to diffuse toxic goiter. The diagnosis of hyperthyroidism is based on clinical signs and symptoms as well as confirmation of excessive thyroid gland function, as demonstrated by appropriate tests (Tables 22-9 and 22-10). The diagnosis of hyperthyroidism during pregnancy is difficult, since an estrogen-induced increase in T_4-binding globulin results in an increased T_4 level. Passive transfer of antibody across the placenta may produce transient neonatal Graves' disease.

Signs and Symptoms

Signs and symptoms of hyperthyroidism reflect the impact of excess amounts of T_3 or T_4, or both, on the speed of biochemical reactions, total body oxygen consumption, and energy (heat) production[36] (Table 22-11). The patient suffers from the consistent presence of anxiety, as well as weight loss despite high-calorie intake. Fatigue, diaphoresis, skeletal muscle weakness, and heat intolerance are characteristic. The appearance or worsening of angina pectoris or congestive heart failure or the unexpected onset of congestive heart failure or atrial fibrillation may reflect undiagnosed hyperthyroidism, especially in an elderly patient in whom the increased amount of thyroid hormones is sufficient only to aggravate underlying heart disease. Mild to moderate hyperthyroidism

may be difficult to diagnose clinically during pregnancy since many normal parturients experience tachycardia, heat intolerance, and emotional instability. In overt hyperthyroidism, a hyperdynamic circulation characterized by tachycardia, tachydysrhythmias, and increased cardiac output suggests excessive activity of the sympathetic nervous system, as well as a compensatory attempt to eliminate excess heat. The sensitivity of beta receptors is increased in the hyperthyroid patient. Adrenal cortex hyperplasia reflects an increased production and utilization of cortisol. Exophthalmus is due to an infiltrative process that involves retrobulbar fat and the eyelids. Retrobulbar edema can be so severe that the optic nerve is compressed, with resultant blindness. The patient with hyperthyroidism may exhibit increased bone resorption and associated hypercalciuria.

Treatment

The three principal treatments of hyperthyroidism are antithyroid drugs, subtotal thyroidectomy, or radioactive iodine. Regardless of the therapy selected, the patient with hyperthyroidism must be followed indefinitely, usually with TSH measurements to see whether hypothyroidism develops, or with T_4 measurements to determine whether hyperthyroidism recurs. Hyperthyroidism that develops during pregnancy often requires no treatment because it is mild or resolves spontaneously.

Table 22-11. Signs and Symptoms of Hyperthyroidism

Sign/Symptom	Incidence (% of Patients)
Goiter	100
Tachycardia	100
Anxiety	99
Tremor	97
Heat intolerance	89
Fatigue	88
Weight loss	85
Eye signs	71
Skeletal muscle weakness	70
Atrial fibrillation	10

Antithyroid Drugs

The initial medical management of the patient with hyperthyroidism is usually with antithyroid drugs, such as propylthiouracil and methimazole. These drugs principally inhibit oxidation of inorganic iodine and its incorporation into tyrosine, rendering most patients euthyroid within 1 to 6 months. A rare but significant complication of treatment with these drugs is agranulocytosis. Intraoperative bleeding owing to drug-induced thrombocytopenia or hypoprothrombinemia has been described in patients being treated with propylthiouracil.[37,38] Traditionally, antithyroid drugs are continued for 1 year, followed by discontinuation, which results in a lasting remission in about 30% of patients. Hypothyroidism is a risk of antithyroid drug therapy, accounting for the common practice of decreasing the dose after a euthyroid state is achieved or adding a small amount of oral T_4 to the daily dose of antithyroid drug.

Beta antagonist drugs such as propranolol are valuable adjuncts in the treatment of hyperthyroidism, acting to ameliorate many of the symptoms of excessive sympathetic nervous system activity (tachycardia, diaphoresis, tremor).[39] The efficacy of propranolol is attributed to beta blockade and to the ability of this drug to interfere with the conversion of T_4 to T_3 in the circulation and tissues.[40] Propranolol does not interfere with the release or synthesis of thyroid hormones. Nadolol, which has a longer duration of action than propranolol, is effective in controlling sympathetic nervous system manifestations of hyperthyroidism with a single daily oral dose.[41]

Subtotal Thyroidectomy

Subtotal thyroidectomy, for reasons that are not clear, induces remission in most patients with Graves' disease. Preoperative preparation of the patient with hyperthyroidism who is scheduled for subtotal thyroidectomy is with a beta antagonist such as propranolol (average oral dose 160 mg·d^{-1}).[42,43] In an emergency, the patient can be prepared for surgery in less than 1 hour with the intravenous administration of propranolol, whereas elective preparation can be achieved within 24 hours.[42] Before the use of beta antagonist therapy, patients were prepared for subtotal thyroidectomy using antithyroid drugs and potassium iodide, a process that required several weeks.

Possible complications of subtotal thyroidectomy include incomplete control or recurrence of hyperthyroidism, hypothyroidism, damage to the recurrent laryngeal nerve, and tracheal compression. The most common nerve injury after subtotal thyroidectomy is damage to the abductor fibers of the recurrent laryngeal nerves. This type of nerve damage, when unilateral, is characterized by hoarseness and by a paralyzed vocal cord that assumes an intermediate position. Bilateral recurrent nerve injury results in aphonia and paralyzed vocal cords, which can flap together, producing airway obstruction during inspiration. Selective injury of the adductor fibers of the recurrent laryngeal nerves leaves the adductor fibers unopposed, and pulmonary aspiration is a hazard. In view of the possibility of damage to these nerves, it would seem prudent to evaluate vocal cord movement at the conclusion of surgery for a subtotal thyroidectomy. This can be accomplished by indirect or direct laryngoscopy and by asking the patient to phonate by saying "e." Symptoms attributed to laryngeal nerve injury may actually be due to laryngeal edema, most likely reflecting surgical trauma. Airway obstruction occurring soon after tracheal extubation despite normal vocal cord function should suggest the diagnosis of tracheomalacia, reflecting weakening of the tracheal rings by chronic pressure from a goiter. The appearance of airway obstruction during the early postoperative period, as in the postanesthesia care unit, may be due to tracheal compression at the operative site by a hematoma.

Hypoparathyroidism resulting from the accidental removal of the parathyroid glands rarely occurs after subtotal thyroidectomy. If damage to the parathyroid glands does occur, hypocalcemia typically develops 24 to 72 hours postoperatively but may be manifested as early as 1 to 3 hours after surgery. Laryngeal muscles are the most sensitive to hypocalcemia, and inspiratory stridor progressing to laryngospasm may be the first suggestion of the presence of surgically induced hypoparathyroidism. Treatment consists of the prompt intravenous administration of calcium, until laryngeal stridor ceases.

Radioactive Iodine

Radioactive iodine therapy reliably renders the hyperthyroid patient euthyroid, without the possible risks associated with anesthesia and surgery. The incidence of thyroid cancer is not increased by this treatment, and no genetic damage has been documented. The principal side effect of radioactive iodine therapy is hypothyroidism, which may be delayed and subtle in onset. Radioactive iodine is not used during pregnancy because of potential radiation-induced damage to the fetus. There is almost universal agreement that radioactive iodine therapy is the treatment of choice in the patient older than 40 years of age.

Thyroid Storm

Thyroid storm (thyrotoxicosis) is an abrupt exacerbation of hyperthyroidism caused by the sudden excessive release of thyroid gland hormones into the circulation. Hyperthermia, tachycardia, congestive heart failure, dehydration, and shock are likely. Thyroid storm associated with surgery can occur intraoperatively but is more likely to occur 6 to 18 hours after surgery. When thyroid storm occurs during the perioperative period, it may mimic malignant hyperthermia.[44] Treatment of thyroid storm is with an infusion of cooled crystalloid solutions and continuous infusion of esmolol, to maintain the heart rate at an acceptable level.[45] When hypotension is persistent, the administration of cortisol (100 to 200 mg IV) may be considered. Dexamethasone may inhibit the conversion of T_4 to T_3, an effect that is additive to propylthiouracil. Aspirin may displace T_4 from its carrier protein and is not recommended for lowering body temperature. It is also important to treat any suspected infection. Ultimately, drugs such as propylthiouracil and sodium iodide are administered to prevent the synthesis and release of thyroid hormone.

Management of Anesthesia

Elective surgery should probably be deferred until the patient has been rendered euthyroid and the hyperdynamic cardiovascular system has been controlled with a beta antagonist, as evidenced by an acceptable resting heart rate. Clearly, all drugs being administered to manage the hyperthyroid state should be continued through the perioperative period. When surgery cannot be delayed in a symptomatic hyperthyroid patient, the continuous infusion of esmolol (100 to 300 $\mu g \cdot kg^{-1} \cdot min^{-1}$ IV) may be useful for the control of cardiovascular responses evoked by sympathetic nervous system stimulation.[45] Poor control of hyperthyroidism plus surgery or parturition are associated with an increased risk of the development of thyroid storm.

Preoperative Medication

Anxiety relief is often provided by the oral administration of a benzodiazepine. The use of an anticholinergic drug is not recommended, since such a drug could interfere with the body's normal heat-regulating mechanism and contribute to an increase in heart rate. Evaluation of the upper airway for evidence of obstruction is an important part of the preoperative preparation. In this regard, computed tomography may be helpful in evaluating airway anatomy.

Induction of Anesthesia

Induction of anesthesia is acceptably achieved with a number of intravenous induction drugs. Thiopental is an attractive selection because its thiourea structure lends antithyroid activity to the drug. Nevertheless, it is unlikely that a significant antithyroid effect will be produced by an induction dose of this drug. Ketamine is not a likely selection because it can stimulate the sympathetic nervous system. Indeed, tachycardia and hypertension have been described after administration of ketamine to euthyroid patients being treated with thyroid hormone replacement.[46] Assuming the absence of airway obstruction from an enlarged goiter, the administration of succinylcholine or of a nondepolarizing muscle relaxant that will not affect the cardiovascular system is useful to facilitate intubation of the trachea.

Maintenance of Anesthesia

Goals during maintenance of anesthesia for a hyperthyroid patient are to avoid the administration of drugs that stimulate the sympathetic nervous system and to provide sufficient anesthetic depression to prevent an exaggerated response to surgical stimulation.[47] The possibility of organ toxicity owing to altered or accelerated drug metabolism in the presence of hyperthyroidism must also be considered when selecting drugs for maintenance of anesthesia.

In an animal model rendered hyperthyroid, the administration of halothane, enflurane, and isoflurane was followed by evidence of hepatic centrilobular necrosis in some animals, with the greatest incidence (92%) in animals exposed to halothane.[48] Three of six patients in whom unexplained hepatitis

developed after exposure to halothane and in whom antibodies developed against a metabolite of halothane were also being treated with thyroid hormones.[49] These data in animals and humans suggest that treatment with thyroid hormones such as T_3 may predispose to halothane-induced hepatic dysfunction. Nevertheless, liver function tests are not altered postoperatively in previously hyperthyroid patients rendered euthyroid before undergoing surgery and anesthesia that includes administration of halothane or enflurane.[50] An undocumented but potential concern with enflurane and sevoflurane would be nephrotoxicity from increased production of fluoride owing to accelerated metabolism of these drugs.

Despite animal evidence of hepatic necrosis after exposure to volatile anesthetics (desflurane and sevoflurane not evaluated), the ability of isoflurane to offset adverse sympathetic nervous system responses to surgical stimulation, yet not sensitize the myocardium to catecholamines, makes this an attractive selection to combine with nitrous oxide for maintenance of anesthesia in the hyperthyroid patient. Nitrous oxide combined with a short-acting opioid is an alternative to administration of a volatile drug, but it has the disadvantage of not reliably suppressing sympathetic nervous system activity.

It is a clinical impression that anesthetic requirements (MAC) are increased in the hyperthyroid patient. Nevertheless, a controlled animal study does not confirm a clinically significant change in halothane MAC in association with altered thyroid gland function[51] (Fig. 22-4). The discrepancy between clinical impression and objective data may reflect the impact of increased cardiac output, which is characteristic of hyperthyroidism, on the rate of increase in the alveolar partial pressure of an inhaled anesthetic. For example, increased cardiac output accelerates the uptake of an inhaled anesthetic, resulting in the need to increase the inspired (delivered) concentration of the anesthetic (perceived clinically as an increased anesthetic requirement) so as to achieve a brain partial pressure (MAC) similar to that achieved with a lower inspired concentration in the euthyroid patient. Likewise, accelerated metabolism of the anesthetic drug does not alter the partial pressure of the drug needed in the brain to produce the desired pharmacologic effect. Another factor that should be considered when evaluating anesthetic requirements in the presence of altered thyroid gland function is body temperature. For example, an increase in body temperature, as could accompany thyroid storm, would be expected to increase MAC by about 5% for each degree that body temperature increases about 37°C.

Monitoring during maintenance of anesthesia in the hyperthyroid patient is directed at early recognition of increased activity of the thyroid gland, suggesting the onset of thyroid storm. Constant monitoring of body temperature is particularly useful; methods to lower body temperature, including a cooling mattress and cold crystalloid solutions for intravenous infusion, are recommended. The electrocardiogram may show tachycardia or cardiac dysrhythmias, or both, indicating the

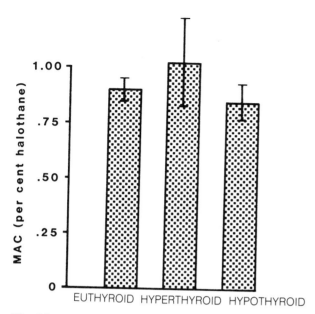

Fig. 22-4. The MAC of halothane in dogs rendered hyperthyroid or hypothyroid is not significantly different from the value in euthyroid animals. Mean ± SD. (Data from Babad AA, Eger EI. The effects of hyperthyroidism and hypothyroidism on halothane and oxygen requirements in dogs. Anesthesiology 1968;29:1087–93.)

need for the intraoperative administration of a beta antagonist (continuous intravenous infusion of esmolol) or lidocaine. The patient with exophthalmos is susceptible to corneal ulceration and drying, emphasizing the need to protect the eyes during the perioperative period.

The selection of a muscle relaxant should include consideration of the potential impact of this drug on the sympathetic nervous system. Pancuronium is not a likely selection, in view of the ability of this drug to increase heart rate and thereby mimic sympathetic nervous system stimulation. Administration of a muscle relaxant with minimal effects on the cardiovascular system is useful. Conceivably, a prolonged response could occur when a traditional dose of muscle relaxant is administered to the patient with co-existing skeletal muscle weakness. For this reason, it may be prudent to decrease the initial dose of muscle relaxant and closely monitor the effect produced at the neuromuscular junction using a peripheral nerve stimulator. Antagonism of neuromuscular blockade with an anticholinesterase drug combined with an anticholinergic drug introduces the concern for drug-induced tachycardia. Although experience is too limited to make a recommendation, it would seem unwarranted to avoid pharmacologic antagonism of a nondepolarizing muscle relaxant in a hyperthyroid patient. Perhaps glycopyrrolate, which has less chronotropic effect

than atropine, would be a more appropriate anticholinergic drug selection.

Treatment of hypotension with a sympathomimetic drug must consider the possibility of the exaggerated responsiveness of the hyperthyroid patient to endogenous or exogenous catecholamines. For this reason, a decreased dose of a direct-acting vasopressor, such as phenylephrine, may be a more logical selection than ephedrine, which acts in part by provoking the release of catecholamines.

Regional Anesthesia

Regional anesthesia with its associated blockade of the sympathetic nervous system is a potentially useful selection for the hyperthyroid patient, assuming there is no evidence of high-output congestive heart failure. A continuous epidural anesthetic may be preferable to spinal anesthesia because of the slower onset of sympathetic nervous system blockade, making severe hypotension less likely.[52] If hypotension occurs, a decreased dose of phenylephrine is recommended, keeping in mind the possible hypersensitivity of these patients to a sympathomimetic drug. Epinephrine should not be added to the local anesthetic solution, as systemic absorption of this catecholamine could produce an exaggerated circulatory response. Increased anxiety and associated activation of the sympathetic nervous system can be treated in the awake patient with the intravenous administration of a benzodiazepine such as midazolam.

Hypothyroidism

Hypothyroidism is a generic term for all conditions in which body tissues are exposed to decreased circulating concentrations of T_3 and T_4, which is estimated to be present in 0.5% to 0.8% of the adult population.[34] The etiology of hypothyroidism is primary because of destruction of the thyroid gland (adequate TSH) or secondary because of central nervous system dysfunction (Table 22-12). Chronic thyroiditis (Hashimoto's thyroiditis) is the most common cause of hypothyroidism, exhibited as an autoimmune disease characterized by progressive destruction of the thyroid gland. The presence of other autoimmune diseases (myasthenia gravis, adrenal insufficiency, premature ovarian failure) should direct attention to the thyroid gland. Other causes of hypothyroidism include drug ablative therapy and hypothalamic or pituitary insufficiency. Hypogonadism that presents as either amenorrhea or impotence almost invariably develops before pituitary hypothyroidism.

The diagnosis of hypothyroidism is based on clinical signs and symptoms plus confirmation of decreased thyroid gland function, as demonstrated by appropriate tests (Table 22-9). Subclinical hypothyroidism manifested only as an increased plasma TSH concentration is present in about 5% of the popu-

Table 22-12. Etiology of Hypothyroidism

Primary Hypothyroidism
  Thyroid gland destruction
    Chronic thyroiditis (Hashimoto's thyroiditis)
    Previous subtotal thyroidectomy
    Previous radioactive iodine therapy
    Irradiation of the neck
  Thyroid hormone deficiency
    Antithyroid drugs
    Excess iodide (inhibits release)
    Dietary iodine deficiency

Secondary Hypothyroidism
  Hypothalamic dysfunction
    Thyrotropin releasing hormone deficiency
  Anterior pituitary dysfunction
    Thyroid stimulating hormone deficiency

lation, with a prevalence of 13.2% in otherwise healthy elderly patients, especially females.[34] Circulating concentrations of TSH are increased in patients with primary hypothyroidism and are decreased in those with secondary (pituitary) hypothyroidism (Table 22-10).

Signs and Symptoms

The onset of hypothyroidism in the adult patient is insidious and may go unrecognized. An adult with diffuse enlargement of the thyroid gland should have antibody measurements to determine the presence of chronic thyroiditis and associated hypothyroidism. Characteristically, there is a generalized decrease in metabolic activity in the patients. Lethargy is prominent, and intolerance to cold is likely to be present. Bradycardia and decreased stroke volume are responsible for a decrease in cardiac output of up to 40%. The decreased cardiac output, combined with an increase in systemic vascular resistance and decreased blood volume, results in a prolonged circulation time and narrow pulse pressure. Peripheral vasoconstriction is characteristic, leading to cool, dry skin. Presumably, vasoconstriction represents an attempt to decrease loss of body heat. Many of the cardiac manifestations of hypothyroidism (cardiomegaly, pleural effusion, ascites, peripheral edema) mimic congestive heart failure. Overt congestive heart failure is unlikely, however, and, if present, may indicate co-existing heart disease or an unrecognized myocardial infarction. There is often atrophy of the adrenal cortex and an associated decrease in the production of cortisol. Inappropriate secretion of antidiuretic hormone by a hypothyroid patient can result in hyponatremia, owing to an impaired ability of renal tubules to excrete free water. Cardiovascular impairment is minimal to absent in the patient with subclinical hypothyroidism.

Treatment

The treatment of hypothyroidism consists of oral administration of T_4. Optimal therapy is characterized by the disappearance of all symptoms of hypothyroidism and a normal plasma TSH level. The patient with ischemic heart disease and hypothyroidism may not tolerate even modest amounts of T_4 without the development of angina pectoris. If angina pectoris appears or worsens during T_4 therapy, coronary angiography and revascularization surgery can be safely undertaken before adequate T_4 therapy is achieved.[53–55] It is not unusual to encounter patients previously started on thyroid hormone replacement without convincing laboratory confirmation of hypothyroidism. Confirmation of the diagnosis may require discontinuing treatment for about 5 weeks and measuring a plasma TSH level, which if elevated, verifies the initial diagnosis.

Myxedema Coma

Myxedema coma is a rare complication of hypothyroidism manifesting as profound lethargy or coma, spontaneous hypothermia (less than 35°C), hypoventilation, and congestive heart failure. Sepsis in an elderly patient or exposure to cold may be the initiating event. Treatment is with intravenous administration of T_3 (exerts a physiologic effect within 6 hours) and cortisol, if adrenal insufficiency is suspected. Digitalis as used to treat congestive heart failure is used sparingly, because the hypothyroid patient's heart cannot easily perform increased myocardial contractile work. Fluid replacement is important, remembering that these patients may be vulnerable to water intoxication and hyponatremia.

Management of Anesthesia

Elective surgery should probably be deferred in the patient with symptomatic hypothyroidism. Nevertheless, controlled clinical studies do not confirm an increased risk when patients with mild to moderate hypothyroidism undergo elective surgery.[56,57] There are no controlled studies to support the position that most hypothyroid patients (1) are unusually sensitive to inhaled anesthetic drugs and opioids, (2) have a prolonged recovery, and (3) experience a higher incidence of cardiovascular complications. Certainly, when ischemic heart disease becomes life-threatening, the evidence is compelling that surgical revascularization can be safely accomplished before beginning treatment of the hypothyroidism.[53–55] Considering the likely presence of subclinical hypothyroidism in many patients who undergo uneventful anesthesia, as well as the lack of increased morbidity in patients with mild to moderate hypothyroidism, there is little evidence to support delaying elective surgery in these patients. Nevertheless, a high index of suspicion for possible adverse effects, including exaggerated ef-

Table 22-13.   Possible Adverse Responses of the Hypothyroid Patient During the Perioperative Period

Increased sensitivity to depressant drugs
Hypodynamic cardiovascular system
    Decreased heart rate
    Decreased cardiac output
Slowed metabolism of drugs
Unresponsive baroreceptor reflexes
Impaired ventilatory responses to arterial hypoxemia or hypercarbia
Hypovolemia
Delayed gastric emptying time
Hyponatremia
Hypothermia
Anemia
Hypoglycemia
Adrenal insufficiency

fects of depressant drugs, would still seem warranted[58] (Table 22-13).

Preoperative Medication

Preoperative medication for the hypothyroid patient should emphasize the value of the preoperative visit and resultant psychological support. Opioid premedication has been administered safely, but there is a historical concern that depressant effects of these drugs may be exaggerated in the hypothyroid patient. Supplemental cortisol may be considered if there is concern that surgical stress could unmask decreased adrenal function that may accompany hypothyroidism. In some patients, it may be better to administer sedative and anticholinergic drugs intravenously after the patient arrives in the operating room, so that any unexpected effect can be promptly recognized and treated.

Induction of Anesthesia

Induction of anesthesia is often accomplished with the intravenous administration of ketamine, with the presumption that the inherent support of the cardiovascular system by this drug will be beneficial. Thiopental has also been used for induction of anesthesia in the hypothyroid patient without apparent excessive cardiovascular depression.[58] Even ketamine, in the absence of an active sympathetic nervous system, might produce unexpected cardiovascular depression. There is, however, no evidence of decreased responsiveness of the hypothyroid patient to exogenous catecholamines. In the severely hypothyroid patient, the inhalation of nitrous oxide might be sufficient to produce unresponsiveness. Intubation of the trachea is facilitated by succinylcholine or a nondepolarizing muscle relaxant, keeping in mind that co-existing skeletal muscle weakness could be associated with an exaggerated muscle relaxant effect.

Maintenance of Anesthesia

Maintenance of anesthesia for the hypothyroid patient is often achieved by inhalation of nitrous oxide plus supplementation, if necessary, with a short-acting opioid, benzodiazepine, or ketamine.[59] A volatile anesthetic may not be recommended in the overtly symptomatic hypothyroid patient, for fear of inducing exaggerated cardiac depression. Furthermore, vasodilation produced by any anesthetic drug in the presence of hypovolemia or attenuated baroreceptor reflex responses, or both, could result in abrupt decreases in blood pressure, suggesting increased sensitivity to the drug. Nevertheless, hypothyroidism does not appear to decrease significantly the anesthetic requirement (MAC) for a volatile drug[51] (Fig. 22-4). Failure of MAC to change may reflect maintenance of the cerebral metabolic oxygen requirement, independent of thyroid activity.[58] The clinical impression that MAC is decreased most likely reflects a decrease in cardiac output that accelerates the establishment of an anesthetizing brain partial pressure of the drug, manifested by the rapid induction of anesthesia. Furthermore, a decrease in body temperature below 37°C would be expected to decrease MAC for inhaled drugs and slow hepatic metabolism and renal clearance of injected drugs.

Maintaining skeletal muscle paralysis to provide surgical working conditions, while at the same time minimizing the dose of anesthetic drugs, is an appropriate goal for management of the hypothyroid patient. Furthermore, controlled ventilation of the lungs is recommended, in view of the tendency for the hypothyroid patient to hypoventilate. Decreased production of carbon dioxide associated with a decreased metabolic rate could make the hypothyroid patient vulnerable to an excessive decrease in $PaCO_2$ during mechanical ventilation of the lungs. Because of mild cardiovascular stimulating effects, pancuronium is often selected for the production of skeletal muscle paralysis in the hypothyroid patient. An intermediate-acting muscle relaxant is also acceptable and is perhaps less likely to produce prolonged neuromuscular blockade. Indeed, decreased skeletal muscle activity associated with hypothyroidism suggests the possibility of a prolonged response, when a traditional dose of muscle relaxant is administered to a hypothyroid patient. Antagonism of the nondepolarizing neuromuscular blockade with an anticholinesterase drug combined with an anticholinergic drug does not pose a known hazard to the hypothyroid patient.

Monitoring of the hypothyroid patient is directed at prompt recognition of exaggerated cardiovascular depression (perhaps reflecting the onset of congestive heart failure) and the detection of the onset of hypothermia. Continuous recording of blood pressure with a catheter placed in a peripheral artery, as well as measurement of cardiac filling pressures, is recommended for invasive operations that may be either prolonged or associated with significant blood loss, or both. Measurement of central venous pressure is helpful for guiding the rate of intravenous fluid infusion. In addition, glucose solutions used for intravenous fluid replacement should contain sodium, to decrease the likelihood of hyponatremia owing to impaired clearance of free water. Hypotension requiring treatment with infusion of fluids or administration of a sympathomimetic drug may introduce the risk of evoking congestive heart failure. For example, administration of an alpha adrenergic agonist, such as phenylephrine, could adversely increase systemic vascular resistance in the presence of a heart that cannot reliably increase myocardial contractility. By contrast, a drug with beta agonist effects could result in cardiac dysrhythmias. A useful approach in the treatment of hypotension may therefore be small doses of ephedrine (2.5 to 5 mg IV) administered during monitoring of cardiac filling pressures and continuous observation of the electrocardiogram. The possibility of acute adrenal insufficiency is a consideration when hypotension persists despite treatment with fluids and sympathomimetic drugs. Maintenance of body temperature is facilitated by increasing the temperature of the operating room and warming the inhaled gases. In addition, the passage of intravenous fluids through a blood warmer may be helpful.

Recovery from the sedative effects of anesthetic drugs may be delayed in the hypothyroid patient, resulting in the need for prolonged observation during the postoperative period. Indeed, prolonged postoperative somnolence and an inability to wean from mechanical support of ventilation have been described in a previously undiagnosed hypothyroid patient[60] (Fig. 22-5). In another report, acute postoperative hypothyroidism manifested as hypothermia, delayed awakening, and hypoventilation despite documented normal thyroid function 1 month earlier. This case emphasizes that a severe nonthyroid illness (gastric ulcer perforation) can precipitate acute thyroid gland dysfunction in a vulnerable patient (removal of a thyroid adenoma 20 years earlier).[61] Removal of the tracheal tube is deferred until the patient is responding appropriately and the body temperature is close to 37°C. Concern about possible increased sensitivity to the effects of opioids is a consideration in the management of postoperative pain, perhaps with emphasis on the use of a nonopioid analgesic. Despite these concerns, a comparison of patients with mild to moderate hypothyroidism with euthyroid patients failed to demonstrate any difference with respect to the lowest body temperature or blood pressure intraoperatively, the incidence of cardiac dysrhythmias, the need for vasopressors, time to tracheal extubation, and the need for postoperative ventilatory support.[56]

Regional Anesthesia

Regional anesthesia is an appropriate selection for the hypothyroid patient, provided that intravascular fluid volume is well maintained. Although supporting evidence is not available, theoretically the dose of local anesthetic necessary for performance of a peripheral nerve block could be decreased. Furthermore, metabolism of an amide local anesthetic that is absorbed into the systemic circulation could be slowed, possibly predisposing the hypothyroid patient to the development of drug-induced systemic toxicity.

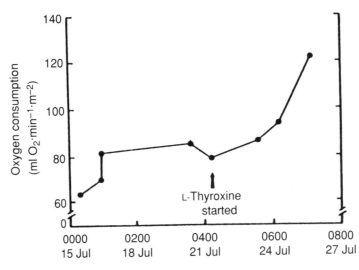

Fig. 22-5. Oxygen consumption in a patient with unsuspected hypothyroidism who underwent elective orthopaedic surgery complicated by hypotension and by the need for mechanical ventilation of the lungs during the postoperative period. Institution of thyroid replacement therapy restored vital signs and ventilation to normal. (From Levelle JP, Jopling MW, Sklar GS. Perioperative hypothyroidism: An unusual postanesthetic diagnosis. Anesthesiology 1985;63:195–7, with permission.)

PARATHYROID GLAND DYSFUNCTION

The four parathyroid glands located behind the upper and lower poles of the thyroid gland produce a polypeptide hormone known as parathyroid hormone (parathormone). Parathyroid hormone is released into the circulation by a negative feedback mechanism dependent on the plasma calcium concentration. For example, hypocalcemia stimulates the release of parathyroid hormone whereas hypercalcemia suppresses both the synthesis and release of this hormone. Parathyroid hormone maintains a normal plasma calcium concentration (4.5 to 5.5 mEq·L^{-1}) by promoting the movement of calcium across three interfaces represented by the gastrointestinal tract, renal tubules, and bone.

Hyperparathyroidism

Hyperparathyroidism is present when secretion of parathyroid hormone is increased. The plasma calcium concentration may be increased, decreased, or unchanged. Hyperparathyroidism is classified as primary, secondary, or ectopic.

Primary Hyperparathyroidism

Primary hyperparathyroidism results from excessive secretion of parathyroid hormone due to a benign parathyroid adenoma, carcinoma of a parathyroid gland, or hyperplasia of the parathyroid glands. A benign parathyroid adenoma is responsible for primary hyperparathyroidism in about 90% of patients; carcinoma of a parathyroid gland is responsible in less than 5%. Hyperplasia usually involves all four parathyroid glands, although not all the glands may be enlarged to the same degree. Hyperparathyroidism owing to an adenoma or hyperplasia is the most common presenting symptom in multiple endocrine neoplasia type I.

An increased plasma calcium concentration (greater than 5.5 mEq·L^{-1}) is the most valuable diagnostic indicator of primary hyperparathyroidism. Marked hypercalcemia (greater than 7.5 mEq·L^{-1}) is most likely to occur in the patient with cancer of a parathyroid gland. As the disease progresses, an increased plasma creatinine concentration may reflect associated renal dysfunction. An increase in the plasma chloride level (greater than 102 mEq·L^{-1}) is most likely due to the influence of parathyroid hormone on renal excretion of bicarbonate, producing a mild metabolic acidosis. Urinary excretion of cyclic adenosine monophosphate is increased in the patient with primary hyperparathyroidism. Measurement of the plasma parathyroid hormone concentration is not always sufficiently reliable to confirm the diagnosis of primary hyperparathyroidism.

Signs and Symptoms

Hypercalcemia is responsible for the broad spectrum of signs and symptoms affecting multiple organ systems that accompany primary hyperparathyroidism (Table 22-14). A modest increase in the plasma calcium concentration discovered incidentally in an ambulatory patient is most often due to a parathyroid adenoma, whereas marked hypercalcemia is more likely due to cancer. Skeletal muscle weakness and hypotonia is the most frequent complaint; it may be so severe as to suggest the presence of myasthenia gravis. Loss of skeletal muscle strength and skeletal muscle mass is most notable in the proximal musculature of the lower extremity. Renal stones, especially in the presence of polyuria and polydipsia, must arouse suspicion of hypercalcemia owing to hyperparathyroidism. Anemia, even in the absence of renal dysfunction, is a consequence of primary hyperparathyroidism. Hypertension is frequent, and the electrocardiogram may reveal a prolonged P-R interval, while the Q-T interval is often shortened. Cardiac rhythm, however, is usually normal. Peptic ulcer disease is common and may reflect potentiation of gastric acid secretion by calcium. Acute and chronic pancreatitis is associated with primary hyperparathyroidism. Even in the absence of peptic ulcer disease or pancreatitis, abdominal pain that often accompanies hypercalcemia can mimic an acute surgical abdomen. The classic skeletal consequence of primary hyper-

Table 22-14.   Signs and Symptoms of Hypercalcemia Due to Hyperparathyroidism

System	Signs/Symptoms
Neuromuscular	Skeletal muscle weakness
Renal	Renal stones Polyuria and polydipsia Decreased glomerular filtration rate
Hematopoietic	Anemia
Cardiac	Hypertension Prolonged P-R interval Short Q-T interval
Gastrointestinal	Abdominal pain Vomiting Peptic ulcer Pancreatitis
Skeletal	Skeletal demineralization Pathologic fractures Collapse of vertebral bodies
Nervous system	Somnolence Psychosis Decreased pain sensation
Ocular	Calcifications (band keratopathy) Conjunctivitis

parathyroidism is osteitis fibrosa cystica, which reflects accelerated osteoclastic activity. Radiographic evidence of skeletal involvement includes generalized osteopenia, subcortical bone resorption in the phalanges and distal ends of the clavicles, and the appearance of bone cysts. Bone pain and pathologic fractures may be present. There may be deficits of memory and cerebration, with or without personality changes or mood disturbances, including hallucinations. Loss of sensation for pain and vibration can occur.

Treatment

Hypercalcemia that is symptomatic is aggressively treated with diuresis (saline 150 ml·h^{-1} plus furosemide 1 to 2 mg·kg^{-1} IV) in the presence of central venous pressure monitoring to decrease the likelihood of fluid overload. Plicamycin (25 μg·kg^{-1} IV) inhibits the osteoclastic activity of parathyroid hormone, producing a prompt (12 to 36 hours) and sustained (3 to 5 days) lowering of the plasma calcium concentration. The toxic effects of plicamycin include thrombocytopenia and damage to the liver or kidneys, or both. Hemodialysis can also be used to lower promptly the plasma calcium concentration. Calcitonin is effective for prompt lowering of the plasma calcium concentration, but the effects of this hormone are transient. A thiazide diuretic is not recommended, as these drugs may increase the plasma calcium concentration unpredictably, presumably reflecting increased renal absorption of calcium. Rarely, hypercalcemia cannot be medically managed; in these cases, emergency parathyroidectomy is required.

Definitive treatment of primary hyperparathyroidism is surgical removal of the diseased or abnormal portions of the parathyroid glands. Successful surgical treatment is reflected by a normalization of the plasma calcium concentration within 3 to 4 days and a decrease in the urinary excretion of cyclic adenosine monophosphate. Postoperatively, the first potential complication is hypocalcemic tetany. Hypomagnesemia that occurs postoperatively aggravates manifestations of hypocalcemia and renders it refractory to treatment. Acute arthritis may occur following parathyroidectomy. Hyperchloremic metabolic acidosis, in association with deterioration of renal function, may occur transiently after parathyroidectomy.

Management of Anesthesia

There is no evidence that a specific anesthetic drug or technique is indicated in the patient with primary hyperparathyroidism undergoing surgical treatment. Maintenance of hydration and urine output is important in the perioperative management of hypercalcemia. The existence of somnolence before the induction of anesthesia introduces the possibility that intraoperative anesthetic requirements could be decreased. Ketamine might be an unlikely selection in the patient with personality changes related to hypercalcemia. The possibility of co-existing renal dysfunction is a consideration in the

selection of enflurane or sevoflurane. Co-existing skeletal muscle weakness suggests the possibility of decreased requirements for muscle relaxants, whereas hypercalcemia might be expected to antagonize the effects of a nondepolarizing muscle relaxant. Indeed, there is a report of sensitivity to succinylcholine and resistance to atracurium in a patient with hyperparathyroidism.[62] In view of the unpredictable response to muscle relaxants, it is probably important to decrease the initial dose of these drugs and to monitor the response produced at the neuromuscular junction by using a peripheral nerve stimulator. Monitoring of the electrocardiogram for manifestations of adverse cardiac effects of hypercalcemia is often recommended, although there is evidence that the Q-T interval may not be a reliable index of changes in the plasma calcium concentration during anesthesia.[63] Careful positioning of the hyperparathyroid patient is necessary because of the likely presence of osteoporosis and associated vulnerability to pathologic fractures.

Secondary Hyperparathyroidism

Secondary hyperparathyroidism reflects an appropriate compensatory response of the parathyroid glands to secrete more parathyroid hormone to counteract a disease process that produces hypocalcemia. For example, chronic renal disease impairs the elimination of phosphorus and decreases the hydroxylation of vitamin D, resulting in hypocalcemia and a compensatory hyperplasia of the parathyroid glands with an increased release of parathyroid hormone. Because secondary hyperparathyroidism is adaptive rather than autonomous, it seldom produces hypercalcemia. Treatment of secondary hyperparathyroidism is best directed at control of the underlying disease, as achieved by normalizing the serum phosphate concentration in the patient with renal disease by the administration of an oral phosphate binder.

On occasion, transient hypercalcemia may follow otherwise successful renal transplantation. This response reflects the inability of previously hyperactive parathyroid glands to adapt quickly to normal renal excretion of calcium and phosphorus, as well as to hydroxylation of vitamin D. The parathyroid glands will usually return to normal size and function with time, although parathyroidectomy is occasionally necessary.

Ectopic Hyperparathyroidism

Ectopic hyperparathyroidism (humoral hypercalcemia of malignancy, pseudohyperparathyroidism) is due to the secretion of parathyroid hormone, or a substance with similar endocrine effects, by tissues other than the parathyroid glands.[64] Carcinoma of the lung, breast, pancreas, or kidney, and lymphoproliferative disease are the most likely ectopic sites for parathyroid hormone secretion. Ectopic hyperparathyroidism is more likely than primary hyperparathyroidism to be associated with anemia and an increased plasma akaline phosphatase concentration. A role for prostaglandins in the production of hypercalcemia in these patients is suggested by the calcium-lowering effects produced by indomethacin, which is an inhibitor of prostaglandin synthesis.

Hypoparathyroidism

Hypoparathyroidism is present when secretion of parathyroid hormone is deficient or peripheral tissues are resistant to the effects of the hormone (Table 22-15). Absence of parathyroid hormone is almost always iatrogenic, reflecting inadvertent removal of the parathyroid glands as during thyroidectomy. Pseudohypoparathyroidism is a congenital disorder in which the release of parathyroid hormone is intact, but the kidneys are unable to respond to the hormone. An affected patient is characterized by mental retardation, calcification of the basal ganglia, obesity, short stature, and short metacarpals and metatarsals. A decreased plasma calcium concentration (less than 4.5 mEq·L^{-1}) is the most valuable diagnostic indicator of hypoparathyroidism.

Signs and Symptoms

Hypocalcemia is responsible for the signs and symptoms of hypoparathyroidism. Clinical manifestations of hypocalcemia depend on the rapidity of onset of the electrolyte abnormality.

Acute Hypocalcemia

An acute onset of hypocalcemia, as can occur after accidental removal of the parathyroid glands during a thyroidectomy, is likely to be manifested as perioral paresthesias, restlessness, and neuromuscular irritability, as evidenced by a positive Chvostek sign or Trousseau sign. A positive Chvostek sign consists of facial muscle twitching, produced by manual tapping over the area of the facial nerve at the angle of the mandible. Nevertheless, Chvostek sign is positive in the absence of hypocalcemia in 10% to 15% of patients. A positive Trousseau sign is carpopedal spasm produced by 3 minutes of limb ischemia, by means of a tourniquet. Inspiratory stridor reflects neuromuscular irritability of the intrinsic laryngeal musculature.

Chronic Hypocalcemia

Chronic hypocalcemia is associated with complaints of fatigue and skeletal muscle cramps that may be associated with a prolonged Q-T interval on the electrocardiogram. The QRS complex, P-R interval, and cardiac rhythm usually remain normal. Neurologic changes include lethargy, cerebration deficits, and personality changes reminiscent of hyperparathyroidism. Chronic hypocalcemia is associated with the formation of cataracts, calcification involving the subcutaneous tissues and basal ganglia, and thickening of the skull. Chronic renal failure is the most common cause of hypocalcemia.

Treatment

Treatment of acute hypocalcemia consists of an infusion of calcium (10 ml of 10% calcium gluconate IV), until signs of neuromuscular irritability disappear. For treatment of hypoparathyroidism not complicated by symptomatic hypocalcemia, the approach is administration of oral calcium and vitamin D. An exogenous parathyroid hormone replacement preparation is not yet practical for clinical use. Thiazide diuretics may be useful, as these drugs cause sodium depletion without proportional potassium excretion, thus tending to increase the plasma calcium concentration.

Management of Anesthesia

Management of anesthesia for the hypoparathyroid patient is determined by the impact of perioperative events on the plasma calcium concentration (see the section, Hypocalcemia, in Chapter 21).

DiGeorge Syndrome

DiGeorge syndrome (congenital thymic hypoplasia) is characterized by hypoplasia or aplasia of the parathyroid glands and thymus gland, resulting in secondary hypocalcemia and a propensity for the development of infections due to defects in cell-mediated immunity.[65] Neonatal tetany is usually present. Associated anomalies are often vascular, including right aortic arch, persistent truncus arteriosus, and tetralogy of Fallot.

Table 22-15.   Etiology of Hypoparathyroidism

Decreased or Absent Parathyroid Hormone
  Accidental removal of parathyroid glands during thyroidectomy
  Parathyroidectomy to treat hyperplasia
  Idiopathic (DiGeorge syndrome)

Resistance of Peripheral Tissues to the Effects of Parathyroid Hormone
  Congenital
    Pseudohypoparathyroidism
  Acquired
    Hypomagnesemia
    Chronic renal failure
    Malabsorption
    Anticonvulsive therapy (phenytoin)

Unknown
  Osteoblastic metastases
  Acute pancreatitis

Micrognathia may interfere with adequate exposure of the glottic opening during direct laryngoscopy. Iatrogenic hyperventilation and associated respiratory alkalosis, as may occur during anesthesia, could accentuate co-existing hypocalcemia. The response to a neuromuscular blocking drug could be altered in the presence of hypocalcemia. Hemodynamic instability may occur if the hypoparathyroid patient is made acutely hypocalcemic. Ability to measure plasma concentrations of calcium, particularly the ionized fraction, is helpful in the perioperative management of these patients. Thymic transplantation may be recommended in the infant who experiences repeated infections.

ADRENAL GLAND DYSFUNCTION

The adrenal glands consist of the adrenal cortex and adrenal medulla. The body's adjustments to the upright posture and responses to stress, as produced by hemorrhage, sepsis, anesthesia, and surgery, are dependent on normal function of the adrenal glands.

The adrenal cortex is responsible for the synthesis of three groups of hormones classified as glucocorticoids, mineralocorticoids, and androgens (Table 22-16). Cortisol is the most important glucocorticoid secreted by the adrenal cortex. The

daily endogenous cortisol production is estimated to be 20 mg. Cortisol is the only hormone produced by the adrenal cortex that is essential for life. Maintenance of blood pressure by cortisol reflects the importance of this hormone in facilitating the conversion of norepinephrine to epinephrine in the adrenal medulla. Hyperglycemia in response to cortisol reflects gluconeogenesis and an inhibition of the peripheral use of glucose by cells. Retention of sodium and excretion of potassium are facilitated by cortisol. The anti-inflammatory effect of cortisol and other glucocorticoids is particularly evident in the presence of high plasma concentrations.

The principal endogenous mineralocorticoid is aldosterone. Secretion and synthesis of aldosterone by the adrenal cortex are regulated by the renin-angiotensin system and the plasma concentration of potassium. For example, renin release from the juxtaglomerular cells of the kidneys, in response to hypotension, hyponatremia, or hypovolemia, results in conversion of angiotensinogen to angiotensin I. Angiotensin I is converted to angiotensin II, which acts as a potent stimulus for the release of aldosterone from the adrenal cortex. In addition, aldosterone secretion is stimulated by hyperkalemia, whereas hypokalemia suppresses its release. Aldosterone regulates extracellular fluid volume by promoting resorption of sodium by the renal tubules. In addition, aldosterone promotes renal tubular excretion of potassium.

The adrenal medulla is a specialized part of the sympathetic nervous system that is capable of synthesizing norepinephrine and epinephrine. The major portion of norepinephrine synthesized in the adrenal medulla is methylated to epinephrine, such that 75% of the catecholamine output from the adrenal medulla is epinephrine. The production of epinephrine is regulated by cortisol, which flows through the adrenal medulla from the adrenal cortex to activate the enzyme, phenylethanolamine N-methyltransferase, necessary for the methylation of norepinephrine to epinephrine. As a result, function of the adrenal medulla is regulated by the adrenal cortex. Considering the many cardiovascular and metabolic effects of epinephrine, it is ironic that this hormone, unlike cortisol, does not need to be replaced in the adrenalectomized or addisonian patient (Table 22-17).

The half-time of norepinephrine and epinephrine in the circulation is less than 1 minute, reflecting their prompt enzymatic breakdown by monoamine oxidase and catechol-o-methyltransferase. Vanillylmandelic acid comprises about 80% of the urinary metabolites of norepinephrine and epinephrine (Table 22-18). By virtue of its ability to stimulate both alpha and beta adrenergic receptors, epinephrine has important effects on the cardiovascular system, ventilation, and metabolism (Table 22-17). Norepinephrine exerts effects on the cardiovascular system and metabolism by virtue of its stimulation of alpha-adrenergic receptors (Table 22-17). Beta stimulation

Table 22-16.   Endogenous and Synthetic Corticosteroids

	Glucocorticoid Potency[a] (Anti-inflammatory Effects)	Mineralocorticoid Potency[a] (Salt-Retaining Effects)	Equivalent Oral or IV Dose[a] (mg)
Cortisol	1	1	20[b]
Cortisone	0.8	0.8	25
Prednisolone	4	0.8	5
Prednisone	4	0.8	5
Methylprednisolone	5	0	4
Betamethasone	25	0	0.75
Dexamethasone	25	0	0.75
Triamcinolone	5	0	4
Corticosterone	0.35	15	—
Fludrocortisone	10	125	—
Aldosterone	0	3000	—

[a] Potencies and equivalent doses are compared with cortisol.
[b] Assumed daily endogenous cortisol production.

Table 22-17. Comparative Effects of Epinephrine and Norepinephrine

	Epinephrine	Norepinephrine
Heart rate	Minimal increase	Moderate decrease
Stroke volume	Moderate increase	Minimal decrease
Cardiac output	Marked increase	No change to minimal to moderate decrease
Cardiac dysrhythmias	Yes	Yes
Systolic blood pressure	Marked increase	Marked increase
Diastolic blood pressure	No change to minimal decrease	Moderate increase
Mean arterial pressure	Minimal increase	Moderate increase
Systemic vascular resistance	Minimal decrease	Moderate to marked increase
Renal blood flow	Moderate to marked decrease	Moderate to marked decrease
Skin blood flow	Moderate decrease	Moderate decrease
Skeletal muscle blood flow	Marked increase	No change to minimal decrease
Airway resistance	Marked decrease	No change
Blood glucose concentration	Marked increase	No change to minimal increase

produced by norepinephrine on the heart is masked by the predominant alpha stimulation produced on the peripheral vasculature. The only important disease process associated with the adrenal medulla is pheochromocytoma. Adrenal medulla insufficiency is not known to occur.

Table 22-18. Urinary Excretion of Catecholamines and Catecholamine Metabolites

	Daily Urinary Excretion	
	Normal	Pheochromocytoma
Total metanephrines	0.1–1.6 mg	2.5–4 mg
Vanillylmandelic acid	1.8 mg	10–250 mg
Norepinephrine	<100 µg	—
Epinephrine	<1 µg	—
Total catecholamines	4–126 µg	200–4000 µg

Hyperadrenocorticism

Hyperadrenocorticism (Cushing's disease) may reflect (1) overproduction of adrenocorticotropic hormone (ACTH) by the anterior pituitary (about two-thirds of cases), (2) ectopic production of ACTH by malignant tumors (especially carcinoma of the lung, kidney, pancreas), (3) excess production of cortisol by a benign or malignant tumor of the adrenal cortex, or (4) exogenous (pharmacologic) administration of cortisol or related drugs. The usual cause of excess ACTH production by the anterior pituitary is a basophilic adenoma, although excess production of corticotropin releasing factor in the hypothalamus could also be the mechanism. A benign adrenal adenoma often secretes only cortisol, whereas adrenal carcinoma almost always produces androgens as well, resulting in hirsutism and defeminization.

The most useful test for the diagnosis of hyperadrenocorticism is measurement of the plasma cortisol concentration the morning after a midnight dose of dexamethasone. Dexamethasone will suppress the plasma cortisol concentration in normal patients, but not in those with hyperadrenocorticism. If the plasma cortisol concentration is less than 5 µg·dl^{-1}, hyperadrenocorticism can be excluded, whereas a value of about 5 µg·dl^{-1} suggests the need for further evaluation to exclude this syndrome. In the patient with hyperadrenocorticism, the urinary cortisol excretion over 24 hours is usually greater than 150 µg, and there is a loss of the diurnal rhythm in the plasma cortisol concentration (normal 10 to 25 µg·ml^{-1} in the morning and 2 to 10 µg·ml^{-1} in the evening). An increased plasma concentration of ACTH suggests a pituitary gland tumor or an ectopic hormone-producing tumor. An extremely high plasma concentration of ACTH is evidence for an ectopic, rather than pituitary gland, source of excess production. Furthermore, in contrast to the gradual onset of symptoms seen with excess anterior pituitary production of ACTH, the clinical presentation in patients with ectopic production of ACTH is that of acute hyperadrenocorticism dominated by mineralocorticoid (hypokalemic alkalosis and skeletal muscle weakness) rather than glucocorticoid effects (rarely a cushingoid appearance). Magnetic resonance imaging is the most sensitive technique for pituitary imaging. Computed tomography demonstrating large adrenal glands in a patient with chronic adrenal insufficiency suggests metastatic tumor or active tuberculosis adrenalitis.

Signs and Symptoms

The diagnosis of hyperadrenocorticism is suggested by several clinical findings (Table 22-19). The affected patient is likely to be hypertensive and to exhibit hyperglycemia, hypokalemia, and skeletal muscle weakness. Obesity is usually present in association with increased skin pigmentation, plethoric and round facies ("moon facies"), and a characteristic accumulation of fat between the scapulae ("buffalo hump").

Table 22-19.   Signs and Symptoms
of Hyperadrenocorticism

Hypertension
Hypokalemia
Hyperglycemia
Skeletal muscle weakness
Osteoporosis
Obesity
Hirsutism
Menstrual disturbances
Poor wound healing
Susceptibility to infection

Osteoporosis reflects cortisol-induced loss of protein from bone. Shortening of the thoracic spine may reflect vertebral body collapse from osteoporosis. Menstrual irregularities are common. Hirsutism is present when hyperadrenocorticism is due to excess secretion of ACTH, reflecting the ability of this hormone to stimulate the release of androgens, as well as cortisol. There is poor wound healing and increased susceptibility to bacterial and fungal infection.

Treatment

Transsphenoidal microadenomectomy is the preferred treatment for hyperadrenocorticism, owing to excess secretion of ACTH by the anterior pituitary. Preoperative treatment with metyrapone serves to inhibit the synthesis of cortisol. In children, external radiation rather than microadenomectomy may be preferred. Bilateral adrenalectomy is necessary when the anterior pituitary tumor is large. Nelson syndrome (hyperpigmentation of the skin and chromophobe tumor of the anterior pituitary) develops in 10% to 40% of patients who have undergone bilateral adrenalectomy. Surgical removal is the treatment of choice for an adrenal adenoma or carcinoma.

Management of Anesthesia

Management of anesthesia for the patient with hyperadrenocorticism must take into consideration the physiologic effects of excess cortisol secretion[66] (Table 22-19). Preoperative evaluation of blood pressure, electrolyte balance, and blood glucose concentration is especially important. Osteoporosis is a consideration in positioning for the operative procedure.

The choice of drugs for preoperative medication, induction of anesthesia, and maintenance of anesthesia is not influenced by the presence of hyperadrenocorticism. Etomidate may transiently decrease the synthesis and release of cortisol by the adrenal cortex, but a therapeutic role for this drug in the presence of hyperadrenocorticism seems unlikely.[67] Surgical stimulation will predictably increase the release of cortisol from the adrenal cortex. It seems unlikely that this stress-induced release would produce a different effect from that in a

normal patient. Furthermore, an attempt to decrease adrenal cortex activity with an opioid, barbiturate, or volatile anesthetic is probably futile, since any drug-induced inhibition will likely be overridden by surgical stimulation. Even regional anesthesia may not be effective in the prevention of increased cortisol secretion during surgery. The dose of muscle relaxant should probably be decreased initially, in view of skeletal muscle weakness, which frequently accompanies hyperadrenocorticism. In addition, the presence of hypokalemia could influence the response to a nondepolarizing muscle relaxant. Mechanical ventilation of the lungs during surgery is recommended, as skeletal muscle weakness, with or without coexisting hypokalemia, may decrease strength in the muscles of breathing. Regional anesthesia is acceptable, but the likely presence of osteoporosis, with possible vertebral body collapse, is a consideration.

The plasma cortisol concentration decreases promptly after microadenomectomy or bilateral adrenalectomy, for which replacement therapy is recommended. In this regard, a continuous infusion of cortisol ($100\ mg \cdot d^{-1}$ IV) may be initiated intraoperatively. Likewise, the patient with metastatic disease involving the adrenal glands may show the development of acute adrenal insufficiency, suggesting the need to institute supplemental therapy. Transient diabetes insipidus and meningitis may occur after microadenomectomy. The patient with hypoadrenocorticism, regardless of etiology, is susceptible to water overload and associated hyponatremia.

Hypoadrenocorticism

Hypoadrenocorticism may develop as a result of (1) destruction of the adrenal cortex by hemorrhage, cancer, or granulomatous disease; (2) prolonged exogenous administration of a corticosteroid that suppresses the pituitary-adrenal axis; and (3) deficiency of ACTH. Primary adrenal insufficiency (Addison's disease) reflects the absence of cortisol and aldosterone, owing to the destruction of the adrenal cortex. The most common cause is adrenal hemorrhage in the anticoagulated patient, but insufficiency can also develop as a result of sepsis or accidental or surgical trauma. The adrenal gland is the endocrine gland most often involved in patients who die of acquired immunodeficiency syndrome, although adrenal insufficiency is uncommon in these patients. Secondary adrenal insufficiency occurs in the patient with panhypopituitarism that includes ACTH deficiency. In contrast to primary adrenal insufficiency, manifestations of secondary adrenal insufficiency reflect the absence of cortisol, as aldosterone secretion remains normal. The definitive diagnosis of hypoadrenocorticism requires measurement of the plasma cortisol concentration before and 1 hour after administration of ACTH.

Signs and Symptoms

Primary adrenal insufficiency is manifested as weight loss, skeletal muscle weakness, hypotension, and abdominal or back pain. Pain owing to hemorrhage into the adrenal cortex, as in the anticoagulated patient, may be the only clue to the onset of adrenal insufficiency.[68] The clinical picture may be indistinguishable from shock due to loss of intravascular fluid volume. Blood urea nitrogen is likely to be increased due to hypovolemia and decreased renal blood flow. Hyponatremia, hyperkalemia, hypoglycemia, and hemoconcentration are often present. A useful clue to the diagnosis is the presence of hyperpigmentation principally over the palmar surfaces and pressure points.

Secondary adrenal insufficiency is less likely than primary adrenal insufficiency to be associated with severe hypovolemia or electrolyte derangements, since aldosterone secretion is maintained. Panhypopituitarism, however, may be associated with symptoms due not only to the lack of ACTH but of TSH, gonadotropins, and growth hormone as well.

Treatment

Treatment of life-threatening hypoadrenocorticism consists of the administration of cortisol (100 mg IV), followed by continuous infusion of 10 mg·h^{-1} IV. It is useful to draw a blood sample for analysis of the plasma cortisol concentration before initiation of therapy, although a delay for more specific diagnostic testing is not recommended. Intravenous infusion of glucose in saline, colloid solutions, and in some cases whole blood, is necessary to restore intravascular fluid volume. Replacement therapy for chronic hypoadrenocorticism is with the administration of cortisone (20 to 25 mg orally in the morning and 10 to 15 mg orally in the afternoon). In addition, a mineralocorticoid effect is provided with fludrocortisone (0.05 to 0.1 mg·d^{-1} orally).

Surgery and Suppression of the Pituitary Adrenal Axis

Corticosteroid supplementation should be increased for any patient being treated for chronic hypoadrenocorticism who undergoes a surgical procedure. This recommendation is based on the concern that this patient could be more susceptible to cardiovascular collapse, since the release of additional endogenous cortisol in response to stress is not likely. More controversial is the management of the patient who displays suppression of the pituitary-adrenal axis owing to current or previous administration of a corticosteroid for a disease such as asthma or rheumatoid arthritis, which is unrelated to pathology in the anterior pituitary or adrenal cortex. The precise dose of corticosteroid or duration of therapy with a corticosteroid that will produce suppression of the pituitary-adrenal axis is unknown. Furthermore, recovery of normal pituitary-adrenal axis function may require as long as 12 months after discontinuation of therapy.[69] In addition, documentation of a normal plasma cortisol concentration during the preoperative period does not confirm an intact pituitary-adrenal axis or the ability of the adrenal cortex to release cortisol in response to surgical stress. Intactness of this axis can be confirmed by the plasma cortisol response to ACTH administered intravenously (plasma cortisol concentration doubles within 1 hour if axis intact), but this remains an impractical and infrequently performed preoperative test.[70] Instead, the clinical approach is often to administer empirically a supplemental dose of a corticosteroid during the perioperative period, when surgery is planned in a patient treated with a corticosteroid or in a patient who has been treated for more than 1 month during the 6 to 12 months immediately preceding the surgery. Nevertheless, it should be appreciated that a cause-and-effect relationship between intraoperative hypotension and acute hypoadrenocorticism in a patient previously treated with a corticosteroid has never been documented.[71,72]

In view of possible adverse influences of corticosteroids (retardation of healing, increased susceptibility to infection, gastrointestinal hemorrhage), attempts have been made to rationalize corticosteroid supplementation for the surgical patient considered at risk of the development of acute hypoadrenocorticism and also to define an appropriate but minimal effective dose schedule.[66] A recommended regimen for corticosteroid supplementation during the perioperative period is cortisol (25 mg IV) at induction of anesthesia, followed by a continuous infusion of cortisol (100 mg IV) over the next 24 hours. This regimen maintains the plasma cortisol concentration above a normal level during major surgery in the patient receiving chronic treatment with a corticosteroid unrelated to hypoadrenocorticism and who shows a subnormal response to the preoperative infusion of ACTH[73] (Fig. 22-6). These data provide a rational and physiologic approach to low-dose corticosteroid supplementation during the perioperative period in a patient considered at risk of pituitary-adrenal axis suppression and scheduled for major surgery. It is likely that the patient undergoing a minor operation will need minimal (cortisol 25 mg IV) to no additional corticosteroid supplementation during the perioperative period.

In addition to low-dose intravenous cortisol supplementation, the patient receiving a daily maintenance dose of a corticosteroid should also receive this dose with the preoperative medication on the day of surgery. The maintenance dose should be continued postoperatively. There are no data to support the practice of instituting an increased maintenance dose preoperatively, followed by gradual decreases over several days postoperatively until the original maintenance dose is reached.[74] In those instances in which postoperative events could exaggerate the need for exogenous corticosteroid supplementation, the continuous infusion of cortisol (100 mg every 12 to 24 hours IV) should be sufficient. This recommendation is based on the estimate that endogenous cortisol production during stress introduced by major surgery or extensive burns is 72 to 150 mg·d^{-1}.

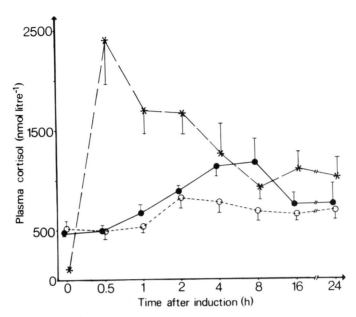

Fig. 22-6. Plasma cortisol concentrations were measured (1) in control patients who had never been treated with corticosteroids (solid symbols), (2) in patients treated chronically with corticosteroids but showing a normal cortisol release response to ACTH (open symbols), and (3) in patients treated chronically with corticosteroids and showing a subnormal cortisol release response to ACTH (asterisks). Only these latter patients were treated with supplemental corticosteroids (cortisol, 25 mg IV, after induction of anesthesia, followed by a continuous infusion of 100 mg IV over the next 24 hours). This approach maintained the plasma cortisol concentration near or above that present in untreated patients. (From Symreng T, Karlberg BE, Kagedal B, Schildt B. Physiological cortisol substitution of long-term steroid treated patients undergoing major surgery. Br J Anaesth 1981;53:949–53, with permission.)

Management of Anesthesia

Management of anesthesia for the patient with known hypoadrenocorticism introduces no unique considerations other than provision of exogenous corticosteroid supplementation and a high index of suspicion for primary adrenal insufficiency, if unexplained intraoperative hypotension occurs. Despite the frequent suggestion that unexplained intraoperative hypotension and even death reflect unrecognized hypoadrenocorticism, there is no evidence that primary adrenal insufficiency is a likely explanation for this response.[71,72] The selection of drugs used for anesthesia or skeletal muscle paralysis is not influenced by the presence of treated hypoadrenocorticism, with the possible exception of etomidate. In this regard, etomidate has been shown to inhibit synthesis of cortisol transiently in normal patients.[67] Typically, the plasma cortisol concentration increases during surgery in response to the surgical stimulus, independent of the anesthetic drugs being administered.

Emergency surgery in the presence of untreated hypoadrenocorticism should be rare. If surgery becomes necessary, however, perioperative management must include administration of a supplemental corticosteroid and intravenous infusion of fluid. Minimal doses of anesthetic drugs should be adminis-

tered, since these patients may be exquisitely sensitive to drug-induced myocardial depression. Invasive monitoring of arterial blood pressure and of cardiac filling pressures is indicated. The plasma concentration of glucose and electrolytes should be measured frequently during the perioperative period. In view of skeletal muscle weakness, the initial dose of muscle relaxant should be reduced and the response produced monitored, using a peripheral nerve stimulator.

Hyperaldosteronism

Primary hyperaldosteronism (Conn syndrome) is present when there is excess secretion of aldosterone from a functional tumor independent of a physiologic stimulus. Secondary hyperaldosteronism is present when increased renin secretion is responsible for the excess secretion of aldosterone. Hyperaldosteronism should be considered in the patient with diastolic hypertension (100 to 125 mmHg) and a plasma potassium concentration of less than 3.5 mEq·L^{-1}. Hypertension reflects aldosterone-induced sodium retention and a resultant increased extracellular fluid volume. Aldosterone promotes renal excretion of potassium, resulting in hypokalemic metabolic alkalosis. Skeletal muscle weakness is presumed to reflect hypokalemia. Hypokalemic nephropathy can result in polyuria and in an inability to concentrate urine optimally.[75] Confirmation of the diagnosis of hyperaldosteronism is the demonstration of an increased plasma concentration of aldosterone and increased urinary potassium excretion (greater than 30 mEq·L^{-1}) despite co-existing hypokalemia. Measurement of the plasma renin activity permits classification of the disease as primary (low renin activity) or secondary (increased renin activity). A syndrome exhibiting all the features of hyperaldosteronism (hypertension, hypokalemia, suppression of the renin-angiotensin system) may result from chronic ingestion of licorice.

Treatment

Initial treatment of hyperaldosteronism consists of supplemental potassium and administration of a competitive aldosterone antagonist, such as spironolactone. Skeletal muscle weakness owing to hypokalemia may require treatment with potassium administered intravenously. Hypertension may require treatment with an antihypertensive drug. Accentuation of hypokalemia from drug-induced diuresis is decreased by using a potassium-sparing diuretic, such as triamterene. Definitive treatment for an aldosterone-secreting tumor is surgical excision. Bilateral adrenalectomy may be necessary if multiple aldosterone-secreting tumors are found.

Management of Anesthesia

Management of anesthesia for the treatment of hyperaldosteronism is facilitated by preoperative correction of hypokalemia and treatment of hypertension. Persistence of hypokalemia may modify responses to nondepolarizing muscle relaxants. Furthermore, it must be appreciated that intraoperative hyperventilation can decrease the plasma potassium concentration. Inhaled or injected drugs are acceptable for maintenance of anesthesia. The use of enflurane or sevoflurane may be questionable, however, if hypokalemic nephropathy and polyuria exist preoperatively.[75] Measurement of cardiac filling pressures through a right atrial or pulmonary artery catheter is important during surgery for adequate evaluation of the intravascular fluid volume and of the response to intravenous infusion of fluids. Indeed, aggressive preoperative preparation can convert the excess intravascular fluid volume status of these patients to unexpected hypovolemia, manifested as hypotension in response to vasodilating anesthetic drugs, positive-pressure ventilation of the lungs, position change, or sudden blood loss. The existence of orthostatic hypotension detected during the preoperative evaluation is a clue to the presence of unexpected hypovolemia in these patients. Acid-base status and plasma electrolyte concentrations should be measured frequently during the perioperative period. Supplementation with exogenous cortisol is probably unnecessary for

surgical excision of a solitary adenoma in the adrenal cortex; bilateral mobilization of the adrenal glands to excise multiple functional tumors, however, may introduce the need for exogenous administration of cortisol. A continuous infusion of cortisol (100 mg IV every 24 hours) may be initiated on an empirical basis if transient hypoadrenocorticism due to surgical manipulation is a consideration.

Hypoaldosteronism

Hyperkalemia in the absence of renal insufficiency suggests the presence of hypoaldosteronism.[76] Heart block secondary to hyperkalemia and postural hypotension with or without hyponatremia may occur. Hyperkalemia is sometimes abruptly enhanced by hyperglycemia. Hyperchloremic metabolic acidosis is a predictable finding.

Isolated deficiency of aldosterone secretion may reflect (1) congenital deficiency of aldosterone synthetase, or (2) hyporeninemia due to a defect in the juxtaglomerular apparatus or treatment with an angiotensin-converting enzyme inhibitor that leads to a loss of angiotensin stimulation. Hyporeninemic hypoaldosteronism typically occurs in a patient older than 45 years of age with chronic renal disease or diabetes mellitus, or both. Indomethacin-induced prostaglandin deficiency is a reversible cause of this syndrome. Treatment of hypoaldosteronism includes liberal sodium intake and daily administration of fludrocortisone.

Pheochromocytoma

Pheochromocytoma is a catecholamine-secreting tumor, which originates in the adrenal medulla or in chromaffin tissue along the paravertebral sympathetic chain, extending from the pelvis to the base of the skull.[77,78] More than 95% of all pheochromocytomas are found in the abdominal cavity, and about 90% originate in the adrenal medulla. An estimated 10% of these tumors involve both adrenal glands, and functional tumors in multiple sites are present in nearly 20% of patients, especially children. Less than 10% of pheochromocytomas are malignant. Pheochromocytoma typically occurs in a patient who is 30 to 50 years of age, although about one-third of reported cases have been in children, principally males. Pheochromocytoma can also occur as part of an autosomal dominant multiglandular neoplastic syndrome designated multiple endocrine neoplasia[78,79] (Table 22-20). Medullary thyroid carcinoma is the most common of the many rare disorders associated with pheochromocytoma. Although less than 0.1% patients with hypertension actually have a pheochromocytoma, nearly 50% of deaths in patients with unsuspected pheochromocytoma occur during anesthesia and surgery or parturition.[80] Pheochromocytoma and associated hypertension and hypermetabolism may mimic other diseases, including malignant hyperthermia.[81]

Table 22-20. Manifestations of Multiple Endocrine Neoplasia (MEN)

Syndrome	Manifestations
MEN type IIa (Sipple syndrome)	Medullary thyroid cancer Parathyroid adenoma Pheochromocytoma
MEN type IIb	Medullary thyroid cancer Mucosal adenomas Marfan appearance Pheochromocytoma
von Hippel-Lindau syndrome	Hemangioblastoma involving the central nervous system Pheochromocytoma

Diagnosis

The diagnosis of pheochromocytoma requires chemical confirmation of excessive catecholamine release. There is a lack of consensus as to the most reliable biochemical marker of a catecholamine-secreting tumor, although comparative studies indicate that measurement of free norepinephrine in a 24-hour urine sample provides a more sensitive index of pheochromocytoma than do catecholamine metabolites (normetanephrine, metanephrine, vanillylmandelic acid [VMA])[82] (Table 22-18). The presence of normotension despite an increased plasma concentration of catecholamines presumably reflects a decrease in the number of alpha receptors (down-regulation) in response to increased circulating concentrations of the neurotransmitter. Clonidine (0.3 mg orally) suppresses the plasma concentration of catecholamines in a hypertensive patient, but not in the patient with a pheochromocytoma[83] (Fig. 22-7). This finding reflects the ability of clonidine to suppress an increase in the plasma catecholamine concentration that results from neurogenic release, but not from the diffusion of excess catecholamines from a pheochromocytoma into the circulation. As such, this clonidine suppression test is useful in distinguishing the patient with essential hypertension and an elevated plasma catecholamine concentration from the patient with hypertension owing to a pheochromocytoma. Computed tomography is considered the initial localizing procedure in the diagnosis of pheochromocytoma.[84]

Signs and Symptoms

The hallmark of pheochromocytoma is paroxysmal hypertension associated with diaphoresis, headache, tremulousness, palpitations, and weight loss, especially in a young to middle-aged adult patient. The triad of diaphoresis, tachycardia, and headache in a hypertensive patient is highly suggestive of pheochromocytoma. Conversely, the absence of this triad virtually rules out the presence of a pheochromocytoma. Flushing is so rare that its presence casts doubt on the diagnosis of pheochromocytoma. Symptoms may last from several minutes to hours and are often followed by fatigue.

Hyperglycemia reflects a predominance of alpha activity (inhibition of insulin release, glycogenolysis) over beta effects (insulin release) produced by catecholamines secreted by the pheochromocytoma. Orthostatic hypotension is a common finding and reflects a decrease in intravascular fluid volume associated with sustained hypertension. A hematocrit greater than 45% may reflect hypovolemia caused by this mechanism. Sustained increases in the plasma catecholamine concentrations can result in focal necrosis of cardiac muscle and the development of a cardiomyopathy. Death resulting from a pheochromocytoma is often due to congestive heart failure, myocardial infarction, or intracerebral hemorrhage.

Treatment

Treatment of pheochromocytoma is surgical excision of the catecholamine-secreting tumor(s). Before surgery is scheduled, however, it is important to establish alpha blockade, to restore the blood volume, to assess end-organ damage, and to treat cardiac dysrhythmias. Preoperatively, alpha blockade is initiated by the administration of phenoxybenzamine or prazosin. Despite its selective postsynaptic alpha-1 receptor antagonist effects, prazosin has been criticized due to its failure to achieve adequate prevention of perioperative hypertensive episodes.[85] Labetalol is a mixed alpha and beta antagonist that may be considered, although a predominance of beta over alpha blockade produced by this drug could be undesirable. Alpha blockade attenuates or prevents catecholamine-induced vasoconstriction, leading to decreased blood pressure. Return to normotension facilitates an increase in intravascular fluid volume, as reflected by a decrease in the hematocrit. Serial monitoring of the hematocrit is a useful method of evaluating the adequacy of intravascular fluid volume expansion, and satisfactory alpha blockade is implied if the hematocrit decreases by about 5%, for example, from 45% to 40%. Normalization of intravascular fluid volume and blood pressure produced by alpha blockade before surgery also decreases the risk of intraoperative hypertension during manipulation of the tumor. In this regard, competitive alpha antagonists (prazosin, labetalol) have not been as effective as phenoxybenzamine in controlling the blood pressure response to massive release of catecholamine intraoperatively, as may occur with manipulation of the tumor. Presumably, irreversible alkylation of alpha receptors by phenoxybenzamine, and not just competitive inhibition, is necessary to ensure that alpha receptors will not respond to the increased plasma concentrations of catecholamines caused by tumor manipulation.[78] For this reason, phenoxybenzamine remains the mainstay of pharmacologic therapy.

Persistence of tachycardia or cardiac dysrhythmias, or both, despite the presence of alpha blockade, is an indication for the preoperative administration of a drug such as propranolol to produce beta blockade. The recommendation that beta

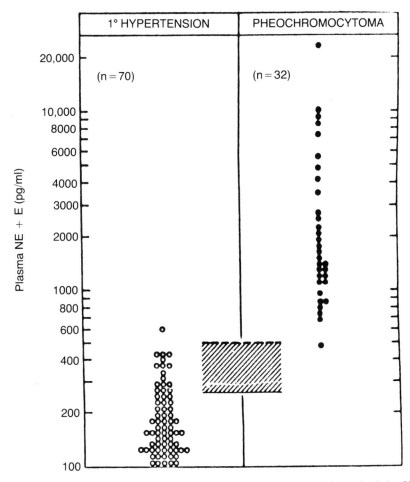

Fig. 22-7. A single dose of clonidine (0.3 mg orally) decreases the plasma concentration of norepinephrine (NE) and epinephrine (E) below 500 pg·ml^{-1} in nearly every patient with essential hypertension. Clonidine does not reliably decrease the plasma concentrations of catecholamines in patients with pheochromocytoma. The cross-hatched area represents the mean ±2 SD of values in a control group of normotensive patients. (From Bravo EL, Gifford RW. Pheochromocytoma: Diagnosis, localization and management. N Engl J Med 1984;311:1298–1303, with permission.)

blockade should not be instituted in the absence of alpha blockade is based on the theoretical concern that a heart depressed by beta blockade might not be able to maintain an adequate cardiac output should unopposed alpha-mediated vasoconstriction from the release of catecholamines result in an abrupt increase in systemic vascular resistance. In addition, the use of a beta antagonist in the presence of a catecholamine-induced cardiomyopathy could precipitate congestive heart failure. Echocardiography may be useful in the recognition of the patient with suspected cardiomyopathy. Hyperglycemia is common preoperatively, although alpha blockade will facilitate the release of insulin and decrease the likelihood of hyperglycemia in the patient with a pheochromocytoma. The preoperative

presence of hypercalcemia may indicate the presence of a multiple endocrine neoplasia that includes hyperparathyroidism[78,79] (Table 22-20).

Management of Anesthesia

Management of anesthesia for the patient requiring excision of a pheochromocytoma is based on the administration of drugs that do not stimulate the sympathetic nervous system plus the use of invasive monitoring techniques to facilitate early and appropriate intervention when catecholamine-induced changes in cardiovascular function occur.[77,78] Continuation of alpha antagonist therapy until the day of surgery is recommended. The argument that this treatment be discontinued preoperatively so as to unmask hypertensive responses during surgical palpation designed to locate the site of the tumor(s) is no longer tenable, in view of the localizing accuracy of computed tomography. Furthermore, even with aggressive pharmacologically induced alpha blockade, most patients show some degree of blood pressure increase during surgical manipulation of the tumor. Concern that sustained alpha blockade could contribute to refractory hypotension when vascular isolation of the tumor is accomplished has not been substantiated by clinical experience. Beta antagonist therapy should also be continued until the day of surgery. The times of significant intraoperative hazard to the patient are (1) during intubation of the trachea, (2) during manipulation of the tumor, and (3) after ligation of the tumor's venous drainage.

Preoperative Medication

Preoperative medication is useful in decreasing the likelihood of anxiety-induced activation of the sympathetic nervous system. Administration of a benzodiazepine, often with scopolamine, is a useful approach. Scopolamine is unlikely to produce an adverse heart rate change and greatly contributes to the sedative effect of preoperative medication. Morphine or any other drug that could release histamine and thus stimulate catecholamine release may be avoided in these patients. If bilateral adrenalectomy is anticipated, supplemental cortisol treatment may be instituted at the time of preoperative medication.

Induction of Anesthesia

The placement of a catheter in a peripheral artery to provide continuous monitoring of blood pressure is useful before proceeding with induction of anesthesia. In the presence of adequate preoperative medication and local anesthesia, this invasive monitor can be placed without the risk of activating the sympathetic nervous system. Induction of anesthesia is most often accomplished with the intravenous administration of a barbiturate, benzodiazepine, etomidate, or propofol. After the onset of unconsciousness, the depth of anesthesia should be increased by ventilation of the lungs with nitrous oxide plus a volatile anesthetic.[86,87] Selection of a volatile anesthetic is based on the ability of these drugs to decrease sympathetic nervous system activity and on their low likelihood of sensitizing the heart to the cardiac dysrhythmic effects of catecholamines. Although the greatest clinical experience is with isoflurane, the ability to rapidly change anesthetic concentrations with desflurane or sevoflurane is an attractive feature of these drugs for the management of anesthesia in the patient with a pheochromocytoma. Halothane is no longer recommended because of its propensity to produce cardiac dysrhythmias in the presence of an increased plasma catecholamine concentration.

Mechanical ventilation of the lungs is facilitated by the production of skeletal muscle paralysis with a nondepolarizing muscle relaxant deemed devoid of vagolytic or histamine releasing effects. Pancuronium is an unlikely selection in view of its known cardiac effects, which could result in an exaggerated blood pressure increase in the patient with a pheochromocytoma.[88] The use of succinylcholine has been questioned, since histamine release or compression of an abdominal tumor by drug-induced skeletal muscle contractions (fasciculations) could provoke the release of catecholamines. Nevertheless, clinical experience has not supported a predictable adverse effect of this drug when administered to a patient with a pheochromocytoma.

Direct laryngoscopy for intubation of the trachea is initiated only after the establishment of a surgical depth of anesthesia with a volatile anesthetic (about 1.3 MAC). An adequate depth of anesthesia is necessary to minimize increases in blood pressure associated with intubation of the trachea. It may be helpful to administer lidocaine (1 to 2 mg·kg^{-1} IV) about 1 minute before initiating direct laryngoscopy, as this drug may attenuate the hypertensive response to intubation of the trachea and decrease the likelihood of cardiac dysrhythmias.[89] In addition, the administration of a short-acting opioid (fentanyl, 100 to 200 µg IV; sufentanil, 10 to 20 µg IV) just before starting direct laryngoscopy may attenuate the pressor response. Nitroprusside or phentolamine should be readily available for administration, should persistent hypertension accompany intubation of the trachea. Nitroprusside (1 to 2 µg·kg^{-1} IV) as a rapid injection is effective for treating an acute and persistent increase in blood pressure. An alternative to nitroprusside is phentolamine (1 to 5 mg IV) as an intermittent injection.

Maintenance of Anesthesia

Maintenance of anesthesia is often accomplished with nitrous oxide plus isoflurane.[78] The concentration of isoflurane delivered should be adjusted in response to any change in blood pressure. Maintenance of anesthesia with nitrous oxide and an opioid is an unlikely approach, as these drugs do not suppress hypertensive responses, owing to catecholamine release. In addition, the ability to decrease the depth of anesthesia, in the face of persistent hypotension, is not easily achieved when injected drugs are used for maintenance of anesthesia. Droperidol is not recommended, in view of reports of hypertension following its administration to patients with pheochromocytoma.[90,91] It is speculated that droperidol may antagonize presynaptic dopaminergic receptors that normally inhibit the release of catecholamines, encouraging their release.

A continuous intravenous infusion of nitroprusside will be necessary if hypertension persists despite delivery of a maximum concentration of isoflurane (about 1.5 to 2.0 MAC). Reflex tachycardia accompanying nitroprusside-induced peripheral vasodilation is treated with a continuous intravenous infusion of esmolol.[92,93] A beta antagonist must be used cautiously in the presence of catecholamine-induced cardiomyopathy, as even minimal beta blockade can accentuate left ventricular dysfunction. Cardiac dysrhythmias are initially treated with lidocaine. A decrease in blood pressure may accompany the prompt decrease in circulating catecholamine concentration that occurs during surgical ligation of the veins draining the pheochromocytoma. This decrease in blood pressure is treated by decreasing the concentration of isoflurane delivered, as well as rapid infusion of either crystalloid or colloid solutions, or both. Rarely, a continuous intravenous infusion of phenylephrine or norepinephrine may be required until the peripheral vasculature can adapt to a decreased level of endogenous alpha stimulation. Although experience is limited, there is no evidence to suggest avoidance of reversal of nondepolarizing neuromuscular blockade with an anticholinesterase drug plus an anticholinergic drug, after excision of a pheochromotycoma.

Monitoring

A pulmonary artery catheter is useful in monitoring the status of intravascular fluid volume in the patient with a pheochromocytoma, especially in the presence of a catecholamine-induced cardiomyopathy.[87] In addition, the ability to measure cardiac output by thermodilution is helpful in evaluating cardiac function and the need for intervention with an inotropic or vasodilator drug. A central venous pressure catheter is an alternative to a pulmonary artery catheter, recognizing that left ventricular dysfunction might not be appreciated from this measurement, and thermodilution measurement of cardiac output will not be possible. Monitoring of arterial blood gases and pH, blood glucose concentration, and electrolytes is recommended. Hyperglycemia is common before excision of the pheochromocytoma, whereas hypoglycemia may occur within minutes of the tumor removal as alpha-induced suppression of insulin release wanes.[94]

Postoperative Management

Invasive monitoring is continued during the postoperative period, since increases or decreases in blood pressure are possible. An estimated 50% of patients will remain hypertensive during the postoperative period despite removal of the pheochromocytoma. A high index of suspicion for hypoglycemia is maintained. Relief of postoperative pain, for example, with neuraxial opioids, may contribute to early tracheal extubation in these often young and otherwise healthy patients.

Regional Anesthesia

Regional anesthesia for the excision of a pheochromocytoma has been successfully used.[78] Despite the ability of this anesthetic technique to block the sympathetic nervous system, the postsynaptic alpha receptors can still respond to direct effects of sudden increases in the circulating concentration of catecholamines. A specific disadvantage of a regional anesthetic is the absence of sympathetic nervous system activity if hypotension accompanies vascular isolation of the pheochromocy-

toma. In addition, the ability of an awake or sedated patient to maintain adequate spontaneous alveolar ventilation may be impaired during intra-abdominal manipulation and retraction. The selection of regional anesthesia is practical only if the surgical procedure is performed in the supine position.

DYSFUNCTION OF THE TESTES OR OVARIES

The principal hormone secreted by the testes is testosterone, whereas the principal hormone secreted by the ovaries is progesterone. In the adult, testosterone is responsible for spermatogenesis, and a metabolite, dihydrotestosterone, is responsible for external virilization. Ovulation and normal menses depend on the presence of ovarian hormones.

Klinefelter Syndrome

Klinefelter syndrome is the most common expression of testicular dysfunction, manifested as aspermatogenesis, decreased plasma testosterone concentration, and testicular atrophy. The buccal smear for the Barr body (chromatin lumps) indicates an XXY chromosomal defect diagnostic of the syndrome. Systemic effects of male hypogonadism include anemia, osteoporosis, fatigue, and skeletal muscle weakness.

Physiologic Menopause

The increase in human longevity means that many females live one-third or more of their lives without natural estrogen and progesterone. Menopause is an almost complete cessation of estrogen production, accompanied by amenorrhea, which occurs at an average age of 51 years. The absence of estrogen has short-range (hot flashes), medium-range (vaginal atrophy), and long-range (osteoporosis) manifestations that can be relieved by exogenous estrogen replacement. The most significant medical consequence of menopause is osteoporosis and the risk of skeletal fractures, often involving the spine and hips.[95] Normally, estrogen maintains the balance between bone formation and resorption; in the absence of estrogen, this balance is shifted toward bone resorption.

Premenstrual Syndrome

The abdominal discomfort (cramps) accompanying the ovulatory cycle probably reflects the effect of prostaglandins, accounting for the effectiveness of nonsteroidal anti-inflammatory drugs in relieving pain. Premenstrual syndrome is a constellation of symptoms that appear the week before menstruation. There is no uniquely diagnostic physical finding or laboratory test, and treatment is symptomatic (analgesics, diuretics, vitamins).

Oral Contraception

Oral contraceptives consist of synthetic estrogens and progestins in varying combinations that prevent pregnancy by drug-induced suppression of pituitary gonadotropin secretion. Platelet aggregation is increased by these drugs. In this regard, a decrease in the estrogen content of the pill to the minimal amount that prevents breakthrough bleeding will decrease, but not eliminate, the risk of venous thrombosis, whereas the risk of arterial thrombosis remains unaltered. The risk of arterial thrombosis may be increased after surgery, and a possible association with oral contraceptives has been speculated.[96]

Ovarian Hyperstimulation Syndrome

Exogenous gonadotropin stimulation in association with ovulation induction for in vitro fertilization may be followed within 3 to 10 days by severe ovarian hyperstimulation, manifested as ascites, pleural effusion, oliguria, hemoconcentration, electrolyte abnormalities, hypercoagulability, and hypotension. It is speculated that the production of prostaglandins by the ovarian follicle, as well as an alteration in the renin-angiotensin system, increase capillary permeability. This change allows for edema formation (ascites) and fluid translocation (hypovolemia, oliguria). Hemoconcentration predisposes to increased blood viscosity and thromboembolic phenomena. Capillary leak has been associated with the development of adult respiratory distress syndrome; liver dysfunction has also been noted.

The estimate that 0.4% to 4% of treatment cycles will be associated with the development of severe ovarian hyperstimulation syndrome introduces the possibility that these patients will require anesthesia for termination of pregnancy or laparotomy. The management of anesthesia in the patient with severe ovarian hyperstimulation syndrome is influenced by the presence of hypovolemia and by the impact of ascites on spontaneous ventilation.[97] The presence of ascites and the frequent presence of nausea and vomiting suggest the need to protect the airway with a cuffed tracheal tube. Ketamine may be a useful drug for the induction and maintenance of anesthesia. Monitoring potentially rapid fluid fluxes may be facilitated by measuring cardiac filling pressures, especially if the planned surgery is extensive.

Turner Syndrome

Turner syndrome (gonadal dysgenesis) is due to the absence of a second X chromosome. Manifestations of the syndrome include primary amenorrhea, genital immaturity, and short stature. Additional associated features that may influence the management of anesthesia include hypertension, short neck, high palate, micrognathia, the occasional presence of aortic stenosis or coarctation of the aorta and pectus excavatum, and an absent kidney. Intelligence is usually normal.

Noonan Syndrome

Noonan syndrome (female pseudo-Turner syndrome) resembles Turner syndrome with respect to short stature and facial characteristics. In contrast to Turner syndrome, Noonan syndrome is associated with mental retardation, right-sided cardiac lesions (pulmonic stenosis), and normal chromosomes. The patient with Noonan syndrome is fertile, and anesthesia may be needed for delivery.

Potential anesthesia problems include difficult airway management and technical problems in performing regional anesthesia related to short stature and associated skeletal anomalies (lumbar lordosis, kyphoscoliosis, narrow spinal canal).[98] The decrease in functional residual capacity produced by pregnancy is further exaggerated by the pectus deformity and kyphoscoliosis that are commonly present. Arterial hypoxemia may occur rapidly, in view of the decreased functional residual capacity. Cardiac evaluation is indicated and, if echocardiography demonstrates pulmonic stenosis, it is important to consider the possible detrimental effects of excess intravenous fluid administration, such as before performance of regional anesthesia. Conversely, if the patient is not adequately hydrated before spinal or epidural anesthesia, the hypotension that may occur from sympathetic nervous system blockade can produce an undesirable decrease in right ventricular stroke volume.

Stein-Leventhal Syndrome

Stein-Leventhal syndrome (polycystic ovary syndrome) accounts for up to 10% of cases of primary amenorrhea. Ultrasonography is useful in the recognition of ovarian enlargement. There is increased production of androgens, with hirsutism and increased muscularity. Height is usually normal, and congenital defects are unlikely. In the past, wedge resection of the ovary was used to improve the fertility of these patients. This disorder is currently treated with the antiestrogen drug, clomiphene, which acts by stimulating ovulation. Treatment of hirsutism includes suppression of androgen excess with prednisone. Long intervals of anovulation can be associated with the development of endometrial carcinoma, perhaps reflecting continuous exposure of the endometrium to estrogen unopposed by progesterone.

PITUITARY GLAND DYSFUNCTION

The pituitary gland is located in the sella turcica at the base of the brain; it consists of the anterior pituitary and posterior pituitary. The anterior pituitary secretes six hormones under

Table 22-21. Hypothalamic and Related Pituitary Hormones

Hypothalamic Hormones	Anterior Pituitary Hormones
Growth hormone-releasing hormone	Growth hormone
Growth hormone release inhibiting hormone	Growth hormone
Prolactin release inhibitory factor (dopamine)	Prolactin
Gonadotropin releasing hormone	Follicle stimulating hormone Luteinizing hormone
Corticotropin releasing hormone	Adrenocorticotropic hormone
Thyrotropin releasing hormone	Thyroid stimulating hormone

Hypothalamus Synthesis Site	Posterior Pituitary Hormones
Osmoreceptors	Antidiuretic hormone Oxytocin

the control of the hypothalamus (Table 22-21). In this regard, the hypothalamus controls the function of the anterior pituitary by means of vascular connections (hormones travel by the hypophyseal portal veins, to reach the anterior pituitary). The posterior pituitary is composed of terminal endings of neurons that originate in the hypothalamus. Antidiuretic hormone (ADH) and oxytocin are synthesized in the hypothalamus and are subsequently transported along the hypothalamic neuronal axons for storage in the posterior pituitary. Stimulus for the release of these hormones from the posterior pituitary arises from osmoreceptors in the hypothalamus that sense plasma osmolarity.

Overproduction of anterior pituitary hormones is most often reflected by hypersecretion of ACTH by a pituitary adenoma manifested as Cushing syndrome. Hypersecretion of other trophic hormones rarely occurs. Underproduction of a single anterior pituitary hormone (monotropic deficiency) is less common than generalized pituitary hypofunction (panhypopituitarism). The pituitary gland is the only endocrine gland in which a tumor, most often a chromophobe adenoma, causes destruction by compression of the gland against the bony confines of the sella turcica. Metastatic tumor, most often from the breast or lung, also occasionally produces hypofunction. Endocrine features of panhypopituitarism are highly variable and depend on the rate at which the deficiency develops and on the age of the patient. For example, gonadotropin deficiency (amenorrhea, impotence) is typically the first manifestation of global pituitary dysfunction. Hypoadrenocorticism occurs 4 to 14 days after hypophysectomy, whereas hypothyroidism is

unlikely to be manifested before 4 weeks. Computed tomography and magnetic resonance imaging are useful in the radiologic assessment of the pituitary.

Acromegaly

Acromegaly is due to excess secretion of growth hormone in an adult, most often from an adenoma in the anterior pituitary gland. Failure of the plasma growth hormone concentration to decrease 1 to 2 hours after the ingestion of 75 to 100 g of glucose is presumptive evidence of acromegaly, as is a growth hormone concentration greater than 3 ng·ml^{-1}. A skull radiograph and computed tomography are useful in detecting enlargement of the sella turcica, which is characteristic of an anterior pituitary adenoma.

Signs and Symptoms

Manifestations of acromegaly reflect parasellar extension of the anterior pituitary adenoma and peripheral effects produced by the presence of excess growth hormone (Table 22-22). Headache and papilledema reflect increased intracranial pressure due to expansion of the anterior pituitary adenoma. Visual disturbances are due to compression of the optic chiasm by the expanding overgrowth of surrounding tissues. Overgrowth of soft tissues of the upper airway (enlargement of the tongue and epiglottis) and increased length of the mandible may make upper airway management difficult.[99-101] Polypoid masses reflect overgrowth of pharyngeal tissue, making the upper airway susceptible to obstruction. Hoarseness and abnormal movement of the vocal cords or paralysis of a recurrent laryngeal nerve may be due to stretching by overgrowth of the cartilaginous structures. In addition, involvement of the cricoarytenoid joints can result in alterations in the voice, owing to

Table 22-22. Manifestations of Acromegaly

Parasellar
  Enlarged sella turcica
  Headache
  Visual field defects
  Rhinorrhea

Excess Growth Hormone
  Skeletal overgrowth (prognathism)
  Soft tissue overgrowth (lips, tongue, epiglottis, vocal cords)
  Connective tissue overgrowth (recurrent laryngeal nerve paralysis)
  Peripheral neuropathy (carpal tunnel syndrome)
  Visceromegaly
  Glucose intolerance
  Osteoarthritis
  Osteoporosis
  Hyperhydrosis
  Skeletal muscle weaknes

impaired movement of the vocal cords. The subglottic diameter may be decreased in the acromegalic patient. Stridor or a history of dyspnea is suggestive of acromegalic involvement of the upper airway.

Peripheral neuropathy is common and most likely reflects trapping of nerves by skeletal, connective, and soft tissue overgrowth. Flow through the ulnar artery may be compromised in the patient exhibiting symptoms of carpal tunnel syndrome. Even in the absence of symptoms of carpal tunnel syndrome, about one-half of patients with acromegaly have inadequate collateral blood flow through the ulnar artery in at least one hand. Glucose intolerance and, on occasion, diabetes mellitus, requiring treatment with insulin, reflects the effects of growth hormone on carbohydrate metabolism. The incidence of hypertension, ischemic heart disease, osteoarthritis, and osteoporosis seems to be increased. Lung volumes are increased, and the ventilation-to-perfusion mismatch may be enhanced. The skin becomes thick and oily, skeletal muscle weakness may be prominent, and complaints of fatigue are common.

Treatment

Transsphenoidal surgical excision of the pituitary adenoma is the preferred initial therapy.[102] When the adenoma has extended beyond the sella turcica, surgery or irradiation is no longer feasible, and medical treatment with suppressive drug therapy (bromocriptine) may be an option.

Management of Anesthesia

Management of anesthesia for the patient with acromegaly is complicated by changes induced by excess secretion of growth hormone (Table 22-22). Particularly important are changes in the upper airway.[99–101,103] Distorted facial anatomy may interfere with the placement of a face mask. Enlargement of the tongue and epiglottis predisposes to upper airway obstruction and interferes with visualization of the vocal cords by direct laryngoscopy. The distance between the lips and vocal cords is increased by overgrowth of the mandible. The glottic opening may be narrowed, owing to enlargement of the vocal cords, which combined with subglottic narrowing may necessitate the use of a smaller internal diameter tracheal tube than would have been predicted on the basis of the age or size of the patient. Nasal turbinate enlargement may preclude the passage of a nasopharyngeal or nasotracheal airway. The preoperative history of dyspnea on exertion or the presence of hoarseness or stridor, or both, suggests involvement of the larynx by acromegaly. In this instance, indirect laryngoscopy may be indicated to quantitate the extent of vocal cord dysfunction. When difficulty in placing a tube in the trachea is anticipated, it may be prudent to consider tracheal intubation with the patient awake, preferably using a fiberoptic laryngoscope. Anticipation of the possible need to insert a small-diameter tracheal tube and minimization of the mechanical trauma to the upper airway and vocal cords are important considerations, as additional edema can result in airway obstruction after removal of the tube from the trachea. In placing a catheter in the radial artery, it is important to consider the possibility of inadequate collateral circulation at the wrist. Monitoring of the plasma glucose concentration is useful if diabetes mellitus accompanies acromegaly. The dose of nondepolarizing muscle relaxant is guided by the use of a peripheral nerve stimulator, particularly if skeletal muscle weakness exists before the induction of anesthesia. Acromegaly does not influence the selection of drugs for maintenance of anesthesia. Skeletal changes that accompany acromegaly may make performance of regional anesthesia either technically difficult or unreliable.

Diabetes Insipidus

Diabetes insipidus reflects the absence of ADH owing to destruction of the posterior pituitary (neurogenic diabetes insipidus) or failure of the renal tubules to respond to ADH (nephrogenic diabetes insipidus). Neurogenic and nephrogenic diabetes insipidus are differentiated on the basis of the response to desmopressin, which produces concentration of the urine in the presence of neurogenic, but not nephrogenic, diabetes insipidus. Classic manifestations of diabetes insipidus are polydipsia and a high output of poorly concentrated urine despite increased plasma osmolarity. Diabetes insipidus that develops during or immediately after pituitary gland surgery is generally due to reversible trauma of the posterior pituitary and is therefore transient. Initial treatment of diabetes insipidus consists of intravenous infusion of electrolyte solutions, if oral intake cannot offset polyuria. Chlorpropamide, an oral hypoglycemic drug, potentiates the effect of ADH on renal tubules and may be useful in the treatment of nephrogenic diabetes insipidus. Treatment of neurogenic diabetes insipidus is with vasopressin administered intramuscularly ever 2 to 4 days or by intranasal administration of DDAVP. Management of anesthesia for patients with diabetes insipidus should include monitoring of urine output and plasma electrolyte concentrations during the perioperative period.

Inappropriate Secretion of Antidiuretic Hormone

Inappropriate secretion of ADH can occur in the presence of diverse pathologic processes, including intracranial tumors, hypothyroidism, porphyria, and carcinoma of the lung, particularly undifferentiated small cell carcinoma. Inappropriate secretion of ADH is also alleged to occur in virtually all patients after surgery. An inappropriately increased urinary sodium concentration and osmolarity in the presence of hyponatremia and decreased plasma osmolarity are virtually diagnostic of inappropriate ADH secretion. Hyponatremia is due to dilution, reflecting expansion of intravascular fluid volume secondary to hormone-induced resorption of water by the renal tubules. Abrupt decreases in the plasma concentration of sodium (especially below 110 mEq·L^{-1}) can lead to cerebral edema and seizures.

Treatment of excess secretion of ADH consists of restricted fluid intake (about 500 ml·d^{-1}), antagonism of the effects of ADH on the renal tubules by the administration of demeclocycline, and infusion of sodium chloride. Often restriction of fluid intake is sufficient treatment for inappropriate ADH hormone secretion not associated with symptoms secondary to hyponatremia. Restriction of fluid intake and administration of demeclocycline, however, are not immediately effective in the management of the patient manifesting acute neurologic symptoms due to hyponatremia. In this patient, the intravenous infusion of hypertonic saline sufficient to increase the plasma concentration of sodium 0.5 mEq·L^{-1}·h^{-1} is recommended. Overly rapid correction of chronic hyponatremia has been associated with a fatal neurologic disorder known as central pontine myelinolysis.[104]

REFERENCES

1. The Carter Center of Emory University: Closing the gap: The problem of diabetes mellitus in the United States. Diabetes Care 1985;8:391–6

2. Herold KC, Rubenstein AH. Immunosuppression for insulin-dependent diabetes. N Engl J Med 1988;318:701–3

3. Stewart WJ, McSweeney SM, Kellett MA, et al. Increased risk of severe protamine reactions in NPH insulin-dependent diabetics undergoing cardiac catheterization. Circulation 1984;70:788–92

4. Holman PR, Dornan TL, Mayon-White V, et al. Prevention of deterioration of renal and sensory-nerve function by more intensive management of insulin-dependent diabetic patients: A two-year randomized prospective study. Lancet 1983;1:204–6

5. Chase HP, Jackson WE, Hoops SL, Cockerham RS, Archer PG, O'Brien D. Glucose control and the renal and retinal complications of insulin-dependent diabetes. JAMA 1989;261:1155–60

6. Mecklenburg RS, Benson EA, Benson JW, et al. Long-term metabolic control with insulin pump therapy—report of experience with 127 patients. N Engl J Med 1985;313:465–9

7. Borland LM, Cook DR. Anesthesia for organ transplantation. In: Stoelting RK, Barash PG, Gallagher TJ, eds. Advances in Anesthesia. Chicago. Year Book Medical Publishers 1986;1–36

8. Gluck SL, Klahr S. Enlarging our view of the diabetic kidney. N Engl J Med 1991;324:1662–3

9. Watkins PJ, Mackay JD. Cardiac denervation in diabetic neuropathy. Ann Intern Med 1980;92:304–7

10. Burgos LG, Ebert TJ, Asiddao C, et al. Increased intraoperative cardiovascular morbidity in diabetics with autonomic neuropathy. Anesthesiology 1989;70:591–7

11. Mordes D, Kreutner K, Metzger W, Colwell JA. Dangers of

12. Oppenheimer SM, Hoffbrand BI, Oswald GA, et al. Diabetes mellitus and early mortality from stroke. Br Med J 1985;291:1014–5

13. Watkins PJ. Diabetic autonomic neuropathy. N Engl J Med 1990;322:1078–9

14. Tsueda K, Huang KC, Dumond SW, Wieman TJ, Thomas MH, Heine MF. Cardiac sympathetic tone in anaesthetized diabetics. Can J Anaesth 1991;38:20–3

15. O'Sullivan JJ, Conroy RM, MacDonald K, McKenna TJ, Maurer BJ. Silent ischaemia in diabetic men with autonomic neuropathy. Br Heart J 1991;66:313–5

16. Ewing DJ, Campbell IW, Clarke BP. Assessment of cardiovascular effects of diabetic autonomic neuropathy and prognostic implications. Ann Intern Med 1980;92:308–11

17. Ciccarelli LL, Ford CM, Tsueda K. Autonomic neuropathy in a diabetic patient with renal failure. Anesthesiology 1986;64:283–7

18. Page MM, Watkins PJ. Cardiorespiratory arrest and diabetic autonomic neuropathy. Lancet 1978;1:14–6

19. Ewing DJ, Campbell IW, Clarke BF. The natural history of diabetic autonomic neuropathy. Q J Med 1980;49:95–108

20. Wright RA, Clemente R, Wathen R. Diabetic gastroparesis: An abnormality of gastric emptying of solids. Am J Med Sci 1985;289:240–2

21. Reissell E, Orko R, Maunuksela E-L, Lindgren L. Predictability of difficult laryngoscopy in patients with long-term diabetes mellitus. Anaesthesia 1990;43:1024–7

22. Hogan K, Rusy D, Springman SR. Difficult laryngoscopy and diabetes mellitus. Anesth Analg 1988;67:1162–5

23. Nathan DM. Hemoglobin A$_{1c}$—infatuation or the real thing? N Engl J Med 1990;323:1062–4

24. Eastwood DW. Anterior spinal artery syndrome after epidural anesthesia in a pregnant diabetic patient with scleredema. Anesth Analg 1991;73:90–1

25. Hirsch IB, Magill JB, Cryer PE, White PF. Perioperative management of surgical patients with diabetes mellitus. Anesthesiology 1991;74:346–59

26. Alberti KGMM. Diabetes and surgery. Anesthesiology 1991;74:209–11

27. Walts LF, Miller J, Davidson MB, Brown J. Perioperative management of diabetes mellitus. Anesthesiology 1981;55:104–9

28. Diltser M, Camu F. Glucose homeostasis and insulin secretion during isoflurane anesthesia in humans. Anesthesiology 1988;68:880–6

29. Lucas LF, Tsueda K. Cardiovascular depression after brachial plexus block in two diabetic patients with renal failure. Anesthesiology 1990;73:1032–5

30. Wulfson HD, Dalton B. Hyperosmolar hyperglycemic nonketotic coma in a patient undergoing emergency cholecystectomy. Anesthesiology 1974;41:286–90

31. VanHeerden JA, Edis AJ, Service FJ. The surgical aspects of insulinomas. Ann Surg 1979;189:677–82

32. Muier JJ, Endres SM, Offord K, et al. Glucose management in patients undergoing operation for insulinoma removal. Anesthesiology 1983;59:371–5

33. Pulver JJ, Cullen BF, Miller DR, Valenta LJ. Use of the artificial

beta cell during anesthesia for surgical removal of an insulinoma. Anesth Analg 1980;59:950–2

34. Cooper DS. Subclinical hypothyroidism. JAMA 1987;258:246–7

35. Sawin CT, Castelli WP, Hershman JM, et al. The aging thyroid: Thyroid deficiency in the Framingham study. Arch Intern Med 1985;145:1386–92

36. Ingbar SH. The thyroid gland. In: Williams Textbook of Endocrinology. 7th Ed. Wilson JD, Foster DW, eds. Philadelphia. WB Saunders 1985;682–815

37. Gotta AW, Sullivan CA, Seaman J, Jean-Gilles B. Prolonged intraoperative bleeding caused by propylthiouracil-induced hypoprothrombinemia. Anesthesiology 1972;37:562–3

38. Ikeda S, Schweiss JF. Excessive blood loss during operation in the patient treated with propylthiouracil. Can Anaesth Soc J 1982;29:477–80

39. Feek CM, Sawers JS, Irvine WJ, et al. Combination of potassium iodide and propranolol in preparation of patients with Graves' disease for thyroid surgery. N Engl J Med 1980;302:883–5

40. Verhoeeven RP, Visser TJ, Doctor R, et al. Plasma thyroxine, 3,3′, 5′-triiodothyronine during beta-adrenergic blockade in hyperthyroidism. J Clin Endocrinol Metab 1977;44:1002–5

41. Hamilton WFD, Forrest AL, Gunn A, et al. Beta-adrenoreceptor blockade and anesthesia for thyroidectomy. Anaesthesia 1984;39:335–42

42. Lee TC, Coffey RJ, Currier BM, Ma X-P, Canary JJ. Propranolol and thyroidectomy in the treatment of thyrotoxicosis. Ann Surg 1982;195:766–71

43. Lennquist S, Jortso E, Anderberg B, Smeds S. Beta blockers compared with antithyroid drugs as preoperative treatment in hyperthyroidism: Drug tolerance, complications, and postoperative thyroid function. Surgery 1985;98:1141–6

44. Peters KR, Nance P, Wingard DW. Malignant hyperthyroidism or malignant hyperthermia? Anesth Analg 1981;60:613–5

45. Thorne AC, Bedford RF. Esmolol for perioperative management of thyrotoxic goiter. Anesthesiology 1989;71:291–4

46. Kaplan JA, Cooperman LH. Alarming reactions to ketamine in patients taking thyroid medication-treatment with propranolol. Anesthesiology 1971;35:229–30

47. Stehling LC. Anesthetic management of the patient with hyperthyroidism. Anesthesiology 1974;41:585–95

48. Berman ML, Kuhnert L, Phythyon JM, Holaday DA. Isoflurane and enflurane-induced hepatic necrosis in triiodythyronine-pretreated rats. Anesthesiology 1983;58:1–5

49. Hubbard AK, Roth TP, Gandolfi AJ, Brown BR, Webster NR, Nunn JF. Halothane hepatitis patients generate an antibody response toward a covalently bound metabolite of halothane. Anesthesiology 1988;68:791–6

50. Seino H, Dohi S, Aiyoshi Y, et al. Postoperative hepatic dysfunction after halothane or enflurane anesthesia in patients with hyperthyroidism. Anesthesiology 1986;64:122–5

51. Babab AA, Eger EI. The effects of hyperthyroidism and hypothyroidism on halothane and oxygen requirements in dogs. Anesthesiology 1966;29:1087–93

52. Halpern SH. Anaesthesia for caesarean section in patients with uncontrolled hyperthyroidism. Can J Anaesth 1989;36:454–9

53. Drucker DJ, Burrow GN. Cardiovascular surgery in the hypothyroid patient. Arch Intern Med 1985;145:1585–7

54. Ellyin F, Fuh C-Y, Singh SP, et al. Hypothyroidism with angina pectoris: a clinical dilemma. Postgrad Med J 1986;79:93–7

55. Hay ID, Duick DS, Vlietstra RE, Maloney JD, Pluth JR. Thyroxine therapy in hypothyroid patients undergoing coronary revascularization: A retrospective analysis. Ann Intern Med 1981;95:456–7

56. Weinberg AD, Brennan MD, Gorman CA, Marsch HM, O'Fallon WM. Outcome of anesthesia and surgery in hypothyroid patients. Arch Intern Med 1983;143:893–7

57. Ladenson PW, Levin AA, Ridgway EC, et al. Complications of surgery in hypothyroid patients. Am J Med 1984;77:261–7

58. Murkin JM. Anesthesia and hypothyroidism: A review of thyroxine physiology, pharmacology, and anesthetic implications. Anesth Analg 1982;61:371–83

59. Kim JM, Hackman L. Anesthesia for untreated hypothyroidism: Report of three cases. Anesth Analg 1977;56:299–302

60. Levelle JP, Jopling MW, Sklar GS. Perioperative hypothyroidism: An unusual postanesthetic diagnosis. Anesthesiology 1985;63:195–7

61. Mogensen T, Hjortso N-C. Acute hypothyroidism in a severely ill surgical patient. Can J Anaesth 1988;35:74–5

62. Al-Mohaya S, Naguib M, Abdelatif M, Farag H. Abnormal responses to muscle relaxants in a patient with primary hyperparathyroidism. Anesthesiology 1986;65:554–6

63. Drop LJ, Cullen DJ. Comparative effects of calcium chloride and calcium gluceptate. Br J Anaesth 1980;52:501–5

64. Burtis WJ, Wu TL, Insogna KL, et al. Humoral hypercalcemia of malignancy. Ann Intern Med 1988;108:454–60

65. Flashburg MH, Dunbar BS, August G, Watson D. Anesthesia for surgery in an infant with DiGeorge syndrome. Anesthesiology 1983;58:479–80

66. Weatherill D. Spence AA. Anaesthesia and disorders of the adrenal cortex. Br J Anaesth 1984;56:741–7

67. Owen H, Spence AA. Etomidate. Br J Anaesth 1984;56:555–7

68. Fitzpatrick PM, Swensen SJ. Report of an unusual case of postoperative adrenal hemorrhage in a young man. Am J Med 1989;86:487–9

69. Libertino JA. Surgery of adrenal disorders. Surg Clin North Am 1988;68:1027–33

70. May ME, Carey RM. Rapid adrenocorticotropic hormone test in practice. Am J Med 1985;79:679–85

71. Knudsen L, Christiansen LA, Lorentzen JE. Hypotension during and after operation in glucocorticoid-treated patients. Br J Anaesth 1981;53:295–301

72. Kehlet H. A rational approach to dosage and preparation of parenteral glucocorticoid substitution therapy during surgical procedures. Acta Anaesthesiol Scand 1975;19:260–4

73. Symreng T, Karlberg BE, Kagedal B, Schildt B. Physiological cortisol substitution of long-term steroid-treated patients undergoing major surgery. Br J Anaesth 1981;53:949–53

74. Udelsman R, Ramp J, Gallucci WT, et al. Adaptation during surgical stress. A reevaluation of the role of glucocorticoids. J Clin Invest 1986;77:1377–81

75. Gangat Y, Triner L, Baer L, Puchner P. Primary aldosteronism with uncommon complications. Anesthesiology 1976;45:542–4

76. Holland OB. Hypoaldosteronism—disease or normal response. N Engl J Med 1991;324:488–9

77. Hull CJ. Phaeochromocytoma. Diagnosis, preoperative preparation and anaesthetic management. Br J Anaesth 1986;58:1453–8

78. Pullerits J, Ein S, Balfe JW. Anaesthesia for phaeochromocytoma. Can J Anaesth 1988;35:526–34

79. Thomas JL, Bernardino ME. Pheochromocytoma in multiple endocrine adenomatosis. JAMA 1981;245:1467–9

80. Kirkendahl WM, Leighty RD, Culp DA. Diagnosis and treatment of patients with pheochromocytoma. Arch Intern Med 1965; 115:529–36

81. Allen GC, Rosenberg H. Phaeochromocytoma presenting as acute malignant hyperthermia—a diagnostic challenge. Can J Anaesth 1990;37:593–5

82. Duncan MW, Compton P, Lazarus L, Smythe GA. Measurement of neorepinephrine and 3,4-dihydroxyphenylglycol in urine and plasma for the diagnosis of pheochromocytoma. N Engl J Med 1988;319:136–42

83. Bravo EL, Gifford RW. Pheochromocytoma: Diagnosis, localization and management. N Engl J Med 1984;311:1298–1303

84. Feldman JM. Diagnosis and management of pheochromocytoma. Hosp Pract 1989;24:175–83

85. Nicholson JP, Vaugh ED, Pickering TG, et al. Pheochromocytoma and prazosin. Ann Intern Med 1983;99:477–9

86. Janeczki GF, Ivankovich AD, Glisson SN, et al. Enflurane anesthesia for surgical removal for pheochromocytoma. Anesth Analg 1977;56:62–7

87. Mihm FG. Pulmonary artery pressure monitoring in patients with pheochromocytoma. Anesth Analg 1983;62:1129–33

88. Jones RB, Hill AB. Severe hypertension associated with pancuronium in a patient with a phaeochromocytoma. Can Anaesth Soc J 1981;28:394–6

89. El-Naggar M, Suerte E, Rosenthal E. Sodium nitroprusside and lidocaine in the anaesthetic management of phaeochromocytoma. Can Anaesth Soc J 1977;24:353–9

90. Sumikawa K, Amakata Y. The pressor effect of droperidol on a patient with pheochromocytoma. Anesthesiology 1977;46:359–61

91. Bitter DA. Innovar-induced hypertensive crises in patients with pheochromocytoma. Anesthesiology 1979;50:366–9

92. Nicholas E, Deutschman CS, Allo M, Rock P. Use of esmolol in the intraoperative management of pheochromocytoma. Anesth Analg 1988;67:1114–7

93. Zakowski M, Kaufman B, Berguson P, Tissot M, Yarmush L, Turndorf H. Esmolol use during resection of pheochromocytoma: Report of three cases. Anesthesiology 1989;70:875–7

94. Levin H, Heefetz M. Phaeochromocytoma and severe protracted postoperative hypoglycaemia. Can J Anaesth 1990;37: 477–8

95. Osteoporosis. NIH Consensus Conference. JAMA 1984;252: 799–801

96. Ratnoff OD, Kaufman R. Arterial thrombosis in oral contraceptive users. Arch Intern Med 1982;142:447

97. Reed AP, Tausk H, Reynolds H. Anesthetic considerations for severe ovarian hyperstimulation syndrome. Anesthesiology 1990;73:1275–7

98. Dadabhoy ZP, Winnie AP. Regional anesthesia for cesarean section in a parturient with Noonan's syndrome. Anesthesiology 1988;68:636–8

99. Kitahata LM. Airway difficulties associated with anaesthesia in acromegaly. Br J Anaesth 1971;43:1187–90

100. Hassan SZ, Matz G, Lawrence AM, Collins PA. Laryngeal stenosis in acromegaly. Anesth Analg 1976;55:57–60

101. Southwick JP, Katz J. Unusual airway difficulty in the acromegalic patient—indications for tracheostomy. Anesthesiology 1979;51:72–3

102. Melmed S. Acromegaly. N Engl J Med 1990;322:966–75

103. Compkin TV. Radial artery cannulation, potential hazard in patients with acromegaly. Anaesthesia 1980;35:1008–9

104. Sterns RH, Riggs JE, Schochet SS. Osmotic demyelination syndrome following correction of hyponatremia. N Engl J Med 1986; 314:1535–42

23

Metabolic and Nutritional Disorders

The presence of metabolic or nutritional disorders can influence the management of anesthesia (Table 23-1). Absence of a specific enzyme is often the reason for the rare occurrence of a metabolic disorder, whereas excess caloric intake is the likely cause of the most common nutritional disorder, obesity.

PORPHYRIAS

The porphyrias are a group of inborn errors of metabolism characterized by the overproduction of porphyrin compounds and their precursors. Porphyrin synthesis is required for the production of heme, a component of hemoglobin, and cytochromes (including P-450) necessary for drug metabolism. The rate of heme synthesis from glycine and acetate is controlled by the enzyme aminolevulinic acid (ALA) synthetase in the mitochondria (Fig. 23-1). Abnormalities in porphyrin metabolism are due to abnormalities in enzymatic activity in this heme synthesis pathway. Porphyrias are classified as hepatic or erythropoietic, reflecting the major sites of heme production in bone marrow and the liver (Table 23-2). Although specific genetic and enzymatic defects are present throughout life, clinical manifestations usually occur after puberty and are characterized by acute attacks separated by long latent periods.

Acute Intermittent Porphyria

Acute intermittent porphyria is the most serious form of the hepatic porphyrias. This disease is an inborn error of porphyrin metabolism, affecting both the central and peripheral nervous systems. Transmission is as an autosomal dominant trait. The metabolic defect is most likely due to increased ALA synthetase activity and to a decrease in uroprophyrino-

gen synthetase activity (Fig. 23-1). As a result of these changes in enzymatic activity, excessive amounts of porphobilinogen are accumulated.

The diagnosis of acute intermittent porphyria is suggested by the demonstration of increased urinary excretion of ALA acid and porphobilinogen during an acute attack. Clinically, it may be observed that the urine turns black on standing, reflecting the increased urinary excretion of porphobilinogen. Urinary excretion of porphobilinogen may not be increased between attacks.

Signs and Symptoms

Severe abdominal pain (mistaken for acute appendicitis, cholecystitis, renal colic) and neurotoxicity occurring in females, especially at the expected time of menstruation, may reflect acute intermittent porphyria. Neurotoxicity may be manifested as dysfunction of the cerebral cortex (psychoses), hypothalamus (syndrome of inappropriate release of antidiuretic hormone, hyponatremia), cranial nerves (bulbar paresis with difficulty in swallowing and aspiration), autonomic nervous system (tachycardia, orthostatic hypotension, hypertension), and peripheral nerves (pain, paresis). Involvement of the intercostal nerves and phrenic nerves may result in hypoventilation. A history of previous negative surgical explorations in a search for the etiology of abdominal pain is possible.

Prevention and Treatment

It is important for the patient with a known risk of porphyria to avoid events and medications capable of provoking an acute attack. For example, starvation, dehydration, and sepsis may trigger an acute attack. A role for female hormones is suggested by the greater severity and frequency of this disease in females, its almost total absence before puberty, and its frequent exacerbation during pregnancy. Classically, barbitu-

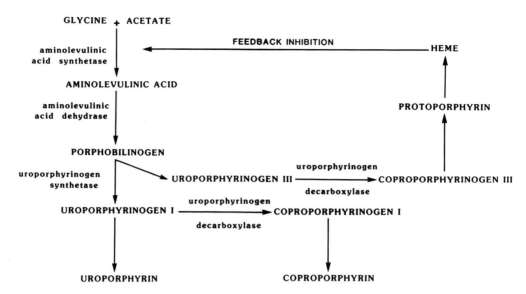

Fig. 23-1. Synthesis of heme begins with the formation of aminolevulinic acid from glycine and acetate. Excess amounts of aminolevulinic acid and porphobilinogen, as seen in acute intermittent porphyria, result from the stimulation of aminolevulinic acid synthetase activity and from decreased uroporphyrinogen synthetase activity. Decreased activity of uroporphyrinogen decarboxylase can lead to an accumulation of uroporphyrin, which is believed to cause porphyria cutanea tarda.

Table 23-1. Metabolic and Nutritional Disorders

Metabolic
  Porphyria
  Gout
  Pseudogout
  Hyperlipidemia
  Carbohydrate metabolism disorders
  Amino acid metabolism disorders
  Mucopolysaccharidoses
  Gangliosidoses

Nutritional
  Morbid obesity
  Obesity hypoventilation syndrome
  Malnutrition
  Anorexia nervosa
  Vitamin imbalance disorders

Table 23-2. Classification of Porphyria

Hepatic Porphyrias
  Acute intermittent porphyria
  Porphyria cutanea tarda
  Variegate porphyria
  Hereditary coproporphyria

Erythropoietic Porphyrias
  Erythropoietic uroporphyria
  Erythropoietic protoporphyria

Table 23-3. Safe and Unsafe Drugs for Administration to a Patient With Acute Intermittent Porphyria

Safe Drugs	Unsafe Drugs
Anticholinergics	Barbiturates
Anticholinesterases	Ethyl alcohol
Depolarizing and nondepolarizing muscle relaxants	Etomidate
	Phenytoin
Droperidol	Pentazocine
Opioids	Corticosteroids
Nitrous oxide	Imipramine
Volatile anesthetics	Tolbutamide
Propofol	Benzodiazepines(?)
Benzodiazepines(?)	Ketamine(?)
Ketamine(?)	

rates have been associated with provoking acute exacerbations of the disease. It is speculated that this class of drugs may increase ALA synthetase activity, leading to increased porphyrin synthesis in a susceptible person. Several other drugs in addition to barbiturates have been incriminated as triggering events for an acute attack (Table 23-3).

Treatment of acute intermittent porphyria includes prompt administration of hematim (3 to 4 mg·kg^{-1} IV over 20 minutes) and glucose (20 g·h^{-1}). Hematin is a powerful repressor of ALA synthetase activity, decreasing urinary excretion of porpholinogen to normal levels in 24 to 48 hours, paralleled by a decrease in pain. Established peripheral neuropathies are not promptly reversed, but their progression is halted by this therapy. Hematin infusion may result in a prolonged partial thromboplastin time, prothrombin time, and fibrinolysis. Opioids may be necessary for the management of pain; a beta antagonist will be useful for the control of excessive sympathetic nervous system activity. Rapidly progressive weakness of the muscles of breathing may necessitate tracheal intubation and mechanical support of ventilation. Nasogastric suction will be necessary if bulbar involvement results in weakened swallowing.

Management of Anesthesia

Management of anesthesia in the patient with a diagnosis of acute intermittent porphyria is designed to avoid administration of drugs that might provoke an acute attack. In this regard, it would seem prudent to provide anesthesia with "safe" drugs (Table 23-3). Barbiturates are avoided, although attacks do not always follow administration of these drugs to patients with known acute intermittent porphyria.[1-3] Ketamine has been used safely in these patients, although concern about its use has been expressed.[4] Propofol has been administered to patients with porphyria, without evidence of exacerbation of the disease.[5,6] The selection of a regional anesthetic may be avoided, for fear that a neurologic deficit produced by porphyria may be incorrectly attributed to the anesthetic. An uneventful spinal anesthetic with bupivacaine for a cesarean section has been reported.[1] Perioperative monitoring should consider the frequent presence of autonomic nervous system dysfunction and the possibility of labile blood pressure. Frequent neurologic evaluation will aid in the management of ventilation in the patient with bulbar involvement.

Porphyria Cutanea Tarda

Porphyria cutanea tarda is due to an enzymatic defect (decreased hepatic activity of uroporphyrinogen decarboxylase) transmitted as an autosomal dominant trait (Fig. 23-1). ALA synthetase activity is not important, and drugs capable of precipitating attacks of other forms of porphyria do not provoke an attack of porphyria cutanea tarda. Likewise, neurotoxicity does not accompany this form of porphyria.

Signs and symptoms of porphyria cutanea tarda most often appear as photosensitivity in males older than 35 years of age. Alcohol abuse is frequently present; abstinence from alcohol can produce a dramatic remission in a symptomatic patient. The patient's skin is often very friable. Porphyrin accumulation in the liver is associated with hepatocellular necrosis.

Anesthesia is not a hazard in the affected patient, assuming that protection from ultraviolet light is provided and excessive pressure on the skin from a face mask and tape is avoided. The choice of drugs for anesthesia should take into consideration the likely presence of co-existing liver disease.

Variegate Porphyria

Variegate porphyria affects both sexes with onset occurring between the age of 10 and 30 years. Transmission occurs as an autosomal dominant trait. Photosensitivity and neurotoxicity are characteristic. The skin is fragile, and bullae frequently develop. As with acute intermittent porphyria, triggering drugs should be avoided. Treatment of variegate porphyria is as described for acute intermittent porphyria.

Hereditary Coproporphyria

Hereditary coproporphyria, like variegate porphyria, is associated with neurotoxicity. Inheritance is as an autosomal dominant trait. Increased fecal excretion of coproporphyrinogen is characteristic. The treatment and management of anesthesia are similar to that described for acute intermittent porphyria.

Erythropoietic Uroporphyria

Erythropoietic uroporphyria is a rare form of porphyria, transmitted as an autosomal recessive trait. In contrast to porphyrin synthesis in the liver, porphyrin synthesis in the erythropoietic system is responsive to changes in hematocrit and tissue oxygenation. Hemolytic anemia, bone marrow hyperplasia, and splenomegaly are often present. Repeated infections are common, and photosensitivity is severe. The urine of an affected patient turns red when exposed to light. Neurotoxicity and abdominal pain do not occur, and the administration of a barbiturate does not adversely alter the course of the disease. Death usually occurs in early childhood.

Erythropoietic Protoporphyria

Erythropoietic protoporphyria is a more common, but less debilitating, form of erythropoietic porphyria. Signs and symptoms include photosensitivity, vesicular eruptions, urticaria, and edema. In an occasional patient, cholelithiasis develops secondary to increased excretion of protoporphyrin. The administration of a barbiturate does not adversely affect the course of the disease, and survival to adulthood is common.

GOUT

Gout is a disorder of purine metabolism that may be classified as either primary or secondary. Primary gout is due to an inherited metabolic defect that leads to an overproduction of uric acid. Secondary gout is hyperuricemia due to an identifiable cause, such as chemotherapeutic drugs used in the treatment of leukemia, leading to the rapid lysis of purine-containing tissues. Gout is characterized by hyperuricemia with recurrent episodes of acute arthritis owing to deposition of urate crystals in joints. Deposition of urate crystals typically initiates an inflammatory response that causes pain and limited motion of the joints. At least one-half of the initial attacks of gout are confined to the first metatarsophalangeal joint. Persistent hyperuricemia also results in deposition of urate crystals in extra-articular locations, manifested most often as nephrolithiasis. Urate crystal deposition can also occur in the myocardium, aortic valve, and extradural spinal regions. The incidence of hypertension, ischemic heart disease, and diabetes mellitus are increased in patients with gout.

The treatment of gout is designed to decrease the plasma concentration of uric acid by administration of a uricosuric drug (probenecid) or inhibition of the conversion of purines to uric acid by xanthine oxidase (allopurinol). Colchicine, which lacks any effect on purine metabolism, is considered the drug of choice for the management of acute gouty arthritis. It relieves joint pain, presumably by modifying leukocyte migration and phagocytosis. The side effects of colchicine include vomiting and diarrhea. Large doses of colchicine can produce hepatorenal dysfunction and agranulocytosis.

Management of Anesthesia

Management of anesthesia in the presence of gout includes prehydration to facilitate the continued renal elimination of uric acid. Sodium bicarbonate to alkalinize the urine also facilitates the excretion of uric acid. As lactate can decrease the renal tubular secretion of uric acid, the use of lactated Ringer's solution may not be wise, although this is unproved. Despite appropriate precautions, acute attacks of gout often follow surgical procedures for no apparent reason in afflicted patients.

Extra-articular manifestations of gout, as well as side effects of drugs used to control the disease, deserve consideration when formulating the plan for management of anesthesia. Renal function should be evaluated, as clinical manifestations of gout usually increase with deteriorating renal function. An abnormality detected on the electrocardiogram could reflect urate deposits in the myocardium. The increased incidence of hypertension, ischemic heart disease, and diabetes mellitus should be borne in mind. Although rare, adverse renal and hepatic effects can be associated with probenecid and colchicine. Limited temporomandibular joint motion from gouty arthritis, if present, can make direct laryngoscopy for intubation of the trachea a difficult procedure.

LESCH-NYHAN SYNDROME

Lesch-Nyhan syndrome is a genetically determined disorder of purine metabolism that occurs exclusively in males. Biochemically, the defect is characterized by decreased or absent activity of hypoxanthine-guanine phosphoribosyl transferase, leading to excess purine production and increased uric acid concentrations throughout the body. Clinically, the patient is often mentally retarded and exhibits a characteristic spasticity and self-mutilation pattern. Self-mutilation usually involves trauma to the perioral tissues, and subsequent scarification may present difficulties with direct laryngoscopy for tracheal intubation. Seizure disorders associated with this syndrome are often treated with a benzodiazepine. Athetoid dysphagia may increase the likelihood of aspiration if vomiting occurs. Malnutrition is often present. Hyperuricemia is associated with nephropathy, urinary tract calculi, and arthritis. Death is often due to renal failure.

Management of anesthesia is influenced by co-existing renal dysfunction and by possible impaired metabolism of drugs administered during anesthesia.[7] The presence of a spastic skeletal muscle disorder suggests caution in the use of succinylcholine. The sympathetic nervous system response to stress is enchanced, suggesting caution in the administration of exogenous catecholamines to these patients.

HYPERLIPOPROTEINEMIA

An abnormal increase in the blood concentration of lipids, cholesterol, and/or triglycerides is termed hyperlipoproteinemia. This term is more correct than hyperlipidemia because it emphasizes the importance of lipoproteins in the pathophysiology of atherosclerosis. The electrophoretic pattern produced by lipoproteins in the plasma is used to classify hyperlipoproteinemia into six categories[8] (Table 23-4). Lipoproteins are classified as chylomicrons, very-low-density lipoproteins, intermediate-density lipoproteins, low-density lipoproteins, and high-density lipoproteins. There is an inverse relationship between high-density lipoproteins and ischemic heart disease. No absolute levels of cholesterol or triglycerides have been found to be diagnostic of hyperlipoproteinemia, but a patient

Table 23-4.   Characteristics of Hyperlipoproteinemias

	Cholesterol	Triglyceride	Xanthomas	Risk of Ischemic Heart Disease
Familial lipoprotein lipase deficiency (hyperchylomicronemia)	Normal	Increased	Eruptive	Very low
Familial dysbetalipoproteinemia	Increased	Increased	Palmar Planar Tendon	Very high
Familial hypercholesterolemia	Increased	Normal to increased	Tendon	Very high
Familial hypertriglyceridemia	Normal	Increased	Eruptive	Low
Familial combined hyperlipidemia	Markedly increased	Markedly increased	Palmar Planar Tendon	High
Polygenic hypercholesterolemia	Increased	Normal	Tendon	Moderate

with a blood cholesterol level above the 90th percentile for gender and age is considered at increased risk of the development of atherosclerosis.[9] The role of an increased concentration of triglycerides in the development of ischemic heart disease is controversial.[10]

Treatment

Treatment of hyperlipoproteineimias includes diet and drug therapy[11,12] (Table 23-5). Drug therapy is ineffective unless an appropriate diet and weight loss are maintained. Aggressive treatment of hypercholesterolemia with diet and drugs can retard or reverse the growth of atherosclerotic lesions in coronary arteries or bypass grafts.[13] As the use of lovastatin may impair liver function, the patient should be followed periodically with liver function tests. Nicotinic acid may be associated with flushing and pruritus and may also cause hepatic dysfunction. Impaired glucose tolerance and increased uric acid levels may accompany treatment with nicotinic acid. Clofibrate is an alternative when patients do not tolerate nicotinic acid. Nau-

sea, myalgias, and gallstone formation may accompany treatment with this drug.

Management of anesthesia in the presence of hyperlipoproteinemia is influenced by the possible presence of ischemic heart disease.[8] Familial lipoprotein lipase deficiency is not associated with an increased risk of ischemic heart disease, but hepatosplenomegaly may develop. The effects of drugs used in the treatment of hyperlipoproteinemia, especially hepatic toxicity, are important to consider. The risk of thrombosis and tissue necrosis in association with an indwelling arterial catheter may be increased in an affected patient.[14]

CARNITINE DEFICIENCY

Carnitine deficiency is a rare condition associated with lipid storage disorders, manifested in a systemic form and myopathic form. Systemic carnitine deficiency is characterized by recurrent attacks of vomiting, diarrhea, and encephalopathy

Table 23-5.   Treatment of Hyperlipoproteinemia

	Caloric Restriction	Decreased Fat	Cholesterol Restriction	Drugs
Hypertriglyceridemia	+ + +	+	+	Nicotinic acid Clofibrate
Hypercholesterolemia Hypertriglyceridemia	+ +	+ +	+	Nicotinic acid Clofibrate
Hypercholesterolemia	+	+ + +	+ + +	Cholestyramine and nicotinic acid Lovastatin Colestipol Gemfibrozil

associated with metabolic acidosis, hypoglycemia, hyperammonemia, coagulation disorders, and increased liver transaminase enzymes. Myopathic carnitine deficiency is characterized clinically by skeletal muscle weakness and cardiomyopathy. Carnitine is the essential cofactor in the enzymatic transport of long-chain fatty acids into the mitochondria, in which they are oxidized.

Management of Anesthesia

Preoperative evaluation of a patient with systemic carnitine deficiency includes assessment of the patient's neurologic status and blood glucose concentration.[15] Cardiac evaluation is intended to determine the presence of cardiomyopathy. It is recommended that these patients receive their usual daily dose of carnitine on the morning of surgery. An intravenous infusion of glucose is initiated preoperatively and maintained throughout the perioperative period, as guided by measurement of the blood glucose concentration. The administration of succinylcholine in the presence of skeletal muscle myopathy may be questionable.

The patient who requires emergency surgery in the presence of a metabolic crisis is prepared with the intravenous infusion of a glucose-containing solution.[15] Electrolyte and acid-base derangements may require correction. Carnitine should be administered intravenously if the patient's neurologic function does not improve with glucose. Hypoprothrombinemia may require treatment with fresh frozen plasma.

DISORDERS OF CARBOHYDRATE METABOLISM

Disorders of carbohydrate metabolism usually reflect a genetically determined enzymatic defect (Table 23-6). The defect can result in either a deficiency or an excess of a precursor or end product of metabolism that is normally involved in the formation of glycogen from glucose. In some instances, an alternate metabolic pathway is used. Ultimately, signs and symptoms of a specific disorder of carbohydrate metabolism reflect the effects produced by an alteration in the amounts of

Table 23-6. Disorders of Carbohydrate Metabolism

von Gierke's disease
Pompe's disease
McArdle's disease
Galactosemia
Fructose 1,6-diphosphate deficiency
Pyruvate dehydrogenase deficiency

precursor or end product of metabolism, which occur as a result of the enzymatic defect.

von Gierke's Disease

von Gierke's disease is due to the enzymatic lack of glucose 6-phosphatase, resulting in an inability of the liver to convert glycogen to glucose. Hypoglycemia can be severe, and oral feedings are required every 2 to 3 hours to maintain an acceptable blood glucose concentration. Seizures, mental retardation, and growth retardation are likely. Hepatomegaly is due to the accumulation of glycogen in the liver. A hemorrhagic diathesis can be due to platelet dysfunction. Survival beyond 2 years of age is unusual, although the surgical creation of a portacaval shunt may be of benefit in an occasional patient.

Management of anesthesia includes provision of exogenous glucose to prevent potentially unrecognized intraoperative hypoglycemia.[16] Monitoring of arterial pH in addition to the blood glucose concentration is indicated, as these patients often become acidotic because of an inability to convert lactic acid to glycogen. In this regard, lactate-containing solutions for intravenous infusion are avoided, to prevent metabolic acidosis from lactate administration during the perioperative period.

Pompe's Disease

Pompe's disease is due to a specific glucosidase enzyme deficiency that results in glycogen deposits in smooth, striated, and cardiac muscle. Myocardial involvement is the most prominent feature, often manifested clinically as congestive heart failure. Echocardiography may demonstrate cardiac hypertrophy and outflow tract obstruction (subaortic stenosis) owing to interventricular septal enlargement. A large, protruding, glycogen-infiltrated tongue and poor skeletal muscle tone predispose the patient to upper airway obstruction. Impaired neurologic function manifests as a decreased cough and gag reflex and incoordination of swallowing. Aspiration and atelectasis are common.

Management of anesthesia must consider potential upper airway obstruction when the patient is rendered unconscious. A volatile anesthetic may produce unexpected and exaggerated cardiac depression, especially if congestive heart failure is present. Either decreased preload or afterload or increased heart rate and myocardial contractility, or both, may precipitate subaortic stenosis. In view of skeletal muscle involvement, it may be wise to avoid administration of succinylcholine to these patients. A diagnostic skeletal muscle biopsy in the lower extremity has been performed using regional anesthesia.[17]

McArdle's Disease

McArdle's disease is caused by a selective deficiency of phosphorylase enzyme in skeletal muscle. Myoglobinuria leading to renal failure can occur, emphasizing the potential value of adequate hydration during the perioperative period. Mannitol may be considered if oliguria occurs despite volume replacement. The propensity for the development of myoglobinuria raises a question about the use of succinylcholine, although this concern has not been substantiated by clinical experience. Since repeated episodes of skeletal muscle ischemia can lead to skeletal muscle atrophy, the intraoperative use of a tourniquet on an extremity is not recommended. Infusion of glucose-containing solutions is intended to prevent adverse effects from unrecognized intraoperative hypoglycemia.

Galactosemia

Galactosemia is due to a deficiency of galactokinase and to an inability to convert galactose to glucose. As a result, galactose accumulates in various tissues, leading to the development of cataracts, cirrhosis of the liver, and mental retardation. Furthermore, elevated plasma galactose levels can suppress the release of glucose from the liver, causing hypoglycemia.

Galactosemia can be mild, with no symptoms until childhood, or can result in hepatic failure and death in infancy. Treatment consists of the avoidance of foods, such as milk, which are high in lactose content. In the absence of hypoglycemia or hepatic dysfunction, there are no specific considerations for the management of anesthesia.

Fructose 1,6-Diphosphatase Deficiency

Fructose 1,6-diphosphatase deficiency means that the liver is unable to achieve efficient conversion of fructose, lactate, glycerol, and amino acids to glucose. When liver glycogen stores are depleted by starvation, hypoglycemia and metabolic acidosis are likely. Hepatomegaly, fatty liver infiltration, and skeletal muscle hypotonia are common.

Administration of sufficient glucose during the perioperative period is essential.[18] The use of lactate-containing intravenous solutions is questionable, as these patients are unable to convert lactate to glucose. As a result, metabolic acidosis could be produced by infusion of lactated Ringer's solution.

Pyruvate Dehydrogenase Deficiency

Pyruvate dehydrogenase deficiency results in an inability to convert pyruvate to acetyl coenzyme A, with the subsequent development of chronic metabolic (lactic) acidosis due to accu-

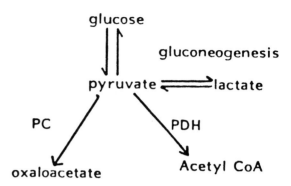

Fig. 23-2. Enzymatic reactions involving pyruvate, lactate, pyruvate dehydrogenase (PDH), and pyruvate carboxylase (PC). (From Dierdorf SF, McNiece WL. Anaesthesia and pyruvate dehydrogenase deficiency. Can Anaesth Soc J 1983;30:413–6, with permission.)

mulation of pyruvate and lactate[19] (Fig. 23-2). Management of anesthesia includes avoidance of events that could contribute to lactic acidosis, such as decreased cardiac output or hypothermia. The use of lactate-containing intravenous solutions is questionable, as their administration could increase the plasma lactate concentration. Lactic acidosis may be accentuated by a carbohydrate load, as delivered by glucose-containing solutions. The selection of drugs for induction and maintenance of anesthesia is influenced by possible drug-induced inhibitory effects on gluconeogenesis, which could enhance co-existing metabolic acidosis. The use of opioids has been recommended for these patients, but excessive depression of ventilation persisting into the postoperative period is possible. Overall, experience is too limited to justify recommendations as to optimal selection of drugs for anesthesia.

DISORDERS OF AMINO ACID METABOLISM

Although there are more than 70 known disorders of amino acid metabolism, most are rare. Classic manifestations include mental retardation, seizures, and amino aciduria (Table 23-7). Metabolic acidosis, hyperammonemia, hepatic failure, and thromboembolism can also occur. Management of anesthesia in patients with these types of disorders is directed toward maintenance of intravascular fluid volume and acid-base homeostasis. Use of anesthetics, such as enflurane, ketamine, and possibly propofol, may be questionable, in view of the likely presence of seizure disorders in these patients.

Table 23-7. Disorders of Amino Acid Metabolism

Disorder	Retardation	Seizures	Metabolic Acidosis	Hyper-ammonemia	Hepatic Failure	Thromboembolism	Other
Phenylketonuria	Yes	Yes	No	No	No	No	
Homocystinuria	Yes/No	Yes	No	No	No	Yes	
Hypervalinemia	Yes	Yes	Yes	No	No	No	Hypoglycemia
Citrullinemia	Yes	Yes	No	Yes	Yes	No	
Branched chain aciduria (maple syrup urine disease)	Yes	Yes	Yes	No	Yes	Yes	
Methylmalonyl-coenzyme A mutase deficiency			Yes	Yes			Avoid nitrous oxide?
Isoleucinemia	Yes	Yes	Yes	Yes	Yes	No	
Methioninemia	Yes	No	No	No	No	No	Thermal instability
Histidinuria	Yes	Yes/No	No	No	No	No	Erythrocyte fragility
Neutral aminoaciduria (Hartnup's disease)	Yes/No		Yes	No	No	No	Dermatitis
Arginemia	Yes		No	Yes	Yes	No	

Phenylketonuria

Phenylketonuria is the prototype of disorders attributable to abnormal amino acid metabolism. Phenylalanine accumulates due to an enzymatic deficiency of phenylalanine hydroxylase. Clinical features include mental retardation and seizures. The skin may be friable and vulnerable to damage from pressure or friction created by adhesive materials.

Homocystinuria

Homocystinuria is due to failure of transsulfuration of precursors of cysteine, an important constituent of crosslinkages in collagen. Manifestations of the disease reflect weakened collagen and include dislocation of the lens, osteoporosis, kyphoscoliosis, brittle light-colored hair, and malar flush.[20] Mental retardation may be prominent. The diagnosis is confirmed by the demonstration of homocystine in the urine, as evidenced by the development of a characteristic magenta color in response to the addition of nitroprusside. Thromboembolism can be life-threatening and is presumed to reflect activation of the Hageman factor by homocystine, resulting in increased platelet adhesiveness. Attempts to minimize the likelihood of thromboembolism during the perioperative period should include the administration of pyridoxine, which decreases platelet adhesiveness; preoperative hydration; infusion of dextran; and early ambulation.[20]

Maple Syrup Urine Disease

Maple syrup urine disease is a rare inborn error of metabolism that results from defective carboxylation of branched-chain amino acids. In the absence of adequate enzymatic activity, consumption of foods containing branched-chain amino acids results in the accumulation of these amino acids and keto acids in the tissues and blood. The increased level of leucine is usually greater than that of isoleucine or valine, since leucine is the predominant amino acid in most proteins. These materials give the urine the odor of maple syrup.

Growth failure and psychomotor retardation are often the consequence of the chronic metabolic imbalance. Infection or fasting commonly results in acute metabolic decompensation, with increased plasma levels of branched-chain amino acids and keto acids due to the breakdown of endogenous protein. The elevated plasma level of keto acids contributes to the production of metabolic acidosis. Hypoglycemia is a possibility, presumably reflecting the ability of an increased plasma leucine concentration to stimulate the release of insulin. A potentially fatal encephalopathy may accompany this disease.

Treatment is directed at decreasing the plasma levels of

branched-chain amino acids and keto acids with peritoneal dialysis or hemodialysis. Parenteral nutrition, using a preparation devoid of branched-chain amino acids, may also be effective.[21]

Management of Anesthesia

Surgery and anesthesia introduce a number of hazards in the patient with maple syrup urine disease.[22] For example, catabolism of body proteins produced by surgery or infection could result in an elevated blood concentration of branched-chain amino acids. Even blood in the gastrointestinal tract, as can occur after a tonsillectomy, produces an added metabolic load in patients with this metabolic defect. Accumulation of branched-chain amino acids in the circulation can produce neurologic deterioration during the perioperative period. The danger of hypoglycemia in an affected patient is exacerbated by the period of starvation that precedes an elective operation. Therefore, it is important to begin an intravenous infusion of glucose preoperatively and to measure the blood glucose concentration intraoperatively. Measurement of arterial pH is necessary to detect metabolic acidosis, due to the accumulation of keto acids. Significant metabolic acidosis during the perioperative period may necessitate treatment with sodium bicarbonate.

Methylmalonyl-Coenzyme A Mutase Deficiency

Methylmalonyl-coenzyme A (MM-CoA) mutase deficiency is an inborn error of branched-chain amino acid metabolism that can result in the formation of methylmalonic acidemia. Acute treatment includes intravenous administration of crystalloid solution with sodium bicarbonate. Events during the perioperative period that increase protein catabolism (starvation, bleeding into the gastrointestinal tract, stress response, tissue destruction) may predispose to acidosis. Nitrous oxide may predispose to methylmalonic acidemia in susceptible patients, reflecting inhibition of a cobalamin coenzyme by this drug. The impact of preoperative starvation on amino acid metabolism and intravascular fluid volume is lessened by permitting fluid intake up to a few hours before the induction of anesthesia. Generous administration of intravenous fluids and glucose is also useful in minimizing hypovolemia and protein catabolism. Experience with anesthesia is limited, and recommendations are based more on theory (avoid nitrous oxide) than on clinical experience.[23]

MUCOPOLYSACCHARIDOSES

Mucopolysaccharidoses represent a group of hereditary disorders involving lysosomal enzymatic defects affecting the degradation of mucopolysaccharides, present ubiquitously in connective tissue. Nearly every organ of the body, especially the brain, heart, liver, and spleen, shows an accumulation of incompletely catabolized mucopolysaccharides. Since deposition of mucopolysaccharides occurs over time, the magnitude of organ involvement increases with age. Seven recognized syndromes are considered to represent mucopolysaccharidoses[24] (Table 23-8). Hurler syndrome is considered the prototypical defect, characterized by the most rapid progression, usually leading to death before 10 years of age. No definitive therapy is available for the affected patient. Indications for surgery are often for the repair of an inguinal or umbilical hernia.

Management of Anesthesia

Preoperative evaluation of the patient with Hurler syndrome (or its equivalent) includes assessment of pulmonary, cardiac, and hepatic function. Pulmonary infection is common and may necessitate treatment before elective surgery. The presence of upper airway obstruction due to accumulation of mucopolysaccharides in the tongue and nasopharyngeal tissues indicates the possibility of technical difficulty in visualizing the glottic opening during direct laryngoscopy for intubation of the trachea.[24,25] Micrognathia, a short neck, and restricted motion at the temporomandibular joint may further increase the difficulty in performing tracheal intubation. Hypoplasia of the odontoid and atlantoaxial subluxation, resulting in instability of the cervical spine, may also occur.[26,27] For all these reasons, intubation of the trachea by means of a fiberoptic laryngoscope may be considered.[25]

General anesthesia is often preferred over regional anesthesia, considering the likely presence of mental retardation and young age of these patients. Co-existing cardiac valve disease, such as aortic regurgitation, or the presence of cardiomyopathy or ischemic heart disease reflecting infiltration of cardiac structures by mucopolysaccharides may influence the choice and dose of anesthetic drugs and muscle relaxants. Depressant effects of opioids are a consideration if obstructive or restrictive ventilatory defects reflect copious airway secretions or skeletal deformities involving the vertebrae and thorax. Pulmonary hypertension may complicate chronic obstructive pulmonary disease in an affected patient.

GANGLIOSIDOSES

Gangliosidoses are diseases characterized by an abnormality of sphingolecithin metabolism, which results in damage to nerve membranes (Table 23-9).

Gaucher's Disease

Gaucher's disease is an autosomal recessive disorder caused by an inherited deficiency of the enzyme (glucocerebrosidase) necessary for the degradation of lipids containing

Table 23-8. Mucopolysaccharidoses

Type	Eponym	Incidence	Clinical Features
I (H)	Hurler	1/100,000	Progressive involvement of heart, skeleton, and airways Progressive mental retardation Possible cervical spine involvement
I (S) (formerly V)	Scheie	1/500,000	Cardiac valve involvement likely Slowly progressive skeletal and airway involvement Intellect usually normal
I (HG)	Hurler/Scheie	1/115,000	Mental retardation Micrognathia common
II	Hunter	1/110,000	Mild to severe forms Slowly progressive
III (A to D)	Sanfilippo	1/24,000(?)	Progressive mental retardation Several enzyme deficiencies
IV (A, B)	Morquio	Rare	Intellect usually normal Odontoid hypoplasia common Pectus carinatum common Aortic valve disease common
VI	Maroteaux-Lamy	Rare	Intellect usually normal Possible odontoid hypoplasia

sugars (glycolipids). In the absence of this enzyme, the extremely insoluble glucocerebroside accumulates in tissues, producing hepatosplenomegaly and bone lesions. The disease varies greatly in severity; mild forms of the disease are encountered frequently, particularly among Ashkenazic Jews. Intravenous infusion of glucocerebroside is an effective but expensive treatment.

MORBID OBESITY

Obesity is the most common nutritional disorder in the United States. It affects about 25% of the population, defined as a body weight 20% above the ideal weight.[28] A measure of obesity is the body mass index, in which a value of 28 for a male and 27 for a female corresponds to 20% above the ideal weight (Table 23-10). The prevalence of obesity increases with age, with an incidence of about 60% in black females older than 45 years of age. It is likely that obese patients who report a failure to lose weight despite dieting in fact greatly underestimate their caloric intake and overestimate their physical activity.[28] There is evidence that genetic factors are present in the pathogenesis of obesity (adopted children more closely resemble biologic parents than their adoptive parents, in terms of obesity), although there is also an interaction between the environment and a predisposition to obesity.[29] Hypothyroidism is rarely a cause of obesity. Males tend to accumulate abdominal fat, which is broken down by the more active form of lipoprotein lipase. In this regard, a male tends to lose weight more readily than a female, who accumulates hip fat. It is likely that caloric restriction initiates a defense system that decreases energy expenditure, which leads to slower weight loss during periods of caloric restriction and more rapid weight gain during periods of increased caloric intake.

Table 23-9. Gangliosidoses

Tay-Sachs disease
Niemann-Pick disease
Gaucher's disease

Table 23-10. Calculation of Body Mass Index

$$\text{Body mass index (BMI)} = \frac{\text{weight (kg)}}{\text{height}^2 \text{ (m)}}$$

Example: A 150-kg, 1.8-m-tall patient has a BMI of 47 (more than 100% above ideal body weight). A similar patient weighing 80 kg has a BMI equal to 25.

Treatment

Decreased dietary intake of saturated fat and increased intake of vegetables, to provide about 1200 cal·d^{-1}, combined with an exercise program (brisk walking for 30 min·d^{-1}) results in weight loss of about 0.07 kg·d^{-1}. One year after adhering to such a program, the average patient regains one-third of the weight lost.[30] A weight loss of only 5 to 10 kg may decrease blood pressure and plasma lipid concentrations and enhance the control of diabetes mellitus.[31]

Very-low-calorie liquid protein diets (400 to 800 cal·d^{-1}) are designed to provide an average weight loss of 20 to 25 kg during a 12-week period. Careful medical supervision of the patient on this type of diet is indicated (Table 23-11). A patient with a body mass index greater than 42 (100% above ideal weight) may be considered for gastroplasty. The objective of this operation is to create a small gastric pouch (about 50 ml) that will limit food intake. Earlier surgical procedures, such as jejunoileal small bowel bypass surgery, have been abandoned because of unacceptable postoperative complications that included fatty liver infiltration, diarrhea, electrolyte disturbances, vitamin B_{12} deficiency, nephrolithiasis, and cholelithiasis.[32] Postsurgical complications of gastroplasty include rupture of the suture line, gastric ulcer, esophagitis, and nausea. Drug-induced appetite suppression is associated with drowsiness and with a relapse rate after discontinuation of medication exceeding that associated with nonpharmacologic approaches.

Adverse Effects

Obesity is associated with increased morbidity and mortality and is a well-established cause of hypertension, lipid abnormalities, and diabetes mellitus (Table 23-12). These changes may be categorized as cardiovascular, ventilation, hepatic, and metabolic.

Cardiovascular

Cardiac output and blood volume are increased in the obese patient. This is not surprising, as each kilogram of fat contains 3000 meters of blood vessels.[33] Cardiac output is estimated to increase 0.1 L·min^{-1} for each kilogram of weight gain re-

Table 23-11. Medical Supervision of Very-Low-Calorie Diets

Heart rate and blood pressure
Serum electrolyte and uric acid concentrations
Complete and differential blood count
Electrocardiogram
Increased incidence of gallstones

Table 23-12. Adverse Effects of Obesity

Systemic hypertension
Hypercholesterolemia
Hypertriglyceridemia
Diabetes mellitus
Ischemic heart diease
Cardiomegaly
Pulmonary hypertension
Congestive heart failure
Restrictive ventilation defect
Arterial hypoxemia
Sleep apnea
Fatty liver infiltration
Osteoarthritis

lated to adipose tissue. This increased cardiac output is due to increased stroke volume, as the resting heart rate in an obese person remains normal or even low. Cardiomegaly and hypertension most likely reflect increased cardiac output. Normotension in an obese patient implies decreased systemic vascular resistance. Pulmonary hypertension is common and most likely reflects chronic arterial hypoxemia or increased pulmonary blood volume, or both. The risk of ischemic heart disease is doubled in the obese patient. The increased demands placed on the cardiovascular system by obesity decrease the reserve of the cardiovascular system and limit exercise tolerance.

Ventilation

Obesity imposes a restrictive ventilation defect because of the weight added to the thoracic cage, as well as the abdominal weight impeding motion of the diaphragm, especially with the assumption of the supine position. Fatty infiltration of the muscles of breathing further diminishes ventilation and limits exercise tolerance. There is a predictable decrease in PaO_2 associated with obesity, presumably reflecting ventilation-to-perfusion mismatching, which is accentuated by decreased lung volumes and capacities (expiratory reserve volume, vital capacity, function residual capacity) due to the compressive effects on the chest and abdomen produced by obesity.[34] In contrast to decreased PaO_2, $PaCO_2$, as well as the ventilatory response to carbon dixoide, remains within a normal range in the obese patient, reflecting the high diffusing capacity and favorable characteristics of the dissociation curve for carbon dioxide. The margin of reserve is small; administration of a ventilatory depressant drug, especially with the assumption of the supine position, may lead to carbon dioxide accumulation in an obese patient. Obese patients typically breathe rapidly and shallowly, as this pattern results in the least oxygen cost of breathing.

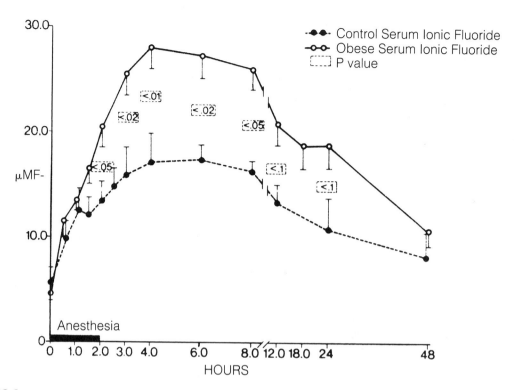

Fig. 23-3. Plasma fluoride concentrations (μMF $-$) (mean $\pm$ SE) were measured in obese and nonobese adults during and after anesthesia that included enflurane. Plasma fluoride concentrations were significantly higher both during and after anesthesia in obese compared with nonobese patients. (From Bentley JB, Vaughn RW, Miller MS, et al. Serum inorganic fluoride levels in obese patients during and after enflurane anesthesia. Anesth Analg 1979;58:409–12, with permission.)

Hepatic

Abnormal liver function tests and fatty liver infiltration are frequent findings in the obese patient. There is evidence that volatile anesthetics are defluorinated to a greater extent in the obese compared with nonobese patients[35–37] (Fig. 23-3). Reductive metabolism of halothane must occur for fluoride to appear as a metabolite. This introduces the concern that fatty liver infiltration, associated with morbid obesity, can result in hepatocyte hypoxia and favor reductive pathways for halothane metabolism, leading to the production of hepatotoxic reactive intermediary metabolites. Nevertheless, there is no evidence of enhanced hepatocyte damage based on liver function tests performed in obese patients receiving halothane.[37] The risk of the development of gallbladder and biliary tract disease is increased threefold in the obese patient, perhaps reflecting abnormal cholesterol metabolism.

Metabolic

Glucose tolerance curves are often abnormal, and the incidence of diabetes mellitus is increased severalfold in the obese patient. This finding is consistent with the resistance of peripheral tissues to the effects of insulin in the presence of increased adipose tissue. Oxygen consumption and carbon dioxide production are increased, placing an increased workload on the heart and lungs of an obese patient. Other metabolic consequences of obesity include hypercholesterolemia and hypertriglyceridemia.

Management of Anesthesia

Management of anesthesia is influenced by obesity-induced alterations in physiologic function (Table 23-12). Possible interactions with appetite suppressants are a consideration. The volume of distribution of drugs may be altered, since fat contains less water than is found in other tissues, leading to a decrease in total body water content in the obese patient.

Induction of Anesthesia

The obese patient is likely to be at increased risk of pulmonary aspiration, considering the increased incidence of gastroesophageal reflux and hiatal hernia in this patient population.

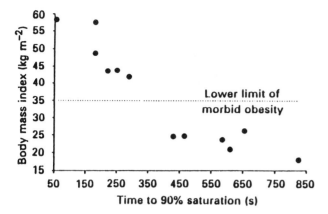

Fig. 23-4. Arterial oxygen saturation decreases to 90% most rapidly in morbidly obese patients, as quantitated by the body mass index. (From Berthoud MC, Peacock JE, Reilly CS. Effectiveness of preoxygenation in morbidly obese patients. Br J Anaesth 1991;67:464–6, with permission.)

Furthermore, gastric acidity, gastric fluid volume, and intragastric pressure are likely to be increased.[38] Mandibular and cervical mobility can be decreased in the obese patient because of the increased amount of soft tissue. This limitation of motion can present problems in airway maintenance and intubation of the trachea. For these reasons, the preoperative administration of an H-2 receptor antagonist or metoclopramide, or both, may be considered in an effort to increase gastric fluid pH and decrease gastric fluid volume. In addition, rapid induction of anesthesia during cricoid pressure, followed by prompt intubation of the trachea with a cuffed tube, is often selected to minimize the risk of pulmonary aspiration. In predetermined patients, awake intubation of the trachea, most often using a fiberoptic laryngoscope, may be selected. A low functional residual capacity predisposes the obese patient to a rapid decrease in PaO_2 during any period of apnea, such as may accompany direct laryngoscopy for intubation of the trachea[39] (Fig. 23-4). This risk of rapid desaturation emphasizes the importance of maximizing the oxygen content in the lungs, before initiating direct laryngoscopy and monitoring arterial oxygen saturation continuously with a pulse oximeter. Decreased functional residual capacity also leads to decreased mixing time for any inhaled drug, accelerating the rate of increase in the alveolar concentration of that drug.

Maintenance of Anesthesia

The best choice of drugs or techniques for maintenance of anesthesia in an obese patient is unclear. An increased incidence of fatty liver infiltration suggests caution in the selection of drugs associated with postoperative liver dysfunction. In-

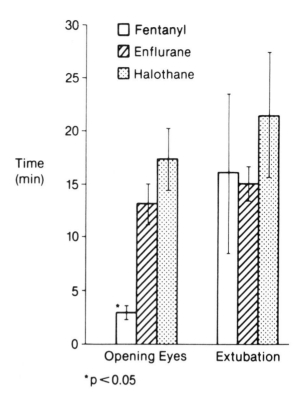

*$p < 0.05$

Fig. 23-5. Awakening time (mean $\pm$ SE) was measured in obese patients anesthetized with nitrous oxide plus fentanyl, enflurane, or halothane, for gastric stapling operations. The time to opening eyes on command was shortest in patients receiving fentanyl, whereas time to extubation of the trachea was similar in all three anesthesia study groups. (From Cork RC, Vaughn RW, Bentley JB. General anesthesia for morbidly obese patients—an examination of postoperative outcomes. Anesthesiology 1981;54:310–3, with permission.)

creased defluorination of volatile anesthetics in the obese patient, however, has not been shown to result in hepatic or renal dysfunction[35–37] (Fig. 23-3). The possibility of prolonged responses to drugs stored in fat (volatile anesthetics, opioids, barbiturates) is not supported by delayed awakening from anesthesia in the obese patient[40] (Fig. 23-5). Nevertheless, the volume of distribution and elimination half-time of sufentanil administered to obese patients is prolonged, reflecting the high lipid solubility of this opioid.[42] Spinal and epidural anesthesia may be technically difficult in the obese patient, as bony landmarks are obscured. Increased pressure in the epidural space secondary to engorged epidural veins may make predictability of the sensory anesthetic level difficult. It would seem prudent to decrease the initial dose of local anesthetic administered for regional anesthesia when body weight is greatly increased due to excess adipose tissue.

Management of Ventilation

Controlled ventilation of the lungs using a large tidal volume is often selected in the management of the obese patient, in an attempt to offset the decreased functional residual capacity and PaO_2 accompanying obesity. The response of the obese patient to positive end-expiratory pressure is unpredictable. It is possible that positive end-expiratory pressure could so decrease cardiac output as to offset the benefits of improved ventilation-to-perfusion matching. The prone and head-down positions can further decrease chest wall compliance and PaO_2 in the obese patient. Assumption of the supine position by a spontaneously breathing obese patient can so decrease PaO_2 as to cause cardiac arrest. Clearly, monitoring arterial hemoglobin oxygen saturation and arterial blood gases is useful in evaluating the adequacy of oxygenation and ventilation during the perioperative period.

Postoperative Complications

Postoperative morbidity and mortality in the obese patient is increased compared to the nonobese patient. Wound infection is twice as common. The likelihood of deep vein thrombosis and the risk of pulmonary embolism are increased, emphasizing the possible importance of early postoperative ambulation. Pulmonary complications are frequent, especially after abdominal surgery. The semisitting position is often used during the postoperative period in an attempt to decrease the likelihood of arterial hypoxemia. Arterial oxygenation should be closely monitored and supplemental oxygen provided as indicated by the PaO_2 value. The maximum decrease in PaO_2 typically occurs 2 to 3 days postoperatively.[42]

OBESITY HYPOVENTILATION SYNDROME

Obesity hypoventilation syndrome, or pickwickian syndrome, occurs in about 8% of obese patients.[43] These patients exhibit massive obesity, episodic daytime somnolence, and hypoventilation. Documentation of an increased $PaCO_2$ in a massively obese patient suggests either the presence of the obesity hypoventilation syndrome or severe underlying lung disease. Ultimately, hypoventilation leads to respiratory acidosis, arterial hypoxemia, polycythemia, pulmonary hypertension, and right ventricular failure. Weight loss is associated with decreased $PaCO_2$. The etiology of obesity hypoventilation syndrome is unclear, but it may represent a disorder of the central nervous system regulation of ventilation or an inability of the muscles of breathing to respond to neural impulses, or both. Obstructive sleep apnea associated with this syndrome has been treated effectively by the application of continuous positive airway pressure through a nasal airway.[43]

BULIMIA NERVOSA

Bulimia nervosa is characterized by episodes of binge eating. It occurs most often in females and leads to obesity despite the occasional practice of self-induced vomiting. Hypokalemia may reflect self-induced vomiting or excessive use of diuretics and laxatives. Peridontal disease is common, perhaps as a result of increased intake of carbohydrates or the presence of acid in the mouth after self-induced vomiting, or both. An elevated serum amylase concentration is likely and may be associated with benign parotid enlargement. Mental depression and alcohol and drug abuse are frequent in this patient group. Treatment of bulimia nervosa is with a tricyclic antidepressant, which seems to act much like a conventional appetite suppressant.

ANOREXIA NERVOSA

Anorexia nervosa is a psychiatric disease characterized by a striking decrease in physical activity and marked diminution of food intake in the obsessive pursuit of thinness. Bulimic symptoms may be part of the anorexia nervosa syndrome. Females are most often affected, and weight loss exceeds 25% of normal body weight despite the patient's perception that she is obese. Endocrine abnormalities, especially amenorrhea, are secondary to starvation; these problems normalize with improved nutrition. Decreased body temperature, orthostatic hypotension, bradycardia, and cardiac dysrhythmias may reflect alterations in autonomic nervous system activity. Cardiac changes include decreased cardiac muscle mass and myocardial contractility. Changes on the electrocardiogram are common and include T wave inversion, ST depression, and a prolonged Q-T interval. Sudden death has been attributed to cardiac dysrhythmias in this patient population.[44] Leukopenia occurs frequently, and thrombocytopenia and anemia may also be present. Bone density is decreased owing to poor nutrition and decreased estrogen levels. Electrolyte abnormalities are unusual, although hypokalemia may occur in the patient who self-induces vomiting or abuses diuretics or laxatives, or both. Occasionally patients exhibit fatty liver infiltration and altered liver function tests. Gastric emptying time is prolonged.

Treatment of anorexia nervosa consists of restoration of body weight, which may require enteral nutrition. Tricyclic antidepressants are not effective, because they act as appetite suppressants. Cyproheptadine is an appetite stimulant that may be useful in these patients.[45] Despite treatment, mortality is 7% to 10%, usually as the result of starvation or suicide.

Management of Anesthesia

Despite the frequency of anorexia nervosa, there is a paucity of information relating to the management of anesthesia for the patient with this eating disorder. The preoperative evaluation is based on the known pathophysiologic effects evoked by starvation. The electrocardiogram is useful in detecting evidence of cardiac dysfunction. Electrolyte abnormalities, hypovolemia owing to dehydration, and delayed gastric emptying are preoperative considerations. Intraoperative cardiac dysrhythmias in a patient with anorexia nervosa have been attributed to the presence of hypokalemia, prolonged Q-T interval indicated by the electrocardiogram, and possible imbalance of the autonomic nervous system.[46] Reversal of neuromuscular blockade and changes in $PaCO_2$ could contribute to the potential for the development of cardiac dysrhythmias in these patients. Experience is too limited to permit recommendations regarding specific anesthetic drugs, muscle relaxants, or anesthetic techniques in the presence of anorexia nervosa.

MALNUTRITION

Malnutrition is a medically definable syndrome that is responsive to caloric support, provided by enteral or total parenteral nutrition (hyperalimentation).[47] More than 90% of malnourished patients are identified by a plasma albumin concentration below 3 g·dl^{-1} and a transferrin level below 200 mg·dl^{-1}. Skin test anergy (immunosuppression) also accompanies malnutrition. Fatty liver infiltration is commonly associated with malnutrition.

Critically ill patients often experience negative caloric intake complicated by hypermetabolic states due to increased caloric needs produced by trauma, fever, sepsis, and wound healing. It is estimated that an intake of 1500 to 2000 cal·d^{-1} is necessary to maintain basic energy requirements. An increase in body temperature of 1°C will increase daily energy (caloric) requirements by about 15%. Multiple fractures increase energy needs by about 25% and major burns by about 100%. A large tumor, by virtue of its growth and metabolism, requires fuels that can exceed 100% of the basal caloric requirements. Postoperatively, patients experience increased protein breakdown and decreased protein synthesis.[48]

Treatment

It is often recommended that patients who have lost more than 20% of their body weight be treated nutritionally before undergoing an elective operation.[49] A patient who is unable to eat or absorb food 1 week postoperatively may require parenteral nutrition. When the gastrointestinal tract is functioning, enteral nutrition can be provided by means of nasogas-

tric or gastrostomy tube feedings. Continuous drip (100 to 120 ml·h^{-1}) is the most frequent way to administer enteral feedings. Complications of enteral feedings are infrequent but may include hyperglycemia leading to osmotic diuresis and hypovolemia. Exogenous insulin administration is a consideration when the blood glucose concentration exceeds 250 mg·dl^{-1}. The high osmolarity of elemental diets (550 to 850 mOsm·L^{-1}) is often a cause of diarrhea.

Total parenteral nutrition is indicated when the gastrointestinal tract is not functioning. Total parenteral nutrition using an isotonic solution delivered through a peripheral vein is acceptable when the patient requires less than 2000 cal·d^{-1}, and the anticipated need for nutritional support is less than 2 weeks. When caloric requirements exceed 2000 cal·d^{-1} or prolonged nutritional support is required, a venous catheter is placed in the subclavian vein to permit infusion of a hypertonic parenteral solution (about 1900 mOsm·L^{-1}) in a volume of about 40 ml·kg^{-1}·d^{-1}.

Potential complications of total parenteral nutrition are numerous (Table 23-13). Blood glucose concentration is monitored as hyperglycemia (above 250 mg·dl^{-1}) may require treatment with exogenous insulin, whereas hypoglycemia may occur if the parenteral nutrition solution infusion is abruptly discontinued (mechanical obstruction in delivery tubing) while elevated circulating endogenous concentrations of insulin persist. Hyperchloremic metabolic acidosis may occur because of the liberation of hydrochloric acid during the metabolism of amino acids present in most parenteral nutrition solutions. Parenteral feeding of patients with compromised cardiac function is associated with the risk of congestive heart failure owing to fluid overload. Increased production of carbon dioxide resulting from metabolism of large amounts of glucose may result in the need to initiate mechanical ventilation of the lungs or failure to wean a patient from long-term ventilator support.[50] Parenteral nutrition solutions can support growth of bacteria and fungi, and catheter-related sepsis is a constant threat. In view of the risk of contamination, the use of a hyper-

Table 23-13. Complications Associated With Total Parenteral Nutrition

Hyperglycemia
Nonketotic hyperosmolar hyperglycemic coma
Hypoglycemia
Hyperchloremic metabolic acidosis
Fluid overload
Increased carbon dioxide production
Catheter-related sepsis
Electrolyte abnormalities
Renal dysfunction
Hepatic dysfunction
Thombosis of central veins

alimentation catheter for administration of medications, withdrawal of blood samples, or monitoring of central venous pressure, as during the perioperative period, is not recommended. Electrolyte abnormalities may include hypokalemia, hypomagnesemia, hypocalcemia, and hypophosphatemia. If intravenous hyperalimentation is continued during surgery, there should probably be a corresponding decrease in the infusion rates of other intravenous fluids so as to minimize the risk of fluid overload.

DISORDERS RELATED TO VITAMIN IMBALANCE

Vitamin deficiencies are largely of historic interest. Nevertheless, it is conceivable that administration of anesthesia for surgery will be required in a patient with a co-existing nutritional deficiency of one or more of the essential vitamins. This is most likely to occur in the chronic alcoholic patient. Although no specific anesthetic drug or techniques can be recommended, it is important to appreciate the changes related to vitamin deficiencies to ensure proper medical judgments during the perioperative period.

Thiamine

Thiamine (vitamin B_1) deficiency (beriberi) is most likely to occur in a chronic alcoholic patient who has a decreased dietary intake of thiamine. Decreased systemic vascular resistance and increased cardiac output may result in high-output cardiac failure in the thiamine-deficient patient. This form of congestive heart failure is similar to the hyperdynamic heart failure that may occur in a patient with a large arteriovenous shunt. It may be difficult to differentiate congestive heart failure due to thiamine deficiency from the cardiomyopathy that may accompany chronic alcoholism. Memory loss (Korsakoff's psychosis) and skeletal muscle weakness may develop. Polyneuropathy with demyelination, paresthesias, and sensory deficits (glove and stocking distribution) are characteristic. Destruction of the peripheral sympathetic nervous system could impair compensatory vasomotor responses that might occur during the perioperative period as exaggerated decreases in blood pressure in response to hemorrhage, positive-pressure ventilation of the lungs, or sudden changes in body position. Treatment of thiamine deficiency consists of the administration of an intravenous preparation of this vitamin.

Ascorbic Acid

Deficiency of ascorbic acid (vitamin C) produces a clinical picture known as scurvy. Ascorbic acid is required for the conversion of proline to hydroxyproline in the production of normal collagen. When ascorbic acid is deficient, manifestations of abnormal ground substance are seen in all tissues. Indeed, capillary fragility, exhibited as petechial hemorrhages, is prominent in the patient with ascorbic acid deficiency. Hemorrhage into the joints and skeletal muscles can result. The failure of odontoblastic activity results in loosened teeth and gangrenous alveolar margins. Fibroblast activity is deficient, resulting in poor wound healing and decreased strength of a new surgical wound. A catabolic state associated with a negative nitrogen balance and potassium deficiency is also characteristic. Iron deficiency anemia is frequent, but the presence of macrocytic anemia suggests a concomitant folic acid deficiency. There are no special considerations for the management of anesthesia.

Nicotinic Acid

A deficiency of nicotinic acid (niacin) produces pellagra (black tongue). Nicotinic acid is part of nicotinamide adenine dinucleotide phosphate, an important component of cellular oxidation-reduction reactions. The body does not depend on exogenous nicotinic acid, as this vitamin can be manufactured from tryptophan. The patient with a carcinoid tumor can show the development of pellagra, since available tryptophan is diverted to the formation of serotonin, rather than nicotinic acid. A diet with a high maize content can lead to a nicotinic acid deficiency, as corn contains large amounts of leucine, which interferes with metabolism of tryptophan. Other causes of pellagra include malabsorption syndromes and chronic alcoholism.

Mental confusion, irritability, and peripheral neuropathy are characteristic of nicotinic acid deficiency. Administration of nicotinic acid usually reverses central nervous system dysfunction in less than 24 hours. Gastrointestinal symptoms include achlorhydria and severe diarrhea, which can lead to hypovolemia and loss of electrolytes. Vesicular dermatitis involving the mucous membranes is also characteristic. Manifestations of dermatitis include stomatitis, glossitis, excessive salivation, and urethritis. There are no specific recommendations regarding the management of anesthesia.

Vitamin A

A deficiency of vitamin A can result from dietary lack of foodstuffs that contain this vitamin (leafy vegetables, animal liver) or from malabsorption syndromes. Clinical manifestations of vitamin A deficiency include loss of night vision, conjunctival drying, and corneal destruction. Anemia from depressed hemoglobin synthesis is frequent. Management of anesthesia may include frequent application of artificial tears and keeping the patient's eyes closed during the intraoperative period.

An excess of vitamin A can produce irritability, hydrocephalus, hepatosplenomegaly, and anemia. Cranial symptoms can be caused by intracranial hypertension secondary to cerebral sinus obstruction.

Vitamin D

Nutritional rickets is due to decreased availability of the active form of vitamin D. Gastrointestinal absorption of calcium is impaired when vitamin D is absent; there is also a tendency for the development of hypocalcemia. This tendency is balanced by parathyroid hormone activity, which increases in response to a low plasma calcium concentration. The osteolytic activity of parathyroid hormone restores the plasma calcium concentration to a near-normal level, at the expense of older bone, which becomes demineralized. New bone formation, which is dependent on the plasma calcium concentrations, takes place in a normal manner. Therefore, changes in the skeleton characteristic of rickets reflect unimpaired formation of new bone and the breakdown of old bone. Thoracic kyphosis from this mechanism may be so severe as to produce hypoventilation. Laboratory studies in the presence of vitamin D deficiency show a normal or low plasma calcium concentration, a low plasma phosphate level, an increased plasma alkaline phosphatase concentration, and a low urinary excretion of calcium.

Vitamin K

Vitamin K is synthesized by bacteria residing in the gastrointestinal tract. Prolonged antibiotic therapy can eliminate these bacteria, leading to a prolonged prothrombin time. Since vitamin K is fat soluble, a deficiency of this substance is likely whenever there is failure of fat absorption from the gastrointestinal tract. Decreased absorption of vitamin K from the gastrointestinal tract is most likely to occur when bile salts are excluded from the intestine.

REFERENCES

1. McNeill MJ, Bennet A. Use of regional anaesthesia in a patient with acute porphyria. Br J Anaesth 1990;64:371–3
2. Mustajoki P, Heinonen J. General anesthesia in "inducible" porphyrias. Anesthesiology 1980;53:15–20
3. Salvin SA, Christoforides C. Thiopental administration in acute intermittent porphyria without adverse effect. Anesthesiology 1976;44:77–9
4. Bancroft GH, Lauria JI. Ketamine induction for cesarean section in a patient with acute intermittent porphyria and achondroplastic dwarfism. Anesthesiology 1983;59:143–4
5. Meissner PN, Harrison GG, Hift RJ. Propofol as an I.V. anaesthetic induction agent in variegate porphyria. Br J Anaesth 1991;66:60–5
6. Kantor G, Rolbin SH. Acute intermittent porphyria and Caesarean delivery. Can J Anaesth 1992;39:282–5
7. Larson LO, Wilkins RG. Anesthesia and the Lesch-Nyhan syndrome. Anesthesiology 1985;63:197–9
8. Grundy SM. Cholesterol and coronary heart disease. A new era. JAMA 1986;256:2849–58
9. National Institutes of Health Consensus Development Conference. Lowering blood cholesterol to prevent heart disease. JAMA 1985;253:2080–6
10. Consensus Conference: Treatment of hypertriglyceridemia. JAMA 1984;251:1196–9
11. Kushi LH, Lew RA, Stare FJ, et al. Diet and 20-year mortality from coronary heart disease: The Ireland-Boston Diet-Heart Study. N Engl J Med 1985;312:811–16
12. Arntzenius AC, Kromhut D, Barth JD, et al. Diet lipoproteins and the progression of coronary atherosclerosis: The Leiden Intervention Trial. N Engl J Med 1985;312:805–10
13. Blankenhorn DH, Nessim SA, Johnson RL, et al. Beneficial effects of combined colestipol-niacin therapy on coronary atherosclerosis and coronary venous bypass grafts. JAMA 1987;257:3233–7
14. Cannon BW, Meshier WT. Extremity amputation following radial artery cannulation in a patient with hyperlipoproteinemia type V. Anesthesiology 1982;56:222–3
15. Rowe RW, Helander E. Anesthetic management of a patient with systemic carnitine deficiency. Anesth Analg 1990;71:295–7
16. Edelstine G, Hirshman CA. Hyperthermia and ketoacidosis during anesthesia in a child with glycogen-storage disease. Anesthesiology 1980;52:90–2
17. Rosen KR, Broadman LM. Anaesthesia for diagnostic muscle biopsy in an infant with Pompe's disease. Can Anaesth Soc J 1986;33:790–4
18. Hashimoto Y, Watanabe H, Satou M. Anaesthetic management of a patient with hereditary fructose-1, 6-diphosphate deficiency. Anesth Analg 1978;57:503–6
19. Dierdorf SF, McNiece WL. Anaesthesia and pyruvate dehydrogenase deficiency. Can Anaesth Soc J 1983;30:413–6
20. Parris WCV, Quimby CW. Anesthetic considerations for the patient with homocystinuria. Anesth Analg 1982;61:70–1
21. Berry GT, Heidenreich R, Kaplan P, et al. Branched-chain amino acid-free parenteral nutrition in the treatment of acute metabolic decompensation in patients with maple syrup urine disease. N Engl J Med 1991;324:175–8
22. Delaney A, Gal TJ. Hazards of anesthesia and operation in maple-syrup-urine disease. Anesthesiology 1976;44:83–6
23. Sharar SR, Haberkern CM, Jack R, Scott CR. Anesthetic management of a child with methylmalonyl-coenzyme A mutase deficiency. Anesth Analg 1991;73:499–501
24. Herrick IA, Rhine EJ. The mucopolysaccharidoses and anaesthesia: A report of clinical experience. Can J Anaesth 1988;35:67–73
25. Wilder RT, Belani KG. Fiberoptic intubation complicated by pulmonary edema in a 12-year old child with Hurler syndrome. Anesthesiology 1990;72:205–7
26. Birkinshaw KJ. Anaesthesia in a patient with an unstable neck: Morquio syndrome. Anaesthesia 1975;30:46–9
27. Jones AEP, Croley TF. Morquio syndrome and anesthesia. Anesthesiology 1979;51:261–2

28. Lichtman SW, Pisarska K, Berman ER, et al. Discrepancy between self-reported and actual caloric intake and exercise in obese subjects. N Engl J Med 1992;327:1893–8

29. Stunkard AJ, Sorensen TIA, Hanis C, et al. An adoption study of human obesity. N Engl J Med 1986;314:193–8

30. Brownell KD, Jeffery RW. Improving long-term weight loss: Pushing the limits of treatment. Behav Ther 1987;18:353–7

31. Kaplan RM, Hartwell SL, Wilson DK, et al. Effects of diet and exercise interventions on control and quality of life in non-insulin-dependent diabetes mellitus. J Gen Intern Med 1987;2:220–6

32. Hocking MP, Duerson MC, O'Leary JP, Woodward ER. Jejunoileal bypass for morbid obesity. Late follow-up in 100 cases. N Engl J Med 1983;308:995–9

33. Fisher A, Waterhouse TD, Adams AP. Obesity: Its relation to anaesthesia. Anaesthesia 1975;30:633–47

34. Vaughn RW, Cork RC, Hollander D. The effect of massive weight loss on arterial oxygenation and pulmonary function tests. Anesthesiology 1981;54:325–8

35. Bentley JB, Vaughan RW, Miller MS, et al. Serum inorganic fluoride levels in obese patients during and after enflurane anesthesia. Anesth Analg 1979;58:409–12

36. Bentley JB, Vaughan RW, Gandolfi AJ, Cork RC. Halothane biotransformation in obese and nonobese patients. Anesthesiology 1982;57:94–7

37. Nawaf K, Stoelting RK. SGOT values following evidence of reductive biotransformation of halothane in man. Anesthesiology 1979;51:185–6

38. Vaughan RW, Baker S, Wise L. Volume and pH of gastric juice in obese patients. Anesthesiology 1975;43:686–9

39. Berthoud MC, Peacock JE, Reilly CS. Effectiveness of preoxygenation in morbidly obese patients. Br J Anaesth 1991;67:464–6

40. Cork RC, Vaughan RW, Bentley JB. General anesthesia for morbidly obese patients—an examination of postoperative outcomes. Anesthesiology 1981;54:310–3

41. Schwartz AE, Matteo RS, Ornstein E, Young WL, Myers KJ. Pharmacokinetics of sufentanil in obese patients. Anesth Analg 1991;73:790–3

42. Vaughan RW, Wise L. Postoperative arterial blood gas measurements in obese patients: Effect of position on gas exchange. Ann Surg 1975;182:705–9

43. Rapoport DM, Sorkin B, Garay SM, Goldring RM. Reversal of the "Pickwickian syndrome" by long-term use of nocturnal nasal-airway pressure. N Engl J Med 1982;307:931–3

44. Isner JM, Roberts WL, Heymsfield SB, Yager J. Anorexia nervosa and sudden death. Ann Intern Med 1985;102:49–52

45. Halmi KA, Eckert E, LaDu TJ, et al. Anorexia nervosa: Treatment efficacy of cyproheptadine and amitriptyline. Arch Gen Psychiatry 1986;43:177–82

46. Arnold DE, Rose RJ, Stoddard P. Intraoperative cardiac dysrhythmias in a patient with bulimic anorexia nervosa. Anesthesiology 1987;67:1003–5

47. Powell-Tuck J, Goode AW. Principles of enteral and parenteral nutrition. Br J Anaesth 1981;53:169–80

48. Carli F, Ramachandra V, Gandy J, et al. Effect of general anaesthesia on whole body protein turnover in patients undergoing elective surgery. Br J Anaesth 1990;65:373–9

49. Michel L, Serrano A, Malt RA. Nutritional support of hospitalized patients. N Engl J Med 1981;304:1147–52

50. Askanazi J, Nordenstrom J, Rosenbaum SH, et al. Nutrition for the patient with respiratory failure: Glucose vs. fat. Anesthesiology 1981;54:373–7

24
Anemia

Anemia, like fever, is a sign of disease manifested clinically as a numerical deficiency of erythrocytes (RBCs).[1] There is no single laboratory value that defines anemia. Indeed, hematocrit may be unchanged despite acute blood loss, while in the parturient the decreased hematocrit reflects an increase in plasma volume and not anemia. Nevertheless, in adults, anemia is usually defined as a hemoglobin concentration of less than 11.5 $g \cdot dl^{-1}$ (hematocrit 36%) for females and a hemoglobin concentration of less than 12.5 $g \cdot dl^{-1}$ (hematocrit 40%) for males. Decreases in hematocrit that exceed 1% every 24 hours can only be explained by acute blood loss or intravascular hemolysis.

The most important adverse effect of anemia is decreased tissue oxygen delivery, owing to the associated decrease in arterial content of oxygen (CaO_2). For example, a decrease in the hemoglobin concentration from 15 $g \cdot dl^{-1}$ to 10 $g \cdot dl^{-1}$ results in a 33% decrease in CaO_2 (Table 24-1). Increasing the PaO_2 above 100 mmHg has only a minor effect in increasing the CaO_2. Compensation for decreased CaO_2 is accomplished by a righward shift of the oxyhemoglobin dissociation curve (facilitates release of oxygen from hemoglobin to tissues) and an increase in cardiac output as a reflection of decreased blood viscosity (Fig. 24-1). Furthermore, when oxygen delivery to the tissues is inadequate, the kidneys release erythropoietin, which subsequently stimulates erythroid precursors in the bone marrow to produce additional RBCs. Fatigue and decreased exercise tolerance reflect the inability of the cardiac output to increase further and maintain tissue oxygenation, especially in anemic patients who become physically active. Anemia has many causes; the most common forms are (1) iron deficiency anemia, (2) anemia of chronic disease, and (3) thalassemia[1] (Fig. 24-2).

IRON DEFICIENCY ANEMIA

Nutritional deficiency of iron is a cause of anemia only in infants and small children. In adults, iron deficiency anemia can only reflect depletion of iron stores owing to chronic blood loss, most likely from the gastrointestinal tract or from the female genital tract, for example, during menstruation. Parturients are susceptible to the development of iron deficiency anemia because of increased RBC mass during gestation, as well as the needs of the fetus for iron. The symptoms of iron deficiency anemia depend on the actual hemoglobin concentration.

Patients experiencing chronic blood loss may not be able to absorb sufficient iron from the gastrointestinal tract to form hemoglobin as rapidly as RBCs are lost. As a result, RBCs are often produced with too little hemoglobin, giving rise to microcytic hypochronic anemia. Nevertheless, most cases of iron deficiency anemia in the United States are mild, exhibiting a hemoglobin concentration of 9 to 12 $g \cdot dl^{-1}$. Indeed, the actual existence of hypochromia in patients with iron deficiency anemia has been questioned.[1] The absence of stainable iron in a bone marrow aspirate is confirmatory for iron deficiency. Alternatively, the demonstration of a decreased plasma ferritin concentration serves as an available cost-effective test for the presence of iron deficiency.

Treatment of iron deficiency anemia is with ferrous iron salts, such as ferrous sulfate administered orally. Iron stores are replenished slowly. Therapy should be continued for at least 1 year after the source of blood loss that led to iron deficiency anemia is corrected. A favorable response to iron therapy is characterized by an increase in the hemoglobin concentration of about 2 $g \cdot dl^{-1}$ in 3 weeks or a return of the hemoglobin concentration to normal in 6 weeks. Continued bleeding will be reflected by reticulocytosis and failure of the hemoglobin concentration to increase in response to iron therapy. In the future, recombinant human erythropoietin may be used to treat drug-induced anemia or to improve the hematocrit before elective surgery.

Management of Anesthesia

A minimum acceptable hemoglobin concentration that should be present before proceeding with elective surgery in the patient with chronic anemia cannot be recommended.

Table 24-1.   Calculation of Arterial Oxygen Content

$$CaO_2 = (Hb \times 1.39)SaO_2 + PaO_2(0.003)$$

CaO_2 = arterial oxygen content (ml·dl^{-1})

Hb = hemoglobin (g·dl^{-1})

1.39 = oxygen bound to hemoglobin (ml·g^{-1})

SaO_2 = saturation of hemoglobin with oxygen (%)

PaO_2 = arterial partial pressure of oxygen (mmHg)

0.003 = disssolved oxygen (ml·mmHg^{-1}·dl^{-1})

Example: Hb = 15 g·dl^{-1}, SaO_2 100%, PaO_2 100 mmHg

CaO_2 = (15 × 1.39)100 + 100(0.003)

= 20.85 + 0.3

= 21.15 ml·dl^{-1}

Example: Hb = 10 g·dl^{-1}, SaO_2 100%, PaO_2 100 mmHg

CaO_2 = (10 × 1.39)100 + 100(0.003)

= 13.9 + 0.3

= 14.2 ml·dl^{-1}

Example: Hb = 10 g·dl^{-1}, SaO_2 100%, PaO_2 500 mmHg

CaO_2 = (10 × 1.39)100 + 500(0.003)

= 13.9 + 1.5

= 15.4 ml·dl^{-1}

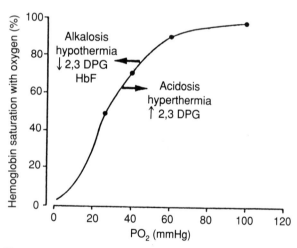

Fig. 24-1. The oxyhemoglobin dissociation curve describes the relationship between the SaO_2 and the PO_2. The PaO_2 at which SaO_2 is 50% is designated the P_{50} (normal 26 mmHg). An increase in the P_{50} reflects a shift of the oxyhemoglobin dissociation curve to the right (increased levels of 2,3-diphosphoglycerate in RBCs, acidosis, increased body temperature); thus, binding of oxygen to hemoglobin is less avid, facilitating its release to peripheral tissues. A decrease in the P_{50} reflects a shift of the oxyhemoglobin dissociation curve to the left (decreased levels of 2,3-diphosphoglycerate in the RBCs, alkalosis, decreased body temperature); thus, binding of oxygen to hemoglobin is more avid, impairing its release to peripheral tissues. Mixed venous blood has a $S\bar{v}O_2$ of about 75% and a corresponding $P\bar{v}O_2$ close to 40 mmHg. When the SaO_2 is about 90%, the corresponding PaO_2 is close to 60 mmHg.

Although a hemoglobin concentration of 10 g·dl^{-1} is frequently quoted as a guideline, there is no evidence that a hemoglobin value below this level indicates a need for perioperative transfusion of RBCs.[2] Furthermore, there is no evidence that postoperative morbidity (wound healing, infection) is adversely affected when surgery is performed in the presence of mild to moderate anemia.[3] Transfusion of RBCs is intended only to increase oxygen-carrying capacity, and not for volume expansion or improved wound healing. The decision to transfuse to a specific hemoglobin level preoperatively must be individualized, taking into consideration several factors (Table 24-2). The ability of the cardiovascular system to compensate for decreases in CaO_2 by increasing the cardiac output is an important compensatory mechanism by maintaining tissue oxygen delivery, especially in the acutely anemic patient. Increased 2,3-diphosphoglycerate concentrations in RBCs are principally responsible for maintaining oxygen-carrying capacity in the presence of chronic anemia. In this regard, cardiac output does not increase in chronically anemic patients until the hemoglobin concentration decreases to about 7 g·dl^{-1}.[4] In vitro data suggest that peak oxygen-carrying capacity occurs at a hematocrit of 30%. Below this hematocrit, oxygen-carrying capacity declines as a result of decreased oxygen-carrying capacity. Above this hematocrit, oxygen-carrying capacity may decline as a result of decreased blood flow due to increased blood viscosity. The clinical desirability of a hematocrit close to 30%, however, has not been confirmed.[4] Preoperative transfusion of packed RBCs can be used to increase the hemoglobin concentration, but it should be recognized that about 24 hours are needed to restore intravascular fluid volume. Compared with a similar volume of whole blood, packed RBCs produce about twice the increase in hemoglobin concentration.

If elective surgery is performed in the presence of chronic anemia, it would seem prudent to minimize the likelihood of significant changes that could interfere further with oxygen delivery to the tissues. For example, drug-induced decreases in cardiac output or a leftward shift of the oxyhemoglobin dissociation curve owing to respiratory alkalosis from iatrogenic hyperventilation of the lungs could interfere with oxygen delivery to the tissues. Decreased body temperature also shifts the oxyhemoglobin dissociation curve to the left. Decreased tissue oxygen requirements may accompany the depressant effects of anesthetics and hypothermia, offsetting to an unpredictable degree the decreased oxygen delivery to the tissues that may accompany anesthesia.

Inhaled anesthetics may be less soluble in the plasma of an anemic patient, reflecting the decrease in lipid-rich RBCs.[5,6] As a result, establishment of the arterial partial pressure of the anesthetic in the plasma of an anemic patient might be accelerated. Nevertheless, the effect of decreased solubility of an inhaled anesthetic owing to anemia is probably offset by the impact of increased cardiac output. Therefore, it seems unlikely that clinically detectable differences in the rate of in-

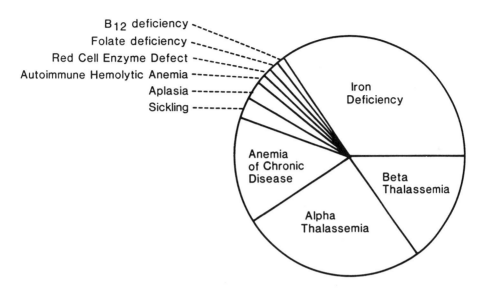

Anemia
Distribution of Causes

Fig. 24-2. Estimate of the prevalence of different types of anemia in the United States. (From Beutler E. The common anemias. JAMA 1988;259:2433–6, with permission.)

duction of anesthesia or vulnerability to an anesthetic overdose would occur in an anemic patient compared with a normal patient. Hemodynamic responses to halothane, as reflected by measurements in chronically anemic animals, are characterized by a higher heart rate, lower systemic vascular resistance, and unchanged mean arterial pressure, as compared with normal animals[2] (Fig. 24-3). Intraoperative blood loss should most likely be replaced with whole blood or packed RBCs, when there is co-existing anemia or cardiovascular or cerebrovascular disease, especially if the hemoglobin concentration decreases acutely to less than 7 g·dl^{-1}.[2] During the postoperative period, it is important to minimize the occur-

Table 24-2. Basis for Decision
to Transfuse Preoperatively

Duration of anemia
Etiology of anemia
Intravascular fluid volume
Urgency of surgery
Likely blood loss during surgery
Co-existing diseases
    Myocardial ischemia
    Lung disease
    Cerebrovascular disease
    Peripheral vascular disease

rence of shivering or increases in body temperature, since these changes could increase total body oxygen requirements.

ANEMIA OF CHRONIC DISEASE

Anemia of chronic disease is one of the most common forms of anemia (Table 24-3). There is nothing characteristic about the appearance of the RBCs, and the underlying mechanism for the development of anemia is unknown. The diagnosis of anemia of chronic disease remains largely one of exclusion. Iron accumulates in the reticuloendothelial system, and there appears to be a block in the release of iron from these cells to the developing erythroblasts. Attempts to treat this form of anemia by iron replacement are uniformly ineffective. In general, however, this form of anemia is mild, only rarely requiring treatment with blood transfusions. Identifying and treating the underlying disease is the most effective therapy for associated anemia.

THALASSEMIA

Thalassemia designates a number of inherited disorders characterized by decreased rates of synthesis or failure of synthesis of structurally normal hemoglobin. Severe thalas-

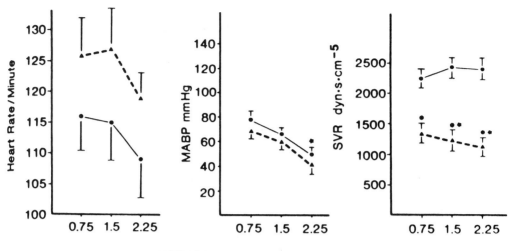

Fig. 24-3. The hemodynamic effects of increasing doses of halothane were determined in chronically anemic (dashed lines) and normal (solid lines) dogs. Anemic dogs showed a significantly lower SVR (systemic vascular resistance) at each dose of halothane, as compared with controls. (From Barrera M, Miletich DJ, Albrecht RF, Hoffman WG. Hemodynamic consequences of halothane anesthesia during chronic anemia. Anesthesiology 1984;61:36–42, with permission.)

semia (thalassemia major) is rare, whereas mild forms of this disease (thalassemia minor) are common. No treatment is available for this form of anemia, other than blood transfusions.

Beta-Thalassemia Major

Beta-thalassemia major (Cooley's anemia) reflects an inability to form beta globin chains of hemoglobin. As a result, adult hemoglobin A is not formed, and anemia develops during the first year of life, as fetal hemoglobin (two alpha and two gamma chains) disappears. Greek and Italian children are most often affected. Jaundice, hepatosplenomegaly, and susceptibility to infection are likely. Death from cardiac hemochromotosis reflects the need for multiple transfusions in the treatment of chronic anemia. Indeed, supraventricular cardiac dysrhyth-

Table 24-3. Chronic Diseases Associated With Anemia

Infections
Cancer
Connective tissue disorders
Acquired immunodeficiency syndrome
Alcoholic liver disease
Renal failure
Diabetes mellitus

mias and congestive heart failure are common. In this regard, it must be appreciated that these patients are unusually sensitive to the effects of digitalis. Splenectomy may be necessary if hypersplenism leads to pancytopenia. Increased production of RBCs results in characteristic skeletal changes, including cephalofacial deformities and thinning of the cortical bone. Hemothorax may occur as a result of hematopoiesis.[8] Overgrowth of the maxillae can make visualization of the glottis difficult during direct laryngoscopy. Spinal cord compression secondary to massive extramedullary hematopoiesis and destruction of vertebral bodies can occur.[9]

Beta-Thalassemia Minor

Beta-thalassemia minor reflects a heterozygote state (trait) that typically results in mild to no anemia. A relatively normal RBC count distinguishes anemia due to thalassemia minor from iron deficiency anemia. This form of thalassemia is encountered more frequently than previously realized.[1]

Alpha-Thalassemia

Alpha-thalassemia is due to a lack of production of alpha chains of adult hemoglobin. A homozygous form of alpha-thalassemia is incompatible with life, resulting in intrauterine demise (hydrops fetalis) or early neonatal death. Patients who are heterozygous for alpha-thalassemia (trait) characteristically acquire mild hypochromic and microcytic anemia. On occasion, blood transfusion to treat anemia or splenectomy to control hemolysis may be necessary.

ACUTE BLOOD LOSS

Orthostatic hypotension, tachycardia, and low central venous pressure suggest acute blood loss equivalent to at least 20% of the circulating blood volume (Table 24-4). Hematocrit may not reflect anemia due to acute blood loss, since physiologic mechanisms for restoring plasma volume operate slowly. For example, the hematocrit does not decrease to a new plateau value for as long as 3 days after acute blood loss.[10] The obvious treatment of anemia due to acute blood loss is correction of the cause leading to hemorrhage and prompt restoration of intravascular fluid volume with RBCs plus colloid or crystalloid solutions. Volume replacement with crystalloid or colloid is probably equally effective, provided the crystalloid is administered at about 3 ml for every 1 ml of colloid.

Hemorrhagic Shock

Hemorrhagic shock (systolic blood pressure less than 90 mmHg, tachycardia, oliguria, metabolic acidosis, restlessness) is a potential complication of acute blood loss. The fundamental defect in hemorrhagic shock is decreased intravascular fluid volume leading to decreased venous return and cardiac output, with subsequent inadequate tissue perfusion. Increased sympathetic nervous system activity during acute hemorrhage is useful in redirecting blood flow to the brain and heart. Increased sympathetic nervous system activity for prolonged periods, however, with associated arteriolar vasoconstriction, results in a detrimental decrease in renal and splanchnic blood flow, one manifestation of which is oliguria. Furthermore, anaerobic metabolism is increased, manifested as metabolic (lactic) acidosis.

Treatment of hemorrhagic shock is with infusion of whole blood. Crystalloid solutions are also indicated, since interstitial fluid shifts accompany acute hemorrhage. Successful treatment often requires continuous monitoring of blood pressure, cardiac filling pressures, and urine output, to guide the adequacy of intravascular fluid volume replacement. Thermodilution measurement of cardiac output and calculation of systemic vascular resistance are helpful in determining appropriate therapy. In this regard, dopamine or dobutamine may be useful in selected patients, especially when the goals of therapy include a mild inotropic effect plus increased renal blood flow. Vasopressors are used sparingly in the treatment of hemorrhagic shock; however, it may be necessary to support cerebral and cardiac perfusion pressure with a vasopressor, until intravascular fluid volume can be replaced. Persistent metabolic acidosis probably reflects the continued presence of hypovolemia and inadequate oxygen delivery to the tissues.

Management of Anesthesia
Induction and maintenance of anesthesia in the presence of hemorrhagic shock requires invasive monitoring of blood pressure and often includes administration of ketamine. The use of ketamine is supported by the known ability of this drug to stimulate the sympathetic nervous system and by the findings of a study in which survival was greater in acutely hemorrhaged rats anesthetized with ketamine as compared with volatile anesthetics.[11] Nevertheless, other animal evidence suggests that ketamine, in contrast to volatile anesthetics, is associated with inadequate tissue perfusion, as reflected by the development of metabolic acidosis.[12] Clinically, adverse metabolic effects of ketamine may be offset by the benefit of maintaining perfusion pressure to vital organs, until intravascular fluid volume can be restored.

APLASTIC ANEMIA

Aplastic anemia refers to bone marrow failure, characterized by destruction of rapidly growing cells normally present in the marrow. Pancytopenia is the most frequent presentation. The most common etiology is the destruction of bone marrow stem cells by cancer chemotherapeutic drugs. This form of bone marrow depression usually responds to removal of the offending drug and to supportive treatment with transfusions of RBCs until surviving stem cells can repopulate the bone marrow. Other causes of aplastic anemia, which are less responsive to this treatment, include solvents, radiation, viral infections, and immunologic disorders. Chloramphenicol causes aplastic anemia in approximately 1 of every 10,000 to 20,000 treated patients, possibly reflecting a unique genetic susceptibility. Bone marrow transplantation as treatment of aplastic anemia may be considered in selected patients. Immunosuppressive therapy with antilymphocyte globulin or corti-

Table 24-4.   Clinical Signs Associated With Acute Blood Loss

Blood Volume Lost (%)	Signs
10	None
20–30	Orthostatic hypotension Tachycardia
40	Tachycardia Hypotension Tachypnea Diaphoresis

costeroids may be an alternative to bone marrow transplantation.

Fanconi Syndrome

Variations of aplastic anemia occur in pediatric patients. For example, Fanconi syndrome is congenital aplastic anemia plus numerous associated anomalies, including patchy hyperpigmentation, microcephaly, exaggerated tendon reflexes, strabismus, and short stature. Defects of the bones of the radial sides of the forearm and hand are frequent. Cleft palate may be present. Cardiac defects and abnormalities of the genitourinary tract have been observed. There is an increased incidence of malignancy in these patients. Treatment of Fanconi syndrome is with erythrocytes, corticosteroids, and androgens.

Diamond-Blackfan Syndrome

Diamond-Blackfan syndrome is a form of pure erythrocyte aplasia, presenting as severe anemia in the first few months of life. Leukocyte and platelet production is normal. Anomalies associated with this syndrome include neck webbing and abnormalities of the first digit of the hand. These infants are treated with RBCs and corticosteroids. Splenectomy may be required for patients resistant to corticosteroids. An infant form of erythrocyte aplasia is associated with thymomas and myasthenia gravis. This association may reflect an immunologic mechanism or the presence of erythropoietic inhibitory factors. Thymectomy will cure about 30% of patients with this form of anemia.

Management of Anesthesia

Management of anesthesia for patients with aplastic anemia requires an understanding of the disease process and of the drugs being used in its treatment.[13] For example, supplementation with corticosteroids may be necessary during the perioperative period. Anemia may be profound, requiring transfusions of RBCs before the induction of anesthesia. The vulnerability of these patients to infection in the presence of pancytopenia must be appreciated, and care must be taken to avoid iatrogenic infection from equipment used during the perioperative period. Thrombocytopenia introduces the risk of hemorrhage with even minor trauma. Intubation of the trachea should be performed when indicated, but it must be appreciated that trauma associated with this procedure could produce hemorrhage in the airway. The choice of drugs used to produce anesthesia is not influenced by the presence of aplastic anemia, although the possible depressant effect of nitrous oxide on bone marrow is a consideration. Maintenance of PaO_2 close to 100 mmHg and the avoidance of anesthetic-induced decreases in cardiac output are important goals during anesthesia, to ensure optimal tissue oxygenation.

MEGALOBLASTIC ANEMIA

Megaloblastic anemia is most often due to deficiencies of vitamin B_{12} (cobalamin) or of folic acid. Both vitamins must be supplied by the diet, as neither is produced in adequate amounts by intrinsic synthesis.

Vitamin B_{12} Deficiency

Vitamin B_{12} is released from ingested proteins in the stomach by enzymatic proteolysis. Absorption of released B_{12} is dependent on a glycoprotein produced by the gastric parietal cells. This glycoprotein is known as intrinsic factor. Malabsorption of B_{12} from the small intestine, due to disease or surgical resection, is the usual cause of vitamin B_{12} deficiency. In addition, atrophy of the gastric mucosa, presumably due to an autoimmune response, results in the absence of intrinsic factor and subsequent inability to absorb vitamin B_{12}. Pernicious anemia refers to megaloblastic anemia that reflects B_{12} deficiency due to atrophy of the gastric mucosa and to a subsequent lack of intrinsic factor. The demonstration of a decreased plasma vitamin B_{12} concentration confirms the diagnosis of pernicious anemia. Thyroid disorders are more common in patients with pernicious anemia.

In addition to megaloblastic anemia, vitamin B_{12} deficiency is associated with a bilateral peripheral neuropathy due to degeneration of the lateral and posterior columns of the spinal cord. There are symmetric paresthesias with loss of proprioceptive and vibratory sensations, especially in the lower extremities. Gait is unsteady, and deep tendon reflexes are diminished. Memory impairment and mental depression may be prominent. These neurologic deficits are progressive, unless parenteral vitamin B_{12} is provided.

Management of Anesthesia

Management of anesthesia in patients with megaloblastic anemia due to vitamin B_{12} deficiency must consider the need to maintain delivery of oxygenated arterial blood to peripheral tissues. The presence of neurologic changes may detract from the selection of regional anesthetic techniques or the use of a peripheral nerve block. The use of nitrous oxide is questionable, as this drug has been shown to inhibit activity of methionine synthetase by oxidizing the cobalt atom of vitamin B_{12} from an active to an inactive state.[14] Indeed, prolonged inhalation of nitrous oxide results in megaloblastic anemia and in neurologic changes indistinguishable from pernicious anemia.[15,16] Even relatively short exposures to nitrous oxide may produce megaloblastic changes.[17]

Folic Acid

Folic acid deficiency is the most common of the vitamin deficiencies. Since folic acid is essential for maturation of RBCs, it is not surprising that megaloblastic anemia develops when there is dietary deficiency of this vitamin. Manifestations of folic acid deficiency include a smooth tongue, hyperpigmentation, mental depression, and peripheral edema. Peripheral neuropathy may or may not accompany these changes. Liver dysfunction frequently occurs. In severely ill patients, alcoholics, and parturients, megaloblastic anemia is most likely to develop due to deficiencies of folic acid in the diet. Phenytoin and other anticonvulsant drugs, including barbiturates, are associated on rare occasions with megaloblastic anemia, presumably reflecting impaired gastrointestinal absorption of folate. Oral folic acid is effective in reversing megaloblastic anemia due to deficiencies of this substance.

HEMOLYTIC ANEMIAS

Anemia due to intravascular hemolysis is characterized by a rapid decrease in the hematocrit and an elevated plasma concentration of bilirubin. Particles released from hemolyzed RBCs may lead to disseminated intravascular coagulation. Causes of hemolysis include abnormalities of RBC membranes, enzyme defects, and abnormalities in the structure of hemoglobin (see the section, Thalassemia). These changes make RBCs so fragile that they rupture easily as they pass through capillaries, especially in the spleen. Therefore, even though the number of RBCs formed is normal, the life span (normally 90 to 120 days) is so shortened by intravascular hemolysis that anemia results.

Hereditary Spherocytosis

Hereditary spherocytosis is characterized by abnormalities of RBC membranes that permit sodium to enter RBCs at an enhanced rate. Water enters the RBCs as well, resulting in swollen or spherocytic cells. These spherical cells, in contrast to normal biconcave RBCs, cannot be compressed and are vulnerable to rupture (hemolysis) with even slight compression as they pass through the spleen. Anemia, reticulocytosis, and mild jaundice are characteristic expressions of hereditary spherocytosis. Infection or folic acid deficiency may trigger a hemolytic crisis with profound anemia, vomiting, and abdominal pain. Anemia and hyperbilirubinemia may be manifestations of this disease in neonates. Children with this defect may present with chronic mild anemia plus episodic falls in hematocrit, particularly during bacterial infections. In elderly patients who have previously been able to compensate for these abnormalities, anemia may develop in response to the decline in the ability to produce RBCs with age. Cholelithiasis secondary to chronic hemolysis and elevation of the plasma bilirubin concentration are frequent in patients with hereditary spherocytosis.

Treatment of patients with hereditary spherocytosis includes splenectomy, if anemia is severe. Splenectomy greatly reduces hemolysis, returning RBC survival to 80% of normal. Splenectomy may be followed, however, by an increased incidence of bacterial infections (especially pneumococcal) in these patients. Prophylactic pneumococcal vaccine may be indicated for this reason.

Paroxysmal Nocturnal Hemoglobinuria

Paroxysmal nocturnal hemoglobinuria is a rare acquired disorder, characterized by acute episodes of hemolysis superimposed on a background of chronic hemolysis. The defect is an abnormal sensitivity of the RBC membrane to lytic actions of complement proteins. Classically, the patient is a young adult who describes hemoglobinuria on first voiding after awakening. There is a striking predisposition for venous thrombosis, especially involving the hepatic, splenic, portal, and cerebral veins. Progressive diffuse hepatic vein thrombosis (Budd-Chiari syndrome) may be rapidly fatal. Thrombotic episodes have been attributed to direct activation of platelets by complement. Surgery with associated stasis and trauma may accentuate thrombosis. Preoperative hydration and prophylactic administration of RBCs have been advocated.[18] Vigorous attempts to prevent infection are important in decreasing the likelihood of complement activation. There is no evidence that a specific anesthetic technique or combination of drugs is preferable.[18] Because postoperative thrombosis is a hazard, it has been suggested that anticoagulation with coumadin be considered. The use of heparin for anticoagulation is controversial, as low doses may activate the complement pathway.

Glucose-6-Phosphate Dehydrogenase Deficiency

Glucose-6-phosphate dehydrogenase deficiency is the most common of the inherited RBC enzyme disorders.[19] Indeed, this deficiency affects about 10% of black males in the United States. The gene for glucose-6-phosphate dehydrogenase enzyme is on the X chromosome, accounting for the predominance of this enzyme deficiency in males. Chronic hemolytic anemia is the most common clinical manifestation of this deficiency. Drugs that form peroxides by interaction with oxyhemoglobin can trigger hemolysis in these patients (Table 24-5). Normally, these peroxides are inactivated by nicotinamide–adenine dinucleotide phosphate (NADPH) and glutathione, produced by metabolic processes dependent on the enzymatic activity of glucose-6-phosphate dehydrogenase. The onset of disseminated intravascular coagulation may accom-

Table 24-5. Drugs That May Induce Hemolysis in Patients With Glucose-6-Phosphate Dehydrogenase Deficiency

Nonopioid Analgesics
  Phenacetin
  Acetaminophen

Antibiotics
  Nitrofurans
  Penicillin
  Streptomycin
  Chloramphenicol
  Isoniazid

Sulfonamides

Antimalarial Agents

Miscellaneous
  Probenecid
  Quinidine
  Vitamin K analogues
  Methylene blue
  Nitroprusside(?)

pany drug-induced hemolysis. Although drugs used during anesthesia have not been incriminated as triggering agents, the onset of hemolysis and jaundice during the early postoperative period, particularly in a black male, should suggest this diagnosis.[20] There is considerable variability in the hemolytic response to drugs; many drugs, such as aspirin, induce hemolysis only in large doses.

Pyruvate Kinase Deficiency

Pyruvate kinase deficiency is the most common of the enzyme defects in the anaerobic glycolytic pathway of RBCs. The result of this enzyme deficiency is a RBC membrane that is highly permeable to potassium and susceptible to rupture, as evidenced by hemolytic anemia. The accumulation of 2,3-diphosphoglycerate in RBCs causes a shift of the oxyhemoglobin dissociation curve to the right and facilitation of oxygen release from hemoglobin to the peripheral tissues. Splenectomy does not prevent hemolysis but does serve to reduce greatly the rate of RBC destruction. Despite increased permeability of RBC membranes to potassium, the administration of succinylcholine has not been associated with hyperkalemia.

Immune Hemolytic Anemia

Immune hemolytic anemia is characterized by immunologic alterations in the RBC membranes. An important aspect of the evaluation of patients with suspected immune hemolytic anemias is performance of the Coombs test. Coombs antiserum is an antibody to human immunoglobulin G. The direct Coombs test is the addition of antiserum to a sample of blood from the patient. The indirect Coombs test consists of the addition of antiserum to a sample of plasma from the patient, to which have been added RBCs of known antigenicity. Clumping of RBCs in response to the addition of antiserum indicates the presence of antibodies to RBCs and is designated as a positive direct or indirect Coombs test. Immune hemolytic anemia may be due to drugs, diseases, or sensitization of RBCs.

Drug-induced Hemolysis

Alpha-methyldopa causes a time- and dose-dependent production of immunoglobulin G antibodies, directed against Rh antigens on the surfaces on RBCs. Indeed, a positive direct Coombs test is often present in patients being treated with alpha-methyldopa, but hemolysis occurs in less than 1% of patients receiving this drug. The mechanism for drug-induced stimulation of antibody production by alpha-methyldopa is unknown. Treatment consists of withdrawal of the drug, which results in a rapid increase in the hemoglobin concentration, although the direct Coombs test may remain positive for as long as 2 years.

High-dose penicillin therapy can also lead to hemolysis, by attaching to RBCs to form haptens that lead to production of antibodies. Levodopa is another drug that occasionally produces an autoimmune hemolytic anemia.

Disease-induced Hemolysis

Hypersplenism is an example of a disease process that can be associated with hemolysis, anemia, leukopenia, and thrombocytopenia. It is thought that an enlarged spleen has an increased blood flow and vascular surface area, exposing an unusually large proportion of RBCs and platelets to attack by phagocytes. For unknown reasons, hypersplenism produces marked increases in plasma volume, which result in dilutional anemia, in addition to hemolytic anemia. Splenectomy may be necessary when anemia due to hemolysis is severe. If thrombocytopenia is present, it may be desirable to infuse platelets intraoperatively, after the splenic pedicle has been surgically clamped.

Sensitization of RBCs

Sensitization of RBCs is most often manifested as hemolytic disease of the newborn (erythroblastosis fetalis). Hemolysis of fetal RBCs occurs when maternal antibodies against fetal RBCs are produced and cross the placenta. Differences in the maternal and fetal ABO blood groups can cause this form of hemolysis. Severe anemia does not usually occur, however, because ABO antibodies are of the immunoglobulin M class and, as such, do not readily cross the placenta. More often, maternal development of antibodies to Rh antigens occurs after delivery of an Rh-positive infant. During subsequent pregnancies, RBCs of an Rh-positive fetus may undergo significant hemolysis from maternal antibodies directed against Rh antigens. The incidence of the development of maternal anti-Rh antibodies has decreased to less than 1% since the introduction of Rh-immune globulin (RhoGAM). This substance, when given to the mother within 72 hours of delivery, destroys fetal RBCs in the maternal circulation, preventing the subsequent development of sensitization.

Clinical features of hemolytic disease of the newborn are related to anemia and hyperbilirubinemia. The fetus can be examined indirectly during gestation by periodic measurement of the bilirubin level in amniotic fluid samples. A fetus determined to be experiencing severe hemolysis may require intrauterine transfusion or induced delivery. Hemolysis may continue after delivery, requiring transfusion of the infant with RBCs. In addition, exchange transfusions of blood may be necessary to reduce plasma levels of bilirubin in the newborn. Eventually, maternal immunoglobulins against Rh antigens are excreted by the newborn, and hemolysis of the RBCs ceases.

Cold Hemagglutinin Disease

For a discussion of cold hemagglutinin disease, see Chapter 29.

Sickle Cell Disease

Sickle cell disease represents an inherited disorder that ranges in severity from the usually benign sickle cell trait to the debilitating and often fatal sickle cell anemia. All the variants of sickle cell disease share in the possession of various quantities of hemoglobin S (HbS). Hemoglobin S differs from normal adult hemoglobin A (HbA) by the substitution of valine for glutamic acid at the sixth position on the beta chain of the hemoglobin molecule. Confirmation of the presence of HbS is dependent on hemoglobin electrophoretic studies.

Sickle Cell Trait

Sickle cell trait is the heterozygote manifestation of sickle cell disease containing the hemoglobin genotype AS. The incidence of sickle cell trait among African Americans is 8% to 10%. The RBCs of affected persons have a HbS concentration of less than 50%; by far most patients with sickle cell trait are asymptomatic, with the exception of occasional hematuria.

Sickle Cell Anemia

Sickle cell anemia is present when a patient is homozygous for HbS, with RBCs containing 70% to 98% HbS. An estimated 0.2% of African Americans are homozygous for HbS and thus susceptible to the development of sickle cell anemia.

Sickle cell anemia is characterized by (1) chronic hemolysis that is stable and only moderately debilitating, and (2) acute episodic vaso-occlusive crises that cause organ failure. Anemia is relatively well tolerated perhaps because of enhanced oxygen delivery to the tissues by oxyHbS, as reflected by a rightward shift of the oxyhemoglobin dissociation curve (P_{50} = 31 mmHg). In contrast to anemia, a sickle cell crisis is a life-threatening complication of sickle disease.

Pathophysiology

The removal of oxygen from HbS results in deformation of the RBC into a sickle shape. Molecularly, the substitution of valine for glutamine acid provides two reactive sites when HbS releases oxygen. As a result, HbS molecules tend to bond with each other at these reactive sites, forming long aggregates, or tactoids. Tactoids of sickle cells increase the viscosity of blood, leading to stasis of blood flow. An infarctive crisis develops when localized or generalized vascular occlusion occurs, owing to formation of sickle cells. The portal circulation in which the PO_2 is normally low, as in the liver or the kidney, is at unique risk of occlusion. Precipitated HbS inside RBCs damages the RBC membrane, increasing the likelihood of rupture and hemolytic anemia.

The initiating event in the sickle crisis is unknown, nor is it clear why some patients have severe crises and others do not, although increased amounts of hemoglobin F (HbF) may be protective. A clear risk factor for sickling is a low PO_2. For example, a PaO_2 less than 40 mmHg is likely to result in the formation of sickle cells in patients who are homozygous for HbS. By contrast, sickling of RBCs in the patient with sickle cell trait probably does not occur until the PaO_2 decreases to about 20 mmHg. The formation of sickle cells tends to be greater in veins than in arteries, emphasizing the importance of pH. Indeed, the presence of acidosis favors the formation of sickle cells, regardless of the prevailing PO_2. A decrease in body temperature or exposure to cold environmental temperatures also promotes the formation of sickle cells by virtue of vasoconstriction, leading to stasis of blood flow and deoxygenation of HbS. Likewise, a hemoglobin concentration above about 8.5 g·dl^{-1} and dehydration with resulting stasis of blood flow favors formation of sickle cells. Pregnancy may be associated with pregnancy-induced hypertension, urinary tract infection, and low fetal birth weight.[21]

Signs and Symptoms

Clinical manifestations of sickle cell disease are due to chronic hemolysis that produces anemia and jaundice, as well as occlusion of blood vessels with sickle cells. These chronic events are periodically interrupted by acute exacerbations of the disease, which often include excruciating musculoskeletal pain.[22] Indeed, pain is the most common cause of acute morbidity in sickle cell disease and signals underlying sudden bone marrow ischemia or necrosis. In the steady state, the hemoglobin concentration is 5 to 10 g·dl^{-1}. Cardiac output is generally increased in compensation for the prevailing chronic anemia.

Multiple organ dysfunction produced by infarctive events in patients with sickle cell anemia is the major reason that survival beyond 30 years of age is unlikely. For example, cardiomegaly most likely reflects cor pulmonale, owing to repeated pulmonary emboli. An increased alveolar-to-arterial difference for oxygen is often present, presumably reflecting pulmonary infarctive events produced by sickle cells. Because of its low PO$_2$, the renal medulla is a frequent site of vascular occlusion with sickle cells. Infarctive events in the renal medulla lead to papillary necrosis with hematuria, impaired ability to concentrate urine, and ultimately renal failure. Hepatic damage may reflect impaired blood flow as a result of sickling in hepatic sinusoids where the PO$_2$ is low. Increased bilirubin loads from chronic hemolysis are associated with a high incidence of cholelithiasis. The need for periodic blood transfusion may increase the risk of blood-transmitted diseases. In severe cases requiring frequent blood transfusions, the resulting increased iron load may be deposited in the liver as hemosiderin leading to cirrhosis. Left ventricular dysfunction may reflect deposition of excess iron in the heart. Splenomegaly is often present in infants with sickle cell anemia. A gradual decrease in the size of the spleen occurs with repeated thrombosis and infarction; by 6 years of age, most patients with sickle cell anemia are asplenic. The absence of splenic function is associated with decreased production of antibodies and an increased risk of the development of bacterial infection. In this regard, pneumococcal vaccine may be indicated as prophylaxis in adults, whereas children may require supplementary penicillin. Neurologic dysfunction is likely in patients with sickle cell anemia, manifested most often as cerebral infarction in children and as intracranial hemorrhage in adults. Aseptic necrosis of the femoral head may necessitate total hip replacement.

An infarctive crisis may be triggered by trauma or infection, with an associated increase in body temperature. The acute onset of pain, often abdominal in location, may signal the beginning of an infarctive crisis. Episodes of abdominal pain associated with fever and vomiting can mimic surgical disease.

In addition to infarctive events and hemolysis, patients with sickle cell anemia are susceptible to the development of aplastic and sequestration crises. Aplastic crises are characterized by bone marrow depression and by a rapidly declining hematocrit, often in association with a viral infection. Sequestration crises are due to depletion of circulating RBCs by virtue of pooling of these cells in the liver and spleen. A patient experiencing sequestration crisis may become acutely hypovolemic and die.

Treatment

Treatment of a painful infarctive crisis is with hydration and intravenous administration of sodium bicarbonate to produce mild alkalinization of the blood. Pain may require treatment

with an opioid. The use of epidural analgesia, using a local anesthetic or an opioid, or both, may be useful in the patient experiencing a vaso-occlusive crisis, if most of the pain is in the lower abdomen or legs.[23] A partial exchange transfusion with RBCs containing HbA will decrease the concentration of HbS and the extent of HbS polymerization, decreasing the likelihood of further infarctive damage.[24] Sickle crisis occurring at the time of delivery is treated with a partial exchange transfusion. The goal of an exchange transfusion is to increase the HbA concentration to close to 50%. It is probably beneficial to keep the hematocrit below 35% with an exchange transfusion because of the influence of hematocrit on blood viscosity and stasis. A mechanism to stimulate the gene that produces HbF may lessen the severity of sickle cell disease. Indeed, administration of hydroxyurea stimulates HbF production and may result in clinical improvement when HbF levels reach about 20%.[25]

Management of Anesthesia

The possible presence of sickle cell disease must be considered in the preoperative evaluation of every black patient. Sickle cell disease may also be present in persons from certain areas of India and Saudia Arabia. The patient with sickle cell trait probably is not at increased risk during the perioperative period. Conversely, the patient with sickle cell anemia must be given special consideration in the management of anesthesia.

Orthopaedic conditions requiring surgical correction are frequent in the patient with sickle cell anemia. For example, necrosis of the head of the femur is common. The incidence of *Salmonella* osteomyelitis is increased. Leg ulcers are often present, requiring skin grafting. The presence of gallstones is reflected by the frequent need for cholecystectomy in these patients. Priapism is a common occurrence in patients with sickle cell anemia. Renal transplantation may be necessary if renal failure develops.[26] Cardiopulmonary bypass, with its attendant low peripheral blood flow plus hypothermia and acidosis, poses a special peril to the patient with sickle cell anemia.[27]

Preoperative preparation should include the correction of any co-existing infection and achievement of an adequate state of hydration and stable hematologic state. The need for preoperative transfusion of RBCs is determined by the severity of co-existing anemia and by the magnitude of the planned surgery. The goal of preoperative infusion of RBCs is to increase the concentration of HbA to close to 50% and to achieve an hematocrit of about 35%.[28] The hazards of preoperative transfusion include depression of hyperactive bone marrow and increased blood viscosity.

Goals in management of anesthesia include avoidance of acidosis due to hypoventilation of the lungs, maintenance of optimal oxygenation, prevention of circulatory stasis due to improper body positioning or use of tourniquets, and maintenance of normal body temperature.[29] Preoperative medication must not produce excessive depression of ventilation. The concentration of inspired oxygen should be increased, to ensure maintenance of a normal to increased PaO_2. Monitoring of the mixed venous oxygen partial pressure may be helpful in recognizing the patient who is vulnerable to the development of sickle cells and in whom therapeutic measures to increase oxygenation are indicated. Administration of supplemental oxygen may be prudent if a regional anesthetic technique is selected. Prevention of circulatory stasis requires (1) maintenance of cardiovascular stability by the appropriate adjustment of the depth of anesthesia, (2) anticipation and rapid correction of hypotension, and (3) maintenance of intravascular fluid volume by the intravenous infusion of a crystalloid solution. An orthopaedic tourniquet is indicated only when optimal surgical results depend on its use.[30] Hazards introduced by the use of a tourniquet include localized stasis of blood flow, acidosis, and hypoxemia, with the subsequent formation of sickle cells. Overzealous transfusion of RBCs can lead to undesirable increases in viscosity of the blood, predisposing to stasis of blood flow. Maintenance of normal body temperature is important to prevent vasoconstriction and stasis of blood flow.

There is no evidence that one anesthetic drug or combination of drugs is superior for administration to the patient with sickle cell anemia.[31] Indeed, there may be a decrease in the number of circulating sickle cells during and immediately after general anesthesia, regardless of the drugs employed.[32] The use of succinylcholine may be modified by occasional occurrences of decreased plasma cholinesterase activity in these patients.[33] Regional anesthetic techniques have been advocated in preference to general anesthesia, but the same precautions regarding ventilation, oxygenation, hypotension, and stasis of blood flow must be appreciated.[23] Epidural or spinal anesthesia produce compensatory vasoconstriction and a decreased PaO_2 in the nonblocked areas, making these areas possible sites for infarction.[34]

The postoperative period is a crucial time for patients with sickle cell anemia. Incisional pain, the use of analgesics, a high incidence of pulmonary infection, and an expected decrease in PaO_2 all predispose to the formation of sickle cells. Depending on the operative site, PaO_2 may not return to the preoperative level for several days after surgery. Supplemental oxygen and maintenance of intravascular fluid volume and body temperature are important considerations.

Methemoglobinemia

Methemoglobin is HbA in which iron exists in the ferric, rather than the normal ferrous state. The ferric form of iron is unable to bind oxygen. As a result, the oxygen-carrying capacity of arterial blood is decreased. In addition to an inability to combine reversibly with oxygen, methemoglobin shifts the oxyhemoglobin dissociation curve to the left, making it more difficult to release oxygen to the tissues. Normally, the methemoglobin concentration is maintained less than 1% by the action of methemoglobin reductase enzyme. Congenital absence of this enzyme may predispose to the development of methemoglobinemia in a patient being treated with nitrate-containing compounds (nitroglycerin, benzocaine).[35,36]

The diagnosis of methemoglobinemia is suggested by cyanosis in the presence of a normal PaO_2 but low measured SaO_2. Calculation of the SaO_2 based on the measured PaO_2 using a nomogram will not detect the discrepancy between these two values, emphasizing the importance of measuring both PaO_2 and SaO_2 when methemoglobinemia is suspected. The absorbance characteristics of methemoglobin are such that the pulse oximeter reads a SaO_2 of about 85%, regardless of the PaO_2.[37]

Cyanosis is usually present when the plasma methemoglobin concentration is about 15% (1.5 g·dl^{-1}), although symptoms (lethargy, dizziness, and headache) are unlikely at levels less than 20%. Treatment of cyanosis owing to methemoglobinemia is with methylene blue (1 to 2 mg·kg^{-1} IV over 5 minutes), which is effective by transferring electrons from NADPH to methemoglobin. This dose may be repeated every 60 minutes if cyanosis persists, but it must be appreciated that doses in excess of about 7 mg·kg^{-1} may oxidize hemoglobin to methemoglobin. The recurrence of cyanosis several hours later presumably reflects release of nitrates from tissues into the peripheral blood. Methylene blue should not be administered to patients with glucose 6-phosphate dehydrogenase deficiency, as hemolytic anemia may occur.

Sulfhemoglobinemia

Sulfhemoglobinemia resembles methemoglobinemia in that neither form of hemoglobin can carry oxygen, and both conditions are associated with cyanosis, despite the presence of an adequate PaO_2.[38] Drugs that stimulate the formation of methemoglobin are also capable of leading to the production of sulfhemoglobin. Indeed, the most common cause of sulfhemoglobinemia is the oxidation of iron in hemoglobin by drugs. The reason that some patients show the development of sulfhemoglobinemia and others methemoglobinemia is unknown. In contrast to methemoglobin, sulfhemoglobin cannot be reconverted to hemoglobin by methylene blue. The only means of removing sulfhemoglobin is by the eventual destruction of affected RBCs.

LEUKOCYTES

Leukocytes are categorized as neutrophils, lymphocytes, eosinophils, basophils, and monocytes (Table 24-6). Certain clinical disorders alter the normal levels of leukocytes in the peripheral blood.

Table 24-6. Leukocyte Values in Peripheral Blood

	Range (cells·mm^{-3})	Total (%)
Neutrophils	1800–7200	55
Lymphocytes	1500–4000	36
Eosinophils	0–700	2
Basophils	0–150	1
Monocytes	200–900	6
All leukocytes	4300–10,000	100

Neutrophils

Neutrophils (polymorphonuclear leukocytes) are the first line of defense against bacterial infection, as they are attracted to the site of inflammation by the process of chemotaxis. A major chemotaxic stimulus for neutrophils is C5a, which may be produced by activation of the complement system by a combination of bacterial antigen and antibody. A variety of events may impair chemotaxis (Table 24-7). Influenza greatly decreases chemotaxis, perhaps explaining the tendency toward superinfections, particularly pneumonia. The rate at which neutrophils move toward a chemotactic stimulus is decreased by drugs used during anesthesia, including halothane, enflurane, and morphine. The decreased motility of neutrophils toward a chemotactic stimulus could increase the risk of bacterial infection. Nevertheless, there is no evidence that general anesthesia increases the risk of postoperative infection (see Chapter 27). Neutrophilia most often reflects the increased production of cells as a reflection of bacterial infection. Impaired egress of neutrophils from the circulation is produced by exercise and corticosteroids. Neutropenia (neutrophil count less than 1800 cells·mm^{-3}) is common in patients with infectious mononucleosis and acquired immunodeficiency syndrome (AIDS). Chemotherapy may lead to neutropenia as a reflection of direct bone marrow suppression.

The administration of granulocyte colony stimulating factors in an effort to increase granulocyte production is a consideration in the patient with neutropenia, owing to chemotherapy, AIDS, thermal injury, or sepsis. Adverse effects of this treatment with importance for the management of anesthesia include pericardial and pleural effusion and a generalized capillary leak syndrome that may lead to interstitial pulmonary edema and perioperative arterial hypoxemia.[39] Preoperative echocardiography is useful in identifying an otherwise asymptomatic pericardial effusion that may merit treatment. Another complication of treatment with colony stimulating factors is thrombosis around the central venous catheter.

Lymphocytes

Lymphocytes are important in the production of immunoglobulins and in the recognition of foreign proteins. Lymphocytosis is typically associated with a viral infection. Lymphocytopenia is a common finding in AIDS patients.

Eosinophils

Eosinophils contain proteins that are toxic to parasites. Eosinophilia may accompany allergic reactions, fungal infections, and diseases such as polyarteritis nodosa and sarcoidosis. Löffler syndrome is eosinophilia plus pulmonary infiltrates, cough, dyspnea, and elevations in body temperature. Treatment of this syndrome is with corticosteroids. Hypereosinophilic syndrome is associated with cardiomyopathy, ataxis, peripheral neuropathy, and recurrent thromboembolism that may necessitate anticoagulation. Decreases in the circulating plasma eosinophil count is not a common sign of underlying disease.

Basophils and Mast Cells

Basophils are circulating cells, whereas mast cells are predominantly present in tissues. These cells contain granules that release chemical mediators (histamine, leukotrienes) during allergic reactions.

Monocytes

Monocytes, and their tissue counterparts, macrophages, are collectively referred to as the mononuclear phagocytic system (formerly known as the reticuloendothelial system). These cells are important in modifying immune function and may also act as phagocytes. Substances secreted by activated monocytes and macrophages include interleukin-1, tumor necrosis factor, interferon, and transforming growth factor.

Table 24-7. Causes of Impaired Chemotaxis

Diabetes mellitus
Hemodialysis
Rheumatoid arthritis
Alcohol ingestion
Influenza
Anesthetic drugs

POLYCYTHEMIA

Polycythemia is present when the hematocrit exceeds about 55%. Blood viscosity, which is responsible for many of the adverse effects of polycythemia, is determined principally by the hematocrit. Phlebotomy is often used to decrease the hematocrit toward a normal level.

Absolute Polycythemia

Accelerated erythropoiesis owing to secretion of the renal hormone erythropoietin is the most likely cause of an absolute increase in RBC mass. Polycythemia vera is an absolute increase in RBC mass that is unrelated to erythropoietin (see Chapter 28).

Relative Polycythemia

Relative polycythemia reflects increased RBC production in response to a decrease in PaO_2 below about 60 mmHg. Cardiopulmonary disease or ascent to altitude may result in a PaO_2 that stimulates RBC production. Another cause of relative polycythemia is cigarette smoking (smoker's polycythemia). Smoking generates carbon monoxide, leading to carboxyhemoglobin levels of 5% to 7% in those who smoke 1.5 packs of cigarettes daily. In these patients, carboxyhemoglobin is unable to load and transport oxygen, leading to the formation of hemoglobin that unloads oxygen poorly (P_{50} less than 26 mmHg). The end result is tissue hypoxia, which stimulates the secretion of erythropoietin. In addition, many cigarette smokers experience a decrease in plasma volume, contributing further to the increased hematocrit. The diagnosis of smoker's polycythemia is confirmed by measurement of the plasma carboxyhemoglobin level at the end of the day. Since the half-time of carboxyhemoglobin is about 4 hours, a fasting measurement taken in the morning, when the patient has not smoked for several hours, may give a false low result. Cessation of smoking for about 5 days usually corrects the decreased plasma volume, and the hematocrit decreases.

REFERENCES

1. Beutler E. The common anemias. JAMA 1988;259:2433–37
2. Willis JL. Transfusion of red cells. FDA Drug Bull 1988;18:26–7
3. National Institutes of Health Consensus Conference: Perioperative red blood cell transfusion. JAMA 1988;260:2700–4
4. Crosby ET. Perioperative haemotherapy: I Indications for blood component transfusion. Can J Anaesth 1992;39:695–707
5. Ellis DE, Stoelting RK. Individual variations in fluroxene, halothane, and methoxyflurane blood-gas partition coefficients, and the effect of anemia. Anesthesiology 1975;42:748–50
6. Lerman J, Gregory GA, Eger EI. Hematocrit and the solubility of volatile anesthetics in blood. Anesth Analg 1984;63:911–4
7. Barrera M, Miletich DJ, Albrecht RF, Hoffman WE. Hemodynamic consequences of halothane anesthesia during chronic anemia. Anesthesiology 1984;61:36–42
8. Smith PR, Manjoney DL, Teitcher JB, et al. Massive hemothorax due to intrathoracic extramedullary hematopoiesis in a patient with thalassemia intermedia. Chest 1988;94:658–61
9. Jackson DV, Randall ME, Richards F. Spinal cord compression due to extramedullary hematopoiesis in thalassemia: Long term follow-up after radiotherapy. Surg Neurol 1988;29:389–96
10. Adamson J, Hillman RS. Blood volume and plasma protein replacement following acute blood loss in normal man. JAMA 1968;205:609–13
11. Longnecker DE, Sturgill BC. Influence of anesthetic agent on survival following hemorrhage. Anesthesiology 1976;45:516–21
12. Weiskopf RB, Townsley MI, Riordan KK, et al. Comparison of cardiopulmonary responses to graded hemorrhage during enflurane, halothane, isoflurane, and ketamine anesthesia. Anesth Analg 1981;160:481–91
13. Bruce DL, Koepke JA. Anesthetic management of patients with bone-marrow failure. Anesth Analg 1972;51:597–606
14. Koblin DD, Watson JE, Deady JE, et al. Inactivation of methionine synthetase by nitrous oxide in mice. Anesthesiology 1981;54:318–24
15. Kripke BJ, Talarico L, Shah NK, Kelman AD. Hematologic reaction to prolonged exposure to nitrous oxide. Anesthesiology 1977;47:342–8
16. Spence AA. Environmental pollution by inhalation anaesthetics. Br J Anaesth 1987;59:96–109
17. Berger JJ, Modell JH, Sypert GW. Megaloblastic anemia and brief exposure to nitrous oxide—a causal relationship? Anesth Analg 1988;67:197–8
18. Ogen GA. Cholecystectomy in a patient with paroxysmal nocturnal hemoglobinuria: Anesthetic implications and management in the perioperative period. Anesthesiology 1990;72:761–4
19. Beutler E. Glucose-6-phosphate dehydrogenase deficiency. N Engl J Med 1991;324:169–75
20. Shapley JM, Wilson JR. Post-anaesthetic jaundice due to glucose-6-phosphate dehydrogenase deficiency. Can Anaesth Soc J 1973;20:390–2
21. Serjeant GR. Sickle haemoglobin and pregnancy. Br Med J 1983;287:628–31
22. Platt OS, Thorington BD, Brambella DJ, et al. Pain in sickle cell disease: Rates and risk factors. N Engl J Med 1991;325:11–6
23. Finer P, Blair J, Rowe P. Epidural analgesia in the management of labor pain and sickle cell crisis—a case report. Anesthesiology 1988;68:799–800
24. Zarkowsky HS, Gallagher D, Gill FM, et al. Bacteremia in sickle hemoglobinopathies. J Pediatr 1986;109:579–85
25. Charache S, Dover GJ, Moyer MA, et al. Hydroxyurea-induced augmentation of fetal hemoglobin production in patients with sickle cell anemia. Blood 1987;69:109–14
26. Gyasi HK, Zarroug AW, Matthew M, Joshi R, Daar A. Anaesthesia for renal transplantation in sickle cell disease. Can J Anaesth 1990;37:778–85
27. Heiner M, Teasdale SJ, David T, et al. Aorto-coronary bypass in a patient with sickle cell trait. Can Anaesth Soc J 1979;26:428–34
28. Schmalzer EA, Lee JO, Brown AK, et al. Viscosity of mixtures of sickle and normal red cells at varying hematocrit levels: Implications for transfusion. 1987;27:228–36
29. Esseltine DW, Baxter MRN, Bevan JC. Sickle cell states and the anaesthetist. Can J Anaesth 1988;35:385–403
30. Stein RE, Urbaniak J. Use of the tourniquet during surgery in patients with sickle cell hemoglobinopathies. Clin Orthop 1980;151:231–3

31. Homi J, Reynolds J, Skinner A, et al. General anaesthesia in sickle-cell disease. Br Med J 1979;1:1599–1600

32. Maduska AL, Guinee WS, Heaton JA, et al. Sickling dynamics of red blood cells and other physiologic studies during anesthesia. Anesth Analg 1975;54:361–5

33. Hilkovitz G, Jacobson A. Hepatic dysfunction and abnormalities of the serum proteins and serum enzymes in sickle-cell anemia. J Lab Clin Med 1961;57:856–67

34. Bridenbaugh PO, Moore DC, Bridenbaugh LD. Alterations in capillary and venous blood gases after regional-block anesthesia. Anesth Analg 1972;51:280–6

35. Gabel RA, Bunn HF. Hereditary methemoglobinemia as a cause of cyanosis during anesthesia. Anesthesiology 1974;40:516–8

36. Zurick AM, Wagner RH, Starr NJ, et al. Intravenous nitroglycerin, methemoglobinemia, and respiratory distress in a postoperative cardiac surgical patient. Anesthesiology 1984;61:464–6

37. Anderson ST, Hajduczek J, Barker SJ. Benzocaine-induced methemoglobinemia in an adult: Accuracy of pulse oximetry with methemoglobinemia. Anesth Analg 1988;67:1099–1101

38. Schmitter CR. Sulfhemoglobinemia and methemoglobinemia–uncommon causes of cyanosis. Anesthesiology 1975;43:586–7

39. Tobias JD, Furman WL. Anesthetic considerations in patients receiving colony-stimulating factors (G-CSF and GM-CSF). Anesthesiology 1991;75:536–8

Coagulation disorders may be hereditary or acquired (Table 25-1). An understanding of the normal coagulation mechanism is useful in evaluating and managing these patients during the perioperative period.

PHYSIOLOGY OF COAGULATION

Arrest of bleeding from a damaged blood vessel depends on (1) vasoconstriction at the site of injury, (2) the formation of a platelet plug at the site of injury, and (3) activation of the clotting cascade. Hemostasis is a highly localized process in which many steps take place on the surface of platelets and endothelial cells. A break in the endothelium of a blood vessel exposes flowing blood to underlying collagen, microfibrils, and basement membrane. Platelets first adhere to the injury site (platelet membrane receptors bind to specific matrix molecules) and release adenosine diphosphate (ADP), which causes other platelets to aggregate. Thromboxane A_2 may also be released, leading to localized vasoconstriction. While platelet aggregation is progressing, tissue under the vascular injury site initiates the coagulation cascade, characterized by activation of circulating clotting factors (procoagulants) (Table 25-2 and Fig. 25-1). Fibrin and thrombin interact with platelets to fuse the platelet plug. The actomysin contractile system of the platelet causes clot retraction, converting the plug into a tightly formed clot. Adhesion and aggregation of platelets seem to be necessary and sufficient to stem the initial hemorrhage from most vessel breaks, whereas fibrin formation is required for permanent hemostasis.

Coagulation is localized to the site of injury by a number of factors, including dilution of procoagulants in flowing blood, removal of activated factors by the liver, and the action of circulating procoagulant inhibitors. The most important of these inhibitors are antithrombin III and protein C. In addition, release of tissue plasminogen activator (t-PA) by injured tissue serves to convert plasminogen to plasmin. Plasmin causes the breakdown of fibrin into small segments known as fibrin

degradation (split) products, which are normally removed by the mononuclear phagocytic system.

All the plasma procoagulants except von Willebrand factor (vWF) are synthesized in the liver (Table 25-2). The synthesis of factors II, VII, IX, and X is dependent on vitamin K. Factor VIII circulates as part of a factor VIII-vWF complex. The major role of vWF is to promote adhesion of platelets to subendothelial surfaces.

PREOPERATIVE EVALUATION

Preoperative evaluation of a patient for the presence of a coagulation disorder includes the history, physical examination, and performance of appropriate laboratory tests. Careful exclusion of a coagulation defect before the induction of anesthesia facilitates the differential diagnosis of intraoperative bleeding.

History

A properly taken history is vital for the detection of an inherited or acquired coagulation disorder. One of the most important questions to ask preoperatively deals with the hemostatic response to prior surgery. Challenges to the coagulation system during infancy include umbilical cord separation and circumcision. Two common surgical procedures that test the coagulation system during childhood are tonsillectomy and dental extraction. A bleeding problem manifested in infancy or childhood suggests a congenital deficiency of an essential procoagulant. Questions regarding relatives with bleeding disorders should be pursued. The response of the coagulation system to episodes of nonsurgical trauma should also be elicited. A detailed record of drug ingestion (aspirin, oral anticoagulants) as well as questions regarding occupational exposure to toxic substances should be included. A prior history of thromboembolism suggests a hypercoagulable state, perhaps reflecting usage of estrogen-containing contraceptive drugs.

407

Table 25-1. Categorization of
Coagulation Disorders

Hereditary
Hemophilia A
Hemophilia B
von Willebrand's disease
Afibrinogenemia
Factor V deficiency
Factor XIII deficiency
Hereditary hemorrhagic telangiectasia
Protein C deficiency
Antithrombin III deficiency

Acquired
Vitamin K deficiency
Drug-induced hemorrhage
Massive blood transfusion
Postcardiopulmonary bypass
Disseminated intravascular coagulation
Drug-induced platelet dysfunction
Idiopathic thrombocytopenic purpura
Thrombotic thrombocytopenic purpura
Catheter-induced thrombocytopenia

Physical Examination

Physical examination may indicate the presence of petechiae, suggesting thrombocytopenia, abnormal platelet function, or defects in the integrity of the vascular wall. By contrast, subcutaneous bleeding in the presence of a deficiency of a procoagulant is typically manifested as ecchymoses. Likewise, hemarthrosis or deep bleeding into the skeletal muscles is more likely to reflect a procoagulant deficiency than thrombocytopenia or a defect in platelet function.

Laboratory Tests

Preoperative laboratory tests that constitute a screening coagulation profile are useful under the following conditions: (1) the history or physical examination suggests the possibility of a coagulation disorder, (2) anticoagulant or antiplatelet medication is being administered, (3) there is co-existing disease that could alter coagulation (liver disease, renal dysfunction), or (4) the scheduled surgery may alter coagulation (cardiopulmonary bypass, liver transplantation). There is no evidence that preoperative performance of coagulation tests in asymptomatic patients is of any value.[1] When laboratory tests of coagulation are indicated, measurement of bleeding time, platelet count, prothrombin time (PT), partial thromboplastin

Table 25-2. Plasma Procoagulants

Factor	Synonyms	Plasma Concentration (μg·ml^{-1})	Half-time (h)	Minimal Level for Surgical Hemostasis (% of normal)	Stability on Storage in Whole Blood (4C, 21 days)
I	Fibrinogen	2500–3500	95–120	50–100	No change
II	Prothombin	100	65–90	20–40	No change
III	Thromboplastin				
IV	Calcium				
V	Proaccelerin	10	15–24	5–20	Half-time 7 days
VI[a]					
VII	Proconvertin	0.5	4–6	10–20	No change
VIII	Antihemophilic factor	15	10–12	30	Half-time 7 days
IX	Christmas factor	3	18–30	20–25	No change
X	Stuart-Prower factor	10	40–60	10–20	No change
XI	Plasma thromboplastin antecedent	<5	45–60	20–30	Half-time 7 days
XII	Hageman factor	<5	50–70	0	No change
XIII	Fibrin-stabilizing factor	20	72–120	1–3	No change

[a] No factor has been assigned to this numeral.

COMMON PATHWAY OF COAGULATION

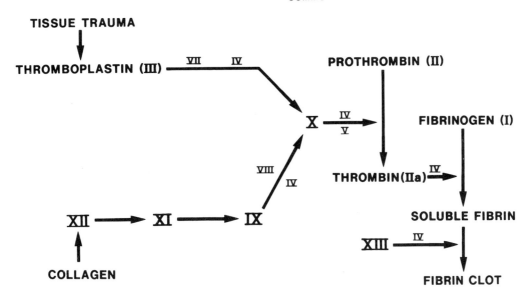

Fig. 25-1. Schematic diagram of the events leading to activation of circulating procoagulants and culminating in the formation of a fibrin clot. Artificial division of the initial steps of the coagulation cascade into an intrinsic and extrinsic coagulation pathway is no longer recommended, in view of the known interrelationships between steps initiated by tissue trauma or collagen on the walls of damaged blood vessels, or both.

time (PTT), and plasma fibrinogen concentration will provide information regarding all phases of coagulation (Table 25-3). Thrombelastography may be considered in selected patients, especially if rapid perioperative evaluation of coagulation is desired.

Table 25-3. Tests of Coagulation

	Normal Value	Measures
Bleeding time (Ivy)	3–10 min	Platelet count, vascular integrity
Platelet count	150,000–400,000 cells·mm^{-3}	
Prothrombin time	12–14 sec	Factors I, II, V, VII, X
Partial thromboplastin time	25–35 sec	Factors I, II, V, VIII, IX, X, XI, XII
Thrombin time	12–20 sec	Factors I, II
Fibrinogen	200–400 mg·dl^{-1}	
Fibrin degradation products	<4 μg·ml^{-1}	
Thrombelastography	See Fig. 25-2	Procoagulants and platelets

Platelet Function

A carefully performed standardized skin bleeding time is the best measure of platelet function. The hallmark of a defect in platelet function is a prolonged bleeding time (greater than 10 minutes) despite a platelet count greater than 100,000 cells·mm^{-3}. Limitations of the bleeding time must be appreciated. For example, bleeding time may be prolonged in the presence of anemia or a platelet count of less than 100,000 cells·mm^{-3}. Factitious prolongation of bleeding time may be caused by patient movement.[2] There is no evidence that skin bleeding time parallels bleeding elsewhere in the body. In fact, aspirin, which prolongs skin bleeding time, has no effect on the duration of bleeding after endoscopic gastric biopsy.[3] Most importantly, no study has established the ability of a bleeding time measurement to predict the risk of hemorrhage in individual patients.[3]

Clot retraction is a qualitative method that evaluates the function of the platelet contractile mechanism. A platelet count estimates only the number, and not the function, of these cells. A platelet count of 50,000 or greater is recommended before undertaking an elective surgical procedure.[3,4] The risk of spontaneous intracranial hemorrhage may be increased when the platelet count is less than 30,000 cells·mm^{-3}.

Table 25-4.   Impact of Anticoagulants on Tests of Coagulation

Anticoagulant	Factors Inhibited	Prothrombin Time	Partial Thromboplastin Time
Heparin			
Low dose	IX	Normal	Prolonged
High dose	II, IX, X	Prolonged	Prolonged
Coumarin			
Low dose	VII	Prolonged	Normal
High dose	II, VII, IX, X	Prolonged	Prolonged

Prothrombin Time

PT is a test that reflects deficiencies of factors I (less than 100 mg·dl^{-1}), II (prothrombin), V, VII, and X. Antagonists of these factors, including heparin (small doses less likely than large doses), coumarin, and fibrin degradation products, can also prolong the PT (Table 25-4). Neither the presence nor the absence of factor VIII activity is reflected by the PT. The normal PT is 12 to 14 seconds; curves based on a commercial standard are often used to express this time as a percentage of the normal response.

Partial Thromboplastin Time

PTT is a test that reflects the presence of a plasma deficiency of all the procoagulants, with the exception of factors VII and XIII. For example, a small dose of a coumarin anticoagulant inhibits factor VII, and the PTT is not prolonged (Table 25-4). Conversely, a small dose of heparin inhibits the activity of factor IX, and the PTT is prolonged (Table 25-4). Ideally, the therapeutic dose of heparin is adjusted to maintain the PTT at about double the normal value of 25 to 35 seconds.

Thrombin Time

Thrombin time reflects abnormalities affecting the conversion of fibrinogen to fibrin. Inhibitors of this conversion, such as heparin and fibrin degradation products, are manifested as a prolonged thrombin time. Fibrin degradation products are the result of the breakdown of fibrinogen and fibrin by plasmin. Elevated plasma concentrations of fibrin degradation products (greater than 4 μg·ml^{-1}) most often accompany secondary fibrinolysis, owing to disseminated intravascular coagulation (DIC). Primary fibrinolysis is rare but has been observed in association with cardiopulmonary bypass, cirrhosis of the liver, and carcinoma of the prostate. A low plasma concentration of fibrinogen most likely due to DIC is also manifested as a prolonged thrombin time.

Thrombelastography

Thrombelastography is a test that evaluates overall clot formation as a dynamic process (unlike standard coagulation tests that measure isolated end points), permitting the diagnosis of a procoagulant deficiency (hemophilia), platelet dysfunction, fibrinolysis (DIC), and hypercoagulation within 30 minutes of obtaining a blood sample[5,6] (Figs. 25-2 and 25-3). In this regard, thrombelastography offers a unique method of monitoring coagulation that is practical for use in the operating room. Coagulation during liver transplantation and after cardiopulmonary bypass may be monitored by thrombelastography. Using this test, it has been demonstrated that progressive blood loss during surgery is associated with a trend toward hypercoagulability.[7] Certainly, the use of fresh frozen plasma or platelets, or both, during moderate or massive blood loss, without docu-

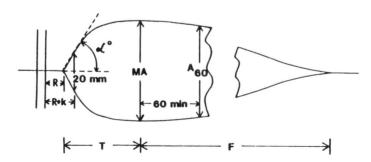

Fig. 25-2.   Variables and normal values measured by thrombelastography. R, reaction time for initial fibrin formation, 6 to 8 minutes; R + K, coagulation time, 10 to 12 minutes; alpha (α°), clot formation rate, greater than 50 degrees; MA, maximum amplitude, 50 to 70 mm; A$_{60}$, amplitude 60 minutes after MA; F, whole blood clot lysis time, greater than 300 minutes. (From Kang YG, Martin DJ, Marquez J, et al. Intraoperative changes in blood coagulation and thrombelastographic monitoring in liver transplantation. Anesth Analg 1985;64:888–96, with permission.)

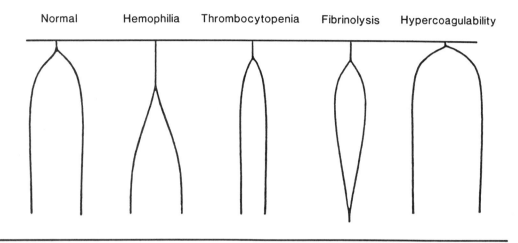

Fig. 25-3. Schematic depiction of coagulopathy as reflected by the thrombelastograph. Compared with the normal thrombelastograph, an absence of coagulation factors (hemophilia) is characterized by a prolonged R and decreased alpha; thrombocytopenia or platelet dysfunction by a prolonged R and decreased MA and alpha; fibrinolysis by decreased MA, alpha, and F; and hypercoagulation by a shortened R and increased MA, alpha, and F. See Figure 25-2 for definition of abbreviations.

mentation of a specific defect, as with thrombelastography, is unwarranted.[7] It is likely that surgical stress, tissue trauma with release of tissue thromboplastin, and increases in the plasma concentration of catecholamines offset any hypercoagulable tendency that results from progressive blood loss.

HEREDITARY COAGULATION DISORDERS

Hereditary (congenital) coagulation disorders are usually due to the absence or decreased presence of a single procoagulant.[8] The three most common hereditary coagulation disorders are hemophilia A (factor VIII deficiency, classic hemophilia), hemophilia B (factor IX deficiency, Christmas disease), and von Willebrand's disease. Knowledge of the deficient or absent procoagulant, of its elimination half-time after exogenous administration, and of the products available for treatment of the coagulation disorder is important in the preoperative evaluation of the affected patient (Table 25-2) (see the section, Transfusion Therapy). Most often, management of coagulation therapy for a patient with a hereditary coagulation disorder undergoing surgery is coordinated with a hematologist.

Hemophilia A

Hemophilia A is an X-linked recessive genetic disorder affecting approximately 1 in 10,000 males that is due to a defective or deficient factor VIII:C molecule, resulting in a hemor-

rhagic tendency. All patients with hemophilia A have a normal plasma concentration of vWF. The female serves as the asymptomatic carrier of the disease. In its most severe form, hemophilia A is a life-threatening and crippling disease. In this regard, there is a direct relationship between the plasma concentration of factor VIII and the severity of bleeding (Table 25-5). For example, spontaneous hemorrhage is likely, when the factor VIII concentration is less than 3% of the normal value (Table 25-5). Indeed, central nervous system bleeding is the major cause of death in patients with hemophilia. Deep tissue bleeding, which may cause nerve compression, hemarthrosis, and hematuria, are common forms of bleeding associated with this coagulation defect.

A useful screening test for hemophilia A is the PTT. This test will be prolonged in all but those with mild disease; for

Table 25-5. Factor VIII Concentrations Necessary for Hemostasis

	Factor VIII Concentration (% of normal)
Spontaneous hemorrhage	1–3
Moderate trauma	4–8
Hemarthrosis and deep skeletal muscle hemorrhage	10–15
Major surgery	>30

example, it is likely to be prolonged when the plasma concentration of factor VIII is less than 50% of normal. The PT is normal in the patient with hemophilia A, as this test does not measure factor VIII activity.

Preoperative Preparation

The goal of preoperative preparation of the patient with hemophilia A is to establish a factor VIII plasma concentration that will ensure hemostasis in the perioperative period (Table 25-5). Calculation of factor VIII replacement therapy is based on the convention that 100% of a procoagulant means there is 1 unit of procoagulant for each milliliter of plasma and that the plasma volume is 40 ml·kg^{-1}. Therefore, a 50-kg patient with less than 1% of procoagulant activity would require 2000 units of factor VIII to increase its concentration to 100% of normal (40 ml·kg^{-1} × 50 kg × 1 unit·ml^{-1}). This dose should be repeated every 12 hours based on a factor VIII elimination half-time of 10 to 12 hours. Ideally, the level of factor VIII should be increased to nearly 100% before elective surgery, such as a dental extraction, and then maintained above 50% for the next 10 to 14 days.[9] A plasma factor VIII concentration greater than 30% of normal is considered adequate for hemostasis after major surgery. Despite achievement of an optimal factor VIII concentration, however, postoperative hemorrhage often occurs, suggesting that other causes may be important.[9] For example, the high incidence of postoperative hemorrhage after knee surgery may reflect the presence of a large surface area of inflamed synovium.

The desired amount of factor VIII:C can be administered as cryoprecipitate or as a heat-treated lypholized concentrate. The risk of disease transmission (hepatitis, acquired immunodeficiency syndrome [AIDS]) is decreased by the use of donor-screened heat-treated concentrates of factor VIII.[10] The availability of recombinant factor VIII provides safe and efficacious treatment of hemophilia A.[11] About 10% of hemophiliacs acquire an antibody inhibitor against factor VIII and hence do not achieve the anticipated factor VIII plasma concentration.

DDAVP (desmopressin) is a synthetic analogue of antidiuretic hormone; it can be administered in the treatment of traumatic hemorrhage in mild to moderate hemophiliacs and even in preparing such patients for minor surgery. DDAVP appears to cause the release of factor VIII:C from endothelial cell storage sites; as such, it cannot be used repeatedly because such stores become depleted. The elimination half-time of the released factor VIII:C is about 12 hours. Because DDAVP also releases t-PA, administration of epsilon aminocaproic acid is recommended as well. Danazol has not proved consistently effective in increasing factor VIII:C concentrations in the patient with hemophilia A.[12]

Management of Anesthesia

Preoperative medication of the patient with hemophilia A is ideally achieved with drugs administered orally. Although the intramuscular injection of drugs is described as acceptable when the plasma factor VIII concentration is at least 35% of normal, it would seem prudent to avoid this route whenever possible.[13] An anticholinergic drug can be administered intravenously before the induction of anesthesia, if it is deemed a necessary part of the anesthetic. Maintenance of anesthesia is most often with general anesthesia, as the risk of uncontrolled bleeding detracts from the selection of a regional anesthetic technique. Nevertheless, the uncomplicated use of an axillary block of the brachial plexus has been described in these patients.[13] Intubation of the trachea need not be avoided, although hemorrhage into the tongue or neck could impair the patency of the upper airway. Selection of anesthetic drugs should consider the likely presence of co-existing liver disease owing to hepatitis from prior blood or factor VIII transfusions. Likewise, the possible presence of the human immunodeficiency virus (HIV) must be considered. Superficial hemorrhage can be controlled by the application of external pressure, until treatment with factor VIII can be initiated.

Hemophilia B

Hemophilia B is an X-linked genetic disorder due to a defective or deficient factor IX molecule resulting in a hemorrhagic tendency. The inheritance pattern and clinical features are indistinguishable from those of hemophilia A. The diagnosis of hemophilia B depends on the demonstration of a low or absent plasma factor IX concentration in the presence of normal factor VIII activity. The PTT will be prolonged in the patient with hemophilia B.

Treatment of hemophilia B is with factor IX concentrate, with the goal of maintaining a plasma concentration of this procoagulant greater than 30% of normal during the perioperative period. The dosing interval of factor IX concentrate is based on an elimination half-time of 24 hours. Fresh frozen plasma (FFP) is no longer considered the first choice as a source for factor IX in the treatment of these patients.[14] Preoperative preparation and management of anesthesia are as described for hemophilia A.

von Willebrand's Disease

von Willebrand's disease is inherited as an autosomal dominant trait affecting both sexes, in contrast to X-linked hemophilia A and B. This coagulation disorder is caused by deficient or defective amounts of vWF in the plasma, which is necessary for adherence of platelets to exposed endothelium. It is likely that factor VIII is two distinct molecules with factor VIII:C and vWF present in the plasma as a complex.[15] The incidence of this defect may be as high as 2% to 3% of the population, although severe (homozygous) von Willebrand's disease is much rarer, with an incidence similar to hemophilia A.[16] Affected patients have a lifelong history of bruising and mild bleeding usually from mucosal surfaces (epistaxis), but they are unaware of a bleeding disorder, until they undergo surgery or experience trauma. Excessive bleeding from surgery or trauma is localized to the site of injury, as hemarthrosis and deep tissue bleeding are uncommon. The diagnosis of von Willebrand's disease is suggested by the patient's history and by the demonstration of a prolonged bleeding time despite a normal platelet count.

The traditional treatment of von Willebrand's disease consists of replacement of vWF with a cryoprecipitate.[16] Alternatively, DDAVP may evoke the release of vWF, serving as an effective treatment in some patients.[17] Because DDAVP seems to enhance fibrinolysis by causing the release of t-PA, the concurrent administration of epsilon aminocaproic acid can be recommended. Pregnancy evokes an increase in the plasma vWF concentration in parturients with mild to moderate forms of this coagulation disorder. Consequently, vaginal delivery can usually be performed without incident.

Afibrinogenemia

Congenital absence of fibrinogen activity may first present as continued bleeding from the stump of the umbilical cord. Minor trauma can precipitate severe hemorrhage, but hemarthroses do not occur. Bleeding time, PT, PTT, and thrombin time are usually prolonged. Quantitative determination of the plasma fibrinogen concentration demonstrates only a trace amount or the total absence of this procoagulant. Treatment is with fibrinogen or cryoprecipitate, to increase the plasma fibrinogen concentration to at least 50 mg·dl^{-1}.

Factor V Deficiency

Factor V deficiency is inherited as an autosomal recessive trait affecting both sexes. Bleeding time, PT, and PTT are prolonged. Bleeding is most often from the mucous membranes, although hemorrhage from accidental trauma or surgery can be extreme. Severe menorrhagia may be a manifestation of this coagulation disorder. Treatment is with FFP to maintain the plasma concentration of factor V within the range of 5% to 20% of normal.[14]

Factor XII Deficiency

Factor XII (Hageman factor) deficiency is not associated with excessive bleeding after trauma or surgery despite prolonged clotting in vitro. In fact, patients with factor XII deficiency may be vulnerable to thromboembolic complications. Congenital deficiency of this factor is suggested when routine preoperative blood coagulation studies demonstrate a prolonged PTT despite a negative bleeding history. No substitution therapy is needed for these patients, even during cardiac surgery.[18] Standard tests to monitor heparin activity depend on in vitro activation of factor XII, making it impossible to monitor heparin activity intraoperatively in these patients. Instead, heparin is given according to weight-based protocols; a normal dose-response relationship is assumed. Alternatively, measurement of the plasma heparin concentration before and after cardiopulmonary bypass confirms maintenance of anticoagulation and its reversal in the factor XII-deficient patient.[18]

Factor XIII Deficiency

Deficiency of factor XIII results in an inability to form insoluble fibrin, manifested at birth as persistent bleeding from the stump of the umbilical cord. In later life, this procoagulant deficiency can result in delayed hemorrhage after accidental trauma or surgery. Central nervous system hemorrhage is common. The position of factor XIII in the coagulation pathway results in normal values of all the routine tests for coagulation (Fig. 25-1). Treatment is with FFP or cryoprecipitate.[14]

Hereditary Hemorrhagic Telangiectasia

Hereditary hemorrhagic telangiectasia (Osler-Weber-Rendu syndrome) is an inherited non-sex-linked disorder, characterized by an abnormal vascular ultrastructure resulting in telangiectasia; arteriovenous fistula formation, especially in the lungs; and the development of aneurysms throughout the cardiovascular system. High-output congestive heart failure may reflect the effect of systemic arteriovenous shunts, whereas arterial hypoxemia and paradoxical air embolism may reflect similar shunts in the lungs. Epistaxis is a common complaint.

Management of anesthesia must take into consideration the possibility of hemorrhage from telangiectatic lesions that may be present in the oropharynx, trachea, and esophagus. Epidural anesthesia has been described for the parturient in labor with Osler-Weber-Rendu syndrome; the risk of neurologic sequelae should be kept in mind, in the event that the bleeding tendency leads to the formation of an epidural hematoma.[19]

May-Hegglin Anomaly

May-Hegglin anomaly is a rare inherited disorder characterized by thrombocytopenia and a bleeding diathesis, manifested commonly as purpura and epistaxis. Tests of platelet function are usually normal, but bleeding time may be prolonged, emphasizing that abnormal bleeding is due to the low platelet count, and not to platelet dysfunction. Since this anomaly is an autosomal dominant trait, a thrombocytopenic fetus would be expected in about one-half of afflicted parturients. Experience with the management of anesthesia in these patients is limited, although spinal anesthesia in a parturient has been described.[20] Preoperative administration of platelet concentrates seems prudent.

Hypercoagulable States

Protein C Deficiency

Protein C is a vitamin K-dependent anticoagulant synthesized in the liver that inhibits activated clotting factors V and VIII and stimulates fibrinolysis.[21] A deficiency of protein C may be inherited or acquired (Table 25-6). Deficiency of protein C most often presents as a tendency for recurrent thromboembolic disease, including myocardial infarction, cerebral infarction, and pulmonary embolism. Thrombosis may be initiated by the events associated with the perioperative period, including endothelial damage, immobility, and stasis of blood flow.[22] Because protein C deficiency does not cause abnormalities in the routine screening coagulation tests (PT, PTT, bleeding time), it is important to maintain a high index of suspicion for the patient who reports either a personal or family history of thromboembolic disease at a young age. Oral anticoagulation is the treatment of choice in the prevention of thrombosis. Regional anesthetic techniques may be useful alternatives to general anesthesia in these patients.[23]

Antithrombin III Deficiency

Antithrombin III (AT-III) inhibits activated clotting factors II and V. Deficiency of AT-III is associated with an increased incidence of thromboembolic disease and resistance to the anticoagulant effects of exogenously administered heparin. Acquired AT-III deficiency may occur in patients being treated with heparin and in those with DIC or severe liver disease. Females who take oral estrogen-containing contraceptives seem to be at increased risk of thromboembolism associated with decreased AT-III levels. The diagnosis of AT-III deficiency is confirmed by measurement of the plasma AT-III concentration. Chronic treatment of AT-III deficiency is with an oral anticoagulant, whereas acute correction is with administration of AT-III, as present in specific concentrate preparations or FFP.

Table 25-6.   Causes of Protein C
Deficiency

Inherited
Acquired
Liver disease
Disseminated intravascular coagulation
Adult respiratory distress syndrome
Postoperative
Postpartum
Hemodialysis

ACQUIRED COAGULATION DISORDERS

Acquired coagulation disorders, in contrast to inherited disorders, are usually due to multiple abnormalities in the coagulation process (Table 25-1).

Vitamin K Deficiency

Vitamin K is necessary in the liver to facilitate the production of gamma-carboxyglutamic acid required for the function of factors II, VII, IX, and X. Vitamin K deficiency occurs in the presence of malnutrition, intestinal malabsorption, antibiotic-induced elimination of intestinal flora necessary for the synthesis of vitamin K, and obstructive jaundice. In obstructive jaundice, bile salts necessary for the absorption of vitamin K from the gastrointestinal tract cannot enter the intestine. The neonate lacks stores of vitamin K and can become deficient in this vitamin, in the absence of supplemental therapy.

The diagnosis of vitamin K deficiency is based on documentation of a prolonged PT in the presence of a normal PTT. Treatment of a coagulation disorder owing to a vitamin K deficiency is determined by the urgency of the situation. For example, treatment with a parenteral vitamin K analogue, such as phytonadione, requires 6 to 24 hours to exert a beneficial effect. If active bleeding is present, the administration of FFP (usually 3 units) is rapidly effective.[14]

Drug-Induced Hemorrhage

Heparin overdose is manifested as subcutaneous hemorrhage and deep tissue hematomas. This anticoagulant is inactivated in the liver and is excreted by the kidneys, explaining the prolonged anticoagulant effects of heparin in the patient with hepatorenal disease. Decreased body temperature is also associated with an enhanced anticoagulant effect of heparin. The PT and PTT are prolonged; bleeding time is normal. Antagonism of an excessive heparin effect is with the intravenous administration of protamine.

An overdose with an oral anticoagulant (coumarin derivative) is manifested as ecchymosis formation, mucosal hemorrhage, and subserosal bleeding into the wall of the gastrointestinal tract. The anticoagulant effect is due to the ability of coumarin to prevent carboxylation of vitamin K to its active form. The PT is markedly prolonged in the presence of a coumarin overdose. Administration of FFP to provide vitamin K is necessary to treat acute hemorrhage owing to coumarin overdose.

Anticoagulation and Regional Anesthesia

The prospect of administering a spinal or epidural anesthetic to a patient who will subsequently receive heparin is a controversial clinical issue. The obvious concern is delayed hemorrhage from a blood vessel that was damaged during the performance of the anesthetic, leading to formation of an epidural or spinal hematoma, with subsequent compression of the spinal cord and the onset of a paraplegia.[24] In this regard, the reported incidence of epidural venous puncture is 1% with a spinal or epidural needle.[25] Trauma, anticoagulation, infusion of urokinase, bleeding diatheses, and intraspinal vascular malformations have been associated with epidural hematoma formation following regional anesthesia, but on rare occasions the hematoma may occur spontaneously without any apparent cause.[26,27] During recent years, more than 30% of reported cases of epidural hematoma have been associated with anticoagulant therapy. Large retrospective reviews of patients receiving epidural or spinal anesthesia, followed in about 1 hour by a dose of heparin sufficient to produce systemic anticoagulation, have not demonstrated the development of a neurologic defect owing to hematoma formation in any patient.[28,29] Despite these reports, it would seem prudent to consider carefully the benefits of regional anesthesia or neuraxial opioids for postoperative pain management relative to the rare risk of hematoma formation. Indeed, the development of a subarachnoid hematoma has been described in a patient undergoing a diagnostic lumbar puncture, later followed by the administration of heparin.[24] In another patient, evidence of epidural hematoma formation occurred within 3 hours after removal of an epidural catheter that had been in place for 48 hours, during which time heparin (5000 units) was administered every 12 hours.[30] It may be prudent to delay surgery, if traumatic needle insertion results in aspiration of blood during the performance of regional anesthesia, with the knowledge that heparin will be required for performance of the surgery. A reasonable period of time to delay surgery cannot be definitely stated, although some would prefer 24 hours.[27] There is, however, no evidence to support or refute the validity of a 24-hour delay. Clearly, monitoring of neurologic function during the early postoperative period is important in the patient considered at risk of epidural hematoma formation, as prompt surgical decompression is essential to prevent permanent sequelae. Prolonged numbness or weakness, paresthesia, and severe back pain should prompt a neurologic evaluation. Magnetic resonance imaging is a useful diagnostic technique for a suspected epidural hematoma.

Even more controversial is the performance of a spinal or epidural anesthetic in a patient who is already anticoagulated. Many are reluctant to administer regional anesthesia to such a patient, even though large series fail to report the occurrence of an epidural hematoma in any patient who was anticoagulated with a coumarin derivative or heparin at the time of the block.[31,32] Likewise, neurologic sequelae have not been observed in patients being treated preoperatively with low-dose heparin. If it is elected to administer a regional anesthetic to an anticoagulated patient, it is presumed that the benefits of this approach outweigh alternative techniques. Postoperative

monitoring of neurologic function for prompt detection of epidural hematoma formation is indicated.

Massive Blood Transfusion

Massive transfusion of stored whole blood (10 units of transfused blood is equivalent to the exchange of one natural blood volume with transfused components) can lead to a coagulation disorder characterized by diffuse microvascular bleeding.[33] The previous assumption that this coagulation disorder represented platelet washout and dilution of procoagulants is probably not entirely accurate. The presence of a coagulation disorder owing to massive blood transfusion is suggested by an abnormal thrombelastograph and a PT and PTT more than 1.8 times control (Fig. 25-3). At this point, circulating plasma concentrations of factors V and VIII are probably less than 20% of normal, and the fibrinogen level is usually less than 50 mg·dl^{-1}. Dilution of procoagulants other than factors V and VIII does not occur during massive blood transfusion, since all other procoagulants are stable in stored blood. Abnormalities of coagulation owing to dilution of factors V and VIII are more likely to occur with infusion of packed RBCs that include a minimal volume of plasma.

The most common reason for coagulopathy in patients receiving massive blood transfusions is the lack of functioning platelets. Platelets in stored blood are probably nonfunctional after 1 to 2 days. Each unit of platelet concentrate administered to an adult can be expected to increase the platelet count by 5000 to 10,000 cells·mm^{-3}. Each unit of platelets also contains 50 to 70 ml of plasma, emphasizing the likely simultaneous delivery of procoagulants with this therapy. There is no justification for prophylactic administration of platelets or FFP in the massively transfused patient.[34,35] The coagulopathy in the massively transfused patient correlates more closely with the duration of the volume deficit than with the total volume of blood transfused.[36] Therefore, the most important factor in preventing this coagulopathy is prompt replacement of intravascular fluid volume.

Emergency Transfusion

Most patients can tolerate an acute decrease in hemoglobin concentration, as long as intravascular fluid volume is maintained, such as with the intravenous administration of crystalloids or colloids. In those occasional situations in which an acute decrease in oxygen-carrying capacity will pose an increased risk (ischemic heart disease, cerebrovascular disease), type-specific blood can be administered while waiting for the completion of a complete cross-match (takes about 5 minutes to determine the ABO type and Rh type of a patient). When no delay is acceptable, it is permissible to administer type O Rh-negative whole blood. Switching immediately back to type A or type B blood can cause hemolysis after multiple units of type O whole blood have been administered to patients who are other than type O.

Postcardiopulmonary Bypass

Excessive bleeding after cardiopulmonary bypass is most often due to an acquired platelet function disorder, and not to dilution of procoagulants or heparin overdose.[37] This platelet defect is most likely caused by contact between the platelets and oxygenator. The degree of platelet dysfunction is directly proportional to the duration of cardiopulmonary bypass and is probably related to the level of hypothermia and to the prophylactic use of semisynthetic penicillins and possibly to other drugs such as nitroprusside and nitroglycerin. In most cases, platelet dysfunction is transient, lasting less than 1 hour but, if bleeding persists, the treatment is infusion of platelet concentrates. Administration of DDAVP has not been consistently effective in decreasing bleeding after cardiopulmonary bypass. DDAVP may be effective, however, in decreasing the volume of mediastinal chest tube drainage after cardiopulmonary bypass in a subgroup of patients in whom the thrombelastograph is characterized by a maximum amplitude of less than 50 mm (Figs. 25-2 and 25-3).[5,38]

Disseminated Intravascular Coagulation

DIC is characterized by uncontrolled activation of the coagulation system, with consumption of platelets and procoagulants. Under normal conditions, the deleterious effects of uncontrolled intravascular coagulation are modulated by (1) the dilutional effects of blood flow, (2) endogenous inhibitors of anticoagulation, and (3) removal of clotting factors by the liver. These carefully controlled mechanisms can be overwhelmed by massive tissue damage and shock (Table 25-7).

The diagnosis of DIC is based on the history, clinical picture, and measurement of coagulation tests. The clinical picture is characterized by hemorrhage from wound sites and around sites of placement of intravascular catheters. The uncontrolled generation of thrombin results in arterial and venous thromboses. Consumption of platelets and procoagulants manifests as a prolonged bleeding time, PT, PTT, and decreased plasma fibrinogen concentration. Increased levels of fibrin degradation products reflect the effects of plasmin and secondary fibrinolysis. A thrombelastograph reflects many of the coagulation changes associated with DIC (Fig. 25-3).

The treatment of DIC is directed at correcting the event responsible for initiation of the generalized activation of the coagulation system (Table 25-7). For example, improvement of the cardiac output, restoration of the intravascular fluid volume, emptying the uterus, or treatment of sepsis may be all the therapy required. Improvement is indicated by stabilization of the platelet count and plasma concentration of fibrinogen, as well as a decrease in the circulating concentration of fibrin degradation products. Platelet concentrates and FFP are administered, as indicated by measurement of the platelet count, bleeding time, PT, and PTT. Heparin has been recommended as therapy, but its use in this situation is controversial and ill-defined. Aminocaproic acid or fibrinogen should not be administered in the presence of continuing intravascular coagulation. Aminocaproic acid would inhibit secondary fibrinolysis, which is an intrinsic protective mechanism in patients with persistent DIC.

Drug-Induced Platelet Dysfunction

Aspirin administered to a normal patient irreversibly inhibits cyclooxygenase, which is responsible for the platelet release of ADP, necessary for platelet aggregation. Indeed, prolongation of the bleeding time by 2 to 3 minutes is detectable within 3 hours after the ingestion of 300 mg of aspirin.[39] Some apparently normal patients display marked sensitivity to the effect of aspirin; in these cases, the bleeding time is greatly prolonged, and significant hemorrhage may occur during the perioperative period or after trauma. Uremic patients are especially sensitive to bleeding induced by aspirin. Phenylbutazone and indomethacin inhibit the platelet release reaction similar to aspirin, sodium salicylate has a lesser effect, and acetaminophen does not interfere with release of ADP from platelets.

Platelet dysfunction induced by aspirin persists for the life of the platelet, which may be for several days after discontinuation of aspirin. Therefore, treatment of acute aspirin-induced hemorrhage consists of the transfusion of platelets that can release ADP. In response to this release reaction, platelets that are inhibited by aspirin can aggregate.

Drugs other than aspirin and related nonsteroidal anti-inflammatory drugs may interfere with platelet release of ADP and with subsequent platelet aggregation. For example, alcohol, dextran, and certain antibiotics (carbenicillin, high doses

Table 25-7. Causes of Disseminated Intravascular Coagulation

Crush injury
Hemorrhagic shock
Severe intracranial damage
Extensive surgery
Retained placenta
Burn injury
Hemolytic transfusion reaction
Malignant hyperthermia
Prolonged cardiopulmonary bypass
Gram-negative sepsis
Tumor products
Snake bites

of penicillin, many of the cephalosporins) interfere with platelet aggregation, manifested by a prolonged bleeding time. Volatile anesthetics and nitrous oxide studied using an in vitro model produce a dose-related decrease in ADP-induced platelet aggregation.[40] It is possible that inhaled anesthetics change the surface characteristics of the platelet cell membrane and thus interfere with cohesion. The clinical importance of this effect on platelet aggregation, if any, is unknown.

Aspirin and Elective Surgery

A controversial question deals with the performance of an elective operation in the presence of known aspirin therapy (see the section, Anticoagulation and Regional Anesthesia). Although bleeding time may return to normal within 72 hours after discontinuing aspirin, it may take 7 to 10 days for in vitro tests of platelet aggregation to return to normal.[41] It has been suggested that the upper limit of a bleeding time acceptable for performance of elective surgery is 10 minutes.[42] Despite the concern that operative blood loss could be increased, there is evidence that perioperative blood loss is not increased in patients receiving 1.2 to 3.6 g·d^{-1} of aspirin and undergoing total hip replacement.[39] Likewise, there is no evidence that spinal or epidural anesthesia should be avoided in the patient receiving antiplatelet drugs, although the incidence of blood-tinged cerebrospinal fluid or blood aspirated through the epidural or spinal needle may be increased in such a patient.[43] Although reassuring, there is a report of hematoma formation after regional anesthesia in the presence of aspirin-induced platelet dysfunction.[44] Postoperative neurologic monitoring is of increased importance in the aspirin-treated patient receiving an epidural or spinal anesthetic for prompt detection of signs of spinal cord compression attributable to hematoma formation.

Idiopathic Thrombocytopenic Purpura

Idiopathic thrombocytopenic purpura (ITP), or autoimmune thrombocytopenic purpura, is characterized by persistent thrombocytopenia caused by an antiplatelet immunoglobulin that binds to the platelet membrane, causing its premature destruction.[45] In addition to accelerated destruction, platelets in the patient with ITP may not function normally, as reflected by a prolonged bleeding time. The hallmark of thrombocytopenia is the formation of petechiae, characteristically at sites of increased internal or external pressure (oral mucosa, constricting clothing, legs). Intracranial hemorrhage is the principal cause of mortality in the patient with ITP. Transplacental passage of antiplatelet antibodies may predispose the neonate to spontaneous bleeding, including intracranial hemorrhage.

Otherwise healthy young females are most often afflicted with ITP, although many disease states and drugs may also

Table 25-8. Factors Associated With Thrombocytopenia

Idiopathic
Infectious mononucleosis
Acquired immunodeficiency syndrome
Hodgkin's disease
Systemic lupus erythematosus
Rheumatoid arthritis
Raynaud's phenomenon
Hyperthyroidism
Sepsis
Heparin
Quinidine
Thiazide diuretics

be associated with thrombocytopenia indistinguishable from ITP (Table 25-8). For example, heparin-induced thrombocytopenia may be manifested as a (1) modest nonprogressive decrease in platelet count that requires no intervention, or (2) severe thrombocytopenia often to less than 50,000 cells·mm^{-3} associated with thromboembolism, particularly arterial thromboembolism. A heparin-dependent antiplatelet antibody seems responsible for the severe form of heparin-induced thrombocytopenia, typically manifested 4 to 6 days after the initiation of anticoagulant therapy. Thrombocytopenia may occur 2 to 10 days after whole blood transfusion, occurring most often in a female exposed to alloantigens during a previous pregnancy.

Treatment of ITP is initially with a corticosteroid such as prednisone, which is presumed to interfere with macrophagic attack on platelets and eventually to decrease the amount of antiplatelet antibody produced. Danazol and vincristine may serve as supplemental or alternative drugs to treatment with a corticosteroid. Immunosuppressive therapy must be used cautiously in the parturient or patient with AIDS. If the platelet response to a corticosteroid is inadequate or not sustained, splenectomy is indicated.

It is recommended that corticosteroids be administered preoperatively, to increase the platelet count close to 50,000 cells·mm^{-3} at induction of anesthesia. When surgery must be performed despite a platelet count below 50,000 cells·mm^{-3}, administration of 6 units of platelet concentrates may be recommended at anesthetic induction and after ligation of the splenic pedicle. Management of anesthesia in such cases includes minimization of trauma to the upper airway, as during direct laryngoscopy for intubation of the trachea. Regional anesthesia is rarely selected because of the potential for spontaneous hemorrhage. The efficacy of splenectomy depends on elimination of the platelet-trapping role of the spleen, as well as its function in producing antiplatelet antibodies. Corticosteroids are continued postoperatively, until the platelet count increases. Cesarean section may be recommended when the fetus is affected by ITP in order to decrease the risk of cerebral trauma to the infant, which seems to be most likely if the platelet count is less than 50,000 cells·mm^{-3}.

Thrombotic Thrombocytopenic Purpura

Thrombotic thrombocytopenic purpura (TTP) is characterized by disseminated intravascular aggregation of platelets, presumably reflecting the presence of an abnormal aggregating factor.[46] Clinical manifestations include (1) thrombocytopenia, (2) severe hemolytic anemia, (3) central nervous system disturbances ranging from focal defects to seizures and coma, (4) fever, (5) mild renal dysfunction, and (6) jaundice. Treatment of TTP is with antiplatelet drugs, such as aspirin, and with exchange plasmapheresis, in an effort to provide a necessary absent factor or remove a toxic substance. Mortality from TTP may approach 60% to 80% in the first 10 days of the disease.

Catheter-Induced Thrombocytopenia

Thrombus formation on a catheter placed in the systemic or pulmonary circulation is a predictable event.[47] Catheter thrombogenicity is presumed to reflect the interaction of blood with the physicochemical and textural properties of the catheter. Catheters fabricated from polyvinylchloride have been found to be particularly thrombogenic. For example, it has been demonstrated that a pulmonary artery catheter may induce thrombus formation within 1 to 2 hours after placement, despite the use of a continuous infusion of heparinized saline through the catheter. By contrast, the use of a pulmonary artery catheter with heparin incorporated into the plastic material does not induce thrombus formation.[47] Although symptomatic pulmonary embolism is not a predictable event associated with the use of a thrombogenic pulmonary artery catheter, it would seem logical to minimize the likelihood of thrombus formation if possible. Therefore, the use of a heparin-bonded pulmonary artery catheter may be a useful consideration.

Thrombocytopenia has also been associated with the use of a pulmonary artery catheter.[48] Conceivably, increased platelet consumption owing to thrombus formation on the pulmonary artery catheter may be responsible for thrombocytopenia. In this regard, sequestration of platelets on the pulmonary artery catheter becomes a possible consideration when thrombocytopenia occurs unexpectedly.

TRANSFUSION THERAPY

Most bleeding disorders encountered during the perioperative period are due to surgical transection of blood vessels. Treatment is with stored whole blood or packed erythrocytes (RBCs). The importance of recognizing adverse reactions associated with transfusion therapy is emphasized by the estimate that about two-thirds of RBC transfusions are administered during the perioperative period.[50,51] Blood substitutes such as stroma-free hemoglobin and recombinant coagulation factor preparations free of infection and compatibility problems are likely to transform the future of transfusion medicine practice.

Concern about the transmission of AIDS and hepatitis and a reevaluation of the concept that the patient's hemoglobin concentration should be at least 10 g·dl^{-1} have led to approaches that emphasize autologous transfusion (1 unit withdrawn from the patient every 4 days, with the last unit obtained 3 days preoperatively; acute normovolemic hemodilution by removing 500 to 1000 ml of blood at the start of operation and replacement with crystalloid; intraoperative salvage) or to the use of single donors.[51-54] When blood is withdrawn within a few days preceding surgery, oral iron supplements should be administered. Presumably, treatment with recombinant erythropoietin would also stimulate production of RBCs. Nevertheless, a hemoglobin concentration of about 8 g·dl^{-1} is now being accepted in the patient who predonates blood for elective surgery.[51,54] Donor blood is tested for HIV, hepatitis B, and hepatitis C. There is no evidence that blood from a directed donor is safer than that obtained from a screened volunteer donor.[55] Clearly, the safest transfusion component is the patient's own blood, as it eliminates the possibility of disease transmission and incompatability reactions.

Component Therapy

The advantages of component therapy include (1) precise treatment of a specific coagulation disorder, (2) storage of specific procoagulants under ideal conditions to maintain their biologic activity, (3) minimization of the likelihood of circulatory overload, and (4) avoidance of the transmission of unnecessary donor plasma that may contain undesirable antigens or antibodies.[50,56] A unit of whole blood is 450 ± 45 ml, including anticoagulants. Using citrate–phosphate–dextrose–adenine solution, RBCs can be stored for up to 49 days. Platelets, however, survive poorly in blood stored at 4°C. Whole blood that tests negative for viral diseases is promptly fractionated into multiple components after its collection (Table 25-9).

Packed Erythrocytes

The only acceptable clinical indication for transfusion of packed RBCs is to increase the oxygen-carrying capacity of the blood. In this regard, 1 unit of infused packed RBCs will increase the average adult hemoglobin concentration by about 1 g·dl^{-1}. Adequate oxygen-carrying capacity can be maintained with a hemoglobin concentration of 7 g·dl^{-1} in most adult patients

Table 25-9. Components Available from Whole Blood

Packed red blood cells (350 ml, hematocrit about 55%)
Frozen erythrocytes
Platelet concentrates (50 ml; 5×10^{10} platelets)
Fresh frozen plasma (225 ml; contains all procoagulants, 1 unit·ml^{-1}; fibrinogen 3–4 mg·ml^{-1})
Cryoprecipitate (10 ml; 80–145 units of factor VIII and fibrinogen 250 mg)
Prothrombin complex concentrates
Granulocytes
Immune human globulins

(except for those with unstable angina pectoris), if intravascular fluid volume is maintained.[51] Indeed, in patients with chronic anemia, cardiac output does not change until the hemoglobin concentration decreases to about 7 g·dl^{-1}.[57] Infusion of RBCs is not indicated for the treatment of hypovolemia or with the presumption that wound healing will be improved. The patient who has been transfused on multiple occasions and who has experienced a febrile reaction may benefit from transfusion of leukocyte-poor blood.

Dilution of RBCs in saline decreases the viscosity of the solution (hematocrit may be as high as 70% to 80%), facilitating rapid intravenous infusion and minimizing hemolysis. Calcium-containing crystalloid solutions are not recommended for dilution of RBCs, since small clots may form due to the presence of calcium in excess of the chelating ability of the citrate anticoagulant. Hypotonic solutions, such as 5% dextrose in water, are not used to dilute RBCs, as clumping of the cells or hemolysis may occur.

Frozen Erythrocytes

Frozen RBCs are expensive to prepare and maintain and do not lower the risk of transmission of hepatitis. The principal use for frozen RBCs is to provide access to rare blood types.

Platelets

Platelet transfusions are administered only to control or prevent bleeding associated with documented thrombocytopenia or platelet dysfunction. Prolongation of the bleeding time to at least twice normal is usually an indication for transfusion of platelets. One unit of platelet concentrate will increase the platelet count in the average adult recipient by at least 5000 cells·mm^{-3}. Acute thrombocytopenia in the presence of microvascular bleeding can be considered an indication for platelet transfusion. Prophylactic platelet transfusion to prevent spontaneous bleeding is probably indicated in the patient with a platelet count of less than 10,000 to 20,000 cells·mm^{-3}. The platelet count should probably be increased to at least 50,000 cells·mm^{-3} in the patient scheduled for invasive elective surgery. Controlled studies for such cases have demon-

strated no correlation between the platelet count and bleeding after cardiopulmonary bypass and no detectable benefit from the prophylactic administration of platelets.[58] Most patients who receive rapid replacement of 1 to 2 blood volumes do not bleed as a result of thrombocytopenia.[58]

The principal risks associated with the administration of platelet concentrates are sensitization reactions and the transmission of viral diseases, especially if pooled donor products are administered. The use of single-donor pheresis platelets (can provide the equivalent of 4 to 6 units of platelets), rather than random donor platelets, decreases the risk of disease transmission. Platelets possess HLA antigens on their cell membranes, emphasizing the importance of administering type-specific platelets to decrease the likelihood of a sensitization reaction. Fever, respiratory distress, and the absence of an increase in the platelet count are manifestations of a sensitization reaction.

Unlike other blood products, platelets are stored at room temperature, which may lead to bacterial growth. Fatal septic reactions to platelet transfusions have been reported.[59] Platelet storage time is currently limited to 5 days.

Fresh Frozen Plasma

FFP should be administered only to increase the level of clotting factors in a patient with a documented procoagulant deficiency.[60,61] For example, FFP is indicated in patients with liver disease who are bleeding and have multiple procoagulant defects. All procoagulants except platelets are present in FFP. Each unit of FFP transfused will increase the level of all procoagulants by 2% to 3% in the average adult. If PT and PTT are less than 1.5 times normal, FFP transfusion is rarely indicated. The patient treated with a coumarin derivative who exhibits spontaneous bleeding or who requires emergency surgery may be treated with FFP, to achieve immediate hemostasis. Administration of FFP provides AT-III to the patient who is deficient in this material and in whom heparin anticoagulation is needed. Administration of FFP may prolong the activated coagulation time in the presence of heparin anticoagulation.[62] There is no evidence to support the use of FFP for prophylaxis in the patient receiving a massive blood transfusion or undergoing cardiopulmonary bypass in the absence of a documented procoagulant defect.[63] As a volume expander, FFP is less effective than albumin. Risks of FFP administration include transmission of viral diseases, allergic reactions, and fluid overload.

Cryoprecipitate

Cryoprecipitate is the fraction of plasma that precipitates when FFP is thawed. This fraction can then be frozen and stored for future use. Cryoprecipitate contains high concentrations of factor VIII in a small volume, as well as high concentrations of fibrinogen. Multiple transfusions of cryoprecipitate in the absence of a low fibrinogen concentration may result in hyperfibrinogenemia. The presence of fibrinogen introduces the risk of transmission of viral diseases. Hemolytic anemia may occur if type-specific cryoprecipitate is not administered.

Plasma Volume Expanders

Plasma volume expanders are categorized as colloids, crystalloids, and synthetic derivatives.

Albumin

Albumin is available in 5% and 25% solutions. The 5% solution is most often used when rapid expansion of intravascular fluid volume is indicated. The 25% solution is most often used to treat hypoalbuminemia. Both albumin solutions contain 130 to 160 $mEq \cdot L^{-1}$ of sodium and less than 2 $mEq \cdot L^{-1}$ of potassium. Coagulation factors are not present in albumin solutions; in fact, albumin-induced increases in intravascular fluid volume may dilute the plasma concentrations of procoagulants and hemoglobin. The risk of transmission of hepatitis by albumin is eliminated by heating these solutions to 60°C for 10 hours.

Plasma Protein Fraction

Plasma protein fraction (Plasmanate) is a 5% solution of plasma proteins (83% albumin and 17% gamma globulin) in a saline solution osmotically equivalent to an equal volume of plasma. The sodium and potassium concentration resemble that present in albumin solutions. The most frequent use of this blood component is to increase acutely the intravascular fluid volume. Like albumin, this blood component is heat treated to eliminate the risk of transmission of viral hepatitis. No cross-matching is necessary, and the absence of cellular elements removes the risk of sensitization with repeated infusions. Plasma protein fractions do not contain coagulation factors.

Dextran

Dextran is a branched-chain polysaccharide that can be administered for acute expansion of the intravascular fluid volume. Low-molecular-weight dextran (Rheomacrodex) produces a transient increase in intravascular fluid volume, as this substance leaks out of the vascular bed within 2 to 4 hours. This form of dextran may be used in an attempt to decrease the risk of thromboembolism by decreasing the viscosity of blood and preventing aggregation of platelets. High-molecular-weight dextran is more useful for expanding the intravascular fluid volume but has minimal beneficial effect on the microcirculation; 32% dextran-70 (Hyskon) may be used during hysteroscopy to improve visualization by distending the uterine cavity and to decrease the likelihood of the development of tubal adhesions after reconstructive tubal surgery for infertility. Noncardiogenic pulmonary edema has been attributed to a direct toxic effect of this dextran solution on pulmonary capillaries after its intravascular absorption from the uterus.[64] Clinical ascites has been observed 2 days after intraperitoneal installation of Hyskon.[65] Dextran has been associated with clinical and laboratory abnormalities that include factitious elevations in the blood glucose concentration; agglutination of RBCs, causing difficulty in performing a cross-match for blood; decreased platelet adhesiveness, especially when the amount of dextran exceeds about 1500 ml; and decreased plasma levels of fibrinogen and factors V, VIII, and IX. Rarely, renal failure or an allergic reaction may accompany the administration of dextran. Elimination of dextran is principally by the kidneys.

Hetastarch

Hetastarch (hydroxyethyl starch) is a synthetic colloid solution that is as effective as 5% albumin as an intravascular fluid volume expander. In this regard, hetastarch solutions (20 $ml \cdot kg^{-1}$) are used to expand intravascular fluid volume in the management of acute hypovolemia.[66] Excessive doses of hetastarch decrease the hematocrit and dilute the plasma concentration of platelets and procoagulants. Hetastarch solutions have about the same risk as dextran in producing an allergic reaction. Unlike dextran, hetastarch does not interfere with cross-matching of blood. Hypervolemia is a potential adverse effect, particularly in the patient with impaired renal function, since hetastarch is excreted principally by the kidneys.

Crystalloid

Crystalloid solutions can be administered to treat acute hypovolemia, but 3 to 4 ml must be given for every 1 ml of estimated blood loss. The increase in intravascular fluid volume produced by a crystalloid solution is transient, in view of the rapid translocation of about three-fourths of the infused solution to other tissue compartments.[67] Pulmonary edema is a risk associated with large volume crystalloid infusions. There is continuing controversy as to the preferable solution (colloid versus crystalloid) for acute replacement of intravascular fluid volume.

Complications of Blood Transfusions

Complications of blood transfusions are reflected principally by (1) transmission of viral diseases, (2) transfusion reactions, and (3) metabolic abnormalities produced by inherent characteristics of the stored blood (Table 25-10). Blood transfusion exerts a nonspecific immunosuppressive effect that may be either detrimental in the patient with cancer or therapeutic in the patient undergoing an organ transplant operation.[68]

Table 25-10. Complications of
Blood Transfusion

Transmission of viral diseases
  Hepatitis B
  Hepatitis C
  Acquired immunodeficiency syndrome
  Cytomegalovirus
  Human T cell lymphotropic virus

Transfusion reactions
  Allergic
  Febrile
  Hemolytic
  Delayed hemolytic

Metabolic abnormalities
  Hydrogen
  Potassium
  2,3-Diphosphoglycerate

Hypocalcemia

Microaggregates

Immunosuppression

Hypothermia

Transmission of a Viral Disease

The use of volunteer donors and routine screening for hepatitis B and C virus has significantly decreased the incidence of transfusion-transmitted hepatitis.[53] The current incidence of post-transfusion hepatitis B infection is estimated to be 1:200,000 per unit transfused. The estimate of seroconversion for hepatitis C is less than 3 per 10,000 units transfused. The estimate of the risk of contracting HIV from a single unit of properly screened blood is 1:225,000 per unit transfused.[55] Other estimates of 1:40,000 to 1:60,000 per unit transfused were based on data collected from geographic areas with high prevalence rates of HIV infection, where causes of seroconversion of recipients were sometimes unclear. Cytomegalovirus is transmitted most readily by transfusion of granulocytes from an infected donor to an immunosuppressed seronegative recipient, whereas infection in an otherwise healthy patient is usually asymptomatic. Transmission of human T cell lymphotropic virus may result in leukemia or neurologic disease, many years after transfusion of blood.

Transfusion Reactions

Transfusion reactions are categorized as allergic, febrile, hemolytic, and delayed hemolytic reactions.[50]

Allergic Reactions

Pruritus, erythema, urticaria, and increased body temperature occur in about 1% of patients receiving correctly typed and cross-matched blood. Incompatible plasma proteins are the presumed mechanism. During anesthesia, the first manifestation of an allergic reaction to blood administration may be the appearance of erythema along the pathway of the vein receiving the blood plus urticaria, particularly on the chest, neck, and face. Changes in blood pressure or heart rate rarely occur.

Treatment of a mild allergic reaction (urticarial reaction in the absence of hypotension) to blood consists of the administration of diphenhydramine (0.5 to 1 mg·kg^{-1} IV) and slowing the rate of blood delivery. More severe allergic reactions require discontinuation of the transfusion, as well as the administration of diphenhydramine. Subsequent urticarial reactions to blood can be prevented by the use of washed RBCs or platelets, in an effort to remove the offending protein allergens. Furthermore, in these at-risk patients, prophylactic administration of diphenhydramine may be useful.

A severe allergic reaction to blood is possible in a patient who lacks immunoglobulin A (IgA) in the plasma. Indeed, infusion of as little as 10 ml of blood into an IgA-deficient patient can result in life-threatening anaphylaxis requiring aggressive intervention with a drug such as epinephrine. An IgA deficiency is estimated to occur in 1 in every 700 patients; these patients should receive blood obtained only from an IgA-deficient donor.

A rare manifestation of an allergic reaction to blood is the development of an acute pulmonary hypersensitivity response, characterized by the abrupt onset of fever, dry nonproductive cough, and pulmonary edema, in the absence of evidence of hypervolemia or congestive heart failure.[69] A chest radiograph may demonstrate congestion of the pulmonary vasculature. Hypotension and arterial hypoxemia may occur. It is presumed that leukocyte antibodies in the donor's plasma react with the recipient's leukocytes producing cellular aggregation, microvascular occlusion, and pulmonary capillary leakage.[69] Treatment is symptomatic and includes discontinuation of the transfusion and administration of diphenhydramine.

Febrile Reactions

Febrile reactions typically develop within 4 hours after initiation of a blood transfusion, with a temperature elevation that rarely exceeds 38°C. It is estimated that febrile reactions occur in 1% to 2% of blood recipients. Since temperature elevation may also be an early sign of a hemolytic transfusion reaction, the diagnosis of a nonhemolytic febrile reaction is based on the absence of signs of hemolysis. The most likely cause of a febrile reaction is an interaction between recipient antibodies and donor leukocytes, with the subsequent release of pyrogenic substances from injured cells. Headache, nausea, vomiting, and chest or back pain may accompany the increase in body temperature.

Treatment of a mild febrile reaction is by slowing the rate of blood infusion and administration of an antipyretic such as aspirin or acetaminophen. The shivering that may accompany this reaction in an adult may respond to meperidine (25 mg IV). A severe febrile reaction may necessitate discontinuation of the blood infusion. Diphenhydramine and corticosteroids produce no beneficial effect in the treatment of a febrile reaction to blood. Future febrile reactions can be avoided by the administration of leukocyte-poor (washed) RBCs or HLA-compatible platelets. The use of a Pall filter will provide RBCs depleted of leukocytes.

Hemolytic Reactions

Accidental administration of ABO-incompatible blood results in activation of the complement system, manifesting initially as chills, fever, restlessness, lumbar and substernal pain, and hypotension. Erythema and urticaria are manifestations of an allergic, but not a hemolytic, reaction. With the exception of hypotension, the initial manifestations of a hemolytic blood reaction are masked in an anesthetized patient. Initial manifestations of a hemolytic reaction are followed by evidence of intravascular hemolysis, which includes visible free hemoglobin in a plasma sample, hemoglobinuria, anemia, and hyperbilirubinemia. The simplest screening test is examination of a centrifuged blood sample for free plasma hemoglobin. If there is no plasma discoloration, a serious hemolytic reaction is unlikely. The increase in plasma bilirubin concentration is maximal 3 to 6 hours after the onset of an acute hemolytic reaction. Oliguria that may progress to acute renal failure is presumed to reflect precipitation of stromal and lipid contents of RBCs in distal renal tubules. Free hemoglobin is unlikely to be responsible for renal dysfunction that accompanies intravascular hemolysis. The development of DIC is likely in a severe reaction, presumably reflecting the effect of material released from hemolyzed RBCs.

Treatment of an acute hemolytic reaction begins with the prompt discontinuation of the blood infusion, since the severity of the reaction is directly proportional to the amount of incompatible flood infused. The donor blood and a blood sample from the patient should be sent to the laboratory for a repeat type and cross-match. It is important to maintain urine output by the liberal infusion of crystalloid solutions intravenously, as well as by administration of furosemide or mannitol. Indeed, the deposition of stroma and lipids from hemolyzed RBCs in renal tubules is presumed to be inversely related to urine output. Alkalinization of the urine with the intravenous administration of sodium bicarbonate is based on the concept that hemoglobin degradation products released by hemolysis are more soluble in an alkaline medium. Nevertheless, the clinical value of alkalinization of the urine has not been proved, nor has the use of corticosteroids in the management of a hemolytic reaction.

Delayed Hemolytic Reaction

A delayed hemolytic reaction to transfused blood may occur despite administration of correctly typed and cross-matched donor RBCs. Clinically, jaundice and evidence of intravascular hemolysis are observed 10 to 14 days after the blood transfusion; a decrease in the hematocrit may also occur. A direct positive Coombs test is likely, confirming that the donor RBCs contained an antigen not present on the recipient's cells; the result is delayed production by the host of antibodies that coat and hemolyze any remaining RBCs from the prior transfusion. Treatment is supportive and corticosteroids are of no value.

Metabolic Abnormalities

Metabolic abnormalities produced by the administration of blood are related to changes that occur during storage. For example, the potassium and hydrogen ion content increases and the RBC concentration of 2,3-diphosphoglycerate (2,3-DPG) decreases during storage of whole blood (Table 25-11). The maximum allowable storage time is determined by the type of preservative. The principal value of warming stored whole blood to close to 37°C before infusion is to minimize the decrease in body temperature associated with the administration of blood stored at 4°C. As a guideline, blood warmers should be used in an adult receiving rapid infusion of 2 or more units of stored whole blood.

Hydrogen Ions

Accumulation of hydrogen ions in stored blood reflects the addition of acid-containing preservative solution and continued metabolic function of RBCs. Despite these changes, metabolic acidosis does not accompany even the rapid infusion of large volumes of stored blood. For this reason, administration of sodium bicarbonate is indicated only when the presence of

Table 25-11.   Changes That Occur During Storage of Whole Blood in Citrate–Phosphate–Dextrose

	Days of Storage at 4°C				
	0	7	14	21	28
Viable cells 24 hours after transfusion (%)	100	98	85	80	75
Plasma pH at 37°C	7.20	7.0	6.9	6.84	6.78
2,3-diphosphoglycerate ($\mu M \cdot ml^{-1}$)	4.8	1.2	1	1	1
P_{50} (mmHg)	26	23	20	17	17
Plasma potassium ($mEq \cdot L^{-1}$)	4	12	17	21	23

acidosis is confirmed by measurement of arterial pH. Indeed, metabolic alkalosis, rather than metabolic acidosis, is a frequent accompaniment of massive blood transfusions.[70] This alkalosis is presumed to be partly due to the metabolism of infused citrate to bicarbonate, which could be further exaggerated by infusion of lactated Ringer's solution. Post-transfusion metabolic alkalosis is most likely to occur in the patient with diminished renal function, since the kidneys are responsible for the elimination of bicarbonate.

Potassium

Despite progressive increases in the potassium content of blood with storage, the rapid infusion of even massive amounts of stored blood does not result in hyperkalemia in the patient with normal renal function. It is possible, however, that potassium present in stored whole blood would predispose to hyperkalemia in the patient with impaired or absent renal function. Failure of the plasma potassium concentration to increase predictably most likely reflects the small amount of potassium actually present in 1 unit of stored whole blood. For example, since 1 unit of whole blood contains only 300 ml of plasma,

a measured plasma potassium concentration of 21 mEq·L^{-1} would represent less than 7 mEq of potassium. Transfusion of 10 units of stored whole blood would result in the addition of only about 70 mEq of potassium, an amount unlikely to produce hyperkalemia. In addition, the production of metabolic alkalosis by massive transfusions of whole blood will favor transfer of potassium from plasma into intracellular sites, further offsetting any tendency toward hyperkalemia. A previous suggestion that warming of stored blood before infusion can be important in restoring the integrity of RBCs and favoring entry of potassium back into RBCs has never been supported by evidence. In fact, there is evidence that warming stored blood does not change the concentration of potassium in the plasma that accompanies the transfused blood.[71]

2,3-Diphosphoglycerate

Storage of blood is associated with a progressive decrease in the concentration of 2,3-DPG in the RBCs, resulting in an increased affinity of hemoglobin for oxygen. The resulting leftward shift in the oxyhemoglobin dissociation curve of the recipient after massive blood transfusion is manifested by a de-

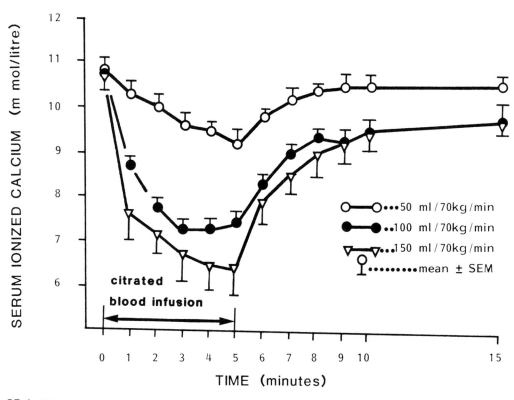

Fig. 25-4. The rate of infusion of citrated whole blood to an adult must exceed 50 ml·70 kg^{-1}·min^{-1} for the serum ionized calcium concentration to decrease. (From Denlinger JK, Nahrwold ML, Gibbs PS, Lecky JH. Hypocalcemia during rapid blood transfusion in anaesthetized man. Br J Anaesth 1976;48:995–1000, with permission.)

creased P_{50}. Conceivably, this change could jeopardize oxygen delivery to the tissues, particularly in the presence of anemia. Nevertheless, the clinical significance of a decreased 2,3-DPG concentration in RBCs has not been confirmed. Furthermore, the higher pH of citrate–phosphate–dextrose anticoagulant, as compared with acid–citrate–dextrose anticoagulant, prevents rapid depletion of 2,3-DPG.

Hypocalcemia

Hypocalcemia owing to binding of calcium by citrate present in transfused stored blood is unlikely, reflecting mobilization of calcium stores in bone and the ability of the liver to metabolize citrate rapidly to bicarbonate. Indeed, the rate of whole blood transfusion to an adult has to exceed 50 ml·70 kg^{-1}·min^{-1} before decreases in the plasma ionized calcium concentration can occur[72] (Fig. 25-4). This finding mitigates against arbitrary administration of calcium intravenously, in the absence of objective indications of hypocalcemia such as prolongation of the Q-T interval on the electrocardiogram or measurement of the plasma ionized calcium concentration. Reversal of hypotension when calcium is administered does not prove the existence of citrate intoxication, since a dose-related positive inotropic effect of calcium can be expected to improve myocardial contractility and thereby blood pressure.

Although hypocalcemia owing to citrate binding of calcium is unlikely in an adult, the same is probably not true in a neonate receiving stored blood. In this regard, supplementation with calcium chloride or calcium gluconate is often recommended. Furthermore, the presence of hypothermia or marked liver dysfunction may interfere with the metabolism of citrate to bicarbonate, predisposing to hypocalcemia.

Hypomagnesemia

Hypomagnesemia, like hypocalcemia, can produce a prolonged Q-T interval on the electrocardiogram, as well as ventricular dysrhythmias after massive transfusion.[73]

Microaggregates

Microaggregates consisting of platelets and leukocytes form during the storage of whole blood, with accumulation becoming significant after 3 to 5 days of storage[74] (Fig. 25-5). An

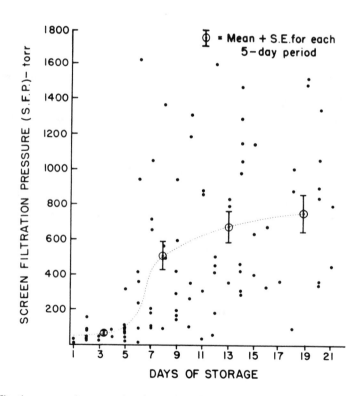

Fig. 25-5. Screen filtration pressure increases after about 5 days of whole blood storage, presumably reflecting the accumulation of significant amounts of microaggregates after this period of storage. (From Harp JR, Wyche MQ, Marshall BE, Wurzel HA. Some factors determining rate of microaggregate formation in stored blood. Anesthesiology 1974;40:398–400, with permission.)

estimated 90% of these microaggregates have diameters within the 10- to 40-μm range. For this reason, micropore filters have been developed to remove these microaggregates, in hopes of decreasing post-transfusion pulmonary dysfunction, which is presumed to reflect pulmonary vascular obstruction of these infused aggregates. Nevertheless, the use of micropore filters has not been conclusively documented to alter the incidence of pulmonary dysfunction after multiple blood transfusions, emphasizing that factors other than microaggregates may be operative.[75] There is no indication to use micropore filters during routine blood transfusions, or even when large volumes of blood are administered. Micropore filters may be useful in preventing febrile transfusion reactions, since these filters remove most of the leukocytes and platelets responsible for these reactions. Micropore filters placed on the arterial side of the cardiopulmonary bypass circuit may be useful in preventing microaggregate emboli in the patient undergoing cardiac surgery. Regardless of the decision as to whether to use a micropore filter, stored blood must always be administered through a 170-μm filter.

REFERENCES

1. Rohrer MJ, Michelotti MC, Nahrwold DL. A prospective evaluation of the efficacy of preoperative coagulation testing. Am Surg 1988;208:554–62
2. Ditto FF, Gibbons JJ. Factitious prolongation of bleeding time associated with patient movement. Anesth Analg 1991;72:710–2
3. George JN, Shattil SJ. The clinical importance of acquired abnormalities of platelet function. N Engl J Med 1991;324:27–39
4. Ramanathan J, Sibai BM, Vu T, Chauhan D. Correlation between bleeding times and platelet counts in women with preeclampsia undergoing cesarean section. Anesthesiology 1989;71:188–91
5. Kang YG, Martin DJ, Marquez J, et al. Intraoperative changes in blood coagulation and thrombelastographic monitoring in liver transplantation. Anesth Analg 1985;64:888–96
6. Mallett SV, Cox DJA. Thrombelastography. Br J Anaesth 1992;69:307–13
7. Tuman KJ, Spiess BD, McCarthy RJ, Ivankovich AD. Comparison of viscolastic measures of coagulation after cardiopulmonary bypass. Anesth Analg 1989;69:69–75
8. Ellison N. Diagnosis and management of bleeding disorders. Anesthesiology 1977;47:171–80
9. Kasper CK, Boylen AL, Iewin NP, et al. Hematologic management of hemophilia A for surgery. JAMA 1985;253:1279–83
10. Goldsmith MT. Hemophilia, beaten on one front, is beset on others. JAMA 1986;256:3200
11. Schwartz RS, Abeldgaard CF, Aledort LM, et al. Human recombinant DNA-derived antihemophilic factor (Factor VIII) in the treatment of hemophilia A. N Engl J Med 1990;323:1800–5
12. Saidi P, Lega BZ, Kim HC, et al. Effect of danazol on clotting factor levels, bleeding incidence, factor infusion requirements, and immune parameters in hemophilia. Blood 1986;68:673–82
13. Sampson JF, Hamstra R, Aldrete JA. Management of hemophiliac patients undergoing surgical procedures. Anesth Analg 1979;58:133–5
14. Consensus Conference. Fresh frozen plasma. Indications and risks. JAMA 1985;253:551–3
15. Fulcher C, Zimmerman T. Characterization of the human factor VIII procoagulant protein with a heterologous precipitating antibody. Proc Natl Acad Sci USA 1982;79:1648–52
16. Cameron CB, Kobrinsky N. Perioperative management of patients with von Willebrand's disease. Can J Anaesth 1990;37:341–7
17. DelaFuente B, Kasper CK, Rickles FR, et al. Response of patients with mild and moderate hemophilia A and von Willebrand's disease to treatment with desmopressin. Ann Intern Med 1985;103:6–11
18. Salmenpera M, Rasi V, Mattila S. Cardiopulmonary bypass in a patient with factor XII deficiency. Anesthesiology 1991;75:539–41
19. Waring PH, Shaw DB, Brumfield CG. Anesthetic management of a parturient with Osler-Weber-Rendu syndrome and rheumatic heart disease. Anesth Analg 1990;71:96–9
20. Kotelko DM. Anaesthesia for caesarean delivery in a patient with May-Hegglin anomaly. Can J Anaesth 1989;36:328–30
21. Clouse LH, Comp PC. The regulation of hemostasis: The protein C system. N Engl J Med 1986;314:1298–1303
22. Sternberg TL, Bailey MK, Lazarchick J, Brahen NH. Protein C deficiency as a cause of pulmonary embolism in the perioperative period. Anesthesiology 1991;74:364–6
23. Wetzel RC, Marsh BR, Yaster M, Casella JF. Anesthetic implications of protein C deficiency. Anesth Analg 1986;65:982–4
24. Owens EL, Kasten GW, Hessel EA. Spinal subarachnoid hematoma after lumbar puncture and heparinization. A case report, review of the literature, and discussion of anesthetic implications. Anesth Analg 1986;65:1201–7
25. Bromage PR. Epidural Analgesia. Philadelphia. WB Saunders 1978;659–60
26. Wittebol MC, VanVeelen CWM. Spontaneous spinal epidural hematoma. Clin Neurol Neurosurg 1984;86:265–70
27. Onishchuk JL, Carlsson C. Epidural hematoma associated with epidural anesthesia: Complications of anticoagulant therapy. Anesthesiology 1992;77:1221–3
28. Rao TLK, El-Etr AA. Anticoagulation following placement of epidural and subarachnoid catheters. Anesthesiology 1981;55:618–20
29. Baron HC, LaRaja RD, Rossi G, Atkinson D. Continuous epidural analgesia in the heparinized vascular surgical patient: A retrospective review of 912 patients. J Vasc Surg 1987;6:144–6
30. Tekkok IH, Cataltepe O, Tahta K, Bertan V. Extradural haematoma after continuous extradural anaesthesia. Br J Anaesth 1991;67:112–5
31. Odoom JA, Sih IL. Epidural analgesia and anticoagulant therapy. Experience with one thousand cases of continuous epidurals. Anaesthesia 1983;38:254–9
32. Waldman SD, Feldstein GS, Waldman HJ, et al. Caudal administration of morphine sulphate in anticoagulated and thrombocytopenic patients. Anesth Analg 1987;66:267–8
33. Ciaverella D, Reed RL, Counts RB, et al. Clotting factor levels and the risk of diffuse microvascular bleeding in the massively transfused patient. Br J Haematol 1987;67:365–9

34. Reed RL, Ciavarella D, Heimbach D, et al. Prophylactic platelet administration during massive transfusion. Ann Surg 1986;203:40–6

35. Murray DJ, Olson J, Strauss R, et al. Coagulation changes during packed red cell replacement of major blood loss. Anesthesiology 1988;69:839–46

36. Harke H, Rahman S. Haemostatic disorders in massive transfusion. Bibl Haematol 1980;46:179–83

37. Harker LA. Bleeding after cardiopulmonary bypass. N Engl J Med 1986;314:1446–8

38. Mongan PD, Hosking MP. A role of desmopressin acetate in patients undergoing coronary artery bypass surgery. A controlled clinical trial with thromboelastographic risk stratification. Anesthesiology 1992;77:38–46

39. Amrein PC, Ellman L, Harris WH. Aspirin-induced prolongation of bleeding and perioperative blood loss. JAMA 1981;245:1825–8

40. Fauss BG, Meadows JC, Bruni CY, Qureshi GD. The in vitro and in vivo effects of isoflurane and nitrous oxide in platelet aggregation. Anesth Analg 1986;65:1170–4

41. Hindman BJ, Koka BV. Usefulness of the post-aspirin bleeding time. Anesthesiology 1986;64:368–70

42. Macdonald R. Aspirin and extradural blocks. Br J Anaesth 1991;66:1–3

43. Horlocker TT, Wedel DJ, Offord KP. Does preoperative antiplatelet therapy increase the risk of hemorrhagic complications associated with regional anesthesia? Anesth Analg 1990;70:631–4

44. Locke GE, Giorgio AJ, Biggers SL, Johnson AP, Sabur F. Acute spinal epidural hematoma secondary to aspirin-induced prolonged bleeding. Surg Neurol 1976;5:293–6

45. McMillan R. Chronic idiopathic thrombocytopenic purpura. N Engl J Med 1981;304:1135–7

46. Crain SM, Choudhury AM. Thrombotic thrombocytopenia. A reappraisal. JAMA 1981;246:1243–6

47. Hoar PF, Wilson RM, Mangano DT, et al. Heparin bonding reduces thrombogenicity of pulmonary-artery catheters. N Engl J Med 1981;305:993–5

48. Richman KA, Kim YL, Marshall BE. Thrombocytopenia and altered platelet kinetics associated with prolonged pulmonary-artery catheterization in the dog. Anesthesiology 1980;53:101–5

49. Snyder EL, Hazzey A, Barash PG, Palermo G. Microaggregate blood filtration in patients with compromised pulmonary function. Transfusion 1982;22:21–5

50. Stehling LC. Recent advances in transfusion therapy. In: Stoelting RK, Barash PG, Gallagher TJ, eds. Advances in Anesthesia. Chicago. Year Book Medical Publishers 1987;4:213–52

51. National Institutes of Health Consensus Conference: Perioperative red blood cell transfusion. JAMA 1988;260:2700–4

52. Oberman HA. Strategies for blood transfusion. Mayo Clin Proc 1988;63:950–6

53. Willis JL. Transfusion of red cells. FDA Drug Bull 1988;18:26–7

54. The use of autologous blood. The national blood resource education program expert panel. JAMA 1990;263:414–7

55. Dodd RY. The risk of transfusion-transmitted infection. N Engl J Med 1992;327:419–20

56. Blajchman MA, Herst R, Perrault RA. Blood component therapy in anaesthetic practice. Can Anaesth Soc J 1983;30:382–9

57. Varat MA, Adolph RJ, Fowler NO. Cardiovascular effects of anemia. Am Heart J 1972;83:41–5

58. Consensus Conference. Platelet transfusion therapy. JAMA 1987;257:1777–80

59. Morrow JF, Braine HG, Kickler TS, Ness PM, Dick JD, Fuller AK. Septic reactions to platelet transfusions. JAMA 1991;266:555–8

60. Consensus Conference. Fresh frozen plasma. Indications and risks. JAMA 1985;253:551–3

61. Bove JR. Fresh frozen plasma: Too few indications—too much use. Anesth Analg 1985;64:849–50

62. Barnette RE, Shupak RC, Pontius J, Rao AK. In vitro effect of fresh frozen plasma on the activated coagulation time in patients undergoing cardiopulmonary bypass. Anesth Analg 1988;67:57–60

63. Roy RC, Stafford MA, Hudspeth AS, Meredith JW. Failure of prophylaxis with fresh frozen plasma after cardiopulmonary bypass. Anesthesiology 1988;69:254–7

64. Mangar D, Gerson JI, Constantine RM, Lenzi V. Pulmonary edema and coagulopathy due to Hyskon (32% dextran-70) administration. Anesth Analg 1989;68:686–7

65. Cleary RE, Howard T, DeZerega GS. Plasma dextran level after abdominal installation of 32% dextran 70: Evidence for prolonged intraperitoneal retention. Am J Obstet Gynecol 1985;152:78–9

66. Puri VK, Howard M, Paidipaty BB, Singh S. Resuscitation in hypovolemia and shock: A prospective study of hydroxyethyl starch and albumin. Crit Care Med 1983;11:518–23

67. Ramsey G. Intravenous volume replacement: Indications and choices. Br Med J 1988;296:1422–3

68. Schriemer PA, Longnecker DE, Mintz PD. The possible immunosuppressive effects of perioperative blood transfusion in cancer patients. Anesthesiology 1988;68:422–8

69. De Wolf AM, Van Den Berg BW, Hoffman HJ, Van Zundert AA. Pulmonary dysfunction during one-lung ventilation caused by HLA-specific antibodies against leukocytes. Anesth Analg 1987;66:463–7

70. Miller RD, Tong MJ, Robbins TO. Effects of massive transfusion of blood on acid-base balance. JAMA 1971;216:1762–5

71. Eurenius S, Smith RM. The effect of warming on the serum potassium content of stored blood. Anesthesiology 1973;38:482–4

72. Denlinger JK, Nahwrold ML, Gibbs PS, Lecky JH. Hypocalcemia during rapid blood transfusion in anaesthetized man. Br J Anaesth 1976;48:995–1000

73. Kulkarni P, Bhattacharya S, Petros AJ. Torsade de pointes and long QT syndrome following major blood transfusion. Anaesthesia 1992;47:125–7

74. Harp JR, Wyche MQ, Marshall BE, Wurzel HA. Some factors determining rate of microaggregate formation in stored blood. Anesthesiology 1974;40:398–400

75. Snyder EL, Hazzey A, Barash PG, Palermo G. Microaggregate blood filtration in patients with compromised pulmonary function. Transfusion 1982;22:21–5

26
Skin and Musculoskeletal Diseases

Diseases of the skin and musculoskeletal systems present obvious effects, as both systems are readily visible. Also, important, however, are the occult systemic effects of the diseases.

EPIDERMOLYSIS BULLOSA

Epidermolysis bullosa is a group of hereditary diseases of the skin that may also involve mucous membranes, particularly of the oropharynx and esophagus. This disease is categorized as simplex, junctional, and dystrophic[1] (Fig. 26-1). In the simplex type, epidermal cells are fragile, and mutations of genes encoding keratin intermediate filament proteins underlie the fragility. In the dystrophic types (incidence about 1 in every 300,000 births), the genetic mutation appears to be in the gene encoding the type of collagen that is the major component of anchoring fibrils.

Signs and Symptoms

Epidermolysis bullosa is characterized by bullae formation (blistering) due to separation within the epidermis, followed by fluid accumulation. Bullae formation is typically initiated when lateral shearing forces are applied to the skin. Pressure applied perpendicular to the skin is not as great a hazard. Bullae formation can occur with even minimal trauma or can occur spontaneously.

The simplex form of epidermolysis bullosa is characterized by a benign course and normal development. By contrast, patients with the junctional form rarely survive beyond early childhood, with most dying from sepsis. Other features that distinguish junctional epidermolysis bullosa from other forms are generalized blistering beginning at birth, absence of scar formation, and generalized mucosal involvement (skin, gastrointestinal, genitourinary, and respiratory). In contrast to the junctional form, manifestations of epidermolysis bullosa dystrophica include severe scarring with fusion of the digits (pseudosyndactyly), constriction of the oral aperture (microstomia), and esophageal strictures. Teeth are often dysplastic. Malnutrition, anemia, electrolyte derangements, and hypoalbuminemia are common, most likely reflecting chronic infection, debilitation, and renal dysfunction. Survival beyond the second decade is unusual. Diseases associated with epidermolysis bullosa include porphyria, amyloidosis, multiple myeloma, diabetes mellitus, and hypercoagulable states. Mitral valve prolapse may accompany epidermolysis bullosa.

Treatment

Treatment of epidermolysis bullosa is symptomatic. Many of these patients will be receiving corticosteroids. Phenytoin has not been proved an effective treatment. Infection of bullae with *Staphylococcus aureus* or with beta hemolytic steptococci is common.

Management of Anesthesia

Management of anesthesia in the patient with epidermolysis bullosa must include consideration of the drugs used to treat the disease.[2] For example, supplemental corticosteroids may be indicated during the perioperative period, if the patient has been chronically treated with these drugs. Avoidance of trauma to the skin and mucous membranes is crucial. Bullae formation can be produced by trauma from tape, blood pressure cuffs, tourniquets, adhesive electrodes (as used to monitor the electrocardiogram or activity at the neuromuscular junction), and rubbing with alcohol wipes. If a blood pressure cuff must be used, it should be padded with a loose cotton

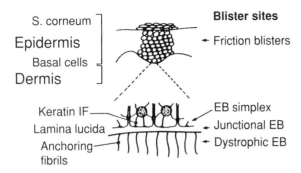

S. corneum
Epidermis
Basal cells
Dermis

Blister sites

→ Friction blisters

Keratin IF
Lamina lucida
Anchoring fibrils

← EB simplex
← Junctional EB
← Dystrophic EB

Fig. 26-1. Schematic drawing of histologic section of skin, indicating sites of cleavage in friction blisters and in the three major types of epidermolysis bullosa (EB). (From Epstein EH. Molecular genetics of epidermolysis bullosa. Science 1992;256:799–803, with permission.)

dressing. Intravenous and intra-arterial catheters should be sutured or held in place with a gauze wrap, rather than taped in place. Pulse oximetry using a nonadhesive sensor is indicated.

Trauma from an anesthetic face mask must be minimized by gentle application against the skin. Lubrication of the patient's face and mask with cortisol ointment can be helpful. Upper airway instrumentation should be minimized, as the squamous epithelium lining the oropharynx and esophagus is more susceptible to trauma than is the columnar epithelium of the trachea. Frictional trauma to the oropharynx, as produced by an oral airway, may result in large intraoral bullae formation and extensive hemorrhage from denuded mucosa. A nasal airway is equally hazardous. An esophageal stethoscope should be avoided, as it can lead to the formation of intraoral or esophageal bullae. Hemorrhage from ruptured oral bullae has been treated successfully by epinephrine-soaked gauze applied to the bullae.

Intubation of the trachea, despite theoretical hazards, has not been associated with laryngeal or tracheal complications in patients with epidermolysis bullosa dystrophica, and its more routine use in these patients has been recommended.[3] Indeed, laryngeal involvement with this form of the disease is rare, and tracheal bullae have not been reported. This finding is consistent with the greater resistance of the columnar epithelium that lines the trachea to disruption compared with the fragile squamous epithelium in the oral cavity. Generous lubrication of the laryngoscope blade with a cortisol ointment and vaseline gel and selection of a smaller size tube than usual is recommended. Chronic scarring of the oral cavity can result in a narrow oral aperture and immobility of the tongue, making tracheal intubation difficult. After tracheal intubation, the tube must be carefully immobilized with a soft cloth bandage, to prevent movement in the oropharynx. Tape is not used to hold the tube in place, and the tube must not exert lateral force at the corners of the mouth. At tracheal extubation, it must be remembered that oropharyngeal suctioning can lead to life-threatening bullae formation. The risk of pulmonary aspiration may be increased by the presence of esophageal strictures. The safety of tracheal intubation in the patient with junctional epidermolysis bullosa involving all mucosa, including the respiratory epithelium, is unproven.[4]

Porphyria cutanea tarda has been reported to occur with increased frequency in patients with epidermolysis bullosa.[5] This type of porphyria does not have the same implications for management of anesthesia as does the presence of acute intermittent porphyria. Ketamine is a useful drug for avoiding airway manipulation when the operative procedure does not require controlled ventilation of the lungs or skeletal muscle relaxation. Despite the presence of dystrophic skeletal muscle, there is no evidence based on clinical experience that these patients are at increased risk of a hyperkalemic response when treated with succinylcholine.[6] There are no known contraindications to the use of an inhaled anesthetic drug in these patients. As an alternative to general anesthesia, regional anesthesia (spinal, epidural, bracheal plexus) has been recommended.[6]

PEMPHIGUS

Pemphigus is a vesiculobullous disease that may involve extensive areas of the skin and mucous membranes. Buccal pemphigus closely resembles the oral manifestations of epidermolysis bullosa dystrophica. Involvement of the oropharynx is present in about 50% of patients with pemphigus. Extensive oropharyngeal involvement makes eating painful, and the patient may reduce oral intake to the point that severe malnutrition develops. Skin denudation and bullae formation can result in significant fluid and protein loss. The risk of secondary infection is great.

Pemphigus is most likely an autoimmune disorder in which circulating antibodies attack antigenic sites on the epidermal cell surface, resulting in destruction of the cell. As with epidermolysis bullosa, there may be an absence of the intercellular bridges that normally prevent the separation of epidermal cells. Therefore, frictional trauma may result in bullae formation. Occasionally, infection or drug sensitivity appear to be the inciting event for bullae formation. Pemphigus vulgaris is the most common variant of pemphigus and is also the most significant because of the high incidence of oral lesions.

Treatment

Treatment with corticosteroids has decreased mortality from this disease from 70% to 5%. Such drugs as azathioprine, methotrexate, cyclophosphamide, and cyclosporine have also been successfully used in the early treatment of pemphigus.

Management of Anesthesia

Management of anesthesia in the patient with pemphigus and epidermolysis bullosa is similar.[2,7] Airway management may be difficult because of co-existing bullae in the oropharynx.[8] Despite obvious concerns, numerous reports of uncomplicated elective tracheal intubation have been described. Likewise, the use of regional anesthesia, although controversial, has been successfully administered to these patients.[9] Ketamine is a useful drug for general anesthesia in selected patients.

Preoperative drug therapy must be considered. In this regard, supplementation of the usual corticosteroid dose may be necessary. Methotrexate produces immunosuppression, hepatorenal dysfunction, and depression of bone marrow activity but is unlikely to alter the activity of plasma cholinesterase enzyme. Azathioprine has been reported to antagonize nondepolarizing neuromuscular blockade, presumably reflecting inhibition of phosphodiesterase enzyme by this drug. Electrolyte derangements may reflect chronic fluid loss through bullous skin lesions.

PSORIASIS

Psoriasis is a common dermatologic disorder characterized by accelerated epidermal growth, resulting in a typical erythematous papule covered with loosely adherent scales. Synthesis of deoxyribonucleic acid in the epidermis of these patients is four times that present in normal epidermis. The skin lesions are symmetrically distributed and typically involve the elbows, knees, hairlines, and presacral regions. An inflammatory asymmetric arthropathy occurs in about 20% of patients with psoriasis. Uveitis and sacroilitis associated with ascending vertebral body disease are common. High cardiac output congestive heart failure has also been observed. Generalized pustular psoriasis is a rare form of the disease that may be complicated by decreased plasma concentrations of albumin, sepsis, and renal failure.

Treatment

Treatment of psoriasis is directed at slowing the rapid proliferation of epidermal cells. Crude coal tar is effective because of its antimitotic action and ability to inhibit enzymes. Topical corticosteroids are also effective, but the disease promptly recurs when treatment is discontinued. Application of corticosteroids under occlusive dressings can result in significant systemic absorption, with associated suppression of endogenous adrenal cortex activity. Systemic therapy with methotrexate, cyclosporine, and folate antagonists may be required for more severe cases. Toxic effects of these drugs include cirrhosis of the liver, renal failure, hypertension, and pneumonitis.

Management of Anesthesia

Management of anesthesia must include consideration of the drugs being used for the treatment of psoriasis. Skin trauma such as venipuncture and surgical incision may accentuate psoriasis in some patients. The patient with psoriasis can have a marked increase in skin blood flow, which could contribute to altered thermoregulation.

MASTOCYTOSIS

Mastocytosis is characterized by an abnormal proliferation of mast cells containing histamine and heparin. When the increase in mast cells occurs in the skin as small red-brown maculae on the trunk and upper extremities, the condition is known as urticaria pigmentosa, usually a benign and asymptomatic form of the disease, which accounts for about 90% of cases of mastocytosis. Children are most often afflicted, and in nearly one-half of patients, the lesions disappear by adulthood. Systemic mastocytosis is present when sites other than skin, most commonly the skeleton, liver, spleen, and lymph nodes, are invaded by mast cells. These abnormal aggregations of mast cells are primarily secretory and can abruptly release vasoactive substances. Some patients with systemic mastocytosis have an aggressive form of the disease that results in severe thrombocytopenia and hemorrhage. These patients often require splenectomy.

Signs and Symptoms

Degranulation of mast cells, with release of histamine, heparin, and prostaglandins into the systemic circulation, can be initiated by trauma, changes in body temperature, or exposure to drugs that stimulate the release of histamine. Often the precipitating event is unknown. The classic symptoms of mastocytosis are thought to be anaphylactoid in origin; manifestations of mast cell degranulation include pruritus, urticaria, and cutaneous flushing. These changes are frequently accompanied by hypotension and tachycardia. Hypotension may be so severe as to be life-threatening.

Symptoms of mastocytosis have traditionally been attributed to the release of histamine from mast cells. Nevertheless, a low incidence of respiratory distress is seen in patients with this syndrome. Furthermore, H-1 and H-2 receptor antagonists may not be protective, suggesting that vasoactive substances in addition to histamine may be involved. For example, there is evidence in some patients that symptoms may be due to overproduction of prostaglandin D2.[10] A bleeding tendency in these patients is unusual, even though mast cells contain heparin.

Management of Anesthesia

Although the reported anesthetic experience in patients with mastocytosis is scant, treatment is directed at mast cell stabilization and avoidance of histamine-releasing drugs.[11] Despite the fact that the intraoperative period is usually benign, there are reports of life-threatening anaphylactoid reactions occurring with even minor surgical procedures, emphasizing the need to have resuscitation drugs such as epinephrine immediately available when anesthetizing these patients.[12,13] Preoperative administration of both H-1 and H-2 antagonists would block receptor uptake of histamine. Nevertheless, these drugs would not influence histamine release from the mast cells. If the action of prostaglandins is suspected in a specific patient, it might be helpful to add a prostaglandin inhibitor such as aspirin to the preoperative preparation.[10] Conversely, aspirin is considered to be contraindicated by some on the basis of an alleged ability of this drug to initiate mast cell degranulation. An obvious goal during the perioperative period is to avoid administering drugs known to be potent stimuli for the release of histamine. Nevertheless, both meperidine and succinylcholine have been administered without adverse effects to these patients.[12] Vecuronium has not been associated with histamine release and may therefore be useful in patients with mastocytosis. Inhaled anesthetic drugs are considered acceptable for administration to the patient with mastocytosis. Propofol has also been used without complication.

ATOPIC DERMATITIS

Atopic dermatitis is the cutaneous manifestation of the atopic state. It is characterized by dry, scaly, eczematous, pruritic patches on the face, neck, and flexor surfaces of the arms or legs. Pruritus is the primary symptom. Systemic antihistamines may be effective in reducing pruritus. Corticosteroids may be indicated for short-term treatment of severe cases. The pulmonary manifestations of the atopic state, such as asthma, hay fever, otitis media, and sinusitis, may influence management of anesthesia.

URTICARIA

Urticaria (hives) is characterized by circumscribed wheals and localized areas of edema produced by extravasation of fluid through the walls of blood vessels. Angioedema describes urticaria involving the mucous membranes, particularly those of the mouth, pharynx, and larynx. Mast cells and basophils regulate the urticarial reaction. When stimulated by certain immunologic (drugs, inhaled allergens) or nonimmunologic events, storage granules in these cells release histamine and other vasoactive substances such as bradykinins. These substances result in the localized vasodilation and transudation of fluid characteristic of urticarial lesions.

Antihistamines are the mainstay of treatment of mild cases of urticaria. Severe urticarial attacks, especially if accompanied by angioedema, may require aggressive treatment with intravenous administration of epinephrine and diphenhydramine.

COLD URTICARIA

Cold urticaria is a rare disease characterized by relatively innocuous cutaneous lesions, which develop on exposure to cold. The pathophysiology appears to be the result of the release of histamine, although other vasoactive mediators, including kinins, have been described. Symptoms are usually limited to local erythematous and pruritic urticarial lesions. A highly sensitive person, however, on exposure to severe cold, may exhibit syncope, laryngeal edema, bronchospasm, and hypotension.[14]

Management of anesthesia should include avoidance of drugs that are likely to cause the release of histamine. Drugs that have been safely administered to these patients include volatile anesthetics, nitrous oxide, and fentanyl.[14] Preoperative administration of diphenhydramine (1 to 1.5 mg·kg^{-1}) and cimetidine (4 to 5 mg·kg^{-1}) has been recommended when an intraoperative reduction in body temperature is unavoidable, as in the patient undergoing cardiac surgery requiring cardiopulmonary bypass.[14] This drug combination will block H-1 and H-2 receptors and thus minimize circulatory effects of cold-induced histamine release. The administration of unwarmed intravenous solutions and the use of any sort of external cooling equipment, such as a surface blanket, would seem unwise.

ERYTHEMA MULTIFORME

Erythema multiforme is an acute recurrent disorder of the skin and mucous membranes characterized by lesions ranging from edematous macules and papules to vesicular or bullous lesions, which may ulcerate. Attacks are associated with viral diseases (especially herpes simplex), hemolytic streptococcal infections, neoplastic processes, collagen vascular diseases, and drug-induced hypersensitivity.

Stevens-Johnson Syndrome

Stevens-Johnson syndrome is a severe manifestation of erythema multiforme associated with multisystem involvement. High fever, tachycardia, and tachypnea may occur. Drugs associated with the onset of this syndrome include antibiotics, analgesics, and over-the-counter cough medications. Corticosteroids are effective in the management of severe cases.

Hazards of administering anesthesia to a patient with Stevens-Johnson syndrome are similar to those encountered in the patient with epidermolysis bullosa.[15] For example, involvement of the respiratory tract can make management of the upper airway and intubation of the trachea difficult. The presence of pulmonary blebs can make these patients vulnerable to pneumothorax, particularly with positive intrathoracic pressure. In addition, the presence of pulmonary blebs might detract from the use of nitrous oxide. Ketamine has been used successfully for anesthesia in these patients.

SCLERODERMA

Scleroderma or progressive systemic sclerosis is characterized by inflammation, vascular sclerosis, and fibrosis of the skin and viscera. Microvascular changes produce tissue fibrosis and organ sclerosis. Injury to vascular endothelial cells results in vascular obliteration and leakage of serum proteins into the interstitial space. These proteins produce tissue edema, lymphatic obstruction, and ultimately fibrosis. In some patients, the disease may evolve into the CREST syndrome (calcinoses, Raynaud's phenomenon, esophageal hypomotility, sclerodactyly, and telangiectasias). Prognosis is poor and is related to the extent of visceral rather than to cutaneous involvement. There is no known effective treatment for this disease. Corticosteroids should not be administered to patients with scleroderma.

The etiology of scleroderma is unknown, but the disease process has the characteristics of both a collagen disease and an autoimmune process. The typical time of onset is at 20 to 40 years of age, and females are most often afflicted. Pregnancy accelerates progression of scleroderma in about half of patients. The incidence of spontaneous abortion, premature labor, and perinatal mortality is high.

Signs and Symptoms

Manifestations of scleroderma occur in the skin and musculoskeletal system, nervous system, cardiovascular system, lungs, kidneys, and gastrointestinal tract.

Skin and Musculoskeletal System
The skin exhibits a mild thickening and a diffuse nonpitting edema. As scleroderma progresses, the skin becomes taut, leading to limited mobility and flexion contractures, especially of the fingers. Skeletal muscles may exhibit a myopathy, manifested as weakness of the proximal muscle groups. The plasma creatine kinase level is typically elevated. Mild inflammatory arthritis may occur, but most of the joint movement limitation is due to the thickened and taut overlying skin. Avascular necrosis of the femoral head may be present.

Nervous System
Peripheral or cranial nerve neuropathy in the presence of scleroderma has been ascribed to nerve compression by thickened connective tissue surrounding nerve sheaths. Facial pain suggestive of trigeminal neuralgia may also occur as a result of this thickening. Keratoconjunctivitis sicca exists in some patients and may predispose to corneal abrasions.

Cardiovascular System
Changes in the myocardium associated with scleroderma reflect sclerosis of smaller coronary arteries and the conduction system, replacement of cardiac muscle with fibrous tissue, and the indirect effects of systemic and pulmonary hypertension. These changes result in cardiac dysrhythmias, cardiac conduction abnormalities, and congestive heart failure. Intimal fibrosis of the pulmonary artery walls is associated with a high incidence of pulmonary hypertension, which may progress to cor pulmonale. Pulmonary hypertension is often present, even in asymptomatic patients. Pericarditis and pericardial effusion, with or without cardiac tamponade, are not an infrequent occurrence. Changes in the peripheral vascular system are common and are characterized by intermittent vasospasm in the small arteries to the digits. Oral or nasal telangiectasias may be present. Raynaud's phenomenon occurs in most cases and may be in the initial manifestation of scleroderma.

Lungs
Effects of scleroderma on the lungs are a major cause of morbidity and mortality. Diffuse interstitial pulmonary fibrosis may occur independent of the vascular changes that lead to pulmonary hypertension. Pulmonary fibrosis causes decreased inspiratory capacity and increased residual volume. Although dermal sclerosis does not decrease chest wall compliance, pulmonary compliance is diminished by fibrosis, and increased airway pressures may be required for adequate ventilation of the lungs. Arterial hypoxemia resulting from decreased diffusion capacity is not unusual in these patients, even at rest.

Kidneys
Renal artery obstruction as a result of arteriolar intimal proliferation leads to reductions in renal blood flow and hypertension. Indeed, sudden development of accelerated hypertension and irreversible renal failure is the most common cause of death in patients with scleroderma. Captopril may improve the impaired renal function that accompanies hypertension in these patients.

Gastrointestinal Tract

Involvement of the gastrointestinal tract by scleroderma may be manifested as dryness of the oral mucosa (xerostomia). Progressive fibrosis of the gastrointestinal tract causes hypomotility of the lower esophagus and small intestine. Dysphagia is a common complaint, due to hypomotility of the esophagus. Lower esophageal sphincter tone is reduced, with subsequent reflux of acidic gastric fluid into the esophagus. Symptoms from the resulting esophagitis can be treated with antacids. Bacterial overgrowth due to intestinal hypomotility can produce a malabsorption syndrome. Indeed, a coagulation disorder may reflect malabsorption of vitamin K from the gastrointestinal tract. Broad-spectrum antibiotics are effective in the treatment of this type of malabsorption syndrome. Intestinal hypomotility may also be manifested clinically as intestinal pseudoobstruction. In this regard, prokinetic drugs are not very effective motor stimulants, whereas a somatostatin analogue, octreotide, may evoke intestinal contractions.

Management of Anesthesia

Preoperative evaluation of the patient with scleroderma should focus attention on the multiple organ systems likely to be involved by the progressive changes associated with this disease.[16,17] Decreased mandibular motion and narrowing of the oral aperture due to taut skin must be appreciated before the induction of anesthesia. The use of a fiberoptic laryngoscope may facilitate endotracheal intubation through a small oral opening. Oral or nasal telangiectasias may bleed profusely if traumatized during placement of a tube in the trachea. Intravenous access may be impeded by dermal thickening. Vasoconstriction may interfere with blood pressure monitoring by auscultation necessitating the use of an ultrasonic blood pressure sensor. Catheterization of a peripheral artery introduces the same concerns present in the patient with Raynaud's phenomenon. Cardiac evaluation, including auscultation of the chest and review of the electrocardiogram, may provide evidence of pulmonary hypertension. Because of chronic systemic hypertension and vasomotor instability, the patient with scleroderma can have a contracted intravascular fluid volume, manifested as hypotension, with vasodilation induced by drugs used for anesthesia. Relaxation of the lower esophageal sphincter makes these patients vulnerable to regurgitation and subsequent pulmonary aspiration, should protective laryngeal reflexes be depressed. For this reason, efforts to increase gastric fluid pH with an antacid or histamine receptor antagonist before the induction of anesthesia may be recommended.

Intraoperatively, decreased pulmonary compliance may necessitate increased positive airway pressure to ensure adequate ventilation of the lungs. Supplemental oxygen is indicated, in view of impaired diffusion capacity and vulnerability for the development of arterial hypoxemia. Indeed, events known to increase pulmonary vascular resistance, such as respiratory acidosis and arterial hypoxemia, must be prevented. An acute increase in central venous pressure during administration of nitrous oxide could reflect pulmonary artery vasoconstriction due to effects of this drug. The eyes should remain protected at all times, in view of the possibility of co-existing keratoconjunctivitis. The role of renal function should be considered in the selection of drugs dependent on this route for clearance from the plasma. Prolonged responses to local anesthetics have been reported, but the explanation or significance of this observation is unclear. Furthermore, regional anesthesia may be technically difficult because of skin and joint changes that accompany scleroderma. Attractive features of regional anesthesia include postoperative analgesia and peripheral vasodilation that improves perfusion to the lower extremities. Other measures to minimize peripheral vasoconstriction include maintenance of operating room temperature above 21°C and administration of warm intravenous fluids. These patients may be sensitive to the ventilatory depressant effects of opioids and postoperative support of ventilation may be required, especially in the presence of severe co-existing pulmonary disease.

PSEUDOXANTHOMA ELASTICUM

Pseudoxanthoma elasticum is a rare hereditary disorder of elastic tissue. Elastic fibers degenerate and calcify with time. The most striking feature of this condition, and often the basis for the diagnosis, is the appearance of angioid streaks in the retina. Substantial loss of visual acuity may result from these changes. Additional impairment of vision may occur when vascular changes predispose to vitreous hemorrhage. Skin changes, consisting of yellowish, rectangular, elevated xanthoma-like lesions, occurring primarily in the neck, axilla, and inguinal regions, are often the earliest recognized clinical features. It is surprising that those tissues most rich in elastic fibers, such as the lungs, aorta, palms, and soles, are not affected by the disease process.

Gastrointestinal hemorrhage is a frequent occurrence in these patients. Degenerative changes in the walls of arteries supplying the gastrointestinal tract are thought to prevent constriction of these vessels in response even to minimal mucosal damage. The incidence of hypertension and ischemic heart disease is increased in these patients. Endocardial calcification may involve the conduction system of the heart, predisposing these patients to cardiac dysrhythmias and sudden death. Involvement of cardiac valves with this disease process is frequent. Calcification of peripheral vessels, particularly of the radial or ulnar arteries, is common. Psychiatric disturbances often accompany this disease.

Management of Anesthesia

Management of anesthesia in the presence of pseudoxanthoma elasticum is based on an appreciation of the abnormalities associated with this disease.[18] Cardiovascular derangements that may occur in these patients are probably the most important considerations. The high incidence of ischemic heart disease should be remembered when establishing limits for acceptable changes in blood pressure and heart rate. Monitoring of the electrocardiogram is particularly important, in view of the potential for the development of cardiac dysrhythmias. The use of an ultrasonic sensor to monitor blood pressure is an acceptable alternative to the placement of an intra-arterial catheter. Trauma to the mucosa of the upper gastrointestinal tract, as may be produced by instrumentation with a gastric tube or esophageal stethoscope, should be minimized. There are no specific recommendations regarding the choice of anesthetic drugs or techniques.

EHLERS-DANLOS SYNDROME

Ehlers-Danlos syndrome consists of a group of inherited connective tissue disorders (at least nine distinct types have been described) due to abnormalities of metabolism in type III collagen. The gastrointestinal tract, uterus, and blood vessels are particularly well-endowed with type III collagen, accounting for complications such as spontaneous rupture of the bowel, uterus, or major blood vessels. Premature labor and excessive bleeding with delivery are common obstetric problems. Dilation of the trachea is often present. The incidence of pneumothorax is increased in these patients. Mitral regurgitation and cardiac conduction abnormalities are possible. Afflicted patients tend to exhibit extensive ecchymosis with even minimal trauma. Nevertheless, a specific coagulation defect has not been identified.

Management of Anesthesia

Management of anesthesia in the patient with Ehlers-Danlos syndrome must consider the cardiorespiratory manifestations of this disease and the propensity for these patients to bleed excessively with interruption of vascular integrity.[19] Prophylactic antibiotics to protect against infective endocarditis may be indicated, in the presence of a cardiac murmur suggestive of mitral regurgitation. Avoidance of intramuscular injections or instrumentation of the nose or esophagus is important, in view of the bleeding tendency. Trauma during direct laryngoscopy for intubation of the trachea must be minimized. Likewise, placement of an arterial or central venous catheter must be tempered with the realization that hematoma formation may be extensive. Extravasation of intravenous fluids due to a displaced venous cannula may go unnoticed because of the extreme distensibility of the skin. Maintenance of low airway pressure during assisted or controlled ventilation of the lungs would seem prudent, in view of the increased incidence of pneumothorax in these patients. There are no specific recommendations for drug choices to provide anesthesia. Regional anesthesia is not recommended, however, because of the tendency of these patients to bleed and form extensive hematomas. Surgical complications include uncontrollable hemorrhage and postoperative wound dehiscence.

POLYMYOSITIS

Polymyositis (dermatomyositis) is a multisystem disease of unknown etiology, manifested as nonsuppurative inflammation of skeletal muscle (inflammatory myopathy). Cutaneous changes include discoloration of the upper eyelids, periorbital edema, a scaly erythematous malar rash, and symmetric erythematous atrophic changes over the extensor surfaces of joints. This characteristic rash has led to the alternate designation of this disease as dermatomyositis. It is speculated that an abnormality of the immune response may be responsible for slowly progressive skeletal muscle damage. The concept that altered cellular immunity causes polymyositis is supported by the fact that 10% to 20% of affected patients have an occult neoplasm.

Signs and Symptoms

Weakness of skeletal muscles typically involves proximal muscle groups, including the flexors of the neck, shoulders, and hips. The patient may have difficulty climbing stairs. Dysphagia, pulmonary aspiration, and pneumonia may result from paresis of pharyngeal and respiratory muscles. Weakness of the intercostal muscles and diaphragm can contribute to ventilatory insufficiency. Necrosis of skeletal muscles results in an elevation of the plasma creatine kinase level that parallels the extent and rapidity of skeletal muscle destruction. There is no evidence that the disease affects the neuromuscular junction.

Heart block secondary to myocardial fibrosis or atrophy of the conduction system, left ventricular dysfunction, and myocarditis can occur. Polymyositis can also be associated with systemic lupus erythematosus, scleroderma, and rheumatoid arthritis. A widespread necrotizing vasculitis may be present in the childhood form of this disease.

Diagnosis and Treatment

The diagnosis of polymyositis is confirmed by proximal skeletal muscle weakness, an elevated plasma creatine kinase concentration, and the presence of the characteristic skin rash. Electromyography may demonstrate a triad consisting of spontaneous fibrillation potentials, decreased amplitude of voluntary contraction potentials, and repetitive potentials on needle insertion. Skeletal muscle biopsy adds support to the clinical diagnosis. Muscular dystrophy or myasthenia gravis can mimic polymyositis. Corticosteroids are considered the treatment of choice, although their efficacy has not been proved in carefully controlled trials. Immunosuppressive therapy with methotrexate, azathioprine, or cyclosporine may be effective when the response to corticosteroids is inadequate. Inclusion body myositis mimics polymyositis, but involvement of distal muscles is characteristic, and these patients are often unresponsive to therapy.

Management of Anesthesia

Management of anesthesia must consider the vulnerability of the patient with polymyosites to pulmonary aspiration. It has been recommended that agents triggering malignant hyperthermia be avoided in these patients, if the plasma creatine kinase concentration is elevated.[21] In view of co-existing skeletal muscle weakness, there is a logical concern that these patients could display abnormal responses to muscle relaxants. Nevertheless, the response to nondepolarizing muscle relaxants (atracurium, vecuronium) and succinylcholine has been described as unchanged in the presence of polymyositis.[20,21] The response to succinylcholine may resemble that observed in the patient with myotonic dystrophy. The possibility of postoperative skeletal muscle weakness, which can lead to ventilatory insufficiency, must be appreciated.

SYSTEMIC LUPUS ERYTHEMATOSUS

Systemic lupus erythematosus is a multisystem chronic inflammatory disease characterized by antinuclear antibody production, most often exhibited in young females. One hypothesis for its pathogenesis is a genetically determined lack of suppression of B lymphocyte function by T lymphocytes, such that the patient's own tissues act as antigens to stimulate the production of antibodies. Stresses such as infection, pregnancy, or surgery may exacerbate the disease. The onset of systemic lupus erythematosus may also be drug induced. Drugs most frequently associated with this syndrome are hydralazine, procainamide, isoniazid, D-penicillamine, alpha methyldopa, and occasionally nonbarbiturate anticonvulsants. Susceptibility to the development of systemic lupus erythematosus, as induced by hydralazine or procainamide, is related to the acetylator phenotype of the patient. In patients who metabolize these drugs slowly (slow acetylators), the disease is more likely to develop. The clinical picture of the drug-induced syndrome is similar to the spontaneous form of the disease, but progression of the disease is usually much slower, and symptoms are milder.

Signs and Symptoms

Clinical manifestations of systemic lupus erythematosus may be categorized as articular and systemic.

Articular

Symmetric arthritis involving the hands, wrists, elbows, knees, and ankles is the most common manifestation of systemic lupus erythematosus, occurring in 90% of patients. Another form of skeletal involvement is avascular necrosis, which most often involves the head or condyle of the femur.

Systemic

Systemic manifestations affect the heart, lungs, kidneys, liver, neuromuscular system, and skin.

Heart

Pericarditis resulting in chest pain and a friction rub is the most common cardiac manifestation of systemic lupus erythematosus. Myocarditis may result in abnormalities of cardiac conduction. Persistent tachycardia and congestive heart failure can develop, with extensive cardiac involvement. Left ventricular dysfunction has been demonstrated in young patients. A noninfectious endocarditis (Libman-Sacks endocarditis) may involve the aortic and mitral valves.

Lungs

Pulmonary involvement of systemic lupus erythematosus may be manifested as lupus pneumonia, characterized by diffuse pulmonary infiltrates, pleural effusion, dry cough, dyspnea, and arterial hypoxemia. Pulmonary function studies in these patients commonly show a restrictive type of pulmonary disease.

Kidneys

The most common renal abnormality is glomerulonephritis with proteinuria, resulting in hypoalbuminemia. Hematuria is a frequent finding. Severe reductions in glomerular filtration rate can terminate in oliguric renal failure.

Liver

Abnormalities of liver function tests may be present in a large number of patients with systemic lupus erythematosus. In some patients, lupoid hepatitis develops, characterized by recurrent jaundice, hepatomegaly, abnormal liver function tests, and hyperglobulinemia. This form of hepatitis may be fatal. In addition, the patient may show signs of an acute abdomen secondary to intestinal ischemia.

Neuromuscular

Psychological changes ranging from mood disturbances suggestive of schizophrenia to signs of organic psychosis with deterioration of intellectual capacity occur in nearly one-half of patients with systemic lupus erythematosus. Myopathy, with weakness of proximal skeletal muscle groups and an elevated plasma creatine kinase concentration, is often present.

Skin

The typical skin lesion associated with systemic lupus erythematosus is an erythematous rash, which develops over the nasal malar area (butterfly rash). This rash is usually transient and often accompanies exacerbations of the disease. Alopecia is another frequent manifestation of exacerbation of the disease.

Laboratory Findings

In addition to the predictable laboratory findings associated with liver and renal dysfunction, the patient with systemic lupus erythematosus may have unexpected laboratory alterations. For example, more than 90% of patients with this disease have a positive antinuclear antibody test. Circulating anticoagulants can be reflected by a prolonged prothrombin time and activated partial thromboplastin time. The patient with circulating anticoagulants often manifests a biologic false positive test for syphilis. Anemia, thrombocytopenia, and leukopenia are common.

Treatment

Anti-inflammatory therapy with aspirin is the usual initial treatment of systemic lupus erythematosus. After initiation of this therapy, some patients have elevated plasma transaminase concentrations, presumably reflecting aspirin-induced hepatitis. Corticosteroids are effective in suppressing glomerulonephritis and adverse changes in the cardiovascular system. Immunosuppressive drugs are often used when the patient does not respond to corticosteroids. Antimalarial drugs, in small doses, may be effective in treating the arthritis and skin rash associated with the disease.

Management of Anesthesia

Management of anesthesia is influenced by drugs used in the treatment of systemic lupus erythematosus and by the magnitude of dysfunction of those organs damaged by the disease.[22] Central nervous system manifestations include seizures, neuropathies, and stroke. Laryngeal involvement, including mucosal ulceration, cricoarytenoid arthritis, and recurrent laryngeal nerve palsy, may be present in as many as 30% of patients.[23]

URBACH-WIETHE DISEASE

Urbach-Wiethe disease (lipoid proteinosis) is a rare recessively inherited multisystem disorder affecting primarily the skin and oral mucosa.[24] A characteristic deposition of a hyaline material in the capillary walls and epithelial basement membrane regions leads to thickening of the skin or mucosa and a predisposition to minor trauma resulting in widespread scarring. Laryngeal scarring is manifested by hoarseness and may cause difficulties with tracheal intubation. Infiltration of the soft tissues and tongue may make direct laryngoscopy difficult, emphasizing the need to consider the use of a flexible fiberoptic laryngoscope. In view of the abnormal oral mucosa, the need for an antisialagogue in the preoperative medication is doubtful. A decreased gag reflex may put these patients at risk of aspiration. A recommendation to avoid epileptogenic anesthetic drugs is based on the propensity of these patients toward the development of epilepsy.[23]

CORNELIA de LANGE SYNDROME

Cornelia de Lange syndrome is a rare disorder believed to be due to hypoplasia of the mesenchyma. The maturation of most organ systems, including the central nervous system, is delayed. There is some growth and mental retardation, hirsutism, and microbrachycephaly. Many of these patients die before 1 year of age, most often due to aspiration. Anesthetic experience is limited but may be characterized by increased sensitivity to depressant drugs, an increased risk of aspiration owing to the common presence of hiatal hernia, and difficult tracheal intubation due to a short neck, small mouth, and high arched palate.[25]

TUMORAL CALCINOSIS

Tumoral calcinosis usually presents as multiple soft tissue masses adjacent to large joints, which appear radiologically as lobulated calcifications. Joint motion is generally unaffected, but the mass may enlarge and interfere with skeletal muscle function. Treatment consists of early and complete excision of the mass. The principal anesthetic consideration is the rare involvement of the hyoid bone, hypothyroid ligament, and cervical intervertebral joints by the disease process, leading to difficult exposure of the glottic opening during direct laryngoscopy.[26]

MUSCULAR DYSTROPHY

Muscular dystrophy is a hereditary disease characterized by painless degeneration and atrophy of skeletal muscles.[27] There is progressive and symmetric skeletal muscle weakness and wasting, but no evidence of muscle denervation (intact sensation and reflexes). Mental retardation is often present. Increased permeability of skeletal muscle membranes precedes clinical evidence of the disease. In order of decreasing frequency, muscular dystrophy can be categorized as pseudohypertrophic (Duchenne), limb-girdle, facioscapulohumeral (Landouzy-Dejerine), nemaline rod myopathy, and oculopharyngeal dystrophy.

Pseudohypertrophic Muscular Dystrophy

Pseudohypertrophic muscular dystrophy is the most common (3 per 10,000 births), and most severe, form of childhood progressive muscular dystrophy. The disease is caused by an X-linked recessive gene, becoming apparent in males aged 2 to 5 years. Initial symptoms (waddling gait, frequent falling, difficulty climbing stairs) reflect involvement of the proximal skeletal muscle groups of the pelvis. Affected skeletal muscles may become larger, as a result of fatty infiltration, accounting for the designation of this disorder as pseudohypertrophic. There is steady deterioration in skeletal muscle strength, resulting in confinement to a wheelchair by 8 to 11 years of age. Kyphoscoliosis may develop, reflecting the unopposed action of antagonists of the dystrophic muscles.[27] Skeletal muscle atrophy can predispose to long bone fractures. The plasma creatine kinase concentration is 30 to 300 times normal, even early in the disease, reflecting skeletal muscle necrosis and the increased permeability of skeletal muscle membranes. Approximately 70% of female carriers of this disease also exhibit an elevated plasma creatine kinase concentration. Skeletal muscle biopsy early in the course of the disease may demonstrate necrosis and phagocytosis of muscle fibers. Death usually occurs at 15 to 25 years of age due to congestive heart failure or pneumonia, or both.

Cardiopulmonary Dysfunction

Degeneration of cardiac muscle invariably accompanies muscular dystrophy. Characteristic changes on the electrocardiogram include a tall R wave in V1, deep Q wave in the limb leads, a short P-R interval, and sinus tachycardia. Mitral regurgitation may be due to papillary muscle dysfunction and to decreased myocardial contractility.

Chronic weakness of inspiratory respiratory muscles and a decreased ability to cough can result in loss of pulmonary reserve and an accumulation of secretions that predisposes to recurrent pneumonia. Respiratory insufficiency often remains covert because impaired skeletal muscle function prevents patients from exceeding their limited breathing capacity. As the disease progresses, kyphoscoliosis can contribute further to a restrictive pattern of lung disease. Sleep apnea is possible

and may contribute to development of pulmonary hypertention (see Chapter 17). An estimated 30% of deaths among patients with this form of muscular dystrophy is due to respiratory causes.[27]

Management of Anesthesia

Preparations for anesthesia in the patient afflicted with pseudohypertrophic muscular dystrophy must take into consideration implications of increased permeability of skeletal muscle membranes and decreased cardiopulmonary reserve.[27] Succinylcholine may be associated with exaggerated potassium release leading to life-threatening cardiac dysrhythmias. Indeed, ventricular fibrillation that occurs during induction of anesthesia that included succinylcholine has been observed in patients later discovered to have pseudohypertrophic muscular dystrophy.[27] Rhabdomyolysis manifested as myoglobinemia can occur. A normal response usually follows the administration of a nondepolarizing muscle relaxant, although the possibility of a prolonged response should be considered when co-existing skeletal muscle weakness is prominent.[28] Dantrolene should be available, as there is an increased incidence of malignant hyperthermia in these patients.[29,30] Malignant hyperthermia has been observed after only a brief period of administration of halothane alone, although most cases have been triggered by succinylcholine or with prolonged inhalation of halothane. Hypomotility of the gastrointestinal tract may delay gastric emptying, which in the presence of weak laryngeal reflexes will increase the risk of pulmonary aspiration. Depressant effects of volatile anesthetics on myocardial contractility can be exaggerated, leading some to recommend the use of opioids in these patients.[31] In this regard, cardiac arrest after induction of anesthesia has been described in afflicted patients.[32] Monitoring is directed at early detection of malignant hyperthermia (capnography, temperature) and cardiac depression. Postoperative pulmonary dysfunction must be anticipated and attempts made to facilitate clearance of secretions. Delayed pulmonary insufficiency may occur up to 36 hours postoperatively, despite apparent recovery to the preoperative level of skeletal muscle strength. Regional anesthesia avoids many of the unique risks of general anesthesia in these patients; during the postoperative period it provides analgesia, which may facilitate chest physiotherapy.[33]

Limb-Girdle Muscular Dystrophy

Limb-girdle muscular dystrophy is a slowly progressive and relatively benign disease. The age of onset varies from the second to fifth decades. The shoulder girdle or hip girdle may be the only skeletal muscle group involved.

Facioscapulohumeral Muscular Dystrophy

Facioscapulohumeral muscular dystrophy is characterized by slowly progressive wasting of facial, pectoral, and shoulder girdle skeletal muscles that begins in adolescence. Eventually, the lower limbs are involved. Early symptoms include difficulty in raising the arms above the head and in smiling. The heart is not involved, and the plasma creatine kinase concentration is seldom elevated. Recovery from atracurium-induced neuromuscular blockade has been described as faster than normal.[34] The course is slow, and longevity is likely.

Nemaline Rod Muscular Dystrophy

Nemaline rod myopathy is an autosomal dominant disease characterized by nonprogressive symmetric skeletal muscle weakness affecting principally proximal skeletal muscles. Diagnosis is confirmed by histologic examination of skeletal muscle demonstrating the presence of rods between normal myofibrils. Affected infants may present with hypotonia, dysphagia, respiratory distress, and cyanosis. Micrognathia and dental malocclusion are common. Other skeletal deformities include kyphoscoliosis and pectus excavatum. Restrictive lung disease may result from myopathy and scoliosis. Cardiac failure has been described.

Intubation of the trachea may be difficult due to associated anatomic abnormalities.[35] Respiratory depressant effects of drugs may be exaggerated in these patients. Bulbar palsy may further complicate anesthetic management due to regurgitation and pulmonary aspiration. Resistance to the effects of succinylcholine has been described in a patient who responded normally to pancuronium. There has been no reported association of nemaline rod myopathy with malignant hyperthermia.

Oculopharyngeal Dystrophy

Oculopharyngeal dystrophy is a rare variant of muscular dystrophy characterized by progressive dysphagia and ptosis. Although experience is limited, these patients may be at risk for aspiration in the perioperative period, and the sensitivity to muscle relaxants may be greatly enhanced.[36]

MYOTONIC DYSTROPHY

Myotonic dystrophy designates a group of hereditary degenerative diseases of skeletal muscles characterized by persistent contracture (myotonia) of skeletal muscles after their stimulation. The electromyographic findings are characterized by a prolonged discharge of repetitive muscle action potentials. The inability of the skeletal muscles to relax after stimulation is diagnostic and results from abnormal calcium metabo-

lism, as the cellular-adenosine triphosphatase system fails to return calcium to the sarcoplasmic reticulum. Unsequestered calcium then remains available to produce sustained skeletal muscle contraction. This accounts for the failure of general anesthesia, regional anesthesia, or muscle relaxants to prevent or relieve contraction of the skeletal muscles. Infiltration of contracted skeletal muscles with local anesthetics may induce relaxation. Quinine (300 to 600 mg IV) has been reported effective in some cases.[37] Warming the ambient air temperature in the operating room reduces the severity of myotonia, as well as the incidence of postoperative shivering, which may precipitate contraction of skeletal muscles. The three important syndromes of myotonic dystrophy are myotonia dystrophica (myotonia atrophica, Steinert's disease), myotonia congenita, and paramyotonia.

Myotonia Dystrophica

Myotonia dystrophica is the most common (2.4 to 5.5 per 100,000 of the population), and most serious, form of myotonic dystrophy afflicting adults.[37–39] This disease is inherited as an autosomal dominant trait, with the onset of symptoms occurring in the second to third decades of life. Treatment is symptomatic and may include the use of phenytoin, quinine, tocainide, or mexiletine. These drugs depress sodium influx into skeletal muscle cells and delay the return of membrane excitability. Death from pneumonia or cardiac failure, or both, usually occurs by the sixth decade, reflecting the progressive involvement of skeletal, cardiac, and smooth muscles. High perioperative morbidity and mortality are caused principally by cardiopulmonary complications.[40]

Signs and Symptoms

Myotonia dystrophica is a multisystem disease, although skeletal muscles are principally afflicted. Typically, the patient shows early facial weakness (expressionless facies), wasting and weakness of sternocleidomastoid muscles, ptosis, dysarthria, and an inability to relax the grip (myotonia). The triad of characteristic features consists of mental retardation, frontal baldness, and cataract formation. Involvement of endocrine glands is manifested as gonadal atrophy, diabetes mellitus, decreased thyroid function, and adrenal insufficiency. Occurrence of central sleep apnea in the patient with myotonic dystrophy is well known and probably accounts for their hypersomnolence. There is an increased incidence of cholelithiasis, especially in males. Exacerbation of symptoms during pregnancy is common, and it is not unusual for uterine atony and retained placenta to accompany vaginal delivery.[41]

Cardiac dysrhythmias and conduction abnormalities presumably reflect myocardial involvement by the myotonic process. First-degree atrioventricular heart block is a common finding on the electrocardiogram before the clinical onset of the disease. Up to 20% of these patients have evidence of mitral valve prolapse on echocardiography. Despite the relatively high incidence of mitral valve prolapse, systemic complications are rare. Reports of sudden death may reflect third-degree atrioventricular heart block. Weakness of pharyngeal and thoracic muscles renders these patients vulnerable to pulmonary aspiration of acidic gastric fluid.

Management of Anesthesia

Management of anesthesia in these patients must consider the likely presence of cardiomyopathy, respiratory muscle weakness, and abnormal responses to drugs used during anesthesia.[42] It should be assumed that even asymptomatic patients have some degree of cardiomyopathy. Therefore, myocardial depression from volatile anesthetic drugs may be exaggerated.[43,44] The need to control cardiac dysrhythmias must be anticipated. Anesthesia and surgery could theoretically aggravate co-existing cardiac conduction blockade by increasing vagal tone or causing transient hypoxia of the conduction system.

The most important potential adverse reaction in these patients is prolonged skeletal muscle contraction after the injection of succinylcholine[37] (Fig. 26-2). Contraction of skeletal muscles can last 2 to 3 minutes and be so severe as to make adequate ventilation of the lungs difficult. Conversely, the response to nondepolarizing muscle relaxants is normal.[45] Theoretically, reversal of neuromuscular blockade could precipitate

skeletal muscle contraction by facilitating depolarization of the neuromuscular junction. Nevertheless, adverse responses do not predictably occur when neostigmine is used to reverse neuromuscular blockade in patients with myotonic dystrophy.[43] Careful titration of neuromuscular blockade and administration of short- or intermediate-acting muscle relaxants may obviate the need for pharmacologic reversal in selected patients.[46]

These patients are very sensitive to the ventilatory depressant effects of barbiturates, opioids, benzodiazepines, and propofol, most likely reflecting central nervous system depression of ventilation by the drug, superimposed on an already weak and atrophic peripheral respiratory musculature. Furthermore, the co-existing hypersomnolence and vulnerability to central sleep apnea may contribute to an increased sensitivity to depressant drugs. Although there is an association between this syndrome and malignant hyperthermia, there are no data to confirm a definite relationship.[38] Postoperatively, local or regional anesthesia is useful for pain relief, and careful nursing surveillance is indicated for several hours.

Myotonia Congenita

Myotonia congenita is transmitted as a mendelian dominant characteristic, manifested at birth or early in childhood. Skeletal muscle involvement is widespread, but there is usually no involvement of other organ systems. The disease does not

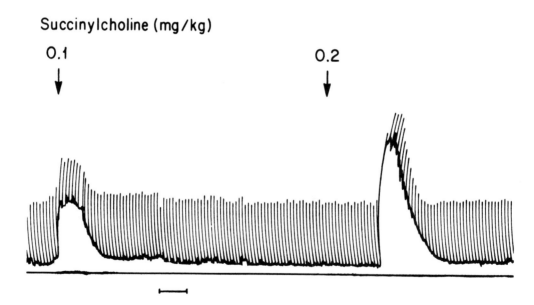

Fig. 26-2. Skeletal muscle contraction after administration of succinylcholine to a patient with myotonia dystrophica, evidenced by the dose-related upward shift of the baseline produced by even small doses of this muscle relaxant. (From Mitchell MM, Ali HH, Savarese JJ. Myotonia and neuromuscular blocking agents. Anesthesiology 1978;49:44–8, with permission.)

progress, nor does it result in a decreased life expectancy. The patient with myotonia congenita responds to quinidine therapy.

Paramyotonia

Paramyotonia is the rarest of the myotonic syndromes. Signs and symptoms are identical to those of myotonia congenita, except that paramyotonia develops only on exposure to cold. It is speculated that paramyotonia is a variant of the hyperkalemic form of familial periodic paralysis (see the section, Familial Periodic Paralysis). The possibility of initiating skeletal muscle contraction by exposure to a decreased ambient temperature in the operating room is undocumented. Nevertheless, logic would suggest that decreased ambient temperatures should be avoided when a patient with this diagnosis requires operation.

FLOPPY INFANT SYNDROME

Floppy infant syndrome is a term used to describe infants who have weak and hypotonic skeletal muscles owing to neuromuscular or non-neuromuscular causes. Diminished cough reflex, aspiration, and recurrent pneumonia are common. Weakness of bulbar musculature may produce difficulty in swallowing and breathing. Progressive weakness and atrophy of skeletal muscles leads to contractures and kyphoscoliosis. Management of anesthesia, as for a skeletal muscle biopsy to confirm the diagnosis, may be associated with an increased sensitivity to nondepolarizing muscle relaxants, hyperkalemia, and cardiac arrest after the administration of succinylcholine. Susceptibility to malignant hyperthermia that may be present in patients with skeletal muscle myopathies limits the use of certain inhaled anesthetics and muscle relaxants. Ketamine is useful for providing surgical anesthesia without depression of ventilation, while avoiding muscle relaxants and other potential triggering drugs for malignant hyperthermia.[47]

HYPEREKPLEXIA

Hyperekplexia (stiff-baby syndrome) is a rare genetic syndrome characterized by intense skeletal muscle rigidity manifested immediately after birth. Similarities between this syndrome and hyperexplexia (exaggerated startle response to sudden noises or movement) are remarkable; they may even be the same disease. Electromyography in a patient with hyperekplexia demonstrates continuous skeletal muscle activity, with only rare periods of quiescence. Choking, vomiting, and difficulty with swallowing are common; motor development is delayed, but intelligence is normal. Skeletal muscle stiffness

or hyperekplexia disappears gradually during the first years of life.

Experience with this syndrome is too limited to make recommendations regarding anesthesia. In a single affected infant, resistance to succinylcholine was observed, whereas the response to pancuronium and neostigmine were considered normal.[48] In this same patient, a substantial increase in the resting tension of skeletal muscles was observed during the onset of action of succinylcholine. Release of potassium was not enhanced after administration of succinylcholine. Responses to volatile anesthetics and nitrous oxide seem predictable in these patients.

TRACHEOMEGALY

Tracheomegaly is characterized by marked dilation of the trachea and bronchi, which is due to a congenital defect of elastic and smooth muscle fibers of the tracheobronchial tree or their destruction after radiotherapy, especially to the head and neck.[49] The diagnosis is confirmed by a tracheal diameter greater than 30 mm on a chest radiograph. Symptoms include chronic productive cough and frequent pulmonary infections, most likely reflecting chronic aspiration. Tracheal and bronchial walls are abnormally flaccid and may collapse, especially during vigorous coughing. Aspiration is a possibility during general anesthesia, especially if maximal inflation of the tracheal tube cuff fails to provide an airtight seal.

MYASTHENIA GRAVIS

Myasthenia gravis is a chronic autoimmune disease involving the neuromuscular junction. The hallmark of the disease is weakness and rapid exhaustion of voluntary skeletal muscles with repetitive use, followed by partial recovery with rest.[50] Skeletal muscles innervated by cranial nerves are especially vulnerable, as reflected by ptosis and diplopia, which may be the initial symptoms of the disease. The incidence is about 1 in every 20,000 adults. Females between 20 and 30 years of age are most often affected, whereas males are often older than 60 years of age when the disease is manifested.

Pathophysiology

The basic defect resulting in skeletal muscle weakness and easy exhaustion is a decrease in the number of available receptors for acetylcholine at the postsynaptic neuromuscular junction[51] (Fig. 26–3). This decrease in available receptors is due to their inactivation or destruction by circulating antibodies. Attachment of these antibodies to receptors for acetylcholine either blocks access for neurotransmitter to receptors or ac-

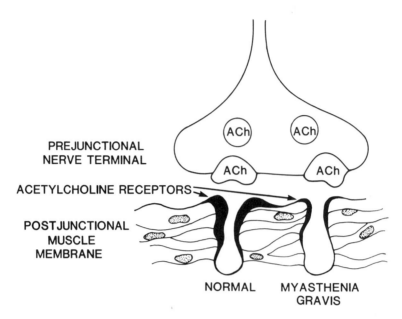

Fig. 26-3. Schematic diagram of the neuromuscular junction, depicting the density of acetylcholine (ACh) receptors on the folds of postjunctional muscle membranes. Compared with normal folds, the density of ACh receptors is greatly reduced in the presence of myasthenia gravis. (Adapted from Drachman DB. Myasthenia gravis. N Engl J Med 1978;298:136–42, with permission.)

celerates degradation of the receptors. An estimated 70% to 80% of functional acetylcholine receptors are lost.[51] This explains the easy exhaustion of a patient with myasthenia gravis and the marked sensitivity to nondepolarizing muscle relaxants.

Receptor binding antibodies are present in the plasma of more than 80% of patients with myasthenia gravis. Indeed, identification of circulating antibodies is a reliable diagnostic test for myasthenia gravis. The origin of this autoimmune type of response is unknown, but a role of the thymus gland is suggested by the association of myasthenia gravis with thymus gland abnormalities. For example, hyperplasia of the thymus gland is present in more than 70% of patients with myasthenia gravis, and 10% to 15% of these patients have thymomas. Indeed, about 75% of patients undergo remission of their myasthenia gravis after thymectomy.

Classification

Myasthenia gravis may be classified on the basis of the skeletal muscles involved and the severity of the symptoms. Type I is limited to involvement of the extraocular muscles. About 10% of patients show signs and symptoms confined to the extraocular muscles and are considered to have ocular myasthenia gravis. Any extension beyond the ocular muscles is likely to involve the bulbar muscles. Patients in whom the

disease has been confined to the ocular muscles for more than 3 years are unlikely to experience any progression in their disease.[50] Type IIA is a slowly progressive and mild form of skeletal muscle weakness that spares the muscles of respiration. The response to anticholinesterase drugs and occasionally corticosteroids is good in these patients. Type IIB is a more severe and rapidly progressive form of skeletal muscle weakness than that which occurs with type IIA. Response to drug therapy is not as good, and muscles of respiration may be involved. Type III is characterized by an acute onset and rapid deterioration of skeletal muscle strength (within 6 months) that is associated with a high mortality. Type IV is a severe form of skeletal muscle weakness that results from progression of type I or II.

Signs and Symptoms

The clinical course of myasthenia gravis is marked by periods of exacerbation and remission. Electromyography demonstrates decreased voltage of the muscle action potential during repetitive stimulation. Ptosis and diplopia from extraocular muscle weakness are the most common initial complaints. Weakness of pharyngeal and laryngeal muscles (bulbar muscles) results in dysphagia, dysarthria, and difficulty in eliminating oral secretions. Skeletal muscle strength may be normal in well-rested patients, but weakness occurs promptly with exercise. Arm, leg, or trunk weakness can occur in any combination and is usually asymmetric in distribution. Skeletal muscle atrophy is unlikely. The patient with myasthenia gravis is at high risk of pulmonary aspiration of gastric contents. Myocarditis may produce cardiomyopathy, atrial fibrillation, and heart block. Myasthenia gravis may be associated with cardiomyopathy. Other diseases often considered autoimmune in origin can occur in association with myasthenia gravis. For example, decreased thyroid function is present in about 10% of patients with myasthenia gravis; rheumatoid arthritis, systemic lupus erythematosus, and pernicious anemia occur more commonly than in patients without myasthenia gravis. About 15% of infants born to mothers with myasthenia gravis demonstrate transient (2 to 4 weeks) skeletal muscles weakness. Infection, electrolyte abnormalities, pregnancy, emotional stress, and surgery may precipitate skeletal muscle weakness or exacerbate co-existing weakness. Antibiotics, particularly the aminoglycosides, can aggravate skeletal muscle weakness associated with myasthenia gravis. Isolated respiratory failure may be the presenting manifestation of myasthenia gravis.[52]

Treatment

Modalities of therapy for myasthenia gravis include anticholinesterase drugs, corticosteroids, immunosuppressants other than corticosteroids, plasmapheresis, and thymectomy. These therapies may be employed singly or in combination. Cyclosporine may be an effective therapy in some patients with myasthenia gravis.

Anticholinesterase Drugs

Neostigmine or pyridostigmine are the anticholinesterase drugs most often selected to treat myasthenia gravis. Presumably, these drugs are effective because they inhibit the enzyme responsible for the hydrolysis of acetylcholine, which serves to increase the amount of neurotransmitter available at the neuromuscular junction. A 15-mg oral dose of neostigmine is equivalent to an intramuscular dose of 1.5 mg and to an intravenous dose of 0.5 mg. Oral pyridostigmine lasts longer (3 to 6 hours) and produces fewer muscarinic side effects than occur with neostigmine. A 60-mg oral dose of pyridostigmine is equivalent to an intramuscular or intravenous dose of 2 mg. Phospholine iodide is an extremely potent anticholinesterase drug reserved for the patient with severe myasthenia gravis.

Excessive anticholinesterase drug effects may result in skeletal muscle weakness known as a cholinergic crisis. The presence of muscarinic side effects (salivation, miosis, bradycardia) plus accentuated skeletal muscle weakness after administration of edrophonium (1 to 2 mg IV) confirms the diagnosis.

Corticosteroids

Various corticosteroids have been used to treat myasthenia gravis, but the best success has been attained with prednisone. The usual daily oral dose is 50 to 100 mg. Presumably, corticosteroids interfere with the production of antibodies responsible for degradation of the cholinergic receptors. Corticosteroids may likewise facilitate neuromuscular transmission. Azothioprine, cyclophosphamide, or plasmapheresis may be effective as well, because of their ability to prevent the production or reduce the circulating concentration of antibodies that react with neuromuscular junction. Assessment of the efficacy of drug therapy is difficult because of the natural variability of the disease.

Plasmapheresis

Plasmapheresis removes circulating antibodies to acetylcholine, resulting in improved skeletal muscle strength, usually within a few treatments. This therapy may be used on an emergency basis in a myasthesic crisis or as preparation for thymectomy.

Thymectomy

Thymectomy is recommended for the patient with drug-resistant myasthenia gravis. Sternotomy permits more complete thymus removal than the transcervical approach. About 75% of these patients demonstrate a marked improvement in skeletal muscle strength after thymectomy, and drug therapy is no longer required.[51] Those patients who fail to show substantial improvement in skeletal muscle strength after thymectomy can often be managed with a reduced dose of anticholinesterase drug, compared with preoperative requirements.

Management of Anesthesia

Anesthesia for the patient with myasthenia gravis is most often required for an elective surgical procedure such as thymectomy.[50]

Preoperative Preparation

Drugs such as opioids should be used with caution, if at all, in the preoperative medication. It is likely that the patient with myasthenia gravis will require ventilatory support after surgery. For this reason, it is useful to advise these patients during the preoperative interview that they will most likely have a tracheal tube in place when they awaken. Preoperatively, criteria that correlate with the likely need for controlled ventilation of the lungs in the postoperative period after a transsternal thymectomy include (1) duration of the disease greater than 6 years, (2) presence of chronic obstructive airway disease unrelated to myasthenia gravis, (3) dose of pyridostigmine greater than 750 mg·d^{-1} during the 48 hours preceding surgery, and (4) preoperative vital capacity less than

2.9 L.[53,54] These criteria are less predictive of the need for postoperative ventilatory support after transcervical thymectomy, suggesting that this less invasive surgical approach has a respiratory sparing effect.

Muscle Relaxants

The response of the patient with myasthenia gravis to muscle relaxants is difficult to predict, although there is general agreement that the initial dose should be titrated against the response at the neuromuscular junction, as monitored with a peripheral nerve stimulator. It is possible that drugs used to treat myasthenia gravis could influence the response to muscle relaxants independent of the disease process. For example, anticholinesterase drugs such as pyridostigmine not only inhibit true cholinesterase but also impair activity of plasma cholinesterase, introducing the possibility of a prolonged response to succinylcholine. Conversely, anticholinesterase drugs would theoretically antagonize the effects of nondepolarizing muscle relaxants. Nevertheless, this response does not seem to occur clinically. Corticosteroid therapy probably does not alter the dose requirements for succinylcholine. Conversely, corticosteroid therapy has been reported to produce resistance to the neuromuscular blocking effects of steroidal muscle relaxants, such as vecuronium.[55]

Controlled measurements in myasthenic patients treated with pyridostigmine demonstrate a resistance to the effects of succinylcholine (ED$_{95}$ about 2.6 times normal)[56] (Fig. 26-4). Because the dose of succinylcholine commonly administered to normal patients (1 to 1.5 mg·kg^{-1}) represents three to five times the ED$_{95}$, it is likely that adequate intubating conditions would be achieved in the patient with myasthenia gravis using these doses. If a rapid onset of neuromuscular blockade was required, however, it is possible that the dose of succinylcholine administered to the patient with myasthenia gravis would need to be increased to 1.5 to 2 mg·kg^{-1}. The mechanism by which the patient with myasthenia gravis is resistant to succinylcholine is unknown, although the decreased number of acetylcholine receptors at the postsynaptic neuromuscular junction may play a role.

In contrast to succinylcholine, the patient with myasthenia gravis may exhibit an exquisite sensitivity to nondepolarizing muscle relaxants. A nonparalyzing dose of nondepolarizing muscle relaxant intended to attenuate succinylcholine-induced fasciculations may produce a profound weakness if inadvertently administered to a patient with unrecognized myasthenia gravis. Controlled data from patients with mild to moderate myasthenia gravis demonstrate the potency of atracurium is increased 1.7 to 1.9 times, compared with the response in normal patients[57] (Fig. 26-5). Patients with myasthenia gravis are also more sensitive to vecuronium.[58] Nevertheless, intermediate-acting muscle relaxants, as well as mivacurium, are eliminated rapidly and can be titrated to achieve the needed degree of skeletal muscle paralysis with confidence that the drug effects can be predictably reversed at the conclusion of surgery.[50]

Induction of Anesthesia

Induction of anesthesia with a short-acting intravenous anesthetic is acceptable for the patient with myasthenia gravis. Logic would suggest, however, that respiratory depressant

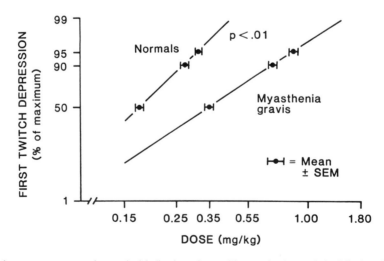

Fig. 26-4. The dose-response curve for succinylcholine in patients with myasthenia gravis is shifted to the right of the curve for normal patients, indicating that myasthenic patients are resistant to the neuromuscular blocking effects of this muscle relaxant. (From Eisenkraft JB, Book WJ, Mann SM, Papatestas AE, Hubbard M. Resistance to succinylcholine in myasthenia gravis: A dose-response study. Anesthesiology 1988;69:760–3, with permission.)

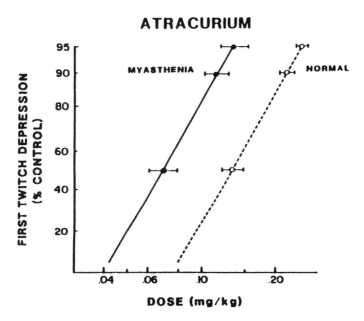

Fig. 26-5. The dose-response curve for atracurium in patients with myasthenia gravis is shifted to the left of the curve for normal patients, indicating that myasthenic patients are sensitive to the neuromuscular blocking effects of this muscle relaxant, and presumably other nondepolarizing muscle relaxants as well. (From Smith CE, Donati F, Bevan DR. Cumulative dose-response curves for atracurium in patients with myasthenia gravis. Can J Anaesth 1989;36:402–6, with permission.)

effects of these drugs could be accentuated. Intubation of the trachea can be accomplished without muscle relaxants in many patients by taking advantage of co-existing skeletal muscle weakness and the relaxing effect of volatile anesthetics on skeletal muscles. Succinylcholine or a short- or intermediate-acting nondepolarizing muscle relaxant can be used to facilitate intubation of the trachea, keeping in mind the need to decrease the initial dose until the response at the neuromuscular junction can be documented with a peripheral nerve stimulator.

Maintenance of Anesthesia

Maintenance of anesthesia is often provided with nitrous oxide plus a volatile anesthetic. Use of a volatile anesthetic may decrease the necessary dose of muscle relaxant or even eliminate the need for its intraoperative administration. Should administration of a nondepolarizing muscle relaxant be necessary, the initial dose should be reduced at least one-half to two-thirds, and the response observed, using a peripheral nerve stimulator. The inherent short duration of action of mivacurium, atracurium, or vecuronium are desirable characteristics when muscle relaxants are administered to these patients, either to facilitate intubation of the trachea or to provide maintenance skeletal muscle relaxation.[58,59] The ability to dissipate the effects of inhaled drugs at the conclusion of anesthesia is important for evaluation of skeletal muscle strength dur-

ing the early postoperative period. Prolonged effects of opioids, especially on ventilation, detract from the use of these drugs for the maintenance of anesthesia. At the conclusion of surgery, it is wise to leave the tracheal tube in place until the patient demonstrates an ability to maintain an adequate level of ventilation. Skeletal muscle strength often seems adequate in the early stages after anesthesia and surgery, only to deteriorate a few hours later. The need to support ventilation of the lungs in the postoperative period should be anticipated for those patients who demonstrate findings in the preoperative evaluation known to correlate with inadequate ventilation after surgery (see the section, Preoperative Preparation).

MYASTHENIC SYNDROME

The myasthenic syndrome (Eaton-Lambert syndrome) is a rare disorder of neuromuscular transmission resembling myasthenia gravis [60,61] (Table 26-1). This syndrome of skeletal muscle weakness, originally described in patients with small cell carcinoma of the lung, has subsequently been described in patients with no evidence of cancer. The myasthenic syndrome is considered to be an autoimmune disease in which immunoglobulin G antibodies to presynaptic calcium channels are produced. Anticholinesterase drugs effective in the treat-

Table 26-1. Comparison of Myasthenic Syndrome and Myasthenia Gravis

	Myasthenic Syndrome	Myasthenia Gravis
Manifestations	Proximal limb weakness (legs > arms) Exercise improves strength Muscle pain common Reflexes absent or decreased	Extraocular, bulbar, and facial muscle weakness Fatigue with exercise Muscle pain uncommon Reflexes normal
Gender	Male > female	Female > male
Co-existing pathology	Small cell carcinoma of the lung	Thymoma
Response to muscle relaxants	Sensitive to succinylcholine and nondepolarizing muscle relaxants Poor response to anticholinesterases	Resistant to succinylcholine Sensitive to nondepolarizing muscle relaxants Good response to anticholinesterases

ment of myasthenia gravis do not produce improvement in the patient with myasthenic syndrome. Conversely, 4-aminopyridine that stimulates the presynaptic release of acetylcholine may improve skeletal muscle strength in the patient with myasthenic syndrome.

Management of Anesthesia

Patients with myasthenic syndrome are sensitive to the effects of both depolarizing and nondepolarizing muscle relaxants.[61] Antagonism of neuromuscular blockade with an anticholinesterase drug may be inadequate. In this regard, the combination of an anticholinesterase with 4-aminopyridine may be the antagonist combination of choice in this condition.[60] The potential presence of myasthenic syndrome and the need to decrease the dose of muscle relaxant should be considered in patients with known carcinoma. Furthermore, this syndrome should be considered in those patients undergoing diagnostic procedures, such as bronchoscopy, mediastinoscopy, or exploratory thoracotomy, for the suspected diagnosis of carcinoma of the lung.

FAMILIAL PERIODIC PARALYSIS

Familial periodic paralysis is characterized by intermittent but acute attacks of skeletal muscle weakness or paralysis, generally sparing only the muscles of respiration (i.e., bulbar musculature). Attacks may last hours or days. Familial periodic paralysis is categorized as hypokalemic or hyperkalemic[62] (Table 26-2). The hyperkalemic form of periodic paralysis is much rarer than the hypokalemic form. It is speculated that paramyotonia is a variant of the hyperkalemic form of familial periodic paralysis (see the section, Paramyotonia).

The fundamental defect in patients with familial periodic paralysis is unknown. It is recognized that the mechanism of the disease is unrelated to an abnormality at the neuromuscular junction. Persistent membrane depolarization during hyperkalemic periodic paralysis is due to a pathologic inward sodium current conducted by sodium channels. Genetic linkage studies indicate that the sodium channel alpha subunit on chromosome 17 contains the hyperkalemic periodic paralysis mutation.[63] Skeletal muscle weakness provoked by a glucose-insulin infusion confirms the presence of the hypokalemic form of

Table 26-2. Clinical Features of Familial Periodic Paralysis

Type	Plasma Potassium Concentration During Symptoms (mEq·L⁻¹)	Precipitating Factors	Other Features
Hypokalemic	<3	Large glucose meals Strenous exercise Glucose-insulin infusions Stress Hypothermia	Cardiac dysrhythmias Signs of hypokalemia on the electrocardiogram
Hyperkalemic	>5.5	Exercise Potassium infusions Metabolic acidosis Hypothermia	Skeletal muscle weakness may be localized to tongue and eyelids

familial periodic paralysis. Conversely, skeletal muscle weakness in response to oral administration of potassium confirms the presence of the hyperkalemic form of familial periodic paralysis. Acetazolamide has been recommended for the treatment of both forms of familial periodic paralysis. Presumably, this drug produces acidosis, which protects against hypokalemic paralysis, while protection in patients with hyperkalemic paralysis is provided by the ability of the drug to promote renal excretion of potassium.

Management of Anesthesia

The nature of the potassium sensitivity in patients with familial periodic paralysis influences the management of anesthesia[62] (Table 26-2). Clearly, the goal for management of anesthesia is avoidance of events that will precipitate skeletal muscle weakness.[62,64] In this regard, large carbohydrate meals should be avoided the day before surgery in patients with the hypokalemic form of familial periodic paralysis. Mannitol should be administered in place of potassium-losing diuretics, should the operative procedure require drug-induced diuresis. Frequent perioperative monitoring (every 15 to 60 minutes) of the plasma potassium concentration is indicated and aggressive intervention (potassium chloride up to 40 mEq·h^{-1} IV) is a consideration. Indeed, hypokalemia may precede the onset of skeletal muscle weakness by several hours, allowing the opportunity to abort these symptoms with potassium supplementation. Recommendations for management of anesthesia in patients with the hyperkalemic form of a familial periodic paralysis include (1) preoperative potassium depletion with furosemide-induced diuresis, (2) prevention of carbohydrate depletion during fasting with the administration of glucose-containing solutions, and (3) avoidance of potassium containing solutions and potassium-releasing drugs such as succinylcholine.[62] As with the hypokalemic form, frequent monitoring of the plasma potassium concentration is indicated, as is the availability of calcium for intravenous administration, should signs of hyperkalemia be seen on the electrocardiogram.

Hypothermia is avoided in patients with familial periodic paralysis, regardless of the nature of the potassium sensitivity. Increasing the ambient temperature of the operating room and warming the inhaled gases and intravenous fluids will minimize decreased body temperature. In patients undergoing cardiopulmonary bypass, it may be necessary to maintain a near-normal body temperature despite the common practice of using systemic hypothermia for these operations.[64] Nondepolarizing muscle relaxants are acceptable for administration to patients with familial periodic paralysis.[62,65]

ALCOHOLIC MYOPATHY

Acute and chronic forms of proximal skeletal muscle weakness occur frequently in the alcoholic patient. Distinction of alcoholic myopathy from alcoholic neuropathy is based on proximal, rather than distal, skeletal muscle involvement; elevation of the plasma creatine kinase concentration; myoglobinuria in acute cases, and rapid recovery after cessation of alcohol consumption.

FREEMAN-SHELDON SYNDROME

Freeman-Sheldon syndrome is a generalized myopathy transmitted as an autosomal dominant trait.[66] Increased tone and fibrosis of facial muscles result in microstomia and pursed lips ("whistling face"), which may be accompanied by micrognathia. Skeletal muscle contractures lead to a short neck and cephalad positioning of the larynx, restrictive lung disease, and kyphoscoliosis. Chronic upper airway obstruction reflects involvement of oral and nasal pharyngeal muscles. Difficulty with swallowing may lead to malnourishment.

Anesthetic considerations include potential difficulty in exposing the glottic opening for intubation of the trachea.[66] Muscle relaxants may not improve intubating conditions if microstomia is due to hypoplasia of facial muscles. Skeletal muscle rigidity has followed the administration of halothane and succinylcholine, suggesting that these patients may be susceptible to malignant hyperthermia. Thickening of subcutaneous tissues may interfere with the achievement of intravenous access.

PRADER-WILLI SYNDROME

Prader-Willi syndrome is manifested at birth as muscular hypotonia, which may be associated with weak swallowing and cough reflexes and upper airway obstruction. Nasogastric feeding may be necessary in infancy. The syndrome progresses during childhood and is characterized by hyperphagia leading to obesity, plus endocrine abnormalities including hypogonadism and diabetes mellitus. The pickwickian syndrome develops in some patients. There is little growth in height and patients remain short. Mental retardation is often severe. There is a high frequency of chromosome 15 deficiency in patients with this syndrome, and an autosomal-recessive mode of inheritance has been proposed. It has been suggested that the incidence of Prader-Willi syndrome is not greatly different from that of the trisomy-21 defect.

Management of Anesthesia

The principal concerns relevant to management of anesthesia for these patients are skeletal muscle hypotonia and altered metabolism of carbohydrates and fat.[67] Weak skeletal musculature is associated with an ineffective cough and an increased incidence of pneumonia. Intraoperative monitoring of the blood glucose concentration and provision of exogenous glucose is necessary, as these patients continue to use circulating glucose to manufacture fat, rather than to meet basal energy needs. The calculation of doses of drugs should consider the decreased skeletal muscle mass and increased fat content in these patients. Although not substantiated, it is predictable that muscle relaxant requirements could be reduced in the presence of skeletal muscle hypotonia. Succinylcholine has been administered without incident to these patients.[67]

Micrognathia, high arched palate, strabismus, a straight ulnar border, and congenital dislocation of the hip may be present. Dental caries associated with enamel defects are common. Chronic regurgitation of gastric contents (rumination) occurs frequently in these patients and may contribute to the development of dental caries and to an increased incidence of perioperative aspiration pneumonitis.[68] Disturbances in thermoregulation, often characterized as intraoperative rises in body temperature and metabolic acidosis, have been observed, although a relationship to malignant hyperthermia has not been established.[67] Seizures are associated with this syndrome, suggesting caution in the use of drugs known to stimulate the central nervous system. Cardiac dysfunction does not seem to accompany this syndrome. Halothane has been used for anesthesia, although other volatile anesthetics would also seem to be acceptable selections.

PRUNE-BELLY SYNDROME

Prune-belly syndrome is characterized by congenital agenesis of the lower central abdominal musculature and by the presence of urinary tract anomalies.[69] Recurrent respiratory infections reflect the impaired ability of these patients to cough effectively. It is unlikely that muscle relaxants will be necessary during the management of anesthesia.

RHEUMATOID ARTHRITIS

Rheumatoid arthritis is a chronic inflammatory disease of unknown etiology, characterized by symmetric polyarthropathy and significant systemic involvement (Table 26-3). Terminal interphalangeal joints are spared, which helps distinguish this disease from osteoarthritis. Rheumatoid arthritis predominates in females; the onset is typically between the ages of 30 to 50 years. Its course is often that of exacerbations and remissions. Rheumatoid nodules are typically present at pressure points, particularly below the elbow. Rheumatoid factor is an anti-immunoglobulin antibody present in up to 90% of patients with rheumatoid arthritis. The presence of rheumatoid factor, however, is not specific, being present in patients with systemic lupus erythematosus, pulmonary fibrosis, and

Table 26-3. Comparison of Rheumatoid Arthritis and Ankylosing Spondylitis

	Rheumatoid Arthritis	Ankylosing Spondylitis
Family history	Rare	Common
Gender	Female (30–50 years old)	Male (20–30 years old)
Joint involvement	Symmetric polyarthropathy	Asymmetric oligoarthropathy
Sacroiliac involvement	No	Yes
Vertebral involvement	Cervical	Total (ascending)
Cardiac changes	Pericardial effusion Aortic regurgitation Cardiac conduction abnormalities Cardiac valve fibrosis Coronary artery arteritis	Cardiomegaly Aortic regurgitation Cardiac conduction abnormalities
Pulmonary changes	Pulmonary fibrosis Pleural effusion	Pulmonary fibrosis
Eyes	Keratoconjunctivitis sicca	Conjunctivitis Uveitis
Rheumatoid factor	Positive	Negative
HLA-B27	Negative	Positive

viral hepatitis. The activation of a cellular immune response in a genetically susceptible host may mark the beginning of rheumatoid arthritis. The cause of this response is unknown but may reflect a viral-induced (Epstein-Barr) activation of B lymphocyte proliferation that culminates in a proliferative synovitis. It is estimated that rheumatoid arthritis affects about 1% of the world's population and that the effect of the disease on human morbidity and mortality has been greatly underestimated.[70]

Signs and Symptoms

The onset of rheumatoid arthritis in the adult may be either acute, producing single or multiple joint involvement, or insidious, generating systemic manifestations that precede overt arthritis by months. In some patients, the clinical onset of the disease may coincide with trauma, a surgical procedure, childbirth, or exposure to extremes of temperature.

Joint Involvement

Morning stiffness is a hallmark of the disease. Multiple joints, particularly in the hands, wrists, and knees, are affected at the same time in a symmetric distribution. Fusiform swelling is typical of the involvement of the proximal interphalangeal joints. Characteristically, these joints are painful and swollen and remain stiff for up to 3 hours after the start of daily activity. Synovitis of the temporomandibular joint may lead to marked limitation of mandibular motion. In patients whose disease is progressive and unremitting, nearly every joint may eventually be affected, although those of the thoracic, lumbar, and sacral spine are almost always spared.

Cervical Spine

In contrast to other sites of the spine, cervical spine involvement by rheumatoid arthritis is frequent and may result in pain and neurologic complications.[71] The abnormality that has received the most attention is atlantoaxial subluxation and consequent separation of the atlanto-odontoid articulation. This deformity is best seen on a lateral radiograph of the neck when, with the neck flexed, the separation of the anterior margin of the odontoid process from the posterior margin of the anterior arch of the atlas can exceed 3 mm. When this separation is severe, the odontoid process may protrude into the foramen magnum and exert pressure on the spinal cord or impair blood flow through the vertebral arteries. Often the odontoid process is eroded, minimizing complications on the spinal cord. Subluxation of the other cervical vertebrae may also occur. Magnetic resonance imaging has confirmed the frequency of cervical spine involvement by rheumatoid arthritis.

Cricoarytenoid Arthritis

Cricoarytenoid arthritis is common in the patient with generalized rheumatoid arthritis. In acute cricoarytenoid arthritis, hoarseness, pain on swallowing, dyspnea, and stridor may accompany tenderness over the larynx. Redness and swelling of the arytenoids can be visualized by direct laryngoscopy. In a chronic state, the patient may be asymptomatic or may manifest variable degrees of hoarseness, dyspnea, and stridor. The presence of cricoarytenoid arthritis may present difficulty in managing these patients, should tracheal intubation be required for the safe conduct of anesthesia.[72]

Systemic Involvement

Many of the systemic manifestations of rheumatoid arthritis are most likely a consequence of vasculitis due to deposition of immune complexes on the walls of small vessels with a subsequent inflammatory reaction. Systemic involvement is usually most obvious in the patient with severe articular disease.

Heart

Pericardial thickening or effusion as reflected by echocardiography is present in about one-third of patients with rheumatoid arthritis. Pericardectomy may be necessary to relieve cardiac tamponade. Cardiac involvement may also be manifested as pericarditis, myocarditis, arteritis involving the coronary arteries, cardiac valve fibrosis, and formation of rheumatoid nodules in the cardiac conduction system. Aortitis with dilation of the aortic root may result in aortic regurgitation.

Lungs

The most common pulmonary manifestation of rheumatoid arthritis is a pleural effusion. Rheumatoid nodules occur in the pulmonary parenchyma and on pleural surfaces. On radiographic examination, these nodules may mimic tuberculosis or neoplasia. Progressive pulmonary fibrosis, associated with cough, dyspnea, and diffuse changes on the chest radiograph, is a rare manifestation. Conversely, asymptomatic diffuse lung involvement characterized by interstitial inflammation and fibrosis may be common.[73] Costochondral involvement may cause restrictive changes with decreased lung volumes and vital capacity. The resulting ventilation-to-perfusion mismatch leads to decreased arterial oxygenation.

Neuromuscular

Loss of strength in skeletal muscles adjacent to joints with active synovitis is common. Peripheral neuropathies are manifested as nerve compression, most often associated with carpal tunnel involvement, but may also be due to entrapment of the ulnar nerve at the elbow or branches of the sural nerve in the tarsal tunnel. Cervical nerve root compression is unlikely to accompany involvement of the cervical vertebrae by rheumatoid arthritis. Another type of neuropathy is a mild distal sensory neuropathy that affects the hands and feet. The most hazardous neuropathy is designated mononeuritis multiplex that accompanies severe disease and is presumed to be caused by deposition of immune complexes in the walls of blood vessels supplying the nerve. Vasculitis in other areas may manifest as myocardial ischemia, cerebral ischemia, and gastrointestinal ischemia.

Blood

The most common hematologic abnormality in the patient with rheumatoid arthritis is mild anemia, partially owing to hemodilution and occasionally due to chronic blood loss aggravated by drugs such as aspirin. Felty syndrome is rheumatoid arthritis with splenomegaly and leukopenia.

Eyes

Keratoconjunctivitis sicca (Sjögren syndrome) occurs in about 10% of patients with rheumatoid arthritis. The cause is lack of tear formation due to impairment of lacrimal gland function.

As a result, the patient experiences a sensation of grittiness with blinking. A similar process may involve the salivary glands, resulting in dryness of the mouth.

Other Systems

Mild abnormalities of liver function are common in the patient with rheumatoid arthritis and may reflect the presence of Sjögren syndrome or the use of salicylates.[74] Rheumatoid arthritis is unlikely to evoke renal dysfunction other than that secondary to amyloidosis or the use of drugs such as phenacetin, gold, or penicillamine.

Treatment

Treatment of rheumatoid arthritis includes efforts to relieve pain, to preserve joint strength and function, and to prevent deformities and attenuation of systemic complications. These objectives may be accomplished by the administration of drugs, utilization of physical therapy, and surgical intervention. Despite improved treatment, there is little evidence that the outcome of rheumatoid arthritis is significantly altered.[75]

Drugs

Drug therapy for rheumatoid arthritis is intended to provide analgesia and to evoke anti-inflammatory, cytotoxic, and immunosuppressive effects. Aspirin is the most important drug for the initial treatment of rheumatoid arthritis. Optimal therapeutic blood levels of 12 to 25 mg·dl^{-1} can be achieved with aspirin (3 to 5 g·d^{-1}). Limiting factors in the use of aspirin are gastrointestinal bleeding, interference with platelet function and occasional hepatic dysfunction. Nonsteroidal anti-inflammatory drugs other than aspirin are probably not more effective but may produce fewer gastrointestinal side effects. An antimalarial drug may be added to the nonsteroidal anti-inflammatory drug regimen in the patient who does not otherwise respond.

Corticosteroids are used extensively for the management of rheumatoid arthritis and are presumably effective in providing symptomatic relief because of their potent anti-inflammatory effects. Nevertheless, these drugs probably neither alter the course of rheumatoid arthritis nor alter the ultimate degree of damage to the joints. The large dose of corticosteroid required is likely to be associated with serious side effects, including suppression of endogenous cortisol release, poor wound healing, increased susceptibility to infection, gastrointestinal bleeding, osteoporosis, and myopathy. Intra-articular administration of a corticosteroid is usually rapidly effective in relieving pain and inflammation, but the risk of infection is great, and repeated injections may result in cartilage destruction and osteonecrosis.

Parenteral gold salts (chrysotherapy) may decrease inflammation and increase the likelihood of remission. Side effects of parenteral gold therapy include eosinophilia, proteinuria, leukopenia, thrombocytopenia, and dermatitis. An oral gold compound, auranofin, is associated with fewer side effects than occur with parenteral therapy. Penicillamine also decreases signs of inflammation and has side effects similar to those with gold therapy. Cytotoxic drugs, including cyclophosphamide, azathioprine, and methotrexate, may be useful when the patient does not respond to more conventional therapy. Cyclophosphamide and azathioprine use is limited by side effects, especially hematologic toxicity and hemorrhagic cystitis. The principal side effect of methotrexate is hepatic toxicity and less often interstitial lung disease and bone marrow toxicity.[76] Sulfasalazine, used in the treatment of ulcerative colitis and Crohn's disease, may be effective in the treatment of rheumatoid arthritis. Plasmapheresis, lymphoplasmapheresis, and total lymphoid irradiation may be useful in an occasional patient in whom the disease is exceptionally aggressive.

Surgery

Surgical treatment of rheumatoid arthritis, such as synovectomy or total replacement of diseased joints, may relieve pain and restore function. Joint stabilization through fusion may be necessary. The release of carpal tunnel compression usually produces relief of symptoms related to median nerve compression.

Management of Anesthesia

Multiple organ involvement and side effects of drugs used in the treatment of rheumatoid arthritis must be appreciated in planning the management of anesthesia. Preoperatively, the patient should be evaluated for airway problems due to the disease process. Compromise of the airway may occur at the cervical spine, temporomandibular joints, and cricoarytenoid joints. For example, flexion deformity of the cervical spine may make it impossible to straighten the neck, and upper airway obstruction is likely when these patients are rendered unconscious. Atlantoaxial subluxation may be present, particularly in those with severe hand deformities and subcutaneous nodules. Radiologic demonstration that the distance from the anterior arch of the atlas to the odontoid process exceeds 3 mm confirms the presence of atlantoaxial subluxation. The importance of atlantoaxial subluxation lies in the fact that the displaced odontoid process can compress the cervical spinal cord or medulla, in addition to occluding the vertebral arteries. In its presence, care must be taken during direct laryngoscopy for intubation of the trachea, to avoid excessive movement of the head and neck, so as to minimize the likelihood of further displacement of the odontoid process and damage to the underlying spinal cord. Certainly, the patient should be evaluated before the induction of anesthesia to determine whether there is interference with vertebral artery blood flow during flexion, extension, or rotation of the head. This may be accomplished by asking the awake patient to demonstrate head movement or positions that can be tolerated without discomfort. Limitation of movement at the temporomandibular joints must be appreciated before the induction of anesthesia. The combination of limited mobility of these joints and of the cervical spine may make visualization of the glottis by direct laryngoscopy difficult or impossible. Intubation of the trachea before induction of anesthesia, using a fiberoptic laryngoscope, may be indicated when preoperative evaluation suggests that direct visualization of the glottis will be difficult. Involvement of the cricoarytenoid joints by arthritic changes is suggested by the presence of hoarseness or stridor preoperatively and by the observation of erythema and edema of the vocal cords during direct laryngoscopy. There may be diminished or even absent movement of these joints, which results in narrowing of the glottic opening.

Preoperative pulmonary function studies plus measurement of arterial blood gases and pH may be indicated if severe lung disease is suspected. The effect of aspirin on clotting should be evaluated. The need for exogenous corticosteroid supplementation must be considered when these drugs are being used for chronic therapy. The presence and implications of anemia should be appreciated. The need for postoperative ventilatory support should be anticipated if severe restrictive lung disease is present preoperatively. Postextubation laryngeal obstruction may occur in the patient with cricoarytenoid arthritis.

SPONDYLARTHROPATHIES

Spondylarthropathies are a group of nonrheumatic arthropathies, which include ankylosing spondylitis (Marie-Strumpell disease), Reiter syndrome, juvenile chronic polyarthropathy, and enteropathic arthropathies. These diseases are characterized by involvement of the sacroiliac joints, peripheral inflammatory arthropathy, and the absence of rheumatoid nodules or rheumatic factor (Table 26-3). The causes of these seronegative spondylarthropathies are unknown, but there is often an association with the human leukocyte antigen (HLA) designated B27.

Ankylosing Spondylitis

A patient with back pain characterized by morning stiffness that improves with exercise, plus radiographic evidence of sacroilitis, has ankylosing spondylitis (Table 26-3). This disease occurs predominantly in males between 20 and 30 years of age. The strong familial incidence is supported by the finding that 90% of patients with this diagnosis are HLA-B27 positive, compared with an incidence of 6% in the normal population.

The disease is often erroneously diagnosed as back pain due to lumbar disc degeneration. Examination of the spine may demonstrate skeletal muscle spasm, loss of lordosis, and decreased mobility involving the entire vertebral column.

Systemic involvement is manifested as weight loss, fatigue, and low-grade fever. Conjunctivitis and uveitis occur in about 25% of patients. A distinctive pulmonary abnormality associated with ankylosing spondylitis is an apical cavity lesion with fibrosis and pleural thickening that mimics tuberculosis. Arthritic involvement of the thoracic vertebral and costovertebral articulations may result in decreased compliance of the chest wall, with an associated decline in vital capacity.

Treatment

Treatment of this disease is with exercises designed to maintain joint mobility, plus anti-inflammatory drugs. Indomethacin or phenylbutazone are commonly used. Bone marrow depression is a potential adverse effect of these drugs. The prognosis is good with early detection and treatment.

Management of Anesthesia

Management of anesthesia in the patient with ankylosing spondylitis is related to (1) the magnitude of upper airway involvement, (2) the presence of a restrictive pattern of lung function due to costochondral rigidity and flexion deformity of the thoracic spine, and (3) the degree of cardiac involvement. Awake intubation of the trachea, either blindly or with the aid of a fiberoptic laryngoscope, may be necessary if spinal column deformity is extensive.[77] Excessive manipulation of the cervical spine could injure the spinal cord. Intraoperatively, ventilation of the lungs should be supported, since the chest wall is stiff and breathing is diaphragmatic. Regional anesthesia is acceptable for peripheral or lower abdominal operative procedures but may be technically difficult due to limited joint mobility and closed interspinous spaces. Sudden or excessive decreases in systemic vascular resistance are poorly tolerated when aortic regurgitation is present.

Reiter's Disease

Reiter's disease occurs in young males and consists of nonspecific urethritis, uveitis, and arthritis. Predisposing factors are a unique genetic makeup (HLA-B27 positive) plus a bacterial infection with *Shigella* or *Chlamydia* organisms. Most of the signs of this disease persist for only a few days, but arthritis progresses to sacroiliitis and spondylitis in about 20% of patients. Cricoarytenoid arthritis can also occur. Hyperkeratotic skin lesions cannot be distinguished from psoriasis, and the two diseases frequently appear to overlap. No cure has been found for Reiter's disease. Symptomatic management is with indomethacin or phenylbutazone.

Juvenile Chronic Polyarthropathy

Pathology of chronic juvenile polyarthropathy is similar to adult rheumatoid arthritis. Growth abnormalities may occur if the arthritis appears before puberty. Hepatic dysfunction may be present, but cardiac involvement is unusual. An acute form of polyarthritis, which presents as fever, rash, lymphadenopathy, and splenomegaly in young children who are negative for rheumatoid factor and HLA-B27, is designated Still's disease. Aspirin is the treatment of choice. Corticosteroids are also effective, but these drugs can produce growth retardation when administered to young patients.

Enteropathic Arthropathies

Approximately 20% of patients with granulomatous ileocolitis or ulcerative colitis show the development of an acute migratory inflammatory polyarthritis, most often involving the large joints of the lower extremities. Remissions occur spontaneously, although subsequent recurrence may parallel exacerbation of the underlying disease. Treatment is directed at control of the underlying gastrointestinal disorder.

Inflammatory bowel disease may also be associated with sacroiliitis and occasionally severe ankylosing spondylitis. There is no correlation between the severity of the bowel disorder and spondylitis. Treatment is as described for ankylosing spondylitis.

A postintestinal bypass syndrome consisting of arthropathy and dermatitis is well documented. The cause is unknown, although immune mechanisms have been implicated.

OSTEOARTHRITIS

Osteoarthritis is a degenerative process affecting the articular cartilage. This process differs from rheumatoid arthritis in that there is minimal inflammatory reaction. The pathogenesis is unclear but may be related to joint trauma. Advancing age and a genetic predisposition are important associated factors. Pain is usually present on motion and relieved by rest. Stiffness tends to disappear rapidly with joint motion, in contrast to the morning stiffness associated with rheumatoid arthritis, which may last several hours.

Characteristically, one joint to several joints are affected by osteoarthritis. The knees and hips are common sites of involvement. Bony enlargements, referred to as Heberden's nodes, are seen at the distal interphalangeal joints. There may be degenerative disease of the vertebral bodies and intervertebral discs, which may be complicated by protrusion of the nucleus pulposus and compression of nerve roots. Degenerative changes are most significant in the middle to lower cervical spine and in the lower lumbar area. Spinal fusion is unusual, in contrast to its common occurrence in ankylosing spondylitis.

Radiographic findings may show narrowing of the intervertebral disc spaces and osteophyte formation.

Treatment

Treatment of osteoarthritis is symptomatic and includes the application of heat and administration of drugs (aspirin, indomethacin) known for their analgesic and anti-inflammatory effects. Symptomatic improvement with application of heat may be due to an increased pain threshold in warm compared with cold tissues. Corticosteroids are not recommended, as they may contribute to degenerative joint changes. Reconstructive joint surgery (total hip or knee replacement) may be recommended when pain is persistent and disabling.

OSTEOPOROSIS

For a discussion of osteoporosis, see Chapter 33.

PAGET'S DISEASE

Paget's disease is characterized by excessive osteoblastic and osteoclastic activity, resulting in abnormally thickened but weak bone. The cause is unknown but may reflect an excess of parathyroid hormone or a deficiency of calcitonin. Radiographic findings include lytic and sclerotic changes, which may involve the skull. There is cortical thickening of long bones. A familial tendency is present, with white males over 40 years of age most frequently affected. Increased bone formation and resorption are associated with an elevated plasma alkaline phosphatase level. In addition to pain and deformity, complications include pathologic fractures, nerve compression, renal calculi, high-output cardiac failure, and hypercalcemia.

Treatment

Calcitonin, which appears to act as a primary inhibitor of bone resorption, is an effective therapeutic agent. Sodium etiodronate, which suppresses osteoblastic and osteoclastic activity, is effective in decreasing pain and the rate of bone turnover. When Paget's disease involves the hip, a replacement arthroplasty may be considered.

OSTEOGENESIS IMPERFECTA

Osteogenesis imperfecta is a rare, autosomal dominant, inherited disease of connective tissue that affects bone, sclera, and the inner ear. Bones are extremely brittle because of defective collagen production. The incidence is higher in females. Clinically, the disease is manifested as one of two forms, osteogenesis imperfecta congenita and osteogenesis imperfecta tarda. In the congenita form, fractures occur in utero, and death usually occurs during the perinatal period. The tarda form typically manifests in childhood or early adolescence with the presence of blue sclera (due to a defective collagen production), fractures with trivial trauma, kyphoscoliosis as a reflection of collapse of vertebral bodies, bowing of the femur and tibia, and the gradual onset of otosclerosis and deafness. Impaired platelet function in these patients may be manifested as a mild bleeding tendency. Increased body temperature with hyperhydrosis may occur in the patient with osteogenesis imperfecta. Increased serum thyroxine concentrations associated with increased oxygen consumption occur in at least 50% of patients with this disease.

Management of Anesthesia

Management of anesthesia is influenced by co-existing orthopaedic deformities and vulnerability to additional fractures during the perioperative period.[78] Intubation of the trachea must be accomplished with minimal manipulation and trauma, as cervical and mandibular fractures may occur. Succinylcholine-induced fasciculations may produce fractures. Dentition is defective and may be vulnerable to easy damage, as during direct laryngoscopy. Awake intubation of the trachea with the use of a fiberoptic laryngoscope may be prudent, if co-existing orthopaedic deformities could make visualization of the glottic opening difficult by direct laryngoscopy. Associated kyphoscoliosis and pectus excavatum may reduce vital capacity, decrease chest wall compliance, and result in arterial hypoxemia due to ventilation-to-perfusion mismatch. An automated blood pressure cuff may be hazardous as overinflation may result in a fracture. Regional anesthesia may be acceptable in selected patients, as it avoids the need for tracheal intubation but may be technically difficult because of kyphoscoliosis. Coagulation status should be evaluated, especially before selecting regional anesthetic techniques. In view of the potential for increased body temperature, it is probably important to monitor temperature continuously. This increase in body temperature is usually mild and not a forerunner of malignant hyperthermia.

McCUNE-ALBRIGHT SYNDROME

McCune-Albright syndrome consists of a triad of physical signs characterized as osseous lesions (polyostotic fibrous dysplasia), melanotic cutaneous macules (café-au-lait spots), and sexual precocity. Conductive and neural deafness occurs when osseous lesions involve the temporal bone, with resultant ossicular or cochlear impingement. Osseous fractures are likely in childhood. In addition to the classic triad, some pa-

tients show endocrine dysfunction, especially hyperthyroidism, hypercortisolism, growth hormone excess, and hypophosphatemia.[79]

FIBRODYSPLASIA OSSIFICANS

Fibrodysplasia ossificans is a rare inherited autosomal dominant disease, usually exhibited before 6 years of age and characterized clinically by interstitial myositis and proliferation of connective tissue. The term myositis ossificans is also applied to this disease, but fibrodysplasia ossificans is more correct, since it is principally a disease of connective tissue rather than of skeletal muscle.[80] Connective tissue undergoes cartilaginous and osteoid transformation, eventually leading to displacement of skeletal muscle mass by ectopic bone formation. Ectopic bone formation typically affects skeletal muscles of the elbow, hip, and knee leading to serious limitation of joint movement. Cervical spine involvement is common, with varying degrees of cervical fusion and the possibility of atlantoaxial subluxation. Temporomandibular joint involvement with obvious implications for intubation of the trachea may occur. Skeletal muscles of the face, larynx, eyes, anterior abdominal wall, diaphragm, and heart usually escape involvement.

In early stages of the disease, fever may occur at the same time that localized lumps appear in affected skeletal muscles. Alkaline phosphatase activity is increased during active phases of the disease. A restrictive pattern of breathing reflects the limitation of rib movement. Progression to respiratory failure is rare, although pneumonia is a common complication. Abnormalities on the electrocardiogram may include ST segment changes and right bundle branch block. Deafness may occur, but mental retardation is unlikely.

Treatment

Treatment directed at halting the progression of the disease is largely unsuccessful, principally because the pathogenesis remains unknown.[80] Corticosteroids, which decrease bone formation by inhibiting periosteal cell proliferation, may provide relief in a few patients, but there is unlikely to be any effect on eventual outcome. Warfarin has been used because of anecdotal reports of subjective improvement in mobility in the patient with ectopic calcification.

MARFAN SYNDROME

Marfan syndrome is a disorder of connective tissue, inherited as an autosomal dominant trait.[81] The incidence is 4 to 6 per 100,000 births, and the mean age of survival is 32 years. Characteristically, these patients have long tubular bones, giving them a tall stature and an "Abe Lincoln" appearance. Additional skeletal abnormalities include a high arched palate, pectus excavatum, kyphoscoliosis, and hyperextensibility of the joints. Early development of pulmonary emphysema is characteristic and may further accentuate the impact of restrictive lung disease related to kyphoscoliosis. There is a high incidence of spontaneous pneumothorax in these patients. Ocular changes characterized by lens dislocation, myopia, and detachment of the retina occur at some time in more than one-half of patients with Marfan syndrome.

Cardiovascular System

Abnormalities that involve the cardiovascular system are responsible for nearly all premature fatalities in patients with Marfan syndrome. Defective tensile strength in the connective tissue of the aorta and the heart valves leads to dilation, dissection, and rupture of the aorta and to prolapse of the cardiac valves, especially of the mitral valve. Mitral regurgitation is a common abnormality, reflecting mitral valve prolapse. The risk of bacterial endocarditis is increased in the presence of valvular heart disease. Cardiac conduction abnormalities, especially bundle branch block, are common. An echocardiogram is particularly useful in detecting cardiac abnormalities in an otherwise asymptomatic patient. Prophylactic beta blocker therapy may be recommended for the patient in whom the thoracic aorta becomes dilated. By contrast, prophylactic surgical replacement of the aortic valve and ascending aorta is indicated for a patient in whom the diameter of the proximal thoracic aorta exceeds 6 cm and in whom substantial aortic regurgitation is present. Extension of an aortic dissection through the sinus of Valsalva into the pericardium can lead to sudden cardiac tamponade. Pregnancy poses a unique risk of rupture or dissection of the aorta in the parturient with Marfan syndrome.

Management of Anesthesia

Preoperative evaluation of the patient with Marfan syndrome should concentrate on cardiopulmonary abnormalities. Prophylactic antibiotics are appropriate if valvular heart disease is present. In most patients, skeletal abnormalities have little impact on the upper airway. Care should be exercised, however, to avoid extreme movements of the mandible, as these patients are susceptible to temporomandibular joint dislocation. In view of the possibility of a weakened wall of the thoracic aorta, it is prudent to avoid sustained elevations of blood pressure, as can occur during laryngoscopy for intubation of the trachea or in response to painful surgical stimulation. A high index of suspicion must be maintained for the development of pneumothorax.

KYPHOSCOLIOSIS

Kyphoscoliosis is a deformity of the costovertebral skeletal structures, characterized by an anterior flexion (kyphosis) and lateral curvature (scoliosis) of the vertebral column. Idiopathic kyphoscoliosis, which accounts for 80% of cases, commonly begins in late childhood and may progress in severity during periods of rapid skeletal growth. The incidence of idiopathic kyphoscoliosis is about 4 per 1000 population. Diseases of the neuromuscular system, such as poliomyelitis, cerebral palsy, and muscular dystrophy, may be associated with kyphoscoliosis. There seems to be a familial predisposition of this disease, with females affected about four times more often than males.

Signs and Symptoms

A curve greater than 40 degrees is considered severe and most likely to be associated with physiologic derangements in cardiac and pulmonary function. Restrictive lung disease and pulmonary hypertension progressing to cor pulmonale are the principal causes of mortality in patients with kyphoscoliosis. As the scoliotic curve worsens, more lung tissue is compressed, resulting in decreased vital capacity and in dyspnea with mild exertion. The work of breathing is increased by abnormal mechanical properties of the thorax and, to a lesser degree, by increased airway resistance resulting from a small lung volumes. The alveolar-to-arterial difference for oxygen is increased. The $PaCO_2$ is usually normal, but relatively minor insults such as bacterial or viral upper respiratory tract infections may result in acute respiratory failure. A poor cough reflex contributes to frequent pulmonary infections. Pulmonary hypertension reflects increased pulmonary vascular resistance due to compression of lung vasculature by the curve in the spine and the pulmonary vascular response to arterial hypoxemia.

Management of Anesthesia

Preoperatively, it is important to assess the severity of the physiologic derangements produced by the skeletal deformity. Pulmonary function tests, with special attention to the vital capacity and forced exhaled volume in 1 second, will reflect the magnitude of restrictive lung disease. Arterial blood gases and pH are helpful in detecting unrecognized arterial hypoxemia or acidosis that could be contributing to pulmonary hypertension. These patients may enter the preoperative period with pneumonia due to chronic aspiration of acidic gastric fluid. Certainly, any reversible component of pulmonary dysfunction, such as bacterial infection or bronchospasm, should be corrected before an elective operation is performed. Preoperative medication with depressant drugs must be administered with caution, if at all, in view of the narrow margin of ventilatory reserve in these patients, as well as the adverse effects on the pulmonary vascular resistance that would occur with respiratory acidosis from hypoventilation.

Intraoperatively, ventilation of the lungs should be controlled to facilitate adequate arterial oxygenation and elimination of carbon dioxide. Adequacy of oxygenation should be confirmed by continuous monitoring of arterial oxygen saturation. Although no specific drug or drug combination can be recommended as superior, it should be remembered that nitrous oxide may increase pulmonary vascular resistance, presumably by direct vasoconstrictive effects on the pulmonary vasculature. Monitoring of central venous pressure may provide an early warning of increased pulmonary vascular resistance produced by nitrous oxide. Signs of malignant hyperthermia (hypercapnia, acidosis, tachycardia, and increased body temperature) must be appreciated, as it has been suggested that there is an increased incidence of this syndrome in patients with scoliosis.[82]

If the surgical procedure is for correction of the spinal curvature, special consideration must be given to intraoperative blood loss and recognition of spinal cord injury. Controlled hypotension, with the combination of a volatile anesthetic and a peripheral vasodilator such as nitroprusside, is effective in reducing blood loss. As the spinal curve is straightened, excess traction on the spinal cord may result in paralysis manifesting during the postoperative period. An intraoperative maneuver designed to detect spinal cord injury is to reverse neuromuscular blockade and discontinue the inhaled anesthetic, until the patient is sufficiently awake to move both legs on request, to confirm that the spinal cord is intact (wake-up test).[83] Inhalation anesthesia is then reestablished and the operation completed. Somatosensory cortical evoked potential monitoring is also useful to confirm an intact spinal cord. The advantage of somatosensory evoked potentials is that the patient need not be awakened intraoperatively. If this approach is used, it must be appreciated that many drugs, including volatile anesthetics, interfere with interpretation of evoked potentials. Therefore, a nitrous oxide–opioid technique is often recommended. In this regard, continuous infusion of the opioid maintains any drug-induced change on evoked potentials at a constant level, making it easier to interpret changes due to spinal cord damage.[84] Unfortunately, postoperative paralysis may still occur despite the absence of any intraoperative abnormality in the somatosensory evoked potentials, emphasizing that this monitor reflects only the sensory (dorsal column function), and not the motor (ventral column), integrity of the spinal cord. For this reason, a wake-up test may still be recommended. In this regard, a wake-up test can often be achieved without use of an opioid antagonist following discontinuation of the continuous opioid infusion. Postoperatively, the major concern is restoration of adequate ventilation. It is likely that slow weaning from the ventilator will be necessary in the patient with severe kyphoscoliosis, regardless of the operative procedure.

DEFORMITIES OF THE STERNUM

Pectus carinatum (outward protuberance of the sternum) and pectus excavatum (inward concavity of the sternum) produce psychological problems, but functional consequences are rare. In general, narrowing of the distance between the posterior sternum and the anterior border of the vertebral bodies to as little as 2 cm (normal is 8 cm in an adult) can be tolerated with respect to cardiopulmonary function. Nevertheless, pectus excavatum may rarely be associated with increased ventricular filling pressures and atrial dysrhythmias, especially during exercise. Obstructive sleep apnea may be more common in young children with pectus excavatum, perhaps reflecting inward movement of a pliable costochondral apparatus due to the effect of negative intrathoracic pressure generated by airway obstruction.

ACHONDROPLASIA

Achondroplasia is the most common cause of dwarfism, occurring predominantly in females, with an incidence of 1.5 per 10,000 births.[85] Transmission is by an autosomal dominant gene, although an estimated 80% of cases represent spontaneous mutation. Indeed, fertility among achondroplastic dwarfs is low. The basic defect is thought to be a decrease in the rate of endochondral ossification, which, coupled with normal periosteal bone formation, leads to short tubular bones. The predicted height for an achondroplastic male is 132 cm and for a female, 122 cm. Kyphoscoliosis and genu varum are common. Premature fusion of the bones at the base of the skull occurs in achondroplasia, resulting in a shortened skull base and small stenotic foramen magnum. This change may result in infantile hydrocephalus or in damage to the cervical cord. For example, central sleep apnea experienced by an achondroplastic dwarf may be a function of brain stem compression from foramen magnum stenosis. Pulmonary hypertension, leading to cor pulmonale, is probably the most common cardiovascular disturbance that develops in dwarfs. Mental and skeletal muscle development are normal, as is life expectancy for those who survive the first year of life.

Management of Anesthesia

Management of anesthesia in the achondroplastic dwarf may be influenced by predictable changes that accompany this disorder (Table 26-4). An achondroplastic dwarf characteristically requires a number of specific procedures, including suboccipital craniectomy for foramen magnum stenosis, laminectomy for spinal column stenosis or nerve root compression, and ventricular peritoneal shunts.[85] Abnormal bone growth is responsible for several potential anesthesia-

Table 26-4.   Characteristics of the Achondroplastic Dwarf That May Influence Management of Anesthesia

Upper airway obstruction
Difficult exposure of glottic opening
Restrictive lung disease
Obstructive sleep apnea
Central sleep apnea
Pulmonary hypertension
Cor pulmonale
Hydrocephalus
Compressive spinal cord and nerve root syndromes
    Foramen magnum stenosis
    Odontoid hypoplasia with cervical instability
    Kyphoscoliosis
Thermal regulation dysfunction (hyperthermia)

related problems.[86,87] A preoperative history of obstructive sleep apnea may predispose to the development of upper airway obstruction after sedation or induction of anesthesia. Facial features characterized by a large protruding forehead, short maxilla, large mandible, flat nose, and large tongue suggest difficulty in attaining a suitable fit with the anesthetic face mask and maintenance of a patent upper airway. Despite these characteristics, clinical experience has not confirmed difficulty in maintaining the upper airway or intubation of the trachea in most of these patients.[86] Hyperextension of the neck during direct laryngoscopy for intubation of the trachea should be avoided, if possible, considering the likely presence of foramen magnum stenosis. The clinical impression of an anatomically abnormal upper airway or cervical spine may be confirmed by computed tomography or magnetic resonance imaging. Weight rather than age is the best guide for predicting the proper size endotracheal tube for these patients.[86] Excess skin and subcutaneous tissue may make establishment of peripheral intravenous lines more difficult. An achondroplastic dwarf undergoing suboccipital craniectomy, especially in the sitting position, is at high risk of venous air embolism, emphasizing the potential value of a right atrial catheter.[88] Placement of a right atrial catheter is technically difficult, however, because of the short neck and difficulty identifying landmarks that may be obscured by excess soft tissues. Monitoring of somatosensory evoked potentials is useful during operations that may be associated with brain stem or spinal cord injury. As with surgery to correct kyphoscoliosis, it is important to remember that somatosensory evoked potentials reflect the integrity of the dorsal, but not ventral, columns of the spinal cord. An achondroplastic dwarf seems to respond normally to drugs used for anesthesia and skeletal muscle relaxation. An anesthetic technique that permits rapid awakening may be desirable for prompt evaluation of neurologic function.

Regional anesthesia in an achondroplastic dwarf may be considered for cesarean section, which is mandated by the small and contracted pelvis in these patients combined with near-normal infant birthweight.[89] Technical difficulties may occur because of kyphoscoliosis and a narrow epidural space and spinal canal. Indeed, the small space present may make it difficult to introduce a catheter or obtain free flow of cerebrospinal fluid. Neurologic changes may occur in later life because of compression of the spinal cord by osteophytes, prolapsed intervertebral discs, or deformed vertebral bodies. There are no data confirming the appropriate dose of local anesthetic for epidural or spinal anesthesia in these patients. For this reason, epidural anesthesia may be preferable to spinal anesthesia, as it permits titration of the local anesthetic dose to achieve a desired sensory level of blockade.

HALLERMANN-STREIFF SYNDROME

Hallermann-Streiff syndrome is characterized by oculomandibulodyscephaly and dwarfism. The nose and mandible are hypoplastic, the teeth brittle, and the temporomandibular joints weak and easily dislocated. These airway abnormalities make direct laryngoscopy for intubation of the trachea both hazardous and difficult. Awake nasotracheal intubation can be difficult if the nares are hypoplastic.[90]

DUTCH-KENTUCKY SYNDROME

Dutch-Kentucky syndrome is a rare inherited disorder characterized by decreased ability to open the mouth due to trismus, as well as flexion deformity of the fingers, which occurs with wrist extension (pseudocampodactyly). Enlarged coronoid processes may be the cause of trismus. Foot deformities and shorter-than-normal stature are frequently present. When these patients require surgery, management of the airway may be facilitated by fiberoptic laryngoscopy.[91,92]

WILLIAMS-BEUREN SYNDROME

Williams-Beuren syndrome is a rare entity characterized by mental retardation, hypercalcemia with associated kidney dysfunction and corneal opacities, kyphoscoliosis, and skeletal muscle hypotonia. Characteristic facies include broad forehead, pointed chin, flattened nasal bridge, large upper lip, and prognathism. Aortic regurgitation is present in more than 50% of these patients. The presence of stenosis of the left subclavian artery can result in unequal blood pressure measurements in the upper extremities.

KLIPPEL-FEIL SYNDROME

Klippel-Feil syndrome is characterized by shortness of the neck, resulting from reduction in the number of cervical vertebrae or fusion of several vertebrae into an osseous mass. Movement of the neck is limited, and associated skeletal abnormalities include spinal canal stenosis or kyphoscoliosis. Mandibular malformations and micrognathia may be present. There is an increased incidence of cardiac and genitourinary anomalies in these patients. Management of anesthesia must consider the risk of neurologic damage during direct laryngoscopy in the presence of cervical spine instability.[93] Preoperative lateral neck radiographs will help evaluate stability of the cervical spine.

ARTHROGRYPOSIS MULTIPLEX CONGENITA

Arthrogryposis multiplex congenita is a rare syndrome characterized by joint contractures and multiple organ congenital abnormalities.[94] Cardiac abnormalities include aortic stenosis, coarctation of the aorta, and cyanotic heart disease. Airway problems are introduced by micrognathia, high arched palate, and cervical spine abnormalities. A decreased skeletal muscle mass may be associated with an increased sensitivity to muscle relaxants. In view of the myopathy associated with this disease, there is an unsubstantiated concern about possible susceptibility to malignant hyperthermia. Regional anesthesia has been successfully conducted, but deformities of the vertebral column may make this technique technically difficult.

REFERENCES

1. Epstein EH. Molecular genetics of epidermolysis bullosa. Science 1992;256:799–803
2. Smith GB, Shribman AJ. Anaesthesia and severe skin disease. Anaesthesia 1984;39:443–55
3. James I, Wark H. Airway management during anesthesia in patients with epidermolysis bullosa dystrophica. Anesthesiology 1982;56:323–6
4. Holzman RS, Worthen HM, Johnson K. Anaesthesia for children with junctional epidermolysis bullosa (letalis). Can J Anaesth 1987;34:395–9
5. Spargo PM, Smith GB. Epidermolysis bullosa and porphyria. Anaesthesia 1989;44:79–83
6. Kelly RE, Koff HD, Rothaus KO, Carter DM, Artusio JF. Brachial plexus anesthesia in eight patients with recessive dystrophic epidermolysis bullosa. Anesth Analg 1987;66:1318–20
7. Jeyaram C, Torda TA. Anesthetic management of cholecystectomy in a patient with buccal pemphigus. Anesthesiology 1974; 40:600–1

8. Drenger B, Zidenbaum M, Reifen E, Leitersdorf E. Severe upper airway obstruction and difficult intubation in acatricial pemphigoid. Anaesthesia 1986;41:1029–31
9. Prasad KK, Chen L. Anesthetic management of a patient with bullous pemphigoid. Anesth Analg 1989;69:537–40
10. Roberts LJ, Sweetman BJ, Lewis RA, et al. Increased production of prostaglandin D2 in patients with systemic mastocytosis. N Engl J Med 1980;303:1400–4
11. Lerno G, Slaats G, Coenen E, Herregods L, Rolly G. Anaesthetic management of systemic mastocytosis. Br J Anaesth 1990;65: 254–7
12. Coleman MA, Liberthson RR, Crone RK, Levine GH. General anesthesia in a child with urticaria pigmentosa. Anesth Analg 1980;59:704–6
13. Hosking MP, Warner MA. Sudden intraoperative hypotension in a patient with asymptomatic urticaria pigmentosa. Anesth Analg 1987;66:344–6
14. Johnston WE, Moss J, Philbin DM, et al. Management of cold urticaria during hypothermic cardiopulmonary bypass. N Engl J Med 1982;306:219–21
15. Cucchira RF, Dawson B. Anesthesia in Stevens-Johnson syndrome: Report of a case. Anesthesiology 1971;35:537–9
16. Younker D, Harrison B. Scleroderma and pregnancy: Anaesthetic considerations. Br J Anaesth 1985;57:1136–9
17. Thompson J, Conklin KA. Anesthetic management of a pregnant patient with scleroderma. Anesthesiology 1983;59:69–71
18. Krechel SLW, Ramirez-Inawant RC, Fabian LW. Anesthetic considerations in pseudoxanthoma elasticum. Anesth Analg 1981;60: 344–7
19. Brighouse D, Guard B. Anaesthesia for caesarean section in a patient with Ehlers-Danlos syndrome type IV. Br J Anaesth 1992; 69:517–9
20. Saarnivaara LHM. Anesthesia for a patient with polymyositis undergoing myectomy of the cricopharyngeal muscle. Anesth Analg 1988;67:701–2
21. Brown S, Shupak RC, Patel C, Calkins JM. Neuromuscular blockade in a patient with active dermatomyositis. Anesthesiology 1992;77:1031–3
22. Davies SR. Systemic lupus erythematosus and the obstetrical patient—implications for the anaesthetist. Can J Anaesth 1991; 38:790–6
23. Espana A, Gutierrez JM, Soria C, et al. Recurrent laryngeal nerve palsy in systemic lupus erythematosus. Neurology (NY) 1990;40:1143–6
24. Kelly JE, Simpson MT, Jonathan D, Hallway TE. Lipoid proteinosis: Urbach-Wiethe disease. Br J Anaesth 1989;63:609–11
25. Sargent WW. Anesthetic management of a patient with Cornelia de Lange syndrome. Anesthesiology 1991;74:1162–3
26. Kasuda H, Akazawa S, Shimizu R, Moriguchi H, Masubuchi M, Miyata M. Difficult endotracheal intubation in a patient with tumoral calcinosis. Anesth Analg 1992;74:159–61
27. Smith CL, Bush GH. Anaesthesia and progressive muscular dystrophy. Br J Anaesth 1985;57:1113–8
28. Wiesel S, Bevan JC, Samuel J, Conati F. Vercuronium neuromuscular blockade in a child with mitochondrial myopathy. Anesth Analg 1991;72:696–9
29. Rosenberg H, Heiman-Patterson T. Duchenne's muscular dys-

trophy and malignant hyperthermia: Another warning. Anesthesiology 1983;59:362

30. Wang JM, Stanley TH. Duchenne muscular dystrophy and malignant hyperthermia-two case reports. Can Anaesth Soc J 1986; 33:492–7

31. Sethna NF, Rockoff MA, Worthen HM, Rosnow JM. Anesthesia-related complications in children with Duchenne muscular dystrophy. Anesthesiology 1988;68:462–5

32. Chalkiadis GA, Branch KG. Cardiac arrest after isoflurane anaesthesia in a patient with Duchenne's muscular dystrophy. Anaesthesia 1990;45:22–6

33. Murat I, Esteve C, Montay G, et al. Pharmacokinetics and cardiovascular effects of bupivacaine during epidural anesthesia in children with Duchenne muscular dystrophy. Anesthesiology 1987; 67:249–52

34. Dresner DL, Ali HH. Anaesthetic management of a patient with facioscapulohumeral muscular dystrophy. Br J Anaesth 1989;62: 331–4

35. Cunliffe M, Burrows FA. Anaesthetic implications of nemaline rod myopathy. Can Anaesth Soc J 1985;32:543–7

36. Landrum AL, Eggers GWN. Oculopharyngeal dystrophy: An approach to anesthetic management. Anesth Analg 1992;75:1043–5

37. Mitchell MM, Ali HH, Savarese JJ. Myotonia and neuromuscular blocking agents. Anesthesiology 1978;49:44–8

38. Mudge BJ, Taylor PB, Vanderspek AFL. Perioperative hazards in myotonic dystrophy. Anaesthesia 1980;35:492–5

39. Aldredge LM. Anaesthetic problems in myotonic dystrophy. A case report and review of the Aberdeen experience comprising 48 general anaesthetics in a further 16 patients. Br J Anaesth 1985;57:1119–30

40. Fall LH, Young WW, Power JA, et al. Severe congestive heart failure and cardiomyopathy as a complication of myotonic dystrophy in pregnancy. Obstet Gynecol 1990;76:481–6

41. Cope DK, Miller JN. Local and spinal anesthesia for cesarean section in a patient with myotonic dystrophy. Anesth Analg 1986; 65:687–90

42. Aldridge LM. Anaesthetic problems in myotonic dystrophy. Br J Anaesth 1985;57:1119–23

43. Ravin M, Newmark Z, Saviello G. Myotonia dystrophica—an anesthetic hazard: Two case reports. Anesth Analg 1975;54: 216–8

44. Meyers MB, Barash PG. Cardiac decompensation during enflurane anesthesia in a patient with myotonia atrophica. Anesth Analg 1976;55:433–6

45. Castano J, Pares N. Anaesthesia for major abdominal surgery in a patient with myotonia dystrophica. Br J Anaesth 1987;59: 1629–31

46. Nightingale P, Healy TEJ, McGuinness K. Dystrophia myotonica and atracurium. Br J Anaesth 1985;57:1131–5

47. Ramchandra DS, Anisya V, Gourie-Deve M. Ketamine monoanaesthesia for diagnostic muscle biopsy in neuromuscular disorders in infancy and childhood: Floppy infant syndrome. Can J Anaesth 1990;37:474–6

48. Cook WP, Kaplan RF. Neuromuscular blockade in a patient with stiff-baby syndrome. Anesthesiology 1986;65:525–8

49. Parris WCV, Johnson AC. Tracheomegaly. Anesthesiology 1982; 56:141–3

50. Baraka A. Anaesthesia and myasthenia gravis. Can J Anaesth 1992;39:476–86

51. Drachman DB. Myasthenia gravis. N Engl J Med 1978;298: 136–42

52. Mier A, Laroche C, Green M. Unsuspected myasthenia gravis presenting as respiratory failure. Thorax 1990;45:422–6

53. Leventhal SR, Orkin FK, Hirsh RA. Prediction of the need for postoperative mechanical ventilation in myasthenia gravis. Anesthesiology 1980;53:26–30

54. Eisenkraft JB, Papatestas AE, Kahn CH, et al. Predicting the need for postoperative mechanical ventilation and myasthenia gravis. Anesthesiology 1986;65:79–82

55. Parr SM, Robinson BJ, Rees D, Galletly DC. Interaction between betamethasone and vecuronium. Br J Anaesth 1991;67:447–51

56. Eisenkraft JB, Book WJ, Mann SM, Papagtestas AE, Hubbard M. Resistance to succinylcholine in myasthenia gravis: A dose-response study. Anesthesiology 1988;69:760–3

57. Smith CE, Donati F, Bevan DR. Cumulative dose-response curves for atracurium in patients with myasthenia gravis. Can J Anaesth 1989;36:402–6

58. Nilsson E, Meretoja OA. Vecuronium dose-response and requirements in patients with myasthenia gravis. Anesthesiology 1990;73:28–31

59. Baraka A, Tabboush Z. Neuromuscular response to succinylcholine-vecuronium sequence in three myasthenic patients undergoing thymectomy. Anesth Analg 1991;72:827–30

60. Telford RJ, Hallway TE. The myasthenia syndrome: Anaesthesia in a patient treated with 3,4-diaminopyradine. Br J Anaesth 1990; 64:363–6

61. Small S, Ali HH, Lennon VA, Brown RH, Carr DB, deArmendi A. Anesthesia for unsuspected Lambert-Eaton myasthenic syndrome with autoantibodies and occult small cell lung carcinoma. Anesthesiology 1992;76:142–5

62. Ashwood EM, Russell WJ, Burrow DD. Hyperkalaemic periodic paralysis. Anaesthesia 1992;47:579–84

63. Koch MC, Ricker K, Otto M, et al. Confirmation of linkage of hyperkalemic periodic paralysis to chromosome 17. J Med Genet 1991;28:583–6

64. Lema G, Urzua J, Moran S, Canessa R. Successful anesthetic management of a patient with hypokalemic familial periodic paralysis undergoing cardiac surgery. Anesthesiology 1991;74:373–5

65. Rooney RT, Shanahan EC, Sun T, Nally B. Atracurium and hypokalemic familial periodic paralysis. Anesth Analg 1988;67:782–3

66. Jones R, Dolcourt JL. Muscle rigidity following halothane anesthesia in two patients with Freeman-Sheldon syndrome. Anesthesiology 1992;77:599–600

67. Yamashita M. Koishi K, Yamaya R, et al. Anaesthetic considerations in the Prader-Willi syndrome: Report of four cases. Can Anaesth Soc J 1983;30:179–84

68. Sloan TB, Kaye CI. Rumination risk of aspiration of gastric contents in the Prader-Willi syndrome. Anesth Analg 1991;73:492–5

69. Hannington-Kiff JG. Prune-belly syndrome and general anaesthesia: Case report. Br J Anaesth 1970;42:649–52

70. Harris ED. Rheumatoid arthritis. Pathophysiology and implications for therapy. N Engl J Med 1990;322:1277–88

71. Smith PH, Sharp J, Kellgren JH. Natural history of rheumatoid cervical subluxations. Ann Rheum Dis 1972;31:222–6

72. Funk D, Raymon F. Rheumatoid arthritis of the cricoarytenoid joints: An airway hazard. Anesth Analg 1975;54:742–5

73. Cervantes-Perez P, Toro-Perez AH, Rodreguez-Jurado P. Pulmonary involvement in rheumatoid arthritis. JAMA 1980;243:1715–9

74. Mills PR, Sturrock RD. Clinical associations between arthritis and liver disease. Ann Rheum Dis 1982;41:295–301

75. Harris ED. Rheumatoid arthritis. Pathophysiology and implications for therapy. N Engl J Med 1990;322:1277–89

76. Weinblatt ME, Coblyn JS, Fox DA, et al. Efficacy of low-dose methotrexate in rheumatoid arthritis. N Engl J Med 1985;312:818–23

77. Munson ES, Cullen SC. Endotracheal intubation in a patient with ankylosing spondylitis of the cervical spine. Anesthesiology 1965;26:365

78. Cho E, Dayan SS, Marx GF. Anaesthesia in a parturient with osteogenesis imperfecta. Br J Anaesth 1992;68:422–3

79. Lee PA, VanDop C, Migeon CJ. McCune-Albright syndrome. Long-term follow-up. JAMA 1986;256:2980–4

80. Newton MC, Allen PW, Ryan DC. Fibrodysplasia ossificans progressiva. Br J Anaesth 1990;64:246–50

81. Pyeritz RE, McKusick VA. The Marfan syndrome. Diagnosis and management. N Engl J Med 1979;300:772–7

82. Kafer ER. Respiratory and cardiovascular functions in scoliosis and the principles of anesthetic management. Anesthesiology 1980;52:339–51

83. Waldman J, Kaufer H, Hensinger RV, et al. Wakeup technique to avoid neurological sequelae during Harrington rod procedure. A case report. Anesth Analg 1977;56:733–5

84. Pathak KS, Brown RH, Nash CL, Cascorbi HF. Continuous opioid infusion for scoliosis fusion surgery. Anesth Analg 1983;62:841–5

85. Berkowitz ID, Raja SN, Bender KS, Kopits SE. Dwarfs: Pathophysiology and anesthetic implications. Anesthesiology 1990;73:739–59

86. Mayhew JF, Katz J, Miner M, et al. Anaesthesia for the achondroplastic dwarf. Can Anaesth Soc J 1986;33:216–21

87. Kalla GN, Fening E, Obiaya MD. Anaesthetic management of achondroplasia. Br J Anaesth 1986;58:117–9

88. Katz J, Mayhew JF. Air embolism in the achondroplastic dwarf. Anesthesiology 1985;63:205–7

89. Cohen SE. Anesthesia for cesarean section in achondroplastic dwarfs. Anesthesiology 1980;52:264–6

90. Ravindran R, Stoops CM. Anesthetic management of a patient with Hallermann-Streiff syndrome. Anesth Analg 1979;58:254–5

91. Browder FH, Lew D, Shahbazian TS. Anesthetic management of a patient with Dutch-Kentucky syndrome. Anesthesiology 1986;65:218–9

92. Vaghadia H, Blackstock D. Anaesthetic implications of the trismus pseudocamptodactylyl (Dutch-Kentucky or Hecht Beals) syndrome. Can J Anaesth 1988;35:80–5

93. Naguib M, Farag H, Ibrahim AEW. Anaesthetic considerations in Klippel-Feil syndrome. Can Anaesth Soc J 1986;33:66–70

94. Quance DR. Anaesthetic management of an obstetrical patient with arthrogryposis multiplex congenita. Can J Anaesth 1988;35:612–4

27

Infectious Diseases

An understanding of the diseases caused by infectious organisms and knowledge of the appropriate treatment of these diseases are important for optimal patient care during surgery and anesthesia.[1] Although infectious diseases are rarely the primary indications for surgery, not infrequently a co-existing infection influences the management of a patient during the perioperative period. Indeed, for a patient who has a known transmissible disease, special attention may be required with respect to the use of disposable equipment. More important, many patients may be carriers of an undiagnosed infectious disease, emphasizing the need to consider all patients as potentially infectious, especially with respect to the handling of blood and other body fluids.[2]

Infection is the most common cause of fever, reflecting the effect of endogenous pyrogens (cytokines) on the hypothalamic setpoint. There is no direct evidence that fever is beneficial to the host. Conversely, high fever may cause seizures in children (6 months to 6 years of age) and altered sensorium in adults. In the elderly or in the patient with cardiopulmonary disease, fever can precipitate cardiac dysrhythmias, myocardial ischemia, and congestive heart failure, reflecting increased oxygen consumption that cannot be met by an increased cardiac output. Significant increases in body temperature should always be treated in young children, in elderly or debilitated patients, and in persons with cardiopulmonary disease. Aspirin-like drugs are used to lower body temperature, owing to an elevated hypothalamic setpoint. If physical cooling methods are used without an antipyretic drug, homeostatic mechanisms will continue to operate in an attempt to increase body temperature, resulting in intense vasoconstriction and shivering.

ANTIBIOTICS

The frequent use of antibiotics in the treatment of bacterial infection necessitates an appreciation of the adverse effects that may be associated with these drugs. Adverse reactions to antibiotics include (1) microbial superinfections, (2) allergic reactions, (3) altered neuromuscular conduction, and (4) direct organ toxicity. It is mandatory that a history of drug allergy be sought before initiating treatment. Penicillin is the antibiotic most often associated with a life-threatening allergic reaction. The incidence of allergic reactions to cephalosporins is less than with penicillin, although possible cross-sensitivity between these two classes of antibiotics probably should prohibit the use of a cephalosporin in a patient with documented systemic allergic symptoms to penicillin. Aminoglycoside antibiotics interfere with the presynaptic release of acetylcholine at the neuromuscular junction. This effect can lead to potentiation of skeletal muscle paralysis, produced by depolarizing and nondepolarizing muscle relaxants. Penicillins, cephalosporins, and erythromycin do not produce effects at the neuromuscular junction, hence are not associated with potentiation of paralysis produced by muscle relaxants. It is important to appreciate that anticholinesterase or calcium-produced antagonism of antibiotic-potentiated neuromuscular blockade may be unreliable.[3] Direct organ toxicity associated with the use of antibiotics includes nephrotoxicity (aminoglycosides, vancomycin, amphotericin B), whereas hypotension during intravenous administration of vancomycin may reflect drug-induced histamine release or a direct myocardial depressant effect of this antibiotic.[4,5] The frequent dependence of antibiotics on renal clearance must be remembered when determining the dose of antibiotic to be administered to a patient with renal insufficiency.

Prophylactic antibiotics are often used for many of the commonly performed surgical procedures. Because of their antimicrobial spectrum and low toxicity, the cephalosporins are likely choices for preoperative prophylaxis when the most common pathogens are normal skin, gastrointestinal, and genitourinary flora. Timing of antibiotic administration should coincide with bacterial inoculation, emphasizing that the prophylactic drug need not be routinely given before the induction of anesthesia. Prolongation of prophylactic antibiotic therapy beyond the first postoperative day probably affords no additional protection.

459

INFECTION DUE TO GRAM-POSITIVE BACTERIA

Organisms categorized as gram-positive bacteria include pneumococci, streptococci, and staphylococci. These organisms are frequently implicated as a cause of infection that may contribute to significant morbidity in the hospitalized patient.

Pneumococci

There are more than 80 distinct serotypes of the *Pneumococcus* genus (*Streptococcus pneumoniae*).[6] These serotypes differ by virtue of the polysaccharide polymers forming their outer capsules. These capsules are crucial to the virulence of pneumococci, since they allow these bacteria to resist phagocytosis. Capsular polysaccharides from the 14 most prevalent serotypes of pneumococci have been incorporated into a pneumococcal vaccine.[7] Pneumococci remain the most important cause of bacterial pneumonia, accounting for about 60% of these infections. Acute otitis media, due to spread of pneumococci from the nasopharynx, is one of the most frequent bacterial infections in children. Indeed, the nasopharynx is the natural habitat of pneumococci. In rare instances, meningitis may reflect the spread of pneumococcal organisms from the middle ear or nasal sinuses. An uncommon pneumococcal syndrome is overwhelming infection after surgical splenectomy.

Penicillin, or another antibiotic with a similar spectrum of activity, remains the drug of choice for treatment of an infection due to pneumococci. Pneumococcal vaccine is indicated in patients at risk of infection, including those with chronic cardiopulmonary disease, cirrhosis of the liver, nephrosis, and sickle cell anemia, and patients who are immunosuppressed.[7] The vaccine may also be useful in the management of the patient with Hodgkin's disease, who is at risk of pneumococcal sepsis after staging laparotomy and splenectomy. It should be appreciated that responses to this vaccine are poor after chemotherapy and radiotherapy.

Streptococci

Streptococci are a diverse group of gram-positive bacteria that reside in humans as part of the normal flora. Based on the composition of their carbohydrate cell walls, streptococci are divided into 18 groups designated as A through H and K through T.

Group A Streptococci

Group A streptococci (*Streptococcus pyogenes*) are one of the most common and ubiquitous of human pathogens. They are responsible for a wide array of infections, the most frequent

Table 27-1.   Infection Due to Group A Streptococci

Pharyngitis ("strep throat") and tonsillitis
Superficial skin infection (impetigo, pyoderma)
Deep skin infection (cellulitis, erysipelas)
Sinusitis
Otitis
Pneumonia
Bacteremia (endocarditis, meningitis, osteomyelitis)
Scarlet fever
Peritonsillar and retropharyngeal abscess
Puerperal sepsis
Nonsuppurative sequelae (acute rheumatic fever, acute glomerulonephritis)

of which are acute pharyngitis and superficial skin infections[8] (Table 27-1).

The most important mode of spread of group A streptococci is by droplets, originating either from asymptomatic nasopharyngeal carriers or from a patient with pharyngitis. Group A streptococci elaborate enzymes that account for the ability of these organisms to produce inflammation and to spread rapidly to adjacent tissues. Among these enzymes are streptolysin O and streptolysin S, which are responsible for hemolysis (reason for designation as beta-hemolytic streptococci) and inactivation of leukocytes. A streptokinase enzyme elaborated by certain streptococci is responsible for promoting fibrinolysis. Elaboration of hyaluronidase enzyme by streptococci facilitates spread of infection into adjacent tissues, due to the ability of this substance to digest hyaluronic acid present in connective tissues.

Group A streptococci are the most common cause of bacterial pharyngitis and tonsillitis. Elaboration of an exotoxin known as erythrogenic toxin is responsible for scarlet fever. Acute rheumatic fever occurs only after pharyngitis caused by group A streptococci. Rheumatic fever is most likely to develop in patients in the 5- to 15-year-old age group. Typically, symptoms of acute rheumatic fever are manifested 1 to 3 weeks after streptococcal infection. Antibodies formed against streptococcal antigens are the most likely mechanism by which prior infection with group A streptococci produces delayed tissue damage. This damage may be manifested as pericarditis, myocarditis, or endocarditis. The mitral and aortic valves are often involved in this disease process. An acute migratory arthritis occurs in more than one-half of patients in whom rheumatic fever develops. Early treatment of pharyngitis due to infection with group A streptococci will prevent subsequent attacks of acute rheumatic fever.[6] Aspirin is effective in controlling the febrile and articular manifestations associated with acute rheumatic fever.

Superficial infection of the epidermis due to group A streptococci is known as impetigo. Impetigo is highly contagious and predisposes to the poststreptococcal infection syndrome known as glomerulonephritis. Surgical wound infection due to streptococci is often manifested as an acute increase of body temperature despite a relatively benign-appearing incision site.

Deep skin infections due to group A streptococci are known as erysipelas and cellulitis. Osteomyelitis, meningitis, and endocarditis are potential complications of group A streptococcal bacteremia. Group A streptococci are the classic cause of postpartum infection.

Penicillin is the drug of choice for treatment of infections due to group A streptococci. Alternative drugs to penicillin include erythromycin and clindamycin. Tetracyclines should not be relied on, since many strains of group A streptococci are resistant to this antibiotic.

Group B Streptococci

Group B streptococci are the most common cause of bacterial sepsis in neonates. Infection due to this organism is most often associated with prematurity and prolonged rupture of the membranes. Pneumonia or meningitis is present in about one-half of the neonates who show infection with this organism. Mortality ranges from 20% to 75%, despite aggressive treatment with antibiotics. Neurologic sequelae are often present in those neonates who survive. Despite the demonstration of a decreased incidence of necrotizing enterocolitis in high-risk infants treated with prophylactic antibiotics, the routine use of this approach is not popular because of the rapid emergence of resistant organisms.

Group D Streptococci

Group D streptococci reside in the gastrointestinal and genitourinary tract. These enterococci are relatively common causes of superficial wound infection, urinary tract infection, peritonitis, endocarditis, and bacteremia. Infection with group D streptococci is most likely in the patient with co-existing disease of the genitourinary or gastrointestinal tract. Treatment of infection due to group D streptococci is difficult, since these organisms are unique among the streptococci in that they are resistant to penicillin.

Staphylococci

The two important species of staphylococci are *Staphylococcus aureus* and *Staphylococcus epidermidis* (formerly *albus*). Unlike pneumococci and streptococci, there is no satisfactory serologic classification of staphylococci.

S. aureus

S. aureus is a widely distributed organism; asymptomatic carriers or persons with staphylococcal lesions act as reservoirs of infection. The incidence of nasal carriage is 15% to 50% in hospital populations. The incidence is even greater in intravenous drug users and in patients with insulin-dependent diabetes mellitus. Contamination of the hands with nasal secretions is the primary mode of transmission.

The most frequent manifestations of *S. aureus* are superficial (conjunctivitis, furuncle, paronychia) and soft tissue (cellulitis, mastitis, surgical incision) infections. These organisms are among the principal causes of septic arthritis and osteomyelitis. Staphylococcal bacteremia may result in endocarditis and meningitis. Staphylococci do not cause pharyngitis and are responsible for less than 10% of all bacterial pneumonias.

Staphylococcal invasion of the gastrointestinal tract may take two forms. In one form, ingestion of staphylococcal enterotoxin results in vomiting and diarrhea within 3 to 6 hours after consumption of food contaminated with *S. aureus*. Characteristically, these symptoms are not accompanied by an increase in body temperature. In the second form, staphylococcal enterocolitis is caused by the intestinal overgrowth of *S. aureus* in patients receiving broad-spectrum oral antibiotics.

S. aureus is usually resistant to penicillin. Effective antibiotics include aminoglycoside and cephalosporin antibiotics, oxacillin, and nafcillin. In addition to therapy with antibiotics, other measures, including removal of such portals of entry as indwelling venous catheters and surgical drainage, may be necessary.

Toxic Shock Syndrome

Toxic shock syndrome is a potentially fatal multisystem illness due to *S. aureus* infection and production of toxins. This syndrome is associated with tampon use during menstruation and with the use of vaginal contraceptive sponges. Toxic shock syndrome may be a complication of staphylococcal pneumonia that follows an influenza-like illness (postinfluenza toxic shock syndrome).[9] Other nonmenstrual cases of toxic shock syndrome have been related to nasal packing, childbirth and abortion, surgical wound infections, and vaginal infections.

Criteria for diagnosis of toxic shock syndrome include fever, diffuse macular erythroderma, and hypotension. Desquamation is a characteristic feature of this syndrome but is not an early finding. Evidence of multisystem involvement may include diarrhea, skeletal muscle myalgia (elevated plasma concentration of creatine kinase), renal dysfunction (elevated plasma creatinine concentration), hepatic dysfunction (elevated plasma concentration of transaminase enzymes and bilirubin), disseminated intravascular coagulation, and thrombocytopenia. Isolation of toxin producing *S. aureus* from secretions of affected patients further supports the diagnosis of toxic shock syndrome.

S. epidermidis

S. epidermidis is an organism of low pathogenic potential, universally present as part of the normal flora of the skin. Because of its ubiquity, *S. epidermidis* is frequently isolated from clinical specimens, including blood cultures. Nevertheless, these organisms are most often skin contaminants rather than true pathogens, producing infections only in patients with severe underlying medical problems.

A frequent manifestation of infection with *S. epidermidis* is bacteremia resulting from infection of an intravenous catheter. Many affected patients have associated persistent low-grade fevers, with periodic marked elevations in body temperature. Signs of thrombophlebitis may or may not be present. Removal of the contaminated intravenous catheter is the most important aspect of therapy.

The most difficult therapeutic problem caused by *S. epidermidis* is infection of a prosthetic heart valve. This infection typically has a subacute course, but eradication of organisms is difficult, due to their resistance to many of the available antibiotics.

INFECTION DUE TO GRAM-NEGATIVE BACTERIA

Clinically important diseases caused by infection with gram-negative bacteria include salmonellosis, shigellosis, cholera, and *Escherichia coli*-induced diarrhea. Manifestations of these diseases are predominantly in the gastrointestinal tract.

Salmonellosis

Gastroenteritis accounts for about two-thirds of all infections with *Salmonella*. Ingestion of these organisms is followed in 8 to 48 hours by abdominal cramps, vomiting, and diarrhea. Abdominal pain is typically periumbilical or is localized to the right lower quadrant. As such, this pain can mimic acute appendicitis, cholecystitis, or a ruptured viscus. Antibiotics are not effective.

Enteric fever (typhoid fever) is characterized by a sustained gram-negative bacteremia and by persistent elevations of body temperature. There may be associated dysfunction of multiple organ systems. Chloramphenicol is the treatment of choice.

Shigellosis

Shigellosis is an acute inflammatory disease of the gastrointestinal tract that ranges in severity from mild nonspecific diarrhea to classic dysentery. Initial manifestations of infection with these gram-negative organisms include fever, abdominal cramps, and watery diarrhea. Treatment is with antibiotics from the tetracycline class.

Cholera

Cholera is an acute diarrheal disease produced by enterotoxin secreted by *Vibrio cholerae* organisms. Humans are the only known hosts, so transmission can occur only through infected human excreta. These organisms are exquisitely sensitive to gastric acid; thus, persons who are achlorhydric or who are taking antacids are most susceptible to cholera.

Diarrhea is massive and watery. Fluid loss may be equivalent to $1 \text{ L} \cdot \text{h}^{-1}$ of isotonic fluid at the peak of the disease. Hypotension and metabolic acidosis reflect large fluid and electrolyte losses. Fever is characteristically absent. Treatment is with fluid and electrolyte replacement and eradication of gram-negative organisms with a tetracycline antibiotic.

Escherichia coli-Induced Diarrhea

E. coli is an important constituent of the normal flora of the gastrointestinal tract. Some strains of *E. coli*, however, are not part of the normal flora and produce diarrhea (traveler's disease) when introduced into the gastrointestinal tract by contaminated food or water. Clinical manifestations include abrupt onset of abdominal cramps and watery diarrhea. Absence of a temperature elevation is in keeping with failure of these organisms to invade other tissues or to produce inflammation. This form of diarrhea cannot be distinguished clinically from shigellosis. The most important aspect of treatment is fluid and electrolyte replacement. A single daily dose of the tetracycline antibiotic doxycyline may be effective in preventing this disease.[10]

INFECTION DUE TO SPORE-FORMING ANAEROBES

Spore-forming gram-positive anaerobes that cause invasive infections are normally found in the lower gastrointestinal tracts of humans and animals and in soil contaminated with their excrement. These organisms are strict anaerobes and are protected from lethal effects of oxygen by formation of spores. The introduction of spores into wounds (puncture wounds, burns, uterine instrumentation, subcutaneous infections in intravenous drug users) sets the stage for the conversion of spores into exotoxin-producing vegetative forms. The species most often responsible for disease in humans are *Clostridium perfringens*, *C. tetani*, and *C. botulinum*. Exotoxins elaborated by vegetative forms of these organisms are the causes of clostridial myonecrosis, tetanus, and botulism, respectively.

Clostridial Myonecrosis

Clostridial myonecrosis (gas gangrene) is due to infection with *C. perfringens*. The incubation period after inoculation with clostridial spores is 8 to 72 hours, after which there is a sudden onset of localized skeletal muscle pain and swelling. Necrosis of skeletal muscles and alterations in the integrity of the capillary membranes are caused by elaboration of an exotoxin (lecithinase) by these organisms. A brownish discharge with a foul odor is characteristic. In addition to the exotoxin, these organisms liberate hydrogen and carbon dioxide, which is responsible for crepitus over involved skeletal muscles, while associated swelling can cause compression of surrounding blood vessels.

Systemic effects of infection with *C. perfringens* are prominent. Tachycardia and fever are followed by hypotension and oliguria. Presumably, these responses reflect a decrease in intravacular fluid volume due to massive tissue edema. Anemia, jaundice, and hemoglobinuria are due to intravascular hemolysis in association with clostridial bacteremia. Renal failure may be a consequence of hemoglobinuria. Treatment of clostridial myonecrosis is immediate surgical debridement of infected tissues. Penicillin or an equivalent antibiotic is administered to eradicate organisms not removed by debridement and to control bacteremia.

Management of Anesthesia

Management of anesthesia for surgical debridement must take into account the multiple physiologic derangements produced by infection with this organism.[11] Preoperatively, important considerations include the status of the intravascular fluid volume, oxygen-carrying capacity of the blood, and renal function. Ketamine is a useful drug for the induction and maintenance of anesthesia. A theoretical hazard to the use of nitrous oxide would be expansion of gas pockets produced by clostridial infection. This seems unlikely, however, since these gas pockets are relatively avascular. Likewise, the release of potassium from necrotic skeletal muscles after administration of succinylcholine seems unlikely, since the involved skeletal muscles are avascular and thus effectively isolated from the circulation. In vitro oxygen exposures to less than 2.5 atmospheres pressure do not inhibit the release of the clostridial exotoxin. Therefore, the delivery of oxygen concentrations greater than those needed to maintain adequate arterial oxygenation during surgery is of no advantage. Renal function needs to be considered if certain long-acting nondepolarizing muscle relaxants are administered during surgical debridement. The use of electrocautery must be questioned, in view of the production of hydrogen gas by clostridial organisms. Regional anesthesia is not recommended because clostridial organisms could be introduced into other sites by the needle used to perform the anesthetic. Furthermore, blockade of the peripheral sympathetic nervous system might be undesirable in the presence of an unstable cardiovascular system.

Postoperatively, these patients are not likely to be sources of cross-infection to other patients, since *C. perfringens* organisms are neutralized when exposed to air. Therefore, strict isolation of these patients is not mandatory.

Tetanus

Tetanus is caused by the gram-positive anaerobic bacillus *C. tetani*. Elaboration of the neurotoxin tetanospasmin by vegetative forms of these organisms is responsible for clinical manifestations of tetanus. With the exception of botulinum toxin, tetanospasmin is the most powerful poison known to humans. Tetanospasmin, when elaborated into wounds, spreads centrally along motor nerves to the spinal cord or enters the systemic circulation to reach the central nervous system. This toxin affects the nervous system in several areas. In the spinal cord, toxin suppresses inhibitory internuncial neurons. As a result, generalized skeletal muscle spasm occurs. In the brain, there is fixation of toxin by gangliosides. The fourth cerebral ventricle is believed to have a selective permeability for tetanospasmin, resulting in early manifestations of trismus and neck rigidity. Sympathetic nervous system hyperactivity may manifest as the disease progresses.[12]

Signs and Symptoms

Trismus is the presenting symptom of tetanus in 75% of patients. The greater strength of the masseter muscles, compared with the opposing digastric and mylohyoid muscles, results in "lockjaw." Indeed, these patients are often first seen by a dentist. Rigidity of the facial muscles results in the characteristic appearance described as the sardonic smile (risus sardonicus). Spasm of laryngeal muscles can occur at any time. Intractable pharyngeal spasm following tracheal extubation has been described in a patient with unrecognized tetanus.[13] Dysphagia may be due to spasm of the pharyngeal muscles. Spasm of the intercostal muscles and the diaphragm interferes with adequate ventilation. The rigidity of abdominal and lumbar muscles accounts for the opisthotonic posture. Skeletal muscle spasms are tonic and clonic in nature, and are excruciatingly painful. Furthermore, the increased skeletal muscle work is associated with dramatic increases in oxygen consumption, and peripheral vasoconstriction can contribute to an increase in body temperature. External stimulation, including sudden exposure to bright light, unexpected sound, or tracheal suction, can precipitate generalized skeletal muscle spasm, leading to ineffective ventilation and death. Hypotension has been attributed to myocarditis. Isolated and unexplained tachycardia may be an early manifestation of hyperactivity of the sympathetic nervous system. More often, this hyperactivity is manifested as a transient hypertension. Sympathetic nervous system responses to external stimuli are exaggerated, as demonstrated by cardiac tachydysrhythmias and labile blood pressure. In addition, excessive sympathetic nervous system activity is associated with intense peripheral vasoconstriction, diaphoresis, and increased urinary excretion of catecholamines. Inappropriate secretion of antidiuretic hormone manifested as hyponatremia, as well as decreased plasma osmolarity may occur.

Treatment

Treatment of patients with tetanus is directed at (1) control of skeletal muscle spasm, (2) prevention of sympathetic nervous system hyperactivity, (3) support of ventilation of the lungs, (4) neutralization of circulating exotoxin, and (5) surgical debridement to eliminate the source of exotoxin. Administration of diazepam (40 to 200 mg $\cdot$ d^{-1} IV) is useful to control skeletal muscle spasm. If skeletal muscle spasm is not controlled by diazepam, administration of a nondepolarizing muscle relaxant and control of ventilation of the lungs with a tube placed in the trachea is necessary. Indeed, early and aggressive protection of the airway is mandatory, as laryngospasm may accompany generalized skeletal muscle spasm. Overactivity of the sympathetic nervous system is best managed with intravenous administration of a beta antagonist such as propranolol or esmolol. Continuous epidural anesthesia has also been used to control tetanus-induced sympathetic nervous system hyperactivity.[14] Neutralization of circulating exotoxin is provided with use of intramuscular human hyperimmune globulin. This neutralization does not alter the symptoms already present but does prevent additional exotoxin from reaching the central nervous system. Penicillin is effective in destroying exotoxin-producing vegetative forms of *C. tetani*.

Management of Anesthesia

General anesthesia with intubation of the trachea is a useful approach for surgical debridement. Such debridement is delayed until several hours after the patient has received antitoxin because free tetanospasmin is mobilized into the circulation during surgical manipulation. Monitoring often includes continuous recording of arterial blood pressure from a catheter in a peripheral artery, as well as measurement of central venous or pulmonary artery occlusion pressure, or both. A volatile anesthetic is useful for the maintenance of anesthesia if excessive sympathetic nervous system activity is present. In view of potential cardiac irritability, it might be prudent to select a volatile anesthetic other than halothane. Drugs such as lidocaine, esmolol, and nitroprusside should be readily available for treatment of excess sympathetic nervous system activity during the perioperative period.

Botulism

Botulism is due to effects of a neurotoxin elaborated by *C. botulinum*. This neurotoxin interferes with presynaptic release of acetylcholine from preganglionic nerve endings and at the neuromuscular junction. The diagnosis of botulism must be considered in any patient who presents with acute symmetric

skeletal muscle weakness or paralysis leading to ventilatory failure. The incubation period is 18 to 36 hours after oral ingestion of food contaminated with these organisms.

INFECTIONS DUE TO SPIROCHETES

Syphilis

Syphilis is a sexually transmitted infection caused by the spirochete *Treponema pallidum*. Humans are the only known hosts. Disease of more than 4 years' duration is rarely transmissible. An untreated parturient, however, can pass syphilis to her fetus, regardless of the stage of her disease.

Signs and Symptoms

Clinical manifestations of syphilis depend on the chronologic stage of the disease. The first clinical sign is the chancre, which develops at the inoculation site after 3 to 4 weeks of incubation. Secondary syphilis, characterized by widespread mucocutaneous lesions, lymphadenopathy, and splenomegaly, develops about 6 weeks after the chancre has healed. During the latent stage, there are no clinical or cerebrospinal fluid abnormalities, but serologic tests are positive.

The tertiary stage of syphilis is characterized by destructive lesions in the central nervous system, peripheral nervous system, and cardiovascular system. Tabes dorsalis (locomotor ataxia) develops 15 to 20 years after the initial infection with syphilis. Posterior root dysfunction and posterior column degeneration result in ataxia with a broad-based gait, hypotonic bladder, and jabbing pains that typically occur in the legs. Sudden attacks of abdominal pain may mimic a surgical abdomen.

Cardiovascular syphilis is most often manifested as aortitis, with dilation of the aortic ring and subsequent aortic regurgitation. An aneurysm due to syphilis almost always involves the ascending thoracic aorta, and only rarely the abdominal aorta. Diagnosis of aortitis due to syphilis should be considered in an adult with isolated aortic regurgitation and positive serologic tests. Linear calcification in the wall of the ascending aorta that is visible on a chest radiograph, as well as a positive serologic test, suggests an aneurysm due to syphilis.

Lyme Disease

Lyme disease (Lyme borreliosis) is caused by the spirochete *Borrelia burgdorferi*, which is transmitted to humans by tick bites.[15] Certain species of mice are critical to the life cycle of the spirochete, and deer appear to be crucial to the tick. Although distribution of the disease is worldwide, its name (Lyme disease) reflects its initial description in a clustering of children in Lyme, Connecticut, who were thought to have juvenile rheumatoid arthritis.

Like other spirochetal infections, Lyme disease is characterized by multisystem involvement and occurrence in clinically distinct stages with manifestations that undergo remissions and exacerbations. Erythema chronicum migrans is the initial unique clinical marker for Lyme disease. This classic cutaneous manifestation begins as an area of redness, which expands to a diameter ranging from 3 to 6 cm. Malaise and fatigue, headache, fever, and chills often accompany skin involvement. Some patients have evidence of meningeal irritation, encephalopathy, lymphadenopathy, and hepatitis. Cranial neuritis, including bilateral facial palsy, may occur. Neurologic abnormalities typically last for months but usually resolve completely. Within several weeks after the onset of illness, in about 8% of patients cardiac involvement develops, most often manifested as fluctuating degrees of atrioventricular heart block lasting 7 to 10 days. Rarely, mild left ventricular dysfunction occurs. Duration of cardiac involvement is usually brief (3 days to 6 weeks), but it may recur. From a few weeks to as long as 2 years after the onset of illness, about 60% of patients develop arthritis. Typically, this arthritis consists of migratory musculoskeletal pain, which may recur for years. In about 10% of patients with arthritis, involvement of the large joints becomes chronic, with erosion of cartilage and bone.

Laboratory abnormalities early during the course of Lyme disease include a high erythrocyte sedimentation rate, elevated plasma concentration of liver transaminase enzymes, and immunoglobulin M proteins. These levels generally return to normal within several weeks. Mild anemia may be present. Renal function tests are not altered. Treatment is initially with tetracyclines, followed by penicillin and erythromycin. Despite antibiotic therapy, nearly one-half of patients continue to experience minor complications such as headache, fatigue, or musculoskeletal pain.

INFECTION DUE TO MYCOBACTERIA

Mycobacterium tuberculosis is an obligate aerobe responsible for tuberculosis. These organisms grow most successfully in tissues with high oxygen concentrations, explaining the increased incidence of tuberculosis in the apices of the lungs. Although the incidence of tuberculosis in the United States seems low, the presence of the disease must be considered in Asian immigrants; in elderly patients, especially those in nursing homes; and in those infected with the human immunodeficiency virus (HIV). A positive tuberculin skin test in an otherwise asymptomatic patient indicates a previous infection. This patient may harbor viable tubercle bacilli, unless antituberculous chemotherapy has been administered.

Almost all cases of tuberculosis are acquired by aerosol transmission. Since most infected patients discharge few organisms, there is a low risk of infection in casual contacts. Infectivity is greatest from patients who have pulmonary cavitary disease or tuberculosis of the larynx. After infected particles have settled on surfaces exposed to ambient conditions, they become essentially noninfectious. More than 90% of patients remain asymptomatic during the initial infection and can be identified only by conversion of the tuberculin skin test. Among symptomatic patients, the most frequent manifestations are fever and nonproductive cough. These symptoms resemble pneumonia caused by infection with *Mycoplasma pneumoniae* (see the section, Infection Due to *Mycoplasma*).

Treatment

A patient who has a positive skin test should receive antituberculous chemotherapy with isoniazid. The major toxicities of isoniazid are on the peripheral nervous system, liver, and possibly the kidneys. Neurotoxicity can be prevented by daily administration of pyridoxine. Hepatotoxicity is most likely to be related to the metabolism of isoniazid by hepatic acetylation. Depending on a genetically determined trait, patients may be characterized as slow or rapid acetylators. Hepatitis appears to be more common in rapid acetylators, consistent with greater production of hydrazine, a potentially hepatotoxic metabolite of isoniazid. A persistent elevation of the plasma transaminase concentration mandates that isoniazid be discontinued; a mild and transient elevation does not require discontinuation. In addition to toxic effects on the liver, metabolites of isoniazid, which contain a hydrazine moiety, may also increase defluorination of volatile anesthetics. Indeed, elevated plasma fluoride levels have been observed after enflurane anesthesia administration to patients who were also being treated with isoniazid.[16]

Other drugs used in the treatment of tuberculosis include streptomycin and rifampin. Adverse effects of rifampin include thrombocytopenia, leukopnia, hemolytic anemia, and renal failure. Hepatitis associated with an elevation of the plasma transaminase concentrations occurs in about 10% of patients receiving rifampin.

SYSTEMIC MYCOTIC INFECTIONS

The three most common systemic mycotic infections are blastomycosis, coccidioidomycosis, and histoplasmosis. All three diseases are caused by a specific fungus that gains entry into the host by inhalation into the lungs. Clinical manifestations resemble tuberculosis and include pulmonary cavitary lesions. Amphotericin B administered intravenously is the drug of choice for the eradication of invading organisms that cause these three fungal diseases. Amphotericin B can produce adverse renal and hematologic reactions. For example, decreased glomerular filtration rate is unavoidable during therapy with this drug. It may be necessary to discontinue amphotericin temporarily, to maintain the plasma creatinine concentration below $3 \, \text{mg} \cdot \text{dl}^{-1}$. Renal tubular acidosis, hypokalemia, and hypomagnesemia occur frequently, and exogenous electrolyte replacement is usually necessary. Adverse hematologic effects are typically manifested as anemia. Fever, chills, and hypotension frequently occur within the first few hours after intravenous administration of amphotericin B. Ventricular fibrillation has been observed after the rapid intravenous infusion of amphotericin.[17] Hepatotoxicity is not produced by this drug.

Sporotrichosis differs from other systemic fungal infections because of its wide geographic distribution. Furthermore, the portal of entry and major site of infection is the skin. Pulmonary cavitary disease is rarely present.

Blastomycosis

Blastomycosis is caused by the fungus *Blastomyces dermatitidis*, which is endemic in the southeastern and south central portions of the United States. Pulmonary involvement is manifested as cavitary disease of the upper lobes. Fever, productive cough, hemoptysis, and simultaneous involvement of other organ systems, particularly the skin and skeleton, are present in many patients. Surgery may be necessary for the treatment of persistent pulmonary cavities or to correct deforming orthopaedic lesions.

Coccidioidomycosis

Coccidioidomycosis is caused by the fungus *Coccidioides immitis*, which is endemic in the southwestern United States. Positive skin tests may be the only evidence of systemic infection with this fungus. Pulmonary cavitary disease is often discovered on routine chest radiographs. The most serious extrapulmonary manifestation of coccidioidomycosis is meningitis. Meningitis due to this organism is an indication for intrathecal administration of amphotericin B. Surgical intervention may be necessary to treat hydrocephalus that has occurred as a result of meningitis. Arthralgia develops in 10% to 20% of patients with coccidioidomycosis.

Histoplasmosis

Histoplasmosis is an infection of the phagocytic cells of the reticuloendothelial system, caused by the fungus *Histoplasma capsulatum*. This fungus is endemic in the eastern and central portions of the United States and grows particularly well in soil contaminated with fecal material from birds. Most patients infected with this fungus are asymptomatic or show symptoms indistinguishable from the common cold. The presence of positive skin tests confirms infection with these organisms.

Chronic cavitary histoplasmosis is predominantly a disease of middle-aged and elderly men who also have chronic obstructive airway disease. Surgical ablation of the pulmonary cavity combined with intravenous administration of amphotericin B may be necessary in the presence of cavitary lung disease. Disseminated histoplasmosis is most likely to occur in an elderly or immunosuppressed patient.

INFECTION DUE TO *MYCOPLASMA*

Mycoplasma pneumoniae, formerly designated pleuropneumonia-like organisms, are the smallest known living organisms. Infection with these organisms produces *Mycoplasma pneumoniae* pneumonia, also known as primary atypical pneumonia. In urban populations, about 20% of all pneumonias are due to these organisms.[18]

Mycoplasma pneumoniae pneumonia is characterized by subacute onset of a nonproductive cough and pharyngitis. Headache, chills, and fever up to 40°C are present in most patients. Congested tympanic membranes are present in 10% to 20% of patients. The peripheral leukocyte count is normal in most patients and helps rule out pneumonia due to bacteria. About 50% of patients show a fourfold or greater increase in the cold agglutinin titer (1:128 or higher). By contrast, low titers (less than 1:32) may occur with infectious mononucleosis and with pneumonias caused by adenovirus or influenza viruses. Infection characteristically spreads slowly throughout a family. Erythromycin or tetracyclines are the antibiotics of choice for eradication of these organisms.

INFECTION DUE TO RICKETTSIAL ORGANISMS

Rocky Mountain spotted fever and Q fever are diseases caused by rickettsial organisms. The antibiotics of choice for eradication of these organisms are chloramphenicol or tetracyclines.

Rocky Mountain Spotted Fever

Rocky Mountain spotted fever is an acute tick-borne illness caused by *Rickettsia rickettsii*. The disease is characterized by the sudden onset of fever, headache, and a rash that begins on the extremities and spreads to the trunk. Rash is the most valuable diagnostic sign. Abdominal pain may be prominent, suggesting the need for surgical exploration. Thrombocytopenia occurs in nearly one-half of patients with this infection. Involvement of the myocardium by rickettsial organisms can be manifested on the electrocardiogram as nonspecific ST segment and T wave changes.

Q Fever

Q fever is an acute systemic infection caused by a rickettsial organism known as *Coxiella burnetii*. Infection with this organism produces a clinical picture similar to that of *Mycoplasma pneumoniae* pneumonia. Q fever differs from other diseases caused by rickettsial organisms in that a rash is absent. Furthermore, infection is airborne from infected feces and not by injection from tick bites. Hepatosplenomegaly, jaundice, abnormal liver function tests, and endocarditis may occur.

VIRAL INFECTIONS OF THE UPPER RESPIRATORY TRACT

Influenza viruses, rhinoviruses, and adenoviruses are responsible for infections of the respiratory tract. These infections can occur in all age groups but are most frequent in the adult population. Transmission of viruses is a common event in hospitals.[19]

Influenza Virus

Infection with influenza virus produces an acute febrile illness associated with myalgia, malaise, and headache. This syndrome is commonly referred to as influenza. The most important reservoir of viral particles are the nasopharyngeal secretions of infected persons. Thus, anesthesia personnel can have frequent contact and contribute to the spread of influenza among the surgical population. Influenza is usually self-limited, unless it is complicated by bacterial infection or the presence of co-existing chronic pulmonary disease. Indeed, pneumonia from secondary bacterial infection is the most common complication occurring after influenza. In this regard, it seems likely that influenza causes damage to the mucosal surfaces of the tracheobronchial tree, which, together with impaired mucociliary transport, promotes colonization with bacteria such as *Pseudomonas aeruginosa*. Severe myositis can be associated with myocarditis. Rarely, Guillain-Barré syndrome can follow infection with influenza A.

Prophylaxis

Influenza immunization must be repeated yearly because antigenic shifts in the virus necessitate production of new vaccines to protect against new epidemic strains. A polyvalent vaccine is often produced that contains antigens from the influenza A and B strains that are expected to predominate. It is estimated that the vaccine is about 60% effective in decreasing deaths from influenza in high-risk patients, including elderly patients and those with chronic cardiovascular or pulmonary disease (children with asthma). Pneumococcal and influenza vaccines may be administered simultaneously if needed. Neurologic complications, including Guillain-Barré syndrome, are no longer associated with the influenza vaccine.

Amantadine is an antiviral drug that specifically inhibits influenza A virus. Administered prophylactically, amantidine is highly effective in preventing influenza A. This drug is also effective in ameliorating symptoms, when administered within the first 48 hours of infection. Side effects that occur in 5% to 10% of patients include insomnia, whereas seizures are a possibility when excessive drug levels result in the patient with renal failure.

Rhinovirus

Rhinovirus is responsible for one-third or more of adult common colds. Transmission is most likely by inoculation from contaminated environmental surfaces or from the skin of infected individuals. Airborne transmission by a cough or sneeze is unlikely. The classic syndrome includes acute coryza, slight fever, and malaise. Infection occurs most often in winter, but the reason for this seasonal incidence is unknown. Postexposure prophylaxis with intranasal interferon may prevent respiratory symptoms in those exposed to infected persons.[20]

Adenovirus

Adenovirus produces an acute febrile disease associated with pharyngitis and cough, which most commonly affects children or semiclosed populations, such as military recruits. Another illness caused by adenovirus is highly contagious pharyngoconjunctival fever, characterized by pharyngitis, conjunctivitis, and fever, which usually affects children and young adults. Epidemic keratoconjunctivitis is easily transmitted by contaminated fingers. When caring for patients known to have adenoviral disease, handwashing and use of gloves should reduce the risk of iatrogenic spread of these organisms.

Respiratory Syncytial Virus

Respiratory syncytial virus is the most frequent cause for infant pneumonia and bronchiolitis. Hospital personnel act as transmitters of infection to children by carrying contaminated secretions on their hands and clothes. The antiviral drug, ribavirin, may be effective in the treatment of respiratory syncytial virus bronchiolitis or pneumonia.

Parainfluenza Virus

Parainfluenza virus is the principal cause of laryngotracheobronchitis in children. Transmission occurs by person-to-person contact or by large droplet spread.

Management of Anesthesia

The decision to proceed with or delay an elective operation that requires general anesthesia in the patient with a concurrent viral upper respiratory tract infection or a recent history of such an infection is an important clinical issue.[21–25] Despite some controversy in the literature, it appears prudent to avoid anesthesia that requires tracheal intubation in the patient with, or recovering from, a viral upper respiratory tract infection.[21] This is particularly appropriate in children, whereas data supporting an increased likelihood of complications in the adult with an upper respiratory tract infection are less convincing.[22] Evidence of an increased incidence of complications when anesthesia is administered to at-risk patients includes a threefold increase in the incidence of intraoperative bronchospasm and laryngospasm in asymptomatic patients with a recent history of an upper respiratory tract infection.[23] Reports of unpredicted perioperative arterial hemoglobin oxygen desaturation in patients with asymptomatic upper respiratory tract infection are supported by data from virus-infected animals demonstrating increased intrapulmonary shunting and perhaps increased oxygen consumption by inflamed lung tissue.[24] Viral infection is associated with exacerbations of asthma and chronic obstructive pulmonary disease. Even in the patient without coexisting lung disease, viral infection of the upper respiratory tract can cause temporary airway hyperresponsiveness, emphasizing the importance of considering the effects of tracheal intubation in these patients.

Concern about the potential increased risk of administering anesthesia to the child with an upper respiratory tract infection has resulted in a recommendation for delaying elective surgical procedures for 2 to 6 weeks.[25] If this recommendation is accepted, the potential safe time period for the administration of a general anesthetic is limited, considering that children, especially those younger than 2 years of age, have five to ten upper respiratory infections each year. The greatest risk of airway complications when anesthesia is administered in the presence of an upper respiratory tract infection seems to be in the child younger than 1 year of age, whereas the risk is much less in the child older than 5 years of age, presumably because of the presence of an anatomically larger airway.

When anesthesia cannot be delayed in the patient with an upper respiratory tract infection, it is helpful to consider potential problems (airway hyperreactivity, decreased arterial hemoglobin oxygen saturation, postoperative laryngeal edema) as described in previous clinical reports.[22–25] In this regard, administration of supplemental oxygen and extension of monitoring with pulse oximetry into the postoperative period is a reasonable consideration. Increased airway responsiveness suggests the need to establish an appropriate suppressant concentration of anesthetic drugs before tracheal intubation. Because vagally mediated reflex bronchoconstriction is an almost universal occurrence, the use of atropine to interrupt this reflex arc before tracheal intubation is a consid-

eration. General anesthesia probably does not increase the incidence of pulmonary complications in the patient with an uncomplicated upper respiratory infection who is undergoing a minor operation (myringotomy) without tracheal intubation.[21] Future developments may include more effective antiviral medications (amantadine shortens the illness but probably not the duration of airway hyperresponsiveness) and the introduction of more selective anticholinergic medications that block muscarinic receptors in airway smooth muscle without blocking muscarinic receptors at other sites.

INFECTION DUE TO HERPES VIRUS

The herpes group of viruses is composed of seven human viruses and multiple animal viruses (Table 27-2). All human herpes viruses replicate primarily in cell nuclei and share the properties of latency and reactivation. Sites of latency vary but include neural ganglion cells and B lymphocytes.

Herpes Simplex Virus

Herpes simplex virus type 1 (HSV-1) and type 2 (HSV-2) are characterized by unique routes of transmission and different clinical manifestations (Table 27-3). Although viral titers are increased and transmission is more likely when lesions are present, asymptomatic excretion of virus particles is common. The spread of infection through contact with oral secretions may be an occupational hazard for health care workers, emphasizing the importance of wearing gloves. After initial infection, the HSV travels along sensory nerve pathways to ganglion cells, where viral DNA remains dormant only to be reactivated by certain events such as decreased immunocompetence. After reactivation, the virus reverses its course and spreads peripherally by sensory nerve pathways.

The most common and significant infection caused by HSV-1 is keratitis, which may lead to destruction of the cornea. Herpetic infection of the digits (whitlow) is possible in personnel who experience sustained direct contact with oral, pharyngeal, or tracheal secretions of infected individuals. Despite pain that occurs with paronychial involvement, it is stressed

Table 27-2.   Human Herpes Viruses

Herpes simplex virus type 1 (HSV-1)
Herpes simplex virus type 2 (HSV-2)
Varicella-zoster
Cytomegalovirus
Epstein-Barr
Human herpesvirus type 6 (HHV-6)
Human herpesvirus type 7 (HHV-7)

Table 27-3. Comparison of Herpes Simplex Viruses

	HSV-1	HSV-2
Route of transmission	Oral	Genital
Manifestations	Oral-labial	Genital
	Ocular	Perianal and anal
	Whitlow	Whitlow
	Encephalitis	

that treatment should not include surgical drainage, as this may cause entrance of the HSV-1 into the deep pulp space and secondary bacterial infection. Infected personnel should refrain from dealing with chronically ill, debilitated, or immunosuppressed patients until the lesions resolve.

Treatment

Acyclovir is the drug of choice in the treatment of HSV infection; it is effective topically, orally, or intravenously. Clearance of acyclovir is dependent on renal excretion, but the overall toxicity of this drug is minimal. Rapid intravenous administration, however, has been associated with renal dysfunction and transient increases in liver function tests. The solution is alkaline and thrombophlebitis is possible after intravenous administration of acyclovir.

Varicella-Zoster Virus

Varicella-zoster virus is the cause of varicella (chickenpox) and herpes zoster (shingles). Varicella in one patient cannot produce herpes zoster in another, but a patient with herpes zoster can acquire varicella. Nosocomial transmission of varicella-zoster virus is possible, and hospitalized patients who are infected should probably be isolated. A susceptible immunocompromised patient who is exposed to an infected person may be treated with varicella-zoster immune globulin as prophylaxis. Acyclovir decreases the severity of varicella in children when therapy is initiated during the first 24 hours of rash.[26]

Herpes Zoster

Herpes zoster follows endogenous reactivation of the virus, which is believed to persist in sensory ganglia in a quiescent state after an initial episode of varicella. The incidence of herpes zoster is dramatically increased in immunosuppressed patients. Indeed, the development of herpes zoster in an asymptomatic carrier of HIV is often a forerunner of impending acquired immunodeficiency syndrome (AIDS). An attack of herpes zoster is often preceded by pain that may persist for several days before the unilateral vesicular lesions appear, most often on the thorax. Individual attacks of herpes zoster are usually limited to one of three dermatomes. The most common complication of herpes zoster is postherpetic neuralgia, which may be severe and refractory to treatment, particularly in the elderly. Encephalitis occurs as a complication of herpes zoster, primarily in immunosuppressed hosts. Acyclovir may shorten the course and decrease the severity of herpes zoster but does not appear to be useful for the treatment of postherpetic neuralgia.[27] Likewise, the administration of corticosteroids for the management of postherpetic neuralgia is of unproven efficacy.[28]

Cytomegalovirus

Cytomegalovirus (CMV) is a ubiquitous virus that plays an important role in many diseases, including a heterophile-negative mononucleosis syndrome and disseminated disease in the immunocompromised host. Transmission occurs by contact with infected secretions or leukocyte-containing blood products. Infection of the parturient may result in damage to the immature fetal central nervous system. Blood transfusion and organ transplantation may also transmit CMV from an asymptomatic donor to a previously uninfected recipient.[29] There is no evidence of risk of transmission of CMV from an infected patient to hospital personnel.[30] A dormant CMV infection may be reactivated in the patient with compromised T lymphocyte function (transplant recipient, AIDS, lymphoma). Matching of seronegative transplant or transfusion recipients with seronegative organ or blood donors may decrease the frequency of CMV transmission. Mononucleosis due to CMV is characterized by fever, adenopathy, splenomegaly, hepatitis, and atypical lymphocytes in the blood. Hepatitis is mild and only rarely progresses to chronic liver disease.

Epstein-Barr Virus

Epstein-Barr virus (EBV) infects most humans; in about one-third of persons, heterophil-positive infectious mononucleosis develops. The most common symptoms are fever, pharyngitis, lymphadenopathy, and hepatosplenomegaly. Hyperplasia of the tonsils and adenoids, or edema of the uvula or epiglottis, can compromise the patency of the upper airway.[31] Mild hepatitis can occur, as evidenced by a moderate increase in the plasma concentration of transaminase enzymes, and jaundice develops in 10% to 20% of patients. Splenic rupture is rare but should be considered when abdominal pain occurs. Autoimmune hemolytic anemia may be present. In fewer than 1% of patients with infectious mononucleosis, encephalitis, meningitis, or Guillain-Barré syndrome develops. Transmission is by oral-to-oral contact, and the incubation period is about 28 days. The diagnosis of infectious mononucleosis is confirmed by the presence of heterophile antibodies. Treatment with acyclovir does not seem to be efficacious in the treatment of infectious mononucleosis due to EBV. EBV persists for life in salivary glands and B lymphocytes and in the presence of immunosuppression may present as a life-threatening B lymphocyte proliferative disorder. A relationship between chronic fatigue syndrome and infection with EBV has been speculated but not proved.

RUBELLA

Rubella is highly contagious, spread by airborne transmission. The teratogenic potential of rubella emphasizes the importance for susceptible hospital personnel to become vaccinated. Treatment with vitamin A decreases morbidity and mortality from measles.[32] Indeed, in almost every known infectious disease, vitamin A deficiency is known to be associated with a greater frequency, severity, or mortality.

CREUTZFELDT-JAKOB DISEASE

Creutzfeldt-Jakob disease is a rare noninflammatory disease of the central nervous system caused by a transmissible slowly infectious pathogen known as a prion (see Chapter 17).

ACQUIRED IMMUNODEFICIENCY SYNDROME

AIDS describes the occurrence of a life-threatening opportunistic infection or Kaposi sarcoma, or both, in a patient who displays profound immunosuppression unrelated to drug therapy or known co-existing disease. The syndrome is initiated by a human T lymphotropic retrovirus known as HIV. As the virus replicates, T lymphocytes are damaged or destroyed, leading to cell-mediated immunodeficiency. Two types of HIV have been identified, with HIV-1 being responsible for most of the cases of AIDS in the United States and Europe, whereas HIV-2 is more prevalent in West Africa. More than 1 million people in the United States are thought to harbor asymptomatic HIV.[33] It is estimated that AIDS will develop in more than 50% of those infected with HIV within 10 years and that AIDS will eventually develop in virtually all remaining HIV-infected persons who do not succumb to some other disease process first. Likewise, although antibody to HIV may be found in immunoglobulin preparations, it is clear that the administration of immunoglobulin preparations does not transmit HIV.

Transmission

Four population groups account for the vast majority of AIDS cases in the United States (Table 27-4). HIV can be isolated from blood, saliva, tears, semen, and cervix secretions. There is evidence that anogenital skin lesions or anorectal mucosal ulcerations increase the rate of HIV acquisition and transmission. Transmission of HIV by routes other than sexual contact, transfusion of blood products, or communal intravenous drug use is virtually unknown. Thus, household, school, or work contacts of patients with HIV infection are at minimal or no risk of infection. There is no evidence of airborne transmission of HIV. HIV may survive for prolonged periods (3 to 7 days) outside the host, yet the virus is quite sensitive to mycobactericidal disinfectants or sodium hypochlorite (bleach) as well as low levels of heat (10 minutes at 56°C).[34] Common hospital sterilization techniques using ethylene oxide, steam, and boiling water kill HIV. An important issue is the possibility of accidental transmission of HIV to health care workers. Data suggest that the risk is very low (0.5% for an accidental needle stick and even less for other routes of exposure), but not nonexistent.[35] For this reason, it is important for health care workers to implement universal blood and body fluid precautions when contact with body fluids is unavoidable[2] (Table 27-5).

The safety of the blood supply is based on (1) screening of donated blood and plasma for antibody to HIV since 1985, (2) heat treatment of clotting factor concentrates, and (3) donor screening on the basis of history. Transmission of HIV by 1 unit of blood that has tested negative by current assays for HIV antibody can occur, but the likelihood is estimated to be 1:225,000 per unit transfused.[36] Virtually all patients in whom AIDS has developed as a result of a contaminated blood transfusion received the transfusion before the testing procedures instituted in 1985. More than 95% of patients receiving HIV-contaminated blood or components that have not been heat treated become infected, and symptomatic AIDS develops in 50% of those infected within 7 years. It is estimated that 80% of hemophiliacs in the United States are infected with HIV from transfusions administered before the availability of HIV testing.

The epidemiology of AIDS shows parallels to that of hepati-

Table 27-4. Population Groups Afflicted With Acquired Immunodeficiency Syndrome

	Total Cases (%)
Homosexual/bisexual males	71
Heterosexual intravenous drugs users	17
Blood transfusions (before 1985)	2
Hemophiliacs	1

Table 27.5 Universal Precautions to Prevent Transmission of Human Immunodeficiency Virus

1. Blood and body fluid precautions should be used for all patients, recognizing that it is not possible to identify infected patients reliably.

2. Use barrier precautions to prevent skin and mucous membrane exposure to blood or body fluids that may contain blood.
   a. Wear gloves.
   b. Wear protective eye shields if droplets likely.
   c. Take care to prevent injury when handling sharp devices—do not recap needles.

3. Health care workers with exudative skin lesions should refrain from direct patient care.

4. Use equipment for cardipulmonary resuscitation that obviates the need for mouth-to-mouth resuscitation.

(Adapted from Recommendations for Prevention of HIV Transmission in Health-Care Setting. MMWR 1987;36:2S, with permission.)

Table 27-6. Neurologic Disorders Associated With Human Immunodeficiency Virus

Disorder	Incidence (%)	Manifestations
Encephalitis	90	Memory loss Ataxia Seizures
Peripheral neuropathy	10–50	Paresthesias Weakness Sensory loss
Myelopathy	11–20	Spastic paresis Incontinence
Aseptic meningitis	5–10	Fever Headache Cranial nerve palsies

tis B. In this regard, the presence of HIV antibody, like the presence of hepatitis B surface antigen, serves as a marker of potentially transmissible infection. Both AIDS and hepatitis B are blood-borne infections that may also be spread by personal intimate contact. In addition, asymptomatic viremia, particularly among potential blood donors, has played a role in the transmission of both AIDS and hepatitis B.

Pathogenesis

Virtually all the immunologic abnormalities associated with AIDS can be explained by the loss of the helper functions carried out by T4 helper lymphocytes. The HIV virus has a high affinity for cells that carry a specific surface molecule (CHD) receptor. This receptor is most prevalent on helper lymphocytes. As a result, the HIV selectively replicates in and destroys T lymphocytes, leaving the host unable to cope with a variety of infectious and neoplastic diseases. Despite the immunosuppression caused by HIV, the infected host is able to mount an immune response to the virus after infection. These antibodies form the basis for most of the diagnostic tests for AIDS but offer little protection to the host against the development of the disease.

Signs and Symptoms

The initial clinical manifestation of HIV infection may include an infectious mononucleosis-like illness or more often an unexplained persistent generalized lymphadenopathy sometimes associated with fever and malaise. Lymph node biopsy typically demonstrates a nonspecific hyperplasia. When lymphadenopathy occurs in a patient with a social history compatible with AIDS, it is regarded as a prodromal phase of AIDS and

has been termed the AIDS-related complex. The most important direct clinical effect of HIV is on the central, peripheral, and autonomic nervous systems, with evidence of subacute encephalitis and dementia manifested in 90% of patients (Table 27-6). Other direct effects of HIV include cardiomyopathy, renal dysfunction often accompanied by proteinuria, adrenal insufficiency, and thrombocytopenia. Weight loss, fatigue, and anemia are common.

More common than the direct effects of HIV is the manifestation of AIDS as a syndrome caused by opportunistic infections (Table 27-7). For example, the initial manifestation of AIDS in about 50% of patients is *Pneumocystis carinii* pneumonia. Typically, interstitial pneumonitis is evident on the chest radiograph, and arterial blood gas measurements show hypoxemia and hypercarbia. Other common opportunistic infections include evidence of HSV activation, recurrent mucosal candidiasis, and disseminated CMV infection. Diarrhea reflects the effect of gastrointestinal pathogens, including *Shigella*. Tuberculosis, syphilis, and lymphoma are not infrequent in the patient with AIDS. Approximately 30% of patients with AIDS present with Kaposi sarcoma.

Laboratory Diagnosis

Typically, the presence of antibody to HIV can be detected by enzyme-linked immunoabsorbent assay (ELISA) approximately 1 to 3 months after infection with the virus. More than 90% of patients with AIDS have antibodies and more than 95% of asymptomatic carriers of the HIV are antibody positive. For all practical purposes, anyone who is HIV antibody positive should be assumed to harbor transmissible virus in the blood and secretions. A blood sample that is positive by ELISA is rechecked with a more specific confirmatory test, usually the

Table 27-7. Infectious Complications of Acquired
Immunodeficiency Syndrome

Infecting Organism	Type of Infection
Bacteria	
Streptococcus	Pneumonia, disseminated infection
Haemophilus influenzae type B	Pneumonia, disseminated infection
Salmonella	Gastroenteritis, disseminated infection
Virus	
Herpes simplex	Recurrent localized infection
Varicella-zoster	Localized disseminated infection
Cytomegalovirus	Pneumonia, retinitis, encephalitis, disseminated infection
Epstein-Barr	Lymphoproliferative disorders
Fungus	
Candida albicans	Mucocutaneous infection, esophagitis, disseminated infection
Aspergillus	Necrotizing bronchopneumonia, disseminated infection
Cryptococcus	Meningitis, disseminated infection
Pneumocystis carinii	Pneumonia
Mycobacteria	Tuberculosis, disseminated infection

Western blot assay. Sensitivity of these two tests exceeds 99%.

Antibody testing for screening blood and organ donors is complicated by the observation that the typical pattern of seroconversion in 1 to 3 months after infection is not always the case. Indeed, seronegativity has been observed to persist for as long as 36 months, during which time the patient is potentially able to transmit the virus.[37] Similarly, an immunosuppressed patient, such as a transplant recipient, may have a greatly delayed antibody response to HIV. In addition, a patient harboring HIV may revert to an antibody-negative status.[38]

Treatment

The only certain barrier to the spread of AIDS is the development of a vaccine; the problem is that many strains, and therefore antigens, for HIV exist. Until an effective vaccine is developed, treatment of AIDS will be dependent on drug therapy. In this regard, zidovudine (azidothymidine, AZT) inhibits the replication of some retroviruses, including HIV, and may therefore be useful in decreasing the risk of development of opportunistic infections. This drug crosses the blood-brain barrier and improves neurologic function in symptomatic patients. The use of AZT is limited by dose-dependent anemia and granulocytopenia and the occasional emergence of resis-

tance to the drug after about 6 months of therapy. Prophylaxis against Pneumocystis carinii pneumonia is provided with trimethoprim-sulfamethoxazole or aerosolized pentamidine.

Management of Anesthesia

Management of anesthesia must assume that all patients are potentially infected with HIV or other blood-borne pathogens.[39,40] In this regard, appropriate barrier precautions should include gloves, masks, and protective eyewear, to prevent contact with blood and body fluids during invasive procedures, including placement of intravascular catheters and intubation of the trachea (Table 27-5). Barrier precautions are particularly important in emergency care settings in which the risk of blood exposure is increased and the infection status of the patient is unknown. Attempts to cap needles after use are not recommended, as accidental needle sticks are a potential risk of this procedure. Health care workers with breaks in normal skin integrity (cuts, dermatitis, acne) should be particularly careful to cover these sites when dealing with AIDS patients. Hands and other contaminated surfaces should be washed immediately if accidental contamination with blood or secretions from these patients occurs. There is no evidence that gowns, hoods, or strict patient isolation are of value; patients with AIDS may be transported to the operating room by the usual routes and personnel. The patient wears a mask only if it is believed that transmission of opportunistic infections will be reduced by this approach.

Lack of evidence for spread of HIV by the airborne route does not eliminate concern regarding anesthesia equipment, since airway secretions can be mixed with blood, which is a medium for transmission.[41] The use of disposable anesthetic circuits, soda lime canisters, and ventilator bellows seems prudent, although routine sterilization should kill HIV. Laryngoscopes and other nondisposable items that have touched mucosal membranes or contacted blood or secretions from an infected patient should remain separated from clean equipment and be thoroughly washed with a detergent and water and either gas or steam sterilized or subjected to appropriate disinfection.[40] Surgeons use disposable drapes and gowns that are discarded in the usual manner for contaminated material. Surgical specimens are labeled to indicate that the patient has AIDS. Instruments are sterilized in the usual manner, and the room is cleaned with a dilute (1:10) solution of sodium hypochlorite, which destroys HIV. Care should be taken to avoid spillage of undiluted sodium hypochlorite, which generates fumes when it contacts proteins, such as those present in dried blood.

Choice of anesthetic drugs, techniques, and monitors is influenced by accompanying systemic manifestations of AIDS and associated opportunistic infections. For example, oxygenation may be impaired by pneumonia due to Pneumocystis carinii. Nutrition may be inadequate and blood volume deficient. Anemia from chronic infection is predictable. Care should be taken in placing vascular catheters and tracheal tubes to avoid introduction of bacteria. An increased index of suspicion for the development of perioperative adrenal insufficiency may be reasonable based on the common involvement of the adrenal glands in patients with AIDS. Postoperatively, these patients are managed in the recovery room according to criteria reserved for management of patients with communicable diseases. Nurses assigned to the care of patients with AIDS should not take care of other patients at the same time.

Cardiopulmonary resuscitation raises obvious concerns that can best be circumvented by avoidance of mouth-to-mouth ventilation. Early use of protective airway devices and intubation of the trachea is indicated. As in the operating room and recovery room, masks, gloves, and glasses are recommended for health care workers.

Any health care worker who is stuck by a needle from a patient with AIDS should undergo serologic testing.[40] Even if the worker is initially seronegative, tests should be repeated every 6 weeks to determine whether transmission has occurred. Most infected persons will seroconvert in 1 to 3 months. At the same time as serologic testing, counseling about the risk of infection and prevention of transmission of HIV to others is undertaken. In addition, the health care worker should be reassured that transmission by a single needle stick is unlikely.[39]

NOSOCOMIAL INFECTION

Nosocomial infection is an infection that occurs during the course of a hospital stay. Common sites and causes include the urinary tract (*E. coli*), respiratory tract (*Klebsiella pneumoniae, Pseudomonas aeruginosa*), and surgical incision sites. Nosocomial pneumonia is an important cause of morbidity and mortality in hospitalized patients, accounting for about 15% of all hospital-acquired infections. In adults, acute bacterial meningitis is often nosocomial, due generally to gram-negative bacteria. Nosocomial infection is often resistant to treatment with antibiotics. Transmission of viruses is a common event in hospitals, and most of these infections involve the respiratory tract. Thorough handwashing between patients is an effective way to reduce the role of hospital personnel in transmitting bacterial and viral infections. Use of gloves, likewise, protects both patients and hospital personnel.

Anesthesia Equipment

The role of bacterial contamination of the anesthesia machine and equipment, and the subsequent development of pulmonary infection and of cross-infection between patients, is controversial.[19,42] It is assumed that equipment used to deliver anesthesia is a potential source of bacterial contamination to the patient. On the basis of this assumption, the use of disposable anesthetic delivery circuits containing built-in bacterial filters has been advocated. Nevertheless, their routine use has not been shown to alter the incidence of postoperative pneumonia or other types of infections, as compared with similar surgical patients receiving anesthesia through circuits without bacterial filters. Furthermore, anesthesia administered to the patient with known colonization of gram-negative bacteria does not produce contamination of the anesthesia machine with significant levels of bacteria.[43] These observations suggest that basic hygienic management of equipment used to deliver anesthetic gases will provide safety from the standpoint of cross-infections between patients and will prevent the development of a nosocomial infection from this source. Bacteria placed in vaporizers containing volatile anesthetics do not survive. The role of anesthesia equipment in transmitting viral illness has not been determined, but airborne transmission of intracellular viruses seems less likely than extracellular bacteria.[19] High humidity in the anesthesia circuit will speed inactivation of viruses. Furthermore, anesthetic concentrations of halogenated volatile anesthetics may inhibit viral replication.[44]

Gram-Negative Bacteremia

About one-half of all primary nosocomial bacteremias are associated with gram-negative bacteria. The most frequent presentation of gram-negative bacteremia is fever, chills, and leukocytosis, without hypotension. Chills and fever may not be apparent in an elderly, debilitated, or immunosuppressed patient.

Spinal Anesthesia and Bacteremia

Selection of spinal anesthesia in the presence of bacteremia is influenced by the concern that the needle might introduce infected blood into the subarachnoid space or epidural space, leading to the development of meningitis or an epidural abscess.[45] Nevertheless, performance of diagnostic lumbar puncture in patients with fever or bacteremia of unknown origin, or both, is not associated with evidence that dural puncture leads to meningitis in these patients. Available data support the conclusion that spinal anesthesia need not be avoided in patients at risk of transient, low-grade, intraoperative bacteremia (urologic and obstetric patients) after dural puncture.[45] Performance of spinal anesthesia or epidural anesthesia in patients with evidence of systemic infection is an acceptable consideration, provided that appropriate antibiotic therapy has begun, and the patient has shown a positive response to therapy, as evidenced by a decrease in body temperature.[45] In those rare cases in which central nervous system infection follows regional anesthesia, it is not appropriate to assume a cause-and-effect relationship between the anesthetic and infection. Indeed, most cases of meningitis and epidural abscess occur spontaneously.

SEPTIC SHOCK

An estimated 500,000 cases of septic shock occur annually in the United States, with a mortality of about 35%. One-half of these cases are caused by gram-negative bacteria and, of these, 50% are associated with a positive blood culture. Aggressive oncologic chemotherapy, immunosuppressive therapy for organ transplantation, and the use of surgical prostheses have contributed to an increased incidence of bloodstream invasion by bacteria. Among patients with positive blood cultures, 25% die of complications directly attributable to the bacteremia and 10% due to the underlying disease. Septic shock can be divided into early (hyperdynamic) and late (hypovolemic) phases[46] (Fig. 27-1).

Early Phase

The early phase of septic shock is characterized by hypotension associated with decreased systemic vascular resistance and increased cardiac output. Fever and hyperventilation are frequently present. Vasodilation is presumed to be due to an endotoxin derived from cell walls of bacteria. This endotoxin acts as an antigenic stimulus, causing the release of vasoactive substances, such as histamine and bradykinin. This phase can last up to 24 hours.

Late Phase

In the late phase of septic shock, cardiac output is decreased. Lactic acidosis develops, reflecting impaired tissue oxygenation, presumably due to decreased cardiac output as well as dilation of peripheral vessels that permits shunting of blood across tissues. There may be damage to vascular smooth muscle, causing substantial loss of intravascular fluid volume. Oliguria is characteristically present. Hematologic abnormalities invariably accompany severe septic shock. For example, there is typically a decrease in the platelet count and prolongation of the prothrombin time and partial thromboplastin time. An increase in the concentration of fibrin degradation

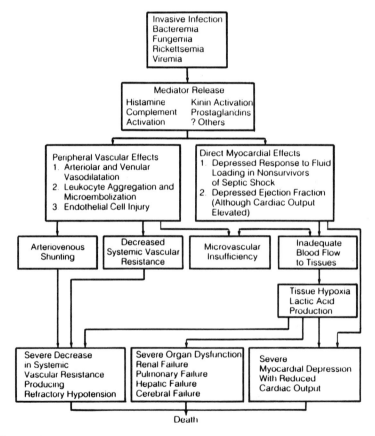

Fig. 27-1. Flow diagram of the pathogenesis of septic shock in humans. (From Parker MM, Parrillo JE. Septic shock. Hemodynamics and pathogenesis. JAMA 1983;250:3324–7, with permission.)

products mirrors the presence of disseminated intravascular coagulation.

Diagnosis

The diagnosis of septic shock is suggested by the development of hypotension (systolic blood pressure less than 90 mmHg) in the presence of peripheral vasodilation and oliguria. This diagnosis should be suspected particularly if these symptoms occur after operations or instrumentation of the genitourinary tract. Changes in the state of consciousness, including confusion and disorientation, can occur as manifestations of gram-negative bacteremia. Measurement of cardiac output and calculation of systemic vascular resistance is helpful in confirming the diagnosis in the early phase. A positive blood culture is diagnostic but is not always present.

Treatment

Treatment of septic shock consists of intravenous administration of antibiotics and repletion of intravascular fluid volume.[47] Antibiotics should be started immediately after blood is drawn for culture and sensitivity. Most often, two antibiotics are selected, with one effective against gram-positive and another against gram-negative bacteria. Clindamycin (25 mg·kg^{-1} IV) is often chosen for protection against gram-positive organisms, and gentamicin (5 mg·kg^{-1} IV) is a frequent choice for eradication of gram-negative bacteria. Antibiotics can be changed if necessary after the results of the blood culture are known. Aggressive intravenous fluid replacement is necessary to restore intravascular fluid volume. In pediatric patients, rapid fluid replacement in excess of 40 ml·kg^{-1} IV during the first hour of treatment is associated with improved survival.[48] Fluid replacement may be guided by measurement of right or left heart filling pressures and urine output. Dopamine is an effective inotropic drug when pharmacologic support of both blood pressure and renal function is necessary. Administration of high doses of methylprednisolone or other corticosteroids for the treatment of septic shock has not been shown to be beneficial and thus cannot be recommended as adjunctive therapy.[49] Immunologic therapy of septic shock is directed against three of the key mediators (endotoxin, tumor necrosis factor, interleukin-1) in the onset of sepsis. Specifically, monoclonal antibodies to endotoxin, monoclonal antibodies to tumor necrosis factor, and a receptor antagonist to interleukin are under investigation.[47,50] In this regard, survival is improved in patients with gram-negative sepsis who are treated with a human monoclonal antibody that binds to the lipid portion of the endotoxin.[52] The cost effectiveness of this therapy, however, remains undocumented, as does the ability to select patients who will most likely benefit from this therapy.[52] Furthermore, this form of therapy is not effective for sepsis owing to gram-positive bacteria.

Surgical intervention may be necessary to treat the source of bacteremia. No specific anesthetic drug has been shown to be ideal in the presence of septic shock. However, administration of ketamine to animals with hemorrhagic shock was associated with less damage to splanchnic organs and increased survival, as compared with animals anesthetized with volatile anesthetics.[53] Conversely, another animal study implies that ketamine-induced peripheral vasoconstriction jeopardizes tissue blood flow, as reflected by the development of metabolic acidosis.[54] Despite these conflicting studies, clinical experience suggests that ketamine is an acceptable drug for induction of anesthesia in the patient requiring an emergency operative procedure in the presence of hypotension due to bacteremia.

INFECTIVE ENDOCARDITIS

Infective endocarditis is a microbial infection that implants on a heart valve or on the wall of the endocardium. Streptococcal organisms account for nearly one-half of cases. Gram-negative bacteria and fungi are rare causes. Morbidity and mortality remain significant despite improvements in antibiotic therapy.

Predisposing Factors

Infective endocarditis cannot occur without preceding bacteremia. Operative procedures that are predictably associated with transient bacteremia include dental treatments resulting in bleeding of the gingiva and surgical procedures or instrumentation of the upper airway, gallbladder, lower gastrointestinal tract, and genitourinary tract. The parenteral injection of a drug, as in the intravenous drug user, or prolonged placement of an indwelling venous catheter, as used for hyperalimentation, can also lead to bacteremia. The patient with a prosthetic heart valve is at greatest risk of the development of infective endocarditis when transient bacteremia occurs. The incidence of infective endocarditis is also increased in the patient with an acquired or congenital heart defect that produces turbulent blood flow. For example, mitral regurgitation, aortic regurgitation, a bicuspid aortic valve, and ventricular septal defect, as is present with tetralogy of Fallot, produce turbulent blood flow and are associated with an increased incidence of infective endocarditis. Patients with aortic or pulmonic stenosis have a lower probability of infection; infective endocarditis rarely develops in patients with mitral stenosis or atrial septal defect.

Antibiotic Prophylaxis

Prophylactic use of antibiotics is recommended in susceptible patients when surgical procedures associated with bacteremia are planned (Table 27-8). Even in the absence of known

Table 27-8. Procedures in Susceptible Patients for Which Antibiotic Prophylaxis Is Recommended

Dental operations associated with gingival bleeding

Operations or procedures performed on the respiratory tract associated with disruption of the respiratory mucosa
  Tonsillectomy and adenoidectomy
  Nasotracheal intubation
  Bronchoscopy

Instrumentation of the gastrointestinal tract or genitourinary tract

Cardiac surgery

Noncardiac surgery in the patient with a prosthetic vascular graft or heart valve

Operations on infected tissues

heart disease, the presence of a diastolic heart murmur must be assumed to represent organic heart disease requiring prophylactic antibiotic therapy during the perioperative period. The patient who is receiving chronic antibiotic therapy because of prior rheumatic fever should also receive additional antibiotics, since doses of antibiotics used for rheumatic fever prophylaxis are probably not adequate to protect against the development of infective endocarditis.

Bactericidal antibiotics are typically chosen to provide prophylaxis against infective endocarditis. Prophylactic antibiotic therapy must be initiated before surgery, as the drug needs to be present in tissues, as well as blood, to provide protection. Furthermore, antibiotic therapy must be continued for 48 to 72 hours after surgery. Specific antibiotic regimens selected should consider the type of bacteria likely to enter the systemic circulation during the operative procedure (Table 27-9).

Alpha-Hemolytic Streptococci

Alpha-hemolytic streptococci are most likely to enter the circulation during dental procedures or surgical manipulation of the upper respiratory tract. Penicillin is highly effective against these organisms (Table 27-9). Vancomycin or erythromycin is selected for the patient with a history of allergy to penicillin. Combined use of penicillin and streptomycin is recommended for the patient with a prosthetic heart valve, as these patients are at greatest risk.

Enterococci

Bacteremia due to enterococci is most likely to follow instrumentation or surgery on the gallbladder, lower gastrointestinal tract, or genitourinary tract. Gram-negative bacteremia may also occur after procedures in these areas, but such organisms rarely produce infective endocarditis. Therefore, prophylaxis is with antibiotics effective against enterococci (Table 27-9).

Staphylococci

Staphylococci are the organisms most likely to invade the circulation during surgery requiring cardiopulmonary bypass. Antibiotics effective against staphylococci include penicillinase-resistant penicillins and cephalosporins (Table 27-9).

Signs and Symptoms

Diagnosis of infective endocarditis must be considered in the patient with a heart murmur, anemia, and fever, particularly if there is a history of co-existing cardiac disease or of a recent surgical procedure, or both. Evidence of systemic embolization, including cerebrovascular occlusion and hematu-

Table 27-9. Infective Endocarditis Prophylaxis

Procedure	Organism	Antibiotic Selection[a]		
		Routine	Allergic to Penicillin	Prosthetic Heart Valve
Dental treatment	Alpha-hemolytic streptococcus	Pencillin	Vancomycin or erythromycin	Penicillin plus streptomycin
Tonsillectomy				
Adenoidectomy				
Nasotracheal intubation				
Bronchoscopy				
Hepatobiliary tract	*Enterococcus*	Penicillin or ampicillin plus gentamicin or streptomycin	Vancomycin	As for routine
Cardiac surgery	*Staphylococcus*	Penicillinase-resistant penicillins or cephalosporins	As for routine	As for routine

[a] Administered intravenously or intramuscularly 30–60 min before the start of surgery.

ria, may reflect dissemination of emboli from vegetations present on a cardiac valve. Congestive heart failure is the most frequent cardiac complication. Acute aortic or mitral regurgitation can reflect destruction or perforation of cardiac valve leaflets. Mitral regurgitation can also be due to rupture of the chordae tendineae. Cardiac conduction abnormalities may indicate extension of valvular infection into the ventricular septum. Cardiac rhythm disturbances, such as ventricular premature beats, may reflect myocarditis.

Operative intervention for valve replacement must be performed in the patient with infective endocarditis in whom intractable congestive heart failure develops. Ideally surgery is delayed until high doses of appropriate antibiotics can be administered, to reduce the likelihood of infection of the new valve.

INFECTIONS OF THE CENTRAL NERVOUS SYSTEM

Infections of the central nervous system are life-threatening emergencies that require prompt and accurate diagnosis and treatment. Computed tomography and magnetic resonance imaging are useful in evaluating the possible presence of space occupying lesions that result from central nervous system infections. Examination of the cerebrospinal fluid (CSF) is important in the differential diagnosis of central nervous system infections. Imaging studies, however, may be needed to exclude an intracranial lesion before a diagnostic lumbar puncture is performed. New chemotherapeutic drugs, especially third-generation cephalosporins, have improved the treatment of central nervous system infections.

Meningitis

Meningitis is manifested as fever, headache, vomiting, nuchal rigidity, and obtundation. Cranial nerve dysfunction involving primarily the third, fourth, sixth, or seventh nerve appears in up to 20% of patients with bacterial meningitis. Seizures may occur and occasionally cerebral edema with associated increased intracranial pressure (ICP) may be present. Coagulopathies ranging from thrombocytopenia to disseminated intravascular coagulation may accompany bacteremia and hypotension in the presence of meningitis.

Characteristic CSF findings in the presence of bacterial meningitis include an increased number of neutrophils, glucose concentration less than 50% of the blood glucose concentration, and increased protein concentration. The definitive diagnosis requires isolation of the causative organisms from the CSF. Meningococcal meningitis is the only form of bacterial meningitis that occurs in an epidemic form. Recurrent episodes of bacterial meningitis are most often the result of ana-tomic defects (traumatic or surgical) that permit access of bacteria into the CSF.

The presence of meningitis enhances the entry of antibiotics into the CSF when these drugs are administered intravenously in high doses. Adjunctive intrathecal therapy with an aminoglycoside antibiotic is useful when meningitis is caused by gram-negative bacteria. When cerebral edema occurs, the conventional methods (diuretics, corticosteroids) to decrease ICP are indicated. Fluid restriction is indicated initially, to minimize the occurrence of cerebral edema. Acute control of seizure activity is often with diazepam, whereas maintenance therapy may be with phenytoin.

Brain Abscess

Brain abscess can result from the direct extension of contiguous infection (paranasal sinuses), retrograde venous spread of infection (chronic otitis), or hematogenous spread (lung abscess, right-to-left intracardiac shunt), typically in the distribution of the middle cerebral artery. Manifestations of brain abscess are most often those of an expanding intracranial mass with obtundation, headache, focal neurologic findings, and seizures. Evidence of increased ICP is somnolence, vomiting, and cranial nerve palsies. Lumbar puncture is not recommended when brain abscess is thought to be present because of the risk of brain herniation. Computed tomography is a highly sensitive method for detecting any abscess greater than 1 cm in diameter and for subsequent confirmation of resolution of the abscess. Magnetic resonance imaging has greater sensitivity than computed tomography for soft tissue lesions and does not require the administration of contrast agents.

Prompt antibiotic therapy, and often surgical aspiration or excision, is necessary in the management of a brain abscess. Emergency surgical decompression is indicated whenever increased ICP leads to evidence of brain herniation. Cerebral edema is managed with diuretics and corticosteroids during the perioperative period. Seizures are a common sequela of a brain abscess.

Epidural Abscess

A lumbar epidural abscess manifests as backache, skeletal muscle weakness, and paralysis. Percussion tenderness and paraspinal muscle spasm over the area and meningismus may be present. Fever is usually an accompanying feature. Infection is most often derived from bloodstream transmission, vertebral osteomyelitis, or contiguous infection. A history of back trauma is present in about 30% of afflicted patients. Introduction of a spinal needle into the lumbar area in the presence of a lumbar epidural abscess can lead to bacterial meningitis. Computed tomography is useful in delineating the site of an epidural abscess. Laminectomy should be performed promptly when an epidural abscess is diagnosed, as irreversible neurologic changes may occur within 24 hours.

BACTERIAL INFECTIONS OF THE UPPER RESPIRATORY TRACT

Bacterial infections of the upper respiratory tract frequently follow processes that impair normal host-defense mechanisms. For example, clearance of pulmonary secretions can be impaired due to the reduced activity of cilia or decreased cough reflexes. Viral respiratory tract infections are often the cause of impaired respiratory defense mechanisms. No infection of the upper respiratory tract is more rapidly progressive or potentially lethal than acute epiglottitis (see Chapter 32).

Acute Sinusitis

Acute sinusitis is characterized by nasal discharge, fever, leukocytosis, and facial pain, which typically increase when the patient leans forward. Viral, allergic, or vasomotor rhinitis is frequently an antecedent event for sinusitis. Nasopharyngeal instrumentation (nasotracheal tubes, nasogastric tubes, nasal packing) in the traumatized patient may predispose to sinusitis.[55] Indeed, sinusitis should be considered when fever occurs without a known focus in the patient with a nasotracheal tube in place.[56] Nasal polyps or deviation of the nasal septum may also predispose to sinusitis by obstructing sinus drainage. Maxillary and frontal sinusitis are more frequent in adults, whereas infection of the ethmoid sinus predominates in children. Maxillary sinusitis is characterized by pain and tenderness over the cheeks. This pain is often referred to the teeth. Frontal sinusitis produces pain and tenderness over the forehead. Patients with ethmoid sinusitis typically complain of pain behind the orbit.

Acute sinusitis responds well to decongestants and analgesics. Although most patients do not require antibiotics, the administration of ampicillin or amoxicillin is often recommended in the patient who fails to respond to decongestants. Sinusitis that leads to intracranial infection, either by bony spread or through the venous channels, requires treatment with high doses of antibiotics and surgical drainage. Administration of anesthesia that includes nitrous oxide to a patient with acute sinusitis introduces the consideration of increased pressure in the sinus, in the event that nitrous oxide enters any air-containing portion of the sinus more rapidly than nitrogen is absorbed. Clinical experience does not support the validity of this theoretical concern.

Acute Otitis Media

Otitis media results when bacteria spread from the nasopharynx to the normally sterile middle ear. Abnormal eustachian tube reflux or obstruction caused by viral or allergic nasopharyngitis may lead to infection. Pain, fever, and hearing loss are the classic presenting manifestations. Diagnosis is based on the presence of a bulging tympanic membrane and obscured bony landmarks. Treatment for acute otitis media includes decongestants, analgesics, and an antibiotic, most often amoxicillin. Although antibiotics are generally administered for 10 days, 5 days of treatment may be equally effective. Myringotomy does not hasten recovery but is indicated for the patient with intractable pain or a poor response to medical therapy. Tympanoplasty tubes may be helpful in children with repeated recurrences of otitis media. Acute mastoiditis was once a common sequela of acute otitis media but is now, with the routine use of antibiotics, an unusual complication. Chronic otitis media is characterized by hearing loss and perforation of the tympanic membrane. A peripheral perforation of the tympanic membrane may be associated with an invasive cholesteatoma.

The differential diagnosis of acute otitis media includes serous otitis media. Serous otitis media differs from the purulent form in that fever and pain are absent. In contrast to purulent otitis media, the tympanic membrane is usually retracted despite the presence of fluid in the middle ear, and the bony landmarks are usually preserved.

Administration of nitrous oxide in the presence of known inflammation or edema of the eustachian tube must consider the blood-gas solubility of this anesthetic relative to air. For example, the middle ear is an air-filled cavity that vents passively by way of the eustachian tube, when the pressure exceeds about 20 cm H_2O. Nitrous oxide diffuses into the middle ear more rapidly than nitrogen leaves, and middle ear pressure may become elevated if decompression through the eustachian tube is not possible. Rupture of the tympanic membrane following anesthesia that included nitrous oxide has been attributed to this mechanism.[57] Conversely, negative middle ear pressure may develop after discontinuation of nitrous oxide, leading to serous otitis.

Pharyngitis

Viruses are the most common cause of pharyngitis, and treatment is symptomatic. Group A streptococci may be responsible for as few as 5% of all cases of pharyngitis but for nearly 40% of cases of tonsillitis.[58] As it is impossible to distinguish clinically between streptococcal and viral pharyngitis, throat cultures are necessary. Antibiotics, most often oral penicillin V or erythromycin, are important for the eradication of infection and prevention of rheumatic fever and local suppurative complications. Because rheumatic fever can be prevented, even if therapy is delayed up to 9 days after the onset of symptoms, treatment need not be initiated until the results of the throat culture are available. Tonsillectomy was once commonly performed in children to prevent recurrent pharyngitis, but this practice has largely been abandoned.

Peritonsillar Abscess

Peritonsillar abscess (quinsy) is a complication of streptococcal tonsillitis. Dysphagia impairs swallowing of saliva, leading to drooling, while pain and edema result in a muffled voice. The affected tonsil is visibly displaced toward the midline, and the soft palate may be edematous. Trismus occurs in some patients. Traditional treatment consists of the parenteral administration of penicillin and surgical drainage. More recently, oral administration of an antibiotic and needle aspiration have produced acceptable results, avoiding the need for hospitalization and operation.[59]

Retropharyngeal Infection

Retropharyngeal infection is most common in childhood because the lymph nodes in this region atrophy during adulthood. Fever, dysphagia, respiratory stridor, and bulging of the posterior wall of the pharynx are present. A lateral radiograph of the neck may demonstrate soft tissue swelling and forward displacement of the larynx. Penicillin is the antibiotic of choice, and surgical drainage is necessary to prevent upper airway obstruction and extension of infection to the mediastinum.

A parapharyngeal infection is characterized by severe trismus, externally visible inflammation behind the angle of the jaw, and medial displacement of the tonsil. Treatment consists of the intravenous administration of penicillin and drainage from behind the angle of the mandible.

Ludwig's Angina

Ludwig's angina is a cellulitis of the submandibular, sublingual, and submental regions. It is most frequently caused by streptococci and is characterized by fever and a rapidly progressive edema of the anterior neck and of the floor of the mouth. Elevation of the tongue impedes swallowing and upper airway obstruction is a potentially fatal complication. Intubation of the trachea may not be possible, necessitating a tracheostomy to preserve the airway. Broad-spectrum antibiotics are indicated, and surgical decompression may be required.

Acute Epiglottitis

For a discussion of acute epiglottitis, see Chapter 32.

PULMONARY PARENCHYMAL INFECTION

Pulmonary parenchymal infections typically develop after an event that impairs normal host-defense mechanisms, such as a viral infection that alters the physical and chemical characteristics of the normally protective mucous secretions in the airway. Indeed, the seasonal increase in viral infections during winter months is typically associated with an increased incidence of bacterial pneumonia. The patient with chronic obstructive pulmonary disease is vulnerable to bacterial infection in the lungs because of impaired mucociliary transport and inefficient cough mechanisms. Cigarette smoke may contribute to an increased incidence of pulmonary infection, by virtue of inhibition of ciliary activity by smoke.

Bacterial Pneumonia

Pneumococci remain the most frequent cause of bacterial pneumonia in adults. Streptococci are also a common cause of bacterial pneumonia. Inhalation of oropharyngeal secretions containing these bacteria, rather than droplet spread from person to person, is responsible for most pneumococcal pneumonias. Inhalation of oropharyngeal secretions often occurs during normal sleep. Nevertheless, bacterial pneumonia is uncommon in healthy patients because of efficient host-defense mechanisms. By contrast, alcoholism, drug abuse, and neurologic disorders are examples of conditions that can impair consciousness and predispose to the inhalation of bacteria-containing secretions and pneumonia. Bacterial pneumonia due to gram-negative bacteria occurs most often in chronically ill and debilitated patients who are confined to bed.

Diagnosis and Treatment

Bacterial pneumonia is characterized by an initial chill, followed by an abrupt increase in body temperature and copious sputum production. Segmental distribution of the infective process results in bronchopneumonia. Lobar pneumonia is present when infection includes more than one segment of a pulmonary lobe or when multiple lobes are involved. Nevertheless, classic physical and radiographic findings of lobar consolidation may be absent. Indeed, dehydration can minimize abnormalities seen on the chest radiograph, in the presence of bacterial pneumonia. Polymorphonuclear leukocytosis is typical, and arterial hypoxemia may occur in severe cases of bacterial pneumonia. Arterial hypoxemia reflects right-to-left shunting of blood due to perfusion of alveoli filled with inflammatory exudate. Microscopic examination of sputum, plus a culture and sensitivity, is necessary for the etiologic diagnosis of pneumonia and the selection of appropriate antibiotic treatment. In addition to antibiotic therapy, adequate hydration through administration of fluids or local humidification of the airways is important for optimizing clearance of secretions.

Bacterial Versus Viral Etiology

It is important to distinguish between bacterial and nonbacterial pneumonia. Nonbacterial pneumonia, such as *Mycoplasma pneumoniae* pneumonia, occurs most frequently in previously healthy and young patients. In contrast to bacterial pneumonia, the presence of a nonbacterial pulmonary infection is suggested by nonproductive cough and the absence of leukocytosis. An interstitial infiltrate on the chest radiograph also suggests a nonbacterial etiology.

Acute Bronchitis Versus Pneumonia

The distinction between acute bronchitis and bacterial pneumonia is anatomic, rather than etiologic, since the same organisms can cause both diseases. The patient with bacterial pneumonia is more likely to develop a high temperature, bacteremia, and arterial hypoxemia. Chest radiographs typically show infiltrates in the patient with pneumonia. Changes associated with chronic lung disease and bronchitis, however, can mimic pulmonary infiltrates.

Legionnaire's Disease

Legionnaire's disease is a form of pneumonia caused by a filamentous gram-negative bacillus designated *Legionella pneumophila*. The disease caused by this organism is characterized by a prodromal myalgia, malaise, and headache, followed within 24 hours by an acute increase in body temperature, as well as tachypnea, nonproductive cough, oliguria, and often obtundation. Clinical and radiographic features are not specific. Mild cases of this disease resemble *Mycoplasma pneumoniae* pneumonia. Erythromycin is the antibiotic of choice for treatment of this disease.

Bronchiectasis

For a discussion of bronchiectasis, see Chapter 13.

Lung Abscess

A lung abscess is most likely to develop after bacterial pneumonia. Alcoholism and poor dental hygiene are frequently present in the patient in whom lung abscess develops. Septic pulmonary embolization, which is most common in the intravenous drug user, may also result in the formation of a lung abscess. A chest radiograph is required to establish the presence of a lung abscess. The finding of an air-fluid level signifies rupture of the abscess into the bronchial tree. Foul-smelling sputum is also characteristic when the lung abscess drains into the bronchial tree. Antibiotics are the mainstay of treatment of a lung abscess. Surgery is indicated only when a complication such as an empyema occurs. Thoracentesis is necessary to establish the diagnosis of empyema, and treatment requires chest tube drainage and antibiotics. Surgical drainage is necessary for the treatment of chronic empyema.

INTRA-ABDOMINAL INFECTION

Peritonitis and subphrenic abscess are examples of intra-abdominal infections that can present during the perioperative period. Both processes can be confused with pneumonia.

Peritonitis

Peritonitis is a localized to diffuse inflammatory process involving the peritoneum. Diffuse inflammation of the peritoneum typically follows a breakdown in the integrity of the gastrointestinal tract, as can occur with appendicitis or diverticulitis, or after trauma. Most likely multiple organisms are contributing to the disease process when peritonitis is due to these events. Acute pancreatitis can also mimic bacterial peritonitis. Likewise, abdominal pain associated with an acute peptic ulcer, cholecystitis, mesenteric artery occlusion, acute porphyria, and diabetic acidosis may suggest peritonitis. Occasionally, bacterial peritonitis develops in patients with systemic lupus erythematosus.

Peritonitis has also been observed in patients with alcoholic cirrhosis of the liver. The most common causative organism in these patients is *E. coli*. For this reason, examination of ascitic fluid is indicated for any patient with cirrhosis in whom abdominal pain or unexplained fever develops. Gentamicin is the drug of choice when *E. coli* is the cause of peritonitis.

Subphrenic Abscess

Subphrenic abscess should be suspected in the patient who has undergone abdominal surgery and subsequently exhibits unexplained fever. The frequent presence of pleural effusion in association with a subphrenic abscess can be attributed incorrectly to bacterial pneumonia. A wide separation between the upper margin of the gastric air bubble and diaphragm, as demonstrated on the chest radiograph, suggests a subphrenic abscess. Leukocytosis is almost always present. Treatment of a subphrenic abscess is with surgical drainage plus antibiotics. The antibiotic can be changed, if indicated, when results of the culture of the abscess fluid are available.

URINARY TRACT INFECTION

Urinary tract infection is the most common of all bacterial infections affecting humans. During the first 50 years of life, this is a disease that predominates in females. Symptoms range from asymptomatic bacteriuria to acute pyelonephritis. Most patients complain of dysuria and frequency. Urinalysis indicates hematuria and the presence of protein. The most frequent etiologic organisms are gram-negative bacteria such as *E. coli*. Ampicillin is usually effective in the treatment of an otherwise uncomplicated urinary tract infection.

Acute bacterial prostatitis is a febrile illness associated with fever, chills, pelvic pain, dysuria, and urinary frequency. The most common causative organisms is *E. coli*. Chronic bacterial prostatitis may require surgical removal of the gland.

FEVER OF UNDETERMINED ORIGIN

Fever of undetermined origin is characterized by temperature increases exceeding 38.3°C on several occasions during at least a 3-week period. Most patients with fever of undetermined origin are subsequently shown to have an infection, neoplasm, or connective tissue disorder. The two major systemic infections to consider are tuberculosis and infective endocarditis. Localized infections to consider include hepatic abscess, subphrenic abscess, and urinary tract infection. Viral infections usually do not produce fevers lasting 3 weeks or longer, the one important exception being infection due to CMV. Ultrasonography and computed tomography are useful for detecting hidden sites of infection, greatly decreasing the number of biopsies required to make a diagnosis.

MUCOCUTANEOUS LYMPH NODE SYNDROME

Mucocutaneous lymph node syndrome (Kawasaki disease) is an acute febrile illness of childhood manifesting most often during the first year of life.[60] The etiology of this disease is not known, although viral and bacterial causes have been speculated. The incidence of this disease is increased in Asian-American children and affects males more often than females. Kawasaki disease generally presents with a prominent necrotizing vasculitis component with aneurysms of the coronary arteries and peripheral arteries. Indeed, coronary artery aneurysms develop in 15% to 25% of children with this disease and may lead to sudden death from cardiac dysrhythmias or myocardial infarction. Fever is associated with conjunctivitis, pharyngitis, erythematous tongue, truncal rash, and cervical lymphadenopathy. Management of anesthesia in these children should consider the possibility of intraoperative myocardial ischemia.[60] Peripheral nerve blocks to provide interruption of sympathetic nervous system activity to inflamed peripheral arteries may be a consideration when the viability of digits is threatened.[61]

INFECTION IN THE IMMUNOSUPPRESSED HOST

The principal cause of morbidity and mortality in an immunosuppressed patient is often infection, rather than the primary illness. In this regard, therapeutic programs that can adversely influence the ability of a patient to withstand infection include antibiotics, radiation therapy, corticosteroids, and cancer chemotherapeutic drugs (see Chapter 28). The major adverse effect of antibiotics is to create a selection process for colonization with organisms resistant to antibiotics. Radiation therapy and treatment with corticosteroids or cancer chemotherapeutic drugs may adversely affect host-immune mechanisms by impairing the function or numbers of neutrophils. The absolute level of circulating neutrophils required to prevent infection is unknown, although the risk of sepsis is increased when the level is less than 1000 cells·mm^{-3}. Neutropenia is the most important factor predisposing to bacterial infection in the presence of cancer, or after organ transplantation. Other conditions that predispose to infection in the immunosuppressed host include malnutrition, diabetes mellitus, uremia, splenectomy, and breaks in the mucocutaneous lining that separates the patient from microbes. In this regard, radiation therapy may damage mucocutaneous surfaces providing a portal of entry for microorganisms. An indirect effect of immunosuppressive therapy, especially in the patient receiving an organ transplant, is the activation of latent CMV or EBV infection.

A common presenting symptom of infection in an immunocompromised patient is fever without localized findings. In this regard, special care must be taken to maintain asepsis during percutaneous introduction of an intravascular catheter or performance of regional anesthesia.[62] The use of an indwelling Hickman-Broviac catheter for venous access, especially in a neutropenic patient may become a source of bacteremia. Most of these catheter infections can be successfully treated with antibiotics, leaving the catheter in place. Prevention of infection in an immunosuppressed patient is improved by avoidance of hospitalization for procedures that can be performed in an outpatient environment and by utilization of indwelling vascular and urinary catheters, only when absolutely necessary.

Pneumonia is the most common infectious cause of death in an immunosuppressed host. A potentially fatal bacteremia may be associated with a trivial-appearing pulmonary infiltrate on the chest radiograph. Fungal infection is a problem in the immunosuppressed host, as reflected by the common presence of candidiasis. Aspergillosis is an airborne fungal infection that rarely occurs in an immunocompetent patient, but in the immunosuppressed patient it is likely to result in bronchopneumonia and bronchitis. The initial manifestations of aspergillosis pneumonia include fever, dyspnea, nonproductive cough, and hemoptysis, with occasional life-threatening hemorrhage.

Rapid and extensive invasion of blood vessels provides access of *Aspergillus* to the circulation, providing a high incidence of spread, particularly to the brain and heart. Cryptococcosis (torulosis) is a systemic fungal disease that may cause pneumonia and meningitis. Treatment of disseminated fungal infection is with intravenous administration of amphotericin B.

Pneumocystis carinii

Pneumocystis carinii is a fungal organism that is a common opportunistic cause of interstitial pneumonia in immunosuppressed patients, especially those with AIDS. This organism may be present in the lungs of healthy persons, suggesting that immunosuppression reactivates latent infection, causing pneumonitis. *Pneumocystis carinii* pneumonia typically presents as sudden onset of fever, nonproductive cough, tachypnea, and progressive dyspnea. The degree of arterial hypoxemia and extent of infiltrate on the chest radiograph correlate best with the breathing rate. The classic radiographic presentation is a diffuse, bilateral symmetric interstitial and alveolar infiltrative pattern that is predominantly perihilar in distribution. Arterial blood gases are a sensitive measurement of pulmonary involvement. The definitive diagnosis entails the demonstration of *Pneumocystis* organisms in airway secretions or lung tissue specimens. A thoracotomy to obtain a lung biopsy may be necessary to establish the diagnosis. During anesthesia, such a patient may require a high inspired concentration of oxygen with or without positive end-expiratory pressure to maintain acceptable arterial oxygenation. Treatment of *Pneumocystis carinii* infection is with intramuscular or intravenous administration of pentamidine. The side effects associated with this drug include facial flushing, hypotension, tachycardia, hypoglycemia, azotemia, and bone marrow suppression. An alternative therapy is with low-toxicity trimethoprim-sulfamethoxazole.

REFERENCES

1. Browne RA, Chernesky MA. Infectious diseases and the anaesthetist. Can J Anaesth 1988;35:655–65
2. Recommendations for prevention of HIV transmission in health care settings. MMWR 1987;36:629–33
3. Sokoll MD, Gergis SD. Antibiotics and neuromuscular function. Anesthesiology 1981;55:148–59
4. Mayhew JF, Deutsch S. Cardiac arrest following administration of vancomycin. Can Anaesth Soc J 1985;32:65–6
5. Symons NLP, Hobbes AFT, Leaver HK. Anaphylactoid reactions to vancomycin during anaesthesia: Two clinical reports. Can Anaesth Soc J 1985;32:178–81.
6. Mufson MA. Pneumococcal infections. JAMA 1981;246:1942–8
7. Shapiro ED, Berg AT, Austrian R, et al. The protective efficacy of polyvalent pneumococcal polysaccharide vaccine. N Engl J Med 1991;325:1453–60
8. Bisno AL. Group A streptococcal infections and acute rheumatic fever. N Engl J Med 1991;325:783–93
9. MacDonald KL, Osterholm MT, Hedberg CW, et al. Toxic shock syndrome. A newly recognized complication of influenza and influenzalike illness. JAMA 1987;157:1053–8
10. Merson MH, Morris GK, Sack DA, et al. Traveler's diarrhea in Mexico. A prospective study of physicians and family members attending a Congress. N Engl J Med 1976;294:1299–1305
11. Laflin MJ, Tobey RE, Reves JG. Anesthetic considerations in patients with gas gangrene. Anesth Analg 1976;55:247–51
12. Tsueda K, Oliver OB, Richter RW. Cardiovascular manifestations of tetanus. Anesthesiology 1974;40:588–92
13. Baronia AK, Singh PK, Dhiman RK. Intractable pharyngeal spasm following tracheal extubation in a patient with undiagnosed tetanus. Anesthesiology 1991;75:1111–2
14. Southorn PA, Blaise GA. Treatment of tetanus-induced autonomic nervous system dysfunction with continuous epidural blockade. Crit Care Med 1986;14:251–2
15. Steere AC. Lyme disease. N Engl J Med 1989;321:586–96
16. Rich SA, Sbordone L, Mazze RI. Metabolism by rat hepatic microsomes of fluorinated ether anesthetics following isoniazid administration. Anesthesiology 1980;53:489–93
17. Craven PC, Gremillion DH. Risk factors of ventricular fibrillation during rapid amphotericin B infusion. Antimicrob Agents Chemother 1985;27:868–71
18. Foy HM, Kenny GE, McMahan R, et al. *Mycoplasma pneumoniae* pneumonia in an urban area: Five years of surveillance. JAMA 1970;214:1666–72
19. duMoulin GC, Hedley-Whyte J. Hospital-associated viral infection and the anesthesiologist. Anesthesiology 1983;59:51–65
20. Hayden FG, Albrecht JK, Kaiser DL, Givaltney JM. Prevention of natural colds by contact prophylaxis with intranasal alpha2-interferon. N Engl J Med 1986;71–5
21. Jacoby DB, Hirshman CA. General anesthesia in patients with viral respiratory infections: An unsound sleep. Anesthesiology 1991;74:969–72
22. Fennelly ME, Hall GM. Anaesthesia and upper respiratory tract infections—a non-existent hazard? Br J Anaesth 1990;64:535–6
23. Tait AR, Knight PR. Intraoperative respiratory complications in patients with upper respiratory tract infections. Can J Anaesth 1987;34:300–3
24. Kinouchi K, Tanigami H, Tashiro C, Nishimura M, Fukumitsu K, Takauchi Y. Duration of apnea in anesthetized infants and children required for desaturation of hemoglobin to 95%. The influence of upper respiratory infection. Anesthesiology 1992;77:1105–7
25. Cohen MM, Cameron CB. Should you cancel the operation when a child has an upper respiratory tract infection? Anesth Analg 1991;72:282–8
26. Dunkle LM, Arvin AM, Whitley RJ, et al. A controlled trial of acyclovir for chickenpox in normal children. N Engl J Med 1991;325:1539–44
27. Surman OS. A double blind placebo controlled study of oral acyclovir in postherpetic neuralgia. Psychosomatics 1990;31:287–91
28. Esmann V, Geil JP, Kroon S, et al. Prednosone does not prevent post-herpetic neuralgia. Lancet 1987;2:126–7
29. Drew WL, Miner RC. Transfusion-related cytomegalovirus infection following noncardiac surgery. JAMA 1982;247:2389–91

30. Balfour CL, Balfour HH. Cytomegalovirus is not an occupational risk for nurses in renal transplant and neonatal units. Results of prospective surveillance study. JAMA 1986;256:1909–14

31. Meyers EF, Krupin B. Anesthetic management of emergency tonsillectomy and adenoidectomy in infectious mononucleosis. Anesthesiology 1975;42:490–1

32. Hussey GD, Klein M. A randomized, controlled trial of vitamin A in children with severe measles. N Engl J Med 1990;323:160–4

33. Estimates of HIV prevalence and projected AIDS cases: Summary of a workshop, October 31–November 1, 1989. MMWR 1990;39:110–6

34. Resnick L, Veren K, Salahuddin SZ, Tondreau S, Markham PD. Stability and inactivation of HTLV-III/LAV under clinical and laboratory environments. JAMA 1986;255:1887–91

35. Chamberland ME, Conley LJ, Bush TJ, Ciesielski CA, Hammett TA, Jaffe HW. Health care workers with AIDS. National Surveillance Update. JAMA 1991;266:3459–62

36. Dodd RY. The risk of transfusion-transmitted infection. N Engl J Med 1992;327:419–20

37. Imagawa DT, Lee MH, Wolinsky SM, et al. Human immunodeficiency virus type 1 infection in homosexual men who remain seronegative for prolonged periods. N Engl J Med 1989;320:1458–64

38. Fazadegan H, Polis MA, Wolinsky SM, et al. Loss of human immunodeficiency virus type 1 (HIV-1) antibodies with evidence of viral infection in asymptomatic homosexual men: A report from the multicenter AIDS Cohort study. Ann Intern Med 1988;108:785–92

39. Recommendations for prevention of HIV transmission in health-care settings. JAMA 1987;258:1293–1305

40. Kunkel SE, Warner MA. Human T-cell lymphotropic virus type III (HTLV-III) infection: How it can affect you, your patients, and your anesthetic practice. Anesthesiology 1987;66:195–207

41. Schwartz D, Schwartz T, Cooper E, Pullerits J. Anaesthesia and the child with HIV infection. Can J Anaesth 1991;38:626–33

42. Feeley TW, Hamilton WK, Xavier B, et al. Sterile anesthetic breathing circuits do not prevent postoperative pulmonary infection. Anesthesiology 1981;54:369–72

43. DuMoulin GC, Saubermann AJ. The anesthesia machine and circle system are not likely to be sources of bacterial contamination. Anesthesiology 1977;47:353–8

44. Knight PR, Bedows E, Nahrwold ML, et al. Alterations in influenza virus pulmonary pathology induced by diethyl ether, halothane, enflurane, and pentobarbital anesthesia in mice. Anesthesiology 1983;58:209–15

45. Chestnut DH. Spinal anesthesia in the febrile patient. Anesthesiology 1992;76:667–9

46. Parker MM, Parrillo JE. Septic shock. Hemodynamics and pathogenesis. JAMA 1983;250:3324–7

47. Rackow EC, Astiz ME. Pathophysiology and treatment of septic shock. JAMA 1991;266:548–54

48. Carcillo JA, Davis AL, Zaritsky A. Role of early fluid resuscitation in pediatric septic shock. JAMA 1991;266:1242–5

49. Bone RC, Fisher CJ, Clemmer TP, et al. A controlled clinical trial of high-dose methylprednisolone in the treatment of severe sepsis and septic shock. N Engl J Med 1987;317:653–8

50. Bone RC. A critical evaluation of new agents for the treatment of sepsis. JAMA 1991;266:1686–91

51. Ziegler EJ, Fisher CJ, Sprung CL. Treatment of gram-negative bacteremia and septic shock with HA-1A human monoclonal antibody against endotoxin. A randomized, double-blind, placebo-controlled trial. N Engl J Med 1991;324:429–36

52. Wenzel RP. Anti-endotoxin monoclonal antibodies—a second look. N Engl J Med 1992;326:1151–2

53. Longnecker DE, Ross DC. Influence of anesthetic on microvascular responses to hemorrhage. Anesthesiology 1979;51:S142

54. Weiskopf RB, Townsley MI, Riordan KK, et al. Comparison of cardiopulmonary responses to graded hemorrhage during enflurane, halothane, isoflurane, and ketamine anesthesia. Anesth Analg 1981;60:481–91

55. Caplan ES, Hoyt NJ. Nosocomial sinusitis. JAMA 1982;247:639–42

56. Hansen M, Paulsen MR, Bendixen DK, Hartmann-Andersen F. Incidence of sinusitis in patients with nasotracheal intubation. Br J Anaesth 1988;61:231–2

57. Perreault L, Normandin N, Plamondon L, et al. Tympanic membrane rupture after anesthesia with nitrous oxide. Anesthesiology 1982;57:325–6

58. Houvinen P, Lahtonen R, Ziegler T, et al. Pharyngitis in adults: The presence and coexistence of viruses and bacterial organisms. Ann Intern Med 1989;110:612–15

59. Ophir D, Bawnik J, Poria Y, et al. Peritonsillar abscess: A prospective evaluation of outpatient management by needle aspiration. Arch Otolaryngol Head Neck Surg 1988;114:661–5

60. McNiece WL, Krishna G. Kawasaki disease—a disease with anesthetic implications. Anesthesiology 1983;58:269–71

61. Edwards WT, Burney RG. Use of repeated nerve blocks in management of an infant with Kawasaki's disease. Anesth Analg 1988;67:1008–10

62. Wiernik PH. The management of infection in the cancer patient. JAMA 1980;244:185–9

28
Cancer

Cancer is the second most frequent cause of death in the United States, exceeded as a cause of mortality only by heart disease. Cancer develops in one of three Americans, and one in five dies of cancer. The number of deaths is increasing as a reflection of a growing elderly population and a decrease in the number of deaths from heart disease. Genes are involved in carcinogenesis by virtue of inherited traits that predispose to cancer (altered metabolism of potentially carcinogenic components, decreased level of immune system function), or mutation of a normal cell gene into an oncogene. Stimulation of oncogene formation by carcinogens (tobacco, alcohol, sunlight) is estimated to be responsible for 80% of cancers in the United States. Tobacco use accounts for more cases of cancer than all other known carcinogens combined. The fundamental event that causes a cell to become malignant is an alteration in the structure of deoxyribonucleic acid (DNA). The responsible mutation occurs in a cell of the target tissue, with that cell becoming the ancestor of the entire tumor cell population. Clonal evolution to even more undifferentiated cells reflects a high mutation rate and contributes to the development of tumors that are resistant to drug, hormone, and antibody therapy. The mutation has no effect on germ cells and is not transmitted genetically.

Cancer cells must evade the host's immune surveillance system, which is designed to seek out and destroy tumor cells. Indeed, most mutant cells stimulate the immune system to form antibodies (see the section, Immunology of Cancer Cells). Some cancer cells may also become metastatic. It seems likely that many cancers reflect activation of genes that restrict growth or activation of genes that promote tumor cell growth. In support of a protective role of the immune system is the increased incidence of cancer in immunosuppressed patients, such as those undergoing organ transplantation.

DIAGNOSIS

Cancer often becomes clinically evident when the tumor bulk compromises the function of vital organs. Initial diagnosis of cancer is by aspiration cytology or biopsy (needle, inci-

sional, excisional). Monoclonal antibodies that recognize antigens for specific cancers (prostate, lung, breast, ovary) may aid in the diagnosis (see the section, Immunology of Cancer Cells). The most commonly used staging system for solid tumors is the TNM system based on tumor size (T), lymph node involvement (N), and distant metastasis (M). This system further groups patients into stages ranging from the best prognosis (stage 1) to poorest prognosis (stage 3 or 4). Tumor invasiveness is related to the release of various tumor mediators that modify the surrounding microenvironment in such a way as to permit neoplastic cells to advance along the lines of least resistance. The lymphatics lack a basement membrane such that regional spread of cancer is influenced by the anatomy of the regional lymphatics. For example, regional lymph node involvement occurs late in squamous cell carcinoma of the vocal cords because this site has few lymphatics, whereas regional lymph node involvement is an early manifestation of supraglottic carcinoma because this region is rich in lymphatics. Imaging techniques including computed tomography and magnetic resonance imaging are used for further delineation of tumor presence and spread.

TREATMENT

Treatment of cancer includes chemotherapy, radiation, and surgery. Surgery is often necessary for the initial diagnosis (biopsy) and subsequent definitive treatment to remove the entire tumor or distant metastases or to reduce tumor mass. Palliative and rehabilitative therapy may require surgery. Adequate relief of cancer pain is mandatory; fear of producing opioid dependence is not a consideration in these cases. Chronic relief of cancer pain may be provided with regional anesthetic techniques or continuous infusion devices that deliver neuraxial opioids. Management of anesthesia for the patient with cancer requires an appreciation of pathophysiologic disturbances that may accompany cancer. Furthermore, the potential adverse effects of chemotherapy may influence management of anesthesia, as well as the patient's physiologic response to the stress of the operative period.

IMMUNOLOGY OF CANCER CELLS

Tumor cells are antigenically different from normal cells and may therefore elicit immune reactions similar to those that cause rejection of histoincompatible allografts. Antigens present in cancer cells but not in normal cells are designated tumor-specific antigens. Conversely, tumor-associated antigens (alpha-fetoprotein, prostate specific antigen, carcinoembryonic antigen) are present in cancer cells and normal cells, but the concentration is greater in tumor cells. Because tumor-associated antigens may be present in normal tissues, the measurement of these antigens may be less useful for the diagnosis of cancer than for monitoring patients with a known malignant disorder.

Antibodies to tumor-associated antigens can be used for the immunodiagnosis of cancer. In this regard, the use of monoclonal antibodies to detect proteins encoded by oncogenes or other types of tumor-associated antigens is a commonly used method of identifying cancer. Monoclonal antibodies to various tumor-associated antigens can be labeled with radioisotopes and injected to monitor the spread of cancer or be used as carriers of immunotoxins or drugs. The enormous antigenic diversity of many forms of cancer makes the development of an effective vaccine a formidable task. Alternatively, attempts may be made to enhance a patient's overall level of immunity with nonspecific immunopotentiators such as BCG (bacillus Calmette-Guérin) and interferons. Most spontaneously occurring tumors appear to be weakly antigenic, whereas other tumors can activate suppressor T cells to dampen the intensity of immune responses to tumor antigens.

PATHOPHYSIOLOGIC DISTURBANCES

Pathophysiologic disturbances that accompany cancer are characterized as paraneoplastic syndromes (Table 28-1). Certain of these disturbances (superior vena cava obstruction, increased intracranial pressure [ICP], pericardial tamponade, renal failure, hypercalcemia) may be manifested as acute life-threatening medical emergencies.

Fever and Weight Loss

Fever may accompany any type of cancer but is particularly likely with metastasis to the liver. Increased body temperature and perhaps lactic acidosis may accompany rapidly prolif-

Table 28-1.   Pathophysiologic Manifestations of Cancer

Fever
Anorexia
Weight loss
Anemia
Thrombocytopenia
Coagulopathies
Neuromuscular abnormalities
Ectopic hormone production
Hypercalcemia
Hyperuricemia
Tumor lysis syndrome
Adrenal insufficiency
Nephrotic syndrome
Ureteral obstruction
Pulmonary osteoarthropathy
Pericardial effusion
Pericardial tamponade
Superior vena cava obstruction
Spinal cord compression
Brain metastases

erating tumors, such as leukemias and lymphomas. Fever may reflect tumor necrosis, inflammation, the release of toxic products by cancer cells, and the production of endogenous pyrogens. Acidosis results from increased anaerobic glycolysis of the hypoxic proliferating tumor cells, especially when hepatic function is concomitantly impaired.

Anorexia and weight loss are frequent occurrences in the patient with cancer, especially carcinoma of the lung. In addition to the psychological effect of cancer on appetite, cancer cells compete with normal tissues for nutrients and may eventually cause nutritive death of normal cells. Hyperalimentation is indicated for nutritional support when malnutrition is severe, especially before elective surgery.

Hematologic Abnormalities

Anemia most likely reflects the direct effects of cancer, such as gastrointestinal ulceration with bleeding or tumor replacement of bone marrow. Cancer chemotherapy is another common cause of bone marrow depression and anemia. Acute hemolytic anemia may accompany lymphoproliferative diseases. Solid tumors, especially metastatic breast cancer, can lead to pancytopenia. In contrast to anemia, an increased amount of erythropoietin, as produced by a hypernephroma or hepatoma, can result in polycythemia. Thrombocytopenia may be due to chemotherapy or the presence of an unrecognized cancer. Disseminated intravascular coagulation may occur in patients with advanced cancer, especially in the presence of hepatic metastases. Recurrent venous thrombosis due to an unknown mechanism is associated with pancreatic cancer.

Neuromuscular Abnormalities

Neuromuscular abnormalities occur in 5% to 10% of patients with cancer. The most common manifestations are skeletal muscle weakness (myasthenic syndrome) associated with carcinoma of the lung.[1] Prolonged responses to depolarizing and nondepolarizing muscle relaxants have been observed in patients with co-existing skeletal muscle weakness, particularly when weakness is associated with an undifferentiated small cell carcinoma of the lung.

Ectopic Hormone Production

Active hormones are produced by a number of tumors, resulting in predictable physiologic effects (Table 28-2).

Hypercalcemia

Cancer is the most common cause of hypercalcemia in hospitalized patients, reflecting local osteolytic activity from bone metastases (especially carcinoma of the breast) or the ectopic hormonal activity associated with tumors that arise from the kidney, lung, pancreas, or ovary. The rapid onset of hypercalcemia that may occur in the patient with cancer may be manifested as lethargy and coma. Polyuria and dehydration may accompany hypercalcemia, which is further exaggerated by bone pain and resulting immobility. Opioids administered to relieve pain can result in further immobility, as well as vomiting or dehydration.

Tumor Lysis Syndrome

Tumor lysis syndrome is caused by the sudden therapeutic destruction of tumor cells, leading to the release of precursors of uric acid, potassium, and phosphate. This syndrome occurs most often after treatment of hematologic neoplasms, such as acute lymphoblastic leukemia. Acute renal failure can accompany hyperuricemia. Likewise, hyperkalemia and resulting cardiac dysrhythmias are more likely in the presence of renal dysfunction. Conversely, hyperphosphatemia can lead to secondary hypocalcemia, which increases the risk of cardiac dysrhythmias from hypokalemia and can cause neuromuscular symptoms such as tetany.

Adrenal Insufficiency

Adrenal insufficiency caused by complete replacement of the adrenal glands by metastatic tumor is rare. More often there is a relative adrenal insufficiency, owing to partial replacement of the adrenal cortex by tumor, or suppression of adrenal cortex function by prolonged treatment with corticosteroids. Adrenal insufficiency is most often seen in the patient with metastatic disease due to melanoma, retroperitoneal tumors, carcinoma of the lung, and carcinoma of the breast.

Table 28-2. Ectopic Hormone Production

Hormone	Associated Cancer	Manifestations
Adrenocorticotropic hormone	Lung (small cell) Thyroid (medullary) Thymoma Carcinoid Non-beta islet cell of pancreas	Cushing syndrome
Antidiuretic hormone	Lung (small cell) Pancreas Lymphomas	Water intoxication
Gonadotropin	Lung (large cell) Ovary Adrenal	Gynecomastia Precocious puberty
Melanocyte stimulating hormone	Lung (small cell)	Hyperpigmentation
Parathyroid hormone	Renal Lung (squamous) Pancreas Ovary	Hyperparathyroidism
Thyroid stimulating hormone	Choriocarcinoma Testicular (embryonal)	Hyperthyroidism
Thyrocalcitonin	Thyroid (medullary)	Hypocalcemia
Insulin	Retroperitoneal tumors	Hypoglycemia

The stress of the perioperative period may unmask adrenal insufficiency. Clinical manifestations include fatigue, dehydration, oliguria, and cardiovascular collapse. Treatment of acute adrenal insufficiency consists of rapid intravenous administration of cortisol, followed by a continuous infusion of cortisol, until oral replacement can be initiated.

Renal Dysfunction

Renal complications of cancer may reflect invasion of the kidney by the tumor, damage from tumor products or chemotherapy. The deposition of tumor antigen-antibody complexes on the glomerular membrane may result in changes considered characteristic of the nephrotic syndrome. Extensive retroperitoneal cancer can lead to bilateral ureteral obstruction and fatal uremia, especially in the patient with carcinoma of the cervix, bladder, or prostate. Percutaneous nephrostomy is indicated if a ureter is totally obstructed. Chemotherapy can destroy large numbers of cells; acute hyperuricemic nephropathy from precipitation of uric acid crystals in the renal tubules is prevented by administration of allopurinol, in combination with hydration and urinary alkalinization. Methotrexate and cisplatin are the chemotherapeutic drugs most often associated with nephrotoxicity. Acute hemorrhagic cystitis is a rare complication of cyclophosphamide therapy.

Acute Respiratory Complications

The acute onset of dyspnea may reflect extension of the tumor or the effects of chemotherapy. Bleomycin-induced interstitial pneumonitis and fibrosis is the most commonly encountered pulmonary complication of chemotherapy. Elderly patients, those with co-existing lung disease, prior use of radiotherapy, or receiving high doses of the drug are at greatest risk of pulmonary toxicity. Pulmonary toxicity rarely occurs when the total dose of bleomycin is less than 150 units·m^{-2}.[2] The most common symptoms of interstitial pneumonitis are the insidious onset of a nonproductive cough, dyspnea, tachypnea, and occasionally fever occurring 4 to 10 weeks after initiation of bleomycin therapy. These symptoms appear in 3% to 6% of patients treated with bleomycin. Incipient toxicity can be detected by measuring the diffusion capacity of the lung for carbon monoxide. The alveolar-to-arterial difference for oxygen is often increased in the affected patient. The appearance of radiographic changes, such as bilateral diffuse pulmonary infiltrates, probably portends irreversible pulmonary fibrosis. In the absence of a biopsy, the clinical and radiographic features of bleomycin-induced pneumonitis may be difficult to distinguish from pneumonia caused by *Pneumocystis carinii*. Corticosteroids are the only treatment for the acute effects of drug-induced pneumonitis, but the interstitial and alveolar fibrosis are irreversible.

Acute Cardiac Complications

Pericardial effusion caused by metastatic invasion of the pericardium can lead to the sudden onset of cardiac tamponade. Carcinoma of the lung seems to be the most common cause of pericardial tamponade. Malignant pericardial effusion is the most common cause of electrical alternans on the electrocardiogram (ECG). Paroxysmal atrial fibrillation or flutter may be an early manifestation of malignant involvement of the pericardium or myocardium. Optimal treatment of malignant pericardial effusion consists of prompt removal of the fluid, followed by surgical creation of a pericardial window (see Chapter 9).

Cardiac toxicity manifested as a life-threatening cardiomyopathy occurs in 1% to 5% of patients treated with doxorubicin or daunorubicin. Cardiotoxicity may be manifested initially as symptoms suggestive of an upper respiratory tract infection (nonproductive cough), followed by rapidly progressive congestive heart failure (CHF), often refractory to cardiac inotropic drugs or mechanical cardiac assistance. Cardiomegaly or pleural effusion, or both, may be evident on the chest radiograph. The QRS voltage on the ECG may be decreased. The patient who has received radiation therapy, particularly to the mediastinum, or the patient who is on concurrent cyclophosphamide therapy seems to be more susceptible to the development of cardiomyopathy.[3] Impairment of left ventricular function for as long as 3 years after discontinuation of doxorubicin has been observed.[4] In contrast to life-threatening cardiomyopathy, about 10% of treated patients show nonspecific and usually benign changes on the ECG (nonspecific ST-T changes, low QRS voltage, atrial or ventricular premature beats) that do not necessarily reflect underlying cardiomyopathy.

Superior Vena Cava Obstruction

Obstruction of the superior vena cava is caused by spread of cancer into the mediastinum or direct invasion of the vessel wall by disease, most often carcinoma of the lung. Engorgement of veins above the waist occurs, particularly in the jugular veins and those in the extremities. Dyspnea and airway obstruction may be present. Edema of the arms and face is usually prominent. Hoarseness may reflect edema of the vocal cords. Increased ICP manifested as nausea, seizures, and decreased level of consciousness is most likely due to increased cerebral venous pressure. Treatment consists of prompt radiation or chemotherapy, as determined by the histopathology of the cancer, so as to decrease the size of the tumor and thus relieve venous and airway obstruction. In this regard, bronchoscopy and mediastinoscopy to obtain a tissue diagnosis can be hazardous, especially in the presence of co-existing airway obstruction and increased pressure in the mediastinal veins.

Spinal Cord Compression

Spinal cord compression results from the presence of a metastatic lesion in the epidural space, most often reflecting carcinoma of the breast, lung, prostate, or lymphoma. Symptoms include pain, skeletal muscle weakness, sensory loss, and autonomic nervous system dysfunction. Myelography may be necessary to visualize the limits of compression, but the associated lumbar puncture may exacerbate the symptoms and necessitate prompt surgical intervention. Computed tomography is an alternative to myelography. Radiation therapy is a useful treatment when neurologic deficits are partial. In this regard, corticosteroids are often administered to minimize any inflammatory reaction and edema that can result from radiation directed to a tumor in the epidural space. Once total paralysis has developed, the results of a surgical laminectomy or of radiation to decompress the spinal cord are equally poor.[5]

Increased Intracranial Pressure

Metastatic brain tumors, most often from the lung and breast, present initially as mental deterioration, focal neurologic defects, and seizures. Computed tomography is the most useful diagnostic test. Treatment of an acute increase in ICP caused by the metastatic lesion includes corticosteroids, diuretics, and mannitol (see Chapter 17). Radiation is the usual palliative treatment, whereas surgery may be considered for the patient with a single metastatic lesion. Intrathecal administration of chemotherapeutic drugs is necessary when the meninges are involved.

MANAGEMENT OF ANESTHESIA

Preoperative evaluation of the patient with cancer requires consideration of the possible known side effects of the disease and an understanding of the adverse effects that may be evoked by cancer chemotherapeutic drugs[3,6,7] (Tables 28-1 and 28-3). Nausea and vomiting are the most common and distressing side effects of chemotherapy and, to some extent, of radiation treatment. Metoclopramide and droperidol may be useful drugs for the control of nausea in these patients during the preoperative period. Tricyclic antidepressants may be useful for potentiating the analgesic effects of opioids, as well as producing some inherent analgesia. Opioids used in the management of cancer-induced pain may be responsible for preoperative sedation.

Clinical tests to detect preoperatively any side effects related to treatment with chemotherapeutic drugs may be useful (Table 28-4). The possible presence of pulmonary and cardiac toxicity is a consideration in the patient being treated with chemotherapeutic drugs known to be associated with this complication. In this regard, the preoperative history of drug-induced pulmonary fibrosis (dyspnea, nonproductive cough) or CHF may influence the subsequence conduct of anesthesia. For example, in the patient treated with bleomycin, it may be helpful to monitor arterial blood gases, as well as SaO_2, and to titrate intravascular fluid replacement, keeping in mind that this patient may be vulnerable to interstitial pulmonary edema, presumably due to impaired lymphatic drainage owing to drug-induced pulmonary fibrosis.[8] The suggestion that bleomycin increases the likelihood of oxygen toxicity in the presence of high inspired concentrations of oxygen is not supported by animal and patient data.[8,9] Nevertheless, it may be prudent to consider administration of colloid solutions to these patients and adjustment of the delivered oxygen concentration to a value that will provide the desired PaO_2 and SaO_2. Support of ventilation of the lungs during the postoperative period is likely to be required, particularly after invasive or prolonged operations, or both, in the patient with preoperative drug-induced pulmonary fibrosis. Likewise, the depressant effects of anesthetic drugs on myocardial contractility may be enhanced in the patient with drug-induced cardiac toxicity. This patient is also more likely to experience postoperative cardiac complications.[4] Signs of central nervous system depression, autonomic nervous system dysfunction, and peripheral neuropathies should be sought in the preoperative evaluation. The presence of renal or hepatic dysfunction may influence the choice of anesthetic drug and muscle relaxant. Although not a consistent observation, the possibility of a prolonged response to succinylcholine is a consideration in the patient being treated with an alkylating chemotherapeutic drug.[4] Preoperatively, correction of nutrient deficiencies, anemia, coagulopathy, and electrolyte abnormalities may be required. Attention to aseptic technique is important, since immunosuppression occurs with most chemotherapeutic drugs. Immunosuppression produced by anesthesia, surgical stimulation, or even transfusion of blood during the perioperative period may exert an as yet undefined effect on the patient's subsequent response to cancer (see the section, Carcinoma of the Colon; see also Chapter 29).

COMMON CANCERS ENCOUNTERED IN CLINICAL PRACTICE

The most frequently encountered cancers in the adult are carcinoma of the lung, breast, colon, and prostate. Lung cancer is the most common malignant tumor in the male, followed by carcinoma of the prostate and colon, whereas in the female the incidence of lung cancer is exceeded only by breast and colon cancer.

Carcinoma of the Lung

Carcinoma of the lung develops in 10% of persons with a history of 40 pack-years of smoking, but it does not develop in 90% of smokers, emphasizing the importance of environmental and genetic factors. The cigarette smoker in whom emphysema develops is at increased risk of lung cancer. Surgical resection is the most effective treatment of lung cancer. Resectability refers to the extent of the disease, whereas operability refers to the medical status of the patient. Five-year survival statistics approach 70% for surgical resection in an asymptomatic patient with early-stage lung cancer detected by a routine chest radiograph.[10] Survival statistics at 5 years are essentially unaffected by traditional adjuvant treatments, including radiation, chemotherapy, and immunotherapy. In advanced disease, radiation therapy is effective in palliation of symptoms (dyspnea, hemoptysis, superior vena cava syndrome) in most patients.

Table 28-3.   Adverse Side Effects Produced

	Immunosuppression	Thrombocytopenia	Leukopenia	Anemia	Cardiac Toxicity	Pulmonary Toxicity
Alkylating agents						
Busulfan (Myleran)	+	+ + +	+ + +	+ + +		+ +
Chlorambucil (Leukeran)	+	+ +	+ +	+ +		+
Cyclophosphamide (Cytoxan)	+ + + +	+	+ +	+		+
Melphalan (Alkeran)	+	+ +	+ +	+ +		+
Thiotepa (Thiotepa)	+	+ + +	+ + +	+ + +		+
Antimetabolites						
Methotrexate (Methotrexate)	+ + +	+ + +	+ + +	+ + +		+
6-Mercaptopurine (Purinethol)	+ + +	+ +	+ +	+ +		
Thioguanine (Thioguanine)	+ + +	+	+ +	+ +		
5-Fluorouracil (Fluorouracil)	+ + + +	+ + +	+ + +	+ + +		
Plant alkaloids						
Vinblastine (Velban)	+ +	+	+ + +	+		
Vincristine (Oncovin)	+ +	+	+ +	+		
Antibiotics						
Doxorubicin (Adriamycin)		+	+ + +	+ +	+ + +	
Daunorubicin (Daunomycin)	+	+ +	+ + +	+ +	+ + +	
Bleomycin (Blenoxane)		+	+	+		+ + +
Mithramycin (Mithracin)	+	+ + + +	+ + + +	+ + +		
Nitrosoureas						
Carmustine (BiCNU)		+ +	+ +	+ +		+
Lomustine (CeeNU)		+ + +	+ + +	+ +		
Enzymes						
L-Asparaginase (Elspar)	+ +	+	+	+		

+, minimal; + +, mild; + + +, moderate; + + + +, marked.
(Adapted from Selvin BL. Cancer chemotherapy: Implications for the anesthesiologist. Anesth Analg 1981;60:425–34, with permission.)

by Cancer + Chemotherapeutic Drugs

Renal Toxicity	Hepatic Toxicity	CNS Toxicity	Peripheral Nervous System Toxicity	Autonomic Nervous System Toxicity	Stomatitis	Plasma Cholinesterase Inhibition	Other
+ +					+	+	Adrenocortical-like effect (+) Hemolytic anemia (+ +)
	+	+				+	Hemolytic anemia (+ +)
+	+				+	+ +	Hemolytic anemia (+ +) Hemorrhagic cystitis (+ + +)
						+	Inappropriate ADH secretion (+)
						+ +	Hemolytic anemia (+ +) Hemolytic anemia (+ +)
+ +	+				+ + +		
+ +	+ + +				+		
	+ + +				+		
		+			+ + +		
			+	+	+		Inappropriate ADH secretion (+)
+		+	+ +	+ +			
	+				+ +		Red urine (+)
					+ +		Red urine (+)
					+ + +		
+ +	+ +	+			+ + +		Coagulation defects (+ + +) Hypocalcemia (+) Hypokalemia (+)
+					+		
	+				+		
+	+ + +	+			+		Hemorrhagic pancreatitis (+) Coagulation defects (+)

Table 28-4.   Preoperative Tests
in the Patient With Cancer

Hematocrit
Platelet count
White blood cell count
Prothrombin time
Electrolytes
Renal function tests
Liver function tests
Blood glucose concentration
Arterial blood gases
Chest radiograph
Electrocardiogram

Carcinoma of the lung is categorized as squamous cell carcinoma, adenocarcinoma, large cell carcinoma, and small cell carcinoma (Table 28-5). Squamous cell lung cancer most often arises in major bronchi and is therefore detectable by sputum cytology. Adenocarcinoma, which predominates in the female, originates in the bronchial glands and mucosal cells, and has a tendency to invade the pleura and evoke a pleural effusion. This form of lung cancer characteristically metastasizes early, especially to the brain, liver, adrenal glands, and bone. Large cell lung cancer metastasizes early and to the brain. Small cell lung cancer exhibits a high frequency of early lymphatic invasion and spread to multiple sites, including the brain, bone, liver, and endocrine glands. Small cell tumors are capable of producing polypeptides that produce endocrine effects. Most patients with symptoms related to lung cancer have occult or overt metastases. Biomarkers of lung cancer (hormones, antigens, monoclonal antibodies) may facilitate the diagnosis

and correlate with progression or successful treatment of the tumor.[10]

Bronchoscopy in combination with bronchial washings or biopsy, or both, is commonly used in the initial evaluation of lung cancer. Peripheral lung lesions are typically diagnosed by percutaneous transthoracic needle biopsy. In the patient with a recently discovered coin lesion, the usual approach is surgical resection, although initial needle biopsy may be preferred in some instances. Computed tomography and magnetic resonance imaging of the head, chest, and abdomen, as well as a gallium bone scan, are carried out to detect metastatic disease. Enlarged mediastinal lymph nodes demonstrated by computed tomography are examined further by mediastinoscopy.

Management of Anesthesia

Management of anesthesia in the patient with carcinoma of the lung includes preoperative consideration of tumor-induced effects that may be manifested as malnutrition, pneumonia, pain, and ectopic endocrine effects, such as hyponatremia (Table 28-2). The propensity of this cancer to metastasize to the brain and bone is of possible significance in evaluation of the patient. When resection of lung tissue is planned, it is important to evaluate underlying pulmonary and cardiac function, especially the presence of pulmonary hypertension.

Mediastinoscopy

Hemorrhage and pneumothorax are the most frequently encountered complications of medistinoscopy. Positive-pressure ventilation of the lungs during mediastinoscopy is recommended to minimize the risk of venous air embolism. The

Table 28-5.   Pathophysiology of Lung Cancer

Type	Incidence (%)	Most Common Site of Metastases at Diagnosis	Five-Year Survival With Surgery (%)	Associated Syndromes
Squamous	30	Mediastinal nodes Brain Liver	30	Hypercalcemia
Adenocarcinoma	29	Mediastinal nodes Brain Bone	17	Osteoarthropathy
Large cell	16	Mediastinal nodes Bone Brain	15	Galoctorrhea Gynecomastia
Small cell	24	Mediastinal nodes Bone Liver	5	Eaton-Lambert syndrome Hyponatremia owing to SIADH Cushing syndrome Hypocalcemia

SIADH, syndrome of inappropriate antidiuretic hormone release.

mediastinoscope can also exert pressure against the right subclavian artery, causing the loss of a pulse distal to the site of compression and an erroneous diagnosis of cardiac arrest. Likewise, unrecognized compression of the right carotid artery may be manifested as a postoperative neurologic deficit. Bradycardia during mediastinoscopy may be due to stretching of the vagus nerve or trachea by the mediastinoscope.

Carcinoma of the Breast

Carcinoma of the breast will develop in about 6% of females in the United States and is the most common cause of death among those between 45 and 50 years of age. Females with fibrocystic disease are not at greater risk of breast cancer. There is an increased risk of breast cancer in a first-degree female family member, presumably reflecting a defect within the genome. The diagnosis of breast cancer is established by excisional biopsy, followed at a later time by a more definitive surgical procedure (mastectomy, wide excision, axillary node dissection) designed to decrease tumor bulk and thus enhance the effectiveness of systemic therapy and radiation. Systemic therapy consists of chemotherapy or hormonal therapy (tamoxifen) intended to eradicate occult micrometastases. A tumor with estrogen binding receptor protein is most likely to respond to depletion of those receptors by tamoxifen or prevention of the synthesis of estrogen by aminoglutethimide. Chemotherapy is indicated in the treatment of the patient with carcinoma of the breast that does not respond to hormonal therapy. Metastases to bone are frequent, emphasizing the importance of a bone scan and measurement of the alkaline phosphatase concentration.

Carcinoma of the Colon

Carcinoma of the colon and rectum (colorectal cancer) is second only to lung cancer as a cause of cancer death in the United States. A 50-year-old person has about a 5% risk of the development of colorectal cancer by 80 years of age and a 2.5% risk of dying from the disease.[11] More than 99% of colorectal cancers are adenocarcinomas, presumably reflecting their origin from an adenomatous polyp. There is a genetic predisposition for this form of cancer, and epidemiologic evidence that dietary habits (low fiber content, red meat consumption) increase the likelihood of the development of colon cancer. Inflammatory bowel disease is likely to be associated with colon cancer, whereas an alleged relationship between cholecystectomy and colorectal cancer has not been confirmed.[12] Most screening efforts are directed at rectal examinations and tests for occult blood in the stool. The intermittent pattern of bleeding from a colorectal cancer limits the usefulness of screening for blood in the stool. Sigmoidoscopic screening is more sensitive than the fecal occult blood test in its ability to detect polyps and cancer, although proximal colonic lesions will still escape detection. Routine endoscopic screening of asymptomatic persons without known risk factors is controversial.[11]

Presenting symptoms of colorectal cancer vary with the anatomic location of the lesion. Because stool is relatively liquid in the right colon, a tumor in this area can become large and greatly narrow the bowel lumen without causing obstructive symptoms. A lesion in the ascending colon frequently ulcerates, resulting in chronic blood loss with associated anemia and fatigue. Stool becomes more concentrated as it passes into the transverse colon, and a tumor in this area may cause abdominal cramping and obstruction. An abdominal radiograph may show a "napkin-ring lesion." The development of cancer in the rectosigmoid colon is associated with narrowing of the stool. Anemia is unusual despite the passage of bright red blood, which is often attributed to hemorrhoids. In the absence of obvious lymph node spread, the 5-year survival rate is 70% to 75% but drops to less than 5% when metastases are present. Colorectal cancer initially spreads to regional lymph nodes and then through the portal venous circulation to the liver, which represents the most common visceral site of metastases. When the primary tumor is in the distal rectum, tumor cells may escape the portal venous system and spread through the paravertebral plexus to the lungs. The median survival time after the detection of distant metastases is 6 to 9 months.

Surgical resection offers the greatest potential for cure in the patient with invasive colorectal cancer. In the presence of metastases, the operative procedure is often more conservative, designed primarily to relieve intestinal obstruction. An abdominal-perineal resection relegates the patient to a permanent sigmoid colostomy. Radiation therapy is an adjuvant to surgical resection of a rectal tumor that is likely to metastasize early by the lymphatic supply of the rectum to the surgically inaccessible pelvic side wall. Unless radiation is needed to shrink the tumor before surgery, it is usually administered postoperatively. Chemotherapy in the treatment of colorectal cancer has been unrewarding.

Management of Anesthesia

Management of anesthesia for surgical resection of a colorectal cancer may be influenced by disease-induced anemia, and the effects of metastases as may be present in the liver or lungs. Chronic large bowel obstruction probably does not increase the risk of aspiration on induction of anesthesia, although extreme abdominal distension could interfere with adequate ventilation and oxygenation. There is evidence that the transfusion of blood during surgical resection for colorectal cancer results in decreased survival time.[13] If true, this could reflect immunosuppression produced by transfused blood, allowing cancer cells to divide more rapidly. The use of a plasma volume expander, rather than blood, as well as reliance on an anesthetic technique that lowers blood pressure, hence intraoperative blood loss, has been proposed in these patients.

Carcinoma of the Prostate

Carcinoma of the prostate is the third leading cause of death among males who die from cancer, exceeded only by lung and colon cancer.[14] The disease may not be recognized until death, when its asymptomatic presence is discovered in as many as 70% of males older than 70 years of age. The plasma concentration of prostate-specific antigen is increased in the presence of prostate cancer.[15] Diffuse induration of the prostate or a discrete nodule, as detected on rectal examination, may be the presenting feature. In other instances, the patient presents with symptoms of urinary obstruction. Less often, the patient presents with symptoms of metastatic disease, such as diffuse bone pain, weight loss, spinal cord compression, or acute renal failure secondary to bilateral hydronephrosis. Metastatic spread is both lymphatic and hematogenous. Hematogenous spread occurs principally to the bones and less so to the lungs and liver. An increased plasma acid phosphatase and alkaline phosphatase concentration is indicative of spread of the tumor beyond the confines of the capsule of the prostate, usually to bone. Osteoblastic lesions may be visible on a skeletal radiograph. It is estimated that about 75% of patients have metastatic disease when the tumor is discovered.

Carcinoma of the prostate that is confined to the gland is usually cured by transurethral resection. Some patients may be considered for more radical treatment, such as radical prostatectomy or radiation. Radical prostatectomy can be performed by either a retropubic or perineal approach. The retropubic approach allows the surgeon to biopsy lymph nodes first and to abort the operation if any of the nodes are positive. Modifications in the surgical technique have decreased the incidence of postresection impotence or incontinence. Radiation therapy can be delivered either by an external beam, using a linear accelerator, or by implantation of radioactive capsules into the gland. Radiation therapy produces impotence less often than surgery, but disabling radiation cystitis or proctitis is possible.

Treatment of metastatic disease is palliative and is based on the fact that prostate cancer is under the trophic influence of androgen hormones. The goal of androgen deprivation can be attained by orchiectomy or by administration of drugs that prevent the synthesis (aminogluthemide), release (leuprolide), or action (flutamide) of androgens.[16] Androgen deprivation produces subjective improvement in about 50% of patients and objective evidence of tumor regression in nearly 50%. There is little benefit in introducing a second hormonal procedure in a patient whose cancer initially responds but then becomes refractory to one form of hormonal therapy. When advanced prostatic cancer becomes resistant to hormonal therapy, incapacitating bone pain may be treated with radiation or chemotherapy. The median survival for patients with metastatic carcinoma of the prostate is 2.5 years.

LESS COMMON CANCERS ENCOUNTERED IN CLINICAL PRACTICE

Head and Neck Cancer

Head and neck cancer accounts for about 5% of all cancers in the United States, with a predominance in males older than 50 years of age. Most patients have a history of excessive cigarette smoking and alcohol abuse. The most common sites of metastasis are lung, liver, and bone. Hypercalcemia may be associated with bone metastases, whereas altered liver function tests presumably reflect alcohol-induced disease. Preoperative nutritional therapy may be indicated before surgical resection of the tumor, which often uses laser technology. The goal of chemotherapy, if selected, is to decrease the bulk of the primary tumor or known metastases, thus enhancing the efficacy of subsequent surgery or radiotherapy. A secondary goal is eradication of subclinical occult micrometastases.

Thyroid Cancer

Thyroid cancer is uncommon but should be considered whenever a thyroid nodule is discovered or whenever there is a history of radiation to the neck in childhood. Papillary thyroid cancer is slow growing, whereas follicular thyroid cancer may be manifested initially as pathologic fractures owing to bone metastases. Medullary thyroid cancer may be associated with pheochromocytoma in an autosomal dominant disorder known as multiple endocrine neoplasia type II (MEN II). This type of thyroid cancer typically produces large amounts of thyrocalcitonin, providing a sensitive measure for the presence of the disease, as well as its cure. Hypocalcemia does not occur despite this increased secretion of thyrocalcitonin. Other clinical manifestations of medullary thyroid cancer include intractable diarrhea and excessive secretion of adrenocorticotropic hormone leading to Cushing syndrome. Undifferentiated cancer of the thyroid is a rapidly growing tumor that may produce tracheal compression.

Diagnosis of thyroid cancer can be made only by an open surgical biopsy. Surgical removal of the thyroid gland with or without a radical neck dissection is the initial treatment of thyroid cancer. After removal of the primary lesion, the patient is usually treated with thyroid replacement. A functional thyroid cancer may take up radioactive iodine, thus responding to high doses of radiation delivered by this approach.

Esophageal Cancer

Excessive alcohol consumption and chronic cigarette smoking are thought to represent independent factors that are responsible for 80% or more of the esophageal cancers in the

United States. Dysphagia and weight loss are the initial symptoms of esophageal cancer in 90% of patients. The disease is usually incurable by the time these symptoms are present. Indeed, the lack of a serosal layer around the esophagus and the presence of an extensive lymphatic system result in rapid spread of the tumor, especially to the liver and lung. Difficulty swallowing may result in regurgitation and the risk of aspiration. The results of primary radiation therapy resemble radical surgery, with a 5-year survival rate of about 5%. Chemotherapy and radiation may be instituted prior to attempting surgical resection. Palliation may include surgical placement of a feeding tube or a polyvinyl esophageal prosthesis. The likelihood of underlying alcohol-induced liver disease, chronic obstructive pulmonary disease from cigarette smoking, and cross-tolerance with other anesthetic drugs is a consideration in the anesthetic management of an affected patient. Furthermore, extensive weight loss often parallels a decrease in intravascular fluid volume, manifested as hypotension during induction or maintenance of anesthesia, or both.

Cardiac Tumors

Cardiac tumors are most often metastatic, whereas primary cardiac tumors are very rare.

Metastatic Cardiac Tumor

Metastatic cardiac tumor is present in about 10% of all patients who die from cancer, but only 5% to 10% of these patients are symptomatic. Tumors most likely to metastasize to the heart include carcinoma of the lung and breast, Kaposi sarcoma, and leukemia. Manifestations of a metastatic cardiac tumor most often reflect pericardial metastases. A malignant pericardial effusion is often hemorrhagic, and cardiac tamponade is possible. The pericardium is sometimes encased in tumor, producing a disorder resembling cardiomyopathy or constrictive pericarditis. Atrial fibrillation may be an early manifestation of malignant involvement of the pericardium. Malignant pericardial effusion is the most common cause of electrical alternans on the ECG. Echocardiography, computed tomography, and magnetic resonance imaging are all useful in the diagnosis of pericardial and cardiac metastases. Treatment is most often related to management of a pericardial effusion that may produce cardiac tamponade.

Primary Benign Tumor

Cardiac myxoma is the most common benign cardiac tumor arising from the epithelium and acting as an intracavitary space-occupying lesion. Most myxomas are pedunculated and originate in the left atrium. Cardiac myxoma may occur as part of a syndrome that includes spotty skin pigmentations and endocrine overreactivity (Cushing syndrome, acromegaly). Manifestations of a cardiac myxoma reflect interference with

Table 28-6. Findings Suggestive of a Cardiac Myxoma

Refractory congestive heart failure
Unexplained cardiac rhythm disturbances
Syncope related to position change
Unexplained systemic or pulmonary emboli
Pulmonary hypertension of unknown cause

filling and emptying of the involved cardiac chamber and release of emboli composed either of myxomatous material or of thrombi that have formed in the tumor (Table 28-6). A left atrial myxoma may mimic mitral valve disease with the development of pulmonary edema. Conversely, a right atrial myxoma will mimic tricuspid valve disease and is associated with impaired venous return and evidence of right heart failure. A right atrial myxoma may be manifested as isolated tricuspid stenosis, dyspnea, and arterial hypoxemia. Any surgically removed emboli should be examined microscopically for myxomatous material. Echocardiography is a useful technique for the noninvasive diagnosis of a cardiac myxoma.[17] Treatment of a cardiac myxoma is surgical excision. Occasionally, associated involvement or damage may necessitate cardiac valve replacement. Because of occasional local recurrence, resection of that portion of the atrial septum from which the tumor arises may be indicated.

Management of Anesthesia

Anesthetic considerations in a patient with a right atrial myxoma include a low cardiac output and arterial hypoxemia owing to obstruction at the tricuspid valve.[17] Symptoms of obstruction to blood flow may be exacerbated by changes in body position. The presence of a right atrial myxoma probably should discourage the placement of a right atrial or pulmonary artery catheter.[17]

Primary Malignant Tumor

A primary malignant tumor of the heart is most often some form of sarcoma and is more apt to occur in the right heart than the left heart. Signs and symptoms reflect intracavitary growth of the tumor, including pulmonary artery outflow obstruction. Sudden onset and rapid progression of refractory CHF, especially right-sided failure, is common, as is syncope. Tumor invasion of the myocardium and compromise of the coronary circulation may resemble myocardial infarction.

Gastric Cancer

The incidence of gastric cancer has decreased dramatically since 1930, when it was the leading cause of cancer-related death among males in the United States. The presenting features of gastric cancer (indigestion, epigastric distress, anorexia) are indistinguishable from a benign peptic ulcer. About 90% of gastric cancers are adenocarcinomas, and about 50% of these occur in the distal portion of the stomach. The cancer is usually far advanced when symptoms such as weight loss and ascites are present. Treatment is surgical resection of the tumor and associated lymph nodes. Even when the disease is incurable, surgical resection of the primary tumor decreases the tumor burden and may improve the response to palliative radiation or chemotherapy, or both.

Liver Cancer

Liver cancer occurs most often in males with cirrhosis of the liver caused by hepatitis B. The initial manifestation is often a painful mass in the right upper quadrant accompanied by weight loss. There is often compression of the inferior vena cava or portal vein, or both, as well as synthesis of abnormal prothrombin molecules, resulting in impaired coagulation. Liver function tests are likely to be abnormal. Computed tomography of the liver can determine the anatomic location of the tumor, although angiography is more useful for distinguishing hepatocellular cancer (hypervascular) from hepatic metastases (hypovascular) and for determining whether the tumor can be resected. Radical surgical resection or alternatively liver transplantation offer the only hope for survival. Most patients with liver cancer are not surgical candidates, however, because of extensive cirrhosis or greatly impaired liver function. Chemotherapy is of limited value, whereas radiation is principally useful for pain relief.

Gallbladder Cancer

Gallbladder cancer is uncommon in the United States, occurring more commonly in females, discovered unexpectedly during performance of cholecystectomy to treat cholelithiasis. The risk of gallbladder cancer in a patient with asymptomatic cholelithiasis is no greater than the operative mortality for cholecystectomy. Therefore, cholecystectomy is not recommended as a prophylactic measure for gallbladder cancer. When gallbladder cancer is invasive at discovery, the 5-year survival rate is less than 5% despite radical surgery, postoperative radiation, and chemotherapy.

Pancreatic Cancer

Pancreatic cancer, despite its low incidence, is the fourth most common cause of cancer-related mortality. Evidence linking this cancer to alcohol abuse, caffeine ingestion, cholelithiasis, or diabetes mellitus is not available, whereas cigarette smoking shows a positive correlation. About 95% of pancreatic cancers are ductal adenocarcinomas, with most occurring in the head of the pancreas. Abdominal pain, anorexia, and weight loss are often insidious initial symptoms. Pain suggests retroperitoneal invasion and infiltration of splanchnic nerves. Jaundice reflects biliary obstruction in the patient with a tumor in the head of the pancreas. Diabetes mellitus is rare in the patient in whom pancreatic cancer develops.

Pancreatic cancer may appear as a localized mass or as a diffuse enlargement of the gland on computed tomography of the abdomen. Biopsy of the lesion is necessary to confirm the diagnosis. Complete surgical resection is the only effective treatment of ductal pancreatic cancer. The patient most likely to have a resectable lesion has a tumor in the head of the pancreas that causes painless jaundice. Extrapancreatic spread eliminates the possibility of a surgical cure. The two most commonly employed resection techniques are total pancreatectomy and pancreatoduodenectomy (Whipple procedure). Total pancreatectomy is technically easier but has the disadvantage of producing diabetes mellitus and malabsorption. Only 10% of patients who undergo complete resection survive 5 years, whereas the median survival for the patient with an unresectable tumor is 5 months. Palliative procedures include surgical diversion of the biliary system, radiation, and chemotherapy. Celiac plexus block with alcohol or phenol is the most effective intervention for treatment of pain owing to pancreatic cancer. Complications of celiac plexus block include hypotension due to sympathetic nervous system denervation, especially in a chronically ill hypovolemic patient. Computed tomography may be used to confirm proper needle placement before injection of any solution intended to act on the celiac plexus.

Renal Cell Carcinoma

Renal cell carcinoma is most often manifested in a male as hematuria, flank pain and a palpable mass. Risk factors include a family history and cigarette smoking. Renal ultrasonography helps identify a renal cyst, whereas computed tomography and magnetic resonance imaging are useful for determining the presence and extent of a renal neoplasm. Evaluation for distant metastases includes a chest radiograph, bone scan, and liver function tests. Altered laboratory values may include eosinophilia and liver function abnormalities. High-output CHF, when it occurs, is presumed to reflect the development of a renal arteriovenous fistula. The only curative therapy for renal adenocarcinoma limited to the kidney is a radical nephrectomy with regional lymphadenectomy. Radical nephrectomy is not helpful in the patient with distant metastases, whereas chemotherapy may show some efficacy, although 5-year survival is less than 5%.

Bladder Cancer

Bladder cancer occurs most often in males and is associated with cigarette smoking and chronic exposure to chemicals, as used in the textile and rubber industries. The most common presenting feature is gross, painless hematuria. Metastatic disease is characterized by involvement of the adjacent lymph nodes and spread to the lungs, liver, and bones.

Treatment of noninvasive bladder cancer includes endoscopic resection and intravesical chemotherapy. Carcinoma in situ of the bladder, unlike that of the uterine cervix, often behaves virulently and may require cystectomy to help prevent muscle invasion and metastatic spread. Traditional treatment for metastatic disease often includes preoperative radiation, followed by cystectomy and chemotherapy. The most common urinary diversion is ureteroileostomy. Alternatively, the creation of an artificial bladder from a segment of colon can obviate the need for external diversion.

Testicular Cancer

Although testicular cancer is rare, it is the most common cancer in young males and represents a tumor that can be cured even when distant metastases are present. Orchiopexy before 2 years of age is recommended for cryptorchidism, to decrease the risk of testicular cancer. The initial manifestation of testicular cancer is usually a painless mass. When the diagnosis is suspected, an inguinal orchiectomy is performed and histologic confirmation determined. A transscrotal biopsy is not performed, as disruption of the scrotum may predispose to a local recurrence and metastatic spread to the inguinal lymphatics. Germ cell cancers, which account for 95% of testicular cancers, can be subdivided into seminomas and nonseminomas. Seminomas often metastasize through the regional lymphatics to the retroperitoneum and mediastinum, whereas nonseminomas also spread hematogenously to the viscera, especially the liver and lungs. Abdominal and pelvic computed tomography are useful in assessing metastatic disease.

The patient with a seminoma that does not extend beyond the retroperitoneal lymph nodes is treated with radiation. Chemotherapy is recommended when the seminoma is advanced. Nonseminomas are not radiosensitive and are treated by retroperitoneal lymph node dissection, often with adjuvant chemotherapy. The side effects of chemotherapy in such a patient may include myelosuppression, anemia, cardiotoxicity, pulmonary toxicity, nephrotoxicity, and peripheral neuropathy.

Carcinoma of the Uterine Cervix

Carcinoma of the uterine cervix is the most common gynecologic cancer in females aged 15 to 34 years. Viruses such as herpes simplex and human papillomavirus may predispose to cervical cancer. Carcinoma in situ as detected by a Papanicolaou (Pap) smear is treated with a cone biopsy, whereas disease that has metastasized is treated with radiation therapy, surgery, and chemotherapy.

Carcinoma of the Uterus

Carcinoma of the uterine endometrium occurs most frequently in females aged 50 to 70 years and may be associated with obesity, hypertension, and diabetes mellitus. Females who smoke heavily may be at decreased risk of endometrial cancer, presumably reflecting decreased estrogen levels caused by cigarette smoking.[19] The most common manifestation of endometrial cancer is vaginal bleeding in a menopausal or perimenopausal female. The initial evaluation may include a fractional dilation and curettage. In the absence of metastatic disease, a total abdominal hysterectomy and bilateral salpingo-oophorectomy with or without radiation is the treatment. Hormonal therapy, usually with progesterone, is useful in the treatment of those with metastatic disease. Chemotherapy for endometrial cancer has not been widely used.

Carcinoma of the Ovary

Carcinoma of the ovary is most likely to develop in females who experience early menopause or who have a family history of ovarian cancer. Advanced disease is usually present when the disease is discovered, often including omental metastases reflecting lymphatic drainage of the ovary through retroperitoneal lymph nodes. Surgery is the treatment for early-stage ovarian cancer, often followed by chemotherapy or radiation. The efficacy of chemotherapy is increased when the tumor mass has been decreased by surgery. Intraperitoneal chemotherapy may be indicated in selected patients.

Cutaneous Melanoma

The incidence of cutaneous melanoma is increasing faster than that of any other cancer.[20] It is estimated that melanoma will develop in 1 in 90 Americans by the year 2000. There is evidence that sunlight (ultraviolet range) is an important environmental factor in the pathogenesis of melanoma. Melanoma is suspected when there is a change in color, size, shape, or surface of a mole. The initial treatment of a suspected lesion is an excisional biopsy. Evidence of metastatic disease is most likely in the lymph nodes, brain, liver, lungs, and bone. Metastatic melanoma is usually incurable, with palliation provided by regional lymph node dissection, radiation, and chemotherapy.

Cancer of the Bone

Multiple Myeloma

Multiple myeloma is the most common malignant tumor of bone in the adult (see Chapter 29).

Osteosarcoma

Osteosarcoma occurs most often in adolescents and typically involves the long bones. A genetic predisposition is suggested by the association of this tumor with retinoblastoma. Computed tomography is used to assess the extent of the primary lesion and the existence of metastatic disease, especially to the lungs. The plasma concentration of alkaline phosphatase is likely to be increased in the presence of metastatic disease. Treatment consists of chemotherapy, followed by surgical excision. The success of chemotherapy may permit limb salvage procedures in selected patients. Pulmonary resection may be indicated in the patient with an isolated metastatic lung lesion.

Ewing's Tumor

Ewing's tumor or sarcoma usually occurs in a patient less than 30 years of age, most often involving the pelvis, femur, and tibia. Metastatic disease is usually present at diagnosis. Treatment consists of surgery, local radiation, and chemotherapy.

Chondrosarcoma

Chondrosarcoma usually involves the pelvis, ribs, or upper end of the femur or humerus in a young adult. This tumor grows slowly and is treated by radical surgical excision.

Lymphoma

Hodgkin's disease is an example of lymphoma that has both an infective (Epstein-Barr virus) and genetic association. Another factor that appears to predispose to the development of a lymphoma is impaired immunity as present in a patient with a transplanted organ or the human immunodeficiency virus-infected patient. A typical onset of Hodgkin's disease is a painless enlarging mass that classically appears in the neck. Pruritus can be generalized and severe. Cyclic increases of body temperature and unexplained weight loss may occur. Superior vena cava obstruction reflects invasion of the mediastinum by tumor. Moderately severe anemia is often present. A chest radiograph may reflect involvement of the lungs in Hodgkin's disease, which also often invades the liver and spleen. Peripheral neuropathies and spinal cord compression may occur as a direct result of tumor growth. Bone marrow and central nervous system involvement is unusual in Hodgkin's disease, but not in other lymphomas.

The most useful diagnostic test in the patient with a suspected lymphoma is a lymph node biopsy. Surgical exploration of the abdomen permits evaluation of the spread of the disease and is the basis for classifying a lymphoma in preparation for selection of the appropriate therapy. Radiation and combination chemotherapy can cure about 50% of patients with Hodgkin's disease.

Leukemia

Leukemia is the uncontrolled production of leukocytes owing to cancerous mutation of lymphogenous cells or myelogenous cells. Lymphocytic leukemias begin in lymph nodes and are named according to the type of hematopoietic cell that is primarily involved. Myeloid leukemias begin as cancerous production of myelogenous cells in bone marrow with spread to extramedullary organs. The principal difference between normal and leukemia cells is the ability of the latter to continue to divide. The result is an expanding mass of cells that infiltrate the bone marrow, rendering the patient functionally aplastic. Anemia may be profound. Eventually, bone marrow failure is the cause of fatal infection or hemorrhage due to thrombocytopenia. In addition to bone marrow, leukemia cells may infiltrate the liver, spleen, lymph nodes, and meninges, producing signs of dysfunction at these sites. Extensive use of nutrients by rapidly proliferating cancerous cells depletes amino acids, leading to patient fatigue and to metabolic starvation of normal tissues.

Treatment

A kilogram of leukemia cells (about 10^{12} cells) appears to be a lethal mass. However, symptoms leading to the diagnosis of leukemia are unlikely until the tumor load is about 10^9 cells. Chemotherapy is intended to decrease the number of tumor cells, so that organomegaly will regress, and function of the bone marrow will improve. Drugs used for chemotherapy are principally those that depress activity of bone marrow, such that hemorrhage and infection become the determinants of maximum acceptable doses. Destruction of tumor cells by chemotherapy produces a uric acid load that may result in urate nephropathy and gouty arthritis. Nutritional support of the patient undergoing chemotherapy may be necessary to prevent hypoalbuminemia and loss of immunocompetence.

Bone Marrow Transplantation

Bone marrow transplantation offers the opportunity for cure of otherwise fatal diseases, including refractory leukemia, aplastic anemia, and primary immunodeficiency syndromes.[21] Autologous bone marrow transplants entail donation of the patient's own marrow for subsequent reinfusion, whereas allogeneic transplants use immunocompatible donors. Regardless of the type of transplant, the recipient must undergo a preoperative regimen designed to achieve functional bone marrow ablation. This is achieved over a 7- to 10-day period, using a combination of chemotherapy and total body radiation.

Donor bone marrow (up to 1500 ml) is harvested by multiple aspirations obtained from the posterior iliac spines and iliac crests. General anesthesia or regional anesthesia is required for the harvest. Nitrous oxide may be avoided in the donor because of potential bone marrow depression associated with use of this drug. Nevertheless, there is no evidence that nitrous oxide administered during bone marrow harvesting adversely affects marrow engraftment and subsequent function. Brief heparinization before removal of bone marrow may influence the selection of spinal or epidural anesthesia. The volume of peripheral blood loss parallels the quantity of marrow harvested, emphasizing the substantial fluid loss that may accompany this procedure. Blood replacement may be necessary, either with autologous blood transfusion or by reinfusion of separated erythrocytes obtained during the harvest. The decision to place a Foley catheter is individualized and is influenced by the donor's general health, anticipated duration of the procedure, and estimated volume of bone marrow to be harvested. Postoperative complications are rare, although discomfort at bone puncture sites is predictable.

Processing of the harvested bone marrow (eradicate malignant cells, removal of incompatible erythrocytes) may take 2 to 12 hours. The condensed bone marrow volume (about 200 ml) is then infused into the recipient through an indwelling central venous line. From the systemic circulation, the marrow stem cells pass into bone marrow, providing the microenvironment necessary for maturation and differentiation. Time to engraftment is usually 10 to 28 days, during which time protective isolation is often used. Engraftment is confirmed by daily peripheral blood cell counts and is verified with bone marrow aspiration and biopsy. While awaiting engraftment, it may be necessary to administer platelets to maintain the count above 20,000 cells·mm^{-3} and erythrocytes to maintain the hematocrit above 25%.

Preoperative complications associated with bone marrow transplantation reflect the need to ablate the recipient's bone marrow with chemotherapy and total body radiation. Total body radiation leads to gastrointestinal toxicity (nausea, vomiting, diarrhea, oral mucositis) and may be followed by pulmonary fibrosis, restrictive cardiomyopathy, and cataract formation at a later date. Chemotherapy also introduces the potential for multiple side effects (Table 28-3). Veno-occlusive disease is a unique complication of high-dose chemotherapy manifested as hyperbilirubinemia, right upper quadrant pain, and weight gain. All transplant recipients are susceptible to bacterial, viral, and fungal infection.

Graft-versus-host disease is a life-threatening complication of bone marrow transplantation that occurs in about 50% of transplanted patients. Manifestations of this complication can reflect dysfunction of any organ system but most often the skin, liver, and gastrointestinal tract are affected[21] (Table 28-7). This reaction occurs when immunocompetent T lymphocytes are injected into an immunosuppressed host and reflects cytotoxic injury to organs and the release of lymphokines. The acute manifestations of graft-versus-host disease commonly occur 10 to 100 days after transplantation, whereas the chronic form of this response tends to occur 100 to 400 days after transplantation and has many characteristics of an autoimmune disease. Treatment of graft-versus-host disease includes the administration of corticosteroids, azathioprine, and cyclosporine.

Table 28-7. Manifestations of Graft-versus-Host Disease

Oral ulceration and mucositis
Esophageal ulceration
Diarrhea with fluid and electrolyte loss
Hepatitis with coagulopathy
Pancytopenia and immunodeficiency
Bronchiolitis obliterans
Interstitial pneumonitis
Pulmonary fibrosis
Renal failure

Acute Lymphoblastic Leukemia

Acute lymphoblastic leukemia accounts for about 15% of all leukemia in adults. Central nervous system dysfunction is common. The affected patient is highly susceptible to life-threatening infections, including those due to *Pneumoncystis carinii* and cytomegalovirus. Chemotherapy may produce a long-lasting remission and occasional cure.

Chronic Lymphocytic Leukemia

Chronic lymphocytic leukemia is a malignant clonal disorder of mature lymphocytes, accounting for about 25% of all leukemia in adults, most often the elderly adult. The diagnosis is confirmed by the presence of lymphocytosis and lymphocytic infiltrates in bone marrow. Signs and symptoms are highly variable, with the extent of bone marrow infiltration often determining the clinical course. Autoimmune hemolytic anemia and hypersplenism that results in pancytopenia and thrombocytopenia may be prominent. Lymph node enlargement may obstruct the ureters.

Recurrent infection may require repeated antibiotic therapy or intravenous infusion of immunoglobulins. Chemotherapy with alkylating drugs is the indicated therapy as corticosteroids do not destroy leukemic lymphocytes. Splenectomy may occasionally be necessary.

Adult T Cell Leukemia

Adult T cell leukemia is a rapidly fatal disease characterized by leukocytosis, hepatosplenomegaly, cutaneous lesions, and hypercalcemia. Lytic bone lesions are the likely explanation for hypercalcemia. A human retrovirus termed human T cell lymphotropic virus type 1 (HTLV-1) has been isolated from affected patients. Opportunistic infections caused by *Pneumocystis carinii* and cytomegalovirus are common, as is central nervous system involvement.

Acute Myeloid Leukemia

Acute myeloid leukemia is an aggressive malignant disease that produces death, often in less than 100 days, if untreated. An increase in acute myeloid leukemia appears to be the result of treatment of other cancers. Fever, weakness, bleeding, and hepatosplenomegaly are characteristic. Chemotherapy may produce complete remission in 65% to 85% of patients. By contrast, therapy-related acute myeloid leukemia does not respond to chemotherapy.

Chronic Myeloid Leukemia

Chronic myeloid leukemia is manifested as massive hepatosplenomegaly, often in the presence of a leukocyte cell count that exceeds $50,000$ cells·mm^{-3}. A high leukocyte count may predispose to vascular occlusion. Anemia and thrombocytopenia may be profound in the affected patient. Hyperuricemia is likely and is treated with allopurinol. Leukopheresis, splenectomy, and chemotherapy are often employed. Traditional treatment of chronic myeloid leukemia is with busulfan, although bone marrow transplantation may now be the treatment of choice in selected patients.

Polycythemia Vera

Polycythemia vera is a myeloproliferative disease in which mutation of a single cell results in increased production of erythrocytes, leukocytes, and platelets.[22] The hemoglobin concentration typically exceeds 18 g·dl^{-1}, and the platelet count may exceed $400,000$ cells·mm^{-3}. Clinical symptoms are due to hyperviscosity of the blood, which leads to stasis of blood flow and an increased incidence of vascular thrombosis, particularly in the cardiovascular and central nervous system (transient ischemic attacks). Evidence of decreased cerebral blood flow is a decreased level of consciousness. Defective platelet function is the most likely mechanism for spontaneous hemorrhage that is occasionally observed in an affected patient. In addition to contributing to transient ischemic attacks, disseminated intravascular platelet aggregation may account for erythromelalgia (plethora) and pruritus described by the patient as often associated with taking a shower. Aspirin does not decrease the incidence of thrombotic events. Splenomegaly is often present.

Treatment of polycythemia vera is phlebotomy, to decrease the hematocrit to about 40%. Surgery performed in the presence of polycythemia is associated with a high incidence of perioperative hemorrhage and postoperative venous thrombosis. In an urgent situation, blood viscosity can be decreased by the intravenous infusion of crystalloid solution or low-molecular-weight dextran.

REFERENCES

1. Wise RP. A myasthenic syndrome complicating bronchial carcinoma. Anaesthesia 1962;17:488–90
2. Batist G, Andrews JL. Pulmonary toxicity of antineoplastic drugs. JAMA 1981;246:1449–53
3. Dillman JB. Safe use of succinylcholine during repeated anesthetics in a patient treated with cyclophosphamide. Anesth Analg 1987;66:351–3
4. Burrows FA, Hickey PR, Colan S. Perioperative complications in patients with anthracycline chemotherapeutic agents. Can Anaesth Soc J 1985;32:149–57
5. Gilbert RW, Kim J-H, Posner JB. Epidural spinal cord compression from metastic tumor: Diagnosis and treatment. Ann Neurol 1978;3:40–51
6. Selvin BL. Cancer chemotherapy: Implications for the anesthesiologist. Anesth Analg 1981;60:425–34
7. Klein DS, Wilds PR. Pulmonary toxicity of antineoplastic agents: Anaesthetic and postoperative implications. Can Anaesth Soc J 1983;30:399–405
8. La Mantia KR, Glick JH, Marshall BE. Supplemental oxygen does not cause respiratory failure in bleomycin-treated surgical patients. Anesthesiology 1984;60:65–7
9. Matalon S, Harper WV, Nickerson PA, Olszowka J. Intravenous bleomycin does not alter the toxic effects of hyperoxia in rabbits. Anesthesiology 1986;64:614–9
10. Tockman MS, Gupta PK, Myers JD, et al. Sensitive and specific monoclonal antibody recognition of human lung cancer antigen on preserved sputum cells: A new approach to early lung cancer detection. J Clin Oncol 1988;6:1685–9
11. Ranshoff DF, Lang CA. Screening for colorectal cancer. N Engl J Med 1991;325:37–41
12. Adami HO, Meirik O, Gustavsson S, et al. Colorectal cancer after cholecystectomy: Absence of risk increase within 11–14 years. Gastroenterology 1983;85:859–63
13. Fielding LP. Red for danger: Blood transfusion and colorectal cancer. Br Med J 1985;291:841–3
14. Gittes RF. Carcinoma of the prostate. N Engl J Med 1991;324:236–45
15. Catalona WJ, Smith DS, Ratliff TL, et al. Measurement of prostate-specific antigen in serum as a screening test for prostate cancer. N Engl J Med 1991;324:1156–61
16. Sogani PC, Vagaiwala MR, Whitmore WF, Jr. Experience with flutamide in patients with advanced prostatic cancer without prior endocrine therapy. Cancer 1984;54:744–81
17. Lebovic S, Koorn R, Reich DL. Role of two dimensional transoesophageal echocardiography in the management of a right ventricular tumor. Can J Anaesth 1991;38:1050–4
18. Moritz HA, Azad SS. Right atrial myxoma: Case report and anaesthetic considerations. Can J Anaesth 1989;36:212–4
19. Lesko SM, Rosenberg L, Kaufman DW, et al. Cigarette smoking and the risk of endometrial cancer. N Engl J Med 1985;313:593–7
20. Koh HK. Cutaneous melanoma. N Engl J Med 1991;325:171–82
21. Stein RA, Messino MJ, Hessel EA. Anaesthetic implications for bone marrow transplant recipients. Can J Anaesth 1990;37:571–8
22. Conley CL. Polycythemia vera. JAMA 1990;263:2481–4

29

Disorders Related to Immune System Dysfunction

The immune system, which consists of a number of lymphoid organs (thymus, lymph nodes, tonsils, spleen) is responsible for protecting against infection and recognizing foreign substances. The immunologically active cells of the immune system are lymphocytes, characterized as B lymphocytes and T lymphocytes (Fig. 29-1).

HUMORAL IMMUNITY

Humoral immunity is mediated by B lymphocytes that differentiate into antibody-producing plasma cells when stimulated by an antigen. An antigen is any substance capable of interacting with B lymphocytes to elicit the formation of antibodies. Proteins are almost always antigenic, and the protein composition of cell membranes determines histocompatibility antigens (HLA), serving to differentiate host cells from foreign tissues. Haptens are small molecules, such as drugs (penicillin), that can combine with a self-protein to induce antibody formation manifested clinically as an allergic reaction.

Antibodies are secreted by plasma cells as a heterogeneous group of plasma proteins designated immunoglobulins (Ig), classified as IgG, IgM, IgA, IgD, and IgE on the basis of electrophoretic and serologic properties (Table 29-1). The principal Ig in the plasma is IgG, and most antibodies are IgG. Antigens that preferentially induce IgE antibodies are designated allergens. All allergens are proteins, but there are no common physicochemical characteristics that distinguish them from other antigens. Radioimmunoassay techniques permit measurement of plasma Ig concentrations. Each plasma cell produces a specific Ig, and the ability to produce antibody to specific antigens is inherited as an autosomal dominant trait.

CELLULAR IMMUNITY

T lymphocytes known as helper T lymphocytes do not produce antibodies but instead regulate antibody production by B lymphocytes. Cellular immunity that may result in rejection of transplanted foreign tissue is mediated by T lymphocytes; on contact with an antigen (HLA), the result is activation of cytotoxic T lymphocytes and production of lymphokines. Lymphokines (interleukin-2, interferons) are non-Ig molecules that amplify and regulate a variety of immune responses. Activity of helper T lymphocytes is balanced by suppressor T lymphocytes, which in turn dampen immune responses. Indeed, what is ultimately detected after exposure to an antigen is the result of a balance between helper (activator) and suppressor immune system responses. For example, an excessive immune response can be due to a defect in suppressor mechanisms (autoimmune diseases), whereas immunodeficiency may result from an exaggerated suppressor response.

COMPLEMENT SYSTEM

The complement system, composed of 18 plasma proteins, serves as the principal humoral effector of immunologically induced inflammation. Complement activation can be initiated

501

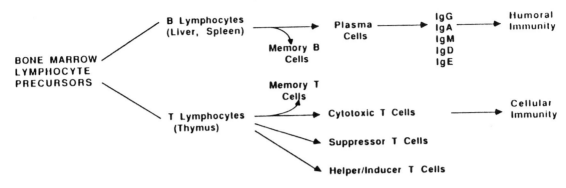

Fig. 29-1. Schematic depiction of the immune system.

by either the classical pathway (antigen-antibody interaction) or the alternative pathway (bacterial polysaccharides)[1] (Fig. 29-2). Although both pathways result in the formation of the same critical component, C3, each pathway appears to have a distinct role in protecting the body, either against autoimmune disease (classical pathway) or against infection (alternative pathway). The products of complement activation are responsible for a number of events, including the release of vasoactive substances from mast cells that leads to increased capillary permeability. This increased permeability permits more antibody to gain access to the site of inflammation. In addition, active components of the complement system attract leukocytes to the inflamed area, facilitating the phagocytosis and lysis of the bacterial cell walls. A deficiency of the protein (C1 inhibitor protein) that normally regulates the progression of the complement cascade is associated with uncontrolled accumulation of the components of the complement system (see the section, Hereditary Angioedema).

INTERFERONS

Interferons are endogenous proteins whose production can be induced in most body cells by various stimuli. These proteins serve as natural defensive responses to bacteria, vi-

ruses, tumor cells, and antigens. Exogenous administration of interferons may be useful in the treatment of certain types of leukemia, Kaposi sarcoma, type C viral hepatitis, and chronic granulomatous disease.[2]

ALLERGIC REACTIONS

Allergic reactions may be due to an antigen-antibody interaction (anaphylaxis, immune-mediated hypersensitivity), release of chemical mediators in the absence of an antigen-antibody interaction (anaphylactoid), and activation of the complement pathway. An anaphylactoid reaction reflects massive release of histamine from basophils in response to administration of certain drugs (opioids, muscle relaxants, protamine) that possess the inherent ability to displace this vasoactive mediator from cells (see the section, Drug Allergy). This histamine release is independent of an antigen-antibody interaction, emphasizing that such a response may occur in a susceptible patient exposed to the drug for the first time.

Table 29-1. Properties of Human Immunoglobulins

	IgG	IgA	IgM	IgD	IgE
Location	Plasma Amniotic fluid	Plasma Saliva Tears	Plasma	Plasma	Plasma
Plasma concentration (mg·dl^{-1})	550–1900	60–333	45–145	0.3–30	Trace
Half-time (d)	23	6	5	3	2.5
Function	Immunity and defense against infection	Topical defense against infection	Lysis of bacterial cell walls	Not shown	Anaphylaxis

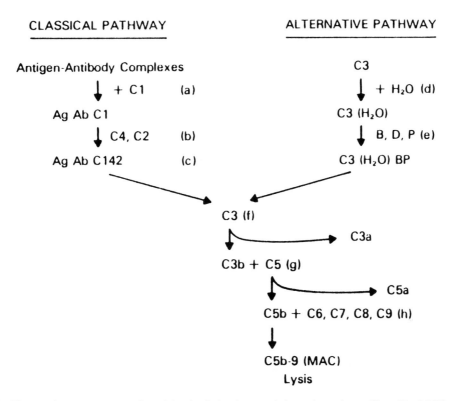

Fig. 29-2. The complement system consists of the classical pathway and alternative pathway. (From Frank MM. Complement in the pathophysiology of human disease. N Engl J Med 1987;316:1525–30, with permission.)

Anaphylaxis

Anaphylaxis is a life-threatening manifestation of an antigen-antibody interaction. This form of an allergic reaction is possible whenever prior exposure to an antigen (drug, food, venom) has evoked the production of antigen-specific IgE antibodies, thus sensitizing the host. Subsequent exposure of the host to the same or chemically similar antigen results in an antigen-antibody interaction that initiates explosive degranulation of mast cells and basophils. Initial manifestations usually occur within 10 minutes of exposure to the antigen. Vasoactive mediators released by degranulation of mast cells and basophils are responsible for the clinical manifestations of anaphylaxis (Table 29-2). An urticarial rash and pruritus are likely in the patient who experiences anaphylaxis. Primary vascular collapse occurs in about 25% of cases of fatal anaphylaxis and is frequently associated with myocardial ischemia and cardiac dysrhythmias.[3] Extravasation of up to 50% of the intravascular fluid volume into the extracellular fluid space reflects the marked increases in capillary permeability.[4] Indeed, hypovolemia is a likely cause of hypotension in these patients, although negative inotropic actions of leukotrienes could also

Table 29-2. Vasoactive Mediators Released During Antigen-Antibody-Induced Degranulation

Vasoactive Mediator	Physiologic Effect
Histamine	Increased capillary permeability Peripheral vasodilation Bronchoconstriction
Leukotrienes	Increased capillary permeability Intense bronchoconstriction Negative inotropy Coronary artery constriction
Prostaglandins	Bronchoconstriction
Eosinophil chemotactic factor	Attraction of eosinophils
Neutrophil chemotactic factor	Attraction of neutrophils
Platelet activating factor	Platelet aggregation and release of vasoactive amines

play a role (Table 29-2). Laryngeal edema, bronchospasm, and arterial hypoxemia may accompany anaphylaxis.

Diagnosis

The diagnosis of anaphylaxis is suggested by the dramatic nature of the clinical manifestations in close temporal relationship to exposure to an antigen. When only a few symptoms are present, however, the response may mimic pulmonary embolism, acute myocardial infarction, aspiration, or a vasovagal reaction. Anesthetic drugs may alter vasoactive mediator release, possibly delaying early recognition of anaphylaxis.[5] Conversely, it is conceivable that blockade of the innervation of the adrenal glands could accentuate the symptoms of anaphylaxis by preventing the endogenous release of catecholamines. Importantly, hypotension may be the only manifestation of anaphylaxis in the patient rendered unconscious by general anesthesia[6] (Table 29-3). Indeed, large studies of anaphylaxis that occurs intraoperatively document the overwhelming predominance of cardiovascular collapse in affected patients.[4,7]

The initial in vivo response of the plasma IgE concentration during anaphylaxis is a decrease reflecting the complexing of antibody with newly injected antigen[8] (Fig. 29-3). After this initial decrease, there is often an overshoot of the plasma IgE

Table 29-3. Incidence of Clinical Signs of Anaphylaxis in Anesthetized Patients

Sign	Patients (%)
Circulatory collapse	68[a]
Widespread flush	55
Edema	26
Bronchospasm	23
Cardiac arrest	11

[a] Only sign in 10% of patients.

(Data from Laxenaire MC, Moneret-Vautrin DA, Boileau S, Moeller R. Adverse reactions to intravenous agents in anaesthesia in France. Klin Wochenchr 1982;60:1006–9.)

concentration. The absence of changes in the plasma concentration of complement proteins supports the occurrence of an allergic reaction due to anaphylaxis. Further biochemical proof of anaphylaxis is provided by an increase in the plasma tryptase concentration in a blood sample collected 15 to 60 minutes after the suspected allergic drug reaction.[9] Tryptase is a neutral protease stored in mast cells that is liberated into blood only if mast cell degranulation occurs. An increased plasma histamine concentration, measured in a blood sample obtained within minutes of a suspected allergic drug reaction, also provides evidence of anaphylaxis.

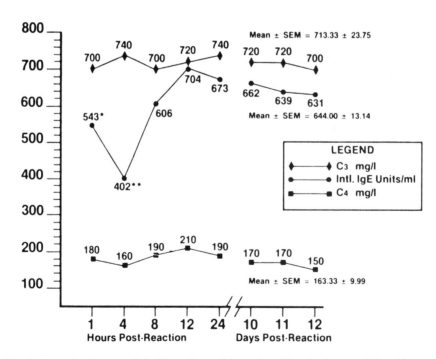

Fig. 29-3. A patient experiencing an anaphylactic reaction to thiopental manifested a decrease followed by an overshoot in the plasma concentration of immunoglobulin E (IgE). Concentrations of complement proteins C3 and C4 were unchanged. (From Lilly JK, Hoy RH. Thiopental anaphylaxis and reagin involvement. Anesthesiology 1980;53:335–7, with permission.)

Identification of the offending antigen is provided by a positive intradermal test (wheal and flare greater than 4 mm in diameter) that confirms the presence of specific IgE antibodies. This test, however, has an inherent risk, emphasizing the need to begin with injection of dilute preservative-free solutions of the suspected antigen (10 to 20 μl). The radioallergosorbent test (RAST) and enzyme-linked immunosorbent assay (ELISA) are commercially available antigen preparations that will combine with antibodies in the patient's plasma that are specific for the test antigen.[10] Detection of drug-specific antibodies by RAST analysis of serum obtained preoperatively from patients experiencing subsequent intraoperative fatal drug-induced allergic reactions (presumed on the basis of nonspecific findings) has been used to confirm the provisional postmortem diagnosis.[10] Two patients were documented to be allergic both to succinylcholine and to thiopental based on RAST analysis of their serum.[10]

Treatment

The three immediate goals in the treatment of anaphylaxis are reversal of arterial hypoxemia, replacement of intravascular fluid, and inhibition of further cellular degranulation with release of vasoactive mediators[11] (Table 29-4). Often 1 to 4 L of balanced salt solution or colloid solution, or both, must be infused rapidly to restore intravascular fluid volume and blood pressure. When anaphylaxis is life-threatening, epinephrine is indicated in doses of 10 to 100 μg IV.[12] Indeed, early intervention with intravenous administration of epinephrine is critical in reversing the life-threatening events characteristic of anaphylaxis. Epinephrine by increasing intracellular concentrations of cyclic adenosine monophosphate (cAMP) serves to restore membrane permeability and thus decrease release of vasoactive mediators. The beta agonist effects of epinephrine also serve to relax bronchial smooth muscle. The dose of epinephrine should be doubled and repeated every 1 to 3 minutes, until a satisfactory blood pressure response is obtained. This titration approach decreases the likelihood of undesirable overshoots in blood pressure by epinephrine. When anaphylaxis is not life-threatening, subcutaneous epinephrine (0.3 to 0.5 mg; 1:1000 dilution) is the standard adult dose.

Administration of an antihistamine such as diphenhydramine (50 to 100 mg IV) to an adult will compete for membrane receptor sites normally occupied by histamine and perhaps decrease manifestations of anaphylaxis, such a hypotension, edema, pruritus, and bronchospasm. There is no evidence,

Table 29-4. Treatment of an Anaphylactic Reaction

Supplemental oxygen
Balanced salt solution or colloid
Epinephrine
Diphenhydramine
Beta-2 agonist
Corticosteroid

however, that administration of an antihistamine is effective in treating anaphylaxis, once mediators have been released. Furthermore, bronchospasm or negative inotropic effects owing to leukotrienes will not be influenced by antihistamines. Anecdotal reports of reversal of life-threatening cardiovascular collapse following intravenous administration of cimetidine are suspect considering the possible beneficial effects of H-2 stimulation (inotropy, chronotropy, coronary vasodilation).[13,14] Furthermore, H-2 receptor stimulation exerts a negative feedback action to diminish further release of vasoactive mediators from basophils and mast cells. Beta-2 agonists such as albuterol delivered by a metered dose inhaler have replaced aminophylline in the treatment of bronchospasm associated with anaphylaxis.

Corticosteroids (cortisol or methylprednisolone) are often administered intravenously to the patient experiencing life-threatening anaphylaxis. Although these drugs have no known action on degranulation or antigen-antibody interaction, the favorable effects of corticosteroids may reflect an enhancement of the beta effects of other drugs and inhibition of the release of arachidonic acid responsible for the production of leukotrienes and prostaglandins. Corticosteroids may be uniquely beneficial in the patient experiencing a life-threatening allergic reaction due to activation of the complement system.

Allergic Rhinitis

Allergic rhinitis is an IgE-mediated inflammatory disease involving the nasal mucous membranes. Symptoms usually begin in childhood and are often seasonal when pollen (antigen) comes into direct contact with the respiratory tract mucosa, leading to the release of vasoactive mediators from submucosal mast cells. Nasal pruritus, rhinorrhea, lacrimation, and sneezing are common symptoms. These symptoms may be aggravated by nonspecific irritants such as cigarette smoke. Complicating inflammatory or infectious sinusitis may result in maxillofrontal headache, postnasal discharge, and persistent nasal stuffiness. Increased numbers of eosinophils in nasal secretions are often present, whereas increased numbers of eosinophils may be present in the peripheral blood of the patient with either allergic or nonallergic rhinitis. Atopic dermatitis is often associated with allergic rhinitis. Viral upper respiratory tract infection and hormonally related rhinitis (premenstrual or during pregnancy) may mimic allergic rhinitis, presenting a dilemma in the preoperative evaluation of the patient scheduled for elective surgery. In contrast to allergic rhinitis, symptoms of a viral respiratory tract infection are usually short-lived (less than 7 days) and include fever and the presence of neutrophils in nasal secretions.

Treatment

Treatment of allergic rhinitis includes avoidance of offending allergens, the use of antihistamines, and administration of allergen-specific immunotherapy. Terfenadine is an H-1 antagonist that has minimal sedative effects and is effective in the treatment of seasonal allergic rhinitis. In addition, a sympathomimetic drug (pseudoephedrine, phenylpropanolamine) may be useful for symptomatic relief. Increased blood pressure and heart rate may accompany the use of sympathomimetics for this purpose. Nasal inhalation of cromolyn or corticosteroids, or both may be useful for resistant cases. Nasal corticosteroids do not suppress the adrenal glands.

Allergic Conjunctivitis

Allergic conjunctivitis is the ocular equivalent of allergic rhinitis and reflects local mediator release as a result of an antigen-antibody interaction. Pruritus is usually a prominent symptom, and a history of allergic rhinitis is almost always present. Many topical preparations used to treat allergic conjunctivitis contain a combination of an antihistamine and a vasoconstrictor.

Allergic Asthma

Allergic asthma is manifested as reversible airway obstruction and bronchospasm accompanied by inflammation of the airways and increased bronchial smooth muscle reactivity (see Chapter 14). The response is triggered by specific allergens and may be aggravated by a viral infection, smoke, air pollution (sulfur dioxide), food preservatives (sodium metabisulfite), and certain drugs (aspirin, nonsteroidal anti-inflammatory drugs). Symptoms are highly variable but usually include wheezing, cough, and dyspnea. Treatment includes the administration of beta-2 agonists, corticosteroids, and cromlyn.

Food Allergy

Food allergy results from antibody-mediated degranulation of gastrointestinal tract mast cells, when exposed to a specific antigen. Abdominal pain and diarrhea are likely. Systemic anaphylaxis may occur within minutes or hours. Intraoperative anaphylactic reactions after the administration of protamine to neutralize heparin may be more likely in the patient allergic to seafood, emphasizing the derivation of this drug from salmon sperm.[15]

Drug Allergy

It is estimated that about 200,000 hospitalized patients experience allergic drug reactions annually in the United States, with another 50,000 annually hospitalized for the treatment of drug allergy.[16] Penicillin accounts for 90% of all allergic drug reactions and is responsible for 97% of all fatal anaphylactic drug reactions.[3] Drug sensitivity has been implicated in 4.3% of anesthetic-related deaths reported in the United Kingdom.[17,18] In Australia, such reactions occur once every 5000

to 25,000 anesthetics, with a 3.4% mortality.[17,18] The incidence of allergic drug reactions during anesthesia seems to be increasing, presumably reflecting the frequent administration of several drugs to the same patient, as well as cross-sensitivity between drugs. Allergic reactions to drugs may reflect anaphylaxis, drug-induced release of histamine (anaphylactoid), or activation of the complement system. In the same patient, more than one mechanism may be involved in the production of an allergic drug reaction. Regardless of the mechanism responsible for a life-threatening allergic drug reaction, the manifestations and treatment are identical (Tables 29-3 and 29-4).

It is not possible to predict reliably which patient is likely to experience anaphylaxis after administration of a drug that is usually innocuous. Nevertheless, patients with a history of allergy (asthma, food, drugs) have an increased incidence of anaphylaxis, primarily as a reflection of a genetic predisposition to form increased amounts of IgE antibodies. A patient allergic to penicillin has a three- to fourfold greater risk of experiencing an allergic reaction to any drug.[19] A history of allergy to specific drugs as elicited in the preoperative evaluation is helpful, but it must be appreciated that prior uneventful exposure to a drug such as thiopental does not eliminate the possibility of anaphylaxis on a subsequent exposure.[17,20–24] Initial injection of a small test dose of drug is more likely to unmask an idiosyncratic reaction than to prevent anaphylaxis. For example, 5 mg of protamine is equivalent to 60×10^{15} molecules. Although the severity of anaphylaxis is likely to be related to the total dose of antigen injected, the rarity of an allergic drug reaction does not support the routine use of test doses of drugs during the perioperative period.[25,26] Conversely, the magnitude of histamine release produced on reexposure to a drug that previously resulted in an anaphylactoid reaction can be decreased by reducing the dose of the drug and slowing its rate of infusion.[23] Since histamine is the principal vasoactive mediator released during an anaphylactoid reaction, it may be useful to provide prophylaxis during the preoperative period, to a patient who, on the basis of history, is deemed likely to display such a reaction. Prophylaxis may include a corticosteroid, and an H-1 and H-2 receptor antagonist, although severe allergic reactions can still occur.[27]

Allergic drug reactions must be distinguished from drug intolerance, idiosyncratic reactions, and drug toxicity (Table 29-5). The occurrence of an undesirable pharmacologic effect at a low dose of the drug reflects intolerance, whereas an idiosyncratic reaction is an undesirable response to a drug independent of the dose administered, and not a known pharmacologic effect of the drug. Evidence of histamine release along the vein in which a drug is injected reflects a localized and nonimmunologic release of histamine insufficient to evoke an anaphylactoid reaction. The patient manifesting this localized response should not be labeled as allergic to the drug. It is estimated that the plasma histamine concentration must

Table 29-5. Differential Diagnosis of Drug Allergy versus Drug Toxicity

	Drug Allergy	Drug Toxicity
Mechanism	Antigen-antibody interaction	Dependent on chemical properties of drug
Manifestations	Hypotension Bronchospasm Urticaria	Variable for each drug
Predictability	Poor	Good based on animal and human studies
Prior exposure	Required	Not required
Dose-related	No	Yes
Onset	Usually within 10 minutes	Usually delayed
Incidence	Low	High, especially if dose sufficient

double before hypotension occurs. Pretreatment with H-1 and H-2 receptor antagonists is more effective in controlling symptoms associated with local drug-induced histamine release than that accompanying an anaphylactoid reaction. Presumably, fewer vasoactive mediators are involved in a localized drug-induced response, with histamine the most important.

Perioperative Period

Allergic reactions have been reported with virtually all drugs that may be injected during the administration of anesthesia[7,16,17,23,24,28] (Table 29-6). The exception to this generalization may be ketamine and benzodiazepines.[29] Cardiovascular collapse is the predominant manifestation of a life-threatening allergic drug reaction in an anesthetized patient, whereas bronchospasm is present in fewer patients[6,7,28] (Table 29-3).

Table 29-6. Causes of Allergic Reactions During the Perioperative Period

Muscle relaxants
Barbiturates
Propofol
Local anesthetics (especially ester derivatives)
Opioids
Volatile anesthetics (especially halothane)
Protamine
Antibiotics
Blood and plasma volume expanders
Intravascular contrast media
Vascular graft material
Latex-containing medical devices

Muscle Relaxants

Drug-induced allergic reactions during the perioperative period are most often due to muscle relaxants.[30–34] It is estimated that 50% of patients who experience an allergic reaction to a muscle relaxant will also be allergic to another muscle relaxant.[33] Cross-sensitivity between muscle relaxants emphasizes the structural similarities of these drugs, especially the presence of one or more antigenic quarternary ammonium groups. Indeed, IgE antibodies to choline have been detected in patients who have experienced allergic reactions to succinylcholine and other muscle relaxants.[34] Drug-induced histamine release from mast cells and basophils is also a possibility with many of the muscle relaxants, especially when they are rapidly administered intravenously in large doses. Although structural similarities are not present, many patients who experience allergic reactions to succinylcholine are also allergic to penicillin.[31]

Induction Drugs

Allergic reactions after the administration of a barbiturate for the induction of anesthesia are rare (1 in about 30,000 anesthetics) but are often life-threatening. Most reported cases are in patients with a history of allergy (food allergy, rhinitis, asthma) but prior uneventful exposure to the barbiturate during anesthesia.[8,20,21] According to one report, an allergic reaction occurred after induction of anesthesia with thiamylal, despite the chronic uneventful use of an oral barbiturate.[22] As little as 10 µg of thiopental administered intravenously may induce evidence of anaphylaxis in a highly sensitized patient.[20] Allergic reactions may occur after administration of a thiobarbiturate or oxybarbiturate, although in vitro data suggest that methohexital is least likely to evoke the release of histamine.[35]

Life-threatening allergic reactions have occurred after the first or subsequent exposure to propofol.[28] Patients with a history of allergy to other drugs seem uniquely susceptible to propofol allergy, perhaps reflecting the presence of common allergenic groups (phenyl nucleus and isopropyl side chain) in propofol and other chemicals (muscle relaxants, local anesthetics, antibiotics, dermatologic preparations). An allergic reaction to etomidate differs from those of other drugs used for induction of anesthesia, in that symptoms are predominantly cutaneous or gastrointestinal in the absence of cardiopulmonary manifestations.

Local Anesthetics

Local anesthetic-induced allergic reactions are rare despite the frequent use of these drugs and the common labeling of a patient as allergic to a drug in this class. It is estimated that only 1% of all reactions to local anesthetics have an allergic mechanism.[36] The mechanism of an adverse response to a local anesthetic can often be determined by careful questioning of the patient and a review of the past medical record describing the event. For example, the occurrence of hypotension and seizures is characteristic of a systemic reaction due to an excessive blood level of the local anesthetic, as is most likely to occur with accidental intravascular injection during the performance of a regional anesthetic (epidural, brachial plexus, intercostal). This response is often erroneously attributed to an allergic reaction. Tachycardia and hypertension associated with injection of a local anesthetic most likely reflect the systemic absorption of epinephrine that was present in the local anesthetic solution. The rare patient who exhibits urticaria, laryngeal edema, and bronchospasm may well be experiencing a local anesthetic-induced allergic reaction.

An ester local anesthetic metabolized to the highly antigenic compound, para-aminobenzoic acid (PABA), is more likely than an amide local anesthetic that is not metabolized to PABA to evoke an allergic reaction.[37] The local anesthetic solution may also contain methylparaben or propylparaben as preservatives with bacteriostatic and fungistatic properties. The structural similarity of these preservatives to PABA may render them antigenic. As a result, anaphylaxis may be due to prior stimulation of antibody production by the preservative and not the local anesthetic.

A common clinical problem deals with the safety of administering a local anesthetic to a patient with a history of allergy to this class of drugs. It is generally agreed that cross-sensitivity does not exist between ester and amide local anesthetics. Therefore, it should be acceptable to administer an amide local anesthetic to the patient with an allergic history for an ester local anesthetic. The reverse of this recommendation would also be true. It must be remembered, however, that the use of a preservative-free local anesthetic solution is important, since these compounds may be responsible for an allergic reaction incorrectly attributed to the local anesthetic. All factors considered, it would seem reasonable to recommend intradermal testing with a preservative-free alternative local anesthetic in the occasional patient who describes a convincing allergic history and in whom failure to document a safe drug would prevent the use of local or regional anesthesia.

Opioids

Anaphylaxis that occurs after administration of opioids is rare, perhaps reflecting the similarity of these drugs to naturally present substances known as endorphins.[38] Fentanyl has produced signs of allergic responses after systemic or neuraxial administration.[39,40] According to one report, a second injection of fentanyl about 2 hours after the first failed to evoke symptoms of an allergic reaction; this suggests that the initial challenge had produced nearly complete degranulation, so that immediate rechallenge failed to produce any significant additional release of vasoactive mediators.[39] Morphine, but not fentanyl or its related derivatives, may directly evoke the release of histamine from mast cells and basophils, to produce an anaphylactoid reaction in a susceptible patient.

Volatile Anesthetics

Clinical manifestations of halothane hepatitis that suggest a drug-induced allergic reaction include eosinophilia, fever, rash, and prior exposure to halothane (see Chapter 18). More important, the plasma of the patient with a clinical diagnosis of halothane hepatitis may contain antibodies that react with halothane-induced liver antigens (neoantigens).[41] These neoantigens are formed by the covalent interaction of the reactive oxidative trifluoroacetyl halide metabolite of halothane with hepatic microsomal proteins. The acetylation of liver proteins in effect changes these proteins from self to non-self (neoantigens), resulting in the formation of antibodies against this now foreign protein. It is presumed that the subsequent antigen-antibody interaction is responsible for the liver injury associated with halothane hepatitis. The possibility of a genetic susceptibility factor is suggested by case reports of halothane hepatitis in closely related females. A similar oxidative halide metabolite is also produced after exposure to enflurane and isoflurane, emphasizing the possibility of cross-sensitivity between volatile anesthetics in susceptible patients.[42] Nevertheless, considering the magnitude of metabolism of these volatile drugs, it is predictable that the incidence of anesthetic-induced allergic hepatitis would be greatest after halothane, intermediate with enflurane, and least after the administration of isoflurane and desflurane. The development of an ELISA for the detection of antibodies evoked by acetylation of liver proteins would help detect the rare patient who has become sensitized from a prior exposure to a volatile anesthetic (most likely halothane), who is thus at presumed increased risk on subsequent exposure to other volatile anesthetics that are also metabolized to trifluoroacetic acid.[43]

Protamine

Anaphylactic reactions after administration of protamine may be more likely in the patient who is allergic to seafood (protamine is derived from salmon sperm) and in the patient with diabetes mellitus who is treated with a protamine-containing insulin preparation (PZI, NPH).[15,17,44,45] Presumably, small amounts of protamine in certain insulin preparations stimulate production of antibodies such that anaphylaxis occurs when large doses of protamine (antigen) are administered to neutralize the effects of heparin. Nevertheless, there are also data suggesting that the incidence of reactions to protamine is not increased in patients being treated with NPH insulin compared with nondiabetics.[46] Vasectomized or infertile males may have circulating antibodies to spermatozoa, but an increased risk of allergic reactions of protamine is undocumented and seems unlikely, since the antibody titers are very low. Protamine is also capable of directly evoking the release of histamine from cells; in susceptible patients, protamine may activate the complement pathway and evoke the release of thromboxane, leading to bronchoconstriction and pulmonary hypertension.[47] The patient known to be allergic to protamine presents a therapeutic dilemma when neutralization of heparin is required, since an alternative to protamine is not available.[48] Spontaneous dissipation of the anticoagulant effects of heparin is prolonged and may be associated with excessive blood loss, especially after successful weaning from cardiopulmonary bypass.

Antibiotics

Cross-sensitivity between penicillins and cephalosporins suggests caution in the administration of the latter to a patient known to be allergic to penicillin. Nevertheless, the current estimate of cross-sensitivity between these two classes of antibiotics (1.1% to 1.7%) is similar to the incidence of allergy to cephalosporins in the general population.[16] The patient with a history of penicillin-induced anaphylaxis, however, probably should not receive a cephalosporin, whereas the history of a penicillin-induced skin rash does not necessitate the same caution. Vancomycin may produce life-threatening allergic reactions in susceptible patients even when its administration rate is greatly slowed.[49–51]

Blood and Plasma Volume Expanders

Allergic reactions to properly cross-matched blood occur in about 3% of patients with manifestations ranging from pruritus, urticaria, and fever to noncardiogenic pulmonary edema (see Chapter 25). Synthetic plasma protein solutions (dextran, hydroxyethyl starch solutions) have been implicated in anaphylaxis and anaphylactoid reactions, with manifestations ranging from only a cutaneous rash and modest hypotension to shock and bronchospasm. Low-molecular-weight dextran cannot induce antibody formation, but this material may react with antibodies formed previously in response to exposure to polysaccharides of viral or bacterial origin. Dextran may also activate the complement system, producing signs of an allergic reaction.

Intravascular Contrast Media

Iodine in intravascular contrast media, as injected intravenously, for radiologic study, evokes an allergic reaction in about 5% of patients. The risk of an allergic reaction is probably increased in the patient with a history of allergies to other drugs or foods. Many of the allergic reactions to contrast media seem to be anaphylactoid and can be modified by pretreatment with corticosteroids, diphenhydramine, and limitation of the dose of iodine. A protective effect of H-2 receptor stimulation is suggested by a higher occurrence of repeat reactions when cimetidine, an H-2 antagonist, is added to the prophylaxis regimen.[52]

Vascular Graft Material

Profound vasodilation and hypotension accompanied by evidence of disseminated intravascular coagulation has been observed in association with the placement of vascular graft material.[53] Presumably, the plasticizers used to bind and combine the inert graft material together are responsible for the release of vasoactive mediators in rare but susceptible patients. Since transient hypotension is frequent following restoration of blood flow after aortic reconstruction grafting, it is possible that an allergic reaction may not be considered a possible explanation, even if hypotension is more severe or persistent than usual. Treatment consists of replacement of the graft with material produced by a different manufacturer.

Latex-Containing Medical Devices

Unexplained cardiovascular collapse during anesthesia and surgery has been attributed to anaphylaxis triggered by latex (natural rubber).[54–58] Proteins in the latex appear to be the source of antigens, especially if there is contact with mucous membranes. Questions about itching, rash, or wheezing after wearing latex gloves or inflating a toy balloon may be useful in identifying a sensitized patient. In this regard, up to 7% of surgical personnel and as many as 40% of spina bifida patients (perhaps reflecting frequent exposure to latex containing bladder catheters) are latex sensitive.[56,57] Patients in whom latex sensitivity is suspected may be referred to an allergist for appropriate skin testing and, if possible, for RAST evaluation for definitive diagnosis.[54] A feature that appears to distinguish latex-induced allergic reactions from reactions after the intravenous administration of drugs is the delayed onset (typically greater than 40 minutes) after the start of surgery. By contrast, most drug-induced allergic reactions occur within 10 minutes of intravenous administration of the drug. A latex reaction is presumed to require a period of time for the responsible allergenic protein to be eluted from the rubber gloves and absorbed into the circulation in amounts sufficient to cause a systemic reaction. In latex-sensitized patients, latex exposure can be prevented by the use of polyvinyl or neoprene surgical gloves and medical equipment made of either synthetic rubber or plastic.[54]

RESISTANCE TO INFECTION

There is abundant evidence that exposure to anesthesia and surgery alters many facets of immunocompetence.[59] Conceivably, depression of the immune system by anesthesia could increase the likelihood of the development of postoperative infections or of augmentation of a co-existing infection. For example, there is evidence that local and inhaled anesthetics (especially nitrous oxide) produce dose-dependent inhibition of mobilization and migration of polymorphonuclear leukocytes necessary for phagocytosis.[59,60] Nevertheless, the effects produced by these drugs are probably clinically insignificant, considering the usual duration of anesthesia and the doses of drugs administered. Indeed, the incidence of postoperative infection seems more likely to be related to surgical trauma and to an associated release of cortisol and catecholamines that are well known to inhibit phagocytosis. In the absence of surgical stimulation, anesthetic drugs are not predictably associated with increased circulating levels of cortisol or catecholamines. The consensus, based on available information, is that effects of anesthetics on resistance to infection are transient, reversible, and of minor importance, as compared with the prolonged immunosuppressive effects of cortisol and catecholamines released as part of the hormonal response to surgery.[59]

If the hormonal response to surgical stimulation is undesirable with respect to vulnerability to infection, it could be reasoned that light anesthesia, which does not reliably attenuate activity of the sympathetic nervous system, is less desirable than a deeper level of anesthesia. Evidence suggests that about 1.5 MAC halothane or enflurane, or greater than 1 mg·kg^{-1} of morphine, is necessary to prevent the sympathetic nervous system response to surgical skin incision in 50% of patients.[61] A sternal incision requiring cutting of bone seems to need even more anesthesia to block sympathetic nervous system responses. Regional anesthesia may also reduce the hormonal response to surgical stimulation.[60] Despite these observations, there is no evidence that the incidence of postoperative infection can be altered by the depth of anesthesia or by the techniques selected to produce anesthesia.

The possible bacteriostatic effects of anesthetic drugs must also be considered. Local anesthetics have been shown to have such effects on a wide variety of organisms at concentrations achievable with topical application.[60] The clinical implications of this observation are that topical anesthesia, used for bronchoscopy, could reduce the incidence of positive cultures. Conversely, concentrations of local anesthetics in the circulation, in association with regional anesthesia or after intravenous administration, do not alter bacterial growth. Likewise, volatile anesthetics do not have bacteriostatic effects.[60] Liquid volatile anesthetics, however, may be bactericidal. Volatile anesthetics in doses as low as 0.2 MAC produce dose-dependent inhibition of measles virus replication and reduce mortality in mice receiving intranasal influenza virus.[62]

RESISTANCE TO CANCER

Immunocompetence is essential for host resistance to cancer. It is a clinical impression that some patients with the preoperative diagnosis of cancer experience rapid growth of the tumor after anesthesia and surgery. Conceivably, drugs administered to produce anesthesia could enhance tumor cell replication and spread by depressing host resistance. Despite this concern, there is no evidence that short-term effects of anesthetic drugs are of any significance in the resistance of the host to cancer.[63] As with infection, the more important concern is immunosuppression produced by the hormonal response to surgical stimulation. If the hormonal response is indeed undesirable with respect to host resistance to cancer, it would seem logical to suppress this response with either regional or deep general anesthesia. It should be emphasized, however, that there is no evidence to support the validity of this speculation.

In contrast to the concern in patients with cancer, immunosuppression secondary to the hormonal response produced by surgical stimulation could be beneficial for the patient undergoing an organ transplant. Nevertheless, if such benefit does occur, it is probably too small or transient to be of any significance during the early transplant period.

DISORDERS OF THE IMMUNOGLOBULINS

X-Linked Agammaglobulinemia

X-linked agammaglobulinemia (congenital agammaglobulinemia) is a genetically transmitted disease characterized by recurrent bacterial infection, decreased to absent plasma concentrations of all classes of Ig, and an inability to produce antibodies even in response to intense antigenic stimulation[64] (Table 29-1). Infants are born with maternal IgG, so manifestations of the disease are not seen before about 9 months of age. As the name implies, only males are affected, although rare cases with similar clinical features have been described in females. The principal defect appears to be the absence of mature B lymphocytes, such that antibodies cannot be produced (Fig. 29-1). By contrast, T lymphocytes are normal, and cell-mediated immunity (graft rejection) is intact (Fig. 29-1). *Pneumocystitis carinii* pneumonia may be the presenting manifestation of this disease. Recurrent infections may lead to chronic sinusitis and bronchiectasis.

Treatment of X-linked agammaglobulinemia consists of intravenous or intramuscular administration of gamma globulin, to maintain the plasma IgG concentration close to 400 to 500 mg·dl^{-1}.[65] The half-time of IgG used in this manner is about 30 days, which is longer than normal, emphasizing the relationship of the catabolism of IgG to the amount of IgG (Table 29-1). The presence of infection results in more rapid catabolism of IgG. Antibiotics are indicated when bacterial infection occurs.

Acquired Hypoimmunoglobulinemia

Acquired hypoimmunoglobulinemia does not appear to be genetically determined and is usually not manifested until after puberty. Symptoms and treatment are the same as for X-linked agammaglobulinemia. This syndrome is associated with autoimmune diseases and malabsorption syndrome.

Selective Immunoglobulin A Deficiency

Selective IgA deficiency occurs in 1 of every 600 to 800 adults. In this condition, the plasma IgA concentration is less than 5 mg·dl^{-1} but the concentration of other immunoglobulins is normal (Table 29-1). Recurrent sinus and pulmonary infections are the most common symptoms, although many patients are asymptomatic and remain undetected until they are screened as potential blood donors. About 40% of these patients produce anti-IgA antibodies and may experience life-threatening anaphylaxis when transfused with blood containing IgA. Therefore, these patients should only receive blood or blood components obtained from an IgA-deficient donor.

Cold Autoimmune Diseases

Cold autoimmune diseases are characterized by the presence of abnormal circulating proteins that may agglutinate in response to decreases in body temperature[66] (Table 29-7).

Cryoglobulinemia

Cryoglobulinemia is a disorder in which circulating abnormal proteins (cold agglutinins or cryoglobulins) precipitate on exposure to cold, leading to activation of the complement pathway, platelet aggregation, and consumption of clotting factors. Hyperviscosity of the plasma is prominent, and acute renal failure may accompany microvascular thrombosis. Indeed, renal dysfunction eventually occurs in more than 20% of patients. Normally, symptoms occur only when blood temperature decreases below about 33°C.

Management of Anesthesia

Management of anesthesia in the patient with cryoglobulinemia includes maintenance of body temperature above the thermal reactivity of the cryoglobulin during the perioperative period.[67] This goal is facilitated by increasing the ambient temperature of the operating room, using a warming blanket, and ventilating the lungs with warmed and humidified gases. Passing intravenous fluids through a blood warmer before delivery to the patient also decreases the loss of body heat during anesthesia.

The patient scheduled for an operation requiring cardiopulmonary bypass may present a significant challenge.[66] Clearly, the introduction of systemic hypothermia may be contraindicated, while use of cold cardioplegia solutions may cause intracoronary hemagglutination with inadequate distribution of cardioplegia solutions, thrombosis, ischemia, or infarction. An alternative to cold cardioplegia is ischemic arrest for short periods of time. In such patients, preoperative plasmapheresis is effective in greatly decreasing the plasma level of cryoglobulins. Efforts to maintain body temperature above the thermal reactivity of the cryoglobulin must also be maintained into the postoperative period.

Cold Hemagglutinin Disease

Cold hemagglutinin disease is characterized by the presence of IgM autoantibodies in the plasma that react with antigens on erythrocytes. This reaction may activate the complement

Table 29-7.   Cold Autoimmune Diseases

	Thermal Reactivity (°C)	Associated Conditions	Response to Cold Exposure
Cryoglobulinemia	17–33	Macroglobulinemia	Hyperviscosity Platelet aggregation Renal failure
Cold hemagglutinin disease	15–32	None	Acrocyanosis Hemolysis Raynaud's phenomenon
Paroxysmal cold hemoglobinuria	10–15	Syphilis	Hemolysis Jaundice Renal failure
Acquired cold autoimmune disease	4–25	Mycoplasma Mononucleosis Leukemia	Acrocyanosis Hyperviscosity Hemolysis

system, leading to severe intravascular hemolysis. Cold hemagglutinins may predispose to vascular occlusion in exposed, and therefore chilled, areas of the body. The diagnosis of cold hemagglutinin disease is suggested by hemolytic anemia and signs of vascular occlusion. Treatment may include infusion of packed erythrocytes that are warmed to decrease the likelihood of cold hemagglutinin. Exchange transfusions and plasmapheresis may be useful when acute hemolysis is occurring. Occasionally, high doses of corticosteroids are useful in decreasing the degree of hemolysis. Management of anesthesia in a patient with this disorder is as described for cryoglobulinemia.

Multiple Myeloma

Multiple myeloma (plasma cell myeloma) is characterized by the neoplastic proliferation of single-clone immunoglobulin-secreting cells. These cells invade bone marrow, causing thrombocytopenia, neutropenia, anemia, and increased susceptibility to infection. Bone is eroded diffusely, often producing painful fractures and vertebral collapse. Extension into the spinal cord produces extradural compression that may require urgent laminectomy to prevent permanent spinal cord transection. Computed tomography and magnetic resonance imaging are useful in evaluating the extent of bone lesions. Hypercalcemia from destruction of bone can lead to central nervous system depression and renal dysfunction. Deposition of an abnormal protein (Bence Jones protein) in the renal tubules may also contribute to renal dysfunction. Extramedullary sites of malignant plasma cell infiltration include the liver, spleen, nasopharynx, and paranasal sinuses. Inactivation of plasma procoagulants by myeloma protein may interfere with coagulation. This protein may also prolong the bleeding time by interfering with platelet function. Peripheral neuropathy may reflect segmental demyelination. Unexplained high-output congestive heart failure has also been observed in these patients.[68] The impaired immune response is associated with an increased susceptibility to infection.

Treatment

The treatment of multiple myeloma includes the use of chemotherapeutic drugs and corticosteroids, in an effort to decrease proliferation of plasma cells. Prevention of dehydration is important if hypercalcemia is present. Hypercalcemia requires prompt treatment with intravenous infusion of saline and administration of furosemide, while in life-threatening situations the administration of plicamycin may be indicated (see Chapter 21). Bed rest is avoided, as inactivity leads to mobilization of calcium and the formation of venous thrombi due to venous stasis. Localized radiation is used for painful lytic lesions, especially those that produce spinal cord compression. Decompression laminectomy is performed if evidence of spinal

cord compression progresses despite treatment. Plasmapheresis is usually effective in decreasing viscosity of the blood, such as before a blood transfusion to treat anemia. Because the patient with multiple myeloma has functional hypogammaglobulinemia, the administration of gamma globulin may be used to prevent or treat bacterial infection.

Management of Anesthesia

The presence of compression fractures emphasizes the need for caution in positioning such a patient during anesthesia and surgery. Postoperatively, pathologic fractures of the ribs may impair ventilation and predispose to the development of pneumonia. Altered responses to drugs owing to abnormal circulating immunoglobulins plus hypoalbuminemia are a theoretical but undocumented concern.

Waldenström's Macroglobulinemia

Waldenström's macroglobulinemia is due to proliferation of a malignant plasma cell clone that secretes IgM, resulting in a marked increase in plasma viscosity. The bone marrow is infiltrated with malignant lymphocytes, as are the liver, spleen, and lungs. Anemia and an increased incidence of spontaneous hemorrhage are frequent findings in these patients. In contrast to multiple myeloma, Waldenström's macroglobulinemia rarely involves the skeletal system. As a result, renal dysfunction due to hypercalcemia is unlikely to occur.

Treatment of Waldenström's macroglobulinemia consists of plasmapheresis to remove the abnormal protein and diminish the viscosity of the plasma. This is especially important before the transfusion of blood that may abruptly increase the hematocrit and viscosity of the plasma. Chemotherapy is also instituted in an attempt to decrease proliferation of the cells responsible for the production of abnormal immunoglobulins.

Amyloidosis

Amyloidosis encompasses several disorders characterized by the accumulation of insoluble fibrillar proteins (amyloid) in various tissues, including the heart, vascular smooth muscle, kidneys, adrenal glands, gastrointestinal tract, peripheral nerves, and skin.[69] Macroglossia may cause problems in swallowing and speaking and could interfere with visualization of the glottic opening by direct laryngoscopy. Salivary gland involvement with extension into adjacent skeletal muscles can produce upper airway obstruction and mimic angioneurotic edema. Cardiac involvement may be manifested as disturbances in the conduction of the cardiac impulse and the appearance of life-threatening heart block. Renal involvement with amyloid results in the nephrotic syndrome. Amyloid deposition in joints causes pain and limitation of motion. Sensory and motor disturbances may reflect the involvement of peripheral nerves. Carpal tunnel syndrome may occur as a result of median nerve compression. Infiltration of autonomic nervous system nerves is manifested as delayed gastric emptying and postural hypotension. Amyloidosis of the gastrointestinal tract may produce malabsorption, ileus, hemorrhage, and intestinal obstruction. Hepatosplenomegaly is a common finding, but hepatic dysfunction is infrequent. Amyloid deposits may trap factor X or evoke fibrinolysis, leading to an increased likelihood of bleeding.

The development of amyloidosis is frequently associated with multiple myeloma, rheumatoid arthritis, and a prolonged antigenic challenge, as produced by a chronic infection. The diagnosis of amyloidosis is confirmed by biopsy of an involved organ. In this regard, the frequent presence of amyloid deposits in the wall of the rectum makes rectal biopsy an important diagnostic test. Treatment of amyloidosis is generally ineffective, although an occasional patient may benefit from chemotherapy. Cardiac amyloidosis seems particularly resistant to therapy. Renal transplantation may be a consideration in the patient with amyloid-induced renal failure.

Hyperimmunoglobulinemia E Syndrome

Hyperimmunoglobulinemia E (Job) syndrome is a rare disorder characterized by recurrent bacterial infections of the skin, sinuses, and lungs, with IgE plasma concentrations at least 10 times normal and neutrophils having a variable chemotactic defect. Most infections are due to *Staphylococcus aureus*. Bacteremia may occur, and mucocutaneous candidiasis is likely. Despite antibiotic therapy, these patients are likely to present repeatedly for surgical drainage of abscesses. Management of anesthesia must consider the risk of epidural abscess, if an epidural or spinal anesthetic is recommended.[70] A prolonged response to succinylcholine in the absence of an obvious explanation has been described in a patient with this syndrome.[71]

Wiskott-Aldrich Syndrome

Wiskott-Aldrich syndrome is inherited as an X-linked recessive disease, thus affecting only males. The syndrome is characterized by thrombocytopenia, eczema, and increased susceptibility to infection. Thrombocytopenia is the result of rapid platelet destruction caused by an intrinsic defect in the platelet. Presenting features are usually related to thrombocytopenia and associated hemorrhage. The plasma concentration of IgM is often decreased. Treatment consists of platelet transfusions, as thrombocytopenia is resistant to corticosteroids and is not improved by splenectomy.

Ataxia Telangiectasia

Ataxia telangiectasia is characterized by progressive cerebellar ataxia beginning in childhood, recurrent sinus and pulmonary infections, and the subsequent development of telan-giectasia of the bulbar conjuctivae. Most patients are found to have absent or decreased plasma concentrations of IgA and IgE. The function of T lymphocytes may also be impaired, and there is a high incidence of lymphoma in these patients. Skin manifestations may include café-au-lait spots and sclerodermoid changes. Disorders of glucose metabolism may be present. A familial incidence suggests that this disease is inherited as an autosomal recessive disorder.

DISORDERS OF THE COMPLEMENT SYSTEM

Hereditary Angioedema

Hereditary angioedema is a rare autosomal dominant disorder due to decreased functional activity of the plasma protein known as C1 esterase inhibitor (Fig. 29-2). In the absence of this inhibitor, the initial activation of the complement pathway is not regulated, leading to the release of vasoactive mediators (possibly bradykinin) that increase vascular permeability. As such, hereditary angioedema is characterized by episodic and painless edema of the skin (face and limbs) and mucous membranes (respiratory and gastrointestinal tract). Laryngeal edema is the most dangerous manifestation and can lead to airway obstruction and death. Abdominal cramps may reflect edema in the small intestine and, on occasion, falsely suggests the need for an exploratory laparotomy. An attack may occur spontaneously but is more often initiated by trauma, particularly a dental procedure, or conceivably direct laryngoscopy and tracheal intubation. Emotional upset and anxiety have also been associated with the onset of an acute attack. A typical attack lasts 48 to 72 hours. The diagnosis of hereditary angioedema is on the basis of family history, clinical manifestations, and documentation of low or absent plasma levels of C1 esterase inhibitor. About 15% of patients with this disease have normal levels of C1 esterase inhibitor, but the functional activity of the protein is zero.

Medical Management

The medical management of hereditary angioedema includes long-term prophylaxis, short-term prophylaxis, and the treatment of an acute attack.[72]

Long-Term Prophylaxis

Long-term prophylaxis is not necessary in every patient, being reserved for those with a history of repeated debilitating attacks associated with facial and laryngeal edema. The two classes of drugs administered for long-term treatment include antifibrinolytics (aminocaproic acid, tranexamic acid) and anabolic steroids (danazol, stanazolol). Antifibrinolytics are thought to act by inhibiting plasmin activation, whereas anabolic steroids are believed to increase hepatic synthesis of C1 esterase inhibitor. Several days of drug treatment are needed with each of these classes of drugs to achieve a therapeutic effect. Children and parturients are rarely treated because of the harmful side effects (masculanization, hepatic dysfunction) that may accompany the use of these drugs.

Short-Term Prophylaxis

Short-term prophylaxis is indicated for the patient with hereditary angioedema who is not receiving long-term prophylaxis but who is scheduled for a traumatic procedure close to the airway (dental surgery, tracheal intubation). Such therapy can be provided by a 2- to 3-day course of an anabolic steroid before surgery or by the use of fresh frozen plasma, or both. Fresh frozen plasma is a source of C1 esterase inhibitor; 2 units administered on the day before surgery can prevent airway swelling during the intraoperative and postoperative periods. A purified preparation of C1 esterase inhibitor administered intravenously is as effective as fresh frozen plasma and does not introduce the risk of viral hepatitis.[73]

Acute Attack

No specific treatment is available to interrupt an acute attack of hereditary angioedema, and efficacy is difficult to determine, as attacks are self-limited and end unpredictably. The patient is unlikely to respond favorably to epinephrine, corticosteroids, or antihistamines while antifibrinolytic and anabolic steroid therapy is of no major benefit during an acute attack. It is theoretically possible that fresh frozen plasma, in addition to providing C1 esterase inhibitor, would also provide substrates such as C2 and C4, enhancing the acute attack. In practice, however, this does not seem to occur.[74] Alternatively, the purified preparation of C1 esterase inhibitor may be useful in abating symptoms of an acute attack when administered intravenously.[73] Should airway obstruction develop during an acute attack of hereditary angioedema, a tube should be placed in the trachea, until the edema involving the airway subsides.

Management of Anesthesia

The key to management of anesthesia in the patient with hereditary angioedema is adequate preoperative prophylaxis with anabolic steroids or fresh frozen plasma, or both.[72,74] In this regard, it has been recommended that 2 units of fresh frozen plasma be administered the evening before surgery to any patient in whom airway trauma, including tracheal intubation, is anticipated.[72] If the patient is receiving prophylactic therapy, these drugs are continued through the perioperative period. Incidental trauma to the upper airway, as produced by an oropharyngeal airway or suctioning, should be minimized. Intramuscular injections do not seem to cause any unique problems in these patients. A regional anesthetic technique is

a reasonable consideration if its selection will eliminate the predictable need for tracheal intubation. Nevertheless, intubation of the trachea with a cuffed tube should not be avoided in these patients, if its placement will contribute to the safe conduct of the anesthetic. The choice of drugs to produce regional or general anesthesia is not influenced by the presence of hereditary angioedema.

Complement Protein C2 Deficiency

Complement protein C2 deficiency occurs in about 1 of every 10,000 patients. About one-half of these patients have a history of systemic lupus erythematosus or a related disorder such as Henoch-Schönlein purpura. This association may reflect a viral origin for these diseases and complement participation in viral neutralization.

Complement Protein C3 Deficiency

Complement protein C3 deficiency is associated with increased susceptibility to life-threatening bacterial infections. Complement-mediated functions, such as bactericidal activity, chemotaxis, and opsonization, are absent in C3-deficient plasma. A patient who is homozygous for C5–C8 complement protein deficiency may also display increased susceptibility to infection.

AUTOIMMUNE DISEASE

Autoimmune disease occurs when the host's own tissues act as self-antigens to evoke the production of autoantibodies[75] (Table 29-8) (see Chapter 26). The resulting antigen-antibody interaction produces tissue injury. Normally, T lymphocytes are responsible for blocking antibody production to host antigen. Failure of suppressor T lymphocytes to prevent antibody productivity by B lymocytes may result in autoimmune disease. Cyclosporine suppresses immune responses by inhibiting helper T lymphocytes but does not inhibit antigen-induced activation of suppressor T lymphocytes. In this regard, cyclosporine may be useful in the management of an autoimmune disease such as insulin dependent (type 1) diabetes mellitus characterized by the production of autoantibodies to insulin receptors. It is possible that self-antigens are modified by combining with a drug (hydralazine, procainamide) or viruses and then stimulate antibody production. A similar mechanism may occur when streptococcal antigens induce formation of antibodies to heart valves (rheumatic fever) or neuronal tissue (Sydenham's chorea) in a genetically susceptible patient. Myasthenia gravis is characterized by the development of autoantibodies to acetylcholine receptors at the neuromuscular junction. The patient with Graves' disease may produce auto-

Table 29-8.   Examples of Autoimmune Diseases

Organ-Specific Diseases
  Insulin dependent (type 1) diabetes mellitus
  Myasthenia gravis
  Graves' disease
  Thyroiditis
  Addison's disease
  Pernicious anemia
  Male infertility
  Primary biliary cirrhosis
  Chronic active hepatitis
  Crohn's disease
  Autoimmune hemolytic anemia
  Psoriasis

Systemic Diseases
  Rheumtic fever
  Rheumatoid arthritis
  Ankylosing spondylitis
  Systemic lupus erythematosus
  Scleroderma
  Polymyositis
  Goodpasture syndrome
  Chronic graft-versus-host disease
  Hypereosinophilic syndrome
  Lyme disease
  Kawasaki disease
  Immunoglobulin A deficiency
  Hereditary complement deficiency
  Vasculitis
  Sarcoidosis

antibodies that act on receptors, leading to increased synthesis of cAMP. Vasculitis is often part of an autoimmune disease, being limited to a single organ such as the kidneys or becoming generalized.

REFERENCES

1. Frank MM. Complement in the pathophysiology of human disease. N Engl J Med 1987;316:1525–30
2. Baron S, Tyring SK, Fleischmann WR, et al. The interferons: Mechanisms of action and clinical applications. JAMA 1991;266:1375–83
3. Delage C, Irey NS. Anaphylactic deaths: A clinicopathologic study of 43 cases. J Forensic Sci 1972;17:525–30
4. Fisher MM. Anaphylaxis. Dis Mon 1987;33:433–79
5. Kettelkamp NS, Austin DR, Cheek DBC, Downes H, Hirshman C. Inhibition of d-tubocurarine-induced histamine release by halothane. Anesthesiology 1987;66:666–9
6. Laxenaire MC, Moneret-Vautrin DA, Boileau S, Moeller R. Adverse reactions to intravenous agents in anaesthesia in France. Klin Wochenchr 1982;60:1006–9
7. Schatz M, Fung DL. Anaphylactic and anaphylactoid reactions due to anesthetic agents. Clin Rev Allergy 1986;4:215–21
8. Lilly JK, Hoy RH. Thiopental anaphylaxis and reagin involvement. Anesthesiology 1980;53:335–7
9. Laroche D, Vergnaud M-C, Sillard B, Soufarapis H, Bicard H. Biochemical markers of anaphylactoid reactions to drugs. Anesthesiology 1991;75:945–9
10. Fisher MM, Baldo BA, Silbert BS. Anaphylaxis during anesthesia: Use of radioimmunoassays to determine etiology and drugs responsible in fatal cases. Anesthesiology 1991;75:1112–5
11. Sage DJ. Management of acute anaphylactoid reactions. Int Anesthesiol Clin 1985;23:175–86
12. Barach EM, Nowak RM, Lee TG, Tomlanovich MC. Epinephrine for treatment of anaphylactic shock. JAMA 1984;251:2118–22
13. Kelly JS, Prielipp RC. Is cimetidine indicated in the treatment of acute anaphylactic shock? Anesth Analg 1990;71:100–6
14. DeSoto H, Turk P. Cimetidine in anaphylactic shock refractory to standard therapy. Anesth Analg 1989;69:264–5
15. Knape JTA, Schuller JL, deHaan P, et al. An anaphylactic reaction to protamine in a patient allergic to fish. Anesthesiology 1981;55:324–5
16. Pallasch TJ. Principles of pharmacotherapy. III. Drug allergy. Anesth Prog 1988;35:178–89
17. Weiss ME, Adkinson NF, Hirshman CA. Evaluation of allergic drug reactions in the perioperative period. Anesthesiology 1989;71:483–6
18. Fisher MMcD, More DG. The epidemiology and clinical features of anaphylactic reactions in anaesthesia. Anaesth Intensive Care 1981;9:226–34
19. Saxon A, Beall GN, Rohr S, Adelman DC. Immediate hypersensitivity reactions to beta lactam antibiotics. Ann Intern Med 1987;107:204–15
20. Etter MS, Helrich M, Mackenzie CF. Immunoglobulin E fluctuation in thiopental anaphylaxis. Anesthesiology 1980;52:181–3
21. Wyatt R, Watkins J. Reaction to methohexitone. Br J Anaesth 1975;47:119–20
22. Thompson DS, Eason CN, Flacke JW. Thiamylal anaphylaxis. Anesthesiology 1973;39:556–8
23. Beaven MA. Anaphylactoid reactions to anesthetic drugs. (Editorial.) Anesthesiology 1981;55:3–5
24. Moudgil GC. Anaesthesia and allergic drug reactions. Can Anaesth Soc J 1986;33:400–14
25. Oh TE, Horton JM. Adverse reactions to atracurium. Br J Anaesth 1989;62:467
26. Bochner BS, Lichtenstein LM. Current concepts: Anaphylaxis. N Engl J Med 1991;324:1785–91
27. Bruno LA, Smith DS, Bloom MJ, et al. Sudden hypotension with a test dose of chymopapain. Anesth Analg 1984;63:533–5
28. Laxenaire M-C, Mata-Bermejo E, Moneret-Vautrin DA, Gueant J-L. Life-threatening anaphylactoid reactions to propofol. Anesthesiology 1992;77:275–80
29. Mathieu A, Goudsouzian N, Snider MT. Reaction to ketamine: Anaphylactoid or anaphylactic? Br J Anaesth 1975;47:624–7
30. Farmer BC, Sivarajan M. An anaphylactoid response to a small dose of d-tubocurarine. Anesthesiology 1979;51:358–9
31. Ravindran RS, Klemm JE. Anaphylaxis to succinylcholine in a patient allergic to penicillin. Anesth Analg 1980;59:944–5

32. Mishima S, Yamamura T. Anaphylactoid reaction to pancuronium. Anesth Analg 1984;63:865–6

33. Harle DG, Baldo BA, Fisher MM. Cross-reactivity of metocurine, atracurium, vecuronium and fazadinium with IgE antibodies from patients unexposed to these drugs but allergic to other myoneural blocking drugs. Br J Anaesth 1985;57:1073–6

34. Harle DG, Baldo BA, Fisher MM. Detection of IgE antibodies to suxamethonium after anaphylactoid reactions during anaesthesia. Lancet 1984;1:930

35. Hirshman CA, Edelstein RA, Ebertz JM, Hanifin JM. Thiobarbiturate-induced histamine release in human skin mast cells. Anesthesiology 1985;63:353–6

36. DeShazo RD, Nelson HS. An approach to the patient with a history of local anesthetic hypersensitivity: Experience with 90 patients. J Allergy Clin Immunol 1979;63:387–94

37. Brown DT, Beamish D, Wiedsmith JAW. Allergic reaction to an amide local anaesthetic. Br J Anaesth 1981;53:435–7

38. Levy JH, Rockoff MA. Anaphylaxis to meperidine. Anesth Analg 1982;61:301–3

39. Bennett MJ, Anderson LK, McMillan JC, et al. Anaphylactic reaction during anaesthesia associated with positive intradermal skin test to fentanyl. Can Anaesth Soc J 1986;33:75–8

40. Zucker-Pinchoff B, Ramanathan S. Anaphylactic reaction to epidural fentanyl. Anesthesiology 1989;71:599–601

41. Hubbard AK, Roth TP, Gandolfi AJ, Brown BR, Webster NR, Nunn JF. Halothane hepatitis patients generate an antibody response toward a covalently bound metabolite of halothane. Anesthesiology 1988;68:791–6

42. Christ DD, Kenna JG, Kammerer W, Satoh H, Pohl LR. Enflurane metabolism produces covalently bound liver adducts recognized by antibodies from patients with halothane hepatitis. Anesthesiology 1988;69:833–8

43. Martin JL, Kenna JG, Pohl LR. Antibody assays for the detection of patients sensitized to halothane. Anesth Analg 1990;70:154–9

44. Moorthy SS, Pond W, Rowland RG. Severe circulatory shock following protamine (an anaphylactic reaction). Anesth Analg 1980;59:77–8

45. Weiss ME, Nyhan D, Peng Z, et al. Association of protamine IgE and IgG antibodies with life-threatening reactions to intravenous protamine. N Engl J Med 1989;320:886–92

46. Levy JH, Schwieger IM, Zaidan JR, Farey BA, Weintraub WS. Evaluation of patients at risk for protamine reactions. J Thorac Cardiovasc Surg 1989;98:200–4

47. Morel DR, Zapol WM, Thomas ST, et al. C5a and thromboxane generation associated with pulmonary vaso- and bronchoconstriction during protamine reversal of heparin. Anesthesiology 1987; 66:597–604

48. Campbell FW, Goldstein MF, Akins PC. Management of the patient with protamine hypersensitivity for cardiac surgery. Anesthesiology 1984;61:761–4

49. Symons NLP, Hobbes AFT, Leaver HK. Anaphylactoid reactions to vancomycin during anaesthesia: Two clinical reports. Can Anaesth Soc J 1985;32:178–81

50. Mayhew JF, Deutsch S. Cardiac arrest following administration of vancomycin. Can Anaesth Soc J 1985;32:65–6

51. Lyon GD, Bruce DL. Diphenhydramine reversal of vancomycin-induced hypotension. Anesth Analg 1988;67:1109–10

52. Greenberger PA, Patterson R, Tapio CM. Prophylaxis against repeated radiocontrast media reactions in 857 cases. Arch Intern Med 1985;145:2192–2200

53. Roizen MF, Rodgers GM, Valone FH, et al. Anaphylactoid reactions to vascular graft material presenting with vasodilation and subsequent disseminated intravascular coagulation. Anesthesiology 1989;71:331–8

54. Hirshman CA. Latex anaphylaxis. Anesthesiology 1992;77:223–5

55. Calenda E, Durand JP, Petit J, et al. Anaphylactic shock produced by latex. Anesth Analg 1991;72:839–45

56. Sussman GL, Tarlo S, Dolovich J. The spectrum of IgE-mediated responses to latex. JAMA 1991;265:2844–7

57. Moneret-Vautrin DA, Laxenaire MC, Bavoux F. Allergic shock to latex and ethylene oxide during surgery for spina bifida. Anesthesiology 1990;73:556–8

58. Slater JE. Rubber anaphylaxis. N Engl J Med 1989;320:1126–30

59. Walton B. Effects of anaesthesia and surgery on immune status. Br J Anaesth 1979;51:37–43

60. Duncan PG, Cullen BF. Anesthesia and immunology. Anesthesiology 1976;45:522–38

61. Roizen MF, Horrigan RW, Frazer BM. Anesthetic doses blocking adrenergic (stress) and cardiovascular responses to incision—MAC BAR. Anesthesiology 1981;54:390–8

62. Knight PR, Bedows E, Nahrwold ML, et al. Alterations in influenza virus pulmonary pathology induced by diethyl ether, halothane, enflurane, and pentobarbital anesthesia in mice. Anesthesiology 1983;58:209–15

63. Lewis RE, Cruse JM, Hazelwood J. Halothane-induced suppression of cell-mediated immunity in normal and tumor-bearing C3Hf/He mice. Anesth Analg 1980;59:666–71

64. Fosen FS, Cooper MD, Wedgwood RJP. The primary immunodeficiencies. N Engl J Med 1984;311:235–42

65. Buckley RH, Schiff RI. The use of intravenous immune globulin in immunodeficiency diseases. N Engl J Med 1991;325:110–7

66. Park JV, Weiss CI. Cardiopulmonary bypass and myocardial protection: Management problems in cardiac surgical patients with cold autoimmune disease. Anesth Analg 1988;67:75–8

67. Diaz JH, Cooper ES, Ochsner JL. Cardiac surgery in patients with cold autoimmune diseases. Anesth Analg 1984;63:349–52

68. McBride W, Jackman JD, Gammon RS, et al. High-output cardiac failure in patients with multiple myeloma. N Engl J Med 1988; 319:1651–6

69. Mizutani AR, Ward CF. Amyloidosis associated bleeding diatheses in the surgical patient. Can J Anaesth 1990;37:910–2

70. Miller FL, Mann DL. Anesthetic management of a pregnant patient with the hyperimmunoglobulin E (Job's) syndrome. Anesth Analg 1990;70:454–6

71. Guzzi LM, Stamatos JM, Job's syndrome: An unusual response to a common drug. Anesth Analg 1992;75:139–40

72. Wall RT, Frank M, Hahn M. A review of 25 patients with hereditary angioedema requiring surgery. Anesthesiology 1989;71:309–11

73. Gadek JE, Hosea SW, Gelfand JA, et al. Replacement therapy in hereditary angioedema. Successful treatment of acute episodes of angioedema with partly purified C1 inhibitor. N Engl J Med 1980;302:542–6

74. Poppers PJ. Anaesthetic implications of hereditary angioneurotic oedema. Can J Anaesth 1987;34:76–8

75. Dalakas MC. Polymyositis, dermatomyositis, and inclusion-body myositis. N Engl J Med 1991;325:1487–98

30

Psychiatric Illness and Substance Abuse

The prevalence of psychiatric illness increases the likelihood that such disorders will be present as co-existing problems in patients requiring anesthesia. An important consideration is the potential drug interactions introduced by the medications used in the treatment of psychiatric illness. Substance abuse and drug dependence may also be viewed as a psychiatric illness.

MENTAL DEPRESSION

Mental depression is the most common psychiatric disorder (affects 2% to 4% of the adult population), distinguished from normal sadness and grief by the severity and duration of the mood disturbance and the presence of fatigue, loss of appetite, and insomnia. Any patient with depression who has had a manic episode is classified as having bipolar disease or manic-depressive disorder. There is a familial pattern of major depression, and females are affected most often. Among patients with major depression, about 15% commit suicide. The pathophysiologic causes of major depression are unknown, although abnormalities of amine neurotransmitter pathways are the most likely etiologic factors. Cortisol hypersecretion may be present in about 50% of patients with major depressive illness.

The diagnosis of major depression is based on the persistent presence of at least five characteristics and the exclusion of organic causes or a normal reaction to the death of a loved one (Table 30-1). Alcoholism and major depression often occur together; it is presumed that toxic effects on the brain are responsible. Depression and dementia may be difficult to distinguish in an elderly patient. All depressed patients should be evaluated for their potential to commit suicide. In the United States, suicide is the tenth leading cause of death and for

physicians younger than 40 years of age, it ranks first. More than 90% of overdose suicide victims have been under the care of a physician shortly before their death, emphasizing the importance of recognizing at-risk patients. Hopelessness is the most important aspect of depression associated with suicide.

Treatment

Treatment of mental depression is with antidepressant drugs or electroconvulsive therapy (ECT).[1] An estimated 70% to 80% of patients respond to antidepressants, and at least 50% who do not respond to medication respond favorably to ECT. In this regard, ECT is generally reserved for the patient who is resistant to antidepressant drugs or for the patient with a medical contraindication to antidepressant drugs. The patient with mental depression plus psychotic symptoms (delusions, hallucinations, catatonia) requires both an antidepressant and antipsychotic drug. The concept that antidepressants work by increasing the availability of norepinephrine and serotonin is not supported by the fact that these drugs are not effective for 14 to 28 days despite an immediate effect on neurotransmitter uptake. Instead, the effects of these drugs on regulation of neurotransmitter receptor function over several days is a more likely mechanism of the therapeutic effects.

Tricyclic Antidepressants

Tricyclic antidepressants are often administered as the initial treatment of mental depression because their use, unlike monoamine oxidase inhibitors, does not require dietary restriction. Side effects of antidepressant drugs influence drug choice because all these drugs are equally effective if used in

Table 30-1. Characteristics of Major Depression

Depressed mood
Decreased interest in daily activities and physical appearance
Fluctuations in body weight
Insomnia or hypersomnia
Fatigue
Decreased ability to concentrate
Recurrent thoughts of suicide

an adequate dose (Table 30-2). Generally, a drug producing sedation is chosen for the patient describing insomnia. It is useful to minimize drug-induced anticholinergic effects (blurred vision, dry mouth, delayed gastric emptying, urinary retention, tachycardia), especially in an elderly patient or in those with glaucoma or prostate hypertrophy. All tricyclic antidepressants evoke some anticholinergic effects, with the most pronounced effects accompanying the use of amitriptyline and protriptyline. In addition to causing sedative and anticholinergic effects, tricyclic antidepressants can cause cardiovascular abnormalities, including orthostatic hypotension and cardiac dysrhythmias. Tricyclic antidepressants tend to slow both atrial and ventricular depolarization manifested as an increase in the P-R and Q-T interval and widening of the QRS complex on the electrocardiogram. These changes on the electrocardiogram, in the absence of an excessive plasma concentration of the drug, are probably benign and gradually disappear with continued therapy[2] (see the section, Tricyclic Antidepressant Overdose). Previous suggestions that tricyclic antidepressants increase the risk of cardiac dysrhythmias and sudden death have not been substantiated in the absence of drug overdose. Even in the presence of co-existing cardiac dysfunction, tricyclic antidepressants lack adverse effects on left ventricular function and may even possess cardiac antidysrhythmic properties.[3,4] Nevertheless, it is possible that a patient with co-existing heart block or prolonged Q-T interval on the electrocardiogram may be at increased risk of cardiac toxicity. Decreased cardiac toxicity for doxepin has not been confirmed.[5] The polycyclic drug maprotiline has a tendency to cause seizures at the upper therapeutic dose range.[6]

It is usually possible to taper the dose of antidepressant drug in a patient with a primary depressive illness who has been free of symptoms for about 6 months. A few patients require long-term treatment, whereas the patient whose depression is secondary to a treatable medical illness may require only a short course of antidepressant therapy. If tricyclic antidepressant treatment is contraindicated because of the patient's cardiac status, ECT or trazodone treatment may be recommended.

Management of Anesthesia

Treatment with a tricyclic antidepressant need not be discontinued before administration of anesthesia for an elective operation. Alterations in response to drugs administered during the perioperative period, however, should be anticipated in the treated patient. For example, the increased availability of neurotransmitters in the central nervous system can result in increased anesthetic requirements.[7] Likewise, the increased availability of norepinephrine at postsynaptic receptors in the peripheral sympathetic nervous system can be responsible for an exaggerated blood pressure response after administration

Table 30-2. Tricyclic Antidepressants and Related Antidepressants

Drug	Sedative Potency	Anticholinergic Potency	Orthostatic Hypotension	Cardiac Dysrhythmia Potentiation
Tricyclics				
Doxepin	+ + +	+ +	+ +	+ +
Amitriptyline	+ + +	+ + + +	+ + +	+ +
Imipramine	+ +	+ +	+ + +	+ +
Protriptyline	+	+ + +	+	+ +
Nortriptyline	+	+	+	+ +
Desipramine	+	+	+ + +	+ +
Related polycyclics				
Anixaoube	+	+	+ +	+ +
Malprotiline	+ +	+	+ +	+ +
Atypical drugs				
Fluoxetine	+	0	0	+
Trazodone	+ + +	+	+ + +	+
Alprazolam	+ + +	0	0	0

0, none; +, low; + +, moderate; + + +, high; + + + +, marked.

of an indirect-acting vasopressor such as ephedrine. If a vasopressor is required during the perioperative period, a direct-acting drug such as phenylephrine may be useful. If hypertension requires treatment, a peripheral vasodilator such as nitroprusside is effective. The potential for hypertensive crises is greatest during acute treatment (first 14 to 21 days) with tricyclic antidepressants, whereas chronic treatment is associated with down-regulation of receptors and a decreased likelihood of exaggerated blood pressure responses after administration of a sympathomimetic.[8] The electrocardiogram is used to detect cardiac conduction abnormalities produced by tricyclic antidepressants. Atropine may be an appropriate therapy for the initial management of atrioventricular heart block.

Chronic therapy with an antidepressant may alter the response to pancuronium. For example, tachydysrhythmias have been observed after administration of pancuronium to patients anesthetized with halothane who were also receiving imipramine.[9] In dogs chronically treated with imipramine, administration of pancuronium has resulted in tachycardia and ventricular dysrhythmias[9] (Fig. 30-1). Similar cardiac dysrhythmias in dogs did not occur when anesthesia was maintained with enflurane. Presumably, there is an interaction between the tricyclic antidepressant and the anticholinergic or sympathetic nervous system stimulating effect of pancuronium, or both. Theoretically, ketamine might produce a similar adverse response to pancuronium when administered in the presence of a tricyclic antidepressant. The dose of exogenous epinephrine necessary to produce ventricular dysrhythmias during anesthesia with a volatile anesthetic may be decreased by prior acute treatment with imipramine.[10] Therefore, it is conceivable that treatment with a tricyclic antidepressant could also accentuate the arrhythmogenic potential of absorbed epinephrine, as present in the local anesthetic solution injected in the performance of a peripheral nerve block or epidural anesthesia. Conversely, chronic imipramine therapy does not alter the cardiac dysrhythmia potential, presumably because of compensating mechanisms occurring at the sympathetic nerve endings.[11]

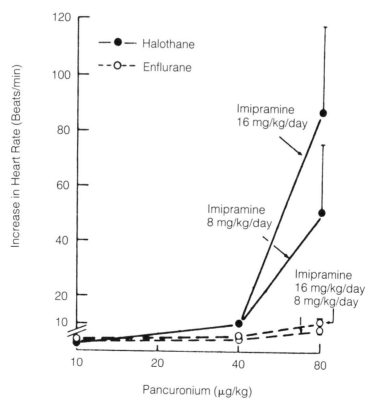

Fig. 30-1. Chronic administration of imipramine is associated with dose-related increases in heart rate after administration of pancuronium to dogs anesthetized with halothane but not enflurane. (From Edwards RP, Miller RD, Roizen MF, et al. Cardiac responses to imipramine and pancuronium during anesthesia with halothane or enflurane. Anesthesiology 1979;50:421–5, with permission.)

Maintenance of anesthesia with enflurane in a patient taking a tricyclic antidepressant is questionable, since both drugs produce evidence of seizure activity on the electroencephalogram (EEG). Indeed, clonic movements during administration of a low inspired concentration of enflurane have been observed in patients receiving amitriptyline.[12] It is speculated that enflurane-induced seizure activity in these patients is enhanced by the presence of amitriptyline. In animals, tricyclic antidepressants augment the analgesic and ventilatory depressant effects of opioids, as well as the sedative effects of barbiturates. If these responses occur in patients as well, it is possible that doses of these drugs should be decreased to avoid exaggerated or prolonged effects, or both.[13] Postoperatively, the likelihood of delerium and confusion might be increased by the additive anticholinergic effects of tricyclic antidepressants and centrally active anticholinergic drugs used for preoperative medication.

Atypical Antidepressant Drugs

Fluoxetine, trazodone, and alprazolam are effective antidepressant drugs but are structurally unrelated to tricyclic or tetracyclic antidepressants. Fluoxetine is relatively free of anticholinergic effects and appears to produce orthostatic hypotension and cardiac conduction disturbances less often than do tricyclic antidepressants. Hypotension, nausea, and sedation are the most common side effects of trazodone. Alprazolam is devoid of cardiac and anticholinergic side effects.

Monoamine Oxidase Inhibitors

The patient who does not respond to tricyclic antidepressants may benefit from treatment with monoamine oxidase inhibitors (MAOI) (phenelzine, isocarboxazid, tranylcypromine). In contrast to tricyclic antidepressants, MAOI have negligible anticholinergic effects and do not sensitize the heart to the arrhythmogenic effects of epinephrine. The principal clinical problem associated with the use of these drugs is the possible occurrence of severe hypertension if a treated patient ingests foods that contain tyramine (cheeses, wines) or receives drugs characterized as sympathomimetics (Table 30-3). Hypertension reflects the inhibition of the enzymatic activity of

monoamine oxidase, which results in increased availability of norepinephrine. Therefore, sympathomimetic drugs such as ephedrine, which act by stimulating the release of norepinephrine, can precipitate hypertension. Likewise, tyramine in foods acts as a potent stimulus for the release of norepinephrine, explaining the association of hypertension if a susceptible patient ingests tyramine-containing food. Orthostatic hypotension is the most common side effect observed in patients being treated with MAOI. The mechanism for this hypotension is unknown, but it may reflect accumulation of a false neurotransmitter such as octopamine, which is less potent than norepinephrine. This mechanism may also explain antihypertensive effects observed with the chronic use of MAOI.

Although uncommon, adverse interactions between MAOI and opioids have been observed.[14,15] Hypertension, hypotension, hyperthermia, depression of ventilation, seizures, and coma may follow the administration of an opioid to the patient being treated with a MAOI. Meperidine has been the most often incriminated opioid, but the same syndrome can occur with other opioids. Explanations for these adverse responses include decreased metabolism of the opioid, mass sympathetic nervous system discharge caused by the opioid, the formation of toxic opioid metabolites, and increased central nervous system concentrations of serotonin.

Management of Anesthesia

In the past, it was recommended that MAOI be discontinued at least 14 to 21 days before elective surgery, to permit the synthesis of a new enzyme.[14,15] This is probably not a realistic recommendation, as discontinuing the MAOI, as before ECT, may put the patient at increased risk of suicide. In fact, there is a growing appreciation that anesthesia can be safely administered to the patient being treated chronically with MAOI.[14–16]

Proceeding with anesthesia and elective surgery in a patient being treated with a MAOI may influence the selection of drugs and doses administered. Opioids should probably be avoided in the preoperative medication of the patient being treated with a MAOI. Likewise, in the absence of a specific indication, the inclusion of an anticholinergic in the preoperative medication is unnecessary. A benzodiazepine is appropriate for relief of preoperative anxiety. Induction of anesthesia can be safely accomplished with drugs administered intravenously, keeping in mind that central nervous system effects and depression of ventilation may be exaggerated. The exception to this generalization would be ketamine, in view of the ability of this drug to stimulate the sympathetic nervous system. The possible decrease in plasma cholinesterase activity associated with phenalzine treatment suggests the need to adjust the dose of succinylcholine.[15] Nitrous oxide combined with a volatile anesthetic is acceptable for maintenance of anesthesia. The selection of a specific volatile anesthetic may be influenced by its ability to evoke cardiac dysrhythmias in the

Table 30-3.   Side Effects of Monoamine Oxidase Inhibitor Treatment

Sedation
Blurred vision
Orthostatic hypotension
Peripheral neuropathy
Hypertension in response to ingestion of tyramine-containing foods
Hyperthermia in response to opioid administration

presence of catecholamines and by the possibility of MAOI-induced hepatic dysfunction, as reflected by liver function tests. It is conceivable, but unproved, that anesthetic requirements would be increased, owing to increased amounts of norepinephrine present in the central nervous system. Fentanyl has been administered intraoperatively to these patients without apparent adverse effect.[14,15] Selection of a nondepolarizing muscle relaxant is not influenced by treatment with MAOI, with the possible exception of pancuronium. Spinal or epidural anesthesia is acceptable, although the potential for these techniques to produce hypotension and the consequent need for a vasopressor may mitigate in favor of general anesthesia.[17] Epinephrine added to the local anesthetic solution should probably be avoided when a regional anesthetic technique is selected.

During anesthesia and surgery, the avoidance of stimulation of the sympathetic nervous system, as produced by arterial hypoxemia, hypercarbia, hypotension, topical cocaine spray, or injection of an indirect-acting vasopressor, is important for decreasing the incidence of hypertension or cardiac dysrhythmias, or both.[18] If a vasopressor is required, a direct-acting agent such as phenylephrine is recommended. Even with this drug, the dose should probably be decreased to minimize the likelihood of an exaggerated hypertensive response. Nevertheless, ephedrine has also been administered without any apparent adverse effect.[15] In this regard, the potential for hypertensive crises is greatest during acute treatment (first 14 to 21 days) with MAOI, whereas chronic treatment is associated with down-regulation of receptors and a decreased likelihood of exaggerated blood pressure responses after administration of a sympathomimetic.[8]

The provision of analgesia during the postoperative period is influenced by the potential adverse interaction between opioids and MAOI. If an opioid is required for postoperative analgesia, morphine or fentanyl is the preferred drug, but the dose should be the least amount necessary to produce pain relief. An alternative to an opioid for provision of postoperative analgesia includes administration of nonopioid analgesics, peripheral nerve blocks with local anesthetics, and the use of transcutaneous electrical nerve stimulation. Neuraxial opioids provide effective analgesia, but experience is too limited to permit a recommendation regarding use of this approach in a patient being treated with MAOI.

Electroconvulsive Therapy

ECT is indicated for the treatment of severe mental depression in a patient who is unresponsive to drugs or who becomes acutely suicidal.[19–21] The only contraindication to ECT is increased intracranial pressure. To minimize memory impairment, ECT is often administered only to the nondominant hemisphere. ECT administered in the brief-pulse waveform uses only one-third to one-fourth the voltage used by ECT administered in the sine waveform. Although the mechanism of action of ECT is unknown, it is likely that therapeutic efficacy is related to the amount of current passed. The previous concept that the therapeutic benefit of ECT depended on the duration of the seizure is not supported by controlled studies.[22] The electrical stimulus produces a grand mal seizure consisting of a brief tonic phase, followed by a more prolonged clonic phase. The EEG shows changes similar to those present during a spontaneous grand mal seizure. Typically, about eight treatments are necessary, with more than 75% of treated patients showing a favorable response.

Side Effects

The side effects of ECT are manifested principally on the cardiovascular and central nervous system[21] (Table 30-4). For example, an initial vagal discharge may lead to bradycardia with a decrease in blood pressure, followed by sympathetic nervous system activation and increased heart rate and blood pressure. These changes may be undesirable in a patient with ischemic heart disease. Indeed, the most common cause of mortality after ECT is myocardial infarction and cardiac dysrhythmias.[23] Ventricular premature beats presumably reflect excess sympathetic nervous system activity. Increased T wave amplitude on the electrocardiogram simulating hyperkalemia may accompany ECT, presumably reflecting an imbalance of autonomic nervous system activity, as electrically induced seizure activity is not known to cause the release of potassium.[24] Venous return to the heart is decreased by the increased intrathoracic pressure that accompanies the seizure or positive-pressure ventilation of the lungs, or both. Cardiac morbidity, which approaches 0.03%, is thought to reflect activation of the sympathetic and parasympathetic nervous system by the electrical shock and resultant seizure.[25] There is evidence, however, that the electrical stimulus, and not the seizure, is responsible for the cardiovascular response to ECT.[26]

Cerebral blood flow increases up to sevenfold, reflecting

Table 30-4. Physiologic Effects of Electroconvulsive Therapy

Parasympathetic nervous system stimulation
Bradycardia
Hypotension
Sympathetic nervous system stimulation
Tachycardia
Hypertension
Cardiac dysrhythmias
Increased cerebral blood flow
Increased intracranial pressure
Increased intraocular pressure
Increased intragastric pressure
Hypoventilation

increased cerebral oxygen consumption in the presence of the seizure. The resulting increase in intracranial pressure is transient but may prohibit the use of ECT in a patient with a known space-occupying lesion or head injury. An elevation in intraocular pressure is an inevitable side effect of an electrically induced seizure and may detract from the use of this therapy in a patient with glaucoma. Increased intragastric pressure also occurs during seizure activity. Transient apnea plus postictal confusion may follow the seizure. The most common long-term effect of ECT is memory impairment.

Management of Anesthesia

Anesthesia is usually administered to ensure patient comfort and safety during ECT.[19] The patient is fasted, but preanesthetic medication is not recommended, as drug-produced sedation could prolong the period of recovery after ECT. Administration of atropine or glycopyrrolate intravenously 1 to 2 minutes before the induction of anesthesia and delivery of the electrical current may be useful for decreasing the likelihood of bradycardia that may accompany ECT. A centrally acting anticholinergic such as atropine may have an additive effect with the central and peripheral anticholinergic effects of tricyclic antidepressants, manifested as delirium and confusion during the postanesthetic period. For this reason, glycopyrrolate may be recommended when ECT is administered to a patient being treated with a tricyclic antidepressant. Nevertheless, many patients have safely undergone ECT without prior administration of an anticholinergic drug.[21] Nitroglycerin ointment applied 45 minutes before ECT decreases the magnitude of treatment-induced hypertension and thus may be useful in the patient considered to be at risk of myocardial ischemia.[27] Likewise, esmolol (100 to 200 mg IV) administered 1 minute before the induction of anesthesia and 2 minutes before ECT is effective in attenuating the increase in blood pressure and heart rate following ECT.[28,29] The duration of seizure activity is shortened by the higher dose of esmolol. Monitoring of the electrocardiogram is useful in recognizing ECT-induced cardiac dysrhythmias.

Methohexital (0.5 to 1 mg·kg^{-1} IV) is a frequent choice for the induction of anesthesia before ECT. Thiopental has no advantage over methohexital and might be associated with a longer recovery time. Indeed, prior treatment of a patient with tricyclic antidepressants or MAOI could enhance the depressant effects of a barbiturate. Propofol (1.5 mg·kg^{-1} IV) is an alternative to methohexital, being associated with a lower blood pressure and heart rate in response to ECT compared with the barbiturate.[30] Recovery time is similar after methohexital and propofol, but an anticonvulsant effect of propofol is suggested by a shortened duration of the electrically induced seizure in patients receiving this drug[30] (Fig. 30-2).

The intravenous injection of succinylcholine promptly after the induction of anesthesia for ECT is intended to attenuate potentially dangerous skeletal muscle contractions and bone

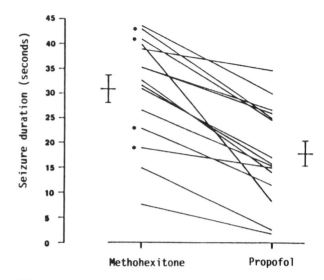

Fig. 30-2. The mean duration of an electrically induced seizure in the same patient was longer in the presence of methohexitone (methohexital) than in the presence of propofol. The lines labeled with an asterisk (*) represent patients receiving treatment with a benzodiazepine. The bars represent mean ± SE for each drug. (From Rampton AJ, Griffin RM, Stuart CS, Durcan JJ, Huddy NC, Abbott MA. Comparison of methohexital and propofol for electroconvulsive therapy: Effects of hemodynamic responses and seizure duration. Anesthesiology 1989;70:412–7, with permission.)

fractures that could be produced by seizure activity. Although the amount of succinylcholine administered varies, a dose of 0.3 to 0.5 mg·kg^{-1} IV is usually sufficient to attenuate contraction of skeletal muscles adequately and still permit visual confirmation of seizure activity. The surest way to document the occurrence of an electrically induced seizure is to record the EEG. Alternatively, the movement of an arm isolated from the circulation with a tourniquet before the administration of succinylcholine is evidence that a seizure has occurred. Pretreatment with a nonparalyzing dose of a nondepolarizing muscle relaxant before the administration of succinylcholine has not been evaluated in these patients. Support of ventilation of the lungs with supplemental oxygen is recommended both before the production of the seizure and until the effects of succinylcholine have dissipated. Denitrogenation of the lungs with oxygen before production of the seizure decreases the likelihood that arterial hypoxemia will develop if it becomes difficult to support ventilation of the lungs in the presence of seizure-induced skeletal muscle contractions. Furthermore, it is important to recognize that apnea lasting up to 2 minutes can follow ECT in the absence of succinylcholine. Monitoring of arterial hemoglobin oxygen saturation with a pulse oximeter is useful in guiding the need for supplemental oxygen and mechanical support of ventilation in the patient undergoing

ECT. The use of a peripheral nerve stimulator will confirm the degree of neuromuscular blockade produced by succinylcholine and will also identify the patient with previously unrecognized atypical cholinesterase enzyme. Since repeated anesthetics will be necessary, it is possible to establish a dose of anesthetic induction drug and succinylcholine that produces the most predictable and desirable effects in each patient. Succinylcholine-induced myalgia is remarkably uncommon, occurring in only about 2% of treated patients undergoing ECT. There is no evidence that succinylcholine-induced release of potassium is increased by ECT.[24]

Occasionally, ECT is necessary in a patient with a permanently implanted artificial cardiac pacemaker. Fortunately, most artificial cardiac pacemakers are shielded and are not adversely affected by the electrical current necessary to produce a seizure. Nevertheless, it would seem prudent to have an appropriate external magnet available to ensure the capability of converting the pacemaker to an asynchronous mode, should malfunction occur. In addition, continuous monitoring of the electrocardiogram, use of a Doppler sensor, and palpation of a peripheral arterial pulse document the uninterrupted function of the artificial cardiac pacemaker.

Safe and successful use of ECT has been described in a patient after successful cardiac transplantation.[31] In such a patient, the lack of vagal innervation to the heart eliminates the risk of bradydysrhythmia. Increased heart rate and blood pressure can still occur as a reflection of catecholamine release in response to the electrically induced seizure.

MANIA

Mania is an autosomal dominant disease with variable penetrance manifesting clinically as a sustained period of mood elevation and in severe cases delusions and hallucinations (Table 30-5). Presumably, there are abnormalities in a neuroendocrine pathway resulting in aberrant regulation of one or more amine neurotransmitter systems. This hypothesis is consistent with the observation that the therapeutic effects of drugs occur over a period of 14 to 28 days rather than immediately, which would be the case if the disease was caused by an excess or deficiency of a specific neurotransmitter.

Table 30-5. Manifestations of Mania

Inflated self-esteem
Decreased need for sleep
Flight of ideas
Short attention span
Increased verbalization

Treatment

Mania necessitates prompt treatment with lithium, which requires about 14 days before improvement is noted. When manic symptoms are severe, lithium is usually administered in combination with an antipsychotic (haloperidol) until the acute symptoms abate, allowing tapering and discontinuation of the antipsychotic.

Lithium

Lithium is efficiently absorbed after oral administration; its therapeutic plasma concentration for acute mania is 1 to 1.2 $mEq \cdot L^{-1}$ and for prophylaxis is 0.6 to 0.8 $mEq \cdot L^{-1}$. Toxicity is likely when the plasma concentration of lithium exceeds 2 $mEq \cdot L^{-1}$ manifested as skeletal muscle weakness, ataxia, sedation, and widening of the QRS complex on the electrocardiogram. Atrioventricular heart block, hypotension, and seizures may accompany severe toxicity. Monitoring of the plasma lithium concentration by flame photometry about 12 hours after the last oral dose is recommended so as to decrease the likelihood of toxicity. The therapeutic effect of lithium is most likely related to an action on the second-messenger system based on phosphatidylinositol turnover. Lithium also affects transmembrane ion pumps and has inhibitory effects on adenylate cyclase.

Lithium inhibits release of thyroid hormones and results in hypothyroidism in about 5% of patients. Long-term administration of lithium occasionally results in a vasopressin-resistant diabetes insipidus-like syndrome (polyuria, polydipsia) that resolves when the drug is discontinued. T wave flattening or inversion on the electrocardiogram may occur, but these changes are considered benign. Cardiac conduction disturbances are rare, although patients with co-existing sinus node dysfunction should probably have an artificial cardiac pacemaker in place before initiating treatment with lithium. Leukocytosis in the range of 10,000 to 14,000 $cells \cdot mm^{-3}$ is possible in the lithium-treated patient.

Lithium is excreted almost entirely by the kidneys. Resorption of lithium occurs at proximal convoluted renal tubules and is inversely related to the concentration of sodium in the glomerular filtrate. For this reason, administration of a loop or thiazide diuretic, which enhances the renal excretion of sodium, will increase the resorption of lithium and thus increase the plasma concentration of lithium by as much as 50%. Administration of sodium-containing solutions or an osmotic diuretic, or both, will favor the renal excretion of lithium in the patient who shows evidence of lithium toxicity.

Carbamazepine

Carbamazepine is an anticonvulsant that is particularly useful in treating the patient who is unresponsive to lithium. Side effects of this drug include leukopenia, aplastic anemia, and hepatotoxicity, emphasizing the importance of performing periodic blood counts and liver functions tests.

Management of Anesthesia

Evidence of lithium toxicity is important to consider in the preoperative evaluation of a treated patient.[32] A recent plasma lithium concentration measurement may be helpful. In view of the potential resorption of lithium in the presence of a decreased sodium concentration, it is reasonable to administer sodium-containing intravenous solutions during the perioperative period. Likewise, stimulation of urine output with a loop or thiazide diuretic could adversely increase the plasma lithium concentration. Inclusion of lithium in the measurement of electrolytes during the perioperative period is reasonable. Likewise, the electrocardiogram is useful for recognizing adverse effects of an excessive plasma lithium concentration on the conduction of cardiac impulses. The association of sedation with lithium therapy suggests that anesthetic requirements for injected and inhaled drugs may be decreased. Indeed, sedative effects of lithium plus the absence of cardiopulmonary depression is the rationale for considering the use of this drug for preoperative medication.[33] Monitoring of neuromuscular blockade is indicated, as the duration of action of succinylcholine and nondepolarizing muscle relaxants may be prolonged in the presence of lithium.[34]

SCHIZOPHRENIA

Schizophrenia is the most common psychotic disorder, accounting for about 20% of all persons treated for mental illness. The hallmark of schizophrenia is psychosis, characterized by delusions, hallucinations, catatonic behavior, and inappropriate affect. The disease is chronic, marked by acute exacerbations and progressive impairment between episodes.

Treatment

Treatment of schizophrenia is with an antipsychotic drug, which most likely exerts its therapeutic effect by inhibition of binding of dopamine at postsynaptic dopamine receptors (Table 30-6). Extrapyramidal symptoms, orthostatic hypotension, and sedation are potential responses that can accompany treatment with an antipsychotic drug. Acute dystonia (contraction of the skeletal muscles of the neck, mouth, and tongue, tremor) responds to the administration of diphenhydramine (25 to 50 mg IV). The most serious side effect of treatment with an antipsychotic drug is tardive dyskinesia, characterized by involuntary choreoathetoid movements. Tardive dyskinesia usually develops after several months of treatment with an antipsychotic drug and may be irreversible, es-

Table 30-6.   Drugs Used in the Treatment of Schizophrenia

Phenothiazines
  Chlorpromazine
  Triflupromazine
  Thioridazine
  Fluphenazine

Thioxanthenes
  Chlorprothixene
  Thiothixene

Butyrophenones
  Haloperidol

Indolones
  Molindone

pecially in an elderly patient. Orthostatic hypotension is more likely when a high dose of antipsychotic drug produces alpha blockade. This may be an important consideration in the management of anesthesia, since intraoperative decreases in blood pressure could be exaggerated, especially with acute blood loss or positive-pressure ventilation of the lungs, since compensatory sympathetic nervous system-mediated vasoconstriction is attenuated by drug-induced alpha blockade. Rarely, an antipsychotic drug may prolong the Q-T interval on the electrocardiogram and predispose to ventricular tachycardia.[35] The presence of sedation preoperatively may parallel decreased anesthetic requirements. Cholestasis was observed early in the clinical use of chlorpromazine but rarely seems to occur with the current use of this drug.

Neuroleptic Malignant Syndrome

Neuroleptic malignant syndrome is an infrequent idiosyncratic reaction to an antipsychotic drug that develops hours to months after exposure to the drug and does not appear to be dose related.[36] Droperidol and metoclopramide administered as a single injection to an otherwise normal patient has also evoked this syndrome.[37] Signs of neuroleptic malignant syndrome appear over a 24- to 72-hour period and include skeletal muscle rigidity, hyperthermia, altered level of consciousness, and autonomic nervous system instability (tachycardia, labile blood pressure, cardiac dysrhythmias, diaphoresis). The patient is usually confused and may experience fluctuating levels of consciousness. Skeletal muscle spasm may so decrease chest wall compliance that mechanical support of ventilation becomes necessary. Skeletal muscle damage may produce an increase in the plasma concentration of creatine kinase. Renal failure may occur from myoglobinuria and dehydration. For unknown reasons, liver function tests are often abnormal. This syndrome is believed to be caused by dopamine blockade in the hypothalamus, basal ganglia, and brain stem, resulting in a disturbance of central thermal regulation. Despite some similarities to malignant hyperthermia, there is no pathophysiologic link between the two syndromes.[38] Indeed, succinylcholine can be safely administered to a patient receiving ECT for the treatment of neuroleptic malignant syndrome without an increased risk of evoking malignant hyperthermia.[39] Nevertheless, in vitro skeletal muscle contracture testing demonstrates responses similar to those present in the patient susceptible to malignant hyperthermia.[40] Skeletal muscle rigidity associated with this syndrome has been treated with dantrolene, dopamine agonists such as bromocriptine, and nondepolarizing muscle relaxants. Mortality may approach 20%, with causes of death including cardiac dysrhythmias, congestive heart failure, hypoventilation, renal failure, and thromboembolism. A patient who resumes treatment with an antipsychotic after recovery from this syndrome is likely to experience a recurrence.

ANXIETY DISORDERS

Anxiety disorders can be a response to exogenous stimuli (situational anxiety, pain, angina pectoris) or endogenous stimuli (Table 30-7). Anxiety resulting from an identifiable stress is usually self-limited and rarely requires pharmacologic treatment. Nevertheless, for the patient whose anxiety is unusually severe, a short course of low-dose benzodiazepine therapy (diazepam 5 mg orally three times daily) is often helpful. A single dose of benzodiazepine may be useful in the treatment of a specific phobia such as a fear of flying. Performance anxiety (stage fright) is a special type of situational anxiety that is better treated with a beta antagonist (propranolol 20 to 40 mg orally) without sedation. Endogenous ligands that have an effect opposite to benzodiazepines (anxiogenic) have been identified and support the hypothesis that an abnormality of the benzodiazepine system is responsible for many anxiety states.

Panic disorders appear to be inherited and are characterized as discrete periods of intense fear that is not triggered by a severe anxiogenic stimulus. This disorder is often accompanied by dyspnea, tachycardia, disphoresis, paresthesias, nausea, chest pain, and a fear of dying. An unexplained observation is that infusion of lactate may provoke a panic attack in a vulnerable patient. A tricyclic antidepressant or MAOI is effective in the treatment of a panic attack. Delayed recovery from anesthesia has been attributed to co-existing hysteria.[41]

AUTISM

Autism is a developmental disorder characterized by disturbances in the rate of development of physical, social, and language skills, although specific cognitive capacities may be present. Abnormal responses to sensory inputs manifest with hyperreactivity that alternates with hyporeactivity. The prevalence of this syndrome is estimated as 4.7 per 10,000 live births, with males affected five times as often as females. Enlarged cerebral ventricles may be present, and seizures frequently begin during late childhood. The cause of this syndrome is unknown, but proposed etiologic factors include viral encephalitis and metabolic disorders. Congenital or familial factors are suggested by the occurrence of autism in twins or siblings. No treatment alters the natural history of the disease and life expectancy is normal. Long-range prognosis is poor, and many patients are classified as mentally retarded. Drug therapy is symptomatic and works best when aimed at controlling specific behaviors.

SUBSTANCE ABUSE AND DRUG OVERDOSE

Substance abuse may be defined as self-administration of drug(s) that deviate(s) from accepted medical or social use, which if sustained can lead to physical and psychological dependence. Dependence is diagnosed when a patient has at least three of nine characteristic symptoms, and some of these symptoms have persisted for at least 1 month or have occurred repeatedly[42] (Table 30-8). Physical dependence has

Table 30-7.   Manifestations of an Anxiety Disorder

Tremor
Dyspnea
Tachycardia
Diaphoresis
Insomnia
Irritability
Polyuria
Fatigue
Diarrhea
Skeletal muscle tension

Table 30-8.   Characteristic Symptoms for Psychoactive Drug Dependence

1. Drug taken in greater dose or for a longer period than intended
2. Unsuccessful attempts to decrease use of drug
3. Increased time spent obtaining the drug
4. Frequent intoxication or withdrawal symptoms
5. Restricted social or work activities because of drug use
6. Continued drug use despite social or physical problems related to drug use
7. Evidence of tolerance to effects of drug
8. Characteristic withdrawal symptoms
9. Drug use to avoid withdrawal symptoms

developed when the presence of the drug in the body is necessary for normal physiologic function and prevention of withdrawal symptoms. Typically, the withdrawal syndrome consists of a rebound in the physiologic systems modified by the drug itself. Tolerance is a state in which tissues become accustomed to the presence of a drug such that increased doses of that drug become necessary to produce similar effects to those observed initially with a smaller dose. The substance abuse patient can manifest cross-tolerance to drugs, making it difficult to predict analgesic or anesthetic requirements.[43,44] Most often, chronic substance abuse results in increased analgesic and anesthetic requirements, whereas additive or even synergistic effects may occur in the presence of acute substance abuse. It is important to recognize the signs of drug withdrawal during the preoperative period. Certainly, acute drug withdrawal should not be attempted during the preoperative period.

Substance abuse is often first suspected or recognized during the medical management of another disorder (hepatitis, acquired immunodeficiency syndrome, pregnancy). The patient almost always has a concomitant personality disorder and displays antisocial traits. Sociopathic characteristics (high school dropout, criminal record, polydrug abuse) seem to predispose to, rather than result from, drug addiction. About 50% of patients admitted to the hospital with factitious disorders are drug abusers, as are some pain patients. Psychiatric consultation is recommended in all cases of substance abuse.

Drug overdose is the leading cause of unconsciousness observed in patients brought to the emergency department; often, more than one class of drugs as well as alcohol have been ingested. Conditions other than drug overdose may result in unconsciousness, emphasizing the importance of laboratory tests (electrolytes, blood glucose concentration, arterial blood gases, renal and liver function tests) in confirming the diagnosis. The depth of central nervous system depression can be estimated on the basis of (1) response to painful stimulation, (2) activity of the gag reflex, (3) presence or absence of hypotension, (4) breathing rate, and (5) size and responsiveness of the pupils. Regardless of the drug(s) ingested, the manifestations are similar; assessment and treatment proceed simultaneously. The first step is to secure the airway and to support ventilation and circulation. Absence of a gag reflex is confirmatory evidence that protective laryngeal reflexes are dangerously depressed. In this situation, a cuffed tracheal tube should be placed, to protect the lungs from aspiration. Body temperature is monitored, as hypothermia frequently accompanies unconsciousness due to a drug overdose. The decision to attempt removal of the ingested substance (gastric lavage, charcoal, forced diuresis, hemodialysis) depends on the drug ingested, the time since ingestion, and the degree of central nervous system depression. Gastric lavage may be beneficial if less than 4 hours have elapsed since ingestion. Gastric lavage or pharmacologic stimulation is contraindicated when the ingested substance is a hydrocarbon or corrosive material or when protective laryngeal reflexes are not intact. After gastric lavage or emesis, activated charcoal can be administered to absorb any drug remaining in the gastrointestinal tract. Hemodialysis may be considered when a potentially fatal dose of drug has been ingested, when there is progressive deterioration of cardiovascular function, or when normal routes of metabolism and renal excretion are impaired. Treatment with hemodialysis is of little value when the ingested drug is highly bound to protein or avidly stored in tissues.

Alcohol

Alcoholism is defined as a primary chronic disease with genetic, psychosocial, and environmental factors that influence its development and manifestations.[45] Alcoholism affects at least 10 million Americans and is responsible for 200,000 deaths annually. Up to one-third of adult patients have medical problems related to alcohol (Table 30-9) (see Chapter 19).

Table 30-9.   Medical Problems Related to Alcoholism

Central Nervous System Effects
  Psychiatric disorders (depression, antisocial behavior)
  Nutritional disorders (Wernicke-Korsakoff syndrome)
  Withdrawal syndrome
  Cerebellar degeneration
  Cerebral atrophy

Cardiovascular Effects
  Dilated cardiomyopathy
  Cardiac dysrhythmias
  Hypertension

Gastrointestinal and Hepatobiliary Effects
  Esophagitis
  Gastritis
  Pancreatitis
  Hepatic cirrhosis (portal hypertension manifested as esophageal varices or hemorrhoids)

Skin and Musculoskeletal Effects
  Spider angiomas
  Myopathy
  Osteoporosis

Endocrine and Metabolic Effects
  Decreased plasma testosterone (impotence)
  Decreased gluconeogenesis (hypoglycemia)
  Ketoacidosis
  Hypoalbuminemia
  Hypomagnesemia

Hematologic Effects
  Thrombocytopenia
  Leukopenia
  Anemia

The diagnosis of alcoholism requires a high index of suspicion combined with nonspecific but suggestive symptoms (gastritis, tremor, history of falling, unexplained episodes of amnesia). The possibility of alcoholism is often overlooked in the elderly.

Male gender and family history of alcohol abuse are the two major risk factors for alcoholism. Adoption studies indicate that male children of alcoholic parents are more likely to become alcoholic, even when raised by a nonalcoholic adoptive parent. Other forms of psychiatric disease such as mental depression or sociopathy are not increased in the offspring of alcoholic parents. Inherited differences in the activity of alcohol dehydrogenase among ethnic groups has not been documented.

Although alcohol appears to produce widespread nonspecific effects on cell membranes, there is evidence that many of its neurologic effects are mediated by actions on the receptor for the inhibitory neurotransmitter, gamma aminobutyric acid (GABA).[45] When GABA binds to the receptor, it causes a chloride channel in the receptor to open, thus hyperpolarizing the neuron and making it less likely to depolarize. Alcohol appears to increase GABA-mediated chloride ion conductance. A shared site of action for alcohol, benzodiazepines, and barbiturates would explain their ability to produce cross-tolerance and cross-dependence.

Treatment

Treatment of alcoholism mandates total abstinence from alcohol ingestion. Disulfiram may be administered as an adjunctive drug along with psychiatric counseling. The unpleasantness of symptoms (flushing, vertigo, diaphoresis, nausea, vomiting) that accompanies alcohol ingestion in the presence of disulfiram is intended to serve as a deterrent to the patient's urge to deviate from alcohol abstinence. These symptoms reflect the accumulation of acetaldehyde from oxidation of alcohol, which cannot be further oxidized because of disulfiram-induced inhibition of aldehyde dehydrogenase activity. Compliance with long-term disulfiram therapy is often poor, and this drug has not been documented to have an advantage over placebo in achieving total alcohol abstinence.[46] Medical contraindications to disulfiram include pregnancy, cardiac dysfunction, hepatic dysfunction, renal dysfunction, and peripheral neuropathies. Emergency treatment of an alcohol-disulfiram interaction includes intravenous infusion of crystalloid solutions and occasionally transient maintenance of blood pressure with a vasopressor.

Overdose

The intoxicating effects of alcohol parallel its blood concentration. In a patient who is not alcoholic, a blood alcohol level of 25 mg·dl^{-1} is associated with impaired cognition and incoordination. At a blood alcohol concentration greater than 100 mg·dl^{-1} signs of vestibular and cerebellar dysfunction (nystagmus, dysarthria, ataxia) increase. Autonomic nervous system dysfunction may result in hypotension, hypothermia, stupor, and ultimately coma. Intoxication with alcohol is usually defined as a blood alcohol concentration greater than 100 mg·dl^{-1}, while levels greater than 500 mg·dl^{-1} are usually fatal, owing to depression of ventilation. The severity of intoxication at a given alcohol blood level is typically greater when the concentration is rising than when it is decreasing, perhaps reflecting acute tolerance. Chronic tolerance from prolonged excessive alcohol ingestion may cause an alcoholic patient to remain sober despite a potentially fatal blood alcohol concentration. The critical aspect of treatment of a life-threatening alcohol overdose is maintenance of ventilation. Hypoglycemia may be profound, if heavy alcohol consumption is associated with food deprivation. It must be appreciated that other central nervous system depressant drugs are often ingested simultaneously with alcohol.

Withdrawal Syndrome

Physiologic dependence on alcohol is manifested as a withdrawal syndrome when the drug is discontinued or when there is a decrease in intake.[45] The earliest and most common withdrawal syndrome is characterized by a generalized tremor that may be accompanied by perceptual disturbances (nightmares, hallucinations), autonomic nervous system hyperactivity (tachycardia, hypertension, cardiac dysrhythmias), nausea, vomiting, insomnia, and a mild confusional state with agitation. These symptoms usually begin within 6 to 8 hours after a substantial decrease in the blood alcohol concentration and are typically most pronounced at 24 to 36 hours. These withdrawal symptoms can be suppressed by the resumption of alcohol ingestion or by the administration of a benzodiazepine, beta antagonist, or alpha-2 agonist. In the clinical situation, diazepam is usually administered to produce sedation; a beta antagonist is included if tachycardia is present as well. The ability of a sympatholytic drug to attenuate these symptoms suggests a role for autonomic nervous system hyperactivity in the etiology of the alcohol withdrawal syndrome.

Delirium Tremens

About 5% of patients experiencing alcohol withdrawal syndrome exhibit delirium tremens, a life-threatening medical emergency. Delirium tremens occurs 2 to 4 days after the cessation of alcohol ingestion as hallucinations, combativeness, hyperthermia, tachycardia, hypertension, hypotension, and grand mal seizures. Treatment must be aggressive, with administration of diazepam (5 to 10 mg IV every 5 minutes, until the patient becomes sedated but remains awake) and a beta antagonist (propranolol, esmolol) to suppress manifestations of sympathetic nervous system hyperactivity (heart rate less than 100 beats·min^{-1}). Protection of the upper airway with a cuffed tracheal tube may be necessary in some patients. Correction of fluid, electrolyte (magnesium, potassium), and metabolic (thiamine) derangements is important. Lidocaine is usually effective when cardiac dysrhythmias occur despite correction of electrolyte abnormalities. Physical restraint may be necessary to minimize the risk of self-injury or injury to others. Despite aggressive treatment, mortality from delirium tremens is about 10%, principally due to hypotension, cardiac dysrhythmias, or seizures.

Wernicke-Korsakoff Syndrome

Wernicke-Korsakoff syndrome reflects the loss of neurons in the cerebellum (Wernicke's encephalopathy) and loss of memory (Korsakoff's psychoses), owing to the lack of thiamine (vitamin B_1), required for the intermediary metabolism of carbohydrates (see Chapter 24). This syndrome is not an alcohol withdrawal syndrome, but its occurrence establishes that the patient is, or has been, physically dependent on alcohol. In addition to ataxia and memory loss, many of these patients exhibit global confusional states, drowsiness, nystagmus, and orthostatic hypotension. An associated peripheral polyneuropathy is almost always present.

Treatment of Wernicke-Korsakoff syndrome consists of intravenous administration of thiamine, with normal dietary intake if possible. Because a carbohydrate load may precipitate this syndrome in a thiamine-depleted patient, it may be useful to administer thiamine before the infusion of glucose to a malnourished or alcoholic patient.

Alcohol and Pregnancy

Alcohol crosses the placenta and as little as 30 ml·d^{-1} of maternal intake may result in decreased birthweight. High doses of alcohol (more than 150 ml·d^{-1}) may result in the fetal alcohol syndrome, characterized by (1) craniofacial dysmorphology, (2) growth retardation, and (3) mental retardation. There is an increased incidence of cardiac malformations, including patent ductus arteriosus and septal defects.

Management of Anesthesia

Management of anesthesia in the patient being treated with disulfiram should consider the potential presence of disulfiram-induced sedation and hepatotoxicity (see Chapter 19; the section, Management of Anesthesia in the Patient with Hepatic Cirrhosis). Decreased drug requirements could reflect additive effects with co-existing sedation or the ability of disulfiram to inhibit metabolism of drugs other than alcohol. For example, disulfiram may result in potentiation of the effects of benzodiazepines. Acute and unexplained hypotension during general anesthesia could reflect inadequate stores of norepinephrine owing to disulfiram-induced inhibition of dopamine beta hydroxylase.[47] This hypotension may respond to ephedrine, but

a direct-acting sympathomimetic, such as phenylephrine, may produce a more predictable response in the presence of norepinephrine depletion. The use of regional anesthesia may be influenced by the occasional patient who is treated with disulfiram and in whom polyneuropathy develops. Alcohol-containing solutions, as used for skin cleansing probably should be avoided in the disulfiram-treated patient.

Cocaine

Cocaine use for nonmedical purposes has evolved from a relatively minor problem into a major public health threat with important economic and social consequences.[48,49] It has been estimated that 30 million Americans have used cocaine and that 5 million use it regularly. Myths associated with cocaine abuse are that it is sexually stimulating, nonaddicting, and physiologically benign. In fact, cocaine is extremely addictive, casual use is impossible once addiction develops, and life-threatening side effects accompany its use. For example, coronary artery vasoconstriction leading to myocardial ischemia and acute myocardial infarction, cardiac dysrhythmias, cerebrovascular accident, seizures, and hyperthermia have been observed.[50,51] These cocaine-induced side effects presumably reflect the ability of this drug to enhance sympathetic nervous system activity principally due to inhibition of norepinephrine uptake into postganglionic nerve endings or direct actions on dopamine receptors, or both. Lung damage and pulmonary edema have been observed in patients who smoke cocaine. Cocaine abuse by the parturient is associated with spontaneous abortion, abruptio placentae, and congenital malformations. Chronic cocaine abuse is associated with nasal septal atrophy, agitated behavior, paranoid thinking, and heightened reflexes. Symptoms associated with cocaine withdrawal include fatigue, mental depression, and increased appetite. Death from cocaine has occurred after all routes of administration (intranasal, oral, intravenous, inhalation by smoking) and is usually due to apnea, seizures, or cardiac dysrhythmias.[52] Persons with decreased plasma cholinesterase enzymatic activity (elderly patients, parturients, severe liver disease) may be at risk of sudden death when using cocaine, because this enzyme is essential for metabolizing the drug.

Overdose

Cocaine overdose evokes overwhelming sympathetic nervous system stimulation of the cardiovascular system. Uncontrolled hypertension may result in pulmonary and cerebral edema, whereas increased circulating levels of catecholamines may induce coronary artery vasoconstriction, spasm, and platelet aggregation. Esmolol as a continuous intravenous infusion at a rate to maintain the heart rate less than 100 beats·min^{-1} has been recommended for control of the excess sympathetic nervous system stimulation that may accompany cocaine overdose.[53] The selective beta-1 effect of esmolol renders hypertension or coronary artery spasm from unopposed alpha-agonist activity less of a risk than with a nonselective beta antagonist such as propranolol. Furthermore, the brief duration of action of esmolol permits titration of its effect as the effects of cocaine wane. For example, the elimination half-time of cocaine after nasal administration is about 1 hour, reflecting its degradation by plasma cholinesterase and hepatic metabolism. Labetalol may be an alternative to esmolol in the treatment of cocaine overdose, although its greater beta than alpha antagonist effects introduce the possibility of relatively unopposed alpha-agonist effects.[54] Diazepam may be effective in terminating cocaine-induced seizures. Active cooling procedures may be necessary if hyperthermia accompanies cocaine overdose.

Management of Anesthesia

Management of anesthesia in the patient acutely intoxicated with cocaine must consider the vulnerability of these patients to myocardial ischemia and cardiac dysrhythmias. Any event or drug likely to increase already enhanced sympathetic nervous system activity must be carefully considered before its selection. In this regard, drugs such as esmolol to control blood pressure and heart rate should be available. It is not surprising that the dysrhythmogenic dose of epinephrine is decreased in animals receiving intravenous cocaine during halothane anesthesia.[55] An increased anesthetic requirement for volatile anesthetics may be present in the acutely intoxicated patient, presumably reflecting an increased concentration of catecholamines in the central nervous system.[56] Thrombocytopenia associated with cocaine abuse may influence the selection of regional anesthesia in these patients.

In the absence of acute intoxication, chronic abuse of cocaine has not been shown to be predictably associated with adverse anesthetic interactions, although the possibility of cardiac dysrhythmias remains a constant concern. It is likely that the rapid metabolism of cocaine reduces the likelihood that an acutely intoxicated patient will present in the operating room. Cocaine ($1.5 \ mg \cdot kg^{-1}$) administered topically before initiating nasotracheal intubation and followed by nitrous oxide–halothane anesthesia is not associated with detectable cardiovascular effects.[57]

Opioids

Contrary to common speculation, opioid dependence rarely develops from the use of these drugs to treat acute postoperative pain. It is possible to become addicted to an opioid, however, in less than 14 days if the drug is administered daily in an ever-increasing dose. Opioids are abused orally, subcutaneously, or intravenously for their euphoric or analgesic effects, or both. Numerous medical problems are encountered

Table 30-10. Medical Problems Associated With Chronic Opioid Abuse

Cellulitis
Superficial skin abscesses
Septic thrombophlebitis
Tetanus
Endocarditis with or without pulmonary emboli
Systemic septic emboli and infarctions
Aspiration pneumonitis
Acquired immunodeficiency syndrome
Adrenal gland dysfunction
Hepatitis
Malaria
Malnutrition
Positive and false positive serology
Transverse myelitis

in the opioid addict, especially the intravenous abuser (Table 30-10). Evidence for these medical problems should be sought in the opioid addict entering the perioperative period. Tolerance may develop to some of the effects of opioids (analgesia, sedation, emesis, euphoria, hypoventilation), but not to others (miosis, constipation). Fortunately, as tolerance increases, so does the lethal dose of opioid. In general, there is a high degree of cross-tolerance between drugs with morphine-like actions, although tolerance can wane rapidly when the addict is withdrawn from the drug.

Overdose

The most obvious manifestation of opioid overdose (usually heroin) is a slow breathing rate with a normal to increased tidal volume. The pupils are usually miotic, although mydriasis may occur if hypoventilation results in severe arterial hypoxemia. Central nervous system manifestations range from dysphoria to unconsciousness, and seizures are unlikely. Pulmonary edema occurs in a high proportion of patients experiencing a heroin overdose. The etiology of pulmonary edema is poorly understood, but arterial hypoxemia, hypotension, neurogenic mechanisms, and drug-related pulmonary endothelial damage are considerations. Gastric atony is a predictable accompaniment of acute opioid overdose. Fatal opioid overdose is most often an outcome of fluctuation in the purity of street products or to the combination of opioids with other central nervous system depressants. Naloxone is the specific opioid antagonist administered to maintain an acceptable breathing rate, usually greater than 12 breaths·min^{-1}.

Withdrawal Syndrome

Although withdrawal from an opioid is rarely life-threatening, it is unpleasant and may complicate management during the perioperative period. In this regard, it is useful to consider

Table 30-11.   Time Course of Opioid Withdrawal
Syndrome

Drug	Onset	Peak Intensity	Duration
Meperidine Dihydromorphine	2–6 h	8–12 h	4–5 d
Codeine Morphine Heroin	6–18 h	36–72 h	7–10 d
Methadone	24–48 h	3–21 d	6–7 wk

the time to onset, peak intensity, and duration of withdrawal after abrupt withdrawal of the opioid[58] (Table 30-11). Opioid withdrawal symptoms develop within seconds after intravenous administration of naloxone. Conversely, it is usually possible to abort the withdrawal syndrome by reinstituting administration of the abused opioid or by substituting methadone (2.5 mg equivalent to 10 mg of morphine). Clonidine may also attenuate opioid withdrawal symptoms presumably by replacing opioid-mediated inhibition (absent during withdrawal) with alpha-2 agonist-mediated inhibition of the sympathetic nervous system in the brain.[59]

Opioid withdrawal symptoms often include manifestations of excess sympathetic nervous system activity (diaphoresis, mydriasis, hypertension, tachycardia). Craving for the drug and anxiety are followed by yawning, lacrimation, rhinorrhea, piloerection (origin of the term "cold turkey"), tremors, skeletal muscle and bone discomfort, and anorexia. Insomnia, abdominal cramps, diarrhea, and hyperthermia may develop. Skeletal muscle spasms and jerking of the legs (origin of the term "kicking the habit") follow, and cardiovascular collapse is possible. Seizures are rare, and their occurrence should introduce the consideration of other etiologies, such as unrecognized barbiturate withdrawal or underlying epilepsy.

Management of Anesthesia

The opioid addict should have the opioid or methadone maintained during the perioperative period. Preoperative medication may also include an opioid.[60] An opioid agonist-antagonist is not an appropriate consideration, as such a drug could precipitate an acute withdrawal reaction. There is no advantage in trying to maintain anesthesia with an opioid, as doses greatly in excess of normal are likely to be required. Furthermore, chronic opioid use leads to cross-tolerance to other central nervous system depressants that may be manifested as a decreased analgesic response to an inhaled anesthetic such as nitrous oxide[61] (Fig. 30-3). Conversely, acute opioid administration decreases anesthetic requirements. Maintenance of anesthesia is most often with a volatile anesthetic, remembering that these patients are likely to have underlying liver dis-

ease. There is a tendency for perioperative hypotension to occur, which may reflect (1) inadequate intravascular fluid volume secondary to chronic infection, fever, or malnutrition; (2) adrenocortical insufficiency and (3) an inadequate opioid concentration in the brain.[62]

Management of anesthesia for the rehabilitated opioid addict, as well as for the patient on antagonist therapy often includes a volatile anesthetic. Regional anesthesia may have a role in some patients, but it is important to remember (1) the tendency for hypotension to occur, (2) the increased incidence of positive serology, (3) the occasional presence of peripheral neuritis and, (4) the rare occurrence of transverse myelitis.

The opioid addict often seems to experience an exaggerated degree of postoperative pain. For reasons that are unclear, satisfactory postoperative analgesia is often achieved when an average dose of meperidine is administered, in addition to the usual daily maintenance dose of methadone or other opioid.

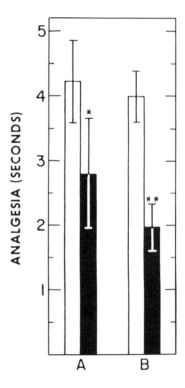

Fig. 30-3. Analgesic effects of nitrous oxide as determined by tail flick latency are decreased in rats (A, Long-Evans rats; B, Sprague-Dawley rats) tolerant to morphine (dark bars) compared to rats not treated with morphine (clear bars). Mean ± SE. *$P < 0.05$ compared with nontolerant rats. **$P < 0.005$ compared with nontolerant rats. (From Berkowitz BA, Finck AD, Hynes MD, Ngai SH. Tolerance to N_2O anesthesia in rats and mice. Anesthesiology 1979;51:309–14, with permission.)

Methadone has minimal analgesic activity with respect to management of postoperative pain. Alternative methods of postoperative pain relief in these patients include continuous regional analgesia with a local anesthetic, neuraxial opioids, and transcutaneous electrical nerve stimulation.

Barbiturates

Chronic barbiturate abuse is not associated with major pathophysiologic changes. These drugs are most commonly abused orally for their euphoric effects, to counter insomnia, and to antagonize stimulant effects of other drugs. Tolerance occurs to most of the actions of these drugs, as well as cross-tolerance to other central nervous system depressants. Although the barbiturate dose required to produce a sedative or euphoric effect increases rapidly, the lethal dose does not increase at the same rate or to the same magnitude. Thus, a barbiturate abuser's margin of error, in contrast to that of the opioid addict, decreases as the barbiturate dose is increased to achieve the desired effect.

Overdose

Central nervous system depression is the principal manifestation of barbiturate overdose.[1] The barbiturate blood level correlates with the degree of central nervous system depression (slurred speech, ataxia, irritability), with very high blood levels resulting in loss of pharyngeal and deep tendon reflexes and the onset of coma. No specific pharmacologic antagonist exists to reverse barbiturate-induced central nervous system depression, and the use of nonspecific stimulants is not encouraged. Depression of ventilation may be profound. As with an opioid overdose, maintenance of the upper airway, protection of the lungs from aspiration, and support of ventilation of the lungs using a cuffed tracheal tube may be necessary. Barbiturate overdose may be associated with hypotension owing to central vasomotor depression, direct myocardial depression, and increased venous capacitance. This hypotension usually responds to an infusion of fluids, although occasionally a vasopressor or inotropic drug is required. Hypothermia is a frequent occurrence and may necessitate aggressive attempts to restore normothermia. Acute renal failure due to hypotension and rhabdomyolysis may occur. Forced diuresis and alkalinization of the urine promote the elimination of phenobarbital but are of lesser value with many of the other barbiturates. Induced emesis or gastric lavage, followed by the administration of activated charcoal, may be helpful in an otherwise awake patient who ingested the drug less than 6 hours previously.

Withdrawal Syndrome

In contrast to opioid withdrawal, the abrupt cessation of excessive barbiturate ingestion is associated with potentially life-threatening responses. The time of onset, peak intensity, and

Table 30-12.   Time Course of Barbiturate Withdrawal Syndrome

Drug	Onset (h)	Peak Intensity (d)	Duration (d)
Pentobarbital	12–24	2–3	7–10
Secobarbital	12–24	2–3	7–10
Phenobarbital	48–72	6–10	10 days or longer

duration of withdrawal symptoms for barbiturates are delayed compared with opioids (Table 30-12). Barbiturate withdrawal symptoms are manifested initially as anxiety, skeletal muscle tremors, hyperreflexia, diaphoresis, tachycardia, and orthostatic hypotension. Cardiovascular collapse and hyperthermia may occur. The most serious problem associated with barbiturate withdrawal is the occurrence of grand mal seizures. Seizures are likely to be caused by an abrupt decrease in the circulating concentration of the drug. Many of the manifestations of barbiturate withdrawal, in particular seizures, are difficult to abort once they develop, in contrast with opioid withdrawal.

Pentobarbital may be administered if evidence of barbiturate withdrawal is manifested. Typically, the initial oral dose is 200 to 400 mg with subsequent doses titrated to effect, since tolerance may disappear very rapidly in these patients. Phenobarbital and diazepam may also be useful in suppressing evidence of barbiturate withdrawal.

Management of Anesthesia

Although few data exist concerning management of anesthesia in the chronic barbiturate abuser, it is predictable that cross-tolerance to depressant effects of anesthetic drugs will occur. For example, mice tolerant to thiopental awaken at a higher barbiturate tissue concentration than do control animals. Similarly, anecdotal reports describe the need for an increased barbiturate dose for induction of anesthesia and for a shorter duration of sleep in the chronic barbiturate abuser.[63] Although acute administration of barbiturates has been shown to decrease anesthetic requirements, there are no reports of increased MAC requirements in the chronic barbiturate abuser. Another concern is that chronic barbiturate abuse will lead to induction of hepatic microsomal enzymes, introducing the potential for drug interactions with concomitantly administered medications (warfarin, digitalis, phenytoin, volatile anesthetics). Venous access is a likely problem in the intravenous barbiturate abuser, as the alkalinity of the injected solution is likely to sclerose veins.

Benzodiazepines

Benzodiazepine addiction probably requires the ingestion of large doses (diazepam 80 to 120 mg for 40 to 50 days). As with barbiturates, tolerance and physical dependence occur with chronic benzodiazepine abuse. Benzodiazepines do not significantly induce microsomal enzymes. Symptoms of withdrawal generally occur later than with barbiturates and are less severe due to the prolonged elimination half-times of most benzodiazepines, as well as the fact that many of these drugs are metabolized to pharmacologically active metabolites that also have prolonged elimination half-times. Anesthetic considerations in the chronic benzodiazepine abuser are similar to those described for the chronic barbiturate abuser.

Overdose

Acute benzodiazepine overdose is much less likely to produce depression of ventilation as compared with barbiturate overdose. It should be recognized, however, that combinations of benzodiazepines and other central nervous system depressants, such as alcohol, have proved to be potentially lethal. Supportive treatment often suffices, whereas a specific benzodiazepine antagonist, flumazenil, will be useful for management of profound overdoses. Seizure activity previously suppressed by benzodiazepines could be unmasked after the administration of flumazenil.

Amphetamines

Amphetamines stimulate the release of catecholamines, resulting in increased cortical alertness with associated appetite suppression and decreased need for sleep. Approved uses of amphetamines are for the treatment of narcolepsy, attention-deficit disorders, and hyperactivity associated with minimal brain dysfunction in children. Tolerance develops to the appetite suppressant effects within a few weeks, making these drugs a poor substitute for a proper diet technique. Physiologic dependence on amphetamines is profound, and daily doses may be increased to several hundred times the therapeutic dose. Chronic abuse of amphetamines results in depletion of body stores of catecholamines. Such depletion may be manifested as somnolence and anxiety or psychotic-like states. Other physiologic abnormalities reported with long-term amphetamine abuse include hypertension, cardiac dysrhythmias, and malnutrition. Amphetamines are most often abused orally or, in the case of methamphetamine, intravenously.

Overdose

Amphetamine overdose causes anxiety, psychotic states, and progressive central nervous system irritability, manifested as hyperactivity, hyperreflexia, and occasionally seizures.[43] Other physiologic effects include increased blood pressure and heart rate, cardiac dysrhythmias, decreased gastrointestinal motility, mydriasis, diaphoresis, and hyperthermia. Metabolic imbalances such as dehydration, lactic acidosis, and ketosis may occur.

The treatment of oral amphetamine overdose is with in-duced emesis or gastric lavage, followed by the administration of activated charcoal and a cathartic. Phenothiazines may antagonize many of the acute central nervous system effects of amphetamines. Similarly, diazepam may be useful to control amphetamine-induced seizures. Acidification of the urine will promote the elimination of amphetamines.

Withdrawal Syndrome

Abrupt cessation of excess amphetamine usage is accompanied by extreme lethargy; mental depression, which may be suicidal; increased appetite; and weight gain. A benzodiazepine is useful in the management of the withdrawal syndrome if sedation is needed, and a beta antagonist may be administered to control sympathetic nervous system hyperactivity. Postamphetamine mental depression may last for months and require treatment with a tricyclic antidepressant such as desimpramine or impramine, which exert the most profound effects on neurotransmitter concentrations of norepinephrine.

Management of Anesthesia

Intraoperatively, the patient who is acutely intoxicated from ingestion of amphetamines may exhibit hypertension, tachycardia, increased body temperature, and elevated requirements for volatile anesthetics. Indeed, in animals, acute intravenous administration of dextroamphetamine produces dose-related increases in body temperature and anesthetic requirements for halothane.[64] On the bases of these observations, it would seem prudent to monitor body temperature during the perioperative period. Furthermore, direct-acting vasopressors and drugs that sensitize the heart to catecholamines must be used with caution in these patients.

Chronic use of amphetamines depletes body stores of catecholamines. This depletion may attenuate responses to indirect-acting vasopressors and may be responsible for the somnolence characteristic of chronic abuse. Indeed, anesthetic requirements for halothane are decreased in animals that have been chronically treated with dextroamphetamine.[64]

Hallucinogens

Hallucinogens, as represented by lysergic acid diethylamide (LSD) and phencyclidine (PCP), are usually ingested orally. Although there is a high degree of psychological dependence, there is no evidence of physical dependence or withdrawal symptoms when LSD is acutely discontinued. Chronic use of hallucinogens is unlikely. The effects of these drugs develop in 1 to 2 hours and last 8 to 12 hours, consisting of visual, auditory, and tactile hallucinations and distortions of surroundings and body image. The ability of the brain to suppress relatively unimportant stimuli is impaired by LSD. Evidence of sympathetic nervous system stimulation includes mydriasis, increased body temperature, hypertension, and tachycardia. Tolerance to behavioral effects of LSD occurs rapidly, whereas tolerance to the cardiovascular effects is less pronounced.

Overdose

Overdose of LSD has not been associated with mortality, although the patient may suffer unrecognized injuries, reflecting the intrinsic analgesic effect of the drug. On rare occasions, LSD produces seizures and apnea. LSD can produce an acute panic reaction, characterized by hyperactivity, mood lability, and, in extreme cases, overt psychosis. The patient is often placed in a calm and quiet environment with minimal external stimuli. No specific antidote exists, although a benzodiazepine may be useful in controlling agitation and anxiety reactions. Supportive care in the form of airway management, ventilation of the lungs, treatment of seizures, and control of the manifestations of sympathetic nervous system hyperactivity is warranted when appropriate. Forced diuresis and acidification of the urine promote elimination of phencyclidine. Forced diuresis introduces the risk of fluid overload and electrolyte abnormalities, especially hypokalemia.

Management of Anesthesia

Anesthesia and surgery have been reported to precipitate panic responses in these patients. In the event that such a response occurs, diazepam is likely to be useful. Exaggerated responses to sympathomimetic drugs would seem likely. Analgesic and presumably ventilatory depressant effects of opioids are prolonged by LSD. Inhibition of plasma cholinesterase activity by LSD is a speculated possibility that seems to have little clinical support.

Marijuana

Marijuana is usually abused by smoking, which increases the bioavailability of the primary psychoactive constituent, tetrahydrocannabinol (THC), over that possible after oral ingestion. Inhalation of marijuana smoke produces euphoria and signs of increased sympathetic nervous system activity and decreased parasympathetic nervous system activity. The most consistent cardiac change is an increased resting heart rate, although orthostatic hypotension may occur. Chronic marijuana abuse leads to increased tar deposits in the lungs, impaired pulmonary defense mechanisms, and decreased pulmonary function. As such, an increased incidence of sinusitis and bronchitis is likely. In predisposed persons, marijuana may evoke seizures. Conjunctival reddening is evidence of dilation of the efferent blood vessels in the iris. Drowsiness is a common side effect. Tolerance to most of the psychoactive effects of THC has been observed. Although physical dependence on marijuana is not believed to occur, abrupt cessation after chronic use is characterized by mild withdrawal symptoms, such as irritability, insomnia, diaphoresis, nausea, vomiting,

and diarrhea. A possible medical indication for THC is its oral administration as an antiemetic in patients receiving cancer chemotherapy.[65]

Management of Anesthesia

Pharmacologic effects of inhaled THC occur within minutes but rarely persist more than 2 to 3 hours, decreasing the likelihood that an acutely intoxicated patient would present in the operating room. Management of anesthesia includes consideration of the known effects of THC on the heart, lungs, and central nervous system. Co-existing drug-induced drowsiness is consistent with animal studies demonstrating decreased dose requirements for volatile anesthetics after intravenous injection of THC.[66,67] Barbiturate and ketamine sleep times are prolonged in THC-treated animals and opioid-induced depression of ventilation is potentiated.[68,69]

Tricyclic Antidepressant Overdose

Deliberate self-administration of an overdose of an antidepressant drug is the most common cause of death from drug ingestion.[70] Since the usual indication for administration of an antidepressant drug is mental depression, it is not surprising that deliberate overdose is a potential occurrence. The potentially lethal dose of these drugs may only be 5 to 10 times the daily therapeutic dose. An overdose principally affects the central nervous system, parasympathetic nervous system, and cardiovascular system. Progression from being alert with mild symptoms to life-threatening changes (seizures, hypoventilation, hypotension, coma) may be extremely rapid. Evidence of an intense anticholinergic effect includes tachycardia, mydriasis, flushed dry skin, urinary retention, and delayed gastric emptying. Cardiovascular toxicity with intractable myocardial depression or ventricular cardiac dysrhythmias, including ventricular fibrillation, are the most common causes of death. The likelihood of seizures and cardiac dysrhythmias is increased when the duration of the QRS complexes on the electrocardiogram exceeds 100 ms.[70] Conversely, the plasma concentration of the ingested antidepressant drug does not predictably correlate with the likely occurrence of cardiac dysrhythmias or seizures. The comatose phase of a tricyclic antidepressant overdose lasts 24 to 72 hours. Even after this phase passes, the risk of life-threatening cardiac dysrhythmias persists for several days, often necessitating the continued monitoring of the electrocardiogram in these patients.

Treatment

Treatment of tricyclic antidepressant overdose in the presence of protective upper airway reflexes is initially with induced emesis or gastric lavage, or both, even if as long as 12 hours have elapsed since drug ingestion, emphasizing the likely presence of a drug-induced delay in gastric emptying.

Table 30-13. Pharmacologic Treatment of Tricyclic Antidepressant Overdose

Side Effect	Treatment
Seizures	Diazepam
	Phenytoin
Cardiac dysrhythmias	Lidocaine
	Phenytoin
Heart block	Isoproterenol
Hypotension	Sympathomimetic
	Inotrope

Depression of ventilation or coma, or both, may require intubation of the trachea and mechanical support of ventilation. Pharmacologic treatment of overdose is directed toward the central nervous system and cardiovascular system (Table 30-13). Alkalinization of the plasma, either by intravenous administration of sodium bicarbonate or by hyperventilation of the lungs, to a pH above 7.45, may attenuate drug-induced cardiotoxicity. Lidocaine is also useful in the treatment of cardiac dysrhythmias. The patient who remains hypotensive after volume expansion and alkalinization may benefit from vasopressor or inotropic support, as guided by measurement of cardiac filling pressures and cardiac output. Diazepam may be useful for control of seizures. Physostigmine is an unpredictable and nonspecific antagonist of tricyclic antidepressant effects on the central nervous system. It must, likewise, be remembered that the duration of action of physostigmine is only 1 to 2 hours; repeated doses of this drug may be necessary owing to a long elimination half-time of the tricyclic antidepressant drug. Hemodialysis and forced diuresis are not effective, since the high lipid solubility of tricyclic antidepressant drugs results in a fixed and slow rate of excretion.

Salicylic Acid Overdose

Symptoms of salicylic acid overdose parallel salicylate blood levels, with a plasma concentration greater than 85 mg·dl^{-1} indicating severe overdose. Hyperventilation is characteristic, reflecting increased carbon dioxide production and direct stimulation of the respiratory center. Resulting respiratory alkalosis favors the water-soluble ionized fraction of salicylic acid, which may undergo renal elimination. Conversely, metabolic acidosis, which may also accompany salicylic acid overdose, favors the lipid-soluble nonionized fraction of the drug, which can leave the blood and enter the tissues, including the brain, where toxic effects are produced. Hypoglycemia may occur from increased peripheral use of glucose or interference with gluconeogenesis. Conversely, hyperglycemia may reflect the effect of epinephrine release secondary to stimulation of the central nervous system by salicylic acid. Noncardiogenic pulmonary edema often occurs during the first 24 hours after salicylic acid overdose. Other manifestations of salicyclic acid overdose include tinnitus, vomiting, hyperthermia, seizures, and coma.

Proper management of salicylic acid overdose includes monitoring of arterial pH, since a decrease in pH to 7.2 doubles the fraction of lipid-soluble drug in the circulation. Indeed, a decreasing plasma salicylate concentration may reflect urinary excretion of salicylic acid or undesirable cellular penetration of this substance secondary to metabolic acidosis. Sodium bicarbonate administration may be necessary to maintain arterial pH above 7.4. Controlled ventilation of the lungs through a tracheal tube is indicated if central nervous system depression and alveolar hyperventilation are prominent. Dehydration and electrolyte disturbances may require treatment. Hemodialysis may be indicated when a potentially lethal plasma concentration (greater than 100 mg·dl^{-1}) of salicylic acid is present.

Acetaminophen Overdose

Acetaminophen overdose is manifested as vomiting, abdominal pain, and life-threatening centrilobular hepatic necrosis. Hepatic necrosis is most likely due to metabolism of acetaminophen to benzoquinonimine, which reacts with and destroys hepatocytes. Normally, this metabolite is inactivated by conjugation with endogenous glutathione, but the increased production owing to the acetaminophen overdose depletes glutathione stores. Depletion of glutathione stores allows this reactive intermediary metabolite to accumulate and destroy hepatocytes. Treatment of acetaminophen overdose is with acetylcysteine, which provides sulhydral groups that act as precursors for glutathione. Indeed, administration of acetylcysteine within 8 hours of acetaminophen overdose protects against the development of hepatotoxicity.[71]

Methyl Alcohol Ingestion

Methyl alcohol (methanol) is metabolized by alcohol dehydrogenase to formaldehyde and formic acid, resulting in metabolic acidosis. A toxic effect, presumably of these metabolites, on the optic nerve is associated with blindness. Severe abdominal pain that mimics a surgical emergency or ureteral colic may occur. Treatment includes attempts to decrease the metabolism of methyl alcohol by intravenous administration of alcohol, which competes with methyl alcohol for the enzyme alcohol dehydrogenase. Alternatively, the activity of alcohol dehydrogenase may be specifically inhibited by administration of methylpyrazole.[72] Metabolic acidosis is treated with intravenous administration of sodium bicarbonate, as guided by measurement of arterial pH. Hemodialysis is also an effective treatment for removing methyl alcohol and for preventing visual and cerebral damage.

Ethylene Glycol Ingestion

Ethylene glycol (antifreeze is about 93% ethylene glycol) is metabolized by alcohol dehydrogenase to glycolic acid resulting in metabolic acidosis. Glycolate is then metabolized to oxalate, which may result in renal failure. Hypocalcemia due to oxalate chelation of calcium may also occur. Treatment of ethylene glycol ingestion is as described for methyl alcohol ingestion. In addition, treatment of hypocalcemia may be necessary.

Petroleum Product Ingestion

Morbidity associated with petroleum product ingestion (gasoline, kerosene, lighter fluid, furniture polish) is usually secondary to pulmonary aspiration during spontaneous vomiting or after induced emesis. Absorption from the gastrointestinal tract is not a likely cause of morbidity. Symptoms of hydrocarbon pneumonitis occur only if aspiration is present and range from coughing and dyspnea with tachypnea to life-threatening adult respiratory distress syndrome. Of those patients in whom hydrocarbon pneumonitis develops, nearly all show radiographic changes within 12 hours of ingestion. Pneumonitis is presumably due to hydrocarbon-induced alterations in physical properties of pulmonary surfactant, leading to atelectasis and airway closure. Gastrointestinal symptoms of petroleum product ingestion include burning of the mouth and throat, nausea, vomiting, and diarrhea. Central nervous system symptoms are usually mild, with unconsciousness or seizures occurring only when aspiration leads to profound arterial hypoxemia. Renal function is not uniquely altered by petroleum product ingestion. Gasoline and glue sniffing have been implicated as causes of sudden and often fatal cardiac dysrhythmias. This may reflect sensitization of the myocardium to endogenous catecholamines.[73]

Induced emesis in the treatment of petroleum product ingestion is not recommended, in view of the risk of pulmonary aspiration. Likewise, intubation of the trachea only to permit gastric lavage is not recommended, since the seal provided by the tracheal tube cuff does not guarantee that aspiration of these low-density liquids will not occur. Activated charcoal and cathartics are not beneficial. The course and severity of hydrocarbon pneumonitis are not altered by administration of corticosteroids. Broad-spectrum antibiotics are indicated if bacterial infection is documented.

Organophosphate Overdose

Organophosphate overdose is most likely to occur when insecticides that are potent inhibitors of the enzyme acetylcholinesterase (true cholinesterase) are ingested, inhaled, or absorbed through the skin.[74] Nerve agents, as developed for chemical warfare, are also inhibitors of this enzyme. Symp-

Table 30-14. Symptoms of Organophosphate (Insecticide) Overdose

Nicotinic Effects (Neuromuscular Junction)
Skeletal muscle fasciculations
Skeletal muscle weakness
Skeletal muscle paralysis (apnea)

Muscarinic Effects
Salivation
Lacrimation
Miosis
Diaphoresis
Bronchospasm
Bradycardia
Hyperperistalsis (diarrhea, urination)

Central Nervous System Effects
Grand mal seizures
Unconsciousness
Apnea
Hyperthermia

toms of organophosphate overdose reflect inhibition (irreversible phosphorylation) of acetylcholinesterase resulting in accumulation of acetylcholine at nicotinic (neuromuscular junction) and cholinergic receptor sites (Table 30-14). The relative intensity of these manifestations is influenced by the route of absorption, with the most intense effects occurring after inhalation. Organophosphate overdose may be followed by delayed peripheral neuropathy involving the distal muscles of the extremities.[74] This neuropathy appears 2 to 5 weeks after the overdose. Skeletal muscle weakness developing 1 to 4 days after organophosphate overdose involves primarily proximal limb muscles, flexors of the neck, certain cranial nerves, and breathing muscles. Death from organophosphate overdose is usually a result of apnea.

Treatment

Treatment of organophosphate overdose includes the administration of anticholinergics, oximes, anticholinesterases, and benzodiazepines (Table 30-15). Atropine is the mainstay of

Table 30-15. Treatment of Organophosphate (Insecticide) Overdose

Drug	Dose
Atropine	2 mg IV until ventilation improves; usual dose for severe toxicity is 15–20 mg during first 3 hours
Pralidoxime	600 mg IV
Diazepam	5–10 mg IV; repeat until seizures are controlled

overdose antidote therapy. The endpoint of atropine therapy is good control of airway secretions and the presence of an adequate tidal volume. Pralidoxime is an oxime that complexes with the organophosphate, resulting in its removal from the acetylcholinesterase enzyme. This drug-induced removal of the organophosphate from acetylcholinesterase reactivates the enzyme, leading to restoration of normal enzymatic inactivation of acetylcholine and reestablishment of normal cholinergic neurotransmission. Diazepam is useful in controlling seizures induced by an organophosphate overdose. Weakness of the muscles of breathing may require mechanical support of ventilation.

Carbon Monoxide Intoxication

Carbon monoxide intoxication is the most frequent immediate cause of death from fire-related smoke inhalation. This colorless, odorless gas exerts its adverse effects by decreasing oxygen delivery to tissues, by virtue of its greater affinity for hemoglobin. Specifically, the affinity of carbon monoxide for oxygen binding sites on hemoglobin is 210 times greater than that of oxygen for the same sites. Because of this affinity, an inspired carbon monoxide concentration of 0.1% in room air produces an equal concentration of oxyhemoglobin and carboxyhemoglobin that results in a 50% decrease in the oxygen-carrying capacity of the blood. Carbon monoxide also produces tissue hypoxia by shifting the oxyhemoglobin dissociation curve to the left. Symptoms of carbon monoxide overdose reflect arterial hypoxemia and include headache, nausea, restlessness, and confusion.

Diagnosis of carbon monoxide intoxication is suggested by the measurement of a low arterial hemoglobin oxygen saturation (SaO_2) in the presence of a normal PaO_2. Calculation of SaO_2 from a nomogram based on the measured PaO_2 will result in an erroneous conclusion. Measurement of the blood carboxyhemoglobin concentration confirms the diagnosis. Carbon monoxide intoxication is considered severe when the blood concentration of carboxyhemoglobin exceeds 40%. It is important to recognize that the presence of a high plasma concentration of carboxyhemoglobin can cause the pulse oximeter to overestimate the actual SaO_2.[75] Despite marked decreases in the oxygen-carrying capacity of the blood, minute ventilation is typically unchanged, since the carotid bodies respond principally to changes in PaO_2 that are likely to be normal in the presence of carbon monoxide intoxication. Therefore, increased minute ventilation may not occur until acidosis develops from tissue hypoxia. Carboxyhemoglobin concentrations in excess of 40% are associated with a classic cherry red appearance and coma.

Treatment

Treatment of carbon monoxide intoxication consists of the inhalation of oxygen, to displace carbon monoxide from hemoglobin. For example, if a patient is breathing room air, the elimination half-time for carboxyhemoglobin is 250 minutes. Administration of 100% oxygen increases the dissociation of carbon monoxide from hemoglobin and decreases this time to about 50 minutes. Inhalation of oxygen in a hyperbaric chamber is reasonable, if the facility for this method of treatment is readily available. It is prudent to administer oxygen initially to any patient who has been exposed to carbon monoxide, especially if inhalation of smoke associated with a fire has occurred.

REFERENCES

1. Potter WZ, Rudorfer MV, Manji H. The pharmacologic treatment of depression. N Engl J Med 1991;325:633–42
2. Thompson TL, Moran MG, Nies AS. Psychotropic drug use in the elderly. N Engl J Med 1983;308:194–8
3. Veith RC, Raskind MA, Caldwell JH, et al. Cardiovascular effects of tricyclic antidepressants in depressed patients with chronic heart disease. N Engl J Med 1982;306:954–9
4. Roose SP, Glassman AH, Giardina E-GV, et al. Nortriptyline in depressed patients with left ventricular impairment. JAMA 1986; 256:521–6
5. Luchins DJ. Review of clinical animal studies comparing the cardiovascular effects of doxepin and other tricyclic antidepressants. Am J Psychiatry 1983;140:1006–11
6. Dessain EC, Schatzberg AF, Woods BT, et al. Maprotiline treatment in depression: A perspective on seizures. Arch Gen Psychiatry 1986;43:86–92
7. Miller RD, Way WL, Eger EI. The effects of alpha-methyldopa, reserpine, guanethidine and iproniazid on minimum alveolar anesthetic requirement (MAC). Anesthesiology 1968;29:1153–8
8. Braverman B, McCarthy RJ, Ivankovich AD. Vasopressor challenges during chronic MAOI or TCA treatment in anesthetized dogs. Life Sci 1987;40:2587–95
9. Edwards RP, Miller RD, Roizen MF, et al. Cardiac responses to imipramine and pancuronium during anesthesia with halothane or enflurane. Anesthesiology 1979;50:421–5
10. Wong KC, Puerto AX, Puerto BA, Blatnick RA. Influence of imipramine and pargyline on the arrhythmogenicity of epinephrine during halothane, enflurane or methoxyflurane anesthesia in dogs. Anesthesiology 1980;53:S25
11. Spiss CK, Smith CM, Maze M. Halothane-epinephrine arrhythmias and adrenergic responsiveness after chronic imipramine administration in dogs. Anesth Analg 1984;63:825–8
12. Sprague DH, Wolf S. Enflurane seizures in patients taking amitriptyline. Anesth Analg 1982;61:67–8
13. Frommer DA, Kulig KW, Marx JA, Rumack B. Tricyclic antidepressant overdose. A review. JAMA 1987;257:521–6
14. El-Ganzouri AR, Ivankovich AD, Braverman B, McCarthy R. Monoamine oxidase inhibitors: Should they be discontinued preoperatively? Anesth Analg 1985;64:592–6
15. Wong KC. Preoperative discontinuation of monoamine oxidase inhibitor therapy: An old wives' tale. Seminars in Anesthesiology 1986;5:145–8

16. Stack CJ, Rogers P, Linter SPK. Monoamine oxidase inhibitors and anaesthesia. Br J Anaesth 1988;60:222–7

17. Wells DG, Bjorksten AR. Monoamine oxidase inhibitors revisited. Can J Anaesth 1989;36:64–74

18. Tordoff SG, Stubbing JF, Linter SPK. Delayed excitatory reaction following interaction of cocaine and monoamine oxidase inhibitor (phenelzine). Br J Anaesth 1991;66:516–8

19. Marks PJ. Electroconvulsive therapy: Physiological and anaesthetic considerations. Can Anaesth Soc J 1984;31:541–8

20. Selvin BL. Electroconvulsive therapy—1987. Anesthesiology 1987;67:367–85

21. Gaines GY, Rees EI. Electroconvulsive therapy and anaesthetic considerations. Anesth Analg 1986;65:1345–56

22. Price TRP, McAllister TW. Response of depressed patients to sequential unilateral nondominant brief-pulse and bilateral sinusoidal ECT. J Clin Psychiatry 1986;47:182–6

23. Gerring JP, Shields HM. The identification and management of patients with a high risk for cardiac arrhythmias during modified ECT. J Clin Psychiatry 1981;43:140–3

24. Khoury GF, Benedetti C. T-wave changes associated with electroconvulsive therapy. Anesth Analg 1989;69:677–9

25. Abrams R. Electroconvulsive Therapy. New York. Oxford University Press 1988

26. Partridge BL, Weinger MB, Hauger R. Is the cardiovascular response to electroconvulsive therapy due to the electricity or the subsequent convulsion? Anesth Analg 1991;72:706–9

27. Lee JT, Erbaugh PH, Stevens WC, Sack RL. Modification of electroconvulsive therapy induced hypertension with nitroglycerin. Anesthesiology 1985;62:793–6

28. Lovac AL, Goto H, Pardo MP, Arakawa K. Comparison of two esmolol bolus doses on the haemodynamic response and seizure duration during electroconvulsive therapy. Can J Anaesth 1991;38:204–9

29. Weinger MB, Partridge BL, Hauger R, Mirow A. Prevention of the cardiovascular and neuroendocrine response to electroconvulsive therapy. I. Effectiveness of pretreatment regimens on hemodynamics. Anesth Analg 1991;73:556–62

30. Rampton AJ, Griffin RM, Stuart CS, Durcan JJ, Huddy NC, Abbott MA. Comparison of methohexital and propofol for electroconvulsive therapy: Effects on hemodynamic responses and seizure duration. Anesthesiology 1989;70:412–7

31. Kellner CH, Monroe RR, Burns C, Bernstein HJ, Crumbley AJ. Electroconvulsive therapy in a patient with a heart transplant. N Engl J Med 1991;325:663

32. Havdala HS, Borison RL, Diamond BI. Potential hazards and applications of lithium in anesthesiology. Anesthesiology 1979;50:534–7

33. Diamond BI, Havdala HS, Borison RL. Potential of lithium as an anesthetic premedicant. Lancet 1977;2:1229–30

34. Hill GE, Wong KC, Hodges MR. Lithium carbonate and neuromuscular blocking agents. Anesthesiology 1977;46:122–6

35. Wilson WH, Weiler SJ. Case report of phenothiazine-induced torsade de pointes. Am J Psychiatry 1984;141:1265–70

36. Guze BH, Baxter LR. Neuroleptic malignant syndrome. N Engl J Med 1985;313:163–6

37. Patel P, Bristow G. Postoperative neuroleptic malignant syndrome. A case report. Can J Anaesth 1987;34:515–8

38. Krivosic-Horber R, Adnet P, Guevart E, Theunynck D, Lestavel P. Neuroleptic malignant syndrome and malignant hyperthermia. Br J Anaesth 1987;59:1554–6

39. Geiduschek J, Cohen SA, Khan A, Cullen BF. Repeated anesthesia for a patient with neuroleptic malignant syndrome. Anesthesiology 1988;68:134–7

40. Caroff SN, Rosenberg H, Fletcher JE, et al. Malignant hyperthermia susceptibility in neuroleptic malignant syndrome. Anesthesiology 1987;67:20–5

41. Adams AP, Goroszeniuk T. Hysteria. A cause of failure to recover from anaesthesia. Anaesthesia 1991;46:932–4

42. Diagnostic and Statistical Manual of Mental Disorders. Washington, DC. American Psychiatric Association 1987

43. Jenkins LC. Anaesthetic problems due to drug abuse and dependence. Can Anaesth Soc J 1972;19:461–77

44. McGoldrick KE. Anesthetic implications of drug abuse. Anesthesiology Review 1980;7:12–7

45. Morse RM, Flavin DK. The definition of alcoholism. JAMA 1992;268:1012–4

46. Fuller RK, Branchey L, Brightwell DR, et al. Disulfiram treatment of alcoholism: A Veterans Administration cooperative study. JAMA 1986;256:1449–53

47. Diaz JH, Hill GE. Hypotension with anesthesia in disulfiram-treated patients. Anesthesiology 1979;51:355–8

48. Cregler LL, Mark H. Medical complications of cocaine abuse. N Engl J Med 1986;315:1495–1500

49. Pollin W. The danger of cocaine. JAMA 1985;254:98

50. Lange RA, Cigarroa RG, Yancy CW, et al. Cocaine-induced coronary-artery vasoconstriction. N Engl J Med 1989;321:1557–62

51. Levine SR, Brust JCM, Futrell N, et al. Cerebrovascular complications of the use of the "crack" form of alkaloidal cocaine. N Engl J Med 1990;323:699–704

52. Kossowsky WA, Lyon AF, Chou AY. Cocaine and ischemic heart disease. Practical Cardiology 1986;12:164–78

53. Pollan S, Tadjziechy M. Esmolol in the management of epinephrine- and cocaine-induced cardiovascular toxicity. Anesth Analg 1989;69:663–4

54. Gay GR, Loper KA. Control of cocaine-induced hypertension with labetalol. Anesth Analg 1988;67:92

55. Koehntop DE, Kiao JC, Van Bergen FH. Effects of pharmacologic alteration of adrenergic mechanisms by cocaine, tropolone, aminophylline, and ketamine on epinephrine-induced arrhythmias during halothane-nitrous oxide anesthesia. Anesthesiology 1977;46:83–9

56. Stoelting RK, Creasser CW, Martz RC. Effects of cocaine administration of halothane MAC in dogs. Anesth Analg 1975;54:422–4

57. Barash P, Kopriva CJ, Langou R, et al. Is cocaine a sympathetic stimulant during general anesthesia? JAMA 1980;243:1437–41

58. Blachly PH. Management of the opiate abstinence syndrome. Am J Psychiatry 1966;122:742–59

59. Gold MS, Pottash AC, Sweeney DR, Kleber HD. Opiate withdrawal using clonidine: A safe, effective, and rapid monopiate treatment. JAMA 1980;243:343–6

60. Giuffrida JG, Bizzarri DV, Saure AC, Sharoff RL. Anesthetic management of drug abusers. Anesth Analg 1970;49:273–82

61. Berkowitz BA, Finck AD, Hynes MD, Ngai SH. Tolerance to N_2O anesthesia in rats and mice. Anesthesiology 1979;51:309–14

62. Marck LC. Hypotension during anesthesia in narcotic addicts. NY State J Med 1966;66:2685–97

63. Lee PKY, Cho MH, Dobkin AB. Effects of alcoholism, morphinism, and barbiturate resistance on induction and maintenance of general anaesthesia. Can Anaesth Soc J 1974;11:366–71

64. Johnston RR, Way WL, Miller RD. Alteration of anesthetic requirements by amphetamine. Anesthesiology 1972;36:357–63

65. Poster DS, Penta JS, Bruno S, Macdonald JS. Tetrahydrocannabinol in clinical oncology. JAMA 1981;245:2047–51

66. Vitez TS, Way WL, Miller RD, Eger EI. Effects of delta-9-tetrahydrocannabinol on cyclopropane MAC in the rat. Anesthesiology 1973;38:525–7

67. Stoelting RK, Martz RC, Gartner J, et al. Effects of delta-9-tetrahydrocannabinol on halothane MAC in dogs. Anesthesiology 1973;38:521–4

68. Johnstone RC, Lief PL, Kulp RA, Smith TC. Combination of delta-9-tetrahydrocannabinol with oxymorphine or pentobarbital. Anesthesiology 1975;42:674–9

69. Siemons AJ, Kalant H, Khanna JM. Effect of cannabis on pentobarbital-induced sleeping time and pentobarbital metabolism in the rat. Biochem Pharmacol 1974;23:447–53

70. Frommer DA, Kulig KW, Marx JA, Rumack B. Tricyclic antidepressant overdose. A review. JAMA 1987;257:521–6

71. Smilkstein MJ, Knapp GL, Kulig KW, Rumack BH. Efficacy of oral N-acetylcysteine in the treatment of acetaminophen overdose. Analysis of the national multicenter study (1976–1985). N Engl J Med 1988;319:1557–62

72. Baud FJ, Galliot M, Astier A, et al. Treatment of ethylene glycol poisoning with intravenous 4-methylpyrazole. N Engl J Med 1988;319:97–100

73. Bass M. Death from sniffing gasoline. (Letter.) N Engl J Med 1978;299:203

74. Davies JE. Changing profile of pesticide poisoning. N Engl J Med 1987;316:807–8

75. Barker SJ, Tremper KK. The effect of carbon monoxide inhalation on pulse oximetry and transcutaneous PO_2. Anesthesiology 1987;66:677–9

31

Physiologic Changes and Diseases Unique to the Parturient

PHYSIOLOGIC CHANGES IN PREGNANCY

Pregnancy and subsequent labor and delivery are accompanied by physiologic changes in multiple organ systems. An appreciation of these changes and their implications as they relate to responses to anesthesia is useful for the management of anesthesia in the parturient and her fetus.

Cardiovascular System

Changes in the cardiovascular system during pregnancy provide for the needs of the developing fetus and prepare the mother for those events that accompany labor and delivery (Table 31-1). An increase in maternal intravascular fluid volume begins in the first trimester and at term results in an average expansion of about 1000 ml (Fig. 31-1). The disproportionate increase in plasma volume accounts for the relative anemia of pregnancy, whereas a maternal hemoglobin concentration less than 11 g·dl^{-1} most likely reflects an iron deficiency anemia. The increased intravascular fluid volume offsets the 400- to 600-ml blood loss that accompanies vaginal delivery and the average 1000-ml blood loss that accompanies cesarean section. The normal nonpregnant intravascular fluid volume is usually reestablished 7 to 14 days postpartum.

Cardiac output is increased about 40% above the nonpregnant level by about the tenth week of gestation and maintained at this level throughout the second and third trimesters, most likely reflecting the effects of placental and ovarian steroids principally on stroke volume. Earlier studies suggesting that cardiac output decreased during the third trimester were in error. Instead, this decrease reflected decreased venous return due to obstruction of the inferior vena cava by the gravid uterus. The onset of labor is associated with additional increases in cardiac output (each uterine contraction can increase cardiac output an additional 20%), whereas the greatest increase (as much as 60% above the prelabor value) occurs early after delivery. The parturient with co-existing heart disease may not be able to increase cardiac output during labor, delivery, and the immediate postpartum period. In this regard, regional anesthesia may protect the compromised cardiovascular system during the peripartum period by attenuating the usual increases in cardiac output.[1]

Systolic blood pressure does not increase above nonpregnant levels during an uncomplicated pregnancy. Since cardiac output is increased, the systemic vascular resistance must decrease for the blood pressure to remain normal. Indeed, diastolic blood pressure usually decreases about 15% during pregnancy.

Supine Hypotension Syndrome

Supine hypotension syndrome (SHS) is a decrease in maternal blood pressure that occurs in about 10% of parturients near term, when they assume the supine position. Diaphoresis, nausea and vomiting, and changes in cerebration may accompany this hypotension. The mechanism for SHS is decreased venous return due to obstruction of the inferior vena cava by the gravid uterus, when the parturient assumes the supine position. Compression of the inferior vena cava is most com-

539

Table 31-1. Changes in the Cardiovascular System

	Average Change from Nonpregnant Value (%)
Intravascular fluid volume	+35
Plasma volume	+45
Erythrocyte volume	+20
Cardiac output	+40
Stroke volume	+30
Heart rate	+15
Peripheral circulation	
Systolic blood pressure	No change
Systemic vascular resistance	−15
Diastolic blood pressure	−15
Central venous pressure	No change
Femoral venous pressure	+15

mon late in pregnancy before the presenting part becomes fixed in the pelvis. Fortunately, most parturients are able to initiate compensatory responses that offset the potential adverse hemodynamic sequelae of this phenomenon. For example, increased venous pressure below the level of the inferior

vena cava obstruction serves to divert venous blood from the lower one-half of the body through the paravertebral venous plexuses to the azygos vein. Flow from the azygos vein enters the superior vena cava and right heart, to maintain venous return, cardiac output, and blood pressure. This compensatory response means that inadvertent intravascular injection of a local anesthetic during an attempted lumbar epidural anesthetic can result in bolus delivery of the drug to the heart. As a result, cardiac depression may be profound. An additional compensatory response that offsets obstruction of the inferior vena cava is an increase in sympathetic nervous system activity and subsequent increase in systemic vascular resistance, permitting maintenance of blood pressure despite a decreased cardiac output. It is important to appreciate that compensatory increases in systemic vascular resistance are impaired by regional anesthetic techniques. Indeed, arterial hypotension is more common and profound during regional anesthesia administered to a parturient, as compared with a nonpregnant patient. Nevertheless, this impairment of compensatory vasoconstriction by regional anesthesia may be less ominous than pain-induced changes, which result in vasoconstriction that includes the uterine vasculature.

In addition to impaired blood flow through the inferior vena cava, angiographic studies have demonstrated compression of the lower abdominal aorta by the gravid uterus, when the parturient assumes the supine position.[2] This compression leads to arterial hypotension in the lower extremities, as well as decreased uterine blood flow. In contrast to compression of the inferior vena cava, obstruction to flow through the abdominal aorta is not associated with maternal symptoms or with a decrease in blood pressure, measured in the upper extremity.

Aortocaval compression results in uteroplacental insufficiency and fetal asphyxia due to decreased uterine blood flow. Even in the presence of a healthy uteroplacental unit, decreased maternal systolic blood pressure to less than 100 mmHg that persists for longer than 10 to 15 minutes may be associated with progressive fetal acidosis and bradycardia.[3] This emphasizes that uterine blood flow and, therefore, placental blood flow varies directly with maternal blood pressure.

The incidence of the SHS can be minimized by nursing the parturient in the lateral position. Measures to increase maternal blood pressure should be instituted whenever (1) systolic blood pressure decreases below 100 mmHg in a previously normotensive parturient, (2) there is a 20% to 30% decrease in blood pressure in a previously hypertensive parturient, or (3) there are fetal heart rate changes suggestive of uteroplacental insufficiency (see the section, Diagnosis and Management of Fetal Distress). Therapeutic measures include intravenous administration of fluids, left uterine displacement, and intravenous administration of ephedrine. Left uterine displacement is effective by moving the gravid uterus off the inferior vena cava or aorta. Displacement of the uterus to the left can

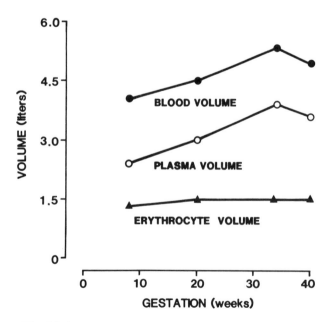

Fig. 31-1. Changes in intravascular fluid volume (blood volume), plasma volume, and erythrocyte volume during progression of normal pregnancy. The disproportionate increase in plasma volume accounts for the relative anemia of pregnancy.

be accomplished manually by lifting and displacing the uterus to the left. Alternatively, the parturient can be positioned by rotating the delivery table 15 degrees to the left or by elevation of the right buttock 10 to 15 cm with a blanket or foam rubber wedge.

Pulmonary System

Changes in the pulmonary system during pregnancy are manifested as alterations in the upper airway, minute ventilation, lung volumes, and arterial oxygenation (Table 31-2 and Fig. 31-2). These changes can influence the selection of tracheal tube sizes and the rate of induction of, and emergence from, anesthesia.

Capillary engorgement of the mucosal lining of the upper respiratory tract can result in difficult nasal breathing and in a propensity toward the development of nose bleeds. Symptoms can be exacerbated by even a mild upper respiratory tract infection or edema associated with pregnancy-induced hypertension. These changes emphasize the need for gentleness during instrumentation of the upper airway. Vigorous oropharyngeal suctioning, placement of a nasal or oral airway, or trauma during direct laryngoscopy can result in hemorrhage and further edema. It may be useful to select a smaller size cuffed tracheal tube (6.5 to 7.0 mm I.D.), since the false vocal cords and arytenoids are often edematous.

An increase in minute ventilation is one of the earliest and most dramatic changes in pulmonary function during preg-

nancy. Minute ventilation is increased about 50% above non-pregnant levels during the first trimester and is maintained at this level for the remainder of the pregnancy. An increased circulating level of progesterone is presumed to be the stimulus for increased minute ventilation. The resting $PaCO_2$ decreases from 40 mmHg to near 30 mmHg during the first trimester, as a reflection of increased minute ventilation. The PaO_2 increases a similar amount. The arterial pH remains near normal because of increased renal excretion of sodium bicarbonate, resulting in about a 4-mEq·L^{-1} decrease in the plasma bicarbonate concentration. Pain associated with labor and delivery results in further hyperventilation, which can be attenuated by epidural analgesia.[4] Opioid-induced depression of ventilation seems to be less in the parturient, perhaps reflecting stimulatory effects of increased circulating concentrations of progesterone.

In contrast to the early appearance of increased minute ventilation, lung volumes do not begin to change until about the fifth month of gestation. With increasing enlargement of the uterus, the diaphragm is forced to assume a more cephalad position. This change is largely responsible for the 20% decrease in expiratory reserve volume and residual volume present at term (Fig. 31-2). As a result of these changes, functional residual capacity is decreased to a similar degree. Other lung volumes and capacities, including vital capacity, are not significantly changed during pregnancy.

The combination of increased minute ventilation and decreased functional residual capacity speeds the rate at which denitrogenation occurs in the term parturient compared with the nonpregnant patient[5] (Fig. 31-3). These changes also speed the rate at which a change in the alveolar concentration of an inhaled anesthetic can be achieved. Induction of anesthesia, emergence from anesthesia, and changes in the depth of anesthesia are notably faster in the parturient. In addition, dose requirements for volatile anesthetic drugs may be reduced during pregnancy.[6] The combination of accelerated onset and decreased anesthetic requirements makes the parturient susceptible to an anesthetic overdose. For example, a low concentration of an inhaled anesthetic may result in loss of protective upper airway reflexes during the administration of an inspired concentration of anesthetic that is usually considered safe.

Induction of general anesthesia in the parturient may be associated with a marked decrease in the PaO_2 if apnea is prolonged, as during intubation of the trachea. This tendency for a rapid decrease in arterial oxygenation reflects a decreased oxygen reserve secondary to a reduction in functional residual capacity. The near 20% increase in oxygen consumption present near term also contributes to a decreased oxygen reserve. These changes emphasize the potential value of pre-oxygenation before any anticipated period of apnea in a parturi-

Table 31-2. Changes in the Pulmonary System

	Average Change from Nonpregnant Value (%)
Minute ventilation	+50
Tidal volume	+40
Breathing rate	+10
PaO_2	+10 mmHg
$PaCO_2$	−10 mmHg
pHa	No change
Total lung capacity	No change
Vital capacity	No change
Functional residual capacity	−20%
Expiratory reserve volume	−20%
Residual volume	−20%
Airway resistance	−35%
Oxygen consumption	+20%

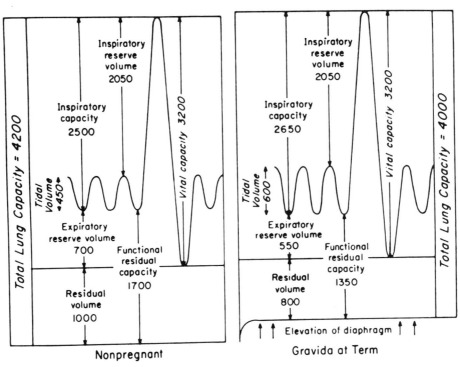

Fig. 31-2. Comparison of lung volumes and capacities in the nonpregnant patient and in the gravida at term. (From Bonica JJ. Principles and Practice of Obstetric Analgesia and Anesthesia. Philadelphia, FA Davis 1976, with permission.)

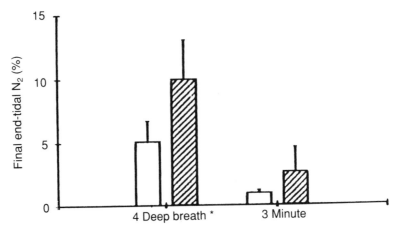

Fig. 31-3. End-tidal nitrogen (N_2) concentration (%) after 3 minutes of tidal breathing or four deep breaths of 100% oxygen in parturients (open bars) and nonparturients (cross-hatched bars). *P (0.0001 vs 3 min); *P (0.001 vs pregnant). (From Norris MC, Kirkland MR, Torjman MC, Goldberg ME. Denitrogenation in pregnancy. Can J Anaesth 1989;36:523–5, with permission.)

ent. In order to maximize the fetal benefit of preoxygenation, the maternal inhalation of oxygen may need to be continued for about 6 minutes, since this is the estimated time required for maternal to fetal equilibration. A mean increase in the umbilical vein PO_2 from 22 mmHg to 28 mmHg can be expected in the fetus of a parturient breathing oxygen for this period of time. The parturient's PaO_2 often exceeds 100 mmHg breathing room air, reflecting the presence of chronic hyperventilation. Assumption of the supine position may result in a decrease in the PaO_2, presumably reflecting a decrease in cardiac output owing to aortocaval compression. Since it is not possible to predict the susceptibility of an individual parturient to aortocaval compression, it would seem prudent to provide left uterine displacement routinely and to administer supplemental oxygen when regional anesthesia is used.

Nervous System

Anesthetic requirements for methoxyflurane, halothane, and isoflurane are reduced 25% to 40% in gravid animals at term.[6] It is presumed, but not documented, that similar changes occur for nitrous oxide requirements. There is evidence that treatment of animals with progesterone can decrease halothane MAC, suggesting that the sedative effect of this hormone may also explain the decreased anesthetic requirement in parturients[7] (Fig. 31-4). Nevertheless, in animals, anesthetic requirements return to nonpregnant values within 5 days postpartum, while the plasma concentration of progesterone remains elevated, suggesting that the mechanism for reduction cannot be attributed entirely to progesterone.[8] Regardless of the mechanism, the important clinical implication is that the alveolar concentration of an inhaled anesthetic that would not produce unconsciousness in a nonpregnant patient may approximate an anesthetizing concentration in a parturient. This degree of central nervous system depression may also impair protective upper airway reflexes and subject the parturient to hazards of pulmonary aspiration.

Increased intra-abdominal pressure as pregnancy progresses, plus shunting of blood through the paravertebral venous plexuses due to compression of the inferior vena cava, results in engorgement of epidural veins. This engorgement decreases the the size of the epidural space and by compression may also reduce the volume of cerebrospinal fluid in the subarachnoid space. These engorged veins also exert a pumping-like effect, resulting in the spread of a local anesthetic placed in the epidural space over more segments than would normally be expected. Furthermore, high pressure in the epidural space may facilitate the transfer of a local anesthetic into the cerebrospinal fluid and favor the action of the drug directly on the spinal cord. In addition, each spinal nerve root is accompanied by an epidural vein as it passes out of the intervertebral foramina. If this vein is swollen, it may decrease the size of the foramina and reduce the escape of drugs that have been injected into the epidural space. Even exaggerated lumbar lordosis of pregnancy may contribute to the cephalad spread of a local anesthetic. These changes are consistent with the 30% to 50% reductions in dose requirements of local anesthetics necessary for epidural or subarachnoid anesthesia at term, as compared with nonpregnant patients.[9] The observation of exaggerated spread of local anesthetics placed in the epidural space as early as the first trimester suggests a role of biochemical and mechanical changes.[10] For example, a reduced plasma concentration of bicarbonate in compensation for hyperventilation could reduce buffer capacity and contribute to

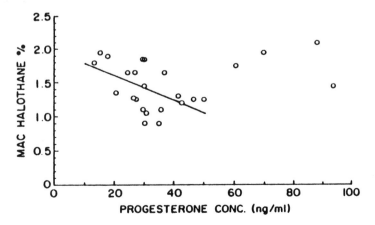

Fig. 31-4. Halothane anesthetic requirements are inversely related to the plasma progesterone concentration. (From Datta S, Migliozzi RP, Flanagan HL, Krieger NR. Chronically administered progesterone decreases halothane requirements in rabbits. Anesth Analg 1989;68:46–50, with permission.)

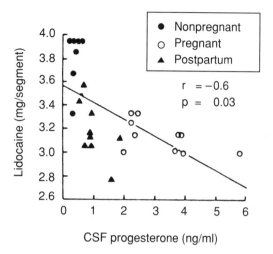

Fig. 31-5. Lidocaine dose requirements (milligrams per segment) are inversely related to the cerebrospinal fluid concentration of progesterone in nonpregnant, pregnant, and postpartum patients. (From Datta S, Hurley RJ, Naulty JS, et al. Plasma and cerebrospinal fluid progesterone concentrations in pregnant and nonpregnant women. Anesth Analg 1986;65:950–4, with permission.)

enhanced actions of a local anesthetic. Likewise, increased plasma and cerebrospinal fluid concentrations of progesterone parallel the augmented dermatomal spread of local anesthetics placed in the subarachnoid space[11] (Fig. 31-5). Despite these observations, there are also data that do not demonstrate a difference in the level of sensory anesthesia achieved, when equal volumes of local anesthetic solution are injected into the epidural space of pregnant and nonpregnant patients, if care is exercised to prevent aortocaval compression.[12]

Kidneys

Renal blood flow and glomerular filtration rate are increased about 50% by the fourth month of gestation. During the third trimester, these values slowly return toward the nonpregnant level. As a reflection of these changes, the normal upper limit of the blood urea nitrogen concentration and plasma creatinine concentration is reduced about 50%.

Liver

The plasma cholinesterase activity is decreased about 25% from the tenth week of gestation to as long as 6 weeks postpartum.[13] This decreased activity is unlikely to be associated with prolongation of the neuromuscular blocking effects of succinylcholine, although occasional unexpected prolonged responses have been observed.[14,15] Acute fatty liver of pregnancy is a rare but potentially fatal disorder that is typically

manifested after about 35 weeks of gestation.[16] Management of anesthesia for a cesarean section using epidural anesthesia has been described in a patient with this disorder.[17]

Gastrointestinal System

Gastrointestinal changes during pregnancy make the parturient vulnerable to regurgitation of gastric contents and to the development of acid pneumonitis, if pulmonary aspiration occurs. For example, the enlarged uterus displaces the pylorus upward and backward, which retards gastric emptying. In addition, progesterone decreases gastrointestinal motility. As a result, gastric emptying time is prolonged, and gastric fluid volume tends to be increased, even in fasting states. Furthermore, the enlarging uterus changes the angle of the gastroesophageal junction, leading to relative incompetence of the physiologic sphincter mechanism. Indeed, lower esophageal sphincter pressure is less and gastric pressure greater in pregnant as compared with nonpregnant patients.[18] As a result, gastric fluid reflux into the esophagus and esophagitis are common in the parturient. These changes emphasize that the parturient is prone to silent regurgitation, even in the absence of sedative drugs or general anesthesia.

The increased risk of pulmonary aspiration of gastric contents is the reason for recommending placement of a cuffed tube in the trachea of every parturient who is going to be rendered unconscious with central nervous system depressant drugs. Only in rare situations, when intubation of the trachea is technically impossible and there is fetal distress necessitating prompt delivery, is general anesthesia in the absence of a cuffed tube in the trachea considered acceptable. In this situation, sustained cricoid pressure should be employed to reduce the possibility of passively regurgitated material entering the hypopharynx. Furthermore, cricoid pressure should prevent excessive gastric distension.

The recognition that pH of inhaled gastric fluid is important in the production and severity of acid pneumonitis is the basis for the administration of oral antacids to parturients during labor and before delivery.[19,20] There is no doubt that oral antacids are effective in increasing the pH of gastric fluid. Nevertheless, it is difficult to confirm benefits of routine use of oral antacids.[21,22] In an attempt to obviate the hazards of inhalation of particulate antacids, the use of a nonparticulate antacid, such as sodium citrate, has been recommended.[23] It is of interest that administration of opioids to provide analgesia during labor slows gastric emptying and prolongs the duration of action of antacids.[24] Frequent antacid administration to patients also receiving opioids could result in accumulating gastric fluid volume. For this reason, when antacids are administered as prophylaxis before general anesthesia they should be administered just before the induction of anesthesia. Considering the potential accumulation of antacids in the stomach, there seems little reason to recommend the routine use of antacids at regular intervals during labor.[24]

Additional drugs for increasing gastric fluid pH and decreasing the gastric fluid volume can be considered. For example, metoclopramide increases lower esophageal sphincter tone and speeds gastric emptying of patients in active labor.[25] In view of its beneficial effects, metoclopramide may be a useful drug to administer to the parturient at high risk of an increased gastric fluid volume (apprehension, opioid analgesia, recent food ingestion, obesity, heartburn indicative of gastric fluid reflux) and requiring general anesthesia. Metoclopramide, however, may not reverse gastric hypomotility due to opioids. In the absence of active labor and an increased gastric fluid volume, metoclopramide has not been shown to result in significant differences in gastric fluid volumes compared with untreated parturients.[26] Indeed, in the absence of active labor, gastric emptying time may not be delayed, as compared with nonpregnant women.[27] For this reason, routine administration of metoclopramide to parturients before elective cesarean section may not be useful. Histamine receptor (H-2) antagonists may also elevate gastric fluid pH predictably in parturients.

PHYSIOLOGY OF THE UTEROPLACENTAL CIRCULATION

The placenta provides for the union of the maternal and fetal circulations for the purpose of physiologic exchange. Maternal blood is delivered to the placenta by the uterine arteries, and fetal blood arrives through two umbilical arteries. Nutrient-rich and waste-free blood is delivered to the fetus through a single umbilical vein. The most important determinants of placental function are uterine blood flow and the placental area available for exchange of nutrients. An acute decrease in placental function interferes with the passage of oxygen to, and carbon dioxide from, the fetus, resulting in fetal hypoxemia and acidosis. A chronic decrease in placental function is associated with delayed fetal growth, reflecting absence of necessary nutrient factors.

Uterine Blood Flow

Uterine blood flow at term is 500 to 700 ml·min^{-1}, which represents about 10% of the maternal cardiac output. Uterine blood flow is not autoregulated; as a result, placental blood flow is directly proportional to mean perfusion pressure (uterine arterial pressure minus uterine venous pressure) and is inversely proportional to uterine vascular resistance. Maintenance of uterine blood flow is critical, as this flow determines the adequacy of placental circulation, and ultimately fetal well-being. Uterine blood flow is reduced by drugs or events that decrease perfusion pressure or that increase uterine vascular resistance. For example, maternal hypotension (SHS) or excessive uterine activity are the events most likely to reduce uterine blood flow acutely. In the presence of a normal placenta, it is estimated that uterine blood flow can decrease about 50% before fetal distress, as reflected by acidosis, is detectable.[28] Alpha agonist drugs such as methoxamine and metaraminol can produce uterine vascular constriction that results in decreased uterine blood flow and development of fetal acidosis[29] (Fig. 31-6). Conversely, ephedrine does not decrease uterine blood flow, despite substantial increases in maternal arterial pressure[29] (Fig. 31-6). Increased uterine vascular resistance, with decreased uterine blood flow, can result from maternal stress or pain that stimulates endogenous release of catecholamines[30] (Fig. 31-7). This response suggests that adequate regional or general anesthesia may be protective to the fetus. During controlled ventilation of the lungs, decreased uterine blood flow may be due to the mechanical effects of positive pressure and not to vasoconstricting effects of a low maternal PaCO$_2$[31] (Fig. 31-8).

Drugs administered to the parturient to produce analgesia and anesthesia during labor and delivery may produce profound effects on uterine blood flow, and, therefore, on fetal well-being. These effects are most likely due to drug-induced changes in maternal blood pressure, rather than to any direct effect on uterine tone or vasculature. Data on the effects of anesthetics on uterine blood flow are almost exclusively from animal models, most often the pregnant ewe. When the inspired concentration of halothane is less than 1%, fetal acid-base status is not adversely affected, suggesting that uterine blood flow is not significantly decreased.[32] A higher inspired concentration of halothane is associated with maternal hypotension and fetal acidosis. Isoflurane and, by inference, other volatile anesthetics, when administered at a concentration comparable to that studied for halothane, have similar effects on uterine blood flow.[33] Thiopental decreases uterine blood flow in proportion to drug-induced decreases in blood pressure. Ketamine, in doses up to 1 mg·kg^{-1} IV, is unlikely to alter uterine blood flow.[34] Higher doses of ketamine may lead to increased uterine tone associated with a decrease in uterine blood flow despite normal to increased maternal blood pressure[34] (Fig. 31-9). Epidural anesthesia with chloroprocaine or bupivacaine does not alter uterine blood flow, if maternal hypotension is avoided.[35,36] Furthermore, the addition of epinephrine to the local anesthetic solution does not seem to influence uterine blood flow.

Passive diffusion is the principal mechanism for the transfer of drugs across the placenta, from the maternal circulation to the fetus. Minimizing the maternal blood concentration of a drug is the most important method for limiting the amount of drug that ultimately reaches the fetus. Furthermore, transfer of a drug to the fetus can be decreased by its intravenous

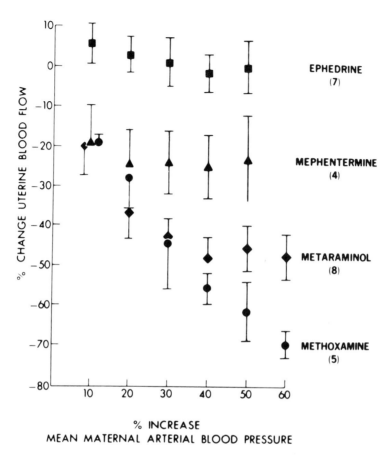

Fig. 31-6. With the exception of ephedrine, uterine blood flow in the pregnant ewe decreases after the administration of a sympathomimetic, despite a concomitant increase in maternal mean arterial blood pressure. (From Ralston D, Shnider SM, deLorimer AA. Effects of equipotent ephedrine, metaraminol, mephentermine, and methoxamine on uterine blood flow in the pregnant ewe. Anesthesiology 1974;40:354–70, with permission.)

injection just before the uterine contraction, since uterine blood flow is markedly decreased during a contraction.

The unique characteristics of the fetal circulation influence the distribution of drugs in the fetus. For example, about 75% of the umbilical venous blood flows through the liver; the remainder of this blood passes through the ductus venosus into the inferior vena cava. As a result of hepatic perfusion, a significant amount of drug can be metabolized. Indeed, hepatic metabolism reduces the concentration of a drug that is eventually delivered by the fetal arterial circulation to vital organs such as the brain and heart. Furthermore, a drug in the portion of the umbilical venous blood that enters the inferior vena cava through the ductus venosus will be diluted by drug-free blood returning from the lower extremities and pelvic viscera of the fetus. Therefore, it is likely that the drug concentration measured in umbilical vein blood will be substantially higher than the concentration delivered to fetal tissues by the arterial

circulation. This is consistent with the observation that maternal depression produced by drugs, such as thiopental or inhaled anesthetics, is not paralleled by similar degrees of fetal central nervous system depression. Indeed, the unique anatomy of the fetal circulation serves to protect the vital organs of the fetus from exposure to a high concentration of drug that may be present in the umbilical venous blood, secondary to passage of these drugs from the maternal circulation. Nevertheless, fetal acidosis is associated with increased myocardial blood flow and cerebral blood flow, with a resulting increased delivery of drugs to these organs during fetal distress. In addition, a lower fetal pH means that weakly basic drugs, such as local anesthetics and opioids that cross the placenta in a nonionized form, will become ionized in the fetal circulation. Since an ionized drug cannot readily cross the placenta back into the maternal circulation, it follows that this drug will accumulate in fetal blood against a concentration gradient. This

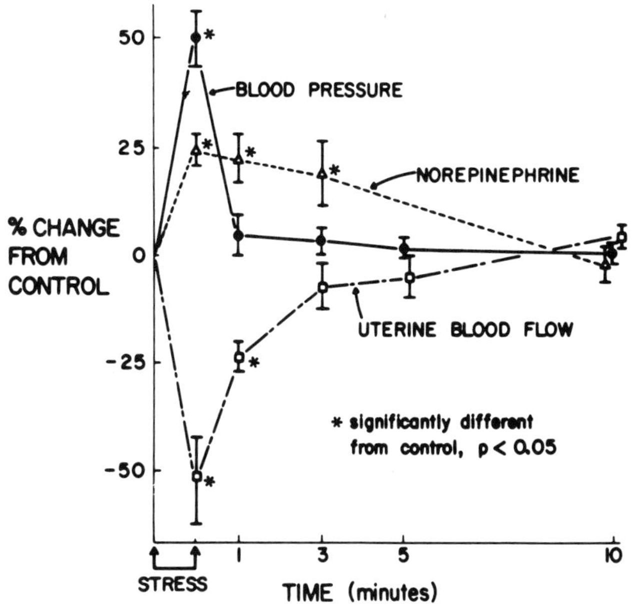

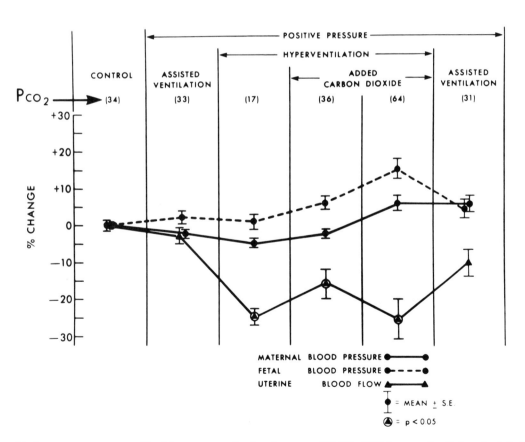

Fig. 31-7. Electrically induced stress in pregnant ewes causes an increase in maternal blood pressure and plasma norepinephrine concentration and a concomitant decrease in maternal uterine blood flow. (From Shnider SM, Wright RG, Levinson G, et al. Uterine blood flow and plasma norepinephrine changes during maternal stress in the pregnant ewe. Anesthesiology 1979;50:524–7, with permission.)

Fig. 31-8. Decreases in uterine blood flow were unrelated to the maternal $PaCO_2$ (PCO_2), suggesting that mechanical effects of positive pressure ventilation of the lungs were responsible. (From Levinson G, Shnider SM, deLorimer AA, Steffenson JL. Effects of maternal hyperventilation on uterine blood flow and fetal oxygenation and acid-base status. Anesthesiology 1974;40:340–7, with permission.)

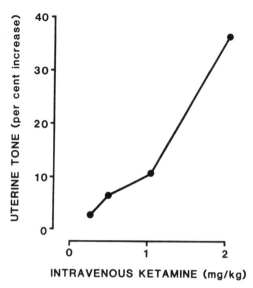

Fig. 31-9. Ketamine produces a dose-related increase in uterine tone, as measured in parturients at term. (Data from Galloon S. Ketamine for obstetric delivery. Anesthesiology 1976;44:522–4.)

phenomenon is known as ion trapping and may explain the higher concentration of lidocaine present in the fetus when acidosis due to fetal distress is present[37] (Fig. 31-10). Furthermore, the conversion of lidocaine to the ionized fraction maintains a concentration gradient from the mother to the fetus for continued passage of nonionized lidocaine to the fetus.

MATERNAL MEDICATION DURING LABOR

Despite the common use of epidural analgesia for pain relief during labor, there is still an occasional role for systemic medication to relieve pain and anxiety. There is no ideal drug, as all systemic medications cross the placenta to some extent

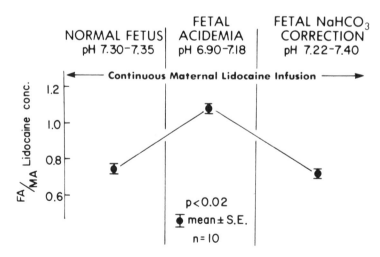

Fig. 31-10. Fetal-to-maternal arterial (FA/MA) lidocaine ratios were increased during fetal acidemia, reflecting ion trapping (acidosis converts lidocaine to the ionized fraction that cannot cross the placenta back into the maternal circulation) of the local anesthetic in the fetus. (From Biehl D, Shnider SM, Levinson G, Callender K. Placental transfer of lidocaine. Effects of fetal acidosis. Anesthesiology 1978;48:409–12, with permission.)

and produce depressant effects on the fetus. The amount of fetal depression depends primarily on the dose of drug and on the route and time of administration before delivery. Drugs likely to be administered as systemic medications are benzodiazepines, opioids, and perhaps ketamine. For example, a low dose of midazolam (0.5 to 1 mg IV) may be useful for relieving anxiety during cesarean section performed with epidural anesthesia. All opioids cross the placenta and may cause neonatal ventilatory depression and altered neurobehavioral status. Meperidine is a popular opioid for administration to the parturient, particularly because the respiratory center of the newborn seems less sensitive to this opioid than morphine.[38] In an occasional parturient, intermittent doses of ketamine (10 to 15 mg IV) can be titrated to produce intense analgesia without producing a loss of consciousness. The onset of action of ketamine is usually within 1 minute, and the duration of effect is 5 to 15 minutes. This low-dose approach is particularly useful for the parturient in whom vaginal delivery is imminent or when regional analgesia is incomplete. Ketamine readily crosses the placenta but in low doses does not cause neonatal depression. Adverse maternal psychological effects may accompany even these low doses of ketamine.

PROGRESS OF LABOR

Progress of labor refers to increasing cervical dilation, effacement, and descent of the presenting fetal part with time[39] (Fig. 31-11). This progress is divided into the first and second stages of labor, depending on the dilation of the cervix. The first stage is further subdivided into a latent and an active phase. The active phase consists of an acceleration phase, phase of maximum slope, and deceleration phase. The onset of regular contractions signals the beginning of the first stage of labor. This stage lasts 7 to 13 hours in a primigravida and 4 to 5 hours in a multigravida. The second stage of labor begins with complete dilation of the cervix.

The progress of labor is unpredictable because it is influenced by many variables, including maternal pain, parity, size and presentation of the fetus, and drugs and techniques used to provide analgesia or anesthesia. Abnormal progress of labor can be classified as slow latent phase, active phase arrest, and arrest of descent (Table 31-3). Excessive sedation or anesthesia is the most common cause for prolongation of the latent phase. The mechanism is decreased uterine activity secondary to depressant drugs. During the active phase, the

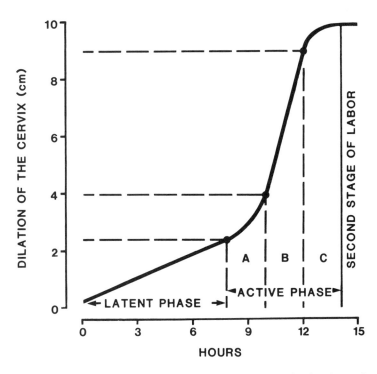

Fig. 31-11. The progress of labor is described as the first stage (latent and active phase) and second stage, depending on the dilation of the cervix. The active phase consists of the accelerated phase (A), the phase of maximum slope (B), and the deceleration phase (C). (Adapted from Friedman EA. Primigravid labor. A graphicostatistical analysis. Obstet Gynecol 1955;6:567–89, with permission.)

Table 31-3.   Abnormal Progress of Labor

	Primigravida	Multigravida
Slow latent phase	>20 hours	>14 hours
Active phase arrest	No dilation of cervix for 2 hours	No dilation of cervix for 2 hours
Arrest of descent	No descent for 1 hour	No descent for 1 hour

most likely causes of delayed progress of labor are cephalopelvic disproportion, fetal malposition, and fetal malpresentation.

The regional anesthetic technique selected to provide analgesia may affect uterine activity and the progress of labor. It is sometimes suggested that the administration of regional analgesia early in the course of labor will slow the progress of labor. It is difficult to confirm this notion, since the early progress of labor is so variable. Indeed, labor can slow during the latent phase in the absence of anesthesia. Furthermore, catecholamines released in response to pain can inhibit coordinated and effective uterine contractions, such that analgesia provided by an appropriate regional anesthetic technique may actually enhance early progress of labor. The impact of anesthesia on the progress of labor is more predictable after labor has become active. For example, during the active phase of the first stage, a T10 sensory level produced by subarachnoid anesthesia or lumbar epidural anesthesia has no significant effect on uterine activity or the progress of labor, provided that fetal malposition or malpresentation is absent and hypotension is avoided.[40,41] By removing the reflex urge of the parturient to bear down, however, regional anesthesia may prolong the second stage of labor. Nevertheless, there is no evidence that labor prolonged by regional anesthesia is harmful to the fetus.

An increased incidence of midforceps deliveries may occur when regional analgesia is administered.[42] Furthermore, relaxation of pelvic musculature interferes with flexion and internal rotation of the fetus, which may predispose to persistent occiput posterior presentations. These problems can be minimized by using a low concentration of local anesthetic for epidural analgesia, to preserve skeletal muscle function, and by withholding perineal doses of the local anesthetic until descent and rotation of the fetus have occurred.

Volatile anesthetics produce dose-related decreases in uterine activity. Indeed, the most reliable way of rapidly producing uterine relaxation is with general anesthesia. Equipotent doses of halothane, enflurane, and isoflurane produce similar degrees of uterine relaxation.[43] The ability to rapidly achieve an anesthetic concentration of desflurane would be an advantage of this drug when rapid uterine relaxation is deemed necessary. Halothane (1% inspired) or enflurane (2%), and presumably the other volatile anesthetics, will relax the uterus but not block the response to oxytocin.

REGIONAL ANALGESIA FOR LABOR AND VAGINAL DELIVERY

Compared with analgesia produced by inhaled or parenteral drugs, the use of regional analgesia for labor and vaginal delivery reduces the likelihood of fetal drug depression and maternal pulmonary aspiration. Rational use of regional anesthetic techniques requires an understanding of the pathways responsible for the transmission of pain during labor and vaginal delivery (Fig. 31-12). For example, pain of labor arises primarily from receptors in uterine and perineal structures. Afferent pain impulses from the cervix and uterus travel in nerves that accompany sympathetic nervous system fibers and enter the spinal cord at T10–L1. Pain pathways from the perineum travel to S2–S4 via the pudendal nerves. Pain during

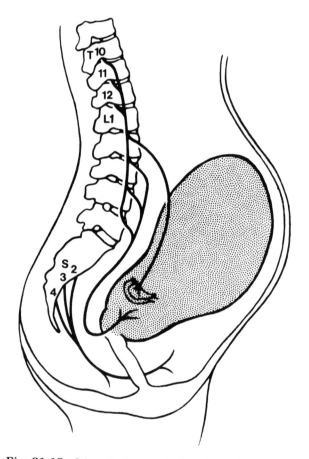

Fig. 31-12. Schematic diagram of pain pathways during parturition. Afferent pain impulses from the cervix and uterus are carried by nerves that accompany sympathetic nervous system fibers and enter the spinal cord at T10–L1. Pain pathways from the perineum travel to S2–S4 through the pudendal nerves.

Table 31-4. Regional Analgesia for Labor and Vaginal Delivery

Technique	Areas of Anesthesia
Paracervical block	Blocks pain impulses that travel via T10–L1
Lumbar epidural analgesia	
Segmental	T10–L1
Standard	T10–S5
Caudal analgesia	T10–S5
Spinal anesthesia	
Saddle	S1–S5
Standard	T10–S5
Pudendal nerve block	S2–S4

the first stage of labor results from dilation of the cervix, contraction of the uterus, and traction on the round ligament. Pain during this first stage of labor is visceral and is referred to dermatomes supplied by spinal cord segments T10–L1. In the second stage of labor, pain is produced by distension of the perineum and stretching of fascia, skin, and subcutaneous tissues. This pain is typically somatic.

The afferent sensory component of pain during labor and vaginal delivery can be interrupted by paracervical, lumbar epidural, caudal, spinal (saddle), and pudendal nerve block anesthesia (Table 31-4). Blocks effective during the first stage of labor include paracervical, lumbar epidural, and caudal. Pain during the second stage of labor is relieved by lumbar epidural, caudal, subarachnoid, or pudendal nerve blocks.

Paracervical Block

Injection of a local anesthetic solution into the fornix of the vagina lateral to the cervix (3 and 9 positions) anesthetizes sensory fibers from the uterus, cervix, and upper vagina. Maternal hypotension does not result, since sympathetic nervous system blockade does not occur. Sensory fibers from the perineum are not blocked; therefore, paracervical block is effective only during the first stage of labor.

The major potential disadvantage of a paracervical block is the 8% to 40% incidence of fetal bradycardia that develops 2 to 10 minutes after injection of the local anesthetic solution.[44] The cause is not clear but is probably related to decreased uterine blood flow secondary to uterine vasoconstriction from the local anesthetic applied in close proximity to the uterine artery, as well as direct cardiac toxicity due to a high fetal blood level of local anesthetic. Because the paracervical area is highly vascular, systemic absorption of local anesthetic is rapid and then readily crosses the placenta to the fetus. In addition, bradycardia produced by a paracervical block is often associated with fetal acidosis. It would seem prudent to avoid this block in the parturient with uteroplacental insufficiency or when there is co-existing fetal distress. Certainly, continuous monitoring of fetal heart rate is useful whenever a paracervical block is administered.

Lumbar Epidural Analgesia

Institution of continuous lumbar epidural analgesia is appropriate when the first stage of labor is well established, as evidenced by dilation of the cervix (6 to 8 cm in a nulipara or 4 to 6 in a multipara) and the presence of strong and regular uterine contractions. Advantages of this technique include (1) the ability to achieve segmental bands of analgesia (T10–T12) during the first stage of labor, when total anesthesia is not required; (2) minimal local anesthetic requirements; and (3) maintenance of pelvic muscle tone, so that rotation of the fetal head is more easily accomplished. Pain during the first stage of labor can be relieved by an injection of 6 to 8 ml of 0.25% bupivacaine into the lumbar epidural space. This low dose of local anesthetic produces a sensory band of analgesia that is unlikely to produce sufficient peripheral sympathetic nervous system blockade to result in maternal hypotension. Nevertheless, parturients should be encouraged to remain in the lateral position. The addition of a small dose of fentanyl (50 to 100 μg) to a dilute concentration of bupivacaine (0.125%) results in a longer duration of analgesia without altering the duration of labor.[45] A similar response has been observed when sufentanil (10 μg·h^{-1}) is added to a 0.125% bupivacaine epidural infusion.[46] The addition of fentanyl to a higher concentration of bupivacaine has not been shown to improve analgesia beyond that achieved with the local anesthetic alone.[47] Additional local anesthetic is injected to provide perineal analgesia as labor progresses. Furthermore, lumbar epidural analgesia can be supplemented to provide adequate anesthesia, should a cesarean section become necessary.

It is a clinical impression that injection of local anesthetic solution into the epidural space during a uterine contraction produces a higher level of anesthesia than if the drug is injected between uterine contractions. Nevertheless, a controlled study failed to document a difference in sensory level whether the local anesthetic was injected during or between uterine contractions.[48] This finding suggests that uterine contractions do not influence the spread of a local anesthetic in the epidural space.

Caudal Analgesia

After placement of a catheter into the sacral epidural space, analgesia is produced by injection of 10 to 12 ml of 0.25% bupivacaine. The advantages of this approach, compared with a continuous lumbar epidural technique, include a lower incidence of inadvertent dural puncture and more profound perineal analgesia. The disadvantages of this technique include (1) difficulty in keeping the sacral area clean; (2) technical difficulties in about 10% of patients, most often reflecting variations in sacral anatomy; (3) extensive peripheral sympathetic nervous system blockade during the first stage of labor; (4) a high incidence of malrotation of the fetal head; (5) possibility of toxic reactions due to vascular absorption of the local anesthetic; and (6) accidental injection into the fetal head. Furthermore, it may not be possible to produce a sufficient level of anesthesia with this technique, should a cesarean section become necessary.

Spinal (Saddle Block) Anesthesia

Spinal anesthesia in the parturient differs from spinal anesthesia in the nonparturient in several ways.[49] For example, a small dose of local anesthetic is needed for spinal anesthesia in the parturient, and the spread of the drug in the cerebrospinal fluid is less predictable. Hypotension and spinal headache are more common in the parturient, and there may be technical difficulty in finding the subarachnoid space, owing to the increased lumbar lordosis that accompanies pregnancy.

Spinal anesthesia is administered immediately before vaginal delivery by injecting a small dose of hyperbaric tetracaine (3 to 5 mg) or lidocaine (25 to 30 mg) into the lumbar subarachnoid space, with the parturient in the sitting position. The sitting position may be maintained for 60 to 90 seconds, if the goal is to achieve principally perineal analgesia (saddle block or area of the body that would be in contact with the saddle). A true saddle block does not produce complete pain relief as afferent fibers from the uterus are not interrupted. In reality, a true saddle block is rarely achieved. The more likely result is sensory blockade that extends to about T10, which prevents pain from uterine contractions. An alternative to injection of a local anesthetic is subarachnoid placement of an opioid combination (fentanyl 25 μg and morphine 0.25 mg) that may provide adequate pain relief during labor, requiring only the addition of a pudendal block for vaginal delivery.[50]

When the sensory level is kept below T10, a spinal anesthetic does not produce significant peripheral sympathetic nervous system blockade and the likelihood of hypotension is reduced. There is an increased need for forceps delivery, when abdominal muscle relaxation is produced by a spinal anesthetic. The major disadvantage, however, is the occasional occurrence of a postspinal headache. Typically, this headache is accentuated by sitting up and relieved by assuming the supine position. Presumably, the cause of headache is cerebrospinal fluid hypotension due to loss of fluid through the hole in the dura produced during performance of the anesthetic. Compared with a nonpregnant patient, a parturient is twice as likely to experience such a headache. The incidence of

postspinal headache can be minimized (incidence 1% or less) by using a small-bore spinal needle (25 gauge). It should be recognized that accidental dural puncture occurs in 1% to 2% of attempted epidural anesthetics. In this event, the dura is punctured with a large-bore needle (17 to 18 gauge); in more than one-half of these patients, severe headaches develop. If a headache persists despite bed rest and hydration, the recommended approach is epidural injection of autologous blood (blood patch).

Complaints of backache may follow performance of an epidural or subarachnoid anesthetic administered for vaginal delivery. Backache is a frequent complaint in the parturient, and the incidence is similar after general anesthesia and regional anesthetic techniques. Backache most likely reflects ligamentous strain from the lordosis of pregnancy. In extreme cases, the muscular efforts of labor may give rise to a prolapsed intervertebral disc, with subsequent nerve root compression, typically manifested as back pain and numbness in the affected segmental area.

The most common type of nerve damage during the postpartum period is caused by compression of the lumbosacral trunk between the descending fetal head and the sacrum. Lumbosacral trunk injuries are characterized by footdrop combined with sensory loss. In addition, compression of the femoral nerve (L2–L4) or lateral femoral cutaneous nerve can occur at the inguinal ligament, resulting in sensory loss over the lateral aspect of the thigh and leg. This compression usually occurs from a prolonged posture in the lithotomy position. The sciatic nerve (L4–S3) divides into the common peroneal nerve and tibial nerve. The common peroneal nerve is superficial as it extends laterally around the head of the fibula and is subject to damage at this area due to compression from positioning in stirrups during vaginal delivery (see Chapter 17). Such damage is manifest by an inability to dorsiflex the great toe, by footdrop, and by sensory loss over the lateral aspect of the leg and the anterior portion of the foot. When neurologic deficits develop during the postpartum period, particularly after lumbar epidural or spinal anesthesia, it is important to establish whether the lesion is within the spinal canal or distal to the intervertebral foramen. The incidence of paresthesias and motor dysfunction after labor and vaginal delivery is about 1.9% per 1000 deliveries.[51] These symptoms resolve within 72 hours with supportive therapy, and the incidence is not influenced by the use of regional anesthesia.

Pudendal Nerve Block

A pudendal nerve block is typically administered transvaginally by the obstetrician just before delivery. Bilateral pudendal nerve blocks using a local anesthetic such as lidocaine (10 ml of 1%) provide satisfactory perineal analgesia for normal vaginal delivery but not for application of forceps. This block is not associated with peripheral sympathetic nervous system blockade, and labor is not prolonged. Unfortunately, even in experienced hands, a successful bilateral pudendal nerve block is achieved in only about 60% of attempts.

INHALATION ANALGESIA FOR VAGINAL DELIVERY

The goal of inhalation analgesia is to maintain the parturient in an awake and cooperative state with intact laryngeal reflexes for the first and second stages of labor. The major risk is the loss of protective airway reflexes due to an inadvertent overdose of inhaled anesthetic made more likely by the reduced functional residual capacity and decreased anesthetic requirements that accompany pregnancy.

Placental transfer of inhaled anesthetics occurs rapidly, as these drugs are lipid soluble and possess a low molecular weight. The degree of neonatal depression is directly proportional to the maternal inspired concentration and duration of administration. Analgesic concentrations of inhaled anesthetics, however, are free from excessive depressant effects on the fetus, even if continued for a prolonged period.[52]

Nitrous oxide must be inhaled for about 50 seconds before effective analgesic concentrations are reached; less than satisfactory analgesia results when nitrous oxide is administered only during uterine contractions. Therefore, more effective inhalation analgesia is obtained by the continuous administration of 30% to 40% nitrous oxide. After delivery, rapid passage of nitrous oxide from blood into alveoli can cause diffusion hypoxia in the newborn infant. Therefore, infants born during administration of nitrous oxide analgesia may benefit from supplemental oxygen for 30 to 60 seconds after delivery.

Intermittent inhalation of methoxyflurane (0.1% to 0.3% inspired) is an alternative to continuous administration of nitrous oxide. An analgesic concentration of methoxyflurane does not dangerously depress maternal laryngeal reflexes, and neonates are not sedated. Both the maternal and neonatal serum fluoride level, however, is increased in a dose-related manner after administration of methoxyflurane.[53,54] Nevertheless, there is no evidence of renal dysfunction in either parturients or neonates. Enflurane (0.5% inspired) provides analgesia during the second stage of labor similar to that achieved with nitrous oxide (30% to 40%).[55]

ANESTHESIA FOR CESAREAN SECTION

Common indications for cesarean section include a previous cesarean section, cephalopelvic disproportion, failure of labor to progress, maternal hemorrhage, and fetal distress. The dictum that a previous cesarean section mandates the same route of delivery for all subsequent pregnancies is no longer strictly followed. In selected patients (prior low segment transverse uterine incision and cephalic presentation), it is acceptable to permit vaginal delivery despite prior cesarean section.[56] Cesarean section may be selected to avoid the potential trauma of a difficult vaginal delivery, as with a breech presentation. Electronic and biochemical monitoring of the fetus has increased the number of fetuses judged to be in jeopardy and in need of rapid delivery by cesarean section, making this operative procedure one of the most frequent of all surgical procedures.[57]

The decision to select general or regional anesthesia to provide anesthesia for cesarean section depends on the desires of the patient and the presence or absence of fetal distress. When fetal distress is present, general anesthesia may be preferable, since anesthesia can be established quickly and maternal hypotension is less likely. Regional anesthesia is more often chosen for elective cesarean section, particularly when maternal awareness is desirable. Furthermore, regional anesthesia minimizes the likelihood of maternal pulmonary aspiration and avoids fetal depression.

General Anesthesia

Preoperative medication may include pharmacologic attempts to increase gastric fluid pH. A nonparticulate antacid is widely used for this purpose. An H-2 receptor antagonist is also effective in increasing gastric fluid pH, but the time required for this drug to act, unlike an antacid, precludes its use when induction of anesthesia is imminent.[58] Furthermore, an H-2 receptor antagonist, unlike antacids, has no effect on pH of gastric fluid present in the stomach at the time the drug is administered. Clearly, an antacid is the logical choice to increase gastric fluid pH when an emergency cesarean section is planned. Metoclopramide could be administered to facilitate gastric emptying before the induction of anesthesia, although the usefulness of this drug in the parturient undergoing elective cesarean section is not established. If an anticholinergic drug is judged to be necessary, glycopyrrolate is useful, since its quaternary ammonium structure prevents significant transfer across lipid barriers such as the placenta. If the cesarean section is elective and the parturient is extremely apprehensive, a benzodiazepine can be administered for the purpose of allaying anxiety.

After preoxygenation, induction of general anesthesia is often accomplished with the administration of thiopental (3 to 5 mg·kg^{-1} IV) plus succinylcholine (1 to 1.5 mg·kg^{-1} IV) to facilitate intubation of the trachea. Cricoid pressure may be applied until the trachea is protected with a cuffed endotracheal tube. The importance of preoxygenation is emphasized by the rapid decrease in maternal arterial oxygenation that can occur during apnea, as associated with direct laryngoscopy for intubation of the trachea. This vulnerability to arterial hypoxemia reflects the decreased functional residual capacity and increased metabolic oxygen requirements associated with pregnancy. The use of a small dose of nondepolarizing muscle relaxant to prevent fasciculations produced by the subsequent administration of succinylcholine is often included in the induction sequence. Thiopental rapidly crosses the placenta, and peak concentrations are present in the umbilical venous blood in about 1 minute. Nevertheless, the fetal brain will not be exposed to high concentrations of the drug, as clearance by the fetal liver and dilution by blood from the viscera and extremities results in delivery of a decreased concentration to the brain.[59] Clearly, there is no advantage to delaying delivery until thiopental has been redistributed from the fetus to the mother.

Difficult (failed) intubation of the parturient's trachea is an important cause of anesthetic-related morbidity and mortality. A management plan is useful when failed intubation occurs, keeping in mind the principal goal is oxygenation without aspiration[60,61] (Table 31-5). Cricoid pressure is considered useful in preventing regurgitation and aspiration.

Table 31-5.   Suggested Approach for Management of a Difficult Airway in the Parturient

Glottic Opening Cannot Be Visualized
   Maintain cricoid pressure
   Summon help
   Repeat direct laryngoscopy
      Optimal head position
      Suction pharynx
      Smaller tracheal tube with stylet
      Temporarily reduce cricoid pressure

If Tracheal Intubation Still Unsuccessful Reapply Cricoid Pressure and Select the Appropriate Option
   Ventilation Possible—Elective Case
      Maintain cricoid pressure
      Allow patient to awaken
      Select an alternative form of anesthesia
         Regional
         Awake tracheal intubation, followed by general anesthesia
   Ventilation Possible—Emergency Case
      Maintain cricoid pressure
      Add an inhalation anesthetic during spontaneous or controlled ventilation
      Expedite delivery and avoid fundal pressure
   Ventilation Impossible
      Maintain cricoid pressure
      Insert an oropharyngeal and/or nasopharyngeal airway
      Summon surgical help
      Cricothyrotomy
      Tracheostomy

(Adapted from Davies JM, Weeks S, Crone LA, Pavlin E. Difficult intubation in the parturient. Can J Anaesth 1989;36:668–74, with permission.)

Maintenance of anesthesia until delivery of the fetus is often with nitrous oxide (50% to 60% inspired) in oxygen plus succinylcholine for skeletal muscle paralysis. The maternal alveolar concentration of nitrous oxide approaches the inspired concentration rapidly, reflecting the reduced functional residual capacity that accompanies pregnancy. It must also be remembered that nitrous oxide is rapidly transferred across the placenta. Nevertheless, the concentration of nitrous oxide delivered to the fetal central nervous system is decreased by tissue uptake and dilution in blood returning from the lower extremities. As a result, fetal central nervous system depression from nitrous oxide is minimal. Nitrous oxide does not produce significant uterine relaxation.

The major disadvantage of using only nitrous oxide until delivery of the infant is patient awareness during the operation. The reported incidence of awareness is 2% to 26%.[62] Maternal amnesia can be ensured by the administration of a low inspired concentration of a volatile anesthetic (halothane 0.5%, enflurane 1.0%, isoflurane 0.75%) with nitrous oxide.[63] A low dose of desflurane is also a consideration. These low doses of volatile drugs do not increase maternal blood loss, alter the response of the uterus to oxytocin, or produce neonatal depression. An additional advantage of using a volatile anesthetic is a decrease in the inspired concentration of nitrous oxide. As a result, fetal oxygenation can be improved by increasing the inspired maternal oxygen concentration. Finally, nitrous oxide supplemented with a volatile anesthetic is associated with a reduced sympathetic nervous system response to surgical stimulation and a better maintenance of uterine blood flow thought to reflect inhibition of endogenous norepinephrine secretion by the volatile anesthetic.[30]

Ventilation of the lungs is controlled; excessive hyperventilation must be avoided, as effects of positive pressure can reduce uterine blood flow. Furthermore, respiratory alkalosis will increase the affinity of maternal hemoglobin for oxygen and thus decrease placental transfer of oxygen to the fetus.

Succinylcholine can be used to provide skeletal muscle relaxation during the operative procedure. Although plasma cholinesterase activity is decreased at term, the clinical response to succinylcholine does not seem to be altered.[14] Administration of succinylcholine to a parturient with unsuspected atypical cholinesterase enzyme, however, will cause prolonged apnea in the neonate who is also homozygous for the atypical enzyme.[64] Alternatives to succinylcholine for maintenance of skeletal muscle relaxation are the short- and intermediate-acting nondepolarizing muscle relaxants. Succinylcholine and nondepolarizing muscle relaxants, when administered in appropriate clinical doses, do not cross the placenta in amounts sufficient to produce effects on the fetus.

There is controversy regarding the optimal time for delivery, when general anesthesia is used for cesarean section. In the absence of maternal hypotension, a time from induction of anesthesia to delivery that approaches 30 minutes is not associated with acidosis in the neonate.[65] More important is a short time to delivery after incision into the uterus has been made. Indeed, Apgar scores are often decreased when the uterine incision to delivery time exceeds 90 seconds. Adverse responses associated with a prolonged time to delivery after uterine incision may reflect impaired uteroplacental blood flow or decreased umbilical vein blood flow, or both, due to manipulation of the uterus. All factors considered, it seems prudent to minimize the times from both induction of anesthesia and uterine incision to delivery.

After delivery, anesthesia can be supplemented with additional volatile drug or an opioid. It would seem reasonable to pass an oral tube into the stomach to evacuate gastric fluid before the conclusion of surgery. The cuffed tube should not be removed from the trachea until the return of maternal laryngeal reflexes has been ensured. It may be important to administer oxygen to the neonate for 30 to 60 seconds to decrease the possibility of arterial hypoxemia due to the rapid elimination of nitrous oxide from the fetal circulation into the lungs.

Regional Anesthesia

Spinal or epidural anesthesia is often selected for an elective cesarean section. This form of anesthesia permits the mother to be awake, minimizes the likelihood of maternal pulmonary aspiration, avoids drug depression from general anesthetics, and permits administration of a high inspired concentration of oxygen to the mother. Selection of a spinal or lumbar epidural technique is based on the relative advantages and disadvantages of each as they relate to the individual parturient. Administration of supplemental oxygen to the parturient during regional anesthesia improves fetal oxygen stores during cesarean section.

Spinal Anesthesia

Advantages of spinal anesthesia include its technical ease and high success rate. Fetal depression from the local anesthetic does not occur, since a small dose is used and absorption of the local anesthetic from the subarachnoid space is minimal. Disadvantages of this technique include (1) difficulty in controlling the sensory level; (2) a high incidence of hypotension, reflecting the abrupt onset of peripheral sympathetic nervous system blockade; (3) nausea and vomiting; and (4) postoperative headache.

The parturient is particularly susceptible to hypotension after completion of a spinal anesthetic. The incidence of hypotension is less in the presence of active labor, compared with the patient who is not in labor. A possible explanation may be the autotransfusion of about 300 ml of blood, which occurs with each uterine contraction. Hypotension is hazardous,

since decreased maternal blood pressure is associated with comparable falls in uterine blood flow and placental perfusion, leading to fetal hypoxemia and acidosis. The incidence and magnitude of hypotension may be minimized by continuous left uterine displacement, intravenous hydration with 500 to 1000 ml of lactated Ringer's solution administered 15 to 30 minutes before performing the anesthetic, and the intramuscular injection of ephedrine (25 to 50 mg) approximately 15 minutes before performing the anesthetic.[66] If hypotension occurs (systolic blood pressure below 100 mmHg in a normotensive parturient or a 30% decrease in a previously hypertensive parturient) despite the above measures, an additional dose of ephedrine (2.5 to 10 mg IV) is indicated. The onset of nausea after a spinal anesthetic should immediately suggest the presence of hypotension, leading to decreased cerebral blood flow. In the absence of hypotension, nausea may be due to traction on the peritoneum or to an imbalance of autonomic nervous system activity due to blockade of the sympathetic nervous system fibers in the presence of intact vagal innervation. If excessive parasympathetic nervous system activity is the cause of nausea, intravenous administration of an anticholinergic drug may be considered. Although glycopyrrolate is less likely than atropine to cross the placenta, fetal heart rate was not significantly altered by either drug administered intravenously.[74]

Technically, the lumbar subarachnoid space is entered with a 25-gauge needle. A convenient guide for judging the appropriate dose of local anesthetic to be injected into the subarachnoid space is based on the height of the parturient (Table 31-6). Despite the traditional clinical reliance on the parturient's height as a guide to the dose of local anesthetic required for spinal anesthesia, data from term parturients fail to verify the relationship between height and maximum cephalad spread of sensory anesthesia[68] (Fig. 31-13). A sensory level of T4–T6 is necessary to ensure adequate anesthesia for performance of the cesarean section. After injection of the local anesthetic solution into the subarachnoid space, the parturient is placed supine, with the right hip elevated to minimize aortocaval compression. Maternal blood pressure must be monitored frequently until delivery of the neonate.

Table 31-6. Dose of Local Anesthetic for Spinal Anesthesia Prior to Cesarean Section

Height (cm)	Tetracaine (mg)	Lidocaine (mg)	Bupivacaine (mg)
<155	7	50	9
155–170	8	60	11
>170	9	70	13

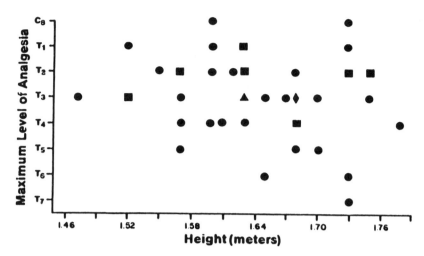

Fig. 31-13. There was no relationship between the height of the parturient and the sensory level of anesthesia produced by the subarachnoid placement of 12 mg of hyperbaric bupivacaine. (From Norris MC. Height, weight, and the spread of subarachnoid hyperbaric bupivacaine in the term parturient. Anesth Analg 1988;67:555–8, with permission.)

Lumbar Epidural Anesthesia

Compared with a spinal anesthetic, the sensory level is more controllable and hypotension less precipitous with a lumbar epidural anesthetic. Presumably, the slower onset of peripheral sympathetic nervous system blockade is responsible for the more gradual decrease in blood pressure. Unlike a spinal anesthetic, an epidural anesthetic requires a dose of local anesthetic associated with significant systemic absorption of the drug. Absorbed local anesthetic, particularly lidocaine or mepivacaine, can cross the placenta and produce detectable effects on the fetus. Nevertheless, an infant whose mother received epidural anesthesia with bupivacaine does not demonstrate a measurable difference from an infant born after a spinal anesthetic. Technically, lumbar epidural anesthesia is more difficult to perform than a spinal anesthetic. Postoperative headache does not occur, since the dura is not punctured.

The bupivacaine concentration injected into the epidural space must be at least 0.5% to ensure adequate anesthesia for the surgical stimulus associated with the performance of a cesarean section. This contrasts with the degree of analgesia acceptable for vaginal delivery produced using 0.25% bupivacaine. Limitation of the concentration of bupivacaine to 0.5% is recommended to minimize the likelihood of cardiotoxicity, should this local anesthetic be accidentally injected intravenously. When a local anesthetic is injected into the epidural space, it is mandatory to administer a test dose to detect unrecognized placement of the epidural catheter into a vein or the subarachnoid space. Administration of 3 ml of local anesthetic solution containing 1:200,000 epinephrine (15 μg) usually produces transient maternal tachycardia if the drug goes intravenously and signs of subarachnoid block if the solu-

tion enters the subarachnoid space. Assuming a negative test dose response and the absence of spinal anesthesia after the test dose, an additional amount of bupivacaine is injected through the lumbar epidural catheter, to produce a T4–T6 sensory level of anesthesia. When rapid onset of analgesia is necessary, 3% 2-chloroprocaine-CE can be used. When chloroprocaine is used, a subarachnoid injection must be avoided, since permanent neurologic damage has been reported after accidental subarachnoid injection of large volumes of this local anesthetic.[69,70] Administration of a local anesthetic, such as bupivacaine, after placement of chloroprocaine in the epidural space, may be less effective. An alternative to chloroprocaine when a rapid onset of analgesia would be desirable is the use of the amide local anesthetic prilocaine, 1% to 3%. Methemoglobinemia after systemic absorption and metabolism of prilocaine is not likely if the total dose of drug placed in the epidural space does not exceed 600 mg. In the past, lidocaine has not been a popular drug because of neurobehavioral changes detectable in neonates of mothers who received this local anesthetic during epidural analgesia or anesthesia. Nevertheless, there is no convincing evidence that these neurobehavioral changes are hazardous, nor have these observations been reproducible.[71] Therefore, lidocaine would seem to be an appropriate alternative either to bupivacaine or to chloroprocaine. There is no evidence that epidural anesthesia in the patient with active genital herpes simplex increases the risk of transmission of the virus into the central nervous system or results in recurrence of the infection.[72]

Postoperative analgesia after cesarean section may be provided by epidural administration of an opioid. For example, epidural morphine (3 to 5 mg) provides intense and prolonged analgesia following a cesarean section.[73] Alternatively, intrathecal administration of morphine (0.1 to 0.5 mg) provides a similar degree of postoperative analgesia that may be even more prolonged than that which follows epidural opioid administration.[73,74] Continuous intravenous infusion of fentanyl may provide a degree of postoperative analgesia similar to that provided by a neuraxial opioid.[75]

ABNORMAL PRESENTATIONS AND MULTIPLE BIRTHS

Presentation of the fetus is determined by the presenting part and that aspect of the fetus felt by manual examination through the cervix. Description of fetal position is based on the relationship of the fetal occiput, chin, or sacrum to the left or right side of the parturient. Approximately 90% of deliveries are cephalic presentations in either the occiput transverse or occiput anterior positions. All other presentations and positions are considered abnormal.

Persistent Occiput Posterior

During active labor the occiput undergoes internal rotation to the occiput anterior position. If this rotation does not occur, the persistent occiput posterior position results, and labor becomes prolonged and painful. For example, severe back pain reflects pressure on the posterior sacral nerves by the fetal occiput. Spontaneous delivery requires more uterine and abdominal work. The incidence of cervical and perineal lacerations and postpartum bleeding is increased. Although spontaneous delivery may occur, it is more likely that manual or forceps rotation and extraction will be necessary. A prolonged second stage of labor or difficult midforceps rotation is associated with increased birth trauma, intracranial hemorrhage, and birth asphyxia in the neonate.

A regional anesthetic technique that relaxes the maternal perineal muscles is best avoided until spontaneous internal rotation of the fetal head occurs. Analgesia can be provided with a segmental (T10–L1) lumbar epidural technique. If back pain persists, analgesia may be extended to the sacral areas by injecting a dilute concentration of bupivacaine (0.125% to 0.25%), which should not paralyze the skeletal muscles necessary for internal rotation of the fetal head. Complete analgesia and perineal relaxation is appropriate when midforceps rotation is planned.

Breech Presentation

Breech rather than a cephalic presentation characterizes about 3.5% of pregnancies. Breech presentations are classified as (1) frank (feet are against the face), (2) complete (but-

tocks with feet along side them present at the cervix, and (3) incomplete or footling (one or both feet present at the cervix). Frank breech is present in about 60% of breech deliveries, complete breech in about 10%, and incomplete breech in about 30%. The causes of breech presentations are unknown. However, conditions that seem to predispose to this presentation include prematurity, placenta previa, multiple gestations, and uterine anomalies. Fetal abnormalities, including hydrocephalus and polyhydramnios, are associated with breech presentations.

Breech deliveries result in increased maternal morbidity. Compared with a cephalic presentation, there is a greater likelihood of cervical lacerations, perineal injury, retained placenta, and shock due to hemorrhage. Neonatal morbidity and mortality are increased. These infants are more likely to experience arterial hypoxemia and acidosis during delivery, due to umbilical cord compression. Prolapse of the umbilical cord occurs in about 10% of complete or incomplete breech presentations, compared with an incidence of 0.5% for cephalic and frank breech presentations, and is thought to reflect failure of the presenting part to fill the lower uterine segment. There is also an increased chance of fetal intracranial hemorrhage due to head trauma during breech deliveries.

Cesarean Delivery

There is a trend to deliver breech presentations by elective cesarean section. If cesarean section is planned, either regional or general anesthesia may be selected. It should be appreciated that during regional anesthesia, there may be difficulty in extracting the infant through the uterine incision. If uterine hypertonus is the cause, it will be necessary to produce general anesthesia rapidly. After intubation of the trachea, administration of a volatile anesthetic will relax the uterus.

Vaginal Delivery

For vaginal delivery of a breech presentation, the parturient must be able to expel the fetus until the umbilicus is visible. The obstetrician then completes the delivery, either manually or with the application of forceps. Analgesia during labor is often provided with intramuscular or intravenous medications, followed by perineal infiltration of a local anesthetic or performance of a pudendal block. Inhalation analgesia may also be administered. Rapid induction of general anesthesia, with intubation of the trachea, may be necessary, if perineal muscle relaxation is inadequate for delivery of the aftercoming fetal head, or if the lower uterine segment contracts and traps the head. An alternative to infiltration and inhalation analgesia is use of lumbar epidural anesthesia. For example, a continuous lumbar epidural technique provides analgesia and maximal perineal relaxation for delivery of the fetal head. Furthermore, the ability of the parturient to push during the delivery can be preserved by using a minimal concentration of local anesthetic (0.25% bupivacaine) and providing constant maternal encouragement. Indeed, the incidence of complete breech extraction is not increased in the presence of epidural analgesia.[76] If uterine relaxation is required for facilitation of a breech extraction during vaginal delivery, it will be necessary to produce general anesthesia.

Multiple Gestations

The incidence of twin gestations is approximately 1 in 90 births. Pregnancy-induced hypertension, anemia, premature labor, breech presentation, and hemorrhage are more common in multiple gestations. Approximately 60% of twins are premature. The large uterus associated with multiple gestations produces more aortocaval compression, predisposing the parturient to a higher incidence of severe supine hypotension. This hypotension may be even further exaggerated if sympathetic nervous system blockade is produced by a spinal or epidural anesthetic. Blood loss during twin delivery is twice that of a single gestation, and manual extraction of the placenta is required twice as often. It must be appreciated that the second twin is more likely to be depressed, presumably reflecting a period of fetal arterial hypoxemia and acidosis due to contraction of the uterus or to premature separation of the placenta, after the first neonate is delivered.

Considerations for the choice of anesthesia in the presence of multiple gestations relate to the frequent occurrence of prematurity and breech presentation. Preparations must be made for the possibility of providing anesthesia for version, extraction, breech delivery, cesarean section, or midforceps delivery. Pudendal block with or without inhalation analgesia introduces minimal depression to the fetus, but maternal analgesia is often inadequate, and relaxation of the perineal muscles is absent. Continuous lumbar epidural anesthesia provides good analgesia and eliminates the need for administration of an opioid to the parturient, which is particularly important for avoiding depression in premature neonates. Segmental lumbar epidural anesthesia with bupivacaine (0.25%) provides adequate analgesia and preserves sufficient abdominal muscle strength, so that the mother may assist in delivery. In addition, forceps deliveries, likely with multiple gestations, are more easily accomplished in the presence of perineal muscle relaxation provided by epidural anesthesia. Intravenous infusion of fluids and left uterine displacement are important in minimizing aortocaval compression when peripheral sympathetic nervous system blockade is produced.

PREGNANCY AND HEART DISEASE

Maternal heart disease is estimated to be present in about 1.6% of all pregnancies. The two most common causes are congenital malformations and acquired valvular heart disease due to rheumatic fever (see Chapters 2 and 3). Many of the signs and symptoms of normal pregnancy can mimic those of cardiac disease. For example, dyspnea associated with interstitial pulmonary edema due to left ventricular failure may be difficult to distinguish from labored breathing typical of normal pregnancy. Leg edema from congestive heart failure can be mistaken for venous stasis due to aortocaval compression. The presence of congestive heart failure is suggested by hepatomegaly and jugular venous distension, as these changes do not accompany a normal pregnancy. It may be difficult to differentiate a heart murmur due to an organic lesion from one due to increased blood flow. Rotation of the maternal heart, which occurs from elevation of the diaphragm as pregnancy progresses, can be mistaken for cardiac hypertrophy.

Pregnancy and labor often result in circulatory changes that may have adverse effects on the already diseased cardiovascular system. For example, cardiac output is increased about 40% during gestation and can be increased an additional 30% to 45% above prelabor values during labor and delivery. After delivery, relief of aortocaval obstruction contributes to increased venous return and central blood volume, resulting in an even further increase in cardiac output above the prelabor value. These increases, well tolerated by the normal heart, may result in congestive heart failure in the presence of co-existing heart disease. Indeed, in nearly 50% of patients with symptoms of heart disease during minimal activity or at rest, congestive heart failure develops during pregnancy. Drugs (lidocaine, propranolol, digoxin) used to treat heart disease readily cross the placenta and may affect the fetus. For example, a maternal blood lidocaine concentration in excess of 5 $\mu g \cdot ml^{-1}$ may be associated with neonatal depression. Propranolol may produce fetal bradycardia and hypoglycemia. The elimination half-time of digoxin is likely to be significantly longer in the fetus. Electrical cardioversion, as used to treat paroxysmal atrial tachycardia, has no adverse fetal effects.

Detection and evaluation of heart disease is crucial for planning management of anesthesia during labor and delivery. For most types of heart disease, no one anesthetic technique is specifically indicated or contraindicated. Nevertheless, analgesia produced by a continuous lumbar epidural technique can minimize adverse effects of increased cardiac output due to pain or anxiety. Inhalation analgesia or anesthesia is usually selected when a sudden decrease in blood pressure would be detrimental.

Invasive monitoring during labor and delivery is probably not necessary in the absence of cardiac symptoms due to co-existing heart disease. Exceptions are parturients with pulmonary hypertension, right-to-left intracardiac shunts, or coarctation of the aorta. In these patients, the ability to measure cardiac output and cardiac filling pressures, as well as to calculate systemic and pulmonary vascular resistance, is helpful. Since the hemodynamic changes seen during labor and delivery can persist into the postpartum period, it is logical to continue invasive cardiac monitoring for several hours after delivery.

Mitral Stenosis

Mitral stenosis is the most common type of cardiac valvular defect present during pregnancy. The parturient with mitral stenosis has an increased incidence of pulmonary edema, atrial fibrillation, and paroxysmal atrial tachycardia. A continuous lumbar epidural anesthetic producing segmental analgesia is useful for labor and vaginal delivery, as this approach minimizes undesirable effects produced by pain on heart rate and cardiac output. Perineal analgesia prevents the parturient's urge to push and eliminates the deleterious effects of a Valsalva maneuver on venous return. General or regional anesthesia can be provided for cesarean section. If general anesthesia is selected, drugs that produce tachycardia and events that increase pulmonary vascular resistance (arterial hypoxemia, hypoventilation) must be avoided (see Chapter 2).

Mitral Regurgitation

Mitral regurgitation is the second most common cardiac valvular defect present during pregnancy. In contrast to the parturient with mitral stenosis, these patients usually tolerate pregnancy well. Indeed, clinical symptoms related to mitral regurgitation do not usually develop until after the age of child-bearing.

Continuous lumbar epidural analgesia is recommended for labor and vaginal delivery, as this technique reduces peripheral vasoconstriction associated with pain and thus helps to maintain forward left ventricular stroke volume. Regional techniques, however, will also increase venous capacitance, such that intravenous fluids may be required to maintain the filling volume of the left ventricle. General anesthesia is acceptable when cesarean section is planned (see Chapter 2).

Aortic Regurgitation

Complications of aortic regurgitation, like those of mitral regurgitation, usually develop after the childbearing years. Therefore, these patients usually have an uneventful pregnancy, although congestive heart failure may develop in a small percentage. The decreased systemic vascular resistance and increased heart rate during pregnancy may reduce both the regurgitant flow and the intensity of the cardiac murmur associated with aortic regurgitation. Conversely, increased systemic vascular resistance associated with pain during labor and vaginal delivery can lead to reduced forward left ventricular stroke volume. As with mitral regurgitation, a continuous lumbar epidural technique is recommended for analgesia during labor and vaginal delivery. General anesthesia is acceptable when cesarean section is planned (see Chapter 2).

Aortic Stenosis

Rarity of aortic stenosis during pregnancy reflects the typical 35- to 40-year latent period between acute rheumatic fever and symptoms of aortic stenosis. The asymptomatic parturient is not at increased risk during labor and delivery. Because of the fixed orifice valve lesion, however, these parturients are vulnerable to decreased stroke volume and hypotension, if systemic vascular resistance is abruptly decreased. Therefore, if a regional technique is selected, a gradual onset of analgesia produced by a continuous lumbar epidural anesthetic is useful. In view of the hazards of hypotension, techniques using systemic medication, pudendal block, and inhalation analgesia are often used for labor and vaginal delivery. General anesthesia is acceptable when cesarean section is planned (see Chapter 2).

Tetralogy of Fallot

Pregnancy increases the morbidity and mortality associated with tetralogy of Fallot. For example, pain during labor and vaginal delivery may increase pulmonary vascular resistance, leading to an increase in the right-to-left intracardiac shunt, with a decrease in pulmonary blood flow and accentuation of arterial hypoxemia. In addition, the normal decrease in systemic vascular resistance that accompanies pregnancy can also increase the right-to-left shunt and accentuate arterial hypoxemia. Indeed, most cardiac complications develop immediately postpartum, when systemic vascular resistance is lowest.

Analgesia for labor and vaginal delivery is often provided with a pudendal block. Regional anesthesia must be used with caution because of the hazards of decreased blood pressure due to peripheral sympathetic nervous system blockade. Therefore, general anesthesia is usually selected for cesarean section (see Chapter 3). Invasive monitoring, including continuous measurement of arterial and cardiac filling pressures, is helpful. Easy access to arterial blood facilitates determination of the PaO_2 and early detection of increased arterial hypoxemia, which can occur if the magnitude of the right-to-left shunt is accentuated by decreased systemic blood pressure. Pulse oximetry will also reflect changes in arterial oxygenation.

Eisenmenger Syndrome

Eisenmenger syndrome consists of obliterative pulmonary vascular disease with resultant pulmonary hypertension, a right-to-left or bidirectional intracardiac shunt, and arterial hypoxemia. This combination of problems is not amenable to surgical correction, and pregnancy is not well tolerated. Indeed, maternal mortality can approach 30%, with the highest comparable mortality about 4% in the parturient with coarctation of the aorta or tetralogy of Fallot.[77]

The major hazards facing a parturient with Eisenmenger syndrome are (1) decreased systemic vascular resistance, which can lead to an increase in the magnitude of the right-to-left intracardiac shunt, and (2) thromboembolism, which may interfere with an already decreased pulmonary blood flow. Indeed, the magnitude of the intracardiac shunt can be accentuated by even normal decreases in systemic vascular resistance that accompany pregnancy or the widespread pulmonary vasoconstriction that accompanies even small pulmonary emboli. The greatest risk to these patients occurs during delivery and immediately postpartum.

Management of Anesthesia

The principle of any technique of analgesia or anesthesia chosen for the patient with Eisenmenger syndrome is to avoid a decrease in systemic vascular resistance or reduction in cardiac output. Likewise, events that could further increase pulmonary vascular resistance (hypercarbia, increased arterial hypoxemia) must be avoided. Meticulous attention is required to prevent infusion of air through tubing used to deliver intravenous fluids, since the possibility of paradoxical air embolism is great.

Vaginal delivery is an acceptable goal. Analgesia provided with a continuous lumbar epidural technique avoids the stress of an exhausting and painful labor. If epidural analgesia is selected, however, it is crucial that decreased systemic vascular resistance be minimized. Epinephrine probably should not be added to the local anesthetic solution, since decreased systemic vascular resistance can be accentuated by the peripheral beta effect of epinephrine absorbed from the epidural space. Alternatively, management of the parturient with Eisenmenger syndrome has been described, using intrathecal morphine to provide analgesia for the first stage of labor, followed by a pudendal nerve block to provide anesthesia for the second stage of labor.[78] Analgesia for vaginal delivery may also be provided with an inhaled drug.

Delivery by cesarean section is most often accomplished using general anesthesia. Extensive peripheral sympathetic nervous system blockade is the major disadvantage of an epidural or spinal anesthetic. Nevertheless, epidural anesthesia has been successfully used for elective cesarean section in these patients.[77] Regardless of the anesthetic technique selected, antibiotics should be given during the perioperative period as protection against infective endocarditis (see Chapter 27). It should be recognized that the arm-to-brain circulation time is rapid due to the right-to-left intracardiac shunt. Therefore, drugs given intravenously will have a rapid onset of action. Ketamine has a theoretical advantage over barbiturates in these patients, since it does not reduce systemic vascular resistance, although an increase in pulmonary vascular resistance is theoretically possible. In contrast to parenteral drugs, the rate of rise of the arterial concentration of an inhaled drug is slow due to decreased pulmonary blood flow.

Despite the slow onset, myocardial depressant and vasodilating actions of volatile drugs emphasize the potential hazards of using these anesthetics in patients with Eisenmenger syndrome. Even nitrous oxide can have adverse effects, as this drug has been shown to increase pulmonary vascular resistance.[79] It must be appreciated that positive-pressure ventilation of the lungs can decrease pulmonary blood flow. Invasive monitoring of arterial and cardiac filling pressures is helpful. Since the right ventricle is at greater risk than the left ventricle for dysfunction, measurement of right atrial pressure is a uniquely useful determination. The value of a pulmonary artery catheter monitoring in these patients is unclear.[80]

Coarctation of the Aorta

Coarctation of the aorta, like aortic stenosis, represents a fixed obstruction to the forward ejection of the left ventricular stroke volume. Increases in cardiac output can be achieved primarily by increases in heart rate. During periods of high demand, as during labor or acute increases in intravascular fluid volume produced by uterine contraction, the heart rate may not be able to increase to the extent necessary to maintain an adequate cardiac output. This sequence of events may result in acute left ventricular failure. Another hazard during labor and vaginal delivery is damage to the vascular wall of the aorta. Specifically, with the increased heart rate and myocardial contractility that accompany the pain of labor, the rate of ejection of blood from the left ventricle will increase and may lead to dissection of the aorta.

Maintenance of heart rate, myocardial contractility, and systemic vascular resistance are important considerations in the management of anesthesia. As with aortic stenosis, analgesia for labor and vaginal delivery is often provided with systemic medications or inhalation analgesia and pudendal block. Likewise, general anesthesia is recommended for cesarean section. Invasive monitoring of arterial and cardiac filling pressures is helpful.

Primary Pulmonary Hypertension

Primary pulmonary hypertension is a disease that predominates in young females (see Chapter 8). Pain during labor and vaginal delivery is especially detrimental because it may further increase pulmonary vascular resistance and decrease venous return. Continuous lumbar epidural anesthesia is useful for preventing pain-induced increases in pulmonary vascular resistance, although careful titration of the local anesthetic is important to minimize any decrease in systemic vascular resistance.[81] The addition of an opioid to the local anesthetic solution may be useful. General anesthesia is often recommended for cesarean section, although epidural anesthesia has also been successfully used.[82] Spinal anesthesia is not recommended for cesarean section because of the potential for sudden decreases in systemic vascular resistance associated with the high sensory level required for this operation.[83] Potential risks of general anesthesia in these patients include increased pulmonary artery pressure during laryngoscopy and tracheal intubation, the adverse effects of positive-pressure ventilation on venous return, and the negative inotropic effects of volatile anesthetics. Nitrous oxide may further increase pulmonary vascular resistance. Predelivery assessment of the effects of vasodilators, inotropes, oxytocin, and fluid administration may be of value during subsequent anesthetic management. In addition to oxygen, the administration of isoproterenol may be useful for decreasing pulmonary vascular resistance.[81] Hemodynamic monitoring, including systemic arterial pressure and pulmonary arterial pressure, is indicated in these patients. Pulmonary artery rupture and thrombosis are a risk with the use of a pulmonary artery catheter in the presence of pulmonary hypertension, but the benefits in these critically ill patients appear to offset the potential hazards.[83] Maternal mortality is more than 50% with most deaths due to congestive heart failure that occurs during labor and the early postpartum period.

Cardiomyopathy of Pregnancy

Left ventricular failure late in the course of pregnancy or during the first 6 weeks postpartum has been termed cardiomyopathy of pregnancy. If such failure persists despite diuretics and digitalis, it is recommended that analgesia for labor and vaginal delivery be provided with a continuous lumbar epidural technique. An acute increase in systemic vascular resistance should be avoided. In about one-half of these parturients, heart failure is transient and recurs only during subsequent pregnancies. In the remaining parturients, idiopathic congestive cardiomyopathy persists and death is likely, especially if another pregnancy is allowed to progress to term.

Dissecting Aneurysm of the Aorta

There is a recognized association between pregnancy and dissecting aneurysm of the aorta. Indeed, nearly 50% of such aneurysms in females younger than 40 years of age occur in association with pregnancy. A continuous lumbar epidural anesthetic is recommended to maintain a pain-free state and a normal to slightly decreased blood pressure in the parturient in whom this disorder is known to have developed.

Prosthetic Valve Replacement

Prosthetic valve replacement usually requires anticoagulation to decrease the likelihood of thromboembolism. Typically, a coumarin anticoagulant is replaced at 6 to 12 weeks of gestation with heparin, which does not cross the placenta. The presence of anticoagulation limits the use of spinal or epidural anesthesia in these patients.

PREGNANCY-INDUCED HYPERTENSION

Pregnancy-induced hypertension (PIH) encompasses a range of disorders collectively and formerly known as toxemia of pregnancy, which includes isolated hypertension (nonproteinuric hypertension), pre-eclampsia (proteinuric hypertension), and eclampsia. Occurring in 5% to 15% of all pregnancies, PIH is a major cause of obstetric and perinatal morbidity and mortality. The three principal mechanisms proposed for the etiology of PIH are (1) vasospasm caused by an abnormal sensitivity of vascular smooth muscle to catecholamines, (2) an antigen-antibody reaction between fetal and maternal tissues in the first trimester that initiates placental vasculitis, and (3) an imbalance in the production of vasoactive prostaglandins (thromboxane A and prostacyclin), leading to vasoconstriction of small arteries and aggregation of platelets. With respect to this last mechanism, it has been demonstrated that administration of aspirin (60 to 150 mg·d^{-1}) during the second and third trimesters decreases the risk of PIH.[84]

Gestational hypertension is characterized by the onset of hypertension, without proteinuria or edema, during the last few weeks of gestation or during the immediate postpartum period.[85] The increased blood pressure is usually mild, and the outcome of pregnancy is not affected appreciably. Blood pressure normalizes during the first few weeks postpartum, but hypertension often recurs during subsequent pregnancies. It is believed that essential hypertension will develop in these females later in life. Chronic hypertension is considered to be present when blood pressure is increased before 20 weeks of gestation and persists for more than 6 weeks postpartum.

Pre-eclampsia is a syndrome exhibited after 20 weeks of gestation, characterized by hypertension, proteinuria, and generalized edema. Symptoms and signs of pre-eclampsia usually abate within 48 hours after delivery. A blood pressure above 140/90 mmHg, with a urine protein loss greater than 2 g·d^{-1}, is sufficient evidence for the diagnosis. Severe pre-eclampsia is indicated by a blood pressure above 160/110 mmHg; urine protein loss greater than 5 g·d^{-1}; and complaints of headache, visual disturbances, and epigastric pain. Hemolysis (H), elevated liver transaminase enzyme activity (EL), and low platelet count (LP) have been characterized as the HELLP syndrome and represent the most severe manifestation of the pre-eclampsia spectrum.[86] Eclampsia is present when convulsions are superimposed on pre-eclampsia. Eclampsia is associated with a maternal mortality of about 10%. Causes of maternal mortality from eclampsia include congestive heart failure and intracranial hemorrhage.

Table 31-7. Manifestations of Pregnancy-Induced Hypertension

Cerebral edema
Grand mal seizures
Cerebral hemorrhage
Hypertension
Congestive heart failure
Decreased colloid oncotic pressure
Arterial hypoxemia
Laryngeal edema
Hepatic dysfunction
Oliguric renal failure
Hypovolemia
Disseminated intravascular coagulation
Decreased uterine blood flow
Premature labor and delivery

Pathophysiology

The pathophysiology of PIH involves nearly every organ system[87] (Table 31-7).

Central Nervous System

The central nervous system is hyperirritable, reflecting cerebral edema due to increased intracellular fluid volume of the brain cells. Grand mal seizures can occur spontaneously or secondary to additional increases in maternal blood pressure. Coma, in association with increased intracranial pressure, may follow. Cerebral hemorrhage accounts for 30% to 40% of deaths in these patients.[87]

Cardiovascular Systems

The peripheral vasculature in the presence of PIH exhibits increased sensitivity to catecholamines, sympathomimetic drugs, and the oxytocics. There is generalized arteriolar vasoconstriction consistent with elevations of maternal blood pressure. Increased afterload can lead to left ventricular failure and pulmonary edema.

Pulmonary System

Reductions of colloid oncotic pressure can result in the interstitial accumulation of fluid in the lungs. Indeed, decreases in the PaO_2 are a frequent occurrence in the presence of PIH. Edema of the upper airway and larynx, which accompanies normal gestation, is exaggerated in these parturients. This change may influence the size of tube chosen for intubation of the trachea.

Hepatorenal System

Hepatic dysfunction is associated with decreased hepatic blood flow and conceivably decreased plasma cholinesterase activity. In addition, progressive decreases in renal blood flow and

glomerular filtration rate may culminate in oliguric renal failure. Increased renal loss of protein leads to decreased colloid oncotic pressure.

Intravascular Fluid Volume

Intravascular fluid volume is often decreased below nonpregnant levels in the presence of PIH. This hypovolemia results in an increased hematocrit that may obscure the presence of anemia.

Coagulation

Abnormalities of the coagulation system may progress to disseminated intravascular coagulation, as manifested by an increased plasma concentration of fibrin degradation products. The platelet count is also frequently reduced in the parturient with PIH, presumably reflecting increased platelet consumption. In the presence of PIH, the bleeding time and platelet count correlate when the platelet count is less than 100,000 cells·mm^{-3}.[88]

Uteroplacental Circulation

Perfusion of the uterus and placenta is reduced in the presence of PIH. Decreased uterine blood flow predisposes to a hyperactive uterus, and premature labor is common. The fetus is at increased risk due to marginal placental function. The neonate is often premature and small for gestational age. As a result, these infants are vulnerable to depression from drugs used to provide maternal analgesia. Meconium aspiration is a common problem in the neonate born to these parturients.

Treatment

Definitive treatment of PIH is delivery of the fetus and placenta. Until delivery is possible, therapy is directed at treating major organ dysfunction. For example, intravenous infusion of fluids is guided by atrial filling pressures and the urine output. Approximately one-third of the fluid infused should consist of 5% albumin to correct decreased colloid oncotic pressure. Digitalis and a renal tubular diuretic are indicated if pulmonary edema and congestive heart failure accompany PIH. Cerebral edema may be managed with an osmotic diuretic, such as mannitol. Sodium restriction is not recommended, as this may lead to sodium depletion and activation of the renin-angiotensin-aldosterone system. Magnesium and antihypertensive drugs are frequently used in the treatment of PIH[85] (Table 31-8).

Magnesium

Magnesium is administered to the parturient with PIH in an attempt to decrease irritability of the central nervous system. Magnesium also decreases hyperactivity at the neuromuscular junction. The mechanism for these effects is the ability of

Table 31-8. Treatment of Pregnancy-Induced Hypertension

Prevent Convulsions

Magnesium sufficient to maintain a serum concentration of 4–6 mEq·L^{-1} (continue 12–24 hours postpartum, as many experience convulsions during this time)

Maintain Diastolic Blood Pressure <110 mmHg

Hydralazine 5–10 mg IV every 20–30 minutes

Diazoxide 30 mg IV, if resistant to hydralazine (arrest of labor and fetal hypoglycemia are risks)

Labetalol (maternal hepatotoxicity a concern)

Calcium channel blockers (may potentiate effects of magnesium, resulting in hypotention)

Nitroprusside and angiotensin-converting enzyme inhibitors not recommended

---

magnesium to decrease the presynaptic release of acetylcholine, as well as to reduce the sensitivity of the postjunctional membranes to acetylcholine. In addition, magnesium has a mild relaxant effect on the vascular and uterine smooth muscle. Uterine relaxation is beneficial, since uterine blood flow is improved.

Clinically, therapeutic effects of magnesium therapy are estimated in terms of its effects on the deep tendon reflexes. Marked depression of patellar reflexes is an indication of impending magnesium toxicity. Periodic determination of the plasma magnesium level is also helpful in adjusting supplemental doses of magnesium, to keep the plasma concentration within a therapeutic range of 4 to 6 mEq·L^{-1}. Commonly, the parturient receives an intravenous loading dose of magnesium 4 g in a 20% solution infused over 5 minutes. The therapeutic plasma concentration is maintained by a continuous infusion of 1 to 2 g·h^{-1}. A plasma magnesium level in excess of the therapeutic range can lead to severe skeletal muscle weakness, with ventilatory failure and cardiac arrest. Administration of intravenous calcium counteracts adverse effects of magnesium. Magnesium is excreted by the kidneys and must be used with caution when renal function is impaired.

Potentiation of both depolarizing and nondepolarizing muscle relaxants by magnesium is clinically significant. This potentiation introduces the need for careful titration of the dose of a muscle relaxant and for monitoring the effects produced at the neuromuscular junction. PIH may be associated with a reduction in the plasma cholinesterase activity that is greater than that normally associated with pregnancy, resulting in potentiation of the effects of succinylcholine independent of magnesium therapy.[89] Doses of sedatives and opioids should be reduced, as magnesium can potentiate their effects. Since magnesium readily crosses the placenta, it seems possible that neonatal skeletal muscle tone could be decreased at birth. Nevertheless, the deleterious effects of maternal magnesium therapy do not occur in the nonasphyxiated full-term neonate, suggesting that depression of ventilation previously attributed to magnesium was due to asphyxia or prematurity, or both. Conversely, hypomagnesemia may cause postpartum neurologic dysfunction, which may be erroneously attributed to the regional anesthetic technique used during labor and delivery.[90]

Antihypertensive Drugs

It is appropriate to initiate therapy with antihypertensive drugs when diastolic blood pressure remains above 110 mmHg. Hydralazine (5 to 10 mg IV) is frequently selected because of its rapid onset, usually within 15 minutes. Additional doses of hydralazine are administered as necessary to maintain diastolic blood pressures close to 90 mmHg. Hydralazine often increases cardiac output, uteroplacental circulation, and renal blood flow.

A continuous intravenous infusion of trimethaphan (0.01%) may be lifesaving for the treatment of a hypertensive crisis in the parturient with PIH. The goal is to reduce maternal diastolic blood pressures to around 90 mmHg; one must remember that a sudden decrease in blood pressure may jeopardize uteroplacental circulation and lead to fetal distress. Fetal heart rate should be continuously monitored during the pharmacologic treatment of a maternal hypertensive crises, to ensure an early warning if the lowered blood pressure is compromising uteroplacental circulation. Diazoxide is not popular in these patients because of the unpredictable magnitude of blood pressure reduction produced by this drug.

Nitroprusside may not be recommended for treatment of hypertensive crises in the parturient. This concern is based on the knowledge that cyanide readily crosses the placenta, introducing the possibility of fetal cyanide toxicity. Indeed, the fetus has less thiosulfate substrate for rhodanase detoxication of cyanide than does the adult and may therefore be uniquely vulnerable to the development of cyanide toxicity from a nitroprusside infusion.[91] Nevertheless, deliberate hypotension with nitroprusside has been used to facilitate surgery for control of intracranial aneurysms in parturients, with no apparent adverse effect on the fetus. Indeed, a 20% decrease in blood pressure for 1 hour, produced with an average dose of nitroprusside (1 μg·kg^{-1}·min^{-1}) administered to an animal model, had no adverse effects on the fetus.[91] Conversely, a similar decrease in blood pressure in animals requiring an average dose of nitroprusside (25 μg·kg^{-1}·min^{-1}) produced cyanide toxicity and in utero fetal death. Perhaps short-term use of nitroprusside in low doses is acceptable for treatment of the hypertensive parturient.

Management of Anesthesia

Vaginal delivery in the presence of PIH and in the absence of fetal distress is acceptable. A continuous lumbar epidural technique is a useful method of analgesia for labor and vaginal delivery for the volume-repleted pre-eclamptic patient, under good medical control. Epidural analgesia negates the need for maternal opioids and thus their possible adverse effects on a preterm fetus. The absence of maternal pushing reduces the likelihood of associated blood pressure increases. Furthermore, vasodilating effects produced by epidural anesthesia improve placental blood flow and could conceivably increase renal blood flow.

Before continuous lumbar epidural anesthesia is instituted, the patient should be hydrated with intravenous fluid (1 to 2 L of lactated Ringer's solution), as guided by central venous pressure monitoring. Furthermore, coagulation studies should be performed before placement of a lumbar epidural catheter, particularly if the pre-eclampsia is severe. Initially, a segmental band of anesthesia (T10–L1) will provide analgesia for uterine contractions. As the second stage of labor is entered, the lumbar epidural anesthetic can be extended to provide perineal analgesia. Because of hypersensitivity of the maternal vasculature to catecholamines, it would seem prudent not to add epinephrine to the local anesthetic solution used for the epidural anesthetic. Nevertheless, the use of epinephrine-containing local anesthetic solutions has not produced adverse circulatory responses in these patients.[92]

If vaginal delivery is imminent, a spinal anesthetic limited to the sacral area is an acceptable approach. As with a lumbar epidural technique, institution of intravenous hydration before performance of spinal anesthesia is desirable. The disadvantage of spinal anesthesia is the possible rapid onset of peripheral sympathetic nervous system blockade and hypotension, in the event that the sensory level extends above T10. Should systolic blood pressure decrease more than 30% from the preblock value, treatment is with left uterine displacement and an increased rate of fluid infusion. If hypotension persists, a small dose of ephedrine (2.5 mg IV) is appropriate.

Cesarean section is often necessary in the parturient with PIH. The indication for cesarean section is fetal distress, reflecting progressive deterioration of the uteroplacental circulation. General anesthesia is usually preferred when an emergency cesarean section is necessary. Extensive peripheral sympathetic nervous system blockade that may accompany epidural or spinal anesthesia could make management of blood pressure difficult in these patients during cesarean section. Before induction of anesthesia, an attempt is made to restore intravascular fluid volume. Continuous monitoring of intra-arterial pressure, cardiac filling pressures, urine output, and fetal heart rate is useful. Induction of anesthesia is often with thiopental (3 to 5 mg·kg^{-1}) plus succinylcholine (1 to 1.5 mg·kg^{-1}), to facilitate placement of a cuffed tube in the trachea. Cricoid pressure is provided by an assistant until the trachea is protected by a cuffed tube. The use of a defasciculating dose of a nondepolarizing muscle relaxant before the administration of succinylcholine may not be necessary, since magnesium therapy is likely to attenuate fasciculations produced by succinylcholine. Exaggerated edema of the upper airway structures may interfere with visualization of the glottic opening (swollen tongue and epiglottis), and laryngeal swelling may result in the need to insert a smaller endotracheal tube than anticipated. In patients with impaired coagulation, laryngoscopy could evoke profuse bleeding. Blood pressure increases that predictably accompany direct laryngoscopy and intubation of the trachea might be exaggerated in these parturients, increasing the likelihood of cerebral hemorrhage or pulmonary edema. A short duration of laryngoscopy is helpful for minimizing the magnitude and duration of the blood pressure increase. Hydralazine (5 to 10 mg IV), administered 10 to 15 minutes before the induction of anesthesia, or nitroglycerin (1 to 2 μg·kg^{-1} IV), just before starting direct laryngoscopy, has also been recommended for attenuating these blood pressure responses.[93] A volatile anesthetic (0.5 MAC) can be used before intubation of the trachea and during anesthetic maintenance both to attenuate and to treat hypertension. Potentiation of muscle relaxants by magnesium must be remembered, and a peripheral nerve stimulator used to monitor activity of the neuromuscular junction. Removal of the cuffed tube from the trachea at the conclusion of surgery should be considered only after return of the upper airway reflexes. The use of a synthetic oxytocic to treat uterine atony after delivery must be done cautiously, in view of the hypersensitive peripheral vasculature predictably present in these parturients.

PREGNANCY AND DIABETES MELLITUS

Insulin requirements in the parturient with diabetes mellitus change markedly during pregnancy. For example, less insulin is needed during the first trimester and more in the second trimester. Maternal insulin requirements drop precipitously during the postpartum period. Insulin does not cross the placenta. Conversely, oral hypoglycemic drugs readily cross the placenta and can induce hypoglycemia in the neonate.

Glucose levels during pregnancy in nondiabetic parturients are lower than nonpregnant levels. Therefore, blood glucose concentrations are often maintained at a lower than normal level in the parturient with diabetes mellitus. Accomplishment of this goal may require multiple injections of insulin and rigid adherence to diet. The diabetic parturient is at increased risk of the development of ketoacidosis during the second and third trimesters. PIH is also more common in the presence of diabetes mellitus. Neonates born to diabetic mothers are often large for gestational age and are at increased risk of the development of respiratory distress syndrome.

The goal is to ensure the continuation of pregnancy to near term, to permit maximal fetal lung maturation. Elective cesarean section is often performed in an attempt to avoid the high incidence of fetal death that occurs late in the third trimester, presumably due to placental insufficiency. The best choice of anesthesia is not defined. Fetal acidosis after cesarean section has been reported with epidural or spinal anesthesia that was complicated by maternal hypotension.[94,95] Indeed, there is a suggestion that fetal outcome is better after cesarean section performed under general anesthesia.[95] Nevertheless, regional anesthetic techniques in diabetic parturients provide the advantages of (1) avoiding hyperglycemic responses to surgery, (2) monitoring the central nervous system status of the mother, and (3) providing anesthesia without added drug depression should operative delivery be difficult and prolonged. Regardless of the technique selected for anesthesia, the blood glucose concentration should be checked in the early neonatal period of an infant born to a diabetic parturient.

MYASTHENIA GRAVIS AND PREGNANCY

The course of myasthenia gravis during gestation is highly variable and unpredictable.[96] Exacerbations are most likely to take place during the first trimester or within the first 10 days of the postpartum period. Anticholinesterase drugs should be continued during pregnancy and labor. Theoretically, these drugs would increase uterine contractility, but an increased incidence of spontaneous abortion or premature labor does not occur.

Myasthenia gravis does not affect the course of labor. The use of sedatives should be avoided, in view of the limited margin of reserve in these patients. A continuous lumbar epidural anesthetic is acceptable for labor and vaginal delivery. Outlet forceps are frequently used to shorten the second stage of labor, thereby minimizing the skeletal muscle fatigue associated with expulsive efforts. Regional anesthesia can be used safely for cesarean section, but it must be appreciated that co-existing skeletal muscle weakness may lead to hypoventilation in the presence of a high sensory level.

Neonatal myasthenia gravis can occur transiently in 20% to 30% of babies born to mothers with this disorder. Manifestations usually occur within 24 hours of birth and are characterized by generalized skeletal muscle weakness and an expressionless face. When respiratory efforts are inadequate, a tube should be placed in the trachea and ventilation of the lungs should be mechanically supported. Anticholinesterase therapy in the neonate is usually necessary for about 21 days after birth.

HEMORRHAGE IN THE OBSTETRIC PATIENT

Hemorrhage remains the leading cause of maternal mortality. Although bleeding can occur at any time during pregnancy, third-trimester hemorrhage is most threatening to maternal and fetal well-being[97] (Table 31-9). Placenta previa and abruptio placentae are the major causes of bleeding during the third trimester. Uterine rupture can be responsible for uncontrolled hemorrhage that manifests during active labor. Postpartum hemorrhage occurs after 3% to 5% of all vaginal deliveries and is typically due to retained placenta, uterine atony, or cervical or vaginal lacerations.

Placenta Previa

Placenta previa is an abnormally low implantation of the placenta in the uterus that occurs in up to 1% of full-term pregnancies[97] (Table 31-9). The cause is not known, although

Table 31-9. Differential Diagnosis of Third-Trimester Bleeding

	Placenta Previa	Abruptio Placentae	Uterine Rupture
Clinical features	Painless vaginal bleeding	Abdominal pain Bleeding partially or wholly concealed Uterine irritability Shock Coagulopathy Acute renal failure Fetal distress	Severe abdominal pain Shock Disappearance of fetal heart tones
Predisposing conditions	Advanced age Multiple parity	Multiple parity Uterine anomalies Compression of the inferior vena cava Chronic hypertension	Previous uterine incision Rapid spontaneous delivery Excessive uterine stimulation Cephalopelvic disproportion Multiple parity Polyhydramnios Spontaneous

there is an association with advancing age of the parturient and with high parity.

Placenta previa is classified as (1) complete, in which the entire internal cervical os is covered by placental tissue; (2) partial, in which the internal cervical os is covered by placental tissue when closed, but not when fully dilated; and (3) marginal, in which placental tissue encroaches on or extends to the margin of the internal cervical os. Nearly 50% of parturients with placenta previa have marginal implantations.

The cardinal symptom of placenta previa is painless vaginal bleeding, which usually stops spontaneously. Bleeding typically manifests around week 32, when the lower uterine segment is beginning to form. When this diagnosis is suspected, the position of the placenta should be confirmed by ultrasonography or radioisotope scan. If these tests are not conclusive and vaginal bleeding persists, the diagnosis is made by direct examination of the cervical os. This examination should be done in the delivery room, only after preparations have been taken to replace acute blood loss and to proceed with an emergency cesarean section. The combination of direct examination of the cervical os in a patient who is surgically prepared for an immediate cesarean section is known as a "double setup." When manual examination of the cervical os triggers hemorrhage, it is likely that bleeding will persist until the placenta can be removed. Ketamine is a useful drug for induction of anesthesia in the presence of acute hemorrhage due to placenta previa. It should be remembered, however, that doses of ketamine in excess of 1 mg·kg^{-1} are associated with increased uterine tone.[34] Theoretically, such increases could further decrease an already compromised uteroplacental circulation. Maintenance of anesthesia before delivery is determined by the hemodynamic status of the mother. Often, anesthesia is maintained with 50% nitrous oxide plus succinylcholine, to produce skeletal muscle relaxation. The neonate delivered from a parturient in hemorrhagic shock is likely to be severely acidotic and hypovolemic. Treatment of placenta previa not accompanied by hemorrhage consists of bed rest followed by elective cesarean section.

Abruptio Placentae

Abruptio placentae is premature separation of a normally implanted placenta after 20 weeks of gestation[97] (Table 31-9). The cause is unknown, but the incidence is increased with high parity, uterine anomalies, compression of the inferior vena cava, and occurrence of hypertension during pregnancy. Abruptio placentae accounts for about one-third of third-trimester hemorrhages.

Clinical manifestations of abruptio placentae depend on the site and extent of the placental separation but abdominal pain is almost always present. When the separation involves only placental margins, the escaping blood can appear as vaginal bleeding. Alternatively, a large volume of blood loss can re-main entirely concealed in the uterus. Severe blood loss from abruptio placentae is manifested as maternal hypotension, uterine irritability and hypertonia, plus fetal distress or even demise. Clotting abnormalities, due to unknown causes but resembling disseminated intravascular coagulation, can occur. Therefore, measurements of coagulation status must be obtained in these patients. The classic hematologic picture includes thrombocytopenia, depletion of fibrinogen, and a prolonged plasma thromboplastin time.[97] Acute renal failure may accompany disseminated intravascular coagulation, reflecting fibrin deposition in renal arterioles. Fetal distress reflects loss of functioning placenta and decreased uteroplacental perfusion because of maternal hypotension.

Definitive treatment of abruptio placentae is to empty the uterus. If there are no signs of maternal hypovolemia, if clotting studies are normal, and if there is no evidence of uteroplacental insufficiency, the use of a continuous lumbar epidural technique is useful to provide analgesia for labor and vaginal delivery. When the magnitude of placental separation and resulting hemorrhage is severe, an emergency cesarean section is necessary, using general anesthesia. Ketamine is a useful drug for induction of anesthesia, followed by the addition of 50% nitrous oxide until the fetus is delivered. It is predictable that the neonate born under these circumstances will be acidotic and hypovolemic.

It is not uncommon for blood to dissect between layers of the myometrium after premature separation of the placenta. As a result, the uterus is unable to contract adequately after delivery, and postpartum hemorrhage occurs. Uncontrolled hemorrhage may require an emergency hysterectomy. Bleeding may be exaggerated by a coagulopathy, in which case infusion of fresh frozen plasma and platelets should replace deficient clotting factors. Clotting parameters usually revert to normal within a few hours after delivery of the neonate.

Uterine Rupture

Uterine rupture occurs in up to 0.1% of full-term pregnancies and may be associated with separation of a previous uterine scar, rapid spontaneous delivery, excessive oxytocin stimulation, or multiple parity with cephalopelvic disproportion or an unrecognized transverse presentation.[97] Overall, however, more than 80% of uterine ruptures are spontaneous without an obvious explanation.[97] Furthermore, uterine rupture and dehiscence represent a spectrum ranging from an incomplete rupture or a gradual scar dehiscence to explosive rupture with intraperitoneal extrusion of uterine contents. Manifestations may include (1) severe abdominal pain, often referred to the shoulder due to subdiaphragmatic irritation by intra-abdominal blood; (2) maternal hypotension; and (3) disappearance of fetal heart tones. Occasionally, a parturient with a previous cesarean section is allowed to deliver vaginally. In these patients, continuous lumbar epidural anesthesia has been questioned, since this form of analgesia could mask abdominal pain, which may be the first indication of impending or actual uterine rupture. Nevertheless, this theoretical concern has not been confirmed by clinical experience and with the proper precautions (continuous fetal monitoring, avoidance of oxytocic stimulation of the uterus), epidural analgesia produced by a dilute concentration of local anesthetic may be safely used in a parturient with a previous cesarean section.[97,98]

Retained Placenta

Retained placenta occurs in about 1% of all vaginal deliveries and usually necessitates manual exploration of the uterus. If epidural or subarachnoid anesthesia is not used for vaginal delivery, manual removal of the placenta may be first attempted under continuous inhalation analgesia. General anesthesia, including administration of a volatile anesthetic to provide uterine relaxation, will be necessary if the uterus remains firmly contracted around the placenta. Intubation of the trachea is necessary when general anesthesia is used to relax the uterus. Ketamine, in a dose exceeding 1 mg·kg^{-1}, is not recommended in view of dose-related increases in uterine tone produced by this drug.[34]

Uterine Atony

Uterine atony after vaginal delivery is an important cause of postpartum bleeding and is a potential cause of maternal mortality. A completely atonic uterus may result in a 2000-ml blood loss in 5 minutes. Conditions associated with uterine atony include multiple parity, multiple births, polyhydramnios, a large fetus, and retained placenta. Uterine atony may occur immediately after delivery or may be manifested several hours later. Treatment is with intravenous oxytocin to cause contraction of the uterus. In rare instances, it may be necessary to perform an emergency hysterectomy.

ASHERMAN SYNDROME

Asherman syndrome (traumatic intrauterine synechiae) most often follows postpartum or postabortion curettage. Although infertility is likely, conception can occur and pregnancy is associated with a high incidence of complications, the most serious of which is antepartum and postpartum hemorrhage due to accretion of the placenta. Placenta accreta describes any condition in which the placenta adheres to, invades, or penetrates the uterine myometrium. The diagnosis of placenta accreta usually mandates emergency hysterectomy, which, considering the highly vascular gravid uterus, may be associated with substantial blood loss. For this reason, selection of a regional anesthetic technique with its associated sympathetic

nervous system blockade may be questionable in the laboring parturient with Asherman syndrome and the likely presence of placenta accreta.[99]

AMNIOTIC FLUID EMBOLISM

Amniotic fluid embolism, which is estimated to occur once in every 20,000 to 30,000 deliveries, is signaled by the sudden onset of respiratory distress, profound hypotension, and arterial hypoxemia.[100] The entry of amniotic fluid into the pulmonary circulation results in (1) pulmonary vascular obstruction, with a consequent decrease in cardiac output and blood pressure; (2) pulmonary hypertension, with acute cor pulmonale; and (3) ventilation-to-perfusion mismatch, producing severe arterial hypoxemia. In some instances, a grand mal seizure precedes the appearance of cardiopulmonary symptoms. Excessive bleeding is usually not present initially but develops later in nearly every affected parturient. Hemorrhage is attributed to disseminated intravascular coagulation.

There is no specific treatment for amniotic fluid embolism, other than that directed toward cardiopulmonary resuscitation and replacement of intravascular fluid volume. Arterial hypoxemia is severe, and supplemental oxygen plus intubation of the trachea and controlled ventilation of the lungs will usually be necessary. Positive end-expiratory pressure may be instituted if arterial hypoxemia persists. Corticosteroids have been used but do not seem to be of demonstrable benefit. Mortality from a massive amniotic fluid embolism is more than 80%.

A multiparous parturient who experiences a tumultuous labor is most likely to experience amniotic fluid embolism. Definitive diagnosis is made by demonstrating amniotic fluid material in maternal blood, which has been aspirated from a central venous catheter.[101] Indeed, examination of a blood smear should be performed in every parturient suspected of having an amniotic fluid embolism. Conditions that can mimic amniotic fluid embolism include inhalation of gastric contents, pulmonary embolism, air embolism, and local anesthetic toxicity. Pulmonary aspiration is more likely when bronchospasm accompanies the clinical picture. Indeed, bronchospasm is rare in the parturient who experiences amniotic fluid embolism. Pulmonary embolism is usually accompanied by chest pain.

ANESTHESIA FOR OPERATIONS DURING PREGNANCY

It is estimated that about 50,000 pregnant females in the United States annually undergo an operative procedure requiring anesthesia.[102] The most frequent nonobstetrical procedure is excision of an ovarian cyst. Appendicitis is the second most frequent indication for operative intervention. Treatment of an incompetent cervix (cervical cerclage) requires anesthesia early in pregnancy. There is also the possibility that anesthesia may be unknowingly administered in early undiagnosed pregnancy. The objectives for management of anesthesia in the parturient undergoing a nonobstetric operative procedure is avoidance of teratogenic drugs, avoidance of intrauterine fetal hypoxia and acidosis, and prevention of premature labor.[103,104]

Avoidance of Teratogenic Drugs

Almost all commonly used medications, including drugs used for anesthesia, have been demonstrated to be teratogenic in at least one animal species. For a drug to be teratogenic, it must be given to a susceptible species in an appropriate dose and during a specific period of organ development. Each organ system undergoes a critical stage of development, during which vulnerability to teratogens is greatest. In humans, the critical period of organogenesis is between 15 and 56 days of gestation; however, surveys of females who had received inhalation anesthesia for operations during pregnancy have failed to demonstrate that any anesthetic is teratogenic or induces abortions.[104,105] Nevertheless, sufficient circumstantial evidence of the harmful nature of nitrous oxide exists to suggest caution in administration of this drug during early pregnancy.[104]

There is concern that subteratogenic doses of some psychoactive drugs, such as anesthetics, could produce behavioral and learning defects without causing gross morphologic changes. This concern is based on the fact that development of the central nervous system is not complete even at birth. Therefore, it has been proposed that drugs administered to parturients, including those used for anesthesia during labor and delivery, might produce permanent organ dysfunction. Indeed, short-duration administration of halothane to pregnant rats resulted in learning deficits in offspring of those animals who were exposed during the first and second but not third trimesters.[106] Nevertheless, there is no evidence establishing the validity of the assertion that anesthesia administered to a parturient adversely affects later mental and neurologic development of the offspring.[107] There is no evidence that any anesthetic drug is carcinogenic to the fetus.

Avoidance of Intrauterine Fetal Hypoxia and Acidosis

Intrauterine fetal hypoxia and acidosis are prevented by avoiding maternal hypotension, arterial hypoxemia, and excessive changes in the $PaCO_2$. It must be appreciated that uterine blood flow and thus placental perfusion is pressure dependent. Hazards to the fetus from decreased maternal oxygenation are obvious. Conversely, maternal hyperoxia does

not produce uterine artery vasoconstriction. Furthermore, a high maternal PaO_2 rarely produces a fetal PaO_2 above 45 mmHg. This reflects the high oxygen consumption of the placenta and uneven distribution of maternal and fetal blood flow in the placenta. For this reason, maternal hyperoxia does not produce in utero retrolental fibroplasia or premature closure of the ductus arteriosus. Maternal hyperventilation should be avoided intraoperatively, as positive airway pressure may reduce uterine blood flow and any resulting respiratory alkalosis increases the maternal hemoglobin affinity for oxygen, resulting in release of less oxygen to the fetus at the placenta.

Prevention of Premature Labor

There is no evidence that a specific anesthetic drug or technique is associated with a higher or lower incidence of premature delivery.[105] Indeed, it is the underlying pathology necessitating the operative intervention that determines the onset of premature labor. For example, premature labor occurs in 28% to 40% of patients undergoing a cervical cerclage, whereas orthopaedic, neurosurgical, or plastic surgical procedures are not associated with premature labor. After successful completion of an operative procedure, it is advisable to continue monitoring of the fetal heart rate and maternal uterine activity in the recovery period.

Premature labor can be treated with a selective beta-2 agonist such as terbutaline or ritordine. These drugs relax uterine smooth muscle, resulting in inhibition of uterine contractions. Relaxation of the uterus also contributes to improved uteroplacental blood flow and fetal well-being. It is important to realize that significant maternal side effects, including pulmonary edema, cardiac dysrhythmias, and hypokalemia, can accompany the use of these drugs.[108,109] These drugs cross the placenta and can cause fetal tachycardia and hypoglycemia. The mechanism for alterations in maternal plasma potassium concentrations is not established. It is thought that beta-2 agonists stimulate both glycolysis and insulin release, resulting in shifts of potassium into the intracellular spaces. It is important to be aware that hypokalemia observed during administration of a beta-2 agonist may persist despite potassium chloride supplementation. The plasma potassium concentration will return to preinfusion levels about 30 minutes after the beta-2 agonist infusion is discontinued. Therefore, it may be prudent to discontinue the infusion about 30 minutes before administration of an anesthetic for delivery.[109] Continuous monitoring of the electrocardiogram and avoidance of intraoperative hyperventilation of the lungs are useful principles for management of anesthesia. Intravenous alcohol has also been used to stop premature labor. Maternal and neonatal central nervous system depression are undesirable side effects of this treatment.

Management of Anesthesia

Elective surgery should be deferred until after delivery. When surgery is urgent, it is best to delay the operation until the second and third trimester. Emergency surgery in the first trimester is often performed with lumbar epidural or spinal anesthesia. Spinal anesthesia is useful, as this technique minimizes fetal drug exposure. Nevertheless, there is no evidence that inhaled anesthetics cause adverse responses when administered to the parturient undergoing nonobstetric surgery.[105] Continuous intraoperative monitoring of fetal heart rate after 16 weeks of gestation is helpful in providing early warning of fetal hypoxia and acidosis due to impaired uteroplacental perfusion (see the section, Diagnosis and Management of Fetal Distress). When inhalation anesthesia is chosen, it should be appreciated that a low concentration of a volatile drug is not associated with significant decreases in uterine blood flow because of concomitant decreases in uterine vascular resistance. Although controversial, it may be prudent to avoid administration of nitrous oxide during early pregnancy.[104] Regardless of the anesthetic technique selected, the inspired concentration of oxygen should be probably maintained at about 50%.

DIAGNOSIS AND MANAGEMENT OF FETAL DISTRESS

Fetal distress due to intrauterine hypoxia and acidosis is most likely to occur when uterine blood flow decreases with each uterine contraction. Indeed, a placenta with borderline function before the onset of labor may not be able to maintain fetal well-being when gas transfer across the placenta is further compromised by a decrease in uterine blood flow associated with a vigorous contraction of the uterus.

Electronic Fetal Monitoring

Electronic fetal monitoring permits evaluation of fetal well-being by following changes in fetal heart rate, as recorded using an external monitor (Doppler) or fetal scalp electrode. The basic principle of electronic fetal monitoring is to correlate changes in fetal heart rate with fetal well-being and uterine contractions. For example, fetal well-being is evaluated by determination of beat-to-beat variability of fetal heart rate, as computed from the R-R interval on the fetal electrocardiogram.[110,111] Another method is evaluation of fetal heart rate decelerations associated with contractions of the uterus.[111,112] The three major types of fetal heart rate decelerations are classified as early, late, and variable. Fetal scalp sampling is indicated when an abnormal fetal heart rate pattern persists.

It has been observed that the fetus is usually depressed when one or more fetal scalp pH values are near 7.00.

Beat-to-Beat Variability

Fetal heart rate varies 5 to 20 beats·min^{-1}, with a normal heart rate ranging between 120 to 160 beats·min^{-1}. This normal heart rate variability is thought to reflect the integrity of neural pathways from the fetal cerebral cortex through the medulla, vagus nerve, and cardiac conduction system. Fetal well-being is ensured when beat-to-beat variability is present. Conversely, fetal distress, due to arterial hypoxemia, acidosis, or central nervous system damage, is associated with minimal to absent beat-to-beat variability.

Drugs administered to the parturient may eliminate fetal heart rate variability, even in the absence of fetal distress. Those drugs most frequently associated with loss of beat-to-beat variability are benzodiazepines, opioids, barbiturates, anticholinergics, and local anesthetics, as used for continuous lumbar epidural analgesia. These drug-induced effects do not appear to be deleterious but may cause difficulty in interpretation of fetal heart rate monitoring. In addition, the absence of heart rate variability may be normally present in the premature fetus and during fetal sleep cycles.

Early Decelerations

Early decelerations are characterized by slowing of the fetal heart rate that begins with the onset of an uterine contraction (Fig. 31-14). Slowing becomes maximum at the peak of the contraction, returning to near baseline at its termination. Decreases in heart rate are usually not greater than 20 beats·min^{-1} or below an absolute rate of 100 beats·min^{-1}. This deceleration pattern is thought to be caused by vagal stimulation secondary to compression of the fetal head. Early decelerations are not prevented by increasing fetal oxygenation but are blunted by the administration of atropine. Most important, this fetal heart rate pattern is not associated with fetal distress.

Late Decelerations

Late decelerations are characterized by slowing of the fetal heart rate that begins 10 to 30 seconds after the onset of a uterine contraction. Maximum slowing occurs after the peak intensity of the contraction (Fig. 31-15). A mild late deceleration is classified as a decrease in heart rate less than 20 beats·min^{-1}; profound slowing is considered present when the decrease is more than 40 beats·min^{-1}. Late decelerations are associated with fetal distress, most likely reflecting myocardial hypoxia secondary to uteroplacental insufficiency. Primary factors contributing to the appearance of late decelerations include maternal hypotension, uterine hyperactivity, and chronic uteroplacental insufficiency, as may be due to diabetes mellitus or hypertension. When this pattern persists, there is a predictable correlation with the development of fetal acido-

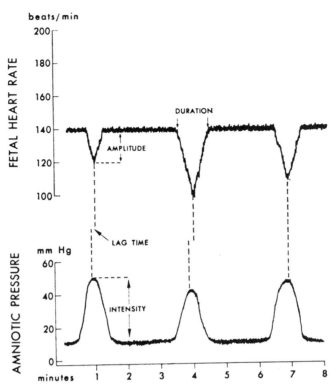

Fig. 31-14. Early decelerations of the fetal heart rate are characterized by a short lag time between the onset of uterine contractions and the beginning of fetal heart rate slowing. Maximum heart rate slowing is usually less than 20 beats·min^{-1} and occurs at the peak intensity of the contraction. Heart rate returns to normal by the time the contraction has ceased. The most likely explanation for this early deceleration is a vagal reflex response to compression of the fetal head. (From Shnider SM. Diagnosis of fetal distress: Fetal heart rate. In: Shnider SM, ed. Obstetrical Anesthesia: Current Concepts and Practice. Baltimore. Williams & Wilkins 1970;197–203, with permission.)

sis.[111,112] Late decelerations can be corrected by improving fetal oxygenation. When beat-to-beat variability of fetal heart rate persists despite late decelerations, the fetus is still likely to be born vigorous.

Variable Decelerations

Variable decelerations are the most common pattern of fetal heart rate changes observed in the intrapartum period. As the term indicates, these decelerations are variable in magnitude, duration, and time of onset relative to an uterine contraction (Fig. 31-16). For example, this pattern may begin before, with, or after the onset of a uterine contraction. Characteristically, deceleration patterns are abrupt in onset and cessation. Fetal heart rate almost invariably falls below 100 beats·min^{-1}. Variable decelerations are thought to be caused by umbilical cord compression. Atropine diminishes the severity of variable decelerations, but administration of oxygen to the mother is without effect. If deceleration patterns are not severe and

repetitive, there are usually only minimal alterations in the fetal acid-base status. Severe variable deceleration patterns that persist for 15 to 30 minutes are associated with fetal acidosis.

EVALUATION OF THE FETUS

It is important to identify intrauterine growth retardation (lower weight than would be expected for gestational age) and prematurity (born less than 37 weeks after the last menstrual period). An infant who is small for gestational age is more likely to become hypoglycemic and septic, and congenital abnormalities occur more frequently. It is postulated that the nutritional deficiency or chronic arterial hypoxemia that results in low birthweight is also responsible for poor neurologic development. Premature neonates have an increased incidence of fetal distress, respiratory distress syndrome, hypovolemia,

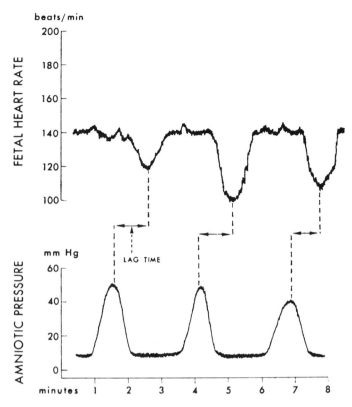

Fig. 31-15. Late decelerations of the fetal heart rate are characterized by a delay (lag time) between the onset of the uterine contraction and the beginning of fetal heart rate slowing. The fetal heart rate does not return to normal until after the contraction has ceased. A mild late deceleration pattern is present when slowing is less than 20 beats·min^{-1}; profound slowing is present when fetal heart rate slows more than 40 beats·min^{-1}. Late fetal heart rate decelerations indicate fetal distress owing to uteroplacental insufficiency. (From Shnider SM. Diagnosis of fetal distress: Fetal heart rate. In Shnider SM, ed. Obstetrical Anesthesia: Current Concepts and Practice. Baltimore. Williams & Wilkins 1979;197–203, with permission.)

hypoglycemia, sepsis, intracranial hemorrhage, and temperature instability; they are also susceptible to the development of retrolental fibroplasia (see Chapter 32). A number of laboratory studies can be used to assess fetal function and maturity. These tests include measurement of maternal urinary estriol excretion and plasma placental lactogen concentrations, analysis of amniotic fluid for lecithin and sphingomyelin levels, and assessment of fetal biparietal diameter by ultrasonography.

Amniotic Fluid Analysis

An index of fetal lung maturity is often obtained before elective cesarean section is performed or induction of labor is undertaken. For example, amniotic fluid, as obtained by abdominal amniocentesis, can be used to assess fetal lung maturity. With maturation of the appropriate enzyme system at

about 35 weeks of gestation, there is an abrupt increase of the lecithin concentration in the amniotic fluid[113] (Fig. 31-17). A ratio of lecithin to sphingomyelin greater than 2 to 3.5, as determined by thin layer chromatography, confirms adequate pulmonary surfactant activity and virtually ensures that the neonate will not develop respiratory distress syndrome. Assessment of fetal lung maturity is especially important in the parturient with diabetes mellitus, for whom the intent is to prolong gestation as long as possible yet initiate delivery before diabetic-associated intrauterine complications become likely.

Ultrasonography

Fetal biparietal diameter, as measured by ultrasound, relates precisely to fetal age. Therefore, ultrasound is frequently used to confirm fetal maturity before elective cesarean section

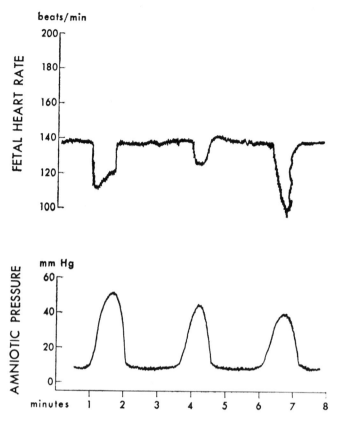

Fig. 31-16. Variable decelerations of the fetal heart rate are characterized by decreases in the heart rate of varying magnitude and duration that do not show a consistent relationship to uterine contractions. This pattern of fetal heart rate slowing is associated with umbilical cord compression. (From Shnider SM. Diagnosis of fetal distress: Fetal heart rate. In Shnider SM, ed. Obstetrical Anesthesia: Current Concepts and Practice. Baltimore. Williams & Wilkins 1970;197–203, with permission.)

and to diagnose intrauterine growth retardation. Ultrasound is also useful in detecting hydramnios, hydrocephaly, anencephaly, and anomalies of the fetal spine.

EVALUATION OF THE NEONATE

The importance of assessment immediately after birth is to identify promptly a depressed neonate who requires active resuscitation. As a guide to identifying and treating the depressed neonate, the Apgar score has not been surpassed.

Apgar Score

The Apgar score assigns a numerical value to five vital signs measured or observed in the neonate 1 minute and 5 minutes after delivery (Table 31-10). Of the five criteria, heart rate

and the quality of the respiratory effort are the most important and color the least informative, in identifying a distressed newborn. A heart rate of less than 100 beats·min^{-1} generally signifies arterial hypoxemia. Disappearance of cyanosis is often rapid when ventilation and circulation are normal. Nevertheless, many healthy neonates still have cyanosis at 1 minute, due to peripheral vasoconstriction in response to a cold ambient temperature in the delivery room. Acidosis and pulmonary vasoconstriction are the most likely causes of persistent cyanosis.

The Apgar score correlates well with acid-base measurements performed immediately after birth. When scores are above 7, neonates are either normal or have a mild respiratory acidosis. Infants with scores of 4 to 6 are moderately depressed; those with scores of 3 or below have combined metabolic and respiratory acidosis. Mild to moderately depressed infants (Apgar scores of 3 to 7) frequently improve in response

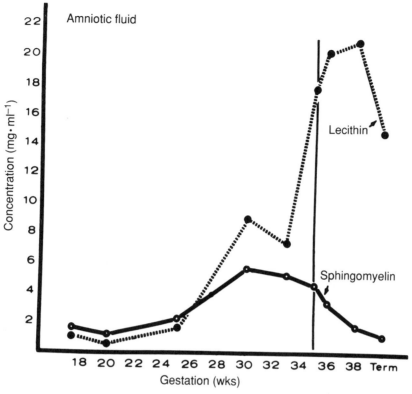

Fig. 31-17. The concentration of lecithin and sphingomyelin in amniotic fluid increases as gestation progresses. An abrupt increase in the lecithin concentration at about 35 weeks of gestation parallels fetal lung maturity. (From Gluck L, Kulovich MV, Barer RC, et al. The diagnosis of the respiratory distress syndrome (RDS) by amniocentesis. Am J Obstet Gynecol 1971;109: 440–5, with permission.)

to oxygen administered by face mask, with or without positive-pressure ventilation of the lungs. Intubation of the trachea and perhaps external cardiac massage is indicated when the Apgar score is less than 3. The Apgar score is not sufficiently sensitive to detect reliably drug-related changes or to provide data necessary to evaluate the subtle effects of obstetric anes-

thetic techniques on neonates (see the section, Neurobehavioral Testing).

Time to Sustained Respiration

The time interval between delivery and the establishment of sustained respiration has been used to identify depressed neonates. A time-to-sustained respiration greater than 90 seconds indicates a depressed neonate and correlates with an Apgar score of 6 or less. Routine determination of the time-to-sustained respiration is not recommended, since this time would be better used by ventilating the neonate's lungs with oxygen.

Neurobehavioral Testing

Neurobehavioral testing (early neonatal neurobehavioral scale) is able to detect subtle or delayed effects of drugs administered during labor and delivery, which are not appreci-

Table 31-10. Evaluation of the Neonate Using the Apgar Score

	0	1	2
Heart rate (beats·min⁻¹)	Absent	<100	>100
Respiratory effort	Absent	Slow Irregular	Crying
Reflex irritability	No response	Grimace	Crying
Muscle tone	Limp	Flexion of extremities	Active
Color	Pale Cyanotic	Body pink Extremities cyanotic	Pink

ated by the Apgar score.[114,115] This testing evaluates the neonate's state of wakefulness, reflex responses, skeletal muscle tone, and responses to sound. Ability of neonates to decrease their responses to stimuli is known as habituation and probably represents the earliest example of processing of information by the cerebral cortex. Habituation has been shown to be impaired by anesthetic drugs administered as maternal systemic medication during labor and delivery. Data demonstrating that neonates born to mothers who had received epidural anesthesia with lidocaine or mepivacaine had lower scores on tests of skeletal muscle strength and tone ("floppy") than did neonates born from mothers receiving epidural anesthesia with bupivacaine have not been reproducible.[114,115] Indeed, more recent data have failed to show any difference between these local anesthetics and lidocaine has regained acceptance as a local anesthetic for obstetric anesthesia.[115] Compared with spinal anesthesia, the use of general anesthesia for elective cesarean sections results in infants who exhibit generalized depression of neurobehavioral testing, despite similar Apgar scores in both groups. Despite the documented decrease in neurobehavioral performance, there is no evidence of prolonged adverse effects on the infant.[115]

Alternatives to neurobehavioral testing to determine the impact of drugs administered to the mother during labor on the neonate are the use of the neurologic and adaptive capacity scores.[116] In contrast to neurobehavioral testing, this score places greater emphasis on skeletal muscle tone, avoids the use of noxious stimuli, and provides a single numerical value that identifies a depressed or vigorous neonate. It is recommended that the neurologic and adaptive capacity be performed initially in the delivery room approximately 15 minutes after birth and repeated 2 hours later. If abnormalities are present, the examination should be repeated at 24 hours.

IMMEDIATE NEONATAL PERIOD

Immediately after delivery, major changes in the neonatal cardiovascular system and respiratory system must occur. For example, with clamping of the umbilical cord at birth, systemic vascular resistance increases, left atrial pressure increases, and flow through the foramen ovale ceases. Expansion of the lungs reduces pulmonary vascular resistance, and the entire right ventricular output is diverted to the lungs. In a normal newborn, an increase in the PaO_2 to above 60 mmHg causes vasoconstriction and functional closure of the ductus arteriosus. When adequate oxygenation and ventilation are not established after delivery, a fetal circulation pattern persists, characterized by increased pulmonary vascular resistance and decreased pulmonary blood flow. Furthermore, the ductus arteriosus and foramen ovale remain open, resulting in a large right-to-left intracardiac shunt, with associated arterial hypoxemia and acidosis.

A high index of suspicion must be maintained for serious abnormalities, which can be present at birth or be manifested shortly after delivery. These include meconium aspiration, choanal stenosis and atresia, diaphragmatic hernia, hypovolemia, hypoglycemia, tracheoesophageal fistula, laryngeal anomalies, and Pierre Robin syndrome (see Chapter 32).

Meconium Aspiration

Meconium is the breakdown product of swallowed amniotic fluid, gastrointestinal cells, and secretions. It is seldom present before 34 weeks of gestation. After about 34 weeks, intrauterine arterial hypoxemia can result in increased gut motility and defecation. Gasping associated with arterial hypoxemia causes the fetus to inhale amniotic fluid and debris into the lungs. If delivery is delayed, meconium will be broken down and excreted from the lung. If birth occurs within 24 hours after aspiration, the meconium will still be present in the major airways and will be distributed to the lung periphery with the onset of breathing. Obstruction of small airways causes ventilation-to-perfusion mismatch. The breathing rate may be more than 100 breaths·min^{-1}, and lung compliance decreases to levels seen in an infant with respiratory distress syndrome. In severe cases, pulmonary hypertension and right-to-left shunting through the patent foramen ovale and ductus arteriosus (persistent fetal circulation) lead to severe arterial hypoxemia. Pneumothorax is also a common problem in the presence of meconium aspiration.

Treatment of meconium aspiration consists of placement of a tube in the trachea immediately after delivery. Suction is applied to the tube by the attendant's mouth, and the tube is removed. If meconium is present in the tube, the trachea is again intubated and suction once more applied. This procedure is repeated until the tube no longer contains meconium. Gentle ventilation of the lungs with oxygen may be necessary between tracheal intubations.

Choanal Stenosis and Atresia

Nasal obstruction should be suspected in any neonate who has good breathing efforts but in whom air entry is absent. Cyanosis develops if these infants are forced to breathe with their mouths closed. Diagnosis of unilateral or bilateral choanal stenosis is made by failure to pass a small catheter through each naris; such failure may reflect congenital (anatomic) obstruction or more commonly functional atresia due to blood, mucus, or meconium. The congenital form of choanal atresia must be treated surgically in the neonatal period. An oral airway may be necessary until surgical correction can be accomplished. Functional choanal atresia is treated by nasal suctioning. Opioids such as heroin often cause congestion of the nasal mucosa and obstruction. Such congestion can be treated with phenylephrine nose drops.

Diaphragmatic Hernia

Severe respiratory distress at birth, associated with cyanosis and a scaphoid abdomen, suggests the diagnosis of diaphragmatic hernia (see Chapter 32). A chest radiograph demonstrates abdominal contents in the thorax. Initial treatment in the delivery room includes intubation of the trachea and ventilation of the lungs with oxygen. A pneumothorax on the side opposite the hernia is likely, if attempts are made to expand the ipsilateral lung.

Hypovolemia

The newborn with a mean arterial pressure below 50 mmHg at birth is likely to be hypovolemic. Poor capillary refill, tachycardia, and tachypnea are present. Hypovolemia frequently follows intrauterine fetal distress, during which greater than normal portions of fetal blood are shunted to the placenta and remain there after delivery and clamping of the umbilical cord. Umbilical cord compression is also frequently associated with hypovolemia.

Hypoglycemia

Hypoglycemia can be manifested as hypotension, tremors, and seizures. Infants with intrauterine growth retardation and those born to diabetic mothers or after severe intrauterine fetal distress are vulnerable to hypoglycemia.

Tracheoesophageal Fistula

Tracheoesophageal fistula should be suspected when polyhydramnios is present (see Chapter 32). An initial diagnosis in the delivery room is suggested when a catheter inserted into the esophagus cannot be passed into the stomach. Copious amounts of oropharyngeal secretions are usually present. A chest radiograph with the catheter in place will confirm the diagnosis.

Laryngeal Anomalies

Stridor is present at birth as a manifestation of both laryngeal anomalies and subglottic stenosis. Insertion of a tube into the trachea beyond the obstruction alleviates the symptoms. Vascular rings are anomalies of the aorta, which may compress the trachea, producing both inspiratory and expiratory obstruction (see Chapter 3). It may be difficult to advance a tracheal tube beyond the obstruction produced by a vascular ring.

Pierre Robin Syndrome

Pierre Robin syndrome is characterized by glossoptosis and micrognathia in all patients and the presence of cleft palate in more than one-half of patients. Respiratory obstruction occurs when the tongue is sucked against the posterior pharyngeal wall by negative intrapharyngeal pressure. Initial treatment in the delivery room consists of the establishment of a patent airway, either by inserting an oral airway or by pulling the tongue forward with a clamp. The prone position also helps displace the tongue away from the posterior pharyngeal wall. A small tube passed through the naris into the posterior pharynx may be required to vent negative intraoral pressures. Under no circumstances should these infants be given muscle relaxants, as paralysis may make ventilation of the lungs impossible in the absence of a tracheal tube.

POSTPARTUM TUBAL LIGATION

Postpartum tubal ligation is the most common type of surgery performed during the early postpartum period.[117] The problem of the risk of aspiration and timing of surgery is resolved to a great extent if the surgery has been anticipated and continuous epidural anesthesia or spinal anesthesia is used for delivery. Residual anesthesia from delivery is used to perform the intra-abdominal procedure, which necessitates a T5 sensory level to ensure patient comfort. When epidural or spinal anesthesia has not been used for delivery, it is common practice to wait 8 to 12 hours postpartum before inducing anesthesia for tubal ligation. This time interval is useful to allow the parturient to reach cardiovascular stability and increase the likelihood of gastric emptying. Nevertheless, there is no demonstrable difference in gastric fluid volume and pH when parturients are studied 1 to 8 hours after vaginal delivery.[117]

If general anesthesia is selected for the patient undergoing a postpartum tubal ligation, many recommend administration of an antacid or H-2 antagonist before induction of anesthesia and subsequent placement of a cuffed tube in the trachea. Spinal anesthesia provides a rapid onset of surgical anesthesia compared with epidural anesthesia and is also technically easier to accomplish. The incidence and severity of hypotension and occurrence of nausea and vomiting are less after postpartum tubal ligation than after cesarean section, reflecting the decreased size of the uterus. Avoiding spinal anesthesia in preference for epidural anesthesia based on a concern that headache may follow the former is questionable, considering the low incidence of this side effect when a small-gauge needle is used to puncture the dura and the likely occurrence of a severe headache if the dura is accidentally punctured during the performance of an epidural anesthetic with a large bore needle.[117]

REFERENCES

1. Ueland K, Hansen JM. Maternal cardiovascular dynamics. III. Labor and delivery under local and caudal analgesia. Am J Obstet Gynecol 1969;103:8–18

2. Eckstein K-L, Marx GF. Aortocaval compression and uterine displacement. Anesthesiology 1974;40:92–6
3. Zilanti SM. Fetal heart rate and pH of fetal capillary blood during epidural analgesia in labor. Obstet Gynecol 1970;36:881–6
4. Fisher A, Prys-Roberts C. Maternal pulmonary gas exchange. A study during normal labor and extradural blockade. Anaesthesia 1968;23:350–6
5. Norris MC, Kirkland MR, Torjman MC, Goldberg ME. Denitrogenation in pregnancy. Can J Anaesth 1989;36:523–5
6. Palahniuk RJ, Shnider SM, Eger EI II. Pregnancy decreases the requirement of inhaled anesthetic agents. Anesthesiology 1974; 41:82–3
7. Datta S, Migliozzi RP, Flanagan HL, Krieger NR. Chronically administered progesterone decreases halothane requirements in rabbits. Anesth Analg 1989;68:46–50
8. Strout DD, Nahrwold ML. Halothane requirement during pregnancy and lactation in rats. Anesthesiology 1981;55:322–3
9. Bromage PR. Spread of analgesic solutions in the epidural space and their site of action: A statistical study. Br J Anaesth 1962; 34:161–78
10. Fagraeus L, Urban BJ, Bromage PR. Spread of epidural analgesia in early pregnancy. Anesthesiology 1983;58:184–7
11. Datta S, Hurley RJ, Naulty JS, et al. Plasma and cerebrospinal fluid progesterone concentrations in pregnant and nonpregnant women. Anesth Analg 1986;65:950–4
12. Grundy EM, Zamora AM, Winnie AP. Comparison of spread of epidural anesthesia in pregnant and nonpregnant women. Anesth Analg 1979;57:544–6
13. Whittaker M. Plasma cholinesterase variants and the anaesthetist. Anaesthesia 1980;35:174–97
14. Blitt CD, Petty WC, Alberternst EE, Wright BJ. Correlation of plasma cholinesterase and duration of action of succinylcholine during pregnancy. Anesth Analg 1977;56:78–81
15. Weissman DB, Ehrenwerth J. Prolonged neuromuscular blockade in a parturient associated with succinylcholine. Anesth Analg 1983;62:44–6
16. Kaplan MM. Acute fatty liver of pregnancy. N Engl J Med 1985; 313:367–70
17. Anatognini JF, Andrews S. Anaesthesia for Caesarean section in a patient with acute fatty liver of pregnancy. Can J Anaesth 1991;38:904–7
18. Brock-Utne JB, Dow TGB, Dimopoulos GE, et al. Gastric and lower oesophageal sphincter (LOS) pressures in early pregnancy. Br J Anaesth 1981;53:381–4
19. Taylor G, Pryse-Davies J. The prophylactic use of antacids in the prevention of the acid-pulmonary aspiration syndrome (Mendelson's syndrome). Lancet 1966;1:288–91
20. Roberts RB, Shirley MA. Reducing the risk of acid aspiration during cesarean section. Anesth Analg 1974;53:859–68
21. Scott DB. Mendelson's syndrome. (Editorial.) Br J Anaesth 1978;50:977–8
22. Hutchinson BR. Acid aspiration syndrome (correspondence). Br J Anaesth 1979;51:75
23. Viegas OJ, Ravindran RS, Shumacker CA. Gastric fluid pH in patients receiving sodium citrate. Anesth Analg 1981;60:521–3
24. O'Sullivan GM, Bullingham RE. Noninvasive assignment by radiotelemetry of antacid effect during labor. Anesth Analg 1985; 64:95–100
25. Howard FA, Sharp DS. Effect of metoclopramide on gastric emptying during labour. Br Med J 1973;1:446–8
26. Cohen SE, Jason J, Talafre M-L, et al. Does metoclopramide decrease the volume of gastric contents in patients undergoing cesarean section? Anesthesiology 1984;61:604–7
27. Macfie AG, Magides AD, Richmond MN, Reilly CS. Gastric emptying in pregnancy. Br J Anaesth 1991;67:54–7
28. Parer JT, Behrman RE. The influence of uterine blood flow on the acid base status of the rhesus monkey. Am J Obstet Gynecol 1970;107:1241–9
29. Ralston D, Shnider SM, deLorimier AA. Effects of equipotent ephedrine, metaraminol, mephentermine, and methoxamine on uterine blood flow on the pregnant ewe. Anesthesiology 1974; 40:354–70
30. Shnider SM, Wright RG, Levinson G, et al. Uterine blood flow and plasma norepinephrine changes during maternal stress in the pregnant ewe. Anesthesiology 1979;50:524–7
31. Levinson G, Shnider SM, deLormier AA, Stefenson JL. Effects of maternal hyperventilation on uterine blood flow and fetal oxygenation and acid-base status. Anesthesiology 1974;40:340–7
32. Cosmi EV, Marx GF. The effect of anesthesia on the acid-base status of the fetus. Anesthesiology 1969;30:238–42
33. Palahniuk RJ, Shnider SM. Maternal and fetal cardiovascular and acid-base changes during halothane and isoflurane anesthesia in the pregnant ewe. Anesthesiology 1974;41:462–72
34. Galloon S. Ketamine for obstetric delivery. Anesthesiology 1976;44:522–4
35. Wallis KL, Shnider SM, Hicks JS, Spivey HT. Epidural anesthesia in the normotensive pregnant ewe: Effects on uterine blood flow and fetal acid-base status. Anesthesiology 1976;44:481–7
36. Jouppila R, Jouppila P, Hollmen A, Juikka J. Effect of segmental extradural analgesia on placental blood flow during normal labour. Br J Anaesth 1978;50:563–7
37. Biehl D, Shnider SM, Levinson G, Callender K. Placental transfer of lidocaine. Effects of fetal acidosis. Anesthesiology 1978; 48:409–12
38. Way WL, Costley EC, Way EL. Respiratory sensitivity of the newborn infant to meperidine and morphine. Clin Pharmacol Ther 1965;6:454–61
39. Friedman EA. Primigravid labor. A graphicostatistical analysis. Obstet Gynecol 1955;6:567–89
40. Johnson WL, Winter WW, Eng M, et al. Effect of pudendal, spinal, and peridural block anesthesia on the second stage of labor. Am J Obstet Gynecol 1972;113:166–75
41. Vasicka A, Kretchmer H. Effect of conduction and inhalation anesthesia on uterine contractions. Am J Obstet Gynecol 1961; 82:600–11
42. Hoult IJ, MacLenna AH, Carrie LES. Lumbar epidural analgesia in labour: Relation to fetal malposition and instrumental delivery. Br Med J 1977;1:14–6
43. Coleman AJ, Downing JW. Enflurane anesthesia for cesarean section. Anesthesiology 1975;43:354–7
44. Paul RH, Freeman RK. Fetal cardiac response to paracervical block anesthesia. Am J Obstet Gynecol 1972;113:592–7
45. Celleno D, Capogna G. Epidural fentanyl plus bupivacaine 0.125 per cent for labour: Analgesic effects. Can J Anaesth 1988;35: 375–8
46. Phillips G. Continuous infusion epidural analgesia in labor: The

effect of adding sufentanil to 0.125% bupivacaine. Anesth Analg 1988;67:462–5

47. Cohen SE, Tan S, Albright GA, Halpern J. Epidural fentanyl/ bupivacaine mixtures for obstetric analgesia. Anesthesiology 1987;67:403–7

48. Sivakumarin C, Ramanthan S, Chalon J, Turndorf H. Uterine contractions and the spread of local anesthetics in the epidural space. Anesth Analg 1982;61:127–9

49. Kestin IG. Spinal anaesthesia in obstetrics. Br J Anaesth 1991; 66:596–607

50. Leighton BL, DeSimone CA, Norris MC, Ben-David B. Intrathecal narcotics for labor revisited: The combination of fentanyl and morphine intrathecally provides rapid onset of profound, prolonged analgesia. Anesth Analg 1989;69:122–5

51. Ong BY, Cohen MM, Esmail A, et al. Paresthesias and motor dysfunction after labor and delivery. Anesth Analg 1987;66: 18–22

52. Clark RB, Cooper JO, Brown WE, Greifenstein FE. The effect of methoxyflurane on the foetus. Br J Anaesth 1970;42:286–94

53. Creasser CW, Stoelting RK, Krishna G, Peterson C. Methoxyflurane metabolism and renal function after methoxyflurane analgesia during labor and delivery. Anesthesiology 1974;41:62–6

54. Clark RB, Beard AG, Thompson DS. Renal function in newborns and mothers exposed to methoxyflurane analgesia for labor and delivery. Anesthesiology 1979;51:464–7

55. Abbound TK, Shnider SM, Wright RG, et al. Enflurane analgesia in obstetrics. Anesth Analg 1981;60:133–7

56. Gellman E, Goldstein MS, Kaplan S, Shapiro WJ. Vaginal delivery after cesarean section. JAMA 1983;249:2935–7

57. Datta S, Alper MH. Anesthesia for cesarean section. Anesthesiology 1980;53:142–60

58. Hodgkinson R, Glassenberg R, Joyce TH, et al. Comparison of cimetidine (Tagamet) with antacid for safety and effectiveness in reducing gastric acidity before elective cesarean section. Anesthesiology 1983;59:86–90

59. Kosaka Y, Takahashi T, Mark LC. Intravenous thiobarbiturate anesthesia for cesarean section. Anesthesiology 1969;31: 489–506

60. Davies JM, Weeks S, Crone LA, Pavlin E. Difficult intubation in the parturient. Can J Anaesth 1989;36:668–74

61. Tunstall ME. Failed intubation in the parturient. Can J Anaesth 1989;36:611–3

62. Crawford JS. Awareness during operative obstetrics under general anaesthesia. Br J Anaesth 1971;43:179–82

63. Warren TM, Datta S, Ostheimer GW, et al. Comparison of the maternal and neonatal effects of halothane, enflurane, and isoflurane during cesarean delivery. Anesth Analg 1983;62:516–20

64. Baraka A, Haroun S, Bassili M. Response of the newborn to succinylcholine injection in homozygotic atypical mothers. Anesthesiology 1975;43:115–6

65. Crawford JS, James FM, Crawley M. A further study of general anaesthesia for cesarean section. Br J Anaesth 1976;48:661–7

66. Gutsche BB. Prophylactic ephedrine preceding spinal analgesia for cesarean section. Anesthesiology 1976;45:462–5

67. Abboud T, Raya J, Sadri S, et al. Fetal and maternal cardiovascular effects of atropine and glycopyrrolate. Anesth Analg 1983; 62:426–30

68. Norris MC. Height, weight, and the spread of subarachnoid

69. Reisner LS, Hochman BN, Plumer MH. Persistent neurologic deficit and adhesive arachnoiditis following intrathecal 2-chloroprocaine injection. Anesth Analg 1980;59:452–4

70. Ravindran RS, Bond VK, Tasch MD, et al. Prolonged neural blockade following regional analgesia with 2-chloroprocaine. Anesth Analg 1980;59:447–51

71. Kuhnert BR, Harrison MJ, Lin PL, Kuhmert PM. Effects of maternal epidural anesthesia on neonatal behavior. Anesth Analg 1984;63:301–8

72. Crosby HT, Halpren SH, Rolbin SH. Epidural anaesthesia for cesarean section in patients with active recurrent genital herpes simplex infections: A retrospective review. Can J Anaesth 1989; 36:701–4

73. Chadwick HS, Ready LB. Intrathecal and epidural morphine sulfate for postcesarean analgesia—a clinical comparison. Anesthesiology 1988;68:925–9

74. Abboud TK, Dror A, Mosaad P, et al. Mini-dose intrathecal morphine for the relief of post-cesarean section pain: Safety, efficacy, and ventilatory responses to carbon dioxide. Anesth Analg 1988;67:137–43

75. Ellis DJ, Millar WL, Reisner LS. A randomized double-blind comparison of epidural versus intravenous fentanyl infusion for analgesia after cesarean section. Anesthesiology 1990;72:981–6

76. Crawford JS. An appraisal of lumbar epidural blockade in patients with singleton fetus presenting by the breech. Br J Obstet Gynaecol 1974;81:867–72

77. Spinnato JA, Kraynack BJ, Cooper MW. Eisenmenger's syndrome in pregnancy: Epidural anesthesia for elective cesarean section. N Engl J Med 1981;304:1215–6

78. Pollack KL, Chestnut DH, Wenstrom KD. Anesthetic management of a parturient with Eisenmenger's syndrome. Anesth Analg 1990;70:212–5

79. Hilgenberg JC, McCammon RL, Stoelting RK. Pulmonary and systemic vascular responses to nitrous oxide in patients with mitral stenosis and pulmonary hypertension. Anesth Analg 1980;59:323–6

80. Robinson S. Pulmonary artery catheters in Eisenmenger's syndrome: Many risks, few benefits. Anesthesiology 1983;58: 588–9

81. Slomka F, Salmeron S, Zetlaoui P, Cohen H, Simonneau G, Samii K. Primary pulmonary hypertension and pregnancy: Anesthetic management for delivery. Anesthesiology 1988;69: 959–61

82. Breen TW, Tanzen JA. Pulmonary hypertension and cardiomyopathy: anaesthetic management for Caesarean section. Can J Anaesth 1991;38:895–9

83. Weeks SK, Smith JB. Obstetric anaesthesia in patients with primary pulmonary hypertension. Can J Anaesth 1991;38:814–6

84. Imperiale TF, Petrulis AS. A meta-analysis of low-dose aspirin for the prevention of pregnancy-induced hypertensive disease. JAMA 1991;266:260–5

85. Cunningham FG, Lindheimer MD. Hypertension in pregnancy. N Engl J Med 1992;326:927–32

86. Patterson KW, O'Toole DP. HELLP syndrome: a case report with guidelines for diagnosis and management. Br J Anaesth 1991;66:513–5

hyperbaric bupivacaine in the term parturient. Anesth Analg 1988;67:555–8

87. Wright JP. Anesthetic considerations in preeclampsia-eclampsia. Anesth Analg 1983;63:590–61

88. Ramanathan J, Sibai BM, Vu T, Chauhan D. Correlation between bleeding times and platelet counts in women with preeclampsia undergoing cesarean section. Anesthesiology 1989;71:188–91

89. Kambam JR, Mouton S, Entman S, Sastry VR, Smith BE. Effect of preeclampsia on plasma cholinesterase activity. Can J Anaesth 1987;34:509–11

90. Ravindran RS, Carrelli A. Neurologic dysfunction of postpartum patients caused by hypomagnesemia. Anesthesiology 1987;66:391–2

91. Rigg D, McDonagh A. Use of sodium nitroprusside for deliberate hypotension during pregnancy. Br J Anaesth 1981;53:985–7

92. Heller PJ, Goodman C. Use of local anesthetics with epinephrine for epidural anesthesia in preeclampsia. Anesthesiology 1986;65:224–6

93. Snyder SW, Wheeler AS, James FM. The use of nitroglycerin to control severe hypertension of pregnancy during cesarean section. Anesthesiology 1979;51:563–4

94. Datta S, Brown WU, Ostheimer GW, et al. Epidural anesthesia for cesarean section in diabetic parturients: Maternal and neonatal acid-base status and bupivacaine concentration. Anesth Analg 1981;60:574–8

95. Datta S, Brown WU. Acid-base status in diabetic mothers and their infants following general or spinal anesthesia for cesarean section. Anesthesiology 1977;47:272–6

96. Rolbin SH, Levinson G, Shnider SM, Wright RG. Anesthetic considerations for myasthenia gravis and pregnancy. Anesth Analg 1978;57:441–7

97. Gatt SP. Anaesthetic management of the obstetric patient with antepartum or intrapartum haemorrhage. In: Ostheimer GW, ed. Clinics in Anaesthesiology. London. WB Saunders 1986;4:373–88

98. Carlsson C, Nybell-Lincahl G, Ingemarsson I. Extradural block in patients who had previously undergone cesarean section. Br J Anaesth 1980;52:827–30

99. Smith CE, Weeks SK. Anesthesia for cesarean section in a patient with Asherman's syndrome. Anesthesiology 1988;68:615–8

100. Sperry K. Amniotic fluid embolism. To understand enigma. JAMA 1986;255:2183–6

101. Schaerf RHM, deCampo T, Civetta JA. Hemodynamic alterations and rapid diagnosis in a case of amniotic fluid embolus. Anesthesiology 1977;46:155–7

102. Brodsky JB, Cohen EN, Brown BW, et al. Surgery during pregnancy and fetal outcome. Am J Obstet Gynecol 1980;138:1165–7

103. Pedersen H, Finster M. Anesthetic risk in the pregnant surgical patient. Anesthesiology 1979;51:439–51

104. Davis AG, Moir DD. Anaesthesia during pregnancy. In: Ostheimer GW, ed. Clinics in Anaesthesiology. London. WB Saunders 1986;4:233–46

105. Duncan PG, Pope WDB, Cohen MM, Greer N. Fetal risk of anesthesia and surgery during pregnancy. Anesthesiology 1986;64:790–4

106. Smith RF, Bowman RE, Katz J. Behavioral effects of exposure to halothane during early development in the rat. Sensitive period during pregnancy. Anesthesiology 1978;49:319–23

107. Committee on Drugs of the American Academy of Pediatrics and the Committee on Obstetrics (Maternal and Fetal Medicine) of the American College of Obstetricians and Gynecologists. Effect of medication during labor and delivery on infant outcome. Pediatrics 1978;62:402–3

108. Ravindran R, Viegas OJ, Padilla LM, LaBlonde P. Anesthetic considerations in pregnant patients receiving terbutaline therapy. Anesth Analg 1980;59:391–2

109. Moravec MA, Hurlbert BJ. Hypokalemia associated with terbutaline administration in obstetrical patients. Anesth Analg 1980;59:917–20

110. Finster M, Petrie RH. Monitoring of the fetus. Anesthesiology 1976;45:198–215

111. Sachs BP, Friedman EA. Antepartum and intrapartum assessment of the fetus: Current status and does it influence outcome? In: Ostheimer GW, ed. Clinics in Anaesthesiology. London. WB Saunders 1986;4:53–66

112. Paul RH, Suidan AK, Yeh SY, et al. Clinical fetal monitoring. VII. The evaluation and significance of intrapartum baseline FHR variability. Am J Obstet Gynecol 1975;123:206–10

113. Gluck L, Kulovich MV, Barer RC, et al. The diagnosis of the respiratory distress syndrome (RDS) by amniocentesis. Am J Obstet Gynecol 1971;109:440–5

114. Scanlon JW, Brown WU, Weiss JB, Alper MH. Neurobehavioral responses of newborn infants after maternal epidural anesthesia. Anesthesiology 1974;40:121–8

115. Corke BC. Neonatal neurobehavior. II. Current clinical status. In: Ostheimer GW, ed. Clinics in Anaesthesiology. London. WB Saunders 1986;4:219–27

116. Amiel-Tison C, Barrier G, Shnider SM, et al. A new neurologic and adaptive capacity scoring system for evaluating obstetric medications in full-term newborns. Anesthesiology 1982;56:340–50

117. Abouleish E. Anaesthesia for postpartum surgery. Clin Anaesthesiol 1986;4:419–28

32

Diseases Common to the Pediatric Patient

The pediatric patient presents unique anatomic, physiologic, and pharmacologic considerations for the management of anesthesia in the presence of diseases that occur exclusively or with increased frequency in this age group. It is important to recognize that neonates (up to 28 days of age) and infants are the age groups in which differences from adult patients are most marked. Neonates are also more likely to experience an adverse perioperative cardiopulmonary event.[1]

ANATOMY OF THE AIRWAY

The large head and tongue, mobile epiglottis, and anterior position of the larynx characteristic of the neonate makes intubation of the trachea easier with the head in a neutral or slightly flexed position than with the head hyperextended (Fig. 32-1). Since the infant's larynx is higher in the neck than in the adult, the infant's tongue obstructs the airway more easily. The cricoid cartilage is the narrowest portion of the larynx in a pediatric patient and necessitates selection of a tracheal tube that minimizes the risk of trauma to the airway and the subsequent development of subglottic edema. For example, a 3.0-mm internal diameter tracheal tube is recommended for a term neonate. As in adults, angulation of the right main stem bronchus favors a right endobronchial intubation if the tracheal tube is inserted beyond the carina. To prevent endobronchial intubation of the neonate's trachea, a convenient guideline for depth of insertion from the lips is a distance of 7 cm for a 1-kg neonate and an additional 1 cm of depth for each kilogram increase in body weight, to a maximum depth of 10 cm for a term neonate. Ultimately, tracheal tube diameter and depth of insertion to result in a midtrachea position of the distal end of the tube are based on age (Table 32-1).

PHYSIOLOGY

Physiologic differences between the pediatric and adult patient are important determinants in the development of working concepts, when administering anesthesia to children.

Respiratory System

Respiratory immaturity of the preterm neonate is well known. In this regard, the production and secretion of surfactant are of paramount importance in normal lung function. Surfactant is a complex of surface-active phospholipids produced exclusively by type II pneumocytes. Although type II pneumocytes begin to differentiate at 24 weeks gestation, a marked synthesis of surfactant does not begin until 34 to 36 weeks gestation.

The single most important difference that physiologically distinguishes the pediatric patient from the adult patient is oxygen consumption. Oxygen consumption of the neonate is greater than $6 \ ml \cdot kg^{-1} \cdot min^{-1}$, which is about twice that of an adult on a weight basis (Table 32-2). To satisfy this increased demand, alveolar ventilation is doubled compared with that in an adult. Carbon dioxide production is also increased in the neonate, but the increased alveolar ventilation results in maintenance of a near-normal $PaCO_2$. Since the tidal volume on a weight basis is similar for the infant and adult, the increased alveolar ventilation is accomplished by an increased breathing rate. The PaO_2 increases rapidly after birth, but several days are needed to achieve levels present in older children. Initially, the low PaO_2 is secondary to a decreased functional residual capacity and perfusion of fluid filled alveoli. Functional residual capacity reaches adult levels (about $30 \ ml \cdot kg^{-1}$) by about 4 days of age (Table 32-2). The control of ventilation is immature in the neonate, as reflected by decreased ventilatory responses to hypoxemia and hypercarbia. Conceivably, the

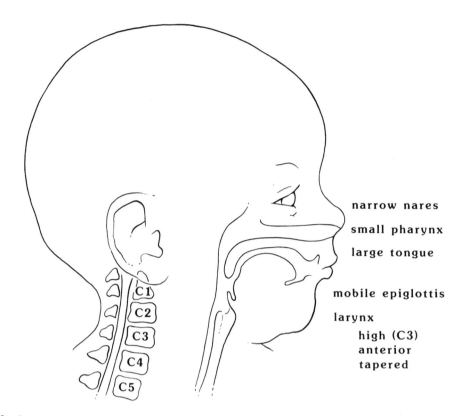

narrow nares

small pharynx

large tongue

mobile epiglottis

larynx
 high (C3)
 anterior
 tapered

Fig. 32-1. Schematic depiction of the anatomic characteristics of the neonate, which may influence the ease of intubation of the trachea during direct laryngoscopy.

Table 32-1. Endotracheal Tube Size

Weight or Age	Internal Diameter[a] (mm)	Distance of Tube Insertion for Midtracheal Position (cm)
1 kg	2.5 uncuffed	7
1.5 kg	3.0 uncuffed	7.5
2 kg	3.0 uncuffed	8
3 kg (preterm)	3.0 uncuffed	9
3 kg (term)	3.0 uncuffed	10
6–12 mo	3.5 uncuffed	11
12–18 mo	3.5 uncuffed	12
18–36 mo	4.0 uncuffed	13
3–5 y	4.5 uncuffed	14
5–6 y	5.0 cuffed	15
6–8 y	5.5 cuffed	16
8–10 y	6.0 cuffed	18
10–12 y	6.5 cuffed	18

[a] Endotracheal tube size for an uncuffed tube should result in an audible air leak when positive airway pressure equivalent to 25 cm H_2O is applied.

Table 32-2. Mean Pulmonary Function Values

	Neonate (3 kg)	Adult (70 kg)
Oxygen consumption (ml·kg^{-1}·min^{-1})	6.4	3.5
Alveolar ventilation (ml·kg^{-1}·min^{-1})	130	60
Carbon dioxide production (ml·kg^{-1}·min^{-1})	6	3
Tidal volume (ml·kg^{-1})	6	6
Breathing frequency (min)	35	15
Vital capacity (ml·kg^{-1})	35	70
Functional residual capacity (ml·kg^{-1})	30	35
Tracheal length (cm)	5.5	12
PaO$_2$ (F$_I$O$_2$ 0.21, mmHg)	65–85	85–95
PaCO$_2$ (mmHg)	30–36	36–44
pH	7.34–7.40	7.36–7.44

combination of ventilatory depression from residual anesthetic plus immature control of ventilation could result in neonatal hypoventilation during the postoperative period.

Cardiovascular System

Birth and the beginning of spontaneous ventilation initiate circulatory changes, permitting the neonate to survive in an extrauterine environment.[2] Fetal circulation is characterized by high pulmonary vascular resistance, low systemic vascular resistance (placenta), and right-to-left shunting of blood through the foramen ovale and ductus arteriosus. Onset of spontaneous ventilation at birth is associated with decreased pulmonary vascular resistance and increased pulmonary blood flow. As left atrial pressure increases, the foramen ovale functionally closes. Anatomic closure of the foramen ovale occurs between 3 months and 1 year of age, although 20% to 30% of adults have a probe patent foramen ovale.[3] Functional closure of the ductus arteriosus normally occurs 10 to 15 hours after birth, with anatomic closure taking place in 4 to 6 weeks. Constriction of the ductus arteriosus occurs in response to the increased PaO_2 that develops after birth. Nevertheless, the ductus arteriosus may reopen during periods of arterial hypoxemia. In addition, certain conditions, such as diaphragmatic hernia, meconium aspiration, pulmonary infection, and polycythemia are associated with high pulmonary vascular resistance and persistence of fetal circulatory patterns.[3] Presumably, high pulmonary vascular resistance results in shunting of desaturated pulmonary arterial blood into the systemic circulation through the ductus arteriosus. The diagnosis of persistent fetal circulation can be confirmed by measurement of the PaO_2 in blood obtained simultaneously from preductal (right radial) and postductal (umbilical, posterior tibial, dorsalis pedis) arteries (Fig. 32-2). A difference of greater than 20 mmHg verifies the diagnosis.

Blood pressure in the neonate varies with gestational age and weight (Table 32-3). In this regard, the neonate is highly dependent on heart rate for maintenance of cardiac output and blood pressure. The vasoconstrictive response of the neonate to hemorrhage is less than that of an adult. For example, a 10% decrease in intravascular fluid volume is likely to cause a 15% to 30% decrease in mean arterial pressure in the neonate. Hypotension that accompanies administration of a volatile anesthetic to a premature neonate is most likely due to decreased intravascular fluid volume or anesthetic overdose, or both.

Distribution of Body Water

Total body water content and extracellular fluid (ECF) volume are increased proportionately in the neonate. The ECF volume is equivalent to about 40% of the body weight of a neonate compared with about 20% in an adult. By 18 to 24 months of age, the proportion of ECF volume relative to body weight is similar to the adult.

The increased metabolic rate characteristic of the neonate results in an accelerated turnover of ECF and dictates meticulous attention to intraoperative fluid replacement. Intraoperative fluid replacement may be considered as maintenance fluid and replacement fluid (Table 32-4). The recommended fluid often contains glucose, although the clinical impression that the pediatric patient is more susceptible than an adult to hypoglycemia during fasting has been challenged.[4,5] Maintenance fluid is best correlated with metabolic rate; replacement fluid requirements should be based on the underlying pathologic process, extent of surgery, and anticipated fluid translocation. Third space translocation of fluid is similar for a neonate and adult. Maintenance fluid requirements for the first 24 hours of life are approximately 75 to 80 ml·kg^{-1}. The preterm neonate has a higher fluid requirement in the first 24 hours equivalent to 100 ml·kg^{-1}. Insensible fluid loss varies greatly. Fever, radiant warmers, increased ambient temperature, and decreased humidity all increase insensible fluid loss. A small

Table 32-3. Mean Circulatory Values for the Neonate

	Weight (kg)				
	0.75	1	2	3	>3
Systolic blood pressure (mmHg)	44	49	54	62	66
Mean arterial pressure (mmHg)	33	34	41	46	50
Heart rate (beats·min^{-1})	—	—	—	120	—
Cardiac index (L·min^{-1}·m^{-2})	—	—	—	4.1	—

Table 32-4. Intraoperative Fluid Therapy for the Pediatric Patient

Surgical Procedure	5% Glucose in Lactated Ringer's Solution[a] (ml·kg^{-1}·h^{-1})		
	Maintenance	Replacement	Total
Minor surgery (herniorrhaphy)	4	2	6
Moderate surgery (pyloromyotomy)	4	4	8
Extensive surgery (bowel resection)	4	6	10

[a] The concentration of glucose in the replacement fluids may be influenced by the duration of surgery. Measurement of the plasma glucose concentration may be useful during prolonged surgical procedures.

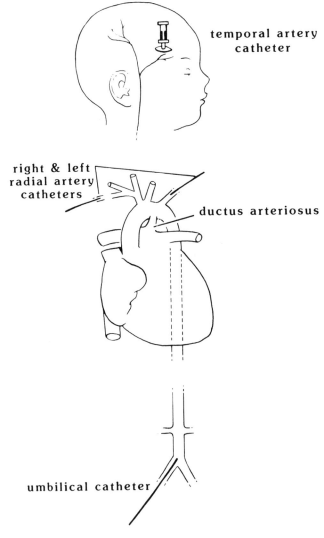

Fig. 32-2. Schematic depiction of sites for sampling of arterial blood relative to the ductus arteriosus.

neonate requires more radiant energy to maintain a neutral thermal environment; as a result, there is greater insensible fluid loss in these patients.

Renal Function

The glomerular filtration rate is greatly decreased in the term neonate but is increased nearly fourfold by 3 to 5 weeks of age (Table 32-5). A preterm neonate may show a delayed increase in the glomerular filtration rate. The neonate is an obligate sodium loser and cannot concentrate urine as effec-

Table 32-5.   Renal Function in the Pediatric Patient

Age	Glomerular Filtration Rate ($ml \cdot min^{-1} \cdot 1.7\ m^{-2}$)
Preterm neonate	16
Term neonate	20
3–5 weeks	60
1 year	80
Adult	120

tively as an adult. Therefore, adequate exogenous sodium and water must be supplied during the perioperative period. Conversely, it must be appreciated that the neonate is likely to excrete a volume load more slowly than an adult and is therefore more susceptible to fluid overload. Decreased renal function can also delay the excretion of drugs dependent on renal clearance for elimination.

Hematology

The characteristics of fetal hemoglobin (HbF) influence oxygen transport. For example, HbF has a P_{50} of 19 mmHg, as compared with 26 mmHg for adult hemoglobin (HbA). The decreased P_{50} for HbF causes a shift of the oxyhemoglobin dissociation curve to the left. The resulting increased affinity of hemoglobin for oxygen is manifested as decreased oxygen release to the peripheral tissues. This decreased release of oxygen to the tissues is offset by the increased oxygen delivery provided by the increased hemoglobin concentration characteristic of a neonate (Table 32-6). By 2 to 3 months of age, however, physiologic anemia results. After 3 months, there is a progressive increase in erythrocyte mass and hematocrit. By 4 to 6 months, the oxyhemoglobin dissociation curve approximates that of an adult. In view of the decreased cardiovascular reserve of the neonate and the leftward shift of the oxyhemoglobin dissociation curve, it may be useful to maintain the neonate's hematocrit close to 40%, rather than the 30% often accepted for older children. Calculation of the estimated erythrocyte mass and of the acceptable erythrocyte loss provides a useful guide for intraoperative blood replacement[6] (Table 32-7). The decision to administer a blood transfusion must be individualized on the basis of the patient's ability to compensate for anemia and the risks of transfusion, recognizing that desirable hemoglobin levels for young patients have not been established.[7]

The need for routine preoperative hemoglobin determination is controversial. There is evidence that routine preoperative hemoglobin determination in patients older than 1 year of age detects only a small number with a hemoglobin concentra-

Table 32-6. Normal Hemogram Values

Age	Hemoglobin (g·dl^{-1})	Hematocrit (%)	Leukocytes (cells·mm^{-3})
1 day	19.0	61	18,000
2 wk	17.3	54	12,000
1 mo	14.2	43	—
2 mo	10.7	31	—
6 mo	12.3	36	10,000
1 y	11.6	35	—
6 y	12.7	38	—
10–12 y	13.0	39	8,000

Table 32-7. Estimation of Acceptable Blood Loss[a]

A 3.2-kg term neonate is scheduled for intra-abdominal surgery. The preoperative hematocrit is 50%. What is the acceptable intraoperative blood loss to maintain the hematocrit at 40%?

Calculations

Estimated blood volume	85 ml·kg^{-1} × 3.2 kg	= 272 ml
Estimated erythrocyte mass	272 ml × 0.5	= 136 ml
Estimated erythrocyte mass to maintain hematocrit at 40%	272 ml × 0.4	= 109 ml
Acceptable intraoperative erythrocyte loss	136 ml − 109 ml	= 27 ml
Acceptable intraoperative blood loss to maintain hematocrit at 40%	27 × 2[b]	= 54 ml

[a] These calculations are only a guideline and do not consider the potential impact of intravenous infusion of crystalloid or colloid solutions on the hematocrit.

[b] Factor to correct the original hematocrit to 50%.

tion of 10 g·dl^{-1} or less.[7] Furthermore, when a low hemoglobin concentration is found, it rarely alters the management of anesthesia or delays the planned surgery. Because of the potential benefit of identifying anemia in infancy, preoperative hemoglobin testing may be justifiable in this age group alone.[8]

Coagulation tests, with the exception of bleeding time, are often abnormal in the neonate. The concentration of vitamin K-dependent factors (II, VII, IX, X) is decreased, leading to a prolonged prothrombin time. The partial thromboplastin time is also prolonged. Fibrinogen and factor V concentrations are similar to levels present in the adult. Despite these laboratory abnormalities, the blood of a term neonate coagulates normally or at an increased rate, presumably because of a deficiency in the amounts of naturally occurring anticoagulants. The acutely ill neonate, however, may have a bleeding diathesis, because of thrombocytopenia or vitamin K factor deficiency.

Thermoregulation

The neonate and infant are vulnerable to hypothermia during the perioperative period. In this age group, body heat is lost more rapidly than in the older child or adult, because of the large body surface area relative to body weight, the thin layer of insulating subcutaneous fat, and a decreased ability to produce heat. Shivering is of little significance in heat production in a neonate, whose primary mechanism is nonshivering thermogenesis mediated by brown fat. Brown fat is a specialized adipose tissue located in the posterior neck and in the interscapular and vertebral areas and surrounding the kidneys

Table 32-8. Neutral and Critical Temperatures

Patient Age	Neutral Temperature (°C)	Critical Temperature (°C)
Preterm neonate	34	28
Term neonate	32	23
Adult	28	1

and adrenal glands. Metabolism in brown fat is stimulated by norepinephrine and results in triglyceride hydrolysis and thermogenesis.

An important mechanism for loss of body heat in the operating room is radiation. To minimize oxygen consumption, the neonate must be in a neutral thermal environment. Neutral temperature is defined as the ambient temperature that results in the least oxygen consumption (Table 32-8). The critical temperature is that ambient temperature below which an unclothed, unanesthetized person cannot maintain a normal core body temperature (Table 32-8). Most operating rooms are below the critical temperature of even a term neonate, and it is imperative that heat loss be minimized. Steps designed to decrease loss of body heat include transporting the neonate in a heated module, increasing the ambient temperature of the operating room, humidifying and warming inspired gases,

using a warm solution to cleanse the skin, warming infused blood and intravenous solutions, and using a heating mattress and radiant warmer. The use of plastic drapes during the transport of a neonate and during surgery will also significantly reduce heat loss.

PHARMACOLOGY

Pharmacologic responses produced by drugs may differ in the pediatric patient compared with the adult patient. Specifically, there may be differences in anesthetic requirements, responses to muscle relaxants, and altered pharmacokinetics of drugs.

Anesthetic Requirements

Fetal animals demonstrate decreased anesthetic requirements. Human full-term neonates require lower concentrations of volatile anesthetics than do infants 1 to 6 months of age. For example, MAC has been shown to be about 25% less in neonates as compared with infants.[9] Furthermore, MAC in preterm neonates less than 32 weeks gestational age is less than MAC in preterm neonates 32 to 37 weeks gestational age, and both of these age groups are less than MAC in full-term neonates[10] (Fig. 32-3). The low anesthetic requirements

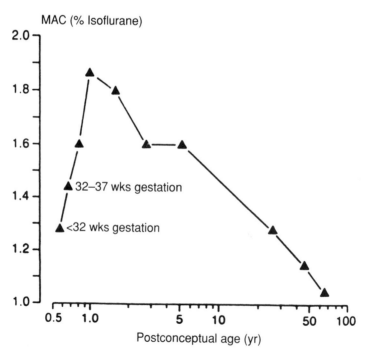

Fig. 32-3. Anesthetic requirements (MAC) of isoflurane and postconceptual age. (From LeDez KM, Lerman J. The minimum alveolar concentration (MAC) of isoflurane in preterm neonates. Anesthesiology 1987;67:301–7, with permission.)

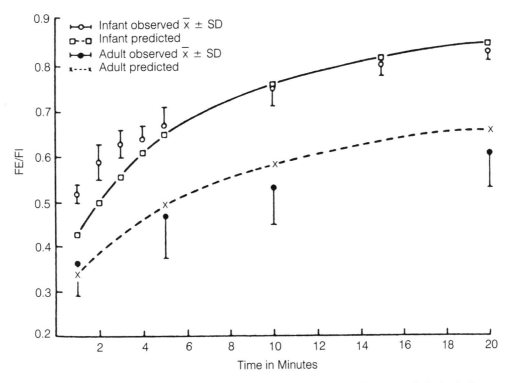

Fig. 32-4. Predicted and observed rates at which the end-tidal halothane concentrations approach the inspired concentration (FE/FI) are more rapid in infants than in adults. (From Brandom DW, Brandom RB, Cook DR. Uptake and distribution of halothane in infants: In vivo measurements and computer simulations. Anesth Analg 1983;62:404–10, with permission.)

of newborns may be related to the immaturity of the central nervous system and to elevated levels of progesterone and beta endorphins.[9] MAC steadily increases until 2 to 3 months of age. After 3 months of age, MAC steadily declines with aging, although there are slight increases at puberty.

Uptake of inhaled anesthetics is more rapid in infants than in older children or adults[11–13] (Fig. 32-4). The infant has a high alveolar ventilation relative to functional residual capacity, which may explain this accelerated uptake. Volatile anesthetics are potent negative inotropes when administered to neonates. Indeed, the neonate and infant are more likely to develop hypotension during administration of a volatile anesthetic.[14,15] Considering these factors, a reduced margin of safety when a volatile anesthetic is administered to an infant is predictable.

An immature blood-brain barrier and decreased ability to metabolize drugs could increase the sensitivity of the neonate to the effects of barbiturates and opioids. As a result, the neonate might require a lower dose of barbiturate for induction of anesthesia.[16] Nevertheless, children between the ages of 5 and 15 years require somewhat higher doses of thiopental

and methohexital than do adults, for induction of anesthesia[17] (Fig. 32-5).

Opioids are often administered to selected pediatric patients for anesthesia. Fentanyl (50 to 75 $\mu g \cdot kg^{-1}$ IV) and sufentanil (5 to 10 $\mu g \cdot kg^{-1}$ IV) produce minimal hemodynamic changes even in a preterm infant.[18] The efficacy of fentanyl and sufentanil is particularly apparent for the infant undergoing cardiac surgery, despite substantial respiratory depression and the possible need for postoperative ventilatory support.

Muscle Relaxants

Morphologic and functional maturation of the neuromuscular junction is not complete until about 2 months of age.[19] The implications of this maturity on the pharmacodynamics of muscle relaxants are not clear. With respect to nondepolarizing muscle relaxants, the data suggest that infants are more sensitive to the effects of these drugs.[20–22] Because of the relatively large volume of distribution, however, the initial dose of a nondepolarizing muscle relaxant, calculated on the basis of the infant's body weight, is not different from that of an adult. Immaturity of hepatic or renal function could prolong

Table 32-9.   Age and Response to Succinylcholine

Age	Mean Depression of Twitch Response (%) After Intravenous Succinylcholine		Time to 90% Twitch Recovery (min)	
	0.5 mg·kg^{-1}	1 mg·kg^{-1}	0.5 mg·kg^{-1}	1 mg·kg^{-1}
1–10 wk	69	85	2.3	4.0
5–7 y	84	100	3.0	4.8

(Data from Cook DR, Fischer CG. Neuromuscular blocking effects of succinylcholine in infants and children. Anesthesiology 1975;42:662–5.)

the duration of action of muscle relaxants that are highly dependent on these mechanisms for their clearance. Age affects recovery from atracurium less than recovery from vecuronium.[23] Antagonism of neuromuscular blockade seems to be reliable and in the infant may be associated with decreased dose requirements for the anticholinesterase drug.[24]

The neonate and infant require more succinylcholine on a body weight basis than do older children, to produce neuromuscular blockade[25] (Table 32-9). This reflects the increased ECF volume characteristic of this age group. Consequently, there is a greater volume of distribution of succinylcholine. As a result, a pediatric patient requires about 2 mg·kg^{-1} IV of succinylcholine to provide conditions for tracheal intubation that are similar to those produced with 1 mg·kg^{-1} IV administered to an adult. Intramuscular administration of succinylcholine may be required when the intravenous route is not available. Intramuscular administration of succinylcholine (4 mg·kg^{-1}) produces satisfactory conditions for intubation of the trachea in most children within 3 to 4 minutes.[26] Pretreatment with atropine administered intravenously will significantly attenuate succinylcholine-induced heart rate slowing in children.[27] Succinylcholine produces only a small change in intragastric pressure in children.[28] Therefore, pretreatment with a nondepolarizing muscle relaxant to prevent initial contraction of abdominal muscles (fasciculations) in response to succinylcholine is not necessary as prophylaxis against regurgitation. The incidence of myoglobinuria in children receiving succinylcholine is increased.

The administration of succinylcholine to pediatric patients may be limited by the undesirable side effects of this drug. Despite the introduction of new nondepolarizing muscle relaxants such as mivacurium, no available alternative drug produces the rapidity of onset of profound skeletal muscle relaxation that is characteristic of succinylcholine.[29]

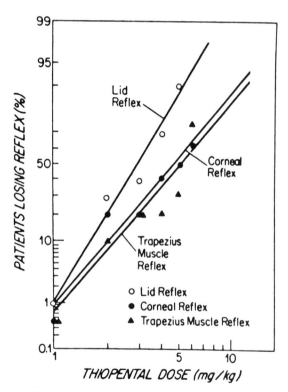

Fig. 32-5. Dose-response curves for loss of various reflex responses 60 seconds after intravenous administration of thiopental to unpremedicated patients 5 to 15 years of age. (From Cote CJ, Gondsouzian NG, Liu LMP, et al. The dose response of intravenous thiopental for the induction of general anesthesia in unpremedicated children. Anesthesiology 1981;55:703–5, with permission.)

PHARMACOKINETICS

Pharmacokinetics differ in neonates and infants as compared with adults. Diminished hepatic and renal clearance of drugs, which is characteristic of the neonate, can produce prolonged drug effects. For many drugs, including theophylline, phenytoin, and diazepam, clearance during the neonatal period is decreased. Clearance rates increase to adult levels by 5 to 6 months of age and during later childhood may even exceed adult rates. Protein binding of many drugs is decreased in the infant, which can result in a higher plasma level of unbound and active drug, leading to increased pharmacologic effects.

MONITORING DURING THE PERIOPERATIVE PERIOD

As in the adult, monitoring of the pediatric patient is directed toward early detection of deviations from accepted norms. Since the neonate and infant have decreased physiologic reserves, early detection of adverse effects of anesthesia and surgery assumes a major role. On the other hand, the use of monitoring devices and techniques must reflect an appreciation of the risk-to-benefit ratio for each monitor. The amount and type of monitoring used depend on the physiologic status of the patient and on the extent of the surgical procedure. Monitoring of neonates and infants during the perioperative period includes continuous display of the electrocardiogram, measurement of blood pressure, measurement of body temperature, the use of a precordial or esophageal stethoscope, and monitoring of systemic oxygenation with a pulse oximeter.

The advantage of a continuous display of the electrocardiogram is the rapid identification of cardiac dysrhythmias. Indeed, changes on the electrocardiogram occurring in a pediatric patient are usually related to cardiac rhythm rather than to myocardial ischemia. As a result, lead II, and not a precordial lead, is the most useful lead to monitor.

Decreased cardiovascular reserve, altered anesthetic requirements, and an exaggerated hypotensive response during general anesthesia make monitoring of the blood pressure of neonates and infants mandatory. A noninvasive blood pressure monitor is dependent on the use of an inflatable cuff, which must be the appropriate size for the arm of the patient. A cuff that is too small will produce an artificially elevated blood pressure; one that is too large will produce a false low reading. The Doppler transducer is an accurate method of noninvasive blood pressure monitoring and has the additional advantage of continuous monitoring of arterial blood flow. Consequently, it serves as a monitor of cardiac rhythm and, to a limited extent, can reflect cardiac output during dysrhythmias. The oscillometric method of noninvasive blood pressure monitoring, as represented by the Dinamapp, is also reliable for the pediatric patient. A catheter placed in a peripheral artery may be the method selected to monitor blood pressure and for obtaining blood samples for analysis of blood gases. The peripheral artery selected for percutaneous placement of the catheter is uniquely important in the neonate. For example, blood sampled from an artery that arises distal to the ductus arteriosus (left radial artery, umbilical artery, posterior tibial artery) may not accurately reflect the PaO_2 being delivered to the retina or brain in the presence of a patent ductus arteriosus (Fig. 32-2). If retinopathy of the newborn is a consideration, a preductal artery, such as the right radial artery, should be cannulated. The temporal artery is also a potential preductal site. This artery, however, has the disadvantage of a risk of embolization of cerebral vasculature by the retrograde flushing of microemboli.

Monitoring of body temperature is used during the perioperative period for the detection of hypothermia and to facilitate recognition of malignant hyperthermia. Hypothermia, as is likely to occur in a neonate or infant during anesthesia, results in increased total body oxygen consumption, depression of ventilation, bradycardia, metabolic acidosis, and hypoglycemia. Sites available for monitoring body temperature include the nasopharynx, esophagus, and rectum. Care must be taken to avoid rectal perforation, if a rectal probe is placed. On a routine basis, the use of a nasopharyngeal or esophageal temperature probe is recommended for a patient who has a tracheal tube in place.

Monitoring the $P_{ET}CO_2$ is reliable in children, although there are some limitations in the neonate and infant. For example, because of the small tidal volume and high inspired gas flow, the exhaled carbon dioxide concentration may be diluted. This dilution would produce a false low $P_{ET}CO_2$. A large gas leak around the tracheal tube will also produce a low $P_{ET}CO_2$.

NEONATAL MEDICAL DISEASES

Significant technologic and medical advances have resulted in improved survival of low-birthweight preterm neonates. Perioperative care of the preterm and term neonate requires a thorough knowledge of the diseases common or unique to this age group (Table 32-10).

Respiratory Distress Syndrome

Respiratory distress syndrome (RDS), or hyaline membrane disease, is responsible for 50% to 75% of deaths that occur in preterm neonates. This syndrome is caused by a deficiency in the alveoli of surface-active phospholipids known as surfactant. The function of surfactant is to maintain alveolar stability. Without surfactant, alveoli collapse, leading to right-to-left intrapulmonary shunting, arterial hypoxemia, and metabolic acidosis. Surfactant is produced by type II pneumocytes. Before 26 weeks gestation, however, there are not enough

Table 32-10.   Neonatal Medical Diseases

Respiratory distress syndrome
Bronchopulmonary dysplasia
Intracranial hemorrhage
Retinopathy of prematurity
Apnea spells
Kernicterus
Hypoglycemia
Sepsis

type II pneumocytes to produce adequate amounts of surfactant. By 35 weeks, there are large numbers of type II cells capable of sufficient surfactant synthesis. Until adequate surfactant can be produced, arterial oxygenation must be maintained using supplemental oxygen, with or without mechanical ventilation of the lungs. Under certain circumstances, antenatal steroids administered to the mother may accelerate maturation of the lungs and prevent the development of RDS in preterm infants. Limited but promising success has been achieved with tracheal administration of human surfactant to preterm infants. The administration of inositol to premature infants with RDS may also improve survival.

During anesthesia in the presence of RDS, the PaO$_2$ should be maintained at its preoperative level. In this regard, volatile anesthetics can alter arterial oxygenation by decreasing cardiac output. Ideally, the PaO$_2$ is monitored from blood obtained from a catheter placed in a preductal artery (Fig. 32-2). For a brief procedure, or when arterial cannulation is not feasible, monitoring of oxygenation using a pulse oximeter is satisfactory. The degree of pulmonary dysfunction in a neonate with RDS is highly variable. The least afflicted neonate may require only supplemental oxygen for a short period of time. A severely afflicted neonate can require mechanical ventilation of the lungs with high inspired oxygen concentrations and positive end-expiratory pressure. Pneumothorax is an ever-present danger and should be considered if oxygenation deteriorates abruptly in a neonate being treated for RDS. An alternative to mechanical ventilation of the lungs of these neonates is high-frequency ventilation.[30] Hypotension is a frequently encountered problem during anesthesia. Administration of albumin (1 g·kg^{-1} IV) to a preterm neonate with RDS is likely to increase the blood volume and glomerular filtration rate. The hematocrit of the neonate is often maintained near 40% to optimize oxygen delivery to the tissues. Fluid administration must be monitored because excess hydration may reopen the ductus arteriosus.

Bronchopulmonary Dysplasia

Bronchopulmonary dysplasia is a chronic pulmonary disorder; it usually afflicts children with a previous history of RDS.[31] Although the precise mechanism is unknown, certain risk factors have been identified. For example, an increased inspired oxygen concentration and positive-pressure ventilation of the lungs, as used for the treatment of RDS, may be etiologic factors. Indeed, 11% to 21% of neonates with RDS requiring supplemental oxygen for more than 24 hours show the development of bronchopulmonary dysplasia.[31] Clinically, infants with bronchopulmonary dysplasia are those with RDS who enter a chronic phase. The more severe the RDS, the greater the degree of bronchopulmonary dysplasia.

Bronchopulmonary dysplasia is characterized by increased airway reactivity and resistance, decreased pulmonary compliance, ventilation-to-perfusion mismatch, decreased arterial oxygenation, and tachypnea.[32] Oxygen consumption is increased by as much as 25%. It should be assumed that children with a prior history of RDS requiring supplemental oxygen and mechanical ventilation of the lungs probably have some degree of residual pulmonary disease. The clinical consequences of this dysfunction are unknown; the prognosis for children surviving the first year of life is good.

The choice of drugs for anesthesia in the patient with bronchopulmonary dysplasia is not as important as management of the airway. For example, management of anesthesia in these children includes intubation of the trachea, delivery of an increased inspired concentration of oxygen, and mechanical ventilation of the lungs. The possible presence of airway hyperreactivity suggests the need to establish a surgical level of anesthesia before instrumentation of the airway is initiated. Although these children may appear clinically well, pulmonary compliance is usually decreased. It should be appreciated, however, that pulmonary dysfunction in these patients will be most marked during the first year of life.

Intracranial Hemorrhage

The four types of intercranial hemorrhage that occur during the neonatal period are subdural, primary subarachnoid, periventricular-intraventricular, and intercellular. The most frequent and important type is periventricular-intraventricular hemorrhage.

The incidence of periventricular-intraventricular hemorrhage is 40% to 45% in neonates less than 35 weeks of gestational age. Newborn prematurity is the single most important risk factor for intracranial hemorrhage. Severe respiratory complications and infections are associated with intracranial hemorrhage. Other factors that predispose preterm neonates to this type of hemorrhage are impaired autoregulation of cerebral blood flow, increased central venous pressure, and immaturity of neonatal cerebral capillary beds. The degree of autoregulation of cerebral blood flow in the normal neonate is unknown, although impaired autoregulation of cerebral blood flow has been demonstrated in the stressed neonate. When autoregulation is impaired, an elevation of blood pressure will cause increased cerebral blood flow, which may result in periventricular-intraventricular hemorrhage. Arterial hypoxemia and hypercapnia during asphyxia associated with delivery can also result in this type of hemorrhage. The diagnosis of periventricular-intraventricular hemorrhage can be made by maintaining a high index of suspicion in the susceptible neonate and by clinical and radiologic features. Clinical features can range from subtle and not easily elicited neurologic aberrations to catastrophic deterioration with rapid onset of coma. Ultrasound scanning and computed tomography provide useful modes for identifying periventricular-intraventricular hemorrhage.

Although the effects of anesthesia on cerebral blood flow in the neonate are unknown, some recommendations can be made concerning the management of anesthesia. Certainly, factors known to precipitate periventricular-intraventricular hemorrhage, such as arterial hypoxemia and hypercapnia, should be avoided. In view of the altered autoregulation of cerebral blood flow, systolic blood pressure should be maintained within the normal range to reduce the risk of cerebral overperfusion. To accomplish these goals, careful monitoring of oxygenation, ventilation, and blood pressure is useful.

Retinopathy of Prematurity

Retinopathy of prematurity (retrolental fibroplasia) is probably due to multiple interacting events. The most significant risk factor is prematurity. The risk of retinopathy is inversely related to birthweight, with significant risk occurring in infants weighing less than 1500 g.[33] Retinal development and maturation is a complicated process. Our understanding of the process and factors that may alter development of retinal vasculature is poor. Under normal circumstances, retinal vasculature develops from the optic disc toward the periphery of the retina. During arterial hyperoxia, retinal vasoconstriction occurs, and normal retinal development is disturbed. When normotoxic conditions return, vascularization of the retina resumes in an abnormal fashion, with resultant neovascularization and scarring. Although 80% to 90% of retinal changes will regress spontaneously, 10% to 20% of children will be left with some visual impairment. Cryotherapy, and possibly laser surgery to ablate the avascular peripheral retina, arrests the progression of the disease in many cases and may decrease visual impairment.

There are many unanswered questions concerning retinopathy. It is not known precisely what magnitude or duration of arterial hyperoxia produces adverse effects on retinal vasculature. Exposure to a PaO_2 greater than 80 mmHg for prolonged periods (premature infants 500 to 1300 g) may be associated with an increased incidence and severity of retinopathy.[33] Although retinopathy may be a result of the interaction between vasoconstriction and an immature retina, it is also possible that the direct effects of oxygen may produce retinal damage. Retinopathy has even occurred in preterm infants who did not receive supplemental oxygen and in infants with cyanotic congenital heart disease. Clearly, arterial hyperoxia is an important risk factor in the development of retinopathy, but prematurity must also be present. The risk of retinopathy is negligible after 44 weeks postconception. Therefore, a preterm infant born after 36 weeks' gestation probably remains at risk of retinopathy until after 8 weeks of age. Retinopathy of prematurity appears not to be a preventable disease caused by the misuse of oxygen, but rather a disease of prematurity in which several factors can injure the retinal vessels.[33]

Management of Anesthesia

Management of anesthesia in patients with retinopathy of prematurity introduces the dilemma of trying to minimize oxygen administration to a group of patients that is also susceptible to arterial hypoxemia. To reduce the risk of retinopathy in a susceptible infant, it is recommended that the PaO_2 be maintained between 60 and 80 mmHg. During anesthesia, it is useful to dilute the concentration of oxygen delivered, using nitrous oxide or air. The concentration of oxygen delivered can be confirmed with an oxygen analyzer. Although it may be desirable to monitor arterial oxygenation in blood sampled from a preductal artery, the use of a pulse oximeter is an acceptable alternative (Fig. 32-2). It should also be appreciated that arterial hypoxemia is a significant threat to the neonate. Certainly, an attempt to prevent arterial hyperoxia must be tempered with the realization that unrecognized arterial hypoxemia can result in irreversible brain damage.

Apnea Spells

Apnea spells are defined as cessation of breathing that lasts at least 20 seconds and produces cyanosis and bradycardia. An estimated 20% to 30% of preterm infants experience apnea spells during the first month of life.[34] The more premature the infant, the greater the likelihood of apnea spells. A preterm infant may also have RDS and bronchopulmonary dysplasia in addition to apnea spells. Inguinal hernia and incarceration of an inguinal hernia are common in the preterm infant. Consequently, many preterm infants require inguinal hernia repair. Even though infant inguinal hernia repair is a minor surgical procedure, up to 33% of such preterm infants have respiratory complications (apnea spells, atelectasis) during the perioperative period.[35] The incidence of postoperative apnea in preterm infants less than 60 weeks postconceptual age undergoing inguinal hernia repair may be increased when the preoperative hematocrit is less than 30%.[36] For these reasons, it is helpful to seek information about prematurity and RDS during the preoperative interview with the parents.

Since all anesthetics, both inhaled and intravenous, affect the control of breathing and contribute to upper airway obstruction, it is likely that the risk of apnea spells will be increased during the postoperative period, especially in preterm infants less than 60 weeks postconceptual age.[35] Regional anesthesia may also be associated with apnea spells.[37] Consequently, a preterm infant with a history of apnea spells is probably not a suitable candidate for outpatient surgery. It is recommended that these patients be monitored in the hospital for at least 12 hours after surgery.[37,38] The risk of postoperative apnea spells seems to be reduced beyond 60 weeks postconception, leading some to recommend postponement of nonessential surgery in a preterm infant to after this age.

Sudden Infant Death Syndrome

Sudden infant death syndrome (SIDS) is the most frequent cause of death in infants between 1 and 12 months of age. Those at increased risk of SIDS include premature infants, infants who have had bronchopulmonary dysplasia, and those with infant apnea syndrome (not to be confused with apnea resulting from prematurity, which disappears as the infant matures). There is no evidence that general anesthesia triggers SIDS.

Kernicterus

Kernicterus is the term applied to a syndrome caused by the toxic effects of unconjugated bilirubin on the central nervous system. The gross clinical features of kernicterus include hypertonicity, opisthotonos, and spasticity. It is also evident that bilirubin encephalopathy can produce more subtle changes, such as dyslexia, hyperactivity, and decreased intellectual development.

Bilirubin is not lipophilic and does not readily cross the blood-brain barrier. Nevertheless, the blood-brain barrier of a neonate, especially a preterm neonate, is immature, which may explain the ability of bilirubin to enter the brain and produce cell damage.[39] In addition, alterations in the blood-brain barrier by arterial hypoxemia, hypercapnia, or acidosis may facilitate the passage of bilirubin into the central nervous system. Rapid changes in cerebral blood flow, such as may occur during exchange transfusion or rapid blood transfusion, may also disrupt the blood-brain barrier and permit the entry of both bound and unbound bilirubin into the central nervous system. The neonate with other diseases, such as RDS and sepsis, may have decreased bilirubin-binding capacity and be at increased risk of kernicterus.

Treatment of hyperbilirubinemia includes phototherapy, exchange blood transfusions, and drugs. Phototherapy converts bilirubin to photobilirubin. Photobilirubin is water soluble and does not bind to albumin. Although exchange blood transfusions are usually performed when the plasma bilirubin concentration exceeds 18 mg·dl^{-1}, other risk factors, such as low birthweight, decreased plasma albumin concentration, acidosis, arterial hypoxemia, and hypothermia, must also be considered and may necessitate an exchange blood transfusion at a lower plasma bilirubin concentration. There are no data concerning effects of anesthesia on the plasma concentration of bilirubin in the preterm infant.

Hypoglycemia

In contrast to the adult, the neonate has a poorly developed system for maintaining an adequate plasma glucose concentration and, therefore, is susceptible to the development of hypoglycemia. By definition, hypoglycemia is a plasma glucose concentration of less than 25 mg·dl^{-1} for a preterm neonate and less than 35 mg·dl^{-1} for a neonate younger than 3 days of age. The plasma glucose concentration at 3 days of age should be greater than 45 mg·dl^{-1} for a term neonate.

Signs of hypoglycemia in the neonate include irritability, seizures, bradycardia, hypotension, and apnea. Many of these signs are nonspecific, and a high index of suspicion must be maintained. Manifestations of hypoglycemia may be attenuated by anesthetic drugs, suggesting the potential value for intraoperative monitoring of the blood glucose concentration in an at-risk neonate. Maintenance of an adequate plasma glucose concentration in the neonate may require intravenous infusion of a solution containing glucose. The immediate treatment of hypoglycemia is administration of glucose (0.5 to 1 g·kg^{-1} IV) or a continuous infusion of glucose (8 mg·kg^{-1}·min^{-1} IV). Hyperglycemia must also be avoided, as a plasma glucose concentration in excess of 125 mg·dl^{-1} can produce osmotic diuresis, with resultant dehydration.

Hypocalcemia

Fetal calcium stores are largely achieved during the last trimester of gestation. A preterm neonate may therefore be susceptible to the development of hypocalcemia. Hypocalcemia in a neonate is defined as a plasma calcium concentration of less than 3.5 mEq·L^{-1} or a plasma ionized calcium concentration of less than 1.5 mEq·L^{-1}. Signs of hypocalcemia are nonspecific and include irritability, hypotension, and seizures. A neonate with hypocalcemia exhibits increased skeletal muscle tone and twitching, in contrast to skeletal muscle hypotonia associated with hypoglycemia.

Hypocalcemia can occur with rapid intraoperative infusion of citrate, as may occur during an exchange transfusion or infusion of citrated blood or fresh frozen plasma. The hypotensive effect of citrate-induced hypocalcemia can be minimized by administration of calcium gluconate (1 to 2 mg IV) for each milliliter of blood transfused.

Sepsis

Sepsis in the neonate is associated with a mortality approaching 50%. Presumably, this high mortality reflects the neonate's immature immune system. The clinical presentation of sepsis in the neonate is nonspecific. Consequently, the evaluation for sepsis has become an integral part of the evaluation of a critically ill neonate. Suggestive signs of sepsis in the neonate include lethargy, skeletal muscle hypotonia, hypoglycemia, and ventilatory distress. In contrast to the adult, increased body temperature or leukocytosis may be absent in the neonate. A positive blood culture is important in confirming the diagnosis. Common sequelae of untreated neonatal sepsis include meningitis and disseminated intravascular coagulation. Most neonates presenting for surgery are already receiving antibiotics, as the risk of sepsis is great. Nevertheless, the occurrence of pulmonary dysfunction during the postoperative period should arouse suspicion as to the possible presence of sepsis.

NEONATAL SURGICAL DISEASES

Neonatal surgical diseases in the first days of life are invariably of an urgent nature[40] (Table 32-11). In addition to the physiologic aberrations produced by the disease process, incomplete adaptation to the extrauterine environment may further complicate perioperative management.

Diaphragmatic Hernia

Diaphragmatic hernia results from incomplete embryologic closure of the diaphragm. The incidence is about 1 in every 5000 live births. Although herniation of abdominal contents into the thorax can occur at several sites, the most common diaphragmatic defect occurs through the left posterolateral pleuroperitoneal canal (foramen of Bochdalek) (Fig. 32-6). Herniation of abdominal contents into the thorax during gestation interferes with normal fetal lung maturation, resulting in varying degrees of pulmonary hypoplasia. The degree of pulmonary hypoplasia is related to the timing of the herniation of abdominal contents into the thorax. Early diaphragmatic herniation will cause more pulmonary hypoplasia, resulting in a less favorable prognosis. Hypoplasia of the left ventricle may also occur, contributing to postnatal cardiac insufficiency. Despite significant progress in pediatric surgery and anesthesia, perioperative mortality is still substantial, with death most often due to pulmonary hypoplasia or persistent pulmonary hypertension.

Signs and Symptoms

Signs and symptoms of diaphragmatic hernia evident soon after birth include scaphoid abdomen, barrel-shaped chest, detection of bowel sounds during auscultation of the chest, and profound arterial hypoxemia. A chest radiograph will show loops of intestine in the thorax and a shift of the mediastinum to the opposite side (Fig. 32-7). Arterial hypoxemia reflects the presence of right-to-left shunting through the ductus arteriosus as a manifestation of persistent fetal circulation. Increased pulmonary vascular resistance is further aggravated by arterial hypoxemia, hypercarbia, and acidosis, ensuring that the ductus arteriosus will remain patient and a fetal pattern of circulation will persist. There is a high incidence of

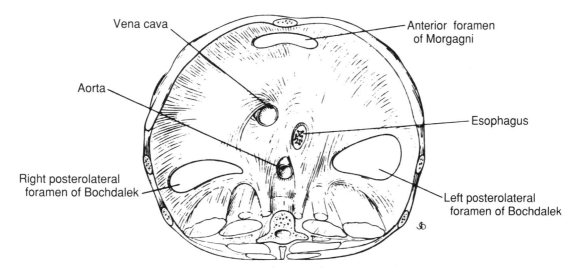

Fig. 32-6. Diaphragmatic hernia with passage of abdominal viscera into the thorax most commonly occurs through the left posterolateral pleuroperitoneal canal (foramen of Bochdalek). (From Smith RM. Anesthesia for Infants and Children. 4th Ed. St. Louis. CV Mosby 1980, with permission.)

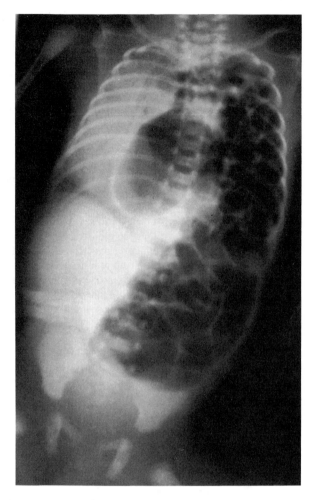

Fig. 32-7. Chest radiograph of a newborn with a diaphragmatic hernia, as evidenced by the loops of intestine in the left thorax, displacement of the mediastinum to the right, and compression of the right lung. Note the dilated stomach contributing to mediastinal displacement.

congenital heart disease and intestinal malrotation in neonates with diaphragmatic hernia.

Treatment

Immediate treatment of a neonate with suspected diaphragmatic hernia includes decompression of the stomach with an orogastric or nasogastric tube and administration of supplemental oxygen. Positive-pressure ventilation by mask should be avoided, as the passage of gas into the esophagus may increase stomach volume and further compromise pulmonary function. Indeed, awake intubation of the trachea should be performed if the need for mechanical ventilation of the lungs is anticipated for any sustained period of time. After intubation of the trachea, positive airway pressure during mechanical ventilation of the lungs should not exceed 25 to 30 cm H_2O,

since excessive airway pressures can result in damage to the normal lung, manifested as pneumothorax.

Although diaphragmatic hernia has been considered a surgical emergency, there is increasing evidence that preoperative stabilization for a period of hours or days may decrease mortality in unstable patients.[41] Preoperative stabilization may include skeletal muscle paralysis, mechanical ventilation of the lungs, intravenous infusion of pulmonary vasodilators (tolazoline, prostaglandin E-1, isoproterenol), and institution of extracorporeal membrane oxygenation.

Management of Anesthesia

Management of anesthesia for a neonate with a diaphragmatic hernia consists of awake intubation of the trachea after preoxygenation. In addition to routine monitors, the right radial or temporal artery (preductal artery) is often cannulated for monitoring of blood pressure, blood gases, and pH. Anesthesia can be induced and maintained with a low concentration of a volatile drug. Nitrous oxide should be avoided, as its diffusion into loops of intestine present in the chest may result in distension of these loops and subsequent compression of functioning lung tissue. If the level of arterial oxygenation permits, the delivered concentration of oxygen can be diluted by adding air to the oxygen until the desired concentration of oxygen is attained, as reflected by an oxygen analyzer. Since prolonged postoperative ventilation of the lungs is required by almost all infants with diaphragmatic hernia, an alternative approach to inhaled drugs for anesthesia is the use of an opioid such as fentanyl plus a muscle relaxant, often pancuronium.[42] This regimen can also be continued during the postoperative period. The advantage of this technique is that the hormonal response to stress can be minimized postoperatively. Mechanical ventilation of the lungs is recommended, but airway pressure should be monitored and maintained below 25 to 30 cm H_2O to minimize the risk of pneumothorax. Reduction of the diaphragmatic hernia is accomplished through an abdominal surgical approach. After reduction of the hernia, an attempt to inflate the hypoplastic lung is not recommended, as it is unlikely to expand, and damage to the normal lung can occur from excessive positive airway pressure. In addition to a hypoplastic lung, these neonates are likely to have an underdeveloped abdominal cavity, such that a tight surgical abdominal closure will cause increased intra-abdominal pressure, with cephalad displacement of the diaphragm, reduced functional residual capacity, and compression of the inferior vena cava. To prevent an excessively tight abdominal surgical closure, it is often necessary to create a ventral hernia, which can be repaired later.

Postoperative Management

Postoperative management of the infant with a diaphragmatic hernia presents significant challenges. The prognosis of these infants is ultimately determined by the degree of pulmonary hypoplasia. There is no effective treatment for pulmonary hypoplasia, other than keeping the infant alive with the hope that lung maturation will occur. Extracorporeal membrane oxygenation has been used successfully for this purpose in these patients.[43]

The postoperative course, after surgical reduction of a diaphragmatic hernia, is often characterized by rapid improvement, followed by sudden deterioration with profound arterial hypoxemia, hypercapnia, and acidosis, resulting in death. The mechanism for this deterioration is the reappearance of a fetal pattern of circulation, with right-to-left shunting through the foramen ovale and ductus arteriosus. If shunting occurs through the ductus arteriosus, there will be a 20 mmHg or greater difference in the PaO_2 measured simultaneously from a sample obtained from a preductal and postductal artery. If shunting is occurring predominantly through the foramen ovale, no such gradient will exist.

Tracheoesophageal Fistula

Survival of the neonate with a tracheoesophageal fistula and no associated defects approaches 100%. Nevertheless, about 20% of neonates with tracheoesophageal fistula have a major co-existing cardiovascular anomaly (ventricular septal defect, tetralogy of Fallot, coarctation of the aorta, atrial septal defect), and 30% to 40% are born preterm. Survival in those infants with other anomalies is reduced. Five types of tracheoesophageal fistula are associated with esophageal atresia (Fig. 32-8). The most common defect consists of a blind upper esophageal pouch and a fistula between the lower esophagus and trachea.

Signs and Symptoms

The diagnosis of tracheoesophageal fistula is usually made soon after birth, when an oral catheter cannot be passed into the stomach, or when the infant exhibits cyanosis and cough-

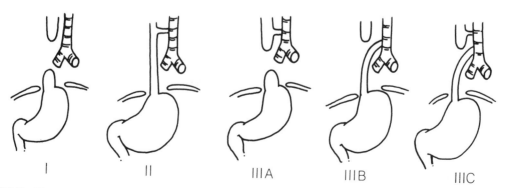

Fig. 32-8. The five types of tracheoesophageal fistula are classified as I, II, IIIA, IIIB, and IIIC, depending on the anatomic characteristics of the trachea and esophagus. A blind upper esophageal pouch and a fistula connecting the stomach to the trachea (IIIB) is the most common type of tracheoesophageal fistula. (From Dierdorf SF, Krishna G. Anesthetic management of neonatal surgical emergencies. Anesth Analg 1981;60:204–15, with permission.)

ing during oral feedings. Pulmonary aspiration is likely to occur. After the diagnosis is suspected, the blind upper pouch must be decompressed and the infant placed in a head-up position. Gastric distension can be of sufficient magnitude to impair diaphragmatic excursion. Should life-threatening gastric distension occur, one-lung ventilation may be necessary until the stomach can be decompressed.[44]

Treatment

The preferred surgical approach for treatment of the newborn with a tracheoesophageal fistula is ligation of the defect and primary anastomosis of the esophageal segments by an extrapleural approach.[44] Infants with this disorder who are premature may exhibit significant associated anomalies or have pneu-

monitis. In these infants, a staged surgical approach with an initial gastrostomy under local anesthesia may be selected. Definitive repair of the tracheoesophageal fistula can then be delayed until the neonate's condition has improved.

Management of Anesthesia

Proper placement of the tracheal tube is critical; it should be above the carina but below the tracheoesophageal fistula. Management of the airway is influenced by the presence or absence of a gastrostomy. By placing the gastrostomy tube into a beaker of water and applying positive airway pressure, one can determine the position of the tracheal tube[40] (Fig. 32-9). For example, absence of bubbling in the beaker during positive airway pressure confirms that the distal end of the

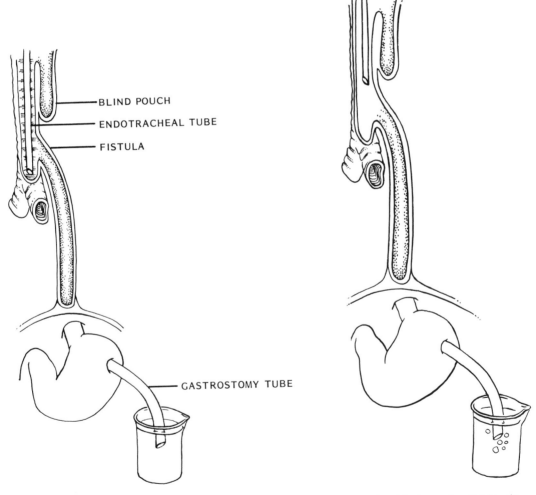

BLIND POUCH

ENDOTRACHEAL TUBE

FISTULA

GASTROSTOMY TUBE

Fig. 32-9. Application of positive airway pressure through a tube correctly positioned in the trachea distal to the tracheoesophageal fistula will not produce bubbling in the beaker of water in which the gastrostomy tube is placed (**A**). Incorrect placement of the tube in the trachea proximal to the tracheoesophageal fistula is detected by the presence of bubbling in the beaker containing the gastrostomy tube when positive airway pressure is applied (**B**). (From Dierdorf SE, Krishna G. Anesthetic management of neonatal surgical emergencies. Anesth Analg 1981;60:204–15, with permission.)

tracheal tube is beyond the fistula. Likewise, it is critical that the tracheal tube be above the carina, as the right lung is compressed during thoracotomy. Accidental intubation of the right main stem bronchus will result in a precipitous decrease in arterial oxygenation, especially during surgical retraction of the lung. If the infant does not have a gastrostomy, care must be exercised to avoid excessive airway pressure and further gastric distension. After tracheal intubation, the use of a pediatric fiberoptic bronchoscope is valuable for confirming the proper position of the tracheal tube.

Selection of anesthetic drugs for administration during surgical correction of tracheoesophageal fistula depends on the physiologic status of the neonate. A volatile anesthetic may be used if the neonate is adequately hydrated. Nitrous oxide should be used with caution in a neonate without a gastrostomy, as diffusion of this gas into the distended stomach would be undesirable. If nitrous oxide is not administered, it may be necessary to dilute the concentration of oxygen delivered with air, to avoid arterial hyperoxia and the risk of retinopathy of prematurity. In addition to routine monitors, a catheter placed in a peripheral artery will permit continuous monitoring of blood pressure, as well as measurement of blood gases and pH. A pulse oximeter is a useful monitor for detecting rapid changes in arterial oxygenation.

A consistent pathologic finding in the neonate with tracheoesophageal fistula is decreased tracheal cartilage. This reduced support can result in tracheal collapse after tracheal extubation, requiring immediate reintubation of the trachea. By contrast, in some neonates, symptomatic tracheal compression develops several months after repair of a tracheoesophageal fistula. Chronic gastroesophageal reflux and aspiration pneumonitis can follow corrective surgery, necessitating antireflux surgical procedures at a later time in life.

Abdominal Wall Defects

Omphalocele and gastroschisis are congenital defects of the anterior abdominal wall, which permit external herniation of abdominal viscera.

Omphalocele

Omphalocele is associated with external herniation of abdominal viscera through the base of the umbilical cord[40] (Fig. 32-10). The incidence is about 1 in every 5000 to 10,000 live

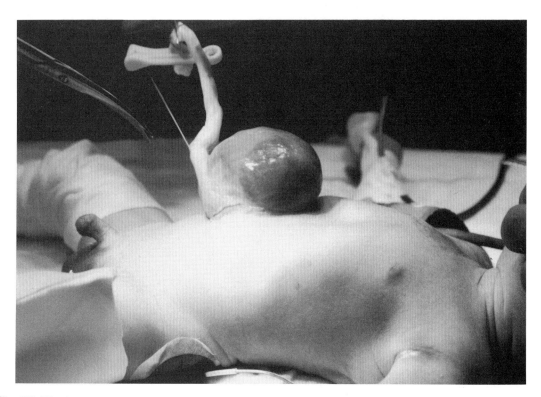

Fig. 32-10. Omphalocele is the herniation of abdominal viscera through the base of the umbilical cord. An intact hernia sac covers the abdominal contents. (From Dierdorf SF, Krishna G. Anesthetic management of neonatal surgical emergencies. Anesth Analg 1981;60:204–15, with permission.)

births, with a male predominance. Omphalocele is associated with a 75% incidence of other congenital defects, including cardiac anomalies, trisomy-21, and Beckwith syndrome (omphalocele, organomegaly, macroglossia, and hypoglycemia). About 33% of neonates with omphalocele are preterm. Cardiac defects and prematurity are the major causes of the 30% mortality in newborns with an omphalocele.

Gastroschisis

Gastroschisis is characterized by external herniation of abdominal viscera through a 2- to 5-cm defect in the anterior abdominal wall, lateral to the normally inserted umbilical cord[40] (Fig. 32-11). Unlike omphalocele, a hernia sac does not cover the herniated abdominal viscera. Gastroschisis is rarely associated with other congenital anomalies. The incidence of preterm birth, however, is higher than in neonates with an omphalocele.

Preoperative Preparation

Considerations in the preoperative preparation of a neonate with omphalocele or gastroschisis are the prevention of infection and minimization of fluid and heat loss from exposed ab-

dominal viscera. Covering exposed viscera with moist dressings and a plastic bowel bag and maintaining a neutral thermal environment are effective methods of decreasing fluid and heat loss. The stomach should be decompressed with an orogastric tube to decrease the risk of regurgitation and pulmonary aspiration. Adequate hydration during the preoperative period is essential. Initial fluid requirements in these neonates are increased, ranging from 6 to 12 ml·kg^{-1}·h^{-1}. These neonates experience considerable protein loss and third-space translocation. Hypovolemia is evidenced by hemoconcentration and metabolic acidosis. The plasma albumin concentration and colloid oncotic pressure are reduced. To maintain normal oncotic pressure, protein-containing solutions should constitute about 25% of the replacement fluids. Sodium bicarbonate administration to correct metabolic acidosis should be guided by arterial pH measurements.

Management of Anesthesia

Important aspects of management of anesthesia for surgical treatment of omphalocele and gastroschisis include maintenance of body temperature and continuation of fluid replace-

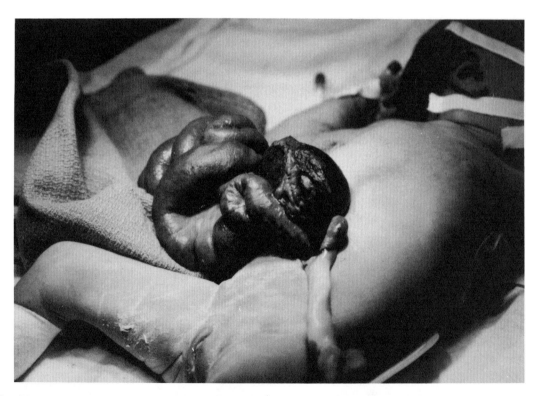

Fig. 32-11. Gastroschisis is the herniation of abdominal viscera through a defect in the abdominal wall lateral to the normally inserted umbilical cord. A hernia sac to cover the abdominal viscera is absent. (From Dierdorf SF, Krishna G. Anesthetic management of neonatal surgical emergencies. Anesth Analg 1981;60:204–15, with permission.)

ment. Awake intubation of the trachea, after decompression of the stomach and preoxygenation, is often recommended. Opioids such as fentanyl or sufentanil or a volatile anesthetic may be used. Because of co-existing hypovolemia, anesthetics must be carefully titrated to avoid hypotension. The use of nitrous oxide may be questioned, as this gas could diffuse into the intestinal tract and interfere with the ease of returning exposed and distended loops of bowel back into the abdomen. If nitrous oxide is not used, the concentration of oxygen delivered is adjusted by dilution with air, a necessity because these often preterm neonates are vulnerable to the development of retinopathy of prematurity. Muscle relaxants must be administered judiciously, as excessive skeletal muscle relaxation may make it difficult to determine whether primary surgical abdominal wall closure is feasible. It must be remembered that these neonates have an underdeveloped abdominal cavity; a tight surgical abdominal closure can result in reduction of diaphragmatic excursion and compression of the inferior vena cava. Monitoring airway pressure is helpful for detecting changes in pulmonary compliance due to abdominal closure. High intra-abdominal pressures interfere with abdominal organ perfusion.[45] If primary surgical abdominal closure is not possible, temporary coverage with a Dacron-reinforced Silastic silo is performed. The hernia is then gradually reduced over 1 to 2 weeks.

Intensive intraoperative and postoperative monitoring is recommended. Direct monitoring of arterial blood gases and pH is valuable for guiding fluid therapy, minimizing the risk of the development of retinopathy of prematurity, and recognizing previously undiagnosed cardiac anomalies. Mechanical ventilation of the lungs is indicated for 24 to 48 hours for most neonates following omphalocele or gastroschisis repair. Refinement of techniques of postoperative mechanical ventilation of the lungs and availability of total parenteral nutrition have increased the survival of infants with omphalocele to about 75%.

Pyloric Stenosis

Pyloric stenosis occurs in about 1 of every 500 live births. It is generally manifested in a male infant 2 to 5 weeks of age. Pyloric stenosis is as common in preterm neonates as it is in term neonates.

Signs and Symptoms

Pyloric stenosis is characterized by persistent vomiting, resulting in the loss of hydrogen ions from the stomach. As hydrogen ions are lost, the kidneys secrete potassium in exchange for hydrogen ions, in an effort to maintain a normal arterial pH. In addition, the kidneys begin exchanging potassium and hydrogen ions for sodium ions, as the infant becomes sodium depleted from vomiting. The result is a dehydrated

infant with a hypokalemic, hypochloremic metabolic alkalosis. Measurement of plasma electrolyte concentrations, arterial blood gases, and pH will help quantitate the degree of metabolic abnormality.

Treatment

Surgical treatment of pyloric stenosis is not an emergency.[46] The patient with pyloric stenosis should be treated initially with intravenous fluids containing sodium and potassium chloride. Surgery is performed electively after 24 to 48 hours of intravenous fluid therapy.

Management of Anesthesia

Pulmonary aspiration of gastric fluid is a definite risk in an infant with pyloric stenosis. This risk is further increased in an infant with pyloric stenosis who has undergone radiographic examination of the upper gastrointestinal tract, using barium. Therefore, the stomach should be emptied as completely as possible with a large-bore catheter, before induction of anesthesia. Awake intubation of the trachea is indicated for the less vigorous infant. Intubation of the trachea after rapid-sequence induction of anesthesia, with intravenous administration of a barbiturate followed by succinylcholine and during continuous cricoid pressure, can be used for a more vigorous infant. Maintenance of anesthesia with a volatile drug, with or without nitrous oxide, is acceptable. Skeletal muscle relaxation, as provided by a muscle relaxant, is usually not needed during maintenance of anesthesia. Mechanical ventilation of the lungs is recommended during the operation. If skeletal muscle relaxation is needed, administration of a short-acting drug such as succinylcholine or mivacurium is a consideration.

Postoperative Management

Postoperative depression of ventilation often occurs in the infant with pyloric stenosis. The cause is unknown but may be related to cerebrospinal fluid alkalosis and intraoperative hyperventilation of the lungs. For this reason, the infant should be fully awake and should display acceptable patterns of ventilation before extubation of the trachea is considered. Hypoglycemia may occur 2 to 3 hours after surgical correction of pyloric stenosis.

Lobar Emphysema

Lobar emphysema is a rare cause of respiratory distress in the neonate. Pathologic causes of congenital lobar emphysema include collapse of bronchi from hypoplasia of supporting cartilage, bronchial stenosis, mucous plugs, obstructing cysts, and vascular compression of bronchi. Acquired lobar emphysema may be a result of bronchopulmonary dysplasia. The left upper and right middle lobes are most commonly affected by lobar emphysema.

Signs and Symptoms

Regardless of the cause of lobar emphysema, the end result is an overdistended lobe that produces compression atelectasis of normal lung tissue, mediastinal shift, and impaired venous blood return, with subsequent arterial hypoxemia and hypotension. About one-half of patients will exhibit evidence of lobar emphysema during the first months of life. Signs and symptoms of labor emphysema include tachypnea, tachycardia, cyanosis, wheezing, and asymmetric breath sounds. A chest radiograph will demonstrate a hyperinflated lobe with mediastinal shift. The presence of bronchovascular markings in the hyperinflated lobe helps differentiate lobar emphysema from pneumothorax.

Management of Anesthesia

Management of anesthesia for surgical lobectomy in the treatment of lobar emphysema must consider cardiovascular and pulmonary changes that can occur with mechanical ventilation of the lungs.[47] In this regard, the infant may be at greatest risk during induction of anesthesia, as positive-pressure ventilation of the lungs before the chest is open may cause rapid expansion of the emphysematous lobe (gas enters but cannot leave), with sudden mediastinal shift and cardiac arrest. For this reason, maintenance of spontaneous breathing with minimal airway pressure may be recommended.[48] General anesthesia may be supplemented with local anesthesia until the chest is opened and the emphysematous lobe delivered. Thereafter, the patient may be paralyzed and the lungs mechanically ventilated. Nitrous oxide should not be used, as its diffusion into the diseased lobe can cause further distension. A severely decompensated infant may require emergency needle aspiration or thoracotomy for decompression of the affected lobe.

Necrotizing Enterocolitis

Necrotizing enterocolitis is primarily a disease of small preterm neonates, resulting in substantial perinatal morbidity and mortality. Neonates at greatest risk are less than 32 weeks gestation and weigh less than 1500 g. Survivors of necrotizing enterocolitis often have significant long-term nutritional and developmental problems.

The etiology of necrotizing enterocolitis is multifactorial. Perinatal asphyxia, infection, umbilical artery catheterization, exchange blood transfusions, hyperosmolar feedings, and cyanotic congenital heart disease have all been implicated. The common feature of this disease is hypoperfusion of the gastrointestinal tract, with subsequent mucosal and bowel wall ischemia. Initial mucosal ischemia may make the bowel more susceptible to bacterial damage and to the effects of hyperosmolar feedings.

Signs and Symptoms

The most common initial signs of necrotizing enterocolitis are abdominal distension and bloody feces. Apnea spells, lethargy, and thermal instability also occur. Hypovolemic shock and metabolic acidosis may occur secondary to generalized peritonitis from multiple bowel perforations. A hemorrhagic diathesis secondary to thrombocytopenia is often present. Bowel gas frequently penetrates the damaged mucosa and enters the submucosal region; as a result, gas may gain access to the mesenteric veins and the portal venous system. Gas in the intestinal submucosa results in the classic pneumatosis intestinalis seen on radiographs of the abdomen. RDS requiring mechanical ventilation of the lungs frequently co-exists.

Treatment

Medical treatment, consisting of gastric decompression, intravenous fluids, and antibiotics, is often successful in the management of the neonate with necrotizing enterocolitis. Surgery is reserved for those neonates in whom medical treatment has failed, as evidenced by peritonitis, bowel perforation, and progressive metabolic acidosis.

Management of Anesthesia

The neonate with necrotizing enterocolitis is frequently hypovolemic and requires vigorous fluid resuscitation with crystalloid and colloid solutions before induction of anesthesia. Blood and platelet transfusions are often necessary. Adequate monitoring of fluid resuscitation is critical. A catheter placed in a peripheral artery provides the ability to measure blood pressure continuously, as well as to monitor arterial blood gases, pH, hematocrit, and electrolytes. It must be appreciated that rapid fluid administration to a preterm neonate may cause intracranial hemorrhage or reopening of the ductus arteriosus.

Volatile anesthetics can produce significant hypotension in these neonates, particularly if hypovolemia is present. Therefore, reduced doses of ketamine, fentanyl, or sufentanil plus a nondepolarizing muscle relaxant may be selected for the maintenance of anesthesia. Nitrous oxide should be avoided, as it may increase the size of gas bubbles in the mesenteric veins and in the portal venous system. Gas embolism can also occur if portal venous gas bubbles traverse the ductus venosus and enter the inferior vena cava.[49] Postoperative mechanical ventilation of the lungs is usually required because of abdominal distension and co-existing RDS.

TRAUMA

Trauma is the leading cause of death in children older than 1 year of age.[50] Blunt head injury from motor vehicle accidents is responsible for most injuries and deaths. Most preventable deaths are due to airway obstruction, pneumothorax, intra-abdominal bleeding, or an expanding intracranial hematoma. The most important indicator of intracranial bleeding and the need for prompt surgical intervention is a decrease in the level of consciousness as documented by a decrease in the Glasgow coma score (see Table 17-4). The Glasgow Coma Scale may need to be modified for the child who is too young to talk. There is a trend toward nonoperative treatment of blunt abdominal injury, based on diagnosis using computed tomography.

NERVOUS SYSTEM

Diseases of the nervous system that afflict pediatric patients include cerebral palsy, hydrocephalus, myelomeningocele, craniostenosis, seizure disorders (epilepsy), trisomy-21 (Down syndrome), neurofibromatosis, and Reye syndrome. Management of these patients during the perioperative period is facilitated by understanding the pathophysiology of these diseases.

Cerebral Palsy

Cerebral palsy includes a group of nonprogressive disorders characterized by central motor deficits resulting from hypoxic or anoxic cerebral damage. Etiologic factors include genetic abnormalities, metabolic defects, or injury to the brain, which may occur during the prenatal period. In addition, mechanical birth trauma, congenital cerebrovascular malformations, intra-uterine and neonatal infections, toxins, prematurity, kernicterus, and hypoglycemia are known causes of cerebral palsy. Cerebral palsy can be due to anatomic disorders, with localized or diffuse atrophy of the cerebral cortex, basal ganglia, and subcortical white matter. Despite the perceived association between a multitude of factors and cerebral palsy, the cause of most cases of cerebral palsy is unknown.[51]

Signs and Symptoms

Cerebral palsy is classified as spastic, extrapyramidal, atonic, and mixed. The most common manifestation is skeletal muscle spasticity. Extrapyramidal cerebral palsy is associated with choreoathetosis and dystonia. Cerebellar ataxia is characteristic of atonic cerebral palsy. Varying degrees of mental retardation and speech defects can accompany cerebral palsy. Seizure disorders can co-exist with cerebral palsy.

Children with cerebral palsy may have varying degrees of spasticity of different skeletal muscle groups, resulting in contractures and fixed deformities of several joints of both the upper and lower extremities. These include fixed flexion and internal rotation deformities of the hip joint due to involved adductor and flexor muscles and plantar flexion of the ankles due to involvement of the Achilles tendon. These children often undergo elective orthopaedic corrective procedures, such as Achilles tendon lengthening, hip adductor and iliopsoas release, and derotational osteotomy of the femur. Stereotactic surgery may be performed in an attempt to reduce skeletal muscle rigidity, spasticity, and dyskinesia. Dental restorations

requiring general anesthesia are frequently necessary in the patient with cerebral palsy. Gastroesophageal reflux is common in children with central nervous system disorders, and antireflux operations are often performed.

Children with cerebral palsy are frequently receiving phenobarbital and phenytoin for control of seizures, and dantrolene for relief of skeletal muscle spasticity. Phenytoin may lead to gingival hyperplasia and megaloblastic anemia. Phenobarbital stimulates hepatic microsomal enzymatic activity and may lead to altered responses to drugs that undergo metabolism in the liver.

Management of Anesthesia

Management of anesthesia in the patient with cerebral palsy includes intubation of the trachea because of the propensity for gastroesophageal reflux and poor function of laryngeal and pharyngeal reflexes. Although patients with cerebral palsy have skeletal muscle spasticity, succinylcholine does not produce abnormal potassium release.[52] Body temperature should be monitored, as these patients may be susceptible to the development of hypothermia during the intraoperative period. Emergence from anesthesia may be quite slow because of the cerebral damage from cerebral palsy and the presence of hypothermia. Extubation of the trachea should be delayed until these children are fully awake and body temperature has returned toward normal. Postoperatively, these children have a high incidence of pulmonary complications.

Hydrocephalus

Hydrocephalus in the pediatric patient is due to an increase in cerebrospinal fluid volume, resulting in enlarged cerebral ventricles and increased intracranial pressure. Hydrocephalus due to overproduction or abnormal absorption of cerebrospinal fluid is classified as nonobstructive or communicating hydrocephalus, as there is no obstruction to the flow of cerebrospinal fluid. Obstructive hydrocephalus is present when there is obstruction to the flow of cerebrospinal fluid and its absorption from the subarachnoid space. This obstruction can be due to congenital, neoplastic, post-traumatic, or postinflammatory lesions. Congenital causes of obstructive hydrocephalus include (1) Arnold-Chiari malformation, in which the basilar subarachnoid pathways are underdeveloped; (2) aqueductal stenosis between the third and fourth ventricles; and (3) Dandy-Walker syndrome, with occlusion at the outlet of the fourth ventricle by a congenital membrane. Ventricular dilation commonly follows periventricular-intraventricular hemorrhage that most often occurs in preterm infants.

Signs and Symptoms

Signs and symptoms of hydrocephalus depend on the age of the child and the rapidity with which the condition occurs. For example, the prominent feature of congenital hydrocephalus is an abnormal enlargement of the head, which may present at birth or may occur soon after birth. Enlargement of the head is usually prominent in the frontal area of the skull. The cranial vault transilluminates in affected areas, and the cranial sutures are separated. Percussion of the skull produces a resonant note. The eyes are often deviated inferiorly. Scalp veins are dilated, and the skin is thin and shiny. Optic atrophy due to compression of the optic nerve can occur in chronic and untreated cases of hydrocephalus. Late-onset hydrocephalus may not produce an enlarged head but instead may cause significant increases in intracranial pressure. Hydrocephalus due to Arnold-Chiari malformation or aqueductal stenosis can lead to medullary and lower cranial nerve dysfunction, resulting in swallowing abnormalities, stridor, and atrophy of the tongue. Hydrocephalic children may have varying degrees of intellectual dysfunction; the dysfunction does not always correlate with the size of the ventricles or the thinness of the cortical mantle. Serial measurement of head circumference, skull radiographs, and computed tomography will confirm the diagnosis.

Treatment

Treatment depends on the mechanism responsible for hydrocephalus. Operative excision of the lesion responsible for obstruction to the flow of cerebrospinal fluid is performed if feasible. A shunting procedure is necessary if the obstruction cannot be surgically relieved. The shunt system employs a one-way valve, which directs flow of cerebrospinal fluid away from the ventricles. Shunting procedures include ventriculocisternostomy (Torkildsen's procedure) and ventriculoatrial and ventriculoperitoneal shunts. Less common are ventriculocholecystostomy, ventriculoureterostomy, and ventriculospinal shunts.

The ventriculoatrial shunt is performed for either nonobstructive or obstructive hydrocephalus. The distal end of the catheter is placed in the right atrium, as indicated by monitoring the changes in venous pressure wave patterns during advancement of the catheter into the atrium from the superior vena cava. Complications from an atrial catheter include thrombosis of the internal jugular vein or superior vena cava, septicemia, meningitis, pleural effusion, pulmonary embolism, and pulmonary hypertension. Furthermore, growth of these children will displace the cardiac end of the catheter into the superior vena cava, necessitating either revision of the shunt or its conversion to a ventriculoperitoneal shunt. Erosion of a ventriculoperitoneal catheter into a bronchus, with the development of a ventriculobronchial fistula, has been described.[53]

Management of Anesthesia

Operative procedures in children with hydrocephalus are likely to be necessary for placement, revision, or removal of a cerebrospinal fluid shunt system. Some of these children will have increased intracranial pressure, for which precautions should be taken during anesthesia. This is particularly important in a child in whom a shunt is to be inserted before craniotomy for excision of an intracranial tumor. For hydrocephalic infants and children with normal intracranial pressure, induction of anesthesia with thiopental plus succinylcholine or a short-acting nondepolarizing muscle relaxant to facilitate intubation of the trachea, followed by maintenance of anesthesia with a volatile anesthetic or an opioid plus nitrous oxide, is acceptable. In the presence of co-existing intracranial hypertension, it may be important to consider the potential for further increases in intracranial pressure to occur in association with administration of succinylcholine.[54] It should be appreciated that sudden hypotension sometimes occurs when tensely distended cerebral ventricles are decompressed. Furthermore, venous air embolism and increased blood loss can occur when large neck veins are opened for placement of an atrial catheter. Postoperatively, these patients are maintained in slight head-up positions, to permit free drainage of cerebrospinal fluid.

During surgery in a child with a ventriculoperitoneal shunt, excessive pressure on the skin of the scalp overlying the shunt should be avoided by rotating the head to the side opposite the shunt. Pressure over the ventricular reservoir can produce skin necrosis and possibly cause shunt malfunction.

Myelomeningocele

The neural tube of the embryo is formed from the ectodermal neural crest. The neural crest deepens to form the neural groove, the margins of which fuse to form the neural tube. Failure of closure of the caudal end of the neural tube can result in (1) spina bifida, characterized by defects of the vertebral arches; (2) meningocele, characterized by a sac that contains meninges; and (3) myelomeningocele, characterized by a sac that contains neural elements.

Signs and Symptoms

Children with a meningocele are usually born without neurologic deficits; those with myelomeningocele are likely to have varying degrees of motor and sensory deficits. For example, a child with a lumbosacral myelomeningocele exhibits flaccid paraplegia; loss of sensation to pinprick; and loss of anal, urethral, and vesicle sphincter tone. Associated congenital anomalies include clubfoot, hydrocephalus, dislocation of the hips, extrophy of the bladder, prolapsed uterus, Klippel-Feil syndrome, and congenital cardiac defects.

In these children, severe dilation of the upper urinary tract may develop, necessitating urinary diversion procedures, such as vesicostomy, cutaneous ureterostomies, and ileal or colon conduits. They are likely to experience recurrent urinary tract infections, which may be complicated by gram-negative sepsis. The need for corrective orthopaedic procedures on the lower extremities is predictable. As these patients mature, they have a tendency toward the development of varying degrees of scoliosis, often requiring posterior spinal fusion. There is a frequent need for replacement or revision of ventriculoperitoneal or ventriculoatrial shunts because of infection of the shunt or its malfunction due to malposition of the distal end of the catheter, reflecting normal patient growth.

Management of Anesthesia

The absence of skin covering a myelomeningocele introduces the risk of infection, necessitating surgical closure within a few hours of birth. Closure is performed during local or general anesthesia. If general anesthesia is selected, awake tracheal intubation may be performed with the child in the lateral decubitus position, to avoid pressure on the meningocele sac. Anesthesia may also be induced with the patient supine if the sac is protected by elevation of the infant on a doughnut-shaped support. Maintenance of anesthesia is with an inhaled anesthetic, delivered using mechanical ventilation of the lungs. The operative procedure is performed with these patients in the prone position. Although succinylcholine may be used to facilitate tracheal intubation, a long-acting nondepolarizing muscle relaxant should be avoided, as the surgeon may need to use a nerve stimulator to identify functional neural elements. Surgical closure of the myelomeningocele sac must be tight enough to prevent leakage of cerebrospinal fluid, as confirmed by raising the pressure in the sac with positive airway pressure. Postoperatively, the neonate should be maintained in the prone position, with a high index of suspicion maintained for the development of increased intracranial pressure.

Older children with myelomeningoceles require numerous corrective procedures, primarily involving the urologic and musculoskeletal systems. Although myelomeningoceles produce both upper and lower motor neuron dysfunction, succinylcholine does not produce a hyperkalemic response.[55] Inhaled anesthetics or opioids may be used for maintenance of anesthesia. Myelomeningocele patients, however, may have abnormal ventilatory responses to hypoxia and hypercarbia. These patients often have gastroesophageal reflux and abnormal vocal cord motility, emphasizing the need to take precautions against aspiration.

Patients with spina bifida have an increased incidence of sensitivity to latex (natural rubber), manifested by intraoperative cardiovascular collapse and bronchospasm.[56] It is possible that chronic exposure to indwelling catheters results in sensitization to latex. A preoperative history of itching, rashes, or wheezing after wearing latex gloves or inflating a toy balloon is suggestive of latex allergy. Latex allergy can be confirmed by the radioallergosorbent test. This test has been recommended as part of the preoperative preparation of the patient with spina bifida.[56] If latex sensitization is present, the use of plastic materials and nonlatex gloves is suggested.

Craniostenosis

Craniostenosis (craniosynostosis) is a congenital disorder resulting in a variety of deformities due to premature closure of one or more cranial sutures. Premature closure of the sagittal suture is the most common. The incidence of craniostenosis is 1 in every 1000 live births.

Signs and Symptoms

Craniostenosis results in deformity of the skull, which may lead to exophthalmus, optic atrophy, blindness, increased intracranial pressure, seizures, and mental retardation. Congenital cardiac defects and hydrocephalus may also be associated with craniostenosis. The shape of the deformed skull depends on the location of the suture that closes prematurely, since the cranial vault can compensate and grow only in areas with patent sutures. A skull radiograph and computed tomography will confirm the diagnosis.

Treatment

Craniectomy is the surgical procedure effective for the treatment of craniostenosis. This operation is usually performed as soon as the diagnosis is confirmed, since prompt correction has fewer complications and better cosmetic results. When multiple cranial sutures are involved, craniectomy is performed as a staged procedure. Craniectomy involves removing linear strips of bone on either side of the involved sutures and extending them across the adjoining normal cranial sutures. The adjacent periosteum is stripped widely to retard new bone formation.

Management of Anesthesia

The possibility of increased intracranial pressure must be considered in children with craniostenosis. Nevertheless, most of these children have normal intracranial pressure, and induction of anesthesia with intravenous administration of thiopental, followed by succinylcholine or a short- or intermediate-acting nondepolarizing muscle relaxant to facilitate intubation of the trachea, is an acceptable approach. The selection of drugs for maintenance of anesthesia should consider the likelihood that the surgeon will infiltrate the incision area with a local anesthetic solution containing epinephrine to minimize the blood loss associated with skin incision. Continuous monitoring of arterial blood pressure through a catheter in a peripheral artery is useful. Sudden and rapidly exsanguinating blood loss from the longitudinal sinus is possible during craniectomy. Most of the blood loss, however, occurs during bone stripping and is gradual. Since most of these patients are positioned prone, care should be taken to prevent pressure damage to the face and eyes. The patient is often tilted into a slight head-up position to minimize blood loss from venous oozing. Depending on the degree of tilt and area of surgery, intraoperative venous air embolism is a distinct possibility; precautions should be taken to prevent, recognize, and acutely treat such an episode.

Postoperatively, blood is likely to ooze into the wound, and these patients often need additional transfusions of blood. They should be closely monitored for the onset of hypotension or of localizing neurologic signs indicative of an epidural hematoma.

Epilepsy

Causes of epilepsy in children are often unknown, but recognized etiologies include metabolic disorders (phenylketonuria, hypoglycemia, kernicterus, tuberous sclerosis) and organic cerebral disorders (brain tumor, cerebral injury) (see Chapter 17). The Lennox-Gastaut syndrome is a severe epileptic encephalopathy (multiple types of seizures) that affects children and constitutes about 5% of childhood epilepsies. It is difficult to control seizures in these patients, even with multiple anticonvulsant drugs, and progressive mental retardation is likely.

Trisomy-21

Trisomy-21 (Down syndrome) occurs in about 0.15% of live births. About 80% of conceptions with trisomy-21 terminate in spontaneous abortion. The abnormality in these patients is due to the presence of an extra (trisomy) twenty-first chromosome. The risk of having a child with trisomy-21 increases with maternal age. For example, the 20-year-old mother has a risk of about 1 in 2000, but the risk increases to about 1 in 400 by age 35, and to 1 in 40 for mothers older than age 45.

Signs and Symptoms

Children with trisomy-21 are readily recognized by their characteristic flat facies with oblique palpebral fissures (hence the old term "mongolism"), single palmar crease (simian crease), and dysplastic middle phalanx of the fifth finger. Several features alter the upper airway in these children. For example, the nasopharynx is narrow, and the tonsils and adenoids unusually large. The tongue is normal at birth but later becomes enlarged due to hypertrophy of the papillae. To compensate for their restricted airways, these children habitually hold their mouths open, with their tongues slightly protruding. Chronic upper airway obstruction, which may lead to arterial hypoxemia, is a result of airway changes characteristic of trisomy-21.

Congenital heart disease occurs in about 40% of patients with trisomy-21. Endocardial cushion defects account for about one-half of the total, and ventricular septal defects occur in about one-fourth of these patients. Other abnormalities include tetralogy of Fallot, patent ductus arteriosus, and atrial septal defect of the secundum type. Surgical correction of congenital heart disease in children with trisomy-21 is associated with increased morbidity (postoperative atelectasis and pneumonia) and mortality, presumably due to increased susceptibility to recurrent infections, and an increased incidence

of co-existing pulmonary hypertension. It has been suggested that impaired development of alveoli and of the pulmonary vasculature, combined with arterial hypoxemia due to chronic upper airway obstruction, predisposes patients with trisomy-21 to preoperative pulmonary hypertension and postoperative pulmonary complications.[57] Congenital duodenal atresia occurs 300 times more frequently in patients with trisomy-21. Microcephaly and small brain mass may be present. Mental retardation in noninstitutionalized patients tends to be mild to moderate, and measurement of social and vocational adjustment tends to be within the low-normal range. Behavioral traits are subject to great individual variability, but infants with trisomy-21 are most often described as being good babies. Later, they are often characterized as content, good-natured, and affectionate. They may also be noted for their extreme stubbornness.

Oblique palpebral fissures and the presence of Brushfield spots (light-colored slightly elevated spots near the periphery of the iris) are characteristic of the eyes in a patient with trisomy-21. There is a high incidence of cataract and strabismus, often necessitating surgical correction. Otitis media and hearing loss are common, necessitating frequent ear examinations and myringotomies.

The skin appears to be too large for the skeleton, especially at the wrists and ankles. Furthermore, these patients are frequently obese. Both factors tend to make venous cannulation more difficult than in average pediatric patients.

Numerous musculoskeletal changes are noted in patients with trisomy-21. For example, about 20% of these patients have an asymptomatic dislocation of the atlas on the axis. Although spinal cord compression is rare, this potential hazard must be remembered if the head and neck are forcefully manipulated during intubation of the trachea.[58] Screening for atlantoaxial instability includes a lateral radiograph of the neck in a flexed, extended, and neutral position. If the distance between the anterior arch of the atlas and the adjacent odontoid process exceeds 5 mm, the diagnosis of atlantoaxial instability is likely.[58] Posterior cervical spine fusion is required for any patient who is symptomatic from this subluxation.

Most hematologic parameters are within normal limits, although polycythemia has been observed. Leukemia occurs in 1% of patients, but an increased incidence of other malignancies is not observed. The plasma concentration of norepinephrine is normal, and the sympathetic nervous system responds appropriately to stress. The pharmacologic response to atropine is unusual in that mydriasis occurs more rapidly in these patients, although the degree and duration of pupillary dilation is normal. Furthermore, cardiovascular responses to atropine are not altered. Thyroid function is normal in these patients.

Management of Anesthesia

Preoperative medication of a patient with trisomy-21 may include an anticholinergic drug, such as atropine or glycopyrrolate, to reduce upper airway secretions. As with other patients with mental retardation, responses to sedatives are unpredictable. Occasionally, a small dose of ketamine injected intramuscularly will facilitate preparation for induction of anesthesia in an obstinate patient. Patency of the upper airway may be difficult to maintain after the patient loses consciousness, reflecting the short neck, small mouth, narrow nasopharynx, and large tongue characteristic of these patients. Nevertheless, tracheal intubation is usually not difficult, keeping in mind that asymptomatic dislocation of the atlas on the axis is present in about 20% of these patients. In the absence of congenital heart disease, most commonly used inhalation or intravenous techniques of general anesthesia are acceptable. Otherwise, the selection of anesthetic drugs is influenced by the pathophysiology of the congenital cardiac lesion (see Chapter 3).

Neurofibromatosis

Neurofibromatosis is a congenital progressive disease of supportive tissues of the nervous system, with an incidence of 1 in every 3000 live births (see Chapter 17). It is estimated that neurofibromatosis will develop in 40% of children with an affected parent.

Reye Syndrome

Reye syndrome, or acute encephalopathy with fatty infiltration of the viscera, causes death because of diffuse cerebral edema, ultimately resulting in brain infarction and herniation. Management of the patient with Reye syndrome is directed toward monitoring and control of intracranial pressure, until natural resolution of the disease process occurs.[59]

Signs and Symptoms
Most cases of Reye syndrome develop in preteen children, after a 3- to 7-day prodromal viral illness involving the respiratory or gastrointestinal tract, or both. Protracted vomiting or neurologic signs associated with increased intracranial pressure herald the onset of Reye syndrome. At the initial physical examination, the child displays a mild fever, tachycardia, tachypnea, and hepatomegaly. Neurologic examination indicates either a lethargic person or a combative one, with hyperactive tendon reflexes. Serial neurologic examinations may demonstrate rapid deterioration in neurologic status.

Laboratory abnormalities include an elevated plasma concentration of liver transaminase enzymes and ammonia. Prothrombin and partial thromboplastin times are prolonged. The plasma glucose concentration is often decreased. Respiratory alkalosis is a frequent finding on measurement of the arterial blood gases and pH. Examination of cerebrospinal fluid typically shows no cellular or protein abnormalities, and glucose concentrations parallel plasma glucose levels.

The brain and liver are the principal organs affected in Reye syndrome, although the kidneys, pancreas, and skeletal muscles may be involved as well. Clinical symptoms and biochemical derangements indicate that both the liver and brain are already injured by the time the patient is first examined. Signs of injury to these organs progress for 3 to 6 days and then resolve rapidly, if cerebral edema does not result in death. A confirmatory liver biopsy is not recommended, in view of the coagulation abnormalities.

Etiology
Reye syndrome is found predominantly in patients younger than 10 years of age.[60] Almost all cases are associated with a prodromal viral illness. Influenza A and B and varicella are the most frequently associated viral infections, but more than a dozen others have also been implicated. There is a striking association between the use of salicylates during these viral illnesses and the development of Reye syndrome. Since discovery of this association and appropriate warnings about the use of salicylates, there has been a steady decline in the incidence of Reye syndrome. Cases associated with influenza tend to be clustered in midwinter. By contrast, varicella-associated cases tend to be sporadic and occur throughout the year. Retrospective studies of autopsies indicate that this may be a relatively new disease, as very few cases compatible with this diagnosis are found in the literature before 1950.

Treatment
Treatment of a mild case of Reye syndrome (plasma ammonia concentration less than 100 $\mu M \cdot L^{-1}$) is directed toward the reversal of associated metabolic derangements. For example, management of these patients includes the administration of intravenous fluids, vitamin K if the prothrombin time is prolonged, oral neomycin, and lactulose.

Treatment of a severe case of Reye syndrome (plasma ammonia concentration greater than 100 $\mu M \cdot L^{-1}$) is similar to that for a patient with increased intracranial pressure (see Chapter 17). Therapeutic and monitoring measures include intubation of the trachea, mechanical ventilation of the lungs, placement of an intracranial pressure monitor, insertion of a central venous or pulmonary artery catheter, and the introduction of a catheter into a peripheral artery. These measures are initiated in the operating room. Intubation of the trachea is performed after intravenous administration of thiopental and a muscle relaxant (succinylcholine questionable, in view of its ability to elevate intracranial pressure transiently) plus hyperventilation of the lungs to lower the $PaCO_2$ to 20 to 25 mmHg. After tracheal intubation, a burr hole is created for placement of a transducer to monitor intracranial pressure. The goal is to maintain intracranial pressure below 15 mmHg and cerebral perfusion pressure above 50 mmHg. Placement of a central venous or pulmonary artery catheter is often accomplished through the basilic vein of the arm, to circumvent the need for the head-down position, which would be necessitated by the use of the subclavian or internal jugular vein. It must be appreciated that even transient head-down positioning may result in sustained increases in intracranial pressure.

Cerebral perfusion pressure may become inadequate because of a decrease in mean arterial blood pressure. The differential diagnosis includes decreased intravascular fluid volume; myocardial depression or vasodilation from barbiturates, or both, as used to lower intracranial pressure; and vasodilation from septic shock. In this situation, measurement of thermodilution cardiac output and cardiac filling pressures by means of a pulmonary artery catheter is useful in making the correct diagnosis and instituting proper therapy. For example, a continuous infusion of dopamine or dobutamine may be necessary to improve cardiac output and restore mean arterial blood pressure to an acceptable level.

Treatment of severe Reye syndrome can be gradually withdrawn when intracranial pressure remains below 15 mmHg for 36 to 48 hours. Intensive treatment of the patient with Reye syndrome, including barbiturate coma and occasionally bifrontal craniectomy, appears to have substantially reduced the mortality associated with this disease. Patients who survive Reye syndrome are likely to recover completely, with no permanent metabolic or neurologic sequelae.

CRANIOFACIAL ABNORMALITIES

Craniofacial abnormalities are of consequence to patients because of cosmetic appearance. Indeed, these patients will often present for major reconstructive surgical procedures. In addition, these abnormalities are important because they may be associated with airway obstruction. Craniofacial abnormalities likely to require surgical correction include (1) cleft lip and palate; (2) mandibular hypoplasia as associated with Pierre Robin, Treacher Collins, and Goldenhar syndromes; and (3) hypertelorism.

Cleft Lip and Palate

Cleft lip and palate, considered together, constitute the third most common congenital anomaly requiring surgical correction at an early age. About 50% of patients have cleft lip and palate, and 14% of patients with cleft lip (with or without cleft palate) and 33% with cleft palate have associated congenital anomalies, which may include congenital heart disease. Infants with cleft lip and palate have problems with deglutition and frequently experience pulmonary aspiration. Furthermore, the incidence of upper respiratory tract infections is increased, resulting in chronic otitis media. Anemia is often present, reflecting poor nutrition due to feeding problems.

Treatment
Surgical treatment of cleft lip (cheiloplasty) is based on variations of a Z-plasty. Treatment of cleft palate (palatoplasty) is performed by midline closure of the cleft, after adequate mobilization of the tissues of the hard and soft palate with bilateral relaxing incisions. Pushback palatoplasty is a procedure performed to add length to the soft palate with a local soft tissue flap. Posterior pharyngeal flap is another procedure, wherein a flap of mucosa and muscle is raised from the posterior pharyngeal wall and attached to the posterior aspect of the soft palate. Cheiloplasty is usually performed when the infant is 2 to 3 months of age, but palatoplasty is delayed until the infant is about 18 months of age.

Management of Anesthesia
Induction of anesthesia for children with cleft lip or cleft palate, or both, depends on the degree of airway abnormality. For example, induction of anesthesia for the patient with no other airway anomalies can be safely accomplished by intravenous administration of a barbiturate or a comparable induction drug, followed by a muscle relaxant to facilitate intubation of the trachea. Conversely, a volatile anesthetic and intubation of the trachea during spontaneous ventilation are recommended for children with associated anomalies such as Pierre Robin syndrome. In an infant with a large cavernous defect of the palate, intubation of the trachea may be difficult, if the blade of the laryngoscope slips into the cleft, presenting problems in manipulating the blade. Insertion of a small piece of gauze or dental roll to fill the gap will reduce the likelihood of this problem. The tracheal tube should be taped to the lower lip in the midline, to minimize distortion of facial anatomy. The use of a preformed tracheal tube (RAE tube) reduces the likelihood of tracheal tube occlusion by the palate retractor during palatoplasty.

Maintenance of anesthesia is most often accomplished with a volatile anesthetic plus nitrous oxide. The presence of associated congenital heart disease may influence the selection of anesthetic drugs and muscle relaxants, as well as the management of ventilation. In addition, the selection of a volatile anesthetic should consider the likelihood that the surgical site will be infiltrated with a local anesthetic solution containing epinephrine. Nevertheless, in contrast to adults, children seem to tolerate high doses of epinephrine without the development of cardiac dysrhythmias during general anesthesia.[61] A high index of suspicion for accidental dislodgement of the tube from the trachea must be maintained during the operative procedure. Capnography is a useful monitor for confirmation of continued tracheal placement of the tube during intraoral surgery. Conjunctivitis and corneal abrasions are hazards; because of this possibility, the eyes are often lubricated with ophthalmic ointment and protected with eye covers. Blood loss requiring transfusion is uncommon during cheiloplasty or palatoplasty.

Postoperative airway problems are common after palatoplasty.[62] For this reason, a suture may be placed through the middle of the tongue and taped to the cheek. In case of airway obstruction, the tongue can be pulled forward with the suture and patency of the upper airway reestablished. Children with other anomalies associated with small oral cavities may also have significant postoperative airway obstruction because of surgical edema. Tracheal intubation for 48 to 72 hours after surgery may be necessary.

Mandibular Hypoplasia

Mandibular hypoplasia is a prominent feature of Pierre Robin, Treacher Collins, and Goldenhar syndromes. In these syndromes, the small mandible leaves little room for the tongue and makes the larynx appear to be anterior. Therefore, upper airway obstruction and difficult intubation of the trachea are likely to result.

Pierre Robin Syndrome

Pierre Robin syndrome consists of micrognathia, usually accompanied by glossoptosis (posterior displacement of the tongue), and cleft palate. Mandibular hypoplasia may be responsible for displacement of the tongue into the pharynx, which subsequently prevents fusion of the palate. Acute upper airway obstruction can occur in the neonate or infant with Pierre Robin syndrome. Feeding problems, failure to thrive, and cyanotic episodes are other early complications of this syndrome. Associated congenital heart disease is frequent. Fortunately, sufficient mandibular growth during early childhood markedly reduces the degree of airway problems in later years.

Treacher Collins Syndrome

Treacher Collins syndrome is the most common of the mandibulofacial dysotoses. Inheritance of this syndrome is as an autosomal dominant trait with variable expression. A lethal prenatal defect occurs frequently, as fetal wastage is common in affected families. Miller syndrome has facial features similar to that of Treacher Collins syndrome as well as severe deformities of the extremities.

Micrognathia results in early airway problems similar to those experienced by the infant with Pierre Robin syndrome. About 30% of children with Treacher Collins syndrome have an associated cleft palate. Congenital heart disease, particularly ventricular septal defect, frequently accompanies this syndrome. Other features include malar hypoplasia, colobomas (notching of the lower eyelids), and an antimongoloid slant of the palpebral fissures. Ear tags and gross deformities of the external ear canals and ossicular chain are common. Mental retardation is not a primary feature of Treacher Collins syndrome but may result from hearing loss. Intubation of the trachea, as in the infant with Pierre Robin syndrome, is difficult and sometimes impossible, especially once full dentition has been achieved. A patient with Treacher Collins syndrome may present for upper airway management, palatoplasty, treatment of chronic otitis media, and correction of a congenital heart defect. In addition, some patients with Treacher Col-

lins syndrome will undergo extensive craniofacial osteotomies for correction of cosmetic deformities (see the section, Hypertelorism).

Goldenhar Syndrome

Goldenhar syndrome is characterized by unilateral mandibular hypoplasia. Associated anomalies include eye, ear, and vertebral abnormalities on the affected side. Ease of tracheal intubation is highly variable. Some patients present little difficulty for intubation of the trachea, whereas for other patients intubation is extremely difficult.

Management of Anesthesia

Management of anesthesia for the patient with Pierre Robin, Treacher Collins, or Goldenhar syndrome begins with evaluation of the upper airway and formulation of a plan for intubation of the trachea. In addition, preoperative assessment should focus on the cardiovascular system and on the level of hemoglobin. Some patients with chronic airway obstruction experience repeated arterial hypoxemia and develop pulmonary hypertension.

The inclusion of an anticholinergic drug in the preoperative medication is recommended to reduce upper airway secretions. Opioids and other ventilatory depressants are often avoided in the preoperative medication. Oral administration of an H-2 receptor antagonist may be a logical addition to the preoperative regimen in infants and children at risk of aspiration during induction of anesthesia and intubation of the trachea. Several approaches to intubation of the trachea may be considered, but alternative methods must be immediately available, including facilities for emergency bronchoscopy, cricothyrotomy, or tracheostomy. Attempts at direct laryngoscopy may be preceded by intravenous administration of atropine, to minimize the likelihood of vagal stimulation and resultant bradycardia. Preoxygenation before initiation of direct laryngoscopy is recommended. Administration of a muscle relaxant to these patients is not recommended until mechanical ventilation of the lungs through a tracheal tube is established. Awake intubation of the trachea can sometimes be accomplished by either the oral or nasal routes after adequate topical anesthesia has been achieved. Awake intubation of the trachea may produce undue trauma to the upper airway and does not eliminate the risk of pulmonary aspiration. More often, intubation of the trachea is accomplished after induction of anesthesia with a volatile anesthetic, provided that a patent upper airway can be maintained until an adequate depth of anesthesia is attained. Spontaneous ventilation is desirable during induction of anesthesia, to ensure continuous airway control and to avoid inflating the child's stomach with air. Direct laryngoscopy should not be attempted until a sufficient depth of anesthesia has been established. Transtracheal injection of lidocaine will reduce the risk of laryngospasm during laryngoscopy. Forward traction on the tongue may facilitate maintenance of a patent upper airway until a sufficient depth of anesthesia can be obtained. Blind nasal intubation of the trachea may also be performed. Tracheal intubation with the aid of a fiberoptic bronchoscope is an alternative technique for tracheal intubation of older children. The laryngeal mask airway may be an alternative when tracheal intubation is impossible.[63] Tracheostomy during local anesthesia may be required when all other attempts to maintain the airway have failed. Tracheostomy in these children may be technically difficult, however, and susceptible to immediate and delayed complications. Certainly, the risks of pneumothorax, bleeding, air embolism, and poor positioning of the tracheostomy site are increased in a struggling child.

Extubation of the trachea after surgery should be delayed until these patients are fully awake and alert. In addition, equipment for reintubation must be immediately available.

Hypertelorism

Hypertelorism is an increased distance between the eyes and is associated with many craniofacial anomalies, such as Crouzon's disease and Apert syndrome. Crouzon's disease consists of hypertelorism, craniostenosis, shallow orbits with marked proptosis, and midface hypoplasia. Apert syndrome is characterized by essentially the same features, with the addition of syndactyly of all extremities. Other anomalies associated with hypertelorism are cleft palate, synostosis of the cervical spine, hearing loss, and mental retardation. In actuality, hypertelorism is representative of many craniofacial disorders amenable to facial reconstructive surgery.

Treatment

Correction of major craniofacial deformities may involve mandibular osteotomies, craniotomy with wide exposure of the frontal lobes, maxillary osteotomies with forward displacement of the maxilla, medial displacement of the orbits, and multiple rib grafts. Such complex operations may require several hours for completion and involve more than 100 separate surgical steps. Surgical correction is often performed in infancy, before ossification of the facial bones occurs.

Management of Anesthesia

Management of anesthesia for craniofacial surgery in children with hypertelorism is a complex undertaking that begins with meticulous preoperative assessment and preparation and extends into the postoperative period for several days. Craniofacial surgery should be attempted only by a qualified team of physicians, under ideal circumstances. There are many potential problems and anesthetic considerations (Table 32-12).

Management of the patient's airway must not interfere with exposure required to perform the corrective surgery. Predict-

Table 32-12.   Anesthetic Considerations in Management of Craniofacial Surgery

Difficult tracheal intubation vs. elective tracheostomy
Excessive blood loss
Hypothermia
Intracranial hypertension
Corneal abrasions
Invasive monitoring
Postoperative mechanical ventilation of the lungs

ably, intubation of the trachea may be difficult. Intraoperatively, the tracheal tube may become dislodged or kinked during maxillary advancement, mandibular osteotomy, or repositioning of the head and neck. In addition, the tracheal tube may be displaced into a main stem bronchus when the neck is flexed, or the tube may be accidently cut by the osteotome. Dry or inadequately humidified inspired gases are likely to lead to mucous plugs in the tracheal tube during these long operations, especially if a small-diameter tube is required.

Establishment of a tracheostomy 3 days before operation is an attractive alternative to translaryngeal intubation of the trachea for some patients. Advantages include reliable control of the airway during and after the operative procedure. In addition, reinstitution of anesthesia is easily accomplished, should it be necessary. Furthermore, performance of the tracheostomy 3 days earlier reduces the likelihood of complications (bleeding, pneumothorax, and subcutaneous emphysema) on the day of the corrective surgery.

Blood loss generally occurs in a steady ooze from multiple osteotomies and bone graft donor sites, averaging about 1.2 blood volumes. Quantitation of blood loss is difficult because of diffuse oozing. Measurement of serial hematocrits, central venous pressure, and urine output are helpful for estimating blood loss and guiding intravenous fluid replacement. The availability of appropriate amounts of whole blood, platelets, and fresh frozen plasma should be confirmed before surgery. Intravenous catheters must be of sufficient number and diameter to permit rapid transfusion of blood.

Blood loss may be reduced by positioning the patient in a 15- to 20-degree head-up position. In addition, controlled hypotension, using nitroprusside during phases of surgery when major hemorrhage is anticipated, is useful. Mean arterial blood pressure, as measured at the level of the circle of Willis, should probably not be decreased below about 50 mmHg during controlled hypotension. Blood must be filtered; warmed; and, if given rapidly to small children, accompanied by calcium gluconate (1 to 2 mg IV for every milliliter of blood infused), to decrease the possibility of citrate intoxication.

Complex craniofacial reconstruction averages 14 hours. Hypothermia during these lengthy operations can be minimized by placing the patient on a warming blanket; warming intravenous fluids and blood; and using warmed, humidified inspired gases. Pressure necrosis and nerve injuries can be minimized by careful positioning and padding, with emphasis on avoiding traction on the patient's brachial plexus. Despite these precautions, peripheral nerve injury may still occur (especially ulnar neuropathy) in the absence of an obvious explanation (see Chapter 17). Venous stasis can be minimized by wrapping the legs with elastic bandages.

Hyperventilation of the lungs to maintain a $PaCO_2$ of 30 to 35 mmHg; maintenance of the head-up position; and administration of furosemide, mannitol, and corticosteroids are used to minimize brain swelling. Free water is limited by administering 5% dextrose in lactated Ringer's solution, at a rate of 4 $ml\cdot kg^{-1}\cdot h^{-1}$. An anesthetic technique that minimizes brain blood volume (nitrous oxide plus an opioid) is useful. Intraoperative brain swelling can be minimized by continuous drainage of lumbar cerebrospinal fluid. Many reconstructive procedures are extracranial, and cerebral edema is not a consideration.

Corneal abrasions are likely in a patient when ocular proptosis is pronounced. Therefore, eye ointment should be used and the eyelids sutured closed. In addition, ocular or orbital manipulations can evoke the oculocardiac reflex. Release of pressure on the orbits, or administration of a small dose of atropine, will rapidly block the reflex.

In addition to routine monitors, a catheter placed in a peripheral artery for continuous measurement of blood pressure is mandatory. Blood from the arterial catheter also permits determination of blood gases, pH, hematocrit, electrolytes, and plasma osmolarity. A central venous pressure catheter and a Foley catheter are helpful for evaluation of the adequacy of intravenous fluid replacement. An end-tidal carbon dioxide monitor is useful for following the adequacy of ventilation and prompt recognition of dislodgment of the tube from the trachea.

Postoperatively, the entire head may be wrapped in a pressure dressing, through which only the tracheal tube protrudes. It is likely that the mouth will be wired shut. Pharyngeal bleeding, laryngeal edema, and increased intracranial pressure may be present. Therefore, no attempt need be made to reverse opioid or muscle relaxant effects at the end of the operation. Indeed, mechanical ventilation of the lungs should be maintained for at least the first night, and often for several days postoperatively.

DISORDERS OF THE UPPER AIRWAY

Numerous pathologic processes may involve the upper airway and respiratory tract of the pediatric patient (Table 32-13).

Table 32-13.   Disorders of the Pediatric Upper Airway

Epiglottitis (supraglottitis)
Laryngotracheobronchitis
Postintubation laryngeal edema
Foreign body aspiration
Laryngeal papillomatosis
Lung abscess

Epiglottitis

Epiglottitis is a short-lived disease that usually presents with characteristic signs and symptoms[64] (Table 32-14). At times, however, classic signs and symptoms are not present, and it may be difficult to differentiate epiglottitis from laryngotracheobronchitis. Epiglottitis can be fatal if upper airway obstruction is not treated promptly. Edema of supraglottic tissues as well as the epiglottis is the reason some prefer the designation of this disease as supraglottitis rather than epiglottitis.

Signs and Symptoms

Classically, children with epiglottitis are 2 to 6 years of age and present with a history of acute difficulty in swallowing, as well as high fever and inspiratory stridor. These signs and symptoms have usually developed over a period of less than 24 hours. In addition, there may be excessive drooling, a muffled voice, neutrophilia, and the characteristic posture of sitting upright and leaning forward. In fact, a change in this posture may cause more airway obstruction. A lateral radiograph of the neck may demonstrate swelling of the epiglottis and aryepiglottic folds. Nevertheless, taking the time to perform the radiograph is not an option if the child is in respiratory distress or if the clinical diagnosis is evident. The definitive diagnosis of epiglottitis is made in the operating room during direct laryngoscopy for intubation of the trachea. The etiologic agent of epiglottitis is most often *Haemophilus influenzae*.

Treatment

It is mandatory that the child with suspected epiglottitis be admitted to the hospital. The history can be quickly obtained and the child examined for signs of upper airway obstruction. An attempt to visualize the epiglottis should not be undertaken until the child is in the operating room and preparations are completed for intubation of the trachea and for possible emergency tracheostomy. It should be remembered that total upper airway obstruction can occur at any time, especially with instrumentation of the upper airway, perhaps reflecting glottic obstruction by the edematous epiglottis, laryngospasm from aspirated saliva, and respiratory muscle fatigue. A physician skilled in intubation of the trachea and positive-pressure ventilation of the lungs with a face mask should accompany the child at all times.

Table 32-14.   Clinical Features of Epiglottitis (Supraglottitis) and Laryngotracheobronchitis

	Epiglottitis	Laryngotracheobronchitis
Age group affected	2–6 years	≤2 years
Incidence	Accounts for 5% of children with stridor	Accounts for about 80% of children with stridor
Etiologic agent	Bacterial (*Haemophilus influenzae*)	Viral
Onset	Rapid over 24 hours	Gradual over 24–72 hours
Signs and symptoms	Inspiratory stridor Pharyngitis Drooling Fever (often >39°C) Lethargic to restless Insists on sitting up and leaning forward Tachypnea Cyanosis	Inspiratory stridor Croupy cough Rhinorrhea Fever (rarely >39°C)
Laboratory	Neutrophilia	Lymphocytosis
Lateral radiograph of the neck	Swollen epiglottis	Narrowing of the subglottic area
Treatment	Oxygen Urgent intubation of the trachea or tracheostomy during general anesthesia Fluids Antibiotics Corticosteroids(?)	Oxygen Aerosolized racemic epinephrine Humidity Fluids Corticosteroids Intubation of the trachea for severe airway obstruction

Definitive treatment of epiglottitis includes the use of appropriate antibiotics and a secured airway, until inflammation of the epiglottis has subsided. Ampicillin is the antibiotic of choice, although chloramphenicol is required for ampicillin-resistant *Haemophilus* strains. Corticosteroids are sometimes advocated to decrease edema, but their effectiveness is unproved. Translaryngeal intubation of the trachea during general anesthesia is the recommended approach for securing the airway.[64] Although epiglottitis is primarily a disease of children, there are an increasing number of reports of epiglottitis in adults. A difference between adult and pediatric epiglottitis may be the appearance of the tissues on physical examination. For example, most children with *H. influenzae* epiglottitis have a striking erythematous ("cherry red") swelling, whereas adults often have only a mild erythema or even a pale watery edematous appearance to the epiglottis. It has been recommended that adult patients be managed in the same manner as children with epiglottitis.[65,66] Nevertheless, there is also an opinion that an adult presenting with acute epiglottitis manifested only as sore throat or difficulty swallowing, or both, need not routinely be subjected to tracheal intubation.[67] Rather, these patients are closely monitored, and provision is made for tracheal intubation of tracheostomy, if respiratory distress becomes evident.

Management of Anesthesia

Induction and maintenance of anesthesia for intubation of the trachea is accomplished with a volatile anesthetic, most often halothane, in oxygen. A high inspired concentration of oxygen, permitted by the use of a volatile anesthetic, facilitates optimal oxygenation in these patients. Before induction of anesthesia, preparations are made for an emergency cricothyrotomy or tracheostomy, which may be required if airway obstruction occurs and translaryngeal intubation of the trachea is not possible. A catheter should be placed in a peripheral vein before induction of anesthesia; administration of atropine (6 to 10 μg·kg^{-1} IV) or glycopyrrolate (3 to 5 μg·kg^{-1} IV) may be useful.

Induction of anesthesia with a volatile anesthetic is begun with the child in the sitting position. After the onset of drowsiness, the child is placed supine, and ventilation of the lungs is assisted as necessary. When an adequate depth of anesthesia has been established, direct laryngoscopy is performed, and a tube is placed in the trachea. After successful intubation of the trachea, a thorough direct laryngoscopy is performed to confirm the diagnosis of epiglottitis. The next step is to replace the orotracheal tube with a nasotracheal tube under direct vision. A nasotracheal tube is preferred, as it is easier to secure and is more comfortable for an awake child. After nasotracheal intubation is accomplished, the child is allowed to awaken from the anesthetic. Usually, intubation of the trachea is required for 48 to 96 hours, although one report has indicated that 8 to 12 hours may be adequate.[68] In some cases, pulmonary edema, pericarditis, meningitis, or septic arthritis may accompany epiglottitis.[64]

Extubation of the trachea may be considered when the body temperature is no longer elevated and other signs such as a decreased neutrophil count have occurred. A clinical sign of resolution of the swelling of the epiglottis is the development of an air leak around the tracheal tube. Regardless of the clinical impression, it is best to take these children to the operating room and to perform direct laryngoscopy under general anesthesia, to confirm that inflammation of the epiglottis and other supraglottic tissues has resolved before extubation of the trachea.

Laryngotracheobronchitis

Laryngotracheobronchitis (croup) is a viral infection of the upper respiratory tract that typically afflicts children younger than 2 years of age[64] (Table 32-14). Parainfluenza, adenovirus, myxovirus, and influenza A virus have been implicated as causative agents. Laryngotracheobronchitis and epiglottitis share certain clinical features and at times are confused with each other[64] (Table 32-14).

Signs and Symptoms

Laryngotracheobronchitis, in contrast to epiglottitis, has a gradual onset over 24 to 72 hours. There are signs of upper respiratory tract infection, such as rhinorrhea and low-grade fever. Leukocyte counts are normal or only slightly elevated with a lymphocytosis. The cough has a characteristic "barking" or "brassy" quality.

Treatment

Treatment of laryngotracheobronchitis includes the use of supplemental oxygen, humidification of inspired gases, and aerosolized racemic epinephrine. For example, hourly treatment with aerosolized racemic epinephrine has been shown to alleviate airway obstruction secondary to laryngotracheobronchitis effectively, thereby reducing the need for intubation of the trachea.[69] Administration of a corticosteroid such as dexamethasone (0.5 to 1.0 mg·kg^{-1} IV) remains controversial therapy. Tracheal intubation is required if physical exhaustion occurs, as evidenced by an increased PaCO$_2$. If tracheal intubation is required, a smaller than normal tracheal tube should be used to minimize edema from intubation. In the event that a smaller than normal tracheal tube fits too tightly in the subglottic area, a tracheostomy may be required. Although laryngotracheobronchitis is generally a short-lived disease, there is evidence that patients with a history of this disease have hyperreactive airways.[70]

Postintubation Laryngeal Edema

Postintubation laryngeal edema is a potential complication of intubation of the trachea in all children, although the incidence is greatest in children between the ages of 1 and 4 years. Studies to delineate the etiology of postintubation laryngeal edema are lacking, but certain predisposing factors seem predictable. For example, mechanical trauma to the airway during intubation of the trachea and placement of a tube that produces a tight fit are possible causes.[71] Postintubation laryngeal edema may be less likely if the size of the tube in the trachea is such that an audible air leak occurs around it during positive airway pressures equivalent to 15 to 25 cm H$_2$O. Another predisposing factor to the development of postintubation laryngeal edema may be a co-existing upper respiratory infection, especially in a neonate or infant in whom any edema secondary to tracheal intubation results in a greater decrease in the cross-sectional area of the trachea, as compared with an older child. Indeed, the incidence of postintubation laryngeal edema seems to be increased in an infant with an upper respiratory infection whose trachea is intubated for an elective operation.[72]

Treatment of postintubation laryngeal edema is with humidification of inspired gases and aerosolized racemic epinephrine, administered hourly until symptoms subside. The dose of racemic epinephrine is 0.05 ml·kg^{-1} (maximum of 0.5 ml) in 2.0 ml saline. For most cases of postintubation laryngeal edema, one or two treatments will produce significant improvement. Reintubation of the trachea or tracheostomy should be required rarely. Although administration of dexamethasone (0.1 to 0.2 mg·kg^{-1} IV) as a single dose has been used for the prevention and treatment of this edema, its efficacy for this condition is undocumented. Indeed, in adults, dexamethasone administered intravenously 1 hour before extubation of the trachea does not influence the incidence of laryngeal edema.

Foreign Body Aspiration

Foreign body aspiration into the airway, with its resultant airway obstruction, can produce a wide range of responses. For example, complete obstruction at the level of the larynx or trachea can result in death from asphyxiation. At the opposite end of the spectrum, passage of a foreign body into a distal airway may elicit only mild symptoms, which may go unnoticed for years. Because of their curiosity and newfound abilities of locomotion, children 1 to 3 years of age are most susceptible to such aspiration.

Signs and Symptoms

Common clinical features of foreign body aspiration are cough, wheezing, and decreased air entry into the affected lung. The most frequent site of aspiration is the right bronchus. Foreign body aspiration often presents with the misdiagnosis of upper respiratory infection, asthma, or pneumonia. Radiographic evaluation provides direct evidence, if the aspirated object is radiopaque. If the aspirated object is radiolucent, indirect evidence can be obtained by demonstrating hyperinflation of the affected lung with atelectasis distal to the foreign body. A chest radiograph during exhalation may accentuate the hyperinflation. Measurement of the PaO_2 is helpful for evaluating the degree of right-to-left intrapulmonary shunting due to airway obstruction.

The type of foreign body aspirated can influence the clinical course. For example, nuts and certain vegetable materials are very irritating to the bronchial tree. Nuts also tend to result in multiple site aspiration. Inert substances, such as plastics, are relatively nonirritating and produce minimal inflammatory reaction.

Treatment

Treatment for an aspirated foreign body requires endoscopic removal. The improved technology of pediatric bronchoscopic equipment has increased the efficacy and safety of this procedure. It is best to remove the foreign body within 24 hours after aspiration. The risks of leaving the foreign body in the airway for longer than 24 hours include migration of the aspirated material, pneumonia, and residual pulmonary disease.

Management of Anesthesia

Few types of cases demand as much flexibility on the part of the anesthesiologist as does the child with an aspirated foreign body. Each case mandates individualization of the technique to fit the clinical situation. Techniques for induction of anesthesia will depend on the severity of airway obstruction. When airway obstruction is present, induction of anesthesia, using only a volatile anesthetic in oxygen, is useful. Induction of anesthesia with a barbiturate or a comparable induction drug, followed by inhalation of a volatile anesthetic, is acceptable if the airway is less tenuous. After an adequate depth of anesthesia has been attained, direct laryngoscopy is performed, and the larynx is sprayed with lidocaine (2 to 4 $mg \cdot kg^{-1}$). Topical anesthesia is effective in preventing laryngospasm when endoscopic manipulation is performed. The administration of atropine (6 to 10 $\mu g \cdot kg^{-1}$ IV) or glycopyrrolate (3 to 5 $\mu g \cdot kg^{-1}$ IV) is useful to reduce the likelihood of bradycardia from vagal stimulation during endoscopy. Muscle relaxants are best avoided during bronchoscopy, as spontaneous ventilation is desirable, providing greater flexibility and additional time for the endoscopist. Furthermore, positive airway pressure could contribute to distal migration of the foreign body, complicating its extraction. In addition, if the foreign body has produced a ball-valve phenomenon, the use of positive-pressure ventilation of the lungs could contribute to hyperinflation, and possibly pneumothorax. During bronchoscopy, anesthesia is maintained with a volatile anesthetic in oxygen. Ventilation through

the bronchoscope can be difficult because of the high resistance to gas flow imposed by the narrow bronchoscope and the large gas leak, which often occurs around the bronchoscope. Therefore, maintenance of spontaneous ventilation is again desirable. Skeletal muscle paralysis produced with succinylcholine or a short-acting nondepolarizing muscle relaxant may be required for removal of the bronchoscope and foreign body, if the object is too large to pass through the moving vocal cords.

Complications that may occur during bronchoscopy include airway obstruction, fragmentation of the foreign body, arterial hypoxemia, and hypercapnia. Trauma to the tracheobronchial tree from the foreign body and instrumentation can result in subglottic edema. After bronchoscopy, inhalation of aerosolized racemic epinephrine and intravenous administration of dexamethasone may reduce subglottic edema. A chest radiograph should be obtained after bronchoscopy for detection of atelectasis or pneumothorax. Postural drainage and chest percussion will enhance clearance of secretions and reduce the subsequent risk of infection.

Laryngeal Papillomatosis

Laryngeal papillomatosis is the most common benign laryngeal tumor of childhood. The likely cause is a tissue response to a virus. Malignant degeneration of juvenile papillomas is rare but can occur in older patients. A change in the character of the voice is the most common symptom of papillomatosis. Most children with papillomatosis present with symptoms before the age of 7 years. Some degree of airway obstruction is present in more than 40% of patients. Papillomas usually regress spontaneously at puberty.

Treatment

Various forms of treatment for laryngeal papillomatosis have been used, including surgical excision, cryosurgery, topical 5-fluorouracil, exogenous interferon, and laser ablation. Since the disease is ultimately self-limiting, the complications of therapy must be avoided. For example, seeding of the distal airways can occur after tracheostomy. Surgical therapy with laser coagulation has been useful. Because papillomas recur, frequent laser coagulation is required until spontaneous remission occurs.

Management of Anesthesia

Management of anesthesia for removal of laryngeal papillomas depends on the severity of airway obstruction. Awake intubation of the trachea is recommended for severe airway obstruction. Certainly, the child with severe airway obstruction should not receive a muscle relaxant in an attempt to facilitate intubation of the trachea. Indeed, in some patients, the glottic opening can be identified only with the child breathing spontaneously. A rigid bronchoscope should be readily available, as this may be the only means of securing an airway in some children. It should be appreciated that the degree of airway obstruction can vary greatly in the same patient between surgical procedures.

Induction and maintenance of anesthesia is often achieved with a volatile anesthetic delivered in a high inspired concentration of oxygen. Surgical therapy for papillomatosis, either by laser ablation or forceps excision, is usually done as a microlaryngoscopic procedure. During microlaryngoscopy, the vocal cords must be quiescent. Skeletal muscle paralysis or deep anesthesia, therefore, is required to produce acceptable operating conditions. A short- or intermediate-acting nondepolarizing muscle relaxant is useful for this purpose. A cuffed tracheal tube of a smaller than predicted diameter should be employed for intubation of the trachea. This will improve visualization of the glottis by the endoscopist. In some instances, an apneic oxygenation technique with temporary removal of the tracheal tube is required. For laser ablation of papillomas, the usual safety precautions concerning laser use should be observed. These precautions may include wrapping the tracheal tube with metallic tape, inflation of the tracheal tube cuff with saline, protection of the patient's face and eyes, and delivery of the lowest supplemental concentration of oxygen compatible with adequate oxygenation, keeping in mind that nitrous oxide may support combustion. After resection of papillomas, the tracheal tube should be removed only when the child is fully awake and laryngeal bleeding has ceased. After extubation of the trachea, inhalation of aerosolized racemic epinephrine and intravenous administration of dexamethasone may reduce subglottic edema.

Lung Abscess

Lung abscess in a child is most likely the result of inhalation of secretions containing disease-producing bacteria. In addition, bronchial obstruction by a tumor may result in a lung abscess distal to the airway obstruction.

Surgical excision of the abscess cavity is indicated for those cases that do not respond to antibiotic therapy. Nevertheless, surgical intervention introduces the risk of rupture of the lung abscess and flooding of the tracheobronchial tree with large amounts of purulent material. Flooding of the lungs can acutely impair ventilation and oxygenation and lead to abscess formation in previously uncontaminated portions of the lung. Isolation of the affected lobe or lung is desirable to minimize this risk. An appropriately sized double-lumen endobronchial tube or bronchial blocker, however, may not be available for use in children. The affected lobe can be effectively blocked with a Fogarty catheter, passed under direct vision through a ventilating bronchoscope.[74] After the Fogarty catheter balloon is inflated, a tracheal tube is positioned in the main stem bronchus of the normal lung. This procedure results in protection

of the normal lung and isolation of the affected lobe of the diseased lung. A high inspired concentration of oxygen is necessary, as one-lung anesthesia produces an increase in the magnitude of right-to-left intrapulmonary shunting, resulting in a decrease in the PaO_2. The $PaCO_2$ is not influenced by one-lung anesthesia if minute ventilation is maintained.

JEUNE SYNDROME

Jeune syndrome is an inherited autosomal recessive disorder that occurs in a neonatal form (asphyxiating thoracic dystrophy) and in a childhood form (diffuse interstitial fibrosis of the kidneys). In its neonatal form, the deformity of the thoracic wall prevents normal intercostal movement, and ventilatory failure ensues. Lung volumes are predictably decreased. Pulmonary hypoplasia and persistent pulmonary hypertension may be present. Even if normoxic at rest, these infants are susceptible to profound arterial hypoxemia when stimulated because of asynchronous rib and abdominal movements. Cor pulmonale is a sequela of chronic arterial hypoxemia. Hepatic fibrosis and myocardial dysfunction have also been observed.

These children may require anesthesia for thoracoplasty, renal transplantation, bronchoscopy, and tracheostomy.[75] Older children undergoing renal transplantation also have the typical thoracic deformity, although it is less severe than in a neonate. During the intraoperative period, peak airway pressure should be minimized to reduce the likelihood of barotrauma. The choice of drugs for anesthesia should include consideration of their impact on pulmonary, cardiovascular, and renal function. An infant undergoing thoracoplasty will require prolonged mechanical support of ventilation.

MALIGNANT HYPERTHERMIA

Malignant hyperthermia is an example of a pharmacogenetic disease. Susceptible patients possess a genetic predisposition for the development of this disease, which is not manifested until they are exposed to triggering agents, such as specific drugs or stressful environmental factors. There are currently three recognized modes of inheritance: autosomal dominant, autosomal recessive or multifactoral, and unclassified. The gene for malignant hyperthermia is located on human chromosome 19, which is also the genetic coding site for the calcium release channel of skeletal muscle sarcoplasmic reticulum (the ryanodine receptor).[76] It is presumed that a defect in the calcium release channel results in malignant hyperthermia susceptibility. Indeed, in swine, a single mutation in the ryanodine receptor gene can account for all cases of malignant hyperthermia. By contrast, a series of different mutations, or even a lack of linkage between malignant hyperthermia and mutations of the ryanodine receptor gene in some patients, indicates a heterogeneous genetic basis for the human syndrome.[76]

Susceptible patients should be thoroughly educated with respect to potential hazards and implications of malignant hyperthermia. Malignant hyperthermia has an estimated incidence of 1 in 12,000 pediatric anesthetics and 1 in 40,000 adult anesthetics. The incidence is higher when succinylcholine is used with other triggering agents.[77] The incidence has an apparent geographic variation, as it is more prevalent in certain areas of the United States. Malignant hyperthermia usually occurs in children and young adults but has been reported at the extremes of age, ranging from 2 months to 70 years. Two-thirds of susceptible patients manifest this syndrome during administration of their first anesthetic and the remaining one-third during administration of subsequent anesthetics.

Signs and Symptoms

Malignant hyperthermia is characterized by signs and symptoms of hypermetabolism (up to 10 times normal). The clinical features of this disorder are nonspecific and include tachycardia, tachypnea, arterial hypoxemia, hypercarbia, metabolic and respiratory acidosis, hyperkalemia, cardiac dysrhythmias, hypotension, skeletal muscle rigidity (trismus or masseter spasm) after the administration of succinylcholine, and increased body temperature.

The earliest signs of malignant hyperthermia are those related to enormous increases in metabolic rate.[78] Increased carbon dioxide production occurs early, emphasizing the value of continuous capnography. Tachycardia is also an early sign of the onset of malignant hyperthermia. Tachycardia reflects the release of epinephrine and norepinephrine, as well as metabolic and respiratory acidosis. Cardiac dysrhythmias, such as ventricular bigeminy, multifocal ventricular premature beats, and ventricular tachycardia, may also occur, especially when hyperkalemia is associated with this syndrome. Skin signs may vary from flushing, caused by vasodilation, to blanching, secondary to intense vasoconstriction.

Susceptible patients may exhibit spasm of the masseter muscles after administration of succinylcholine. This skeletal muscle spasm may be so severe that it is impossible to open the mouth to perform direct laryngoscopy for intubation of the trachea. Conversely, in other patients, drug-induced masseter muscle spasm is mild and transient, or even absent. It is currently recommended that signs of hypermetabolism (metabolic and respiratory acidosis, increased body temperature) should be awaited after masseter spasm is noted before a diagnosis of malignant hyperthermia is contemplated.[79] In the absence of other definitive signs of hypermetabolism, it does not seem justifiable to subject a patient to a skeletal muscle biopsy only on the basis of masseter spasm.[80] It has been suggested, however, that patients in whom masseter spasm develops have a 50% incidence of susceptibility to malignant

hyperthermia.[81,82] Generalized skeletal muscle rigidity during administration of an anesthetic that includes either halothane or succinylcholine, or both, may be a more specific predictor of malignant hyperthermia susceptibility than is masseter spasm after the administration of succinylcholine.[83] Skeletal muscle biopsies are positive for malignant hyperthermia susceptibility in all patients in whom plasma creatinine kinase (CPK) concentrations exceed 20,000 $IU \cdot L^{-1}$ after succinylcholine-induced masseter spasm.[81]

Body temperature elevation is often a late manifestation of malignant hyperthermia. Indeed, diagnosis of malignant hyperthermia should not depend on an increase in body temperature. Nevertheless, the increase in body temperature may be precipitous, increasing at a rate of 0.5°C every 15 minutes, and reaching levels as high as 46°C.

Analysis of arterial and central venous blood will reveal arterial hypoxemia, hypercarbia (100 to 200 mmHg), respiratory and metabolic acidosis (pH 7.15 to 6.80), and marked central venous oxygen desaturation. Hyperkalemia may occur early in the course of the disease, but after normothermia returns, the plasma potassium concentration may drop rapidly. The plasma concentration of transaminase enzymes and CPK will be markedly elevated, although peak levels may not occur for 12 to 24 hours after an acute episode. Plasma and urine myoglobin concentrations (gives urine a color similar to hemoglobin) are also elevated, reflecting massive rhabdomyolysis. Late complications of untreated malignant hyperthermia include disseminated intravascular coagulation, pulmonary edema, and acute renal failure. Central nervous system damage may manifest as blindness, seizures, coma, or paralysis.

Treatment

Successful treatment of malignant hyperthermia depends on early recognition of the diagnosis and institution of a preplanned therapeutic regimen (Table 32-15). Maintenance of appropriate equipment and drugs in a central location within the operating room area will save valuable time. Treatment of malignant hyperthermia can be divided into etiologic and symptomatic. Etiologic treatment is directed at correction of the underlying causative mechanism. Symptomatic therapy is directed toward maintenance of renal function and correction of hyperthermia, acidosis, and arterial hypoxemia.

Etiologic Treatment

Dantrolene, administered intravenously, is the only drug that is reliably effective for the treatment of malignant hyperthermia[76,84] (Table 32-15). Availability of intravenous dantrolene preparations has reduced mortality from malignant hyperthermia from over 70% to less than 5%. Treatment of an acute episode of malignant hyperthermia is with dantrolene (2 to 3

Table 32-15.   Treatment of Malignant Hyperthermia

Etiologic Treatment

Dantrolene (2–3 $mg \cdot kg^{-1}$ IV) as an initial bolus, followed with repeat doses every 5–10 minutes until symptoms are controlled (rarely need total dose >10 $mg \cdot kg^{-1}$)

Prevent recrudescence (dantrolene 1 $mg \cdot kg^{-1}$ IV every 6 hours for 72 hours)

Symptomatic Treatment

Immediately terminate inhaled anesthetics and conclude surgery as soon as possible

Hyperventilate the lungs with 100% oxygen

Initiate active cooling (iced saline 15 $ml \cdot kg^{-1}$ IV every 10 minutes, gastric lavage with iced saline, surface cooling)

Correct metabolic acidosis (sodium bicarbonate 1–2 $mEq \cdot kg^{-1}$ IV based on arterial pH)

Maintain urine output (hydration, mannitol 0.25 $g \cdot kg^{-1}$ IV, furosemide 1 $mg \cdot kg^{-1}$ IV)

Treat cardiac dysrhythmias (procainamide 15 $mg \cdot kg^{-1}$ IV)

Monitor in an intensive care unit (urine output, arterial blood gases, pH, electrolytes)

$mg \cdot kg^{-1}$ IV). This dose is repeated every 5 to 10 minutes to a maximum dose of 10 $mg \cdot kg^{-1}$, depending on the patient's temperature response. Typically, dantrolene (2 to 5 $mg \cdot kg^{-1}$ IV) is required for treatment of an acute episode. Occasionally, a dose greater than 10 $mg \cdot kg^{-1}$ IV may be needed. In addition, dantrolene should be continued in the postoperative period to prevent a possible recrudescence of malignant hyperthermia. One approach is to administer dantrolene (1 $mg \cdot kg^{-1}$ IV) every 6 hours for 72 hours after resolution of the acute episode.

Symptomatic Treatment

Symptomatic treatment for malignant hyperthermia includes immediate termination of the administration of the inhaled anesthetic and prompt conclusion of the surgical procedure (Table 32-15). Under no circumstances should the administration of a volatile anesthetic be continued with the false hope that anesthetic-induced vasodilation will aid in cooling or that high concentrations of these drugs will reduce the metabolic rate. The patient's lungs should be hyperventilated with 100% oxygen and active cooling initiated. Active cooling may be done with surface cooling and intracavitary lavage of the stomach and bladder with a cold saline solution. Intravenous saline solutions infused through peripheral intravenous catheters should also be cooled. Although rarely practical, cooling by extracorporeal circulation with a heat exchanger has been described.[85] Cooling is discontinued when body temperature decreases to 38°C. Other symptomatic therapy includes intravenous administration of sodium bicarbonate to correct metabolic acidosis and hyperkalemia, hydration with saline,

and maintenance of urine output at 2 $ml \cdot kg^{-1} \cdot h^{-1}$ with an osmotic or tubular diuretic. Administration of glucose with regular insulin helps drive potassium intracellularly and provides an exogenous energy source with which to replace depleted cerebral metabolic substrates. Failure to maintain diuresis may result in acute renal failure due to deposition of myoglobin in the renal tubules. Procainamide (15 $mg \cdot kg^{-1}$ IV) can be used for the treatment of ventricular dysrhythmias, which may occur during malignant hyperthermia.

After recovery from an acute episode of malignant hyperthermia, the patient should be closely monitored in an intensive care unit for up to 72 hours. Urine output, arterial blood gases, pH, and serum electrolyte concentrations should be determined frequently. It must be appreciated that malignant hyperthermia may recur in the intensive care unit, in the absence of obvious triggering events.[86]

Identification of Susceptible Patients

The advantage of detecting the patient who is susceptible to malignant hyperthermia before anesthesia is obvious. A detailed medical and family history, with particular reference to previous anesthetic experiences, should be obtained. Prior uneventful anesthetic experiences do not necessarily indicate that the patient is not susceptible. Environmental stress, a consistent trigger of malignant hyperthermia in animals, has also been reported in humans.[87] Therefore, a history of the patient's response to physical exertion may be helpful. Physical examination should focus on the musculoskeletal and cardiac systems. Two distinct myopathic syndromes result in an increased risk of malignant hyperthermia. The first type of myopathy features wasting of the distal ends of the vastus muscles and hypertrophy of the proximal femoris muscles of the thigh. The second myopathy features cryptorchidism, pectus carinatum, kyphosis, lordosis, ptosis, and hypoplastic mandible. The incidence of malignant hyperthermia is increased in patients with Duchenne muscular dystrophy (see Chapter 26). Malignant hyperthermia has also been reported in patients with Burkitt lymphoma, osteogenesis imperfecta, myotonia congenita, neuroleptic malignant syndrome, and myelomeningocele.[88] There is evidence of cardiac muscle involvement in patients who are susceptible to malignant hyperthermia. Cardiac findings include ventricular dysrhythmias and abnormal myocardial imaging with radionuclides.

CPK should be measured in the patient being evaluated for susceptibility to malignant hyperthermia. About 70% of patients susceptible to malignant hyperthermia have elevated resting plasma concentrations of CPK. By contrast, persons in some families with a susceptibility to malignant hyperthermia have normal CPK levels. Other conditions, such as muscular dystrophy and skeletal muscle trauma, also produce elevated CPK levels. For these reasons, measurement of the

CPK level is not a definitive screening test for malignant hyperthermia. Electromyographic changes are seen in 50% of patients susceptible to malignant hyperthermia. These findings include an increased incidence of polyphasic action potentials and fibrillation potentials.

A skeletal muscle biopsy with in vitro isometric contracture testing provides definitive confirmation of susceptibility to malignant hyperthermia. The biopsy is typically taken from the vastus muscle of the thigh, with the patient receiving local or regional anesthesia. Histologic changes in skeletal muscle from a malignant hyperthermia susceptible patient are not diagnostic. Instead, the skeletal muscle specimen must be subjected to isometric contracture testing under the influence of caffeine or halothane, or both. Caffeine and halothane produce exaggerated contracture of skeletal muscle from a patient susceptible to malignant hyperthermia. Since there is some overlap between normal and susceptible patients, an established laboratory should be employed.

There is anticipation that less invasive tests, such as genetic or in vivo phosphorus magnetic resonance imaging, may become useful.[89] Until the reliability of these tests is confirmed, however, muscle biopsy and contracture testing remains the definitive test. Furthermore, not all patients susceptible to malignant hyperthermia demonstrate a genetic linkage based on a mutation of the ryanodine receptor gene.[76]

Management of Anesthesia

No anesthetic regimen has been shown to be reliably safe for the patient who is susceptible to malignant hyperthermia. Nevertheless, certain guidelines should be followed in the management of these patients. Prophylaxis in a patient susceptible to malignant hyperthermia may be provided with the oral administration of dantrolene ($5 \text{ mg} \cdot \text{kg}^{-1}$) in three or four divided doses every 6 hours with the last dose 4 hours preoperatively. This regimen results in a therapeutic plasma concentration of dantrolene at induction of anesthesia for at least the next 6 hours[90] (Fig. 32-12). Alternatively, dantrolene ($2.4 \text{ mg} \cdot \text{kg}^{-1}$ IV) may be administered over 10 to 30 minutes as prophylaxis just prior to the induction of anesthesia and for continued protection, one-half the dose is repeated in 6 hours[91] (Fig. 32-13). Diuresis may accompany intravenous administration of dantrolene, reflecting the addition of mannitol to the dantrolene powder in an effort to make the solution isotonic. For this reason, it is recommended that the patient receiving intravenous dantrolene also have a urinary catheter in place.[92] Large doses of dantrolene administered acutely for prophylaxis against malignant hyperthermia may cause nausea, diarrhea, blurred vision, and skeletal muscle weakness. Drug-induced skeletal muscle weakness may be sufficient to interfere with adequate ventilation or protection of the lungs from aspiration of gastric fluid.[93] In the absence of signs of malignant hyperthermia intraoperatively, it is probably not necessary to continue administration of dantrolene into the postoperative period. Despite prophylaxis with dantrolene, malignant hyperthermia may still develop in an occasional susceptible patient.[94] In view of the potential adverse effects associated with dantrolene therapy, one report suggests that prophylactic use of dantrolene is not necessary in patients suspected to be susceptible to malignant hyperthermia, provided that all known triggering drugs are avoided.[95]

The patient susceptible to malignant hyperthermia should be well sedated before induction of anesthesia. Preoperative medication should not include an anticholinergic drug, to avoid confusion regarding heart rate changes or possible interference with normal body heat loss. All preparations for the treat-

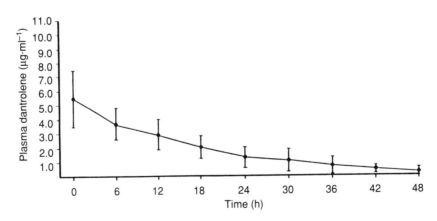

Fig. 32-12. Plasma dantrolene concentration (mean $\pm$ SD) at the induction of anesthesia (0) and for the next 48 hours in patients receiving a total dose of $5 \text{ mg} \cdot \text{kg}^{-1}$ orally in three or four divided doses every 6 hours, with the last dose administered 4 hours preoperatively. (From Allen GC, Cattran CB, Peterson RG, Lalande M. Plasma levels of dantrolene following oral administration in malignant hyperthermia-susceptible patients. Anesthesiology 1988;69:900–4, with permission.)

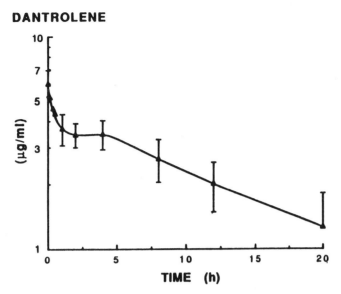

Fig. 32-13. Plasma concentration of dantrolene during the 20 hours following administration of dantrolene (2.4 mg·kg^{-1} IV) to 10 children. (From Lerman J, McLeod ME, Strong HA. Pharmacokinetics of intravenous dantrolene in children. Anesthesiology 1989;70:625–9, with permission.)

ment of malignant hyperthermia must be made before induction of anesthesia (see the section, Treatment). Drugs that can trigger malignant hyperthermia include volatile anesthetics and succinylcholine. Other drugs to be avoided include calcium and potassium. The administration of a calcium entry blocking drug in the presence of dantrolene has been associated with the development of hyperkalemia and myocardial depression.[96] Drugs considered safe for these patients include barbiturates, opioids, benzodiazepines, ketamine, droperidol, and nondepolarizing muscle relaxants (Table 32-16). Prolonged neuromuscular blockade in response to a nondepolariz-

ing muscle relaxant may occur in the patient susceptible to malignant hyperthermia who has been pretreated with dantrolene.[97] Nitrous oxide is probably a safe drug to administer to these patients, although its use has been implicated in the occurrence of malignant hyperthermia.[94] Conceivably, nitrous oxide could influence the course of malignant hyperthermia indirectly through its capacity to stimulate the sympathetic nervous system. Antagonism of nondepolarizing muscle relaxants has not been shown to trigger malignant hyperthermia in susceptible patients. Vasopressors, digitalis, and methylxanthines are acceptable drugs when specific indications for their use are present. No studies confirm that malignant hyperthermia can be triggered by residual concentrations of volatile anesthetics, especially halothane, delivered from a previously used anesthesia machine. Nevertheless, some conservative investigators have advocated the use of a dedicated machine that has never been used to deliver volatile anesthetics, for administration of anesthesia to patients deemed susceptible to malignant hyperthermia. A more practical and acceptable alternative would be to use a conventional anesthesia machine with (1) a disposable anesthesia breathing circuit and a fresh gas outlet hose; (2) new carbon dioxide absorbent; (3) vaporizers removed; and (4) continuous flow of oxygen at 10 L·min^{-1} for 5 to 20 minutes before use of the machine.[98]

Regional anesthesia is an acceptable selection for anesthesia for the patient who is susceptible to malignant hyperthermia. In the past, avoidance of amide local anesthetics was recom-

Table 32-16.   Nontriggering Drugs for Malignant Hyperthermia

Barbiturates
Opioids
Benzodiazepines
Propofol
Etomidate
Droperidol
Nitrous oxide (?)
Nondepolarizing muscle relaxants (? *d*-tubocurarine)
Anticholinesterases
Anticholinergics
Sympathomimetrics
Local anesthetics

mended, as it was believed that these drugs could trigger malignant hyperthermia in a susceptible patient. This opinion seems to be changing, however, and ester, as well as amide local anesthetics, are considered acceptable for production of regional or local anesthesia, as may be necessary for the performance of a skeletal muscle biopsy in these patients.[99] It must be appreciated that regional anesthesia may not protect against triggering of malignant hyperthermia due to stress in a susceptible patient. Therefore, anxiety should be alleviated by sedating these patients during regional anesthesia.

Children otherwise suitable for same-day discharge after elective surgical procedures may be admitted to the hospital for overnight observation solely because they are known or suspected to be susceptible to malignant hyperthermia. There is no evidence to support this practice. Indeed, discharge home after minor surgery is not associated with increased risk in these patients.[100]

FAMILIAL DYSAUTONOMIA

Familial dysautonomia (Riley-Day syndrome) is a rare inherited disorder of the central nervous system, found almost exclusively in children of Eastern European Jewish ancestry. Inheritance of this syndrome is as an autosomal recessive trait, with symptoms appearing in infancy or in early childhood. Approximately 50% of these children die by the age of 4 years, usually as a result of respiratory complications. Nevertheless, as a result of improved treatment of this disease, many afflicted children now survive to adulthood.

Signs and Symptoms

Dysfunction of the autonomic nervous system is the most apparent manifestation of familial dysautonomia. Vasomotor instability is characterized by sudden alterations in blood pressure, ranging from hypertension to hypotension. Orthostatic hypotension with syncope may occur and reflect either defective baroreceptor reflex activity or deficient release of norepinephrine, or both. Indeed, characteristic findings in these patients include failure of the heart rate to increase in response to a decrease in blood pressure and an absence of an increase in the circulating plasma concentration of norepinephrine in response to exercise or on assuming the standing position. Ventilatory responses to arterial hypoxemia and hypercarbia are also depressed. Episodes of hypertension and hyperthermia, often in response to emotional stress, are thought to reflect an exaggerated response to catecholamines (denervation hypersensitivity) and an inability to enlist compensatory parasympathetic nervous system responses. The presence of hypertension distinguishes this disease from Shy-Drager syndrome.

Pain perception is decreased to absent in the affected child. There may be a history of repeated episodes of unrecognized trauma. Split-thickness skin grafts have been harvested from these patients without anesthesia. Corneal anesthesia and the absence of tears predispose to corneal ulcerations. Taste and thermal discrimination are invariably defective, as evidenced by the inability of the patient to distinguish tap water from ice water. In this regard, the tongue is smooth due to the absence of fungiform papillae.

The gag reflex and esophageal motility are markedly impaired, predisposing these patients to recurrent pulmonary aspiration. A vomiting crisis characterized by convulsive retching that occurs as often as every 15 to 20 minutes over a period of 1 to 5 days, in association with hypertension and diaphoresis, is a common reason for hospitalization of the child with familial dysautonomia. Dehydration and pulmonary aspiration of vomitus may occur during these crises. Hematemesis complicates about 25% of these crises, for which surgical intervention may be necessary. Chlorpromazine (0.5 to 1 mg·kg^{-1} IM) may be useful for decreasing anxiety and blood pressure, while also acting as an antiemetic.

Temperature control in the child with familial dysautonomia is erratic. Early morning temperature may be 35°C or lower. Conversely, a mild infection may trigger a marked increase in body temperature and appearance of a febrile seizure. By contrast, a major infection may not be accompanied by a febrile response.

Kyphoscoliosis occurs in nearly 90% of these children, reflecting neuromuscular imbalance. Severe kyphoscoliosis may result in restrictive lung disease, culminating in arterial hypoxemia and pulmonary hypertension. About 40% of these patients have a history of epilepsy, most often attributed to fever. Emotional lability and immature dependent behavior are characteristic of these patients. Mild mental retardation may be secondary to chronic illness, motor incoordination, and sensory deprivation, rather than being a primary feature of the disease.

Management of Anesthesia

Preoperative assessment of the child with familial dysautonomia often includes evaluation of pulmonary function (arterial blood gases, pulmonary function tests), especially if surgery for correction of kyphoscoliosis is being planned. Recurrent aspiration may be accompanied by preoperative evidence of pneumonia. Fluid and electrolyte status are of special interest in the child with a recent history of protracted vomiting. Atropine as administered for preoperative medication does not prevent bradycardia or hypotension during induction of anesthesia in these patients. The use of an opioid in the preoperative medication is not recommended, since these children are relatively insensitive to pain. Furthermore, an opioid may serve to depress further an already blunted ventilatory response to arterial hypoxemia and hypercarbia.

Induction of anesthesia with conventional intravenous drugs is acceptable. Nitrous oxide plus a muscle relaxant are often sufficient for maintenance of anesthesia in patients who are relatively insensitive to pain. Nevertheless, fentanyl anesthesia has also been recommended in these patients.[101] Stimulation as associated with intubation of the trachea may result in exaggerated hypertension. In this regard, intermittent administration of a volatile anesthetic may be useful, keeping in mind that these drugs may produce precipitous hypotension.[101,102] Use of a nondepolarizing muscle relaxant with minimal circulatory effects would seem prudent. Succinylcholine has been administered to these patients, although the risk of increased potassium release in any patient with a progressive neurologic disease is a consideration. Blood pressure is critically dependent on blood volume in these patients, emphasizing the need for prompt monitoring and replacement of fluid loss. Hypotension is treated with the intravenous infusion of crystalloid solutions or the administration of small doses of a direct-acting vasopressor such as phenylephrine, bearing in mind that an exaggerated increase in blood pressure could accompany the administration of a sympathomimetic. Continuous monitoring of blood pressure, cardiac rhythm, and body temperature is important in these patients. Particular care should be taken to avoid a corneal abrasion, in view of the likely decrease in sensation and tear production present in these patients. A central venous or pulmonary artery catheter is helpful during major surgery, particularly when cardiopulmonary function is already marginal. Regional anesthesia does not seem to be an attractive choice, in view of the cardiovascular instability characteristic of this disease.

Postoperative Management

Complications during the postoperative period include persistent vomiting, pulmonary aspiration, hyperthermia, labile blood pressure, arterial hypoxemia, hypoventilation, and seizures. An increased inspired concentration of oxygen should be routinely administered to these patients. Continuous monitoring of arterial oxygenation with pulse oximetry and measurement of arterial blood gases and pH is indicated, if there is any question regarding the adequacy of oxygenation of ventilation. The need for an opioid to produce analgesia is unlikely, as these patients have decreased sensory perception. Chlorpromazine has been a useful drug in controlling nausea, hyperthermia, and elevated blood pressure during the postoperative period.

SOLID TUMORS

Cancer is second only to accidental trauma as a cause of death in children aged 1 to 14 years. Although treatment of acute lymphoblastic leukemia was the first recognized success of pediatric oncology, similar success is now being achieved in the treatment of malignant solid tumors. Dramatic improvements in survival have been achieved with multimodal therapy (coordination of surgery, chemotherapy, and radiotherapy). In addition to anesthesia for primary tumor excision, there is a continually increasing need for anesthesia for patients undergoing diagnostic and supportive procedures.

Solid tumors that develop in infants and children may be intra-abdominal or retroperitoneal in origin. Nearly 60% of intra-abdominal tumors in children reflect leukemia involving the liver and spleen. Conversely, most intra-abdominal tumors in infants are benign and of renal origin. Retroperitoneal solid tumors are also likely to be of renal origin. Two-thirds of these renal masses are cystic lesions, such as hydronephrosis, whereas the remainder are nephroblastomas (Wilms tumors). Neuroblastoma is another example of a solid tumor that tends to occur in the retroperitoneal space.

Neuroblastoma

Neuroblastoma results from malignant proliferation of sympathetic ganglion cell precursors. These tumors may arise anywhere along the sympathetic ganglion chain, but 60% to 75% occur in the adrenal medulla and the retroperitoneal area. Neuroblastoma has an incidence of about 1 in every 10,000 live births. It is estimated that 10% to 20% of solid tumors in children are neuroblastomas. Neuroblastomas most often occur in children less than 1 year of age.

Signs and Symptoms

The child with a neuroblastoma typically presents with a protuberant abdomen, often discovered by a parent. On clinical examination, a neuroblastoma is a large, firm, nodular, sometimes painful, flank mass, usually fixed to the surrounding structures. Ptosis and periorbital ecchymosis secondary to periorbital metastases may be present. Some children present with pulmonary metastases. Paraspinal neuroblastoma may extend through the neural foramina into the epidural space, producing paralysis. Enlarged peripheral lymph nodes, Horner syndrome, complete to partial absence of the iris, and metastatic enlargement of the liver may also be present. A neuroblastoma may secrete vasoactive intestinal peptides, which are responsible for persistent water diarrhea, with loss of fluid and electrolytes. These tumors also synthesize catecholamines, but the incidence of hypertension is low.

Diagnosis

Ultrasonography, computed tomography, and magnetic resonance imaging are the primary diagnostic procedures for the evaluation of abdominal masses in children. Arteriography is helpful in delineating the extent of involvement of the great vessels by the tumor and its resectability. In some cases, the great vessels are entrapped by the tumor, such that attempts at complete resection would risk major blood loss. An inferior vena cavagram may be necessary to demonstrate the extent of involvement of this vessel by the tumor. Urinary excretion of vanillylmandelic acid is increased in most children with neuroblastomas, reflecting the metabolism of catecholamines produced by these tumors. Unfortunately, tumor with distant metastases is present in 50% of children at diagnosis. Indeed, the overall survival rate in children with neuroblastomas is only 30%.

Treatment

Treatment of neuroblastoma consists of surgical removal, including local metastases and involved lymph nodes. If the tumor cannot be resected completely, it is removed by morcellation. An alternative is to treat with chemotherapy or radiation before surgical resection. The child presenting with signs of spinal cord compression and varying degrees of paralysis may require the performance of a myelogram during general anesthesia, followed by emergency laminectomy for removal of the tumor that has extended into the epidural space. Radiation therapy can be given either as a palliative or as a therapeutic measure. Drugs used for chemotherapy, in varied combinations, include cyclophosphamide, vincristine, and doxorubicin. Possible adverse effects of chemotherapy must be considered in the preoperative evaluation of these patients (see Chapter 28).

Management of Anesthesia

Management of anesthesia for resection of a neuroblastoma is as described for the child with a nephroblastoma.

Nephroblastoma

Nephroblastoma (Wilms tumor) accounts for about 10% of solid tumors in children. One-third of these tumors occur in children younger than 1 year of age, and three-fourths are diagnosed by 4 years of age. The incidence is about 1 in every 13,500 births.

Signs and Symptoms

Nephroblastoma typically presents as an asymptomatic flank mass in an otherwise healthy child. The mass is usually accidentally discovered by the parents or the physician during a routine physical examination. Nephroblastomas vary in size and are usually firm, nontender, and free from surrounding structures. Pain, fever, and hematuria are usually late manifestations. These children may exhibit malaise, weight loss, anemia, disturbances of micturition, and symptoms such as vomiting or constipation, due to compression of adjacent portions of the gastrointestinal tract by the tumor. Hypertension may be a manifestation of a nephroblastoma, particularly if the tumor involves both kidneys. Increases in blood pressure are usually mild but, on rare occasions, hypertension may be so

severe that encephalopathy and congestive heart failure develop. Hypertension may reflect renin production by the tumor or indirect stimulation of renin release due to compression of renal vasculature. Secondary hyperaldosteronism and hypokalemia may be present. Hypertension usually disappears after nephrectomy but may recur if metastases develop.

Diagnosis

Radiography of the abdomen demonstrates a renal mass and occasional calcification. Intravenous pyelography shows distortion of the renal collecting system and occasionally absence of excretion by the involved kidney. This diagnostic test also assesses the function of the contralateral kidney. An inferior vena cavagram may indicate tumor invasion of this blood vessel. An arteriogram will show the extent of the tumor and involvement of the contralateral kidney. A chest radiograph or liver scan may demonstrate metastatic disease.

Treatment

Treatment of a nephroblastoma consists of nephrectomy, with or without subsequent radiation and chemotherapy, depending on the stage of involvement. Combined treatment of a nephroblastoma is associated with a survival rate approaching 80%. An extensive tumor may necessitate radical en bloc resection, including portions of the inferior vena cava, pancreas, spleen, and diaphragm. The presence of metastases may require multiple surgical procedures. If the tumor is inoperable on initial exploration or if the patient is in poor clinical condition, radiation therapy is given initially to shrink the tumor; the patient is then reexplored. Prior radiation therapy may produce radiation nephritis of the normal kidney, especially when given in association with chemotherapy.

Bilateral nephroblastomas occur in 3% to 10% of patients. Two-thirds of these tumors occur at the same time; in the remainder, involvement of the contralateral kidney occurs at a later date. Depending on the magnitude of tumor involvement, surgical treatment can consist of bilateral partial nephrectomy or bilateral total nephrectomy, followed by dialysis and eventually renal transplantation.

Management of Anesthesia

The infant or child scheduled for exploration and resection of a neuroblastoma or nephroblastoma will be in varying degrees of general health. For example, if the tumor is diagnosed at a late stage, it is likely that anemia will be severe. In addition, adverse effects related to chemotherapy must be considered (see Chapter 28). Anemia should be corrected to a concentration of about 10 g·dl^{-1}. The child scheduled for surgery after radiation and chemotherapy may have a low platelet count, requiring the transfusion of platelets before induction of anesthesia. An adequate amount of blood should be cross-matched preoperatively, since resection of a neuroblastoma or nephroblastoma may be associated with excessive blood loss. These children need to be well hydrated preoperatively and to have electrolyte and acid-base imbalance corrected, especially in the face of excessive fluid and electrolyte loss due to diarrhea.

In addition to routine monitoring, placement of a catheter in a peripheral artery is recommended to permit constant monitoring of blood pressure, as well as frequent determination of arterial blood gases and pH. Intraoperative hypotension is not uncommon due to the sudden blood loss that is most likely to occur during dissection of the tumor from around major blood vessels. Catheters for infusion of intravenous fluids should be placed in the upper extremity or in the external jugular vein. Lower extremity veins should be avoided, since it may be necessary to ligate or partially resect the inferior vena cava. Measurement of central venous pressure is helpful for evaluating intravascular fluid volume and the adequacy of fluid replacement. Likewise, a Foley catheter to facilitate monitoring urine output will aid in maintaining an optimal intravascular fluid volume.

Precautions should be taken during induction of anesthesia to prevent pulmonary aspiration, particularly if the tumor is producing compression of the gastrointestinal tract. In the child in poor general condition, sudden hypotension may develop during the induction of anesthesia, particularly if intravascular fluid volume has not been restored with preoperative infusion of crystalloid and colloid solutions. Hypertension, as present in some of these children, must be considered, and measures taken for preventing excessive increases in blood pressure during intubation of the trachea. Although this is usually not a troublesome feature in these patients, as compared with the patient with a pheochromocytoma, it is conceivable that a catecholamine-secreting neuroblastoma could cause hypertension similar to that produced by a pheochromocytoma. In addition, hypertension may reflect manipulation of the adrenal medulla during resection of the tumor. Manipulation of the inferior vena cava containing metastatic tumor can result in tumor embolism to the heart or pulmonary artery.[103] This may result in varying degrees of obstruction of blood flow at the level of the right atrium to produce signs characteristic of pulmonary embolism, including precipitous hypotension, cardiac dysrhythmias, and cardiac arrest.

Maintenance of anesthesia is acceptably provided with nitrous oxide plus a volatile anesthetic or opioid. A muscle relaxant is necessary to optimize surgical exposure. The stomach should be decompressed through a nasogastric tube.

ONCOLOGIC EMERGENCIES

Life-threatening syndromes may develop in children with malignancies (see Chapter 28).

Superior Mediastinal Syndrome

Mediastinal lymph nodes that surround the superior vena cava and trachea may produce compression of these structures, if the nodes become invaded by tumor. Although it is desirable to obtain a tissue specimen before initiation of therapy, the severity of airway obstruction may preclude this goal. Since most lymphomas are highly sensitive to radiotherapy, radiation can dramatically reduce the size of the tumor. Unfortunately, radiation may evoke tissue changes that interfere with precise histologic diagnosis.

The risk of anesthesia for the pediatric patient with an untreated mediastinal mass is that ventilation of the lungs may become impossible after the loss of consciousness, even with a properly placed tracheal tube.[104] The inability to ventilate the lungs through a tracheal tube may require emergent insertion of a rigid bronchoscope beyond the site of obstruction.

Spinal Cord Compression

Spinal cord compression by tumor occurs in about 4% of children with cancer. Tumors most likely to produce this effect are sarcomas, neuroblastomas, lymphomas, and leukemias. Definitive treatment requires radiation therapy or surgery.

Tumor Lysis Syndrome

Tumor lysis syndrome occurs 1 to 5 days after initiation of chemotherapy for highly responsive tumors (lymphomas, leukemias) manifested as hyperuricemia, hyperkalemia, and hyperphosphatemia. The syndrome is produced by the sudden systemic overload of uric acid and potassium. Uric acid and phosphate deposition in renal tubules may lead to acute renal failure. Hydration and the administration of allopurinol are frequently instituted in an attempt to prevent the adverse manifestations of this syndrome. Anesthesia may be necessary for insertion of dialysis access catheters.

THERMAL (BURN) INJURY

About 70,000 persons are hospitalized annually in the United States for thermal injury, one-half of whom are children. Of the thermal-related deaths, one-third are children younger than 15 years of age. Survival after thermal injury depends on the age of the patient and on the percentage of body area burned, with younger patients most likely to survive. The extent of thermal injury is estimated by determining the percentage of body surface area affected by the burn. Relative contributions of various portions of the anatomy to body surface area vary with age[105] (Fig. 32-14).

Pathophysiology

Thermal injury produces predictable pathophysiologic responses (Table 32-17). These responses must be considered when formulating a plan for management of anesthesia for a burned patient.

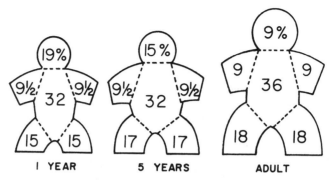

Fig. 32-14. In determining the percentage of body surface area involved by thermal injury, one must consider the age of the patient. (From Smith EI. Acute management of thermal burns in children. Surg Clin North Am 1970;50:807–14, with permission.)

Cardiac Output

Cardiac output decreases dramatically during the immediate postburn period. This initial decrease precedes any measurable loss of intravascular fluid volume and may reflect the presence of a circulating low-molecular-weight myocardial depressant factor.[106] Subsequently, cardiac output is even more profoundly depressed by acute hypovolemia, which occurs as third-space fluid shifts lead to decreased intravascular fluid volume. Although prompt fluid resuscitation results in the return of urine flow within 3 hours, cardiac output remains depressed until the beginning of the second postburn day. Intense vasoconstriction, increased metabolic demands, and hemolysis of erythrocytes further strain the myocardium. Sudden circulatory decompensation may occur if the depressant effects of a volatile anesthetic are superimposed.

After the initial 24 hours of fluid resuscitation, the circulatory system enters a hyperdynamic state that will persist well into the postburn period. Blood pressure and heart rate are increased, and cardiac output stabilizes at about twice normal. Pulmonary artery occlusion pressure will be within a low-normal range, unless high-output congestive heart failure supervenes. Pulmonary edema is rare during the initial few days of fluid resuscitation but is encountered later during the first postburn week, when edema fluid is being resorbed and intravascular fluid volume is maximally increased.

Hypertension

Approximately 30% of children with an extensive thermal injury become hypertensive during the postburn period.[107] The onset of hypertension is usually within the first 2 weeks. Males younger than 10 years of age are at greatest risk of the development of hypertension. Hypertension is usually transient but on occasion may persist for several weeks. Indeed, left untreated, in about 10% of these children hypertensive encephalopathy will develop, characterized by irritability and headache, with or without seizures. The etiology of this hypertension is unknown but may be related to elevated plasma concentrations of catecholamines or activation of the renin-angiotensin system, or both. Treatment with an antihypertensive drug, such as hydralazine or nitroprusside, is indicated in some children.

Intravascular Fluid Volume

Intravascular fluid volume deficits after thermal injury are roughly proportional to the extent and depth of the burn. On the first postburn day, the vascular compartment becomes permeable to plasma proteins, including fibrinogen. This increased permeability exists throughout the vascular system but is most pronounced in the area of the burn. Extravasated plasma proteins exert an osmotic pressure that can hold large volumes of fluid in an extravascular third space. Severe hypo-

Table 32-17. Pathophysiologic Responses Evoked by Burn Injury

Initial decrease in cardiac output, followed by a hyperdynamic circulation
Hypovolemia
Hypertension
Upper airway edema
Chemical pneumonitis
Carbon monoxide poisoning
Increased metabolic rate
Adynamic ileus
Gastric or duodenal ulcer
Oliguria
Initial hyperkalemia, followed by hypokalemia
Hyperglycemia
Hyperviscosity of blood
Hypercoagulable state
Depression of immune function

proteinemia is the primary cause of tissue edema. Pulmonary capillary permeability does not increase unless smoke inhalation occurs. Consequently, colloids do not need to be withheld during the early phases of resuscitation. The loss of fluid from the vascular compartment on the first postburn day is about 4 ml·kg^{-1} for each percentage of body surface burned. For example, in a 40-kg child with a 50% burn, fluids needed for the first 24 hours would be 8000 ml. The most effective restoration of intravascular fluid volume occurs when two-thirds of this fluid is given within the first 8 hours postburn.[108]

On the second postburn day, capillary integrity is largely restored, and fluid and plasma protein losses are markedly decreased. Decreasing amounts of fluid are required to maintain intravascular fluid volume. Further rapid administration of an electrolyte solution at this time results in edema in excess of any gain in circulatory dynamics. Therefore, infusion of crystalloid solutions are sharply reduced after the first postburn day, and colloid solutions are administered.

Airway

Direct thermal injury to the airway, with the exception of steam inhalation, does not occur below the level of the vocal cords, reflecting the low thermal capacity of air and the efficient cooling ability of the upper air passages.[110] Thermal or chemical injury of the upper airway, or both, however, can cause severe edema. Hoarseness, stridor, and tachypnea demand prompt airway evaluation, since swelling of supraglottic tissues can result in sudden, complete upper airway obstruction within hours after the original thermal injury. The airway should be secured before respiratory decompensation occurs, since translaryngeal intubation of the trachea after progression of edema of the airway is likely to be difficult. The small caliber of the pediatric airway accentuates the impact of airway edema on resistance to breathing. If intubation of the trachea is required for a child, a nasotracheal tube is preferred, as a nasal tube is more comfortable and more easily secured than an oral tube.

Tracheostomy is reserved for the patient who shows late pulmonary complications that will require prolonged ventilatory support. Performance of a tracheotomy in a burned child with swelling of the face and neck is a formidable surgical challenge. Early complications of tracheostomy in a burn patient include hemorrhage, pneumothorax, and malposition of the tracheostomy tube; late complications are related to mechanical factors (displacement of the cannula) and to cannula erosion into a blood vessel with massive hemorrhage.

Smoke Inhalation

Inhalation of suspended particles (smoke) and toxic products of incomplete combustion results in chemical pneumonitis similar to that resulting from aspiration of acidic gastric fluid.[110] Most patients with smoke inhalation will have associated face and neck burns or a history of being trapped in a closed space. The smoke inhalation victim often experiences an asymptomatic period, lasting as long as 48 hours before respiratory distress becomes overt. An initial chest radiograph may be clear, but the PaO_2 is consistently decreased while the patient is breathing room air. Production of carbonaceous sputum and detection of wheezes and rales during auscultation of the chest herald impending ventilatory failure.

Treatment of respiratory distress related to smoke inhalation is symptomatic. Administration of warm humidified oxygen and a bronchodilator is indicated. Early institution of positive-pressure ventilation of the lungs with positive end-expiratory pressure should be considered if the PaO_2 is less than 60 mmHg breathing room air. Prophylactic antibiotic administration is not beneficial, and the value of corticosteroids is controversial. Extracorporeal membrane oxygenation has been attempted, but the results have not been encouraging. A catheter placed in a peripheral artery is useful for monitoring the patient with symptomatic smoke inhalation injury. The presence of cardiac dysfunction in association with ventilatory distress is often the indication to place a pulmonary artery catheter.

Carbon Monoxide

Carbon monoxide poisoning often complicates burns that occur in a closed space and is the most common immediate cause of death from fire (see Chapter 30).

Restrictive Thermal Injury

Mechanical factors resulting from thermal injury may interfere with pulmonary function. For example, circumferential burns of the chest and upper abdomen can lead to restricted chest wall motion, as the eschar contracts and hardens. This restriction is further aggravated by ileus and abdominal distension. Escharotomies may be necessary to relieve the restriction.

Metabolism and Thermoregulation

An increased metabolic rate will occur in proportion to the extent of thermal injury. Metabolic rate can be more than doubled in a patient with thermal injury involving 50% of the body surface area. Total parenteral nutrition may be required to meet these increased metabolic requirements. Accompanying this hypermetabolic response, the metabolic thermostat is reset upward, so a burn patient tends to increase skin and core temperature somewhat above normal, regardless of the environmental temperature. Early enteral alimentation of burn patients has several benefits, including attenuation of the hypermetabolic response to the burn injury.[109] Early enteral feeding also maintains intestinal integrity and retards the absorption of bacteria and endotoxins.

Thermoregulatory functions of the skin, including vasoactivity, sweating, piloerection, and insulation, are abolished or diminished by thermal injury. In addition, skin no longer functions as an effective water vapor barrier, resulting in the loss of ion-free water. It is estimated that daily evaporative water loss is equivalent to 4000 ml·m^{-2} of burn surface in a child, compared with 2500 ml·m^{-2} in an adult.[109] Assuming that 0.58 calories is lost for each milliliter of evaporative water loss, a 4000-ml water loss would represent a daily energy loss of about 2400 calories. The failure of occlusive dressings or of increased ambient temperature to lower the metabolic rate substantially confirms that the hypermetabolism of the burn patient does not relate exclusively to loss of water and heat through the area of thermal injury. In the child, intense vasoconstriction in the nonburned areas of skin can result in increased body temperature sufficient to cause a febrile seizure. Conversely, when metabolism and peripheral vasoconstriction are depressed, as during general anesthesia, the child with a thermal injury may experience a rapid decrease in body temperature.

Gastrointestinal Tract

Adynamic ileus is virtually universal after a thermal injury of more than 20% of the body surface area. Therefore, early decompression of the stomach through a nasogastric tube is indicated. Acute ulceration of the stomach or duodenum, known as Curling's ulcer, is the most frequent life-threatening gastrointestinal complication. The precise etiology of Curling's ulcer is unknown; however, the ulcer occurs most frequently in a patient with sepsis or an extensive burn injury, or both. Duodenal ulcer occurs twice as frequently in a child with thermal injury as in an adult (14% versus 7%).[107] Most patients with Curling's ulcer can be managed conservatively with an antacid or H-2 antagonist drug, but an occasional patient may require vagotomy, with or without partial gastrectomy.

Acalculous cholecystitis may occur during the second or third postburn week. Prompt cholecystectomy is indicated for treatment of this complication. A superior mesenteric artery syndrome may occur at the time of maximum weight loss in a burn patient. If conservative therapy fails, duodenojejunostomy or other intra-abdominal surgery may be required.

Renal Function

Immediately after thermal injury, cardiac output and intravascular fluid volume decrease, and plasma catecholamine concentrations increase, resulting in decreased renal blood flow and glomerular filtration rate. Diminished renal blood flow activates the renin-angiotensin-aldosterone system and stimulates the release of antidiuretic hormone. The net effect on renal function is retention of sodium and water and exaggerated losses of potassium, calcium, and magnesium. Later, after adequate fluid resuscitation, renal blood flow and glomerular filtration may increase dramatically.

Hourly urine output remains the most readily available guide to the adequacy of fluid resuscitation. For example, urine output should be about 1.0 ml·kg^{-1}·h^{-1} in an adequately treated child. Renal failure is rare in children who have received adequate fluid resuscitation, unless there are extensive electrical burns or massive thermal injury of skeletal muscles. In the latter circumstance, hemochromogens may be released into the circulation and precipitate in renal tubules, leading to acute tubular necrosis.

Electrolytes

An increase in the plasma concentration of potassium due to tissue necrosis and hemolysis is common during the first 2 postburn days. This is followed over the next several days by marked hypokalemia, due to accentuated renal losses of potassium. Diarrhea and gastric suction will further exaggerate potassium losses. Cardiac dysrhythmias may occur in a hypokalemic patient who receives drugs that promote intracellular movement of potassium (insulin, glucose, sodium bicarbonate) or a drug that opposes myocardial conduction effects of potassium (calcium). Digitalis administration is particularly hazardous in these patients and should not be used prophylactically.

The plasma concentration of ionized calcium may be reduced during the postburn period. Since children are more sensitive than adults to the effects of citrate or potassium, or both, in stored blood, children with extensive thermal injury who are receiving large volumes of rapidly infused whole blood should receive calcium gluconate (1 to 2 mg) for every milliliter of infused blood.

Endocrine Responses

Endocrine responses to thermal injury are characterized by a massive outpouring of adrenocorticotropic hormone, antidiuretic hormone, renin, angiotensin, aldosterone, glucagon, and catecholamines. The plasma concentration of insulin may be either increased or decreased. Nevertheless, the plasma glucose concentration will be elevated, due to an increased concentration of glucagon and catecholamine-induced glycogenolysis in the liver and skeletal muscles. Indeed, glycosuria occurs frequently in the nondiabetic burn patient. The burn patient may be particularly susceptible to the development of nonketotic hyperosmolar coma, especially if total parenteral nutrition is being used.

The maximum increase in the plasma concentration of norepinephrine occurs 3 to 4 days postburn and may remain elevated for several days. The peak plasma concentration of norepinephrine may be 26 times normal.[108] These markedly elevated concentrations produce intense vasoconstriction of the skin and splanchnic vessels. The increased plasma concentration of norepinephrine has been implicated as a causative factor in many of the adverse manifestations of thermal injury in children, including ischemia of the gastrointestinal tract, liver dysfunction, Curling's ulcer, oliguria, disseminated intravascular coagulation, cardiac dysfunction, hypertensive crisis, and elevations of body temperature. Occasionally, a peripheral vasodilator, such as hydralazine, is infused during the early postburn period to offset vasoconstriction and improve tissue perfusion.

Rheology

Blood viscosity increases acutely after thermal injury and remains elevated for several days postburn, even after the hematocrit has returned to normal. After a transient depression, an increase in the plasma concentration of fibrinogen and factors V and VIII persist for several weeks. This hypercoagulable state may give rise to disseminated intravascular coagulation. The diagnosis of disseminated intravascular coagulation is difficult, since the plasma concentration of fibrin split products is almost invariably increased after thermal injury.

Hemolysis of erythrocytes in response to thermal injury is not extensive. Therefore, early transfusion of whole blood or packed erythrocytes, in the absence of other injuries, is rarely necessary. Nevertheless, generalized suppression of erythrocyte production and a decrease in erythrocyte survival time follow thermal injury and may persist well into the postburn period. Therefore, the transfusion of erythrocytes is often needed by about the fifth postburn day, to maintain a hemoglobin concentration above $10 \text{ g} \cdot \text{dl}^{-1}$.

Immunology

Leukocyte function is depressed, and levels of immunoglobulin G and M are low after thermal injury. Sepsis is the most common cause of death in children with thermal injury. Gramnegative bacteremia produces a significantly increased mortality. Pneumonia, suppurative thrombophlebitis, and bacterial invasion of the burn eschar are likely explanations for sepsis. Clearly, aseptic technique must be strictly observed by all persons participating in the care of a burned child.

Liver Function

Liver function tests are frequently abnormal in the burn patient, even when areas of thermal injury are small. Overt liver failure is uncommon, however, unless the postburn course is complicated by hypotension, sepsis, or multiple transfusions of blood. Halothane-associated liver dysfunction in burn patients has not been described.[111]

Management of Anesthesia

Historic information regarding the time and type of burn injury is pertinent for the management of an acutely burned child.[111,112] For example, the time of injury is important, as initial fluid requirements are based on time elapsed since the burn occurred. A child who was trapped in a closed space is likely to have suffered smoke inhalation injury. Electrical burns may produce far more tissue destruction than the surface burns would indicate (see the section, Electrical Burns).

Physical examination should focus on the status of the airway. Head and neck burns, singed nasal hairs, and hoarseness are signs that supraglottic edema may develop or is already present. Carbonaceous sputum, wheezes, or diminished breath sounds suggest the presence of smoke inhalation injury. Abdominal distension may indicate ileus, warranting special precautions during the induction of anesthesia, in order to reduce the risk of pulmonary aspiration. A careful search should be made during the preoperative evaluation for sites suitable for the placement of intravenous catheters and monitoring devices.

Measurement of arterial blood gases and pH and evaluation of the chest radiograph are indicated in the patient suspected of having experienced smoke inhalation. A carboxyhemoglobin level is helpful only for the first few hours after thermal injury. In the presence of carboxyhemoglobin, the pulse oximeter may overestimate saturation of hemoglobin with oxygen, emphasizing the need for caution in relying solely on this monitor in the patient who has recently experienced carbon monoxide exposure.[113] The plasma glucose concentration and osmolarity should be determined, particularly if the patient is receiving total parenteral nutrition. Measures of renal function are indicated after extensive electrical burns. Adequacy of fluid replacement can be judged by urine output, which should be about $1 \text{ ml} \cdot \text{kg}^{-1} \cdot \text{h}^{-1}$. Coagulation profiles should be obtained in the patient in whom extensive intraoperative blood loss is anticipated.

Establishment of intravenous infusion lines may be difficult in the severely burned child. In some instances, it may become necessary to use veins in areas that escaped thermal injury, such as the axilla, the scalp, or the web spaces between the digits. Reliable intravenous catheters of sufficient caliber are essential for the patient undergoing excision of a burn eschar, as large amounts of blood can be lost in a short time. Even split-thickness skin grafts are associated with about 80 ml of blood loss for each 100 cm^2 of skin harvested.[107]

The child with an extensive thermal injury may require intensive monitoring, yet not have an unburned limb available for a blood pressure cuff. A catheter placed into a peripheral artery will occasionally have to be inserted through a burn eschar. Septic complications are likely, such that a catheter placed through the eschar should be removed as soon as possible. Venous cannulation sites are likewise vulnerable to septic complications. Decreased body temperature is exaggerated during the intraoperative period, reflecting the loss of insulating properties of the skin, evaporative loss of water from the eschar, and depression of metabolic rate by general anesthesia. Routine measures for reducing heat loss include the use of warming blankets and radiant overhead warmers. Inspired gases should be warmed and humidified and intravenous fluids administered through a warmer. Ambient temperature of the operating room should be maintained near 25°C. Plastic or paper drapes will reduce evaporative and convective heat losses.

Altered Drug Responses

A number of pathophysiologic alterations produced by burn injury affect drug responses. Immediately after burn injury, organ and tissue blood flow is decreased as a result of hypovolemia, depressed myocardial function, and release of vasoactive substances. Drugs administered by any route other than intravenously will have predictably delayed absorption. Intravenous and inhaled drugs may have increased effects on the brain and heart because of relative increases in blood flow to these organs. After adequate fluid resuscitation, the hypermetabolic phase begins about 48 hours after injury. During this time, oxygen and glucose consumption is markedly increased. The plasma albumin concentration is decreased after burn injury; thus, albumin-bound drugs (benzodiazepines, anticonvulsant drugs) will have an increased free fraction. Conversely, the plasma concentration of alpha-1 acid glycoprotein is increased, so that drugs bound to this protein (muscle relaxants, tricyclic antidepressant drugs) will have a decreased free fraction. Pharmacologic alterations may persist after recovery from burn injury. It has been shown that thiopental requirements are increased in children for more than 1 year after burn injuries[114] (Fig. 32-15). Opioid requirements may also be increased in burn patients.

Of all the classes of drugs, the effects of burn injury on muscle relaxants have been the most extensively studied. The hyperkalemic response to succinylcholine is well known. The risk of hyperkalemia is probably related to the severity of the burn and the time from injury to succinylcholine administration. The greatest risk appears to be between 10 and 50 days after burn injury.[115] Nevertheless, these zones are very poorly defined, and the safest recommendation may be the avoidance of succinylcholine. Several studies have shown that the burn patient develops marked resistance (up to threefold increases in dose requirements) to nondepolarizing muscle relaxants.[112,116–119] (Fig. 32-16). Approximately 30% or more of the body must be burned to produce resistance to nondepolarizing muscle relaxants, manifesting about 10 days after injury, peaking at about 40 days, and declining after about 60 days.[119] Despite this typical time sequence, one report describes prolonged resistance to the effects of a nondepolarizing muscle relaxant lasting 463 days[120] (Fig. 32-17). A pharmacodynamic explanation as the principal mechanism for resistance to effects of nondepolarizing muscle relaxants is documented by the need to achieve a higher plasma drug concentration to produce a given degree of twitch suppression in thermal injured versus nonthermal injured patients[121,122] (Fig. 32-18). It is speculated that a proliferation of extrajunctional cholinergic receptors is responsible for this resistance to the effects produced by nondepolarizing muscle relaxants. This increased number of extrajunctional cholinergic receptors would also increase the available sites for potassium change

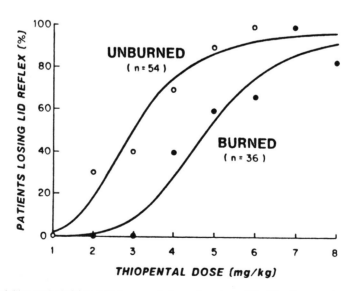

Fig. 32-15. Doses of thiopental administered intravenously to produce loss of the lid reflex were increased in burned children (greater than 15% body surface area burn and more than 1 year after injury) compared with unburned children. (From Cote CJ, Petkau AJ. Thiopental requirements are increased in children reanesthetized at least 1 year after recovery from extensive thermal injury. Anesth Analg 1985;64:1156–60, with permission.)

DOSE RESPONSE CURVES FOR PANCURONIUM

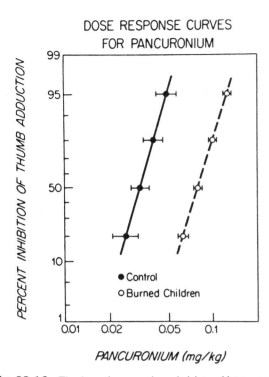

Fig. 32-16. The dose of pancuronium administered intravenously to produce inhibition of thumb adduction is greater in burned children (body surface area burn 4% to 85% and studied 34 ± 7.9 (mean ± SE) days after injury) compared with control children. (From Martyn JAJ, Liu LMP, Szyfelbein SK, et al. The neuromuscular effects of pancuronium in burned children. Anesthesiology 1983;59:561–4, with permission.)

to occur after administration of succinylcholine to a burn injury patient, leading to hyperkalemia. Despite this speculation, there is evidence that thermal injury is not associated with an increase in the number of extrajunctional cholinergic receptors.[123] Instead, an altered affinity of cholinergic receptors for acetylcholine or nondepolarizing muscle relaxants may be the basis for thermal injury-induced resistance to these drugs.

Ketamine has been used for many years as an anesthetic for burn injury patients, especially for dressing changes and escharotomies. This drug can be administered either intravenously or intramuscularly with good effect. Administration of ketamine is often preceded by an anticholinergic drug, as excessive salivation is likely. A single dose of ketamine (2 to 4 $mg \cdot kg^{-1}$ IV) provides excellent somatic analgesia for 15 to 20 minutes. Recovery of consciousness from a single intravenous injection of ketamine is usually rapid, allowing early return to oral nutritional support. Nitrous oxide can be administered to reduce random motion of the limbs, which often accompanies ketamine anesthesia. The incidence of postoperative delirium

after administration of ketamine to pediatric patients appears to be minimal. Nevertheless, if central nervous system effects of ketamine occur, they can be at least partially reversed by the administration of physostigmine (30 $\mu g \cdot kg^{-1}$ IV).[124] Excessive movement during emergence from anesthesia may dislodge skin grafts or promote hemorrhage, resulting in early graft loss. Halothane is the most frequently used inhaled drug for anesthesia in the child with thermal injury. This volatile anesthetic permits maintenance of spontaneous ventilation, as well as administration of a high concentration of oxygen, if necessary. Depth of anesthesia can be adjusted for the surgical stimulus, such that an increased delivered concentration of halothane can be administered during high-intensity stimulation associated with harvesting the skin graft. Application of the skin graft is essentially painless, and the concentration of halothane is decreased during this period. Halothane-associated hepatic dysfunction has not been described in burn injury patients, despite repeated exposures to the drug.[111] Enflurane, isoflurane, and desflurane are acceptable alternatives to halothane, particularly in older patients requiring multiple anesthetics.

ELECTRICAL BURN

A high-voltage electrical current causes tissue damage by conversion to thermal energy.[125] The amount of thermal energy transferred to tissues depends on the voltage of the electrical source, skin resistance of the victim, and the duration of the contact with the source of the electrical current. Tissue damage will be greatest where the electrical current is most concentrated, as occurs at points of entry and exit, and where the involved extremities are narrowest. Visceral injuries due to electrical current is unlikely.

Deep tissue destruction produced by an electrical burn is often extensive, since these tissues cannot dissipate thermal energy as rapidly as more superficial tissues. This makes the extent of damage produced by an electrical current difficult to judge from the extent of superficial injury. Fasciotomies, multiple débridement of wounds, and arteriograms to define the level of viability of affected limbs may be necessary.

At the time of initial electrical injury, cardiopulmonary arrest requiring cardiopulmonary resuscitation may have occurred. Indeed, cardiac dysrhythmias occur in 1 of every 6 patients who experience an electrical burn. These patients should be monitored by continuous displays of the electrocardiogram for at least the first 48 hours postburn.

Renal failure may accompany an electrical burn, reflecting precipitation of myoglobin from injured skeletal muscles in renal tubules. Furthermore, the extent of superficial tissue damage may result in underestimation of the initial fluid requirements. Nevertheless, with recognition of the deep tissue injury accompanying an electrical burn and concurrent admin-

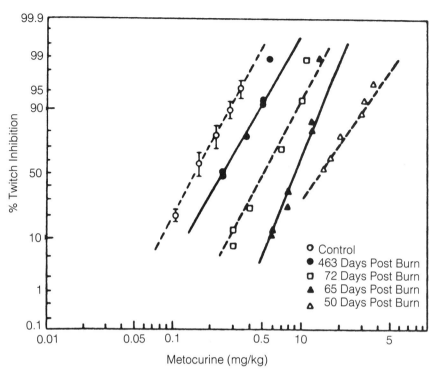

Fig. 32-17. The dose response curve for metocurine administered intravenously to a burned patient is displaced to the right of unburned patients (control) between 50 and 463 days postburn. (From Martyn JAJ, Matteo RS, Szyfelbein SK, Kaplan RF. Unprecedented resistance to neuromuscular blocking effects of metocurine with persistence after complete recovery in a burned patient. Anesth Analg 1982;61:614–6, with permission.)

istration of fluids and diuretics to maintain urine output close to 1 ml·kg^{-1}·h^{-1}, renal failure has become uncommon.

The development of neurologic complications after an electrical burn is common. Peripheral nerve deficits or spinal cord deficits can occur early, reflecting direct injuries of nerves, or later, as a result of perineural scarring or neural ischemia. Neuropathies may involve nerves far removed from points of electrical contact and may progress for several years after injury. Cataract formation is another late sequela of burn injury.

A common type of electrical burn in a child occurs when the child bites through an electrical cord. The resulting burn usually involves the oral commissure. Subsequent scar formation can narrow the oral opening, leading to difficulty in maintaining the upper airway or accomplishing intubation of the trachea during corrective surgery.

Injury due to lightning represents a special form of electrical burn.[126] Lightning tends to flow around the exterior of its victim resulting in superficial flash burns rather than deep tissue thermal injury, as is characteristic of an electrical burn. Transient neurologic deficits and cardiac dysrhythmias are common after an injury due to lightening. Most deaths associated with lightening are due to cardiopulmonary arrest at the time of the initial injury.

SEPARATION OF CONJOINED TWINS

Surgical separation of conjoined twins requires thorough preoperative preparation and discussion among surgeons, pediatricians, and anesthesiologists.[127–129] A detailed rehearsal of the entire procedure, beginning with transportation to the operating room, serves to emphasize the needs and responsibilities of all involved. Preoperative evaluation demonstrates whether there are shared organ systems. Management of anesthesia requires two teams and separate anesthetic machines, delivery systems and ventilators, and monitoring systems. Ultimately, a second operating table will be required.

Awake intubation of the trachea before the administration of a muscle relaxant is often recommended but not mandatory.[127]

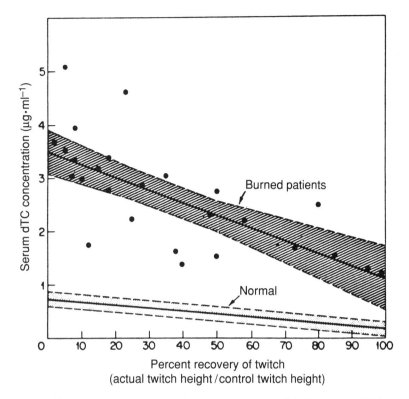

Fig. 32-18. At the same degree of twitch recovery, plasma concentrations of *d*-tubocurarine (*d*Tc) are greater in burned patients than in normal patients. (From Martyn JAJ, Szyfelbein SK, Ali HH, et al. Increased *d*-tubocurarine requirement following major thermal injury. Anesthesiology 1980;52:352–5, with permission.)

Monitoring must be both extensive and invasive (central venous pressure, intra-arterial) to facilitate replacement of blood loss and provide an indication of the adequacy of oxygenation and ventilation. Maintenance of body temperature is important. Monitoring of the plasma concentration of ionized calcium and appropriate replacement is useful for maintaining myocardial contractility and optimizing coagulation.[128] Color coding of all vascular lines, monitors, apparatus, records, and personnel is useful. The presence of cross-circulation means that drugs administered to one infant are likely to produce detectable effects in the other infant. The magnitude of cross-circulation may vary from minute to minute, making the prediction of drug effects even more difficult. Aggressive efforts are required to maintain normothermia. Metabolic acidosis may be prominent and require treatment with sodium bicarbonate. The need for continued support of ventilation of the lungs during the postoperative period is likely.

REFERENCES

1. Cohen MM, Cameron CB, Duncan PG. Pediatric anesthesia morbidity and mortality in the perioperative period. Anesth Analg 1990;70:167–7
2. Pang LM, Mellins RB. Neonatal cardiorespiratory physiology. Anesthesiology 1975;43:171–96
3. Hagen PT, Scholz DG, Edwards WD. Incidence and size of patent foramen ovale during the first 10 decades of life on autopsy study of 965 normal hearts. Mayo Clin Proc 1984;59:17–20
4. Welborn LG, Hannallah RS, McGill WA, et al. Glucose concentrations for routine intravenous infusion in pediatric outpatient surgery. Anesthesiology 1987;67:427–30
5. Sieber FE, Smith DS, Traystman FJ, Wollman H. Glucose: A reevaluation for its intraoperative use. Anesthesiology 1987;67:72–81
6. Furman EB, Roman DG, Lemmer LAS, et al. Specific therapy

in water, electrolyte, and blood volume replacement during pediatric surgery. Anesthesiology 1975;42:187–93

7. Presson RG, Hillier SC. Perioperative fluid and transfusion management. Semin Pediatr Surg 1992;1:22–31

8. Roy WL, Lerman J, McIntrye BG. Is preoperative haemoglobin testing justified in children undergoing minor elective surgery? Can J Anesth 1991;38:700–3

9. Lerman J, Robinson S, Willis MM, Gregory GA. Anesthetic requirement for halothane in young children 0–1 month and 1–6 months of age. Anesthesiology 1983;59:421–4

10. LeDez KM, Lerman J. The minimum alveolar concentration (MAC) of isoflurane in preterm neonates. Anesthesiology 1987; 67:301–7

11. Cook DR. Newborn anaesthesia: Pharmacological considerations. Can Anaesth Soc J 1986;33:38–42

12. Steward DJ, Creighton RE. The uptake and excretion of nitrous oxide in the newborn. Can Anaesth Soc J 1978;25:215–7

13. Brandom BW, Brandom RB, Cook DR. Uptake and distribution of halothane in infants: In vivo measurements and computer simulations. Anesth Analg 1983;62:404–10

14. Friesen RH, Lichtor JL. Cardiovascular effects of inhalation induction with isoflurane in the infants. Anesth Analg 1983;62: 411–4

15. Murray DJ, Forbes RB, Mahoney LT. Comparative hemodynamic depression of halothane versus isoflurane in neonates and infants: An echocardiographic study. Anesth Analg 1992;74: 329–37

16. Westrin P, Jonmarker C, Werner O. Thiopental requirements for induction of anesthesia in neonates and infants one to six months of age. Anesthesiology 1989;71:344–6

17. Cote CJ, Goudsouzian NG, Liu LMP, et al. The dose response of intravenous thiopental for the induction of general anesthesia in unpremedicated children. Anesthesiology 1981;55:703–5

18. Hickey PR, Hansen DD. Fentanyl and sufentanil-oxygen-pancuronium anesthesia for cardiac surgery in infants. Anesth Analg 1984;63:117–24

19. Goudsouzian NG. Maturation of neuromuscular transmission in the infant. Br J Anaesth 1980;50:205–13

20. Fisher DM, O'Keeffe C, Stanski DR, et al. Pharmacokinetics and pharmacodynamics of *d*-tubocurarine in infants, children, and adults. Anesthesiology 1982;57:203–8

21. Goudsouzian NG, Liu LMP, Cote CJ. Comparison of equipotent doses of non-depolarizing muscle relaxants in children. Anesth Analg 1981;60:862–6

22. Brandom BW, Woelfel SK, Cook DR, et al. Clinical pharmacology of atracurium in infants. Anesth Analg 1984;63:309–12

23. Fisher DM, Campbell PC, Spellman MJ, Miller RD. Pharmacokinetics and pharmacodynamics of atracurium in infants and children. Anesthesiology 1990;73:33–7

24. Fisher DM, Cronnelly R, Miller RD, Sharma M. The neuromuscular pharmacology of neostigmine in infants and children. Anesthesiology 1983;59:220–25

25. Cook DR, Fischer CG. Neuromuscular blocking effects of succinylcholine in infants and children. Anesthesiology 1975;42: 662–5

26. Liu LMP, De Cook TH, Goudsouzian NG, et al. Dose response to succinylcholine in children. Anesthesiology 1981;55:599–602

27. Cook DR. Muscle relaxants in infants and children. Anesth Analg 1981;60:335–43

28. Salem MR, Wong AY, Lin YH. The effect of suxamethonium on the intragastric pressure in infants and children. Br J Anaesth 1972;44:166–9

29. Brandom BW, Sarner JB, Woelfel SK, et al. Mivacurium infusion requirements in pediatric surgical patients during nitrous oxide–halothane and during nitrous oxide–narcotic anesthesia. Anesth Analg 1990;71:16–22

30. Froese AB, Butler PO, Fletcher WA. Byford LJ. High-frequency oscillatory ventilation in premature infants with respiratory failure: A preliminary report. Anesth Analg 1987;66:814–8

31. Bancalari E, Gerhardt T. Bronchopulmonary dysplasia. Pediatr Clin North Am 1986;33:1–23

32. Northway WH, Moss RB, Carlisle KB, et al. Late pulmonary sequelae of bronchopulmonary dysplasia. N Engl J Med 1990; 323:1793–9

33. Phelps DL. Retinopathy of prematurity. N Engl J Med 1992; 326:1078–80

34. Gregory GA, Steward DJ. Life-threatening perioperative apnea in the ex-"premie." Anesthesiology 1983;59:495–8

35. Kurth CD, LeBard SE. Association of postoperative apnea, airway obstruction, and hypoxemia in former premature infants. Anesthesiology 1991;75:22–6

36. Welborn LG, Hannallah RS, Luban NLC, Fink R, Tuttimann UE. Anemia and postoperative apnea in former perterm infants. Anesthesiology 1991;74:1003–6

37. Welborn LG, Rice LJ, Hannallah RS, Broadman LM, Ruttimann UE, Fink R. Postoperative apnea in former preterm infants: Prospective comparison of spinal and general anesthesia. Anesthesiology 1990;72:838–42

38. Liu LMP, Cote CJ, Goudsouzian NG, et al. Life-threatening apnea in infants recovering from anesthesia. Anesthesiology 1983;59:506–10

39. Hansen TWR, Bratlid D. Bilirubin and brain toxicity. Acta Paediatr Scand 1986;75:513–22

40. Dierdorf SF, Krishna G. Anesthetic management of neonatal surgical emergencies. Anesth Analg 1981;60:204–15

41. Nakayama DK, Motoyama EK, Tagge EM. Effect of preoperative stabilization on respiratory system compliance and outcome in newborn infants with congenital diaphragmatic hernia. J Pediatr 1991;118:793–9

42. Vacanti JP, Crone RK, Murphy JD, et al. The pulmonary hemodynamic response to perioperative anesthesia in the treatment of high-risk patients with congenital diaphragmatic hernia. J Pediatr Surg 1984;19:672–9

43. Bartlett RH, Toomasian J, Roloff D, et al. Extracorporeal membrane oxygenation (ECMO) in neonatal respiratory failure. 100 cases. Ann Surg 1986;204:236–45

44. Baraka A, Akel S, Haroun S, Yazigi A. One lung ventilation of the newborn with tracheoesophageal fistula. Anesth Analg 1988; 67:189–91

45. Yaster M, Buck JR, Dudgeon DL, et al. Hemodynamic effects of primary closure of omphalocele/gastroschisis in human newborns. Anesthesiology 1988;69:84–8

46. Bissonnette B, Sullivan PJ. Pyloric stenosis. Can J Anaesth 1991;38:668–76

47. Cote CJ. The anesthetic management of congenital lobar emphysema. Anesthesiology 1978;49:296–8
48. Al-Salem AH, Adu-Gyamfi Y, Grant CS. Congenital lobar emphysema. Can J Anaesth 1990;37:377–9
49. Haselby KA, Dierdorf SF, Krishna G, et al. Anaesthetic implications of neonatal necrotizing enterocolitis. Can Anaesth Soc J 1982;29:255–9
50. Jaffe D, Wesson D. Emergency management of blunt trauma in children. N Engl J Med 1991;324:1477–82
51. Nelson KB, Ellenberg JH. Antecedents of cerebral palsy. N Engl J Med 1986;315:81–6
52. Dierdorf SF, McNiece WL, Rao CC, et al. Effect of succinylcholine on plasma potassium in children with cerebral palsy. Anesthesiology 1985;62:88–90
53. Rao CC, Krishna G, Haselby K, et al. Ventriculobronchial fistula complicating a ventriculoperitoneal shunt. Anesthesiology 1977; 47:388–90
54. Minton MD, Grosslight K, Stirt JA, Bedford RF. Increases in intracranial pressure from succinylcholine: Prevention by prior nondepolarizing blockade. Anesthesiology 1986;65:165–9
55. Dierdorf SF, McNiece WL, Rao CC, et al. Failure of succinylcholine to alter plasma potassium in children with myelomeningocele. Anesthesiology 1986;64:272–3
56. Vautrin-Moneret DA, Laxenaire MC, Bavoux F. Allergic shock to latex and ethylene oxide during surgery for spina bifida. Anesthesiology 1990;73:556–8
57. Morray JP, MacGillivray R, Duker G. Increased perioperative risk following repair of congenital heart disease in Down's syndrome. Anesthesiology 1986;65:221–4
58. Williams JP, Somerville GM, Miner ME, Reilly D. Atlanto-axial subluxation and trisomy-21: Another perioperative complication. Anesthesiology 1987;67:253–4
59. Hubert CH. Critical care and anesthetic management of Reye's syndrome. South Med J 1979;72:684–9
60. Barrett MJ, Hurwitz ES, Schonberger LB, Rogers MF. Changing epidemiology of Reye's syndrome in the United States. Pediatrics 1986;77:598–602
61. Karl HW, Swedlow DB, Lee KW, Downes JJ. Epinephrine-halothane interactions in children. Anesthesiology 1983;58:142–5
62. Bell C, Oh TH, Loeffler JR. Massive macroglossia and airway obstruction after cleft palate repair. Anesth Analg 1988;67:71–4
63. Chadd GD, Crane DL, Phillips RM, Tunell WP. Extubation and reintubation guided by the laryngeal mask airway in a child with the Pierre-Robin syndrome. Anesthesiology 1992;76:640–1
64. Diaz JH. Croup and epiglottitis in children. Anesth Analg 1985; 64:621–33
65. Mayo-Smith MF, Hirsch PJ, Wodzinski SF, Schiffman FJ. Acute epiglottitis in adults. N Engl J Med 1986;314:1133–9
66. Muller BJ, Fliegel JE. Acute epiglottis in a 79-year-old man. Can Anaesth Soc J 1985;32:415–7
67. Crosby E, Reid D. Acute epiglottitis in the adult: Is intubation mandatory? Can J Anaesth 1991;38:914–8
68. Phelan PD, Mullins GC, Laundau LI, Duncan AW. The period of nasotracheal intubation in acute epiglottitis. Anaesth Intensive Care 1980;8:402–3
69. Adair JC, Ring WH, Jordan WS, Elwyn RA. Ten-year experience with IPPB in the treatment of acute laryngotracheobronchitis. Anesth Analg 1971;50:649–55
70. Loughlin GM, Taussig LM. Pulmonary function in children with a history of laryngotracheobronchitis. J Pediatr 1979;94:365–9
71. Koka BV, Jeon IS, Andre JM, et al. Postintubation croup in children. Anesth Analg 1977;56:501–5
72. Cohen MM, Cameron CB. Should you cancel the operation when a child has an upper respiratory tract infection? Anesth Analg 1991;72:282–8
73. Darmon J-Y, Rauss A, Dreyfuss D, et al. Evaluation of risk factors for laryngeal edema after tracheal extubation in adults and its prevention by dexamethasone. Anesthesiology 1992;77: 245–51
74. Rao CC, Krishna G, Grosfeld JL, Weber TL. One-lung pediatric anesthesia. Anesth Analg 1981;60:450–2
75. Borland LM. Anesthesia for children with Jeune's syndrome (asphyxiating thoracic dystrophy). Anesthesiology 1987;66: 86–8
76. Mac Lennan DH, Phillips MS. Malignant hyperthermia. Science 1992;256:789–94
77. Ording H. Incidence of malignant hyperthermia in Denmark. Anesth Analg 1985;64:700–4
78. Newbauer KR, Kaufman RD. Another use for mass spectrometry: Detection and monitoring of malignant hyperthermia. Anesth Analg 1985;64:837–9
79. Van der Spek AF, Reynolds PI, Fang WB, Ashton-Miller JA, Stohler CS, Schork MA. Changes in resistance to mouth opening induced by depolarizing and nondepolarizing neuromuscular blockers. Br J Anaesth 1990;64:21–7
80. Saddler JM. Jaw stiffness—an ill understood condition. Br J Anaesth 1991;67:515–6
81. Rosenberg H, Fletcher JE. Masseter muscle rigidity and malignant hyperthermia susceptibility. Anesth Analg 1986;65:161–4
82. Allen GC, Rosenberg H. Malignant hyperthermia susceptibility in adult patients with masseter muscle rigidity. Can J Anaesth 1990;37:31–5
83. Larach MG, Rosenberg H, Larach DR, Broennle AM. Prediction of malignant hyperthermia susceptibility by clinical signs. Anesthesiology 1987;66:547–50
84. Britt BA. Dantrolene. Can Anesth Soc 1984;31:61–75
85. Ryan JF, Donlon JV, Malt RA, et al. Cardiopulmoanry bypass in the treatment of malignant hyperthermia. N Engl J Med 1974; 290:1121–2
86. Mathieu A, Bogosian AJ, Ryan JF, et al. Recrudescence after survival of an initial episode of malignant hyperthermia. Anesthesiology 1979;51:454–5
87. Gronert GA, Thompson RL, Onofrio BM. Human malignant hyperthermia: Awake episodes and correction by dantrolene. Anesth Analg 1980;59:377–8
88. Lees DE, Gadde PL, Macnamara TE. Malignant hyperthermia in association with Burkitt's lymphoma: Report of a third case. Anesth Analg 1980;59:514–5
89. Olgin J, Argov Z, Rosenberg H, et al. Non-invasive evaluation of malignant hyperthermic susceptibility with phosphorus nuclear magnetic resonance spectroscopy. Anesthesiology 1988;68: 507–13
90. Allen GC, Cattrain CB, Peterson RG, Lakende M. Plasma levels of dantrolene following oral administration in malignant hyperthermia-susceptible patients. Anesthesiology 1988;67:900–4

91. Lerman J, McLoen ME, Strong HA. Pharmacokinetics of intravenous dantrolene in children. Anesthesiology 1989;70:625–9

92. Flewellen EH, Nelson TE, Jones WP, et al. Dantrolene dose response in awake man: Implications for management of malignant hyperthermia. Anesthesiology 1983;59:275–80

93. Watson CB, Reierson N, Norfleet EA. Clinically significant muscle weakness induced by oral dantrolene sodium prophylaxis for malignant hyperthermia. Anesthesiology 1986;65:312–4

94. Ruhland G, Hinkle AJ. Malignant hyperthermia after oral and intravenous pretreatment with dantrolene in a patient susceptible to malignant hyperthermia. Anesthesiology 1984;60:159–60

95. Hackl W, Maurtiz W, Winkler M, Sporn P, Steinbereithner K. Anaesthesia in malignant hyperthermia susceptible patients without dantrolene prophylaxis: A report of 30 cases. Acta Anaesthesiol Scand 1990;34:534–7

96. Rubin AS, Zablocki AD. Hyperkalemia, verapamil, and dantrolene. Anesthesiology 1987;66:246–9

97. Dreissen JJ, Wuis EW, Gielen JM. Prolonged vecuronium neuromuscular blockade in a patient receiving orally administered dantrolene. Anesthesiology 1985;62:523–4

98. Beebe JJ, Sessler DI. Preparation of anesthesia machines for patients susceptible to malignant hyperthermia. Anesthesiology 1988;69:395–400

99. Berkowitz A, Rosenberg H. Femoral block with mepivacaine for muscle biopsy in malignant hyperthermia patients. Anesthesiology 1985;62:651–2

100. Yentis SM, Levine MF, Hartley EJ. Should all children with suspected or confirmed malignant hyperthermia susceptibility be admitted after surgery? A 10-year review. Anesth Analg 1992;75:345–50

101. Beilin B, Maayan CH, Vatashsky E, et al. Fentanyl anesthesia in familial dysautonomia. Anesth Analg 1985;64:72–6

102. Stirt JA, Frantz RA, Gunz EF, Conolly ME. Anesthesia, catecholamines, and hemodynamics in autonomic dysfunction. Anesth Analg 1982;61:701–4

103. Milne B, Cervenko FW, Morales A, Salerno TA. Massive intraoperative pulmonary tumor embolus from renal cell carcinoma. Anesthesiology 1981;54:253–5

104. Ferrari LR, Bedford RF. General anesthesia prior to treatment of anterior mediastinal masses in pediatric cancer patients. Anesthesiology 1990;72:991–5

105. Smith EI. Acute management of thermal burns in children. Surg Clin North Am 1970;50:807–14

106. Demling RH. Burns. N Engl J Med 1985;313:1389–98

107. Popp MB, Friedberg DL, MacMillan BG. Clinical characteristics of hypertension in burned children. Ann Surg 1980;191:473–8

108. Pruitt BA. Fluid and electrolyte replacement in the burned patient. Surg Clin North Am 1978;58:1291–1312

109. Deitch EA. The management of burns. N Engl J Med 1990;323:1249–53

110. Fein A, Leff A, Hopewell PC. Pathophysiology and management of the complications resulting from fire and the inhaled products of combustion: A review of the literature. Crit Care Med 1980;8:94–8

111. Boswick JA, Thompson JD, Kershner CJ. Critical care of the burned patient. Anesthesiology 1977;47:164–70

112. Martyn J. Clinical pharmacology and drug therapy in the burned patient. Anesthesiology 1986;65:67–75

113. Barker SJ, Tremper KK. The effect of carbon monoxide inhalation on pulse oximetry and transcutaneous PO_2. Anesthesiology 1987;66:677–9

114. Cote CJ, Petkau AJ. Thiopental requirements may be increased in children reanesthetized at less than one year after recovery from extensive thermal injury. Anesth Analg 1985;64:1156–60

115. Katz RL, Katz LE. Complications associated with the use of muscle relaxants. In: Orkin FK, Cooperman LH, eds. Complications in Anesthesiology. Philadelphia. JB Lippincott 1983;557–9

116. Martyn JAJ, Matteo RS, Grenblatt DJ, et al. Pharmacokinetics of d-tubocurarine in patients with thermal injury. Anesth Analg 1982;61:241–6

117. Martyn JAJ, Liu MLP, Szyfelbein SK, et al. The neuromuscular effects of pancuronium in burned children. Anesthesiology 1983;59:561–4

118. Martyn JAJ, Goudsouzian NG, Matteo RS, et al. Metocurine requirements and plasma concentrations in burned pediatric patients. Br J Anaesth 1983;55:263–8

119. Dwersteg JF, Pavlin EG, Heimbach DM. Patients with burns are resistant to atracurium. Anesthesiology 1986;65:517–20

120. Martyn JAJ, Matteo RS, Szyfelbein SK, Kaplan RF. Unprecedented resistant to neuromuscular blocking effects of metocurine with persistence after complete recovery in a burned patient. Anesth Analg 1982;61:614–7

121. Marathe PH, Dwersteg JF, Pavlin EG, Haschke RH, Heimbach DM, Slattery JT. Effect of thermal injury on the pharmacokinetics and pharmacodynamics of atracurium in humans. Anesthesiology 1989;70:752–5

122. Martyn JAJ, Szyfelbein SK, Ali HH, et al. Increased d-tubocurarine requirement following major thermal injury. Anesthesiology 1980;52:352–5

123. Marathe PH, Haschke RH, Slattery JT, Zucker JR, Pavlin EG. Acetylcholine receptor density and acetylcholinesterase activity in skeletal muscle of rats following thermal injury. Anesthesiology 1989;70:654–9

124. Toro-Mates A, Rendon-Platas AM, Avila-Valdez E, Villarrel-Guzman RA. Physostigmine antagonizes ketamine. Anesth Analg 1980;59:764–7

125. Hunt JL, Mason AD, Masterson TS, Pruitt BA. The pathophysiology of acute electric injuries. J Trauma 1976;16:335–40

126. Cooper MA. Lightening injuries: Prognostic signs for death. Ann Emerg Med 1980;9:134–8

127. Hoshima H, Tanaka O, Obara H, Iwai S. Thoracopagus conjoined twins: Management of anesthetic induction and postoperative chest wall defect. Anesthesiology 1987;66:424–6

128. Georges LS, Smith KW, Wong KC. Anesthetic challenges in separation of craniopagus twins. Anesth Analg 1987;66:783–7

129. Diaz JH, Furman ER. Perioperative management of conjoined twins. Anesthesiology 1987;67:965–73

33

Physiologic Changes and Disorders Unique to Aging

Aging is accompanied by unavoidable alterations in organ function and the responses to drugs. Changes in organ function are manifested as a decreased margin of reserve; in fact, old age can be characterized as a continuation of life with decreasing capacities for adaptation[1] (Fig. 33-1). Decreased organ function can often be demonstrated only by stress testing. For example, cardiac function sufficient for a sedentary life may become inadequate during the perioperative period if anemia or infection occurs. It is important to recognize that there is not necessarily a correlation between biologic and chronologic age.

ORGAN SYSTEM FUNCTION

Aging is associated with progressive declines in central nervous system activity and loss of neurons, particularly in the cerebral cortex. Conduction velocity in peripheral nerves gradually slows with advancing age, and there may be a decreased number of fibers in the spinal cord tracts. These changes are consistent with decreased dose requirements for injected and inhaled anesthetics that accompany aging.

Disturbances in the pattern of sleep characterized by a decrease in slow-wave (stage 4) sleep are common in the elderly patient.[2] For example, the elderly patient spends more time in bed but less time asleep and is more easily aroused from sleep than a younger adult. This increased nighttime wakefulness in the elderly is mirrored by increased daytime fatigue and the likelihood of falling asleep during the day. The elderly patient is less tolerant of phase shifts in the sleep-wake cycle, such as jet lag. Nocturnal respiratory dysfunction (sleep apnea syndrome) is common in elderly patients, especially males (see Chapter 17). These apneic episodes, which last 10 seconds or longer and result in multiple (20 or more nightly) episodes of hypoxemia (arterial hemoglobin oxygen saturation less than 80%), are exacerbated by the use of depressant drugs such as alcohol. Snoring, which is associated with obstructive sleep apnea, increases in prevalence with aging, especially in males. Epidemiologic studies have linked snoring with the development of sleep apnea, hypertension, and cardiovascular disease.[2]

The elderly, especially the very old, are susceptible to delirium as a consequence of almost any physical illness (pneumonia, myocardial infarction) or intoxication with even therapeutic doses of commonly used drugs.[3] Delirium is characterized by acute mental confusion with a sudden onset, often occurring at night. Typically, the severity of the symptoms fluctuates unpredictably during the daytime and peaks at night. Drug ingestion by the elderly patient must be monitored and unnecessary polypharmacy, especially the concurrent use of more than one drug with anticholinergic effects, should be avoided. The duration of delirium is usually less than 1 month, with most patients experiencing a full recovery. It is important to distinguish delirium from dementia (Alzheimer's disease), the only other syndrome characterized by global cognitive impairments[3] (Table 33-1).

Cardiovascular system changes, which accompany aging, often reflect decreased responsiveness to stimulation from the autonomic nervous system, with an associated decrease in the ability of the heart to compensate for stress. Cardiac output tends to decline in parallel with decreased oxygen requirements that accompany aging. Nevertheless, elderly persons who maintain physical fitness may maintain a relatively unchanged cardiac output despite progressive aging.[4] Although resting stroke volume remains relatively unchanged, the ability of the aged heart to increase its cardiac output in response to stress or to compensate for vulnerability to drug-induced decreases in myocardial contractility may be impaired. The aged heart shows less chronotropic response to cate-

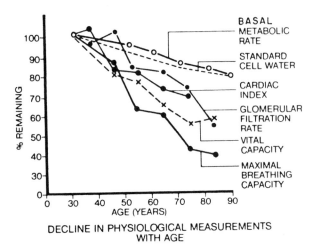

DECLINE IN PHYSIOLOGICAL MEASUREMENTS
WITH AGE

Fig. 33-1. Aging is associated with progressive decreases in function (1% to 1.5% annually) of major organ systems. (From Evans TI. The physiological basis of geriatric general anaesthesia. Anaesth Intensive Care 1973;1:319–28, with permission).

cholamines, perhaps reflecting decreased beta receptor responsiveness, as the density of these receptors is unchanged. Overall, the heart rate decreases with age, suggesting a predominance of parasympathetic nervous system activity or degenerative changes that involve the sinus node or cardiac conduction system, or both. In the sinus node the number of cells declines; by 75 years of age only about 10% of the cells that

Table 33-1. Differential Diagnosis of Delirium and Dementia

	Delirium	Dementia
Onset	Sudden	Insidious
Course over 24 hours	Fluctuating with nocturnal exacerbation	Stable
Consciousness	Decreased	Unchanged
Attention	Globally disordered	Usually normal
Hallucinations	Common	Uncommon
Orientation	Impaired	Impaired
Psychomotor activity	Unpredictable	Usually normal
Speech	Often incoherent	Difficulty finding words
Physical illness or drug toxicity	Common	Uncommon

were present at 20 years of age may remain.[5] This change is consistent with the prevalence of sick sinus syndrome and atrial dysrhythmias often present in elderly patients. Congestive heart failure is a common problem among elderly patients (six times more common in patients older than 65 years of age compared with patients younger than 54 years of age), and is usually associated with hypertension or ischemic heart disease.[5] Blood pressure increases with aging, reflecting the development of thickened elastic fibers in the walls of the large arteries. As a result, blood vessels become poorly compliant and systolic and diastolic blood pressures increase.

Mechanical ventilatory function and the efficiency of gas exchange deteriorate with aging. Mechanical ventilatory function is impaired because of decreased elasticity of the lungs and decreased maximal movement of the thorax. These changes reflect progressive destruction of pulmonary parenchyma and calcification of costochondral cartilages. Increased stiffness of the thoracic cage is accompanied by progressive dorsal kyphosis, with upward and anterior rotation of the ribs and sternum, leading to an increase in the anterior to posterior diameter of the chest and restricted chest expansion. Despite these changes, residual volume and functional residual capacity are increased. The vital capacity and forced vital capacity in 1 second, however, decrease progressively with aging. Progressive reductions in PaO_2 accompany aging, most likely reflecting airway closure and decreased cardiac output, leading to ventilation-to-perfusion mismatching[6] (Fig. 33-2). At rest, the elderly patient may not show symptoms of pulmonary dysfunction, but pulmonary changes produced by surgery, superimposed on the already present changes of aging, can result in severe symptomatology because of the decreased margin of reserve.

Advancing age is associated with a progressive decline in renal blood flow and glomerular filtration rate parallelling decreased cardiac output. As a result, the elderly patient is vulnerable to fluid overload and cumulative effects of drugs that depend on renal clearance (digoxin, antibiotics, certain nondepolarizing muscle relaxants). Despite this deterioration in renal function, the plasma creatinine concentration often does not increase, presumably reflecting the decreased production of creatinine that parallels the decreased skeletal muscle mass that accompanies aging. The decreased urine concentrating ability that accompanies aging means that the elderly patient is less able to concentrate urine after fluid deprivation, and the ability to secrete an acid load is decreased. The elderly patient's ability to conserve sodium is impaired, making this age group vulnerable to hyponatremia, particularly when acute illness leads to decreased oral intake of sodium.

The decreased hepatic blood flow that accompanies aging and parallels cardiac output will possibly influence the clearance of drugs dependent on hepatic metabolism. A decreased rate of gastric emptying may accompany aging. The incidence of diabetes mellitus increases with age, perhaps reflecting de-

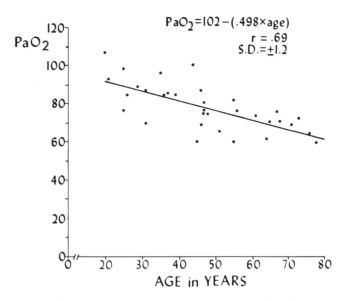

Fig. 33-2. There is an inverse relationship between PaO2 and aging reflected by the formula 102 − (0.498 × age). (From Wahba WM. Body build and preoperative arterial oxygen tensions. Can Anaesth Soc J 1975;22:653–8, with permission.)

creased insulin release or an insensitivity of the receptor to insulin. Subclinical hypothyroidism manifested solely as an increase in the plasma concentration of thyroid stimulating hormone is present in 13.2% of healthy elderly patients, especially females.[7]

PHARMACOKINETICS AND PHARMACODYNAMICS

Age-related changes in pharmacokinetics are most often manifested as an increased elimination half-time of drugs. An increase in the elimination half-time of a drug can reflect decreased renal clearance (digoxin, antibiotics, pancuronium) and hepatic clearance (propranolol, lidocaine, vecuronium) or an increased volume of distribution (diazepam). Events that result in an increased volume of distribution of a drug include increased total body fat content and decreased albumin production that accompany aging. An increase in the elimination half-time will make the elderly patient vulnerable to cumulative drug effects that occur with repeated drug doses. Furthermore, because of age-related alterations in the pharmacokinetics of drugs, the elderly patient is at increased risk of experiencing adverse drug interactions.

Pharmacodynamics depicts the responsiveness of receptors to drugs, as reflected by the pharmacologic response elicited. The number of receptors present in a given tissue is often speculated to decrease with aging. Nevertheless, the density

of beta receptors does not change with aging, whereas the affinity of these receptors for the adrenergic neurotransmitter does decrease. The age-related decrease in MAC for volatile anesthetics reflects a pharmacodynamic effect, although the mechanism is not documented[8] (Fig. 33-3). Conversely, the plasma concentration of pancuronium necessary to produce a specific degree of twitch depression is not altered in the elderly patient, suggesting that changes in the neuromuscular junction do not occur with aging.

MANAGEMENT OF ANESTHESIA

Preoperative evaluation of the elderly patient includes consideration of the likely presence of co-existing diseases independent of the reason for surgery (Table 33-2). In fact, many

Table 33-2. Co-Existing Diseases That Often Accompany Aging

Essential hypertension
Ischemic heart disease
Cardiac conduction disturbances
Congestive heart failure
Chronic pulmonary disease
Diabetes mellitus
Subclinical hypothyroidism
Rheumatoid arthritis
Osteoarthritis

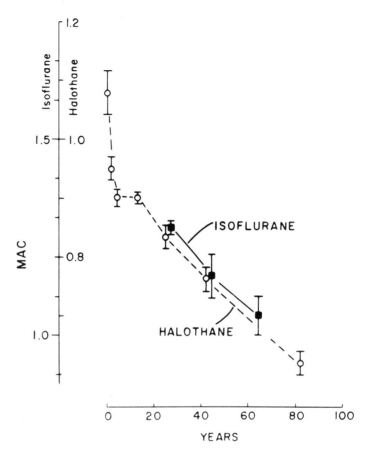

Fig. 33-3. MAC for isoflurane and halothane decreases with increasing age. (From Quasha AL, Eger EI, Tinker JH. Determination and applications of MAC. Anesthesiology 1980;53:315–34, with permission.)

findings that are considered to be typical of aging actually represent disease processes that have a higher incidence among the elderly. Alcoholism may be an unexpected finding in the elderly patient. A recent change in mental function should not be attributed to aging until cardiac or pulmonary disease has been eliminated as an etiology. The hazards of co-existing diseases are emphasized by the increased postoperative mortality in the elderly patient, especially when emergency surgery is necessary. The likelihood of adverse drug interactions is increased by alterations in the pharmacokinetics and pharmacodynamics that accompany aging.[9] Furthermore, the elderly patient is likely to be taking several different drugs, which can result in adverse effects or drug interactions (Table 33-3). Indeed, an estimated 30% of drug prescriptions are written for elderly patients.[10] Anemia and orthostatic hypotension owing to hypovolemia are common preoperative findings in the elderly patient.

Preoperative evaluation of the airway should consider the presence of changes characteristic of aging. For example, the potential presence of vertebrobasilar arterial insufficiency can be evaluated by determining the effect of extension and rotation of the head on mental status. Poor dentition or the presence of dentures may influence the approach to induction of anesthesia. For example, if maintenance of anesthesia by mask is anticipated, it may be useful to ask the edentulous patient to wear dentures to the operating room. Cervical osteoarthritis or rheumatoid arthritis may interfere with visualization of the glottic opening during direct laryngoscopy. Senile atrophy with collagen loss and decreased elasticity makes the skin more sensitive to injury from adhesive tape and monitoring electrodes, as used for recording of the electrocardiogram or eliciting the response to a peripheral nerve stimulator.

Preoperative medication of the elderly patient may be best achieved with a preoperative visit describing the events that are going to occur during the perioperative period. If additional anxiety relief is desired, a benzodiazepine is often selected. Glycopyrrolate, which does not easily cross the blood-brain barrier, is probably less likely to cause undesirable central

Table 33-3. Drugs Commonly Prescribed for the Elderly Patient

Drug	Adverse Effect or Drug Interaction
Diuretics	Hypokalemia
	Hypovolemia
Digitalis	Cardiac dysrhythmias
	Cardiac conduction disturbances
Beta antagonists	Bradycardia
	Congestive heart failure
	Bronchospasm
	Attenuation of autonomic nervous system activity
Centrally acting antihypertensives	Attenuation of autonomic nervous system activity
	Decreased MAC
Tricyclic antidepressants	Anticholinergic effects
	Cardiac dysrhythmias
	Cardiac conduction disturbances
	Increased MAC
Lithium	Cardiac dysrhythmias
	Prolongation of muscle relaxants
Antidysrhythmic agents	Prolongation of muscle relaxants
Antibiotics	Prolongation of muscle relaxants

nervous system effects, if an anticholinergic drug is included in the preoperative medication of the elderly patient.

The selection of drugs and techniques for induction and maintenance of anesthesia in the elderly patient must consider changes in organ function that are likely to accompany aging, as well as altered responses to drugs because of age-related changes in pharmacokinetics or pharmacodynamics. A decreased cardiac output and delayed clearance of drugs may contribute to a delayed onset of effect produced by drugs administered intraoperatively. Furthermore, this delayed onset may be followed by a prolonged pharmacologic effect. In addition, a decreased cardiac output combined with a decreased anesthetic requirement could increase the risk of a volatile anesthetic overdose[8] (Fig. 33-3). Progressive decreases in reactivity of protective upper airway reflexes with aging plus the high incidence of hiatal hernia in the elderly patient may increase the importance of protecting the lungs from aspiration by placement of a cuffed tube in the trachea[11] (Fig. 33-4). There is no evidence that a specific inhaled or injected drug is preferable for maintenance of anesthesia in the elderly patient. An increased heart rate associated with administration of isoflurane is less likely to occur in the elderly compared with the young adult.[12] The possible delayed distribution, metabolism, or clearance of drugs such as thiopental,

opioids, diazepam, and pancuronium must be considered. In contrast to long-acting nondepolarizing muscle relaxants, short- and intermediate-acting drugs are less dependent on renal or hepatic clearance mechanisms and are thus less likely to be influenced by age-related changes in cardiac output. Monitoring of the elderly patient does not introduce unique considerations other than the appreciation that the margin of reserve is decreased in these patients. During the postoperative period, attention to the development of arterial hypoxemia or myocardial ischemia is important. Early ambulation is important in decreasing the likelihood of pneumonia or the development of deep vein thrombosis. Postoperative confusion and impairment of memory may also contribute to morbidity in the geriatric patient.

Regional anesthesia is an acceptable alternative to general anesthesia in selected elderly patients, especially those undergoing transurethral resection of the prostate, gynecologic procedures, inguinal herniorrhaphy, and treatment of hip fractures. A T8 sensory level is desirable for these operative procedures. A prerequisite for selecting a regional anesthetic technique is an alert and cooperative patient. Maintenance of consciousness during surgery permits prompt recognition of acute changes in cerebral function or the onset of angina pectoris. Apprehension despite adequate anesthesia may require intravenous administration of a drug such as midazolam, keeping in mind that the elderly patient may require low doses of this drug, to achieve the desired effect. On occasion, a regional and general anesthetic technique may be combined, as in the elderly patient undergoing hip surgery.

Although unconfirmed by objective measurements, prolongation of spinal anesthesia is thought to reflect decreased vascular absorption of local anesthetic, owing to decreased blood flow in the vessels surrounding the subarachnoid space in an elderly patient with extensive arteriosclerosis. The dose of local anesthetic required to achieve a given sensory level during epidural anesthesia is often perceived to be less with aging, although not all reports describe a linear relationship between dose and age.[13,14] There are also data demonstrating that cephalad spread is more extensive and duration of epidural sensory and motor blockade is shorter in elderly than in younger patients.[15] Decreased dose requirements in the elderly patient are thought to be due in part to anatomic changes in the epidural space, characterized by progressive occlusion of intervertebral foramina with connective tissue. As a result, less local anesthetic solution escapes through the intervertebral foramina, and there is increased spread in the epidural space. This change would also result in an increased surface area for absorption of local anesthetic solution from the epidural space, consistent with the higher peak plasma concentration of lidocaine observed after epidural placement in elderly patients compared with young adults.[14] An exaggerated spread of epidural anesthesia in patients with arteriosclerosis apparently does not occur[16] (Fig. 33-5). There is clinical evi-

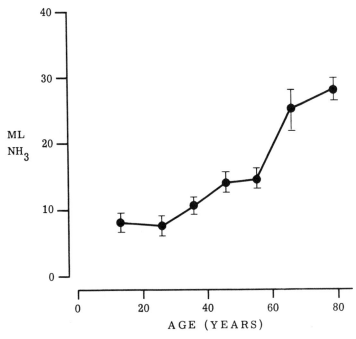

Fig. 33-4. The dose of ammonia gas (milliliters of NH₃) necessary to cause momentary closure of the glottis and a brief pause of inspiration increases with age (especially between 50 and 70 years of age), reflecting decreased sensitivity of the airway. (Data from Pontoppidan H, Beecher HK. Progressive loss of protective reflexes in the airway with the advance of age. JAMA 1960;174: 2209–13.)

dence that regional anesthesia for hip surgery in the elderly patient decreases the magnitude of perioperative blood loss and decreases the incidence of postoperative deep vein thrombosis and pulmonary embolism.[17] Furthermore, regional anesthesia may be associated with less postoperative confusion compared with patients receiving general anesthesia.[18] Anticholinergic medication may contribute to postoperative confusion in the elderly patient, independent of the anesthetic technique.[19]

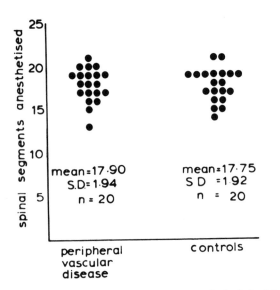

Fig. 33-5. The number of spinal segments anesthetized after injection of bupivacaine into the epidural space is not influenced by the presence of peripheral vascular disease. (From Sharrock NE. Lack of exaggerated spread of epidural anesthesia in patients with arteriosclerosis. Anesthesiology 1977;47:307–8, with permission.)

OSTEOPOROSIS

Osteoporosis is one of the most important disorders associated with aging.[20] More than 1.5 million Americans have fractures and associated pain due to the presence of osteoporosis. During the course of their lifetime, females lose about 50% of their cancellous bone and 30% of their cortical bone and males lose about 30% and 20%, respectively. Cancellous bone is concentrated in the spinal column and at the ends of long bones; these areas are the principal sites of osteoporotic fractures. The tendency for elderly patients to fall is also an important cause of fractures in weakened bones.

Prevention is the only effective approach to the management of osteoporosis. Increased bone mass may be facilitated by weight-bearing exercise. An adequate calcium intake is important. Estrogen replacement therapy continues to be the mainstay of both prevention and treatment in postmenopausal females. Patients who have back pain due to vertebral fractures may benefit from analgesic drug therapy, physical therapy, and perhaps a back brace.

PROGERIA

Progeria (Hutchinson-Gilford syndrome) is characterized by premature aging. This disease is inherited as an autosomal recessive disorder, with clinical manifestations becoming apparent after about 6 months of age. These patients acquire all the diseases of old age during the first or second decades of life. For example, ischemic heart disease, hypertension, cerebrovascular disease, osteoarthritis, and diabetes mellitus are common. The mean survival age is 13 years, with death usually occurring by 25 years of age from congestive heart failure or myocardial infarction.

Management of anesthesia for the patient with progeria is based on changes in organ system function that predictably accompany aging (see the section, Organ System Function).[21] In addition, the presence of mandibular hypoplasia and micrognathia may lead to difficulty in management of the upper airway and intubation of the trachea. The presence of a narrow glottic opening and the need for a small tracheal tube are suggested by the typical high-pitched voice characteristic of these patients. Even minimal laryngeal edema can compromise the patency of the airway. Careful movement and positioning of the patient with progeria are necessary to minimize the likelihood of injury to the thin and fragile extremities.

REFERENCES

1. Evans TI. The physiological basis of geriatric general anaesthesia. Anaesth Intensive Care 1973;1:319–28
2. Prinz PN, Vitiello MV, Raskind MA, Thorpy MJ. Geriatrics: Sleep disorders and aging. N Engl J Med 1990;323:520–6
3. Schor JD, Levkoff SE, Lipsitz LA, et al. Risk factors for delirium in hospitalized elderly. JAMA 1992;267:827–31
4. Craig DB, McLeskey CH, Mitenko PA, et al. Geriatric anaesthesia. Can J Anaesth 1987;34:156–67
5. Wei JY. Age and the cardiovascular system. N Engl J Med 1992;327:1735–9
6. Wahba W. Body build and preoperative arterial oxygen tension. Can Anaesth Soc J 1975;22:653–8
7. Cooper DS. Subclinical hypothyroidism. JAMA 1987;258:246–7
8. Quasha AL, Eger EI, Tinker JH. Determination and applications of MAC. Anesthesiology 1980;53:315–34
9. Greenblatt DJ, Sellers EM, Shader RI. Drug disposition in old age. N Engl J Med 1982;306:1081–8
10. Thompson TL, Moran MG, Nies AS. Psychotropic drug use in the elderly. N Engl J Med 1983;308:136–41
11. Pontoppidan H, Beecher HK. Progressive loss of protective reflexes in the airway with the advance of age. JAMA 1960;174:2209–13
12. Mallow JE, White RD, Cucchiara RF, Tarhan S. Hemodynamic effects of isoflurane and halothane in patients with coronary artery disease. Anesth Analg 1976;55:135–8
13. Park WY, Hagins FM, Rivat EL, Macnamara TE. Age and epidural dose response in adult men. Anesthesiology 1982;56:318–20
14. Finucane BT, Hammonds WD, Welch MB. Influence of age on vascular absorption of lidocaine from the epidural space. Anesth Analg 1987;66:843–6
15. Nydahl P-A, Philipson L, Axelsson K, Johansson J-E. Epidural anesthesia with 0.5% bupivacaine: Influence of age on sensory and motor blockade. Anesth Analg 1991;73:780–6
16. Sharrock NE. Lack of exaggerated spread of epidural anesthesia in patients with arteriosclerosis. Anesthesiology 1977;47:307–8
17. Covert CR, Fox GS. Anaesthesia for hip surgery in the elderly. Can J Anaesth 1989;36:311–9
18. Chung F, Meier R, Lautenschlager E, Carmichael FJ, Chung A. General or spinal anesthesia: Which is better in the elderly? Anesthesiology 1987;67:422–7
19. Berggren D, Gustafson Y, Eriksson B, et al. Postoperative confusion after anesthesia in elderly patients with femoral neck fractures. Anesth Analg 1987;66:497–504
20. Riggs BL, Melton LJ. The prevention and treatment of osteoporosis. N Engl J Med 1992;327:620–7
21. Chapin JW, Kahre J. Progeria and anesthesia. Anesth Analg 1979;58:424–5

Index

Page numbers followed by f indicate figures; those followed by t indicate tables.

Vasoactive mediators, in anaphylaxis, 503, 503t
Vasodilators
in abdominal aortic surgery, 119
in treatment of cardiac tamponade, 110
in treatment of congestive heart failure, 94, 94t
in treatment of COPD, 139
Vasopressin. *See* Antidiuretic hormone (ADH)
Vasospasm
in pregnancy-induced hypertension, 561
in stroke, 204, 204f
Vasospastic angina, in ischemic heart disease evaluation, 4
Vecuronium
cerebral blood flow and, 191
in chronic renal failure, 300–301, 301f
in hepatic cirrhosis, 268, 268f
response to, during anesthesia in dermatomyositis patient, 434
Venous air embolism, in intracranial surgery
detection of, 195
monitoring for, 194
pathophysiology of, 194–195
risk potential for, 194
treatment of, 195f, 195–196
Venous congestion, systemic, in right ventricular failure, 90–91
Venous partial pressure, of oxygen, 175
Venous return, anomalous pulmonary, 48–49
Ventilation
abnormal patterns of, 238–239, 239t
in extracorporeal shock-wave lithotripsy, 307
mechanical. *See* Mechanical ventilation
Ventricles, function of, 89. *See also* Left ventricle; Right ventricle
Ventricular fibrillation, 72
Ventricular premature beats
characteristic appearance of, 71, 71t
conditions associated with, 71t
treatment for, 71–72

Ventricular septal defect, 40f
anesthesia management of, 41
incidence of, 40
signs and symptoms of, 40
treatment of, 40–41
Ventricular septal rupture, surgical treatment of, 12
Ventricular tachycardia, 72
Ventriculoatrial shunt, in hydrocephalus, 600
anesthesia management in, 600
Verapamil therapy
in atrial fibrillation, 70
in paroxysmal supraventricular tachycardia, 70
Vertebrobasilar arterial disease, 197
Vestibular neuronitis, 220
Viral diseases. *See* Viral infections; *specific diseases*
Viral hepatitis
characteristic features of, 257, 257t
clinical course of, 258
cytomegalovirus, 260
Epstein-Barr, 259–260
laboratory tests in, 258
signs and symptoms of, 257–258, 258t
treatment of, 258
type A, 258
type B, 258–259
detection of, 259
prophylaxis for, 259
type C, 259
type D, 259
Viral infections
Creutzfeldt-Jakob disease, 470
herpes virus, 468–470
leading to AIDS. *See* Acquired immunodeficiency syndrome (AIDS); Human immunodeficiency virus (HIV)
rubella, 470
transmission by blood transfusion, 421
of upper respiratory tract, 467
anesthesia management in patient with, 468
Vitamin A
deficiency of, 390
excess of, 390–391
Vitamin B_1 deficiency, 390

Vitamin B_{12} deficiency, 223
anesthesia management in patient with, 399
megaloblastic anemia due to, 399
Vitamin C deficiency, 390
Vitamin D deficiency, 391
Vitamin K
absorption of, liver disease and, 253
deficiency of, 391
causing coagulation process abnormalities, 414
Vitamins, imbalance of, disorders related to, 390–391
Volatile anesthetics. *See* Enflurane; Halothane; Isoflurane
Volume expanders
in coagulation disorders, 420
perioperative allergic reaction to, 509
in treatment of cardiac tamponade, 109–110, 110t
Voluntary deep breathing, for postoperative COPD patient, 145
von Gierke's disease, 380
von Willebrand's disease, 412–413

Wake-up test, in kyphoscoliosis, 453
Waldenström's macroglobulinemia, 512
Wandering atrial pacemaker, 71
Water, electrolyte, and acid-base disturbances, 313–337. *See also* Acid-base disturbances; *specific conditions*
calcium and, 329–331
cell electrophysiology in, 316, 317f
electrolyte distribution and, 315–316, 316t
magnesium and, 331–332
perioperative, etiology of, 313, 314t
potassium and, 321–329
sodium and, 320–321
total body water and, 316–320
Waterston shunt, in treatment of tetralogy of Fallot, 43, 44
Wegener's granulomatosis
anesthesia management in, 125–126
signs and symptoms of, 125, 125t